Quick Review of Surgery

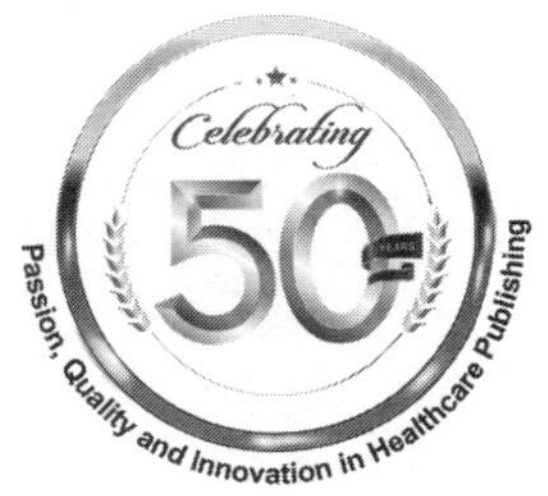

Quick Review of Surgery

Pritesh Kumar Singh

MBBS (MAMC), MS (Surgery), FMAS, FIAGES

Author of Surgery Essence, AIIMS Essence, NEET Essence

Director, 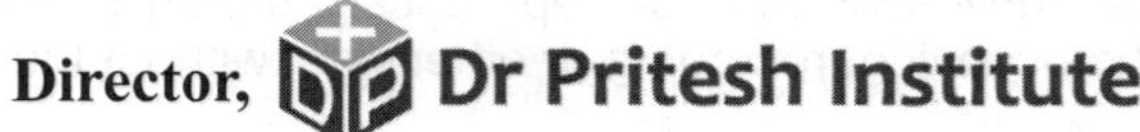 Dr Pritesh Institute

Chief Advisor of Editorial Board—PGMEE, Jaypee Brothers Medical Publishers

Guest Faculty of Surgery, Ningbo University, China

Stavropol State Medical University, Russia

International School of Medicine, Bishkek (Kyrgyzstan)

Avicenna Tajik State Medical University, Tajikistan

Ex. Senior Resident, Lady Hardinge Medical College and
Associated Sucheta Kriplani Hospital
Kalawati Saran Children's Hospital and Ram Manohar Lohia Hospital
New Delhi, India

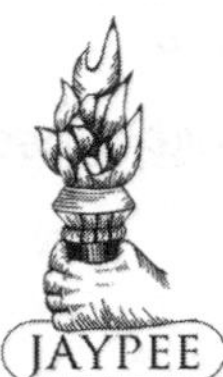

JAYPEE BROTHERS MEDICAL PUBLISHERS

The Health Sciences Publisher

New Delhi | London

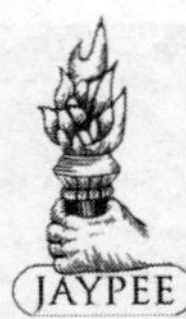 **Jaypee Brothers Medical Publishers (P) Ltd**

Headquarters
Jaypee Brothers Medical Publishers (P) Ltd
4838/24, Ansari Road, Daryaganj
New Delhi 110 002, India
Phone: +91-11-43574357
Fax: +91-11-43574314
Email: jaypee@jaypeebrothers.com

Overseas Office
J.P. Medical Ltd
83 Victoria Street, London
SW1H 0HW (UK)
Phone: +44 20 3170 8910
Fax: +44 (0)20 3008 6180
Email: info@jpmedpub.com

Website: www.jaypeebrothers.com
Website: www.jaypeedigital.com

Quick Review of Surgery

First Edition: **2020**

ISBN 978-93-90020-87-4

Printed at: Sterling Graphics Pvt. Ltd.

Editors

ENDOCRINE SURGERY

- Dr Ashish Jakhetiya (MCh, Surgical Oncology, AIIMS)
- Dr Subham Garg (MCh, Surgical Oncology, TATA)
- Dr Subham Jain (MCh, Surgical Oncology, TATA)
- Dr Niket Harsh (MCh, GI Surgery, AIIMS)

HEPATOBILIARY PANCREATIC SURGERY

- Dr Swati Agarwal (DNB, Surgical Oncology)
- Dr Harsh Shah (MCh, GI Surgery, GB Pant Hospital)
- Dr Vaibhav Varshney (MCh, GI Surgery, GB Pant Hospital)
- Dr Niket Harsh (MCh, GI Surgery, AIIMS)

GASTROINTESTINAL SURGERY

- Dr Vaibhav Varshney (MCh, GI Surgery, GB Pant Hospital)
- Dr Harsh Shah (MCh, GI Surgery, GB Pant Hospital)
- Dr Swati Agarwal (DNB, Surgical Oncology)
- Dr Niket Harsh (MCh, GI Surgery, AIIMS)

UROLOGY

- Dr Gaurav Kochar (MCh, Urology)
- Dr Manoj Kumar Das (MCh, Urology)
- Dr Shiva Navariya (MCh, Urology)
- Dr Animesh Singh (MCh, Urology, AIIMS)

CARDIOTHORACIC VASCULAR SURGERY

- Dr Tarun Raina (MCh, CTVS, GB Pant Hospital)
- Dr Vivek Wadhva (MCh, CTVS, PGI Chandigarh)

PLASTIC SURGERY

- Dr Ritesh Anand (MCh, Plastic Surgery)
- Dr Alok Tiwari (MCh, Plastic Surgery)

NEUROSURGERY

- Dr Amit Kumar Singh (MCh, Neurosurgery, RML Hospital)
- Dr Ishu Bishnoi (MCh, Neurosurgery, GB Pant Hospital)
- Dr Shivender Sobti (MCh, Neurosurgery, RML Hospital)
- Dr Ugan Singh (MCh, Neurosurgery)

HEAD AND NECK

- Dr Ashish Jakhetiya (MCh, Surgical Oncology, AIIMS)
- Dr Subham Garg (MCh, Surgical Oncology, TATA)
- Dr Subham Jain (MCh, Surgical Oncology, TATA)
- Dr Niket Harsh (MCh, GI Surgery, AIIMS)

SURGICAL ONCOLOGY

- Dr Ashish Jakhetiya (MCh, Surgical Oncology, AIIMS)
- Dr Subham Garg (MCh, Surgical Oncology, TATA)
- Dr Subham Jain (MCh, Surgical Oncology, TATA)
- Dr Niket Harsh (MCh, GI Surgery, AIIMS)

GENERAL SURGERY

- Dr Harindra Sandhu (MS, Surgery)
- Dr Mayank Agarwal (MCh, Urology)
- Dr Mohit Garg (MS, Surgery)
- Dr Gunjan Desai (MS, Surgery)

Preface

First of all I would like to thank all my students especially the foreign medical graduates, for their constant suggestions and feedback regarding the launch of the book, *Quick Review of Surgery*.

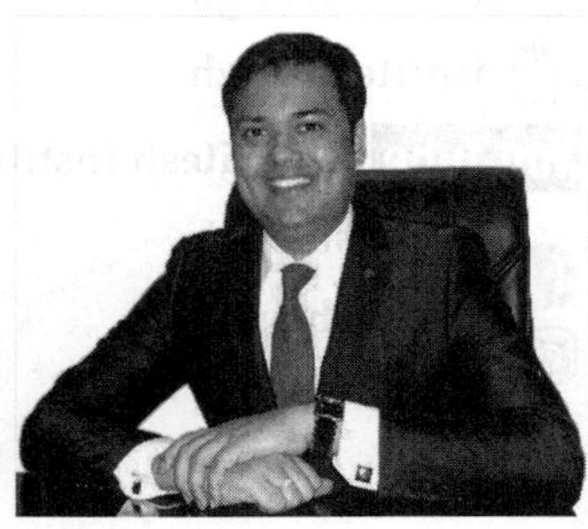

I can proudly say that all my students have contributed a lot to get me to this place, where I am today. They have helped me in becoming a better teacher, a better author and, most importantly, a better human being. I take this opportunity to thank all of you. The happiness you all give me keeps me telling always to work harder, to bring a positive change in the life of my students. This will be reflected in the pages of this book. I always strive to provide a winning edge to my students. This book has become the bestseller chiefly because of the suggestions, love and even critics that I come across and am informed of.

Clearing MCI exam is mandatory to appear for the NEET-PG entrance exam. The pattern of questions of MCI exam is slightly different from NEET-PG. **As an author, I closely follow the types of questions being asked and the change of pattern of questions in the MCI exam**. I am pleased to present the *1st edition of Quick Review of Surgery* replete with new trends in the field of surgery and recent advances. **In MCI exam**, lots of image-based questions are being asked. **To provide to an edge, image-based questions are given in the beginning. Triads, signs, investigation of choices and topics based on "most common" type of questions are included in the annexures to save your precious time and to help you in revision at the most crucial hours.** *Synopsis* of the chapter is given in the beginning to develop concepts about the topics. **The recent questions and their concepts are highlighted and have been written in the way that will help the students to remember and reproduce them in the examination hall.** The information provided is cogent but concise to save the precious time, as we all know the clock is ticking. Time is one thing that can never be recovered once gone. Be careful!

I am passionate about excellence. Excellence in the field of education, and in my efforts to groom my students to make them confident enough that they lose the fear of failure. Being the Director of Dr Pritesh Institute, I follow the same principle in this institute so that the students should be benefited most with an extra edge.

I believe that all my students should know the importance of challenges. Challenges are what make life interesting and overcoming them is what makes life meaningful. For the time being, the only challenge that you should be facing is to pass the MCI exam and secure a good rank in the entrance exam. One of the most important keys to success is having the discipline to do what you know you should do, even when you do not feel like doing it. Nobody ever wrote down a plan to be broke, lazy or stupid. These things happen when you do not have a plan.

My aim, as an author and as a teacher, is to provide students with a learning experience which when amalgamated with perseverance and commitment helps them in achieving goals. I am still not sure about one thing that who is more happy when a student achieves something, the student or the teacher, but I am very sure that the teacher is more satisfied when he sees his students achieving what they deserve and desire. I am working day and night to get that satisfaction and you have to work equally hard so that you do not let me down.

I always tell my students to dream big but not while sleeping. But, these dreams should always be accompanied with intelligence and hard work. To guide your work intelligently, this book and the author, both are there, with you throughout the year. But, the hard work is totally in your hands. Accept responsibility for your life. Know that it is you who will get you where you want to go, no one else.

Extensive revisions have been made to minimize the chances of error but still some mistakes might be there which should be brought to the notice of the author through e-mail address or in writing.

It is a pleasure now to give outlet to the overflowing appreciation and thanks to all my colleagues, friends, teachers and family because this book is the result of encouragement and guidance from all of them.

I am pleased to acknowledge the overwhelming love I have received from my students, who are my ultimate source of inspiration. Wishing you all the best and looking forward for your feedback and suggestions.

✉ drpritesh@drpriteshsurgeryclasses.com

drpriteshsingh

drpriteshsingh

drpriteshsingh

drpriteshsingh

YouTube /Dr Pritesh Institute

drpriteshsingh

drpriteshsingh

www.drpriteshsurgeryclasses.com

Pritesh Kumar Singh

MBBS (MAMC), MS (Surgery), FMAS, FIAGES
Author of Surgery Essence, AIIMS Essence, NEET Essence

**Author of Surgery Essence,
AIIMS Essence, NEET Essence,**

Director, ✚ **Dr Pritesh Institute**

**Chief Advisor of Editorial Board—PGMEE,
Jaypee Brothers Medical Publishers**

Ningbo University, China

Stavropol State Medical University, Russia

International School of Medicine Bishkek (Kyrgyzstan)

Avicenna Tajik State Medical University Tajikistan

www.drpriteshinstitute.com

Acknowledgments

I would like to express my greatest gratitude to the people who have helped and supported me throughout my project.

I wish to thank my parents for their undivided support and interest, who inspired me and encouraged me to go my own way, without whom I would be unable to complete my project.

First of all I would like to thank my beloved wife **Dr Usica Singh,** for her constant support and motivation. She helped me in updating the book from the latest editions of standard textbooks. She helped me throughout this project by giving her valuable advises and feedbacks regarding improvement of the book.

I express my sincere thanks to my friends **Dr Niket Harsh** (MCh, GI Surgery, AIIMS) and **Dr Saurabh Rai** (MS, Orthopedics). They provided me the explanations of difficult and controversial questions.

I am very thankful to **Dr SK Tudu**, Ex. HOD of Surgery, Maulana Azad Medical College, New Delhi, for the valuable help. He was always there to show us the right track when we needed his help. It is with the help of his valuable suggestions, guidance and encouragement, that I was able to complete this project.

I am grateful to **Dr MP Arora,** for the continuous support for the project, from initial advice and contacts in the early stages of conceptual inception and through ongoing advice and encouragement to this day.

I sincerely thank my uncle **Dr SD Maurya** (President SELSI and Ex Professor of Surgery, SNMC, Agra), for his valuable advice and knowledge regarding the surgery subject and surgical skills, which helped me a lot in preparation of certain topics of surgery given in this book.

I wish to express my sincere thanks to **Dr OP Pathania** and **Dr S Thomas** (Principal, VMMC)

I wish to express my sincere thanks to **Dr Manoj Andley,** Professor of Surgery, LHMC, New Delhi, for helping me throughout this project. His caring and fatherly attitude for the unit as well as towards his residents needs a mention. His excellent way of teaching and presentation helped me a lot in making various explanations in the book. His hard working and caring attitude towards patients is source of inspiration for me and surgery residents.

I am very thankful to **Dr Ashok Kumar,** Professor of Surgery, LHMC, New Delhi, for his valuable and indispensable help. His unique ideas regarding presentation of explanations helped me a lot in this project. It is with the help of his valuable suggestions, guidance and encouragement, that I was able to complete this project.

I wish to express my sincere thanks to **Dr Lalit Aggarwal**, **Dr Gyan Saurabh**, **Dr Sudipta Saha**, **Dr P Rahul,** Professor of Surgery, Lady Hardinge Medical College, for guiding me to complete general surgery topics.

I wish to express my sincere thanks to **Dr Pawan Kumar, Dr Priya Hazrah, Dr Nikhil Talwar, Dr Ezaz Siddiqui, Dr Ashish Arsia, Dr Sadan Ali, Dr Jitender, Dr Rajeev Kumar** and **Dr Kusum Meena,** Assistant Professors of Surgery, Lady Hardinge Medical College, for their indispensable contribution.

I would like to thank **Dr UC Garga,** Professor of Radiology, Dr RML Hospital, New Delhi, for his special guidance for radiology and valuable advices for improvement of the book and boosting my morale to bring this project.

I express my extreme gratitude for immense inspiration from my family members specially:

- Dr Avinash Kumar Singh (Urologist)
- Dr Charu Singh (Dermatologist)
- Mr Abhay Kumar Singh (MBA, IMT, Ghaziabad)
- Mrs Deepasha Singh (MBA, IMT, Ghaziabad)
- Mr Ritesh Kumar Singh (B Tech, MBA, Symbiosis, Pune)
- Ms Pratibha Singh (M Tech, Computer Science)
- Ms Monika Singh (B Tech, Computer Science)
- Ms Khushboo Singh (B Tech, Computer Science)
- Mr Rohit Kumar Singh (B Tech, Computer Science)
- Dr Anita Singh (MD, Pediatrics, KGMC, Lucknow)
- Dr Kundan Kumar Patel (DMRD)
- Dr Akanksha Singh (DGO, KGMC)
- Dr Jigyasa Singh (MS, Gynae IMS, BHU)
- Mr Abhishek Kumar Singh (B Tech, IIT Kharagpur)
- Dr Ambuj Kumar Singh (MD Dermatology)
- Mr Rahul Kumar Singh (B Tech)

I would like to thank my friends for their invaluable help and advice from time to time specially:

- **Dr Niket Harsh**
- **Dr Suarabh Rai**

I feel pleasure in conveying my sincere thanks to my friends and colleagues specially:

- Dr Shipra Goel (MD, Microbiology)
- Dr Mayank Agarwal (MCh, GI Surgery, AIIMS)

A special thank of mine goes to **Dr Parul Gautam** (MD, Pathology, MAMC), who helped me in completing the project and exchanged her interesting ideas, thoughts which made this project easy and accurate. Her help for topics related to tumor and pathology is indispensable.

I am equally grateful to my friend **Dr Sushant Bhanja** (MD, Pediatrics), who gave me moral support and guided me in different matters regarding the topics related to Pediatric Surgery. He has been very kind and patient, whilst suggesting me the outlines of this project and correcting my doubts.

I would be failing in my duty if I do not express my thanks to all my friends who have really inspired me to write this book specially:

- Dr Vivek Kumar (MD, Medicine)
- Dr Neha Chaudhary (MD, Pediatrics)
- Dr Harwinder (MS, Orthopedics)
- Dr Nitasha (MS, Ophthalmology)
- Dr Ugan Singh (MCh, Neurosurgery)
- Dr Pragati Meena (MS, Gynae, SMS, Jaipur)
- Dr Bhamini Agal (MS, Gynae, SMS, Jaipur)
- Dr Aniket Malhotra (MD, Pediatrics)
- Dr Anant Pachisia (MD, Anesthesia)
- Dr Anant Shukla (MD, Anesthesia)

I would like to express my sincere thanks to my colleagues at Dr RML Hospital, especially **Dr Amit Kumar Singh** (MCh, Neurosurgery), **Dr Shivender Sobti** (MCh, Neurosurgery), **Dr Humam** (SR, Neurosurgery), **Dr Wazid** (DNB, Neurosurgery), **Dr Uzair** (DNB, Neurosurgery), **Dr Azaz** (DNB, Neurosurgery) and **Dr Neeraj** (DNB, Neurosurgery).

I would like to express my sincere thanks to my colleagues at Lady Hardinge Medical College and Associated Dr RML Hospital, **Dr Sushma Kataria, Dr Gyan Ranjan, Dr Kamal Yadav, Dr Priyank Yadav, Dr Vineet, Dr Munish, Dr Nivedita, Dr Tarun Raina, Dr Sumit Saini** and **Dr Abhinav Veerwal.**

I would like to express my sincere thanks to my colleagues at Lady Hardinge Medical College and Associated Dr RML Hospital, **Dr Meenakshi, Dr Ankur, Dr Prashant, Dr Rigved, Dr Munish Raj, Dr Diwakar Pandey, Dr Vikram Deswal, Dr Gunjan Desai, Dr Vikas, Dr Nikunj Jain, Dr Hari Singh, Dr Vimlesh, Dr Mannu, Dr Anshul, Dr Vikas and Dr Abhijeet Jha, Dr Mayank Aggarwal, Dr Vipul Dogra, Dr Abhishek, Dr Kunjan, Dr Sumit, Dr Kartikey, Dr Rao Bhupender.**

I would like to express my sincere thanks to my colleagues at Lady Hardinge Medical College and Associated Dr RML Hospital, for their valuable advice, specially:

- Dr Divish Saxena (Asst. Prof of Surgery, LMMC, Nagpur)
- Dr Ravindra Gupta (Ex. SR, RML Hospital, MS, Gynae, PMCH)
- Dr Prasad Bhukebag (SR, RML Hospital)
- Dr Ritesh Pathak (SR, RML Hospital)
- Dr Anil Gulwani (MCh, Urology)
- Dr Nitin Sardana (Ex-SR, LHMC)
- Dr Arvinda PS (MCh, GI Surgery)
- Dr Rahul Rai (Ex-SR, LHMC)
- Dr Yogender (SR, LHMC)
- Dr Anand Yadav (Ex-SR, LHMC)
- Dr Shiv Navariya (MCh, Urology)
- Dr Nihar (MCh-Hepatobiliary Surgery SR, LHMC)
- Dr Zuber Khan (FNB, Minimal Invasive Surgery, LHMC)

I would like to express my sincere thanks to my colleagues at Maulana Azad Medical College and Associated LNJP Hospital, for their valuable advice, specially:

- Dr Mohit Garg (MS, Surgery)
- Dr Kamal Kishore Gautam (MS, Surgery)
- Dr Anurag Mishra (Assistant Professor, MAMC)
- Dr Ashish Airen (MS, Surgery)

I would also like to thank **Mr Varish Sharma** and **Mr Anurag Sharma** of MAMC Bookshop for their encouragement for writing this book.

I would like to thank **Dr Ashish Jakhetiya** and **Dr Inderjeet Yadav**, who helped me a lot in gathering different information, collecting data and guiding me from time to time in completing this project. Despite their busy schedules, they gave me different ideas to help make this project unique.

I would like to thank Mr Sahil Mahajan (Senior Manager, Dr Pritesh Institute) and Mr Rajesh Jha (Assistant Manager) for their valuable help.

I would like to express my sincere thanks to **Dr A Najeerul Ameen** (President, All India Foreign Graduates Association) for his constant help and support for the classes in Russia.

I am equally grateful to **Dr M Suresh** (Vice Dean, Stavropol State Medical University, for foreign students) for his valuable help during the classes in Russia.

I am thankful to my student **Dr Anupam** for his constant help and support for the classes in Stavropol State Medical University, Russia.

I feel pleasure in conveying my sincere thanks to **Prof Shakarin V V** (Rector), **Prof Emelynov D N** (Dean) and **Prof Alshuk N A** (Vice Chancellor) of Volgograd State Medical University.

I would like to thank my friend **Dr G Bhanu Prakash** (CEO and Founding Director, Proceum) for his invaluable help and advice from time to time.

I would like to express my sincere thanks to **Dr Jazeer Abdul Khader** (Academic Coordinator for International Students, Guangxi Medical University, China).

I am equally grateful to **Dr Naresh Yadav** and **Dr Sandeep Chouhan** for their constant help and support for the classes in International School of Medicine, Bishkek.

I am thankful to my students **Dr Yogesh Yadav, Dr Anand P Boora, Dr Rakesh Kumar Yadav** and **Dr Yogesh Kumar Yadav** for their constant help and support for the classes in Avicenna Tajik State Medical University, Tajikistan.

Last but not the least I want to thank all my students who appreciated me for my work and motivated me and finally to God who made all the things possible.

I convey my sincere thanks to Jaypee Brothers Medical Publishers (P) Ltd, New Delhi, India, for their efforts and suggestions, especially Shri Jitendar P Vij (Group Chairman), for helping me through my idea.

Contents

★★★★★	Most Important
★★★★	Very Important
★★★	Important

Annexure 1

NAMED CLASSIFICATION FOR TUMORS

Important Tumor Classification	
Chang staging[Q]	Medulloblastoma[Q]
Masaoka staging[Q]	Thymoma[Q]
Shimda index[Q]	Neuroblastoma[Q]
Reiss and **Ellsworth** classification **Esson** prognostic index[Q]	Retinoblastoma[Q]
Bloom-Richardson grading[Q]	CA breast[Q]
Noguchi classification[Q]	Adenocarcinoma lung[Q]
Sullivan modification of **Macfarlane system**[Q]	Adrenocortical carcinoma[Q]
Gleason	CA prostate[Q]
Nevine staging	CA GB[Q]
Duke staging	Colorectal carcinoma[Q]
Robson staging	RCC[Q]
Jackson	CA penis[Q]
Butchart staging	**Mesothelioma**[Q]

Annexure 2

GENES AND CHROMOSOMES

Syndrome	Genes	Locations
Breast/ovarian syndrome	BRCA1	**17**[Q]
	BRCA2[Q]	**13**[Q]
Cowden's disease	PTEN[Q]	**10**[Q]
FAP	APC[Q]	**5**[Q]
HNPCC	hMLH1[Q]	**3**[Q]
	hMSH2[Q]	**2**[Q]
	hMSH6	**2**[Q]
	hPMS1	**2**[Q]
	hPMS2	**7**[Q]
Hereditary papillary RCC	**MET**[Q]	**7**[Q]
Li-Fraumeni	**p53**[Q]	**17**[Q]
	hCHK2	22
MEN-1	MEN1[Q]	**11**[Q]
MEN-2	RET[Q]	**10**[Q]
NF-1	NF1[Q]	**17**[Q]

Contd...

Contd...

Syndrome	Genes	Locations
NF-2	NF2[Q]	22[Q]
Peutz-Jeghers syndrome	STK11[Q]	19[Q]
Retinoblastoma	RB[Q]	13[Q]
Tuberous sclerosis	TSC1[Q]	9[Q]
	TSC2[Q]	16[Q]
VHL syndrome	VHL[Q]	3[Q]
Wilms' tumor	WT[Q]	11[Q]

Name of Incisions	
Lazy 'S', Sistrunk, Modified Blair's	**Parotidectomy**
McBurney's, Grid-Iron, McArthur, Lanz	**Appendectomy**
Pfannenstiel incision	**Caesarean section** **Abdominal hysterectomy**
Chevron incision	**Whipple's procedure** Upper abdominal Malignancies
Cherney incision	**Pelvic surgery** (excellent surgical exposure to the space of Retzius and pelvic side walls)
Kocher's incision	**Open cholecystectomy**
Kustner's incision	Transverse incision made 5 cm above the symphysis pubis but below the anterior superior iliac spine
Maylard incision	• A variation of Pfannenstiel incision • Rectus abdominis muscles are sectioned transversely to permit wider access to the pelvis.
McEvedy's Incision	**Lateral paramedian incision**
Turner-Warwick's incision	• Placed **2 cm above the symphysis pubis** and within the lateral borders of the rectus muscle. • **Good for exposure of retropubic space**.

Annexure 3

LYMPH NODES

Most Common Lymph Nodes Involved	
CA Penis	**Inguinal** LN[Q]
CA Testis	On **right: Inter-aortocaval**[Q] LN On **left: Paraaortic**[Q] LN
CA Bladder	**Obturator**[Q] LN
CA Prostate	**Obturator**[Q] LN

Important Lymph Nodes	
Rotter's nodes[Q]	• **Interpectoral** nodes (**CA breast**)[Q]
Rouvier nodes[Q]	• **Retropharyngeal** nodes (**CA Nasopharynx**)[Q]
Delphian nodes[Q]	• **Pre-cricoid/Pre-tracheal/Pre-laryngeal** lymph nodes[Q]
Irish nodes[Q]	• Nodes in **left axilla** (**CA stomach**)[Q]
Sister Mary Joseph nodes[Q]	• **Periumbilical metastatic cutaneous** nodules
Virchow nodes[Q]	• **Left supraclavicular** node[Q]
Cloquet node[Q]	• **Femoral canal** node[Q]
LN of **Lund**[Q]	• **Cystic** lymph node[Q]
Krouse Lymph node	• **Jugular fossa** lymph node[Q]
Guiliano node	• Sentinel LN in carcinoma breast

Annexure 4

NAMED TRIADS

Important Triads		
Triad	**Seen in**	**Components**
Virchow's Triad[Q]	**Thrombosis**	Hypercoagulability + Stasis + Endothelial injury[Q]
Galezia's Triad[Q]		**Dupuytren's contracture + Retroperitoneal fibrosis + Peyronie's disease** of penis[Q]
Cushing's Triad[Q]	**Intracranial hypertension**	↑ **BP + Bradycardia + ↓ respiratory rate**
Hutchison's Triad[Q]	**Congenital syphilis**	**Hutchison's teeth** (notched upper incisors) **+ Interstitial keratitis + Nerve deafness**[Q]
Trotter's Triad[Q]	**Nasopharyngeal Carcinoma**	**Conductive hearing loss + Immobility** of **homolateral soft palate + Trigeminal neuralgia**[Q]
Saints Triad		Hiatus hernia + Gallstones + Colonic diverticulosis[Q]
Dieulafoy's Triad[Q]	**Acute appendicitis**	**Hypersensitiveness** of skin + Reflex **muscular contraction + tenderness** at MacBurney's point[Q]
Quincke's Triad[Q]	**Hemobilia**	**GI hemorrhage + biliary colic + jaundice**[Q]
Borchardt's Triad[Q]	**Gastric Volvulus**	**Epigastric pain + Inability** to **vomit + Inability** to **pass** a **NG tube**[Q]
Tillaux's Triad[Q]	**Mesenteric cyst**	Soft **fluctuant swelling** in **umbilical region** + Freely **mobile perpendicular** to **mesentery** + Zone of **resonance** all around[Q]
Mackler's Triad[Q]	**Boerhaave's syndrome**	**Thoracic pain + vomiting + cervical subcutaneous emphysema**[Q]
Rigler's Triad[Q]	**Gallstone ileus**	**Small bowel obstruction + Pneumobilia + Ectopic gallstone**[Q]
Whipple's Triad[Q]	**Insulinoma**	**Symptoms** of **hypoglycemia** + S. **glucose <45 mg/dL + Symptomatic relief on glucose ingestion**[Q]
Currarino or ASP triad		<u>A</u>norectal malformations + <u>S</u>acrococcygeal osseous defect + <u>P</u>resacral mass (Anterior sacral meningocele)

Annexure 5

TREATMENT OF CHOICE

Condition	**Treatment of Choice**
Duodenal Atresia	**Duodenoduodenostomy**[Q]
Annular pancreas	**Duodenoduodenostomy**[Q]
Superior mesenteric artery syndrome	**Duodenojejunostomy**[Q]

Enucleation is treatment of choice in	
1. **Hemangioma liver**[Q]	3. **Chylolymphatic cyst**[Q]
2. **Leiomyoma esophagus**[Q]	4. **Insulinoma involving head of pancreas**[Q]

Annexure 6

METASTASIS

Carcinoma Thyroid	
Type	**Mode of spread**
Papillary carcinoma	**Lymphatic**[Q] spread
Follicular carcinoma	**Hematogenous**[Q] spread
Medullary carcinoma	Both **lymphatic** and **hematogenous**[Q] spread
Anaplastic carcinoma	**Direct invasion**[Q]

Carcinoma Thyroid	
Type	**MC site of Metastasis**
Papillary carcinoma	**Lungs**[Q]
Follicular carcinoma	**Bones**[Q]
Medullary carcinoma	**Liver**[Q]
Anaplastic carcinoma	**Lungs**[Q]

Pulsating Secondaries	
1. Follicular carcinoma thyroid[Q]	2. RCC[Q]

Bone Metastasis in Carcinoma Thyroid	
Follicular carcinoma	**Osteolytic** metastasis (**Pulsating secondaries** in **flat bones**)[Q]
Medullary carcinoma	**Osteoblastic** metastasis[Q]

Metastatic Tumors
Metastatic Tumors of Thyroid • Rare, most cases are found in autopsy • MC site of primary: **CA Breast**[Q] > CA Lung • If thyroid metastases is detected pre-mortem, MC site of primary: **RCC**[Q] > CA Breast > CA Lung
Metastatic Tumors to lung, MC primary: CA breast[Q]
Metastatic Tumors to Pancreas • MC site of primary: **RCC**[Q] > Malignant melanoma • On **autopsy**, MC site of primary: **CA lung**[Q]
Metastatic Tumors Adrenal, MC site of primary: **CA Lung**[Q]
Metastatic Tumors to Small Bowel • Metastatic tumors involving small bowel are more common than primary tumors • MC site of primary: Other intra-abdominal organs • MC extra-abdominal source: **Melanoma** > CA Breast > CA Lung
Metastatic Tumors to Skin • MC site of primary in males: **CA Lung**[Q] • MC site of primary in females: **CA Breast**[Q] • **Scalp** is **MC site** for **cutaneous metastatic disease**[Q]
Metastatic Tumors to Liver • MC site of primary: **Colorectal cancer** > **CA lung** > CA Pancreas > CA Breast > CA Stomach
Metastatic Tumors to CNS • MC site of primary for **brain** metastases: **CA Lung**[Q] > CA Breast • MC site of primary for **leptomeningeal metastases**: **CA Breast**[Q]
Metastatic Tumors to esophagus, MC primary: CA lung[Q]

Contd...

Contd...

Metastatic Tumors
Metastatic Tumors to spleen • MC site of primary: **Malignant Melanoma** • MC site of primary for Isolated Secondaries to spleen: **CA ovary**
Metastatic Tumors to Heart • MC primary in **males**: **CA lung**[Q] • MC primary in **females**: **CA breast**[Q]
Metastatic Tumors to Testis • MC site of primary: **CA prostate**[Q] > **CA lung** >**GI malignancies** >**melanoma** >**kidney**
Metastatic Tumors to penis, MC site of primary: CA bladder[Q]

Annexure 7

MOST COMMON SYMPTOMS AND CHEMOTHERAPY

Malignancy	Chemotherapy Regimen
CA breast	**CAF** (**C**yclophosphamide + **A**driamycin + 5-**F**U)[Q]
Hepatoblastoma	**VCF** (**V**incristine + **C**isplatin + 5-**F**U)[Q]
CA gall bladder & Cholangiocarcinoma	**Gemcitabine + Cisplatin**[Q]
CA pancreas	**Gemcitabine**[Q]
CA esophagus & CA stomach	**ECF** (**E**pirubicin + **C**isplatin + 5-**F**U)[Q]
Small intestinal adenocarcinoma	**FOLFOX**
Small bowel carcinoid	**DEF** (**D**acarbazine + **E**pirubicin + 5-**F**U)[Q]
Colorectal carcinoma	**FOLFOX-IV** (**Fol**inic acid/Leucovorin + 5-**F**U + **Ox**aliplatin)[Q]
CA anal canal	**Nigro regimen** (5-FU + Mitomycin-C + Radiation)[Q]
Wilm's tumor	**VCD** (**V**incristine + **C**yclophosphamide + **D**oxorubicin or **D**actinomycin)[Q]
CA bladder	**MVAC** (**M**ethotrexate + **V**inblastine + **A**driamycin + **C**isplatin)[Q]
Testicular tumors	**BEP** (**B**leomycin + **E**toposide + **C**isplatin)[Q]
Rhabdomyosarcoma	**VAC** (**V**incristine + **A**ctinomycin + **C**yclophosphamide)[Q]
Hodgkin's lymphoma	**ABVD** (**A**driamycin + **B**leomycin + **V**inblastine + **D**acarbazine)[Q] **MOPP** (**M**echlorethamine + **O**ncovin or vincristine + **P**rocarbazine + **P**rednisone)[Q]
Non-Hodgkin's lymphoma	**CHOP** (**C**yclophosphamide + **H**ydroxydaunorubicin or Doxorubicin + **O**ncovin or vincristine + **P**rednisone)[Q]

Most Common Symptom	
CA Esophagus	• **Dysphagia** >weight loss[Q]
CA stomach	• **Abdominal pain** >weight loss[Q]
Periampullary carcinoma (including **CA head** of **pancreas**)	• **Jaundice**[Q]
HCC	• **Abdominal pain** >weight loss[Q]
Cholangiocarcinoma	• **Painless progressive jaundice**[Q]
CA Gallbladder	• **Biliary colic**[Q]
CA small bowel	• **Abdominal pain**[Q]
CA colon	• **Abdominal pain**[Q]
CA rectum	• **Bleeding PR**[Q]
CA anal canal	• **Bleeding PR**[Q]

Annexure 8

MOST COMMON SITES

Important Most Common Sites	
• Gastric ulcer[Q]	Lesser curvature (near incisura angularis)
• Peptic ulcer[Q] • Gastric outlet obstruction[Q]	1st part of duodenum
• Small bowel[Q] adenocarcinoma • Atresia[Q]	Duodenum
• Polyps in PJS[Q] • Pneumatosis intestinalis[Q]	Jejunum
• Crohn's disease[Q] • Fistula, perforation and carcinoma in Crohn's disease[Q] • Typhoid ulcer[Q] • Tubercular ulcer[Q] • Small intestinal lymphoma[Q] • Gallstone ileus[Q]	Terminal Ileum
• Amebic colitis[Q] • Bleeding in angiodysplasia[Q] • Bleeding in colonic diverticula[Q]	Cecum and ascending colon
• Ischemic colitis[Q]	Splenic flexure
• Colonic diverticula[Q] • Stricture after ischemic colitis[Q] • Volvulus[Q]	Sigmoid
• Ulcerative colitis[Q] • Colorectal cancer[Q] • Hirschsprung's disease[Q]	Rectum

Annexure 9

NAMED HERNIA

Gibbon's hernia	• Hernia with hydrocele[Q]
Berger's hernia	• Hernia into pouch of Douglas[Q]
Beclard's hernia	• Femoral hernia through opening of saphenous vein[Q]
Amyand's hernia	• Inguinal hernia containing appendix[Q]
Ogilvie's hernia	• Hernia through the defect in conjoint tendon just lateral to where it inserts with the rectus sheath[Q]
Stammer's hernia	• Internal hernia occurring through window in the transverse mesocolon after retrocolic gastrojejunostomy[Q]
Peterson hernia	• Hernia under Roux limb after Roux-en-Y gastric bypass[Q]
Hesselbach's Hernia	• Fatty tissue herniation lateral to the femoral vessels through the lacuna musculorum (lateral compartment of the thigh inferior to the inguinal ligament, for the passage of the iliopsoas muscle)[Q]
Velpeau's Hernia (Prevascular)	• A protrusion of viscera in front of the femoral vessels in the groin[Q]
Serafini's Hernia (Retrovascular)	• The hernial sac emerges behind femoral vessels[Q]
Holthouse hernia	• Inguinal hernia with extension of the loop of intestine along inguinal ligament[Q].

Annexure 10

CHARACTERISTIC RADIOLOGICAL APPEARANCES

Radiological Features	Seen in
• **Apple core lesion** on barium enema	**Carcinoma colon**[Q]
• **Claw appearance** on barium enema	**Intussusception**[Q]
• **Saw tooth appearance**	**Colonic diverticula**
• **Bird beak appearance**	**Achalasia**[Q] (on barium swallow) **Sigmoid volvulus** (on barium enema)
• **Cork screw appearance** • **Rosary bead** appearance • **Pseudodiverticula** appearance	**Diffuse esophageal spasm**[Q]
• **String sign** of Kantor • **Sterlein sign**	**Crohn's disease**[Q] **Tuberculosis**
• **Thumb print** sign	**Ischemic colitis**[Q]
• **Squeeze sign**, **Cushion** sign, **Tenting** sign, **naked fat** sign	**Colonic lipoma**[Q]
• **Rat tail appearance**	**Achalasia**[Q]

Characteristic Appearances	
ADPKD	• **Spider leg** or **Bell deformity**[Q] • **Bubble** or **Swiss cheese** appearance on **IVP**[Q]
Infantile PKD	• **Sunburst pattern** on **IVP**[Q]
Medullary Sponge Kidney	• **Bristles on brush** appearance[Q] • **Bouquet of flower** appearance on **IVP**[Q]
Multicystic Dysplastic Kidney	• **Bunch of grapes** appearance[Q]
Renal Artery Aneurysm	• **Ring like calcification**[Q]
Ectopic Ureteric Orifice	• **Drooping lily sign** on **IVP**[Q]
Retrocaval Ureter	• **Fish hook** or **Reverse 'J' deformity** on **IVP**[Q]
Retroperitoneal Fibrosis	• **Medial pulling** of ureter or **pipestem ureter**[Q] (**Pipestem ureter** is also seen in **TB**)
CA Renal Pelvis	• **Goblet sign** or **stipple sign** on **RGP**[Q]

Radiological Feature	Disease
• **Rim/crescent sign**[Q] • **Soap bubble** appearance[Q]	**Hydronephrosis**
• **Spider leg** appearance[Q]	**Polycystic Kidney**
• **Flower vase** appearance of **ureter**[Q]	**Horse shoe Kidney**
• **Golf hole ureter**[Q]	**TB bladder**
• **Drooping lily sign**[Q]	**Ectopic ureter**
• **Cobra head** or **Adder head** appearance[Q] • **Spring onion** appearance[Q]	**Ureterocele**
• **Egg in cup** appearance[Q]	**Analgesic nephropathy causing papillary necrosis**
• **Thimble bladder**[Q]	**Tubercular chronic cystitis**
• **Sandy patches**[Q]	**Schistosomiasis of bladder**
• **Chalice/ Bergman sign**[Q]	**Ureteric dilatation distal to neoplasm**
• **Fish hook bladder**[Q]	**BPH**

Contd...

Contd...

Radiological Feature	Disease
• B/L **spider leg** appearance[Q] • **Swiss- cheese nephrogram**[Q] • **Sun burst nephrogram**[Q]	Polycystic kidney

Radiological Appearance		
Acute Pancreatitis	**Chronic Pancreatitis**	**CA Pancreas**
• **Renal halo** sign[Q] • **Gasless abdomen**[Q] • **Ground glass appearance**[Q] • **Colon cut off** sign[Q] • **Sentinel loop**[Q]	• **Chain** of lakes appearance[Q] • **String** of pearl appearance[Q] • **Beaded appearance**[Q] • Numerous **irregular calcifications**[Q] are pathognomonic (on X-ray)	• **Double contour** of medial border of duodenal C loop • **Double duct sign**[Q] • **Dilated/widening** of **duodenal C loop**[Q] • **Mucosal irregularity**[Q] • **Scrambled egg appearance** • **Inverted/reverse 3 sign** of **Frostberg**[Q] • **Rose thorning** of **medial wall** of **2**nd part of duodenum[Q] • Antral pad sign

Annexure 11

Suspected Carcinogens	
Carcinogens	**Associated Cancer or Neoplasm**
Alkylating agents	• **Acute myeloid leukemia**[Q], **bladder cancer**[Q]
Androgens	• **Prostate cancer**[Q]
Aromatic amines (dyes)	• **Bladder cancer**[Q]
Arsenic	• Cancer of the **lung**[Q], **skin**[Q]
Asbestos	• Cancer of the **lung**[Q], **pleura**[Q], **peritoneum**[Q]
Benzene	• **Acute myelocytic leukemia**[Q]
Chromium	• **Lung cancer**[Q]
Diethylstilbestrol (prenatal)	• **Vaginal cancer (clear cell)**[Q]
Epstein-Barr virus	• **Burkitt's lymphoma**[Q], **nasal T cell lymphoma**[Q]
Estrogens	• Cancer of the **endometrium, liver, breast**[Q]
Ethyl alcohol	• Cancer of the **breast, liver, esophagus, head & neck**[Q]
Helicobacter pylori	• **Gastric cancer**[Q], **gastric MALT lymphoma**[Q]
Hepatitis B or C virus	• **Liver cancer**[Q]
HIV	• **Non-Hodgkin's lymphoma, Kaposi's sarcoma, squamous cell carcinomas**[Q] (especially of the urogenital tract)
Human papilloma virus	• Cancers of the **cervix, anus, oropharynx**[Q]
Human T cell lymphotropic virus	• **Adult T cell leukemia/lymphoma type 1 (HTLV-1)**[Q]
Immunosuppressive agents (azathioprine, cyclosporine, glucocorticoids)	• **Non-Hodgkin's lymphoma**[Q]
Ionizing radiation (therapeutic or diagnostic)	• **Breast, bladder, thyroid, soft tissue, bone, hematopoietic**[Q]
Nitrogen mustard gas	• Cancer of the **lung, head & neck, nasal sinuses**[Q]
Nickel dust	• Cancer of the **lung, nasal sinuses**[Q]
Diesel exhaust (miners)	• **Lung cancer**[Q]
Phenacetin	• Cancer of the **renal pelvis & bladder**[Q]
Polycyclic hydrocarbons	• Cancer of the **lung, skin (SCC of scrotal skin)**[Q]
Radon gas	• **Lung cancer**[Q]
Schistosomiasis	• **Bladder cancer (squamous cell)**[Q]
Sunlight (ultraviolet)	• **Skin cancer (SCC & melanoma)**[Q]
Tobacco (including smokeless)	• Cancer of the **upper aerodigestive tract, bladder**[Q]
Vinyl chloride	• **Liver cancer (angiosarcoma)**[Q]

Annexure 12

FAMILIAL CANCER SYNDROMES

Familial Cancer Syndromes			
Syndrome	**Genes**	**Locations**	**Cancer Sites and Associated Traits**
Breast/ovarian syndrome	BRCA1	17q21[Q]	Cancer of **breast, ovary, colon, prostate**[Q]
	BRCA2	13q12.3[Q]	Cancer of **breast, ovary, colon, prostate, gallbladder and biliary tree, pancreas, stomach; melanoma**[Q]
Cowden's disease	PTEN	10q23.3[Q]	Cancer of **breast, endometrium, thyroid**[Q]
FAP	APC	5q21[Q]	Cancer of breast, endometrium, thyroid
Familial melanoma	p16	9p21	Melanoma, pancreatic cancer, dysplastic nevi, atypical moles
	CDK4	12q14	
Hereditary diffuse gastric cancer	CDH1	16q22	Gastric cancer
HNPCC	hMLH1[Q]	3p21[Q]	**Colorectal** cancer, **endometrial** cancer, **transitional cell carcinoma** of **ureter** and **renal pelvis, carcinomas** of the **stomach, small bowel, pancreas, ovary**[Q]
	hMSH2[Q]	2p22-21	
	hMSH6	2p16[Q]	
	hPMS1	2q31.1	
	hPMS2	7p22.2[Q]	
Hereditary papillary RCC	MET[Q]	7q31[Q]	Renal cell cancer
Hereditary paraganglioma and pheochromocytoma	SDHB	1p36.1-p35	Paraganglioma, pheochromocytoma
	SDHC	1q21	
	SDHD	11q23	
Juvenile polyposis coli	BMPRIA	10q21-q22	Juvenile polyps of the gastrointestinal tract, gastrointestinal malignancies
	SMAD4/DPC4	18q21.1	
Li-Fraumeni	p53	17p13[Q]	**Breast** cancer, **soft tissue sarcoma, osteosarcoma, brain** tumors, **adrenocortical** carcinoma, **Wilms'** tumor, **phyllodes tumor (breast), pancreatic** cancer, **leukemia, neuroblastoma**[Q]
	hCHK2	22q12.1	
MEN-1	MENIN[Q]	11q13[Q]	**Pancreatic islet cell** tumors, **parathyroid hyperplasia, pituitary adenomas**[Q]
MEN-2	RET[Q]	10q11.2	**Medullary thyroid** cancer, **pheochromocytoma, parathyroid hyperplasia**[Q]
MYH-associated adenomatous polyposis	MYH	1p34.3-p32.1	Cancer of the colon, rectum, breast, stomach
Neurofibromatosis-1	NF1[Q]	17q11[Q]	**Neurofibromas, neurofibrosarcoma, acute myelogenous leukemia, brain** tumors[Q]
Neurofibromatosis -2	NF2[Q]	22q12[Q]	**Acoustic neuromas, meningiomas, gliomas, ependymomas**[Q]
Nevoid basal cell carcinoma	PTC	9q22.3	Basal cell carcinoma
Peutz-Jeghers syndrome	STK11[Q]	19p13.3[Q]	**Gastrointestinal carcinomas, breast** cancer, **testicular** cancer, **pancreatic** cancer, **benign pigmentation** of **skin** and **mucosa**[Q]
Retinoblastoma	RB[Q]	13q14[Q]	**Retinoblastoma, sarcomas, melanoma, malignant neoplasms** of the **brain** and **meninges**[Q]
Tuberous sclerosis	TSC1	9q34	**Multiple hamartomas, RCC, astrocytoma**
	TSC2	16p13	
von Hippel-Lindau syndrome	VHL[Q]	3p25[Q]	**RCC, hemangioblastomas** of **retina** and **CNS, pheochromocytoma**[Q]
Wilms' tumor	WT[Q]	11p13[Q]	**Wilms' tumor, aniridia, genitourinary abnormalities, mental retardation**[Q]

Annexure 13

SUTURES

Suture	Types	Raw material	Tensile strength	Absorption rate
Silk	Braided or twisted **multifilament**; Coated (with wax or silicone) or uncoated	Natural protein Raw silk from silkworm	Loses 20% when wet; 80–100% lost by 6 months	Fibrous encapsulation in body at 2–3 weeks ; **Absorbed** slowly over **1–2 years**[Q]
Catgut	Plain	Collagen derived from healthy **sheep** or cattle	Lost within 7–10 days	**Phagocytosis** and **enzymatic degradation** within **7–10 days**[Q]
Catgut	**Chromic**	Tanned with **chromium salts** to **improve handling** and **resist degradation** in tissue[Q]	Lost within 21–28 days	Phagocytosis and enzymatic degradation **within 90 days**
Polyglactin (Vicryl)	Braided multifilament	Copolymer of **lactide** and **glycolide**[Q] in a ratio of 90:10, coated with polyglactin and calcium stearate	Approx. 60% remains at 2 weeks; 30% remains at 3 weeks	Hydrolysis minimal until 5-6 weeks; Complete absorption **60–90 days**[Q]
Polyglyconate	Monofilament Dyed or undyed	Copolymer of **glycolic acid** and **trimethylene carbonate**[Q]	Approx. 70% remains at 2 weeks; 55% remains at 3 weeks	Hydrolysis minimal until 8–9 weeks; Complete absorption **180 days**[Q]
Poliglecaprone	Monofilament	Copolymer of **glycolite** and **caprolactone**[Q]	21 days maximum	**90–120 days**[Q]
Polyglycolic acid (Dexon)	Braided multifilament Dyed or undyed Coated or Uncoated	Polymer of **polyglycolic acid**[Q]	Approx. 40% remains at 1 weeks; 20% remains at 3 weeks	**Hydrolysis**[Q] minimal at 2 weeks; significant at 4 weeks; Complete absorption **60–90 days**[Q]
Polydioxanone (PDS)	Monofilament dyed or undyed	**Polyester polymer**[Q]	Approx. 70% remains at 2 weeks; 50% remains at 4 weeks; 14% remains at 8 weeks	**Hydrolysis** minimal at 90 days; Complete absorption **180 days**[Q]

Guidelines for Day of Suture Removal by Area			
Body Regions	**Removal**	**Body Regions**	**Removal**
Eyelid	**3–4**	Chest, abdomen	8–10
Eyebrow	**3–5**	Ear	10–14
Nose	**3–5**	**Back**	**12–14**
Lip	**3–4**[Q]	**Extremities**	**12–14**
Face (other)	**3–4**[Q]	**Hand**	10–14
Scalp	**6–8**[Q]	Foot, sole	**12–14**

Annexure 14

NEW DRUGS IN SURGERY

New Drugs in CA Breast	
Ixabepilone	• Used for **anthracycline** and **taxane resistant** breast cancer[Q]
Lapatinib	• Inhibitor of Her-2-neu and EGFR tyrosine kinase • **Second line Her-2-neu therapy**[Q]
Sunitinib	• Approved for **advanced renal cancer** and **refractory metastatic breast cancer**[Q]

New Drugs	
Drug	**Indication**
Imatinib mesylate	• GIST • CML • 1st line treatment for advanced & unresectable **DFSP** (Dermatofibrosarcoma protuberans)
Sunitinib	• **Imatinib resistant GIST** • **Advanced Renal cancer** • **Refractory metastatic breast cancer**[Q]
Sorafenib	• **Unresectable HCC**[Q]
Geftinib	• **Adenocarcinoma lung in non-smoking females**
Lapatinib	• Inhibitor of Her-2-neu and EGFR tyrosine kinase • **Second line Her-2-neu therapy**[Q]
Vandetanib (EGFR inhibitor)	• Only drug approved by US FDA for treatment of **advanced & progressive MTC**.

Annexure 15

INHERITANCE PATTERN

Autosomal Dominant	Autosomal Recessive	X-linked Disorders
• Familial hypercholesterolemia	• Deafness	• **Hemophilia A**[Q] **(recessive)**
• **HNPCC**	• **Albinism**[Q]	• **G6PD deficiency**[Q] **(recessive)**
• **FAP**[Q]	• **Wilson's disease**[Q]	• **Ducchene/Becker muscular dystrophy**[Q] **(recessive)**
• **BRCA1** and **BRCA2** breast cancer	• **Hemochromatosis**[Q]	• Fabry's disease
• Hereditary hemorrhagic telangiectasia	• **Sickle cell anemia**[Q]	• Ocular albinism
• **Marfan's syndrome**[Q]	• **β thalassemia** [Q]	• Testicular feminization
• **Hereditary spherocytosis**[Q]	• **Cystic fibrosis**[Q]	• Chronic granulomatous disease
• **Adult polycystic kidney disease**	• **Hereditary emphysema** (α_1 antitrypsin deficiency)	• **Hypophosphatemic rickets**[Q] **(dominant)**
• **Huntington's chorea**[Q]	• **Homocystinuria**[Q]	• **Fragile-X syndrome**[Q] **(recessive)**
• **Acute intermittent porphyria**[Q]	• **Friedreich's ataxia**[Q]	• **Color blindness**[Q]
• **Osteogenesis imperfecta**[Q]	• **Phenylketonuria**[Q]	
• **von Willebrand's disease**[Q]	• **Fanconi's syndrome**	
• **Myotonic dystrophy**[Q]	• **Gaucher's disease**	
• Familial hypertrophic cardiomyopathy		
• **Neurofibromatosis**[Q]		
• **Tuberous sclerosis**[Q]		
• **Otospongiosis**[Q]		
• **Achondroplasia**[Q]		

Annexure 16

MOST COMMON TYPE OF STONES

Most Common Type of Stones	
Gallbladder	Cholesterol[Q] (**Mixed** if given in the option)
Pancreas	Calcium carbonate[Q]
Kidney	Calcium oxalate[Q]
Primary Bladder Stone	Ammonium urate[Q]
Secondary Bladder Stone	Uric acid >Struvite[Q]
Prostate	Calcium phosphate[Q]
Salivary gland (Submandibular)	Calcium carbonate[Q]

Annexure 17

IDEAL TIME FOR TREATMENT

Ideal time for Treatment	
Undescended testis	6 months[Q]
Hypospadias	6–12 months[Q]
Umbilical hernia	5 years[Q]
Cleft lip	3–6 months[Q]
Cleft palate	6–18 months[Q]
Congenital hydrocele	2 years[Q]

Annexure 18

IMPORTANT NAMES IN THE FIELD OF SURGERY

Father of **surgery** Father of **Indian surgery**	• Sushruta[Q]
Father of **modern surgery**	• Joseph Lister[Q]
Father of **modern neurosurgery**	• Harvey Cushing[Q]
Father of **modern plastic surgery**	• Harold Gillies[Q]
Father of **vascular surgery**	• Rudolph Matas[Q]
Father of **pediatric surgery**	• William Edward Ladd[Q]
Father of **modern urology**	• Hugh Hampton Young[Q]

Annexure 19

INVESTIGATION OF CHOICE

Investigation of Choice		
Barium swallow	**Hiatus hernia**[Q] **Zenker's diverticula**[Q] **Leiomyoma**[Q]	
Barium meal	**Gastric diverticula**[Q]	
Barium meal follow-through	**Small bowel diverticula**[Q]	
Enteroclysis	**Crohn's disease**[Q]	
Barium enema	**Colonic diverticula**[Q]	
CECT	**Diverticulitis**[Q] **Hepatocellular carcinoma**[Q] **(Triple phase CT)** **Mesenteric cyst**[Q] **Renal cell carcinoma**[Q] **GI tuberculosis**[Q] **Retroperitoneal fibrosis**[Q] **Acute pancreatitis**[Q] **Retroperitoneal sarcoma**[Q] **Carcinoma pancreas**[Q] **Renal tuberculosis**[Q] **Pancreatic pseudocyst**[Q] **ADPKD**[Q] **Carcinoma gall bladder**[Q] **GIST**[Q]	
MRI	**Brain tumors**[Q] **Spinal cord tumors**[Q] **Pancoast tumor**[Q] **Soft tissue sarcoma**[Q] **Staging of carcinoma penis**[Q]	
Endoscopy with biopsy	**Barrett's esophagus**[Q] **Carcinoma esophagus**[Q] **Carcinoma stomach**[Q]	
Colonoscopy with biopsy	**Carcinoma colon**[Q]	
Sigmoidoscopy with biopsy	**Carcinoma rectum**[Q]	
Proctoscopy with biopsy	**Carcinoma anal canal**[Q]	
Cystoscopy with biopsy	**Carcinoma bladder**[Q]	
FNAC	**Parotid tumors**[Q] **Thyroid malignancies**[Q]	
Biopsy	**Carcinoma breast** **Skin malignancies**[Q] **Carcinoma penis**[Q] **Oral cavity malignancies**[Q]	
Manometry	**Achalasia cardia**[Q] **Diffuse esophageal spasm**[Q] **Nutcrackers esophagus**[Q]	
24-hours pH monitoring	**GERD**[Q]	
Somatostatin receptor scintigraphy **(IOC for localization)**	**All neuroendocrine tumors of pancreas except insulinoma**[Q] **Carcinoid tumors**[Q]	
Ultrasound	**Gallstones**[Q] **Acute cholecystitis**[Q] **Chronic cholecystitis**[Q]	
MRCP	**CBD stone**[Q] **PSC** **Choledochal cyst**[Q] **Pancreas divisum** **Biliary strictures**[Q] **Chronic pancreatitis**[Q]	

Investigation of Choice	
Acute mesenteric ischemia	• **Angiography**[Q]
Mesenteric venous thrombosis	• **CECT**[Q]
Chronic mesenteric ischemia	• **Aortography**[Q]

Investigation of Choice	
ADPKD **Retroperitoneal Fibrosis**	**CT scan**[Q]
Medullary Sponge Kidney	**IVP**[Q]
VUR	**MCU**[Q]
Retrocaval ureter	**MRI**[Q]
PUJ Obstruction	**DTPA scan**[Q]
Renal structure or surface	**DMSA scan**[Q]

Annexure 20

TUMOR MARKERS

Markers	Associated Cancers	Non-neoplastic Conditions
Hormones		
• **Human chorionic gonadotropin** • **Calcitonin** • **Catecholamines**	• **Trophoblastic tumors**[Q], **nonseminomatous** testicular tumors • **Medullary carcinoma**[Q] of thyroid • **Pheochromocytoma**[Q]	• Pregnancy
Oncofetal Antigens		
• Alpha-Fetoprotein • **CEA**	• **Liver**[Q] cell cancer, **nonseminomatous**[Q] germ cell tumor of testis, **lung**[Q] cancer • Adenocarcinoma of the **colon**[Q], **pancreas**[Q], **lung**[Q], **breast**[Q], **ovary**[Q], **prostate**[Q]	• Cirrhosis, hepatitis • Pancreatitis, hepatitis, inflammatory bowel disease, smoking
Isoenzymes		
• Prostatic acid phosphatase • **Neuron-specific enolase** • Lactate dehydrogenase	• Prostate cancer • **Small cell** cancer of lung[Q], **Neuroblastoma**[Q] • Lymphoma, Ewing sarcoma	• Prostatitis, prostatic hypertrophy • Hepatitis, hemolytic anemia, many others
Specific proteins		
• **Immunoglobulins** • PSA and prostate specific membrane antigen	• **Multiple myeloma**[Q] and other gammopathies • Prostate cancer[Q]	• Infection, MGUS • Prostatitis, prostatic hypertrophy[Q]
Mucins and other Glycoproteins		
• **CA-125** • **CA-19-9** • **CD30** • **CD25**	• **Cancer of ovary**[Q], fallopian tube, **endometrium**[Q], cervix, **breast**[Q], **lung**[Q], **pancreas**[Q] and **colon**[Q] • **Colon**[Q] cancer, **pancreatic**[Q] cancer • **Hodgkin's disease**[Q], anaplastic large cell lymphoma • **Hairy cell leukemia, adult T cell leukemia/lymphoma**[Q]	• **Pregnancy**[Q], **endometriosis**[Q], **PID**[Q], **uterine fibroids**[Q] • **Pancreatitis,** Ulcerative colitis

Annexure 21

MOST COMMON

Indications of Liver Transplantation
• **MC indication** for LT: Cirrhosis from Hepatitis C (**HCV**) [Q]
• **2nd MC indication** for LT: **Alcoholic liver disease**[Q]
• MC indication for LT in **children**: **Biliary atresia**[Q]
• MC **metabolic disorder** requiring LT: **Alpha-1 antitrypsin deficiency**[Q]
• MC indication for LT following **acute liver failure**: **Acetaminophen toxicity**[Q]

Pediatric Tumors	
• **MC malignant** tumor of **infancy** • **MC extracranial solid** tumor in **children** • **MC abdominal** malignancy in **children**	**Neuroblastoma**[Q]
• **MC primary malignant renal** tumor of **childhood**	**Wilms' tumor**[Q]
• **MC renal tumor** of **infancy**	**Congenital mesoblastic nephroma**[Q]
• **MC soft tissue** tumor in **infants** and **children**	**Rhabdomyosarcoma**[Q]
• **MC solid tumor** of childhood	**Brain tumor**[Q]
• **MC cancer** of childhood	**Leukemia**[Q] (30%) >**Brain tumors**[Q] (22%)

MC cancer in males (PLC): **Prostate >Lung >Colorectal**[Q]
MC cancer in females (BLC): **Breast >Lung >Colorectal**[Q]
Cancer deaths in males (LPC): **Lung >Prostate >Colorectal**[Q]
Cancer deaths in females (LBC): **Lung >Breast >Colorectal**[Q]

Annexure 22

MISCELLANEOUS

- **Widest portion** of colon: **Cecum**[Q]
- **Narrowest portion** of colon: **Sigmoid**[Q]
- **MC site** of **colonic rupture** caused **by distal obstruction**: **Cecum**[Q]
- **Colon absorbs water, NaCl**[Q]; **secretes K**[+]**, HCO$_3$ and mucus**[Q]
- **MC site of ischemic colitis: Splenic flexure**

Sarcomas with Lymph Node Metastasis (MARCES)	
• Malignant fibrous histiocytoma[Q]	• Clear cell sarcoma[Q]
• Angiosarcoma[Q]	• Epithelial sarcoma[Q]
• Rhabdomyosarcoma[Q]	• Synovial sarcoma[Q]

Tumors with Spontaneous Regression (NCR MR)	
• Neuroblastoma[Q]	• Malignant melanoma[Q]
• Choriocarcinoma[Q]	• Retinoblastoma[Q]
• Renal cell carcinoma[Q]	

Malignancies associated with Migratory Thrombophlebitis	
• CA pancreas (MC)[Q]	• Prostate cancer[Q]
• CA lung[Q]	• Ovarian cancer[Q]
• GI malignancies[Q]	• Lymphoma[Q]

- **Trousseau's syndrome: Migratory thrombophlebitis**[Q]
- **Trousseau's sign: Carpopedal spasm in hypocalcemia**[Q]
- **Troisier's sign: Palpable left supraclavicular LN (Virchow's node)**[Q]

Perineural Spread is seen in	
1. **Adenoid cystic carcinoma**[Q]	3. **Cholangiocarcinoma**[Q]
2. **CA GB**[Q]	4. **Ductal adenocarcinoma** of pancreas[Q]

Small Round Blue Cell Tumors (WEL PNR)	
• **Wilms' tumor**	• **Primitive neuroectodermal tumor**
• **Ewing's sarcoma**	• **Neuroblastoma**
• **Lymphoma**	• **Rhabdomyosarcoma**
• **Medulloblastoma**	• **Askin tumor**
• **Small cell variant of osteosarcoma**	• **Desmoplastic small cell tumor**

Causes of Postoperative Fever	
Day	**Cause**
2–5 days	• **Atelectasis** of the lung[Q]
3–5 days	• **Superficial** and **deep wound infection**[Q]
5 days	• **Chest infection** including viral respiratory tract infection, **UTI** and **thrombophlebitis**[Q]
> 5 days	• **Wound infection**, anastomotic leakage, intracavitary collections and abscesses[Q]

Increased Cancer Risk in Obese Patients (PEEL CP GO KBC)		
• **Prostate**[Q]	• **Cervix**[Q]	• **Kidney**[Q]
• **Endometrial**[Q]	• **Pancreas**[Q]	• **Bile duct**[Q]
• **Esophagus**[Q]	• **Gallbladder**[Q]	• **Breast**[Q]
• **Liver**[Q]	• **Ovarian**[Q]	• **Colon and rectum**[Q]

Psammoma Bodies (PSM)

1. Papillary carcinoma thyroid[Q]
2. Papillary carcinoma (RCC)[Q]
3. Serous cystadenoma[Q]
4. Meningioma[Q]

Proctoscope	10–12 cm[Q]
Rigid sigmoidoscope	25 cm[Q]
Flexible sigmoidoscope	60 cm[Q]
Colonoscope	160 cm[Q]

• Most radiosensitive **ovarian** tumor	• **Dysgerminoma**[Q]
• Most radiosensitive **brain** tumor	• **Medulloblastoma**[Q]
• Most radiosensitive **testicular** tumor	• **Seminoma**[Q]
• Most radiosensitive **lung** tumor	• **Small cell CA**[Q]
• Most radiosensitive **kidney** tumor	• **Wilms tumor**[Q]
• Most radiosensitive **bone** tumor	• **Ewing's Sarcoma**[Q] and **Multiple myeloma**[Q]

Condition	Seen in
• **Necrolytic erythema migrans**	• **Glucagonoma**
• **Erythema chronicum migrans**	• **Lyme's disease**
• **Erythema infectiosum (fifth disease)**	• **Parvovirus B19**
• **Erythema marginatum**	• **Acute rheumatic fever**

Screening Immunohistochemistry

- **Epithelial Markers**: **Cytokeratin** (positive in **carcinomas**)[Q]
- **Lymphoid Markers**: **CD-45** (positive in **lymphoma**)[Q]
- **Melanocytic Markers**: **S-100** (positive in **melanoma**)[Q]
- **Mesenchymal Markers**: **Vimentin** (positive in **sarcoma**)[Q]
- **Neuroendocrine Markers**: **Chromagranin** and **neuron-specific enolase**[Q]

Annexure 23

FIRST ORGAN TRANSPLANTATION

First **kidney** transplantation (in **identical twins**)	• **Murray**[Q] (1954)
First **liver** transplantation	• **Starzl**[Q] (1963)
First **pancreas** transplantation	• **Kelly & Lillehei**[Q] (1966)
First **heart** transplantation	• **Christian Barnard**[Q] (1967)
First **lung** transplantation	• **Fritz Derom**[Q] (1968)
First **pancreatic islet cell** transplantation	• **Sutherland**[Q] (1974)
First **heart & lung** transplantation	• **Reitz & Shumway**[Q] (1981)
First successful intestinal transplantation	• Deltz (1988)

Annexure 24

SURGICAL POSITIONS

Supine position	• **MC surgical position**, patient lies with back flat on operating room bed
Trendelenburg position	• Same as supine position but the **upper torso is lowered**[Q].
Reverse Trendelenburg position	• Same as supine but **upper torso is raised & legs are lowered**[Q].
Fracture Table Position	• **For hip fracture surgery** • **Upper torso** is in **supine position with unaffected leg raised**. Affected leg is extended with no lower support. The leg is strapped at the ankle and there is padding in the groin to keep pressure on the leg and hip.
Lithotomy position	• Used for **gynecological, anal & urological procedures**[Q]. • **Upper torso is placed in the supine position**, legs are raised and secured, **arms are extended**[Q].
Fowler's position	• Begins with patient in supine position. **Upper torso is slowly raised to a 90° position**[Q].
Semi-Fowler's position	• **Lower torso is in supine position** & **upper torso is bent at a nearly 85° position**. The patient's head is secured by a restraint.
Prone position	• Patient lies with **stomach on the bed**. Abdomen can be raised off the bed.
Jackknife position	• Also called the **Kraske position**[Q] • Patient's abdomen lies flat on the bed. The **bed is scissored so the hip is lifted & legs & head are low**[Q].
Knee-chest position	• Similar to the jackknife except the **legs are bent at the knee at a 90° angle**.
Lateral position	• Also called the **side-lying position**, it is like the jackknife except the patient is on his or her side. Other similar positions are Lateral chest & Lateral kidney.
Lloyd-Davies position	• Common position for **surgical procedures involving the pelvis & lower abdomen**. • **Majority of colorectal & pelvic surgery** is conducted in the **Lloyd-Davis position**[Q].
Kidney position	• **Patient's abdomen is placed over a lift in the operating table** that **bends the body to allow access to the retroperitoneal space**. • A kidney rest is placed under the patient at the location of the lift.
Sims' position	• **Variation of the left lateral position** • Patient will roll to his or her left side. **Keeping the left leg straight, the patient will slide the left hip back and bend the right leg**. This position allows **access to the anus**[Q].

Abdominal Examination Signs		
Sign	**Description**	**Diagnosis**
Aaron sign	**Pain** or pressure **in epigastrium** or **anterior chest** with **persistent firm pressure** applied to **McBurney's point**[Q]	**Acute appendicitis**[Q]
Bassler sign	Sharp pain created by compressing appendix between abdominal wall and iliacus	Chronic appendicitis
Blumberg's sign	Transient abdominal wall **rebound tenderness**[Q]	**Peritoneal inflammation**
Carnett's sign	Loss of abdominal tenderness when abdominal wall muscles are contracted	Intra-abdominal source of abdominal pain
Chandelier sign	Extreme lower abdominal and pelvic pain with movement of cervix	Pelvic inflammatory disease
Claybrook sign	Accentuation of breath and cardiac sounds through abdominal wall	Ruptured abdominal viscus
Courvoisier's sign	**Palpable gallbladder** in presence of **painless jaundice**[Q]	**Periampullary tumor**[Q]
Cruveilhier sign	**Varicose veins** at **umbilicus (caput medusae)**[Q]	**Portal hypertension**[Q]
Danforth sign	Shoulder pain on inspiration	Hemoperitoneum
Fothergill's sign	Abdominal wall mass that does not cross midline and remains palpable when rectus contracted	Rectus muscle hematomas
Mannkopf's sign	Increased pulse when painful abdomen palpated	Absent if malingering
Ransohoff sign	**Yellow discoloration** of **umbilical region**	**Ruptured CBD**[Q]
Ten Horn sign	**Pain** caused by **gentle traction of right testicle**[Q]	**Acute appendicitis**[Q]

Annexure 25

IMPORTANT POINTS ABOUT TUMORS

Breast	• **MC type** of breast cancer: **Adenocarcinoma**[Q] • **MC subtype** of breast cancer: **Invasive ductal cancer**[Q] • **Least common type** of breast cancer: **Papillary**[Q] • **Most malignant** type of breast cancer: **Inflammatory breast cancer**[Q] • Breast cancer associated with **best prognosis: Tubular**[Q] • **MC site** of breast cancer: **Upper outer quadrant**[Q] • **Least common site** of breast cancer: **Lower inner quadrant**[Q] • **MC site of metastasis: Bone (Lumbar vertebra** >Femur >Thoracic vertebra)[Q]
Thyroid	• **MC type** of thyroid cancer: **Papillary** > Follicular >Medullary > Anaplastic[Q] • **MC site of metastasis from papillary** carcinoma: **Lungs**[Q] • MC site of metastasis **from follicular carcinoma: Bones**[Q] (Osteolytic secondaries) • MC site of metastasis **from Medullary carcinoma: Liver**[Q] • MC site of metastasis **from anaplastic carcinoma: Lungs**[Q] • **MC primary** responsible **for metastasis to thyroid: CA breast >CA lung**[Q]
Adrenal	• **MC adrenal tumor: Non-functioning adenoma**[Q]
Liver	• **MC malignancy** of liver: **Metastasis**[Q] • **MC primary malignancy** of liver: **HCC**[Q] • MC primary malignancy of liver **in children: Hepatoblastoma**[Q] • **MC benign tumor** of liver: **Hemangioma**[Q]
Spleen	• **MC neoplasm** of spleen: **Lymphoma** (Non-Hodgkin's lymphoma)[Q] • **MC primary tumor** of spleen: **Hemangioma**[Q] • **MC primary malignant tumor** of spleen: **Angiosarcoma**[Q]
Gallbladder	• **MC site** of CA gallbladder: **Fundus** (60%) > Body (30%) >Neck (10%)[Q] • **Maximum incidence** of CA gallbladder: **India > Pakistan**[Q] • **MC histological type** of CA gallbladder: **Diffuse infiltrative** or **sclerosing**[Q]
Bile Duct	• **MC site** of cholangiocarcinoma: **Hilum** (65%) >Distal (25%) >Intrahepatic (10%)[Q] • **MC histological type** of cholangiocarcinoma: **Diffuse infiltrative** or **sclerosing**[Q]
Pancreas	• **MC site** of carcinoma pancreas: **Head**[Q] • **MC site of gastrinoma: Duodenum** (1st part) > **Pancreas**[Q] • **MC site of insulinoma: Equally distributed in head, body & tail**[Q] • **MC site of glucagonoma & mucinous cystadenoma: Body & tail**[Q] • **MC site of somatostatinoma, PPoma, serous cystadenoma & IPMN: Head**[Q] • **MC site of VIPoma: Tail**[Q]
Esophagus	• **MC type** of carcinoma esophagus: **SCC**[Q] • MC type of carcinoma esophagus **in western population: Adenocarcinoma**[Q] • **MC site of SCC** esophagus: **Middle 1/3rd**[Q] • MC site of **Adenocarcinoma** esophagus: **Lower 1/3rd**[Q] • **MC site of carcinoma esophagus: Middle 1/3rd**[Q]
Stomach	• **MC site of carcinoma stomach, gastric lymphoma: Antrum**[Q] • **MC site of carcinoma stomach in pernicious anemia: Fundus**[Q] • **MC site of diffuse variety of carcinoma stomach: Fundus**[Q]
Small intestine	• **MC tumor of small bowel: Stromal tumor >Adenoma**[Q] • **MC tumor of small bowel in children: Lymphoma**[Q] • **MC malignant tumor** of small bowel: **Adenocarcinoma**[Q] **>Carcinoid** • **MC site of carcinoid, adenoma, lipoma, lymphoma, leiomyoma: Ileum**[Q] • **MC site of adenocarcinoma: Duodenum**[Q]
Colon-Rectum	• **MC site of colorectal cancer: Rectum**[Q] • **Least common site** of colorectal cancer: **Hepatic flexure**[Q] • **MC site of colon cancer: Sigmoid**[Q]

Contd...

Contd...

Appendix	• **MC neoplasm of appendix: Carcinoid tumor**[Q] • **MC malignant neoplasm** of appendix: **Mucinous adenocarcinoma > Adenocarcinoma >Carcinoid tumor**[Q]
Anal canal	• **MC type** of carcinoma anal canal: **SCC>BCC>Melanoma**[Q]
Kidney	• **MC type** of RCC: **Clear cell** carcinoma[Q] • **MC type** of RCC seen **in dialysis associated disease: Papillary** carcinoma[Q] • Type of RCC with **best prognosis: Chromophobe** carcinoma[Q]
Urinary bladder	• **MC type** of carcinoma bladder: **TCC >SCC >Adenocarcinoma**[Q] • **MC benign mesenchymal tumor** of urinary bladder: **Leiomyoma**[Q] • **MC malignant mesenchymal tumor** of urinary bladder: **Leiomyosarcoma**[Q] • **MC malignant mesenchymal tumor** of urinary bladder **in children: Rhabdomyosarcoma**[Q]
Prostate	• **MC type** of carcinoma prostate: **Adenocarcinoma >TCC**[Q] • **MC site** of carcinoma prostate: **Peripheral zone (75%) >Transition zone (15%) >Central zone (10%)**[Q]
Penis & Urethra	• **MC type** of carcinoma penis: **SCC**[Q] • **MC site** of carcinoma penis: **Glans >Prepuce >Shaft (GPS)**[Q] • **MC site of carcinoma male urethra: Bulbomembranous urethra**[Q] • MC type of carcinoma **prostatic urethra: TCC >SCC**[Q] • MC type of carcinoma **penile urethra: SCC >TCC**[Q]
Testis	• MC **histological type** of testicular tumour: **Seminoma**[Q] (**Mixed**[Q] if given in the option) • MC **bilateral primary testicular tumour: Seminoma**[Q] • **Most radiosensitive** testicular tumor: **Seminoma**[Q] • MC testicular tumor in **infant & children up to 3 years: Yolk sac tumour**[Q] • Testicular tumour with **best prognosis: Yolk sac tumour**[Q] • MC testicular tumor in **pre-pubertal children: Teratoma**[Q] • **MC testicular tumor** in **patients >60 years: Lymphoma**[Q] • MC **bilateral testicular tumour: Lymphoma**[Q] • MC **secondary testicular tumour: Lymphoma**[Q] • MC **histologic type** of testicular lymphoma: **DLBL**[Q] • Testicular tumour with **worst prognosis: Hurricane tumour (Type of choriocarcinoma)**[Q]
Scrotum	• **MC benign lesion** of scrotum: **Sebaceous cyst**[Q] • **MC malignant tumor** of scrotum: **SCC**[Q]
Lung	**Adenocarcinoma** • **MC** histological **type**[Q] • MC in **non-smokers, young** patients, **females**[Q] • Located **peripherally**[Q] • **Slow growth** & propensity to **metastasize to opposite lung**[Q] • **Metastasize** more frequently to **CNS**[Q] • Most cells contain **mucin**[Q] • **Noguchi classification**[Q] is used for adenocarcinoma **Squamous Cell Carcinoma** • **MC in smokers**[Q]; MC type in **India**[Q] • MC variety associated with **hypercalcemia** (produces **PTH-rp**)[Q] • **Central**[Q] in distribution • Prone to undergo **central necrosis & cavitation**[Q] • **Pancoast** tumor is histologically **SCC**[Q] • Associated with **best prognosis**[Q]

Contd...

Lung	**Small Cell Carcinoma**	• **Most malignant, central**[Q] in distribution, strongly related to **smoking**[Q] • Associated with **massive hilar** or **mediastinal lymphadenopathy, mediastinal invasion & perihilar mass**[Q] • **MC variety** associated with **paraneoplastic syndrome, hypokalemia & SVC syndrome**[Q] • Most responsive to **chemotherapy** (cisplatin + etoposide) • Shows response to **radiotherapy**[Q] • Hormones produced by small cell carcinoma: **ACTH, AVP** (vasopressin), **calcitonin, ANF**, gastrin releasing peptide[Q]
	Large Cell Carcinoma	• Highly **undifferentiated** with **cavitating nature**[Q] • **Metastasize early** with **poor prognosis**[Q]
Heart		• **MC cardiac tumor: Metastasis**[Q] • **MC primary cardiac tumor: Myxoma**[Q] • MC primary cardiac tumor **in infants & children: Rhabdomyoma**[Q]
Brain		• **MC brain tumor: Metastasis**[Q] • MC **primary** brain tumor: **Meningioma (35%) > Glial tumors (30%)**[Q] • MC **malignant** brain tumor of **children: Medulloblastoma**[Q] • **Most radiosensitive brain tumor: Medulloblastoma**[Q] • **MC astrocytoma in children: Pilocytic astrocytoma**[Q] • **MC astrocytoma in adults: Glioblastoma multiforme**[Q] • **Astrocytoma is supratentorial in adults** & **infratentorial in children**[Q] • **Maximum incidence of calcification** in brain tumor: **Craniopharyngioma (most) >Oligodendroglioma (90%) >Meningioma (25%)**[Q] • **MC pituitary tumor: Adenoma**[Q] (arising from anterior lobe)
Oral cavity		• **MC site of CA oral cavity: Tongue >Lip**[Q] • **MC histological type of CA oral cavity: Squamous cell carcinoma**[Q] • **MC type of cancer in India: CA oral cavity**[Q] • **MC site of CA oral cavity in India: Buccal mucosa**[Q] (38%) > Anterior tongue (16%) >Lower alveolus (15.7%) • **LN metastasis** is **most common in: CA tongue**[Q] >Floor of mouth >Lower alveolus >Buccal mucosa >Upper alveolus >**Hard palate >Lip**[Q]. • **Bilateral lymphatic spread** is common in: **Lower lip**[Q]**, supraglottis**[Q] & **soft palate**[Q].
Salivary gland		• **MC neoplasm of salivary gland: Pleomorphic adenoma**[Q] • **MC malignant tumor** of salivary gland: **Mucoepidermoid carcinoma**[Q] • **MC neoplasm** of salivary gland **in children: Hemangioma**[Q] • **MC malignant tumor** of salivary gland **in children: Mucoepidermoid carcinoma**[Q] • **MC malignant tumor** of **minor salivary glands: Adenoid cystic carcinoma**[Q]
Sarcoma		• **MC site of GIST: Stomach >Small bowel >Colorectum & esophagus**[Q] • **MC soft tissue sarcoma in adults: Liposarcoma >Leiomyosarcoma >Malignant fibrous histiocytoma**[Q] • MC soft tissue sarcoma of **extremities: Malignant fibrous histiocytoma > Liposarcoma**[Q] • MC soft tissue sarcoma of **retroperitoneum: Liposarcoma**[Q] • MC **pediatric** soft tissue sarcoma: **Rhabdomyosarcoma**[Q]
Bone		• **MC site of primary for bone metastasis:** CA **B**reast > CA **P**rostate >**R**CC >CA **L**ung > CA **T**hyroid > CA **B**ladder (**BP** increased by **RL** in **TB**)[Q] • **MC site of bone metastasis: Thoracic vertebra**[Q] • **MC cause of osteoblastic secondaries in males: CA Prostate**[Q] • **MC cause of osteolytic secondaries in males: RCC**[Q] • **Lytic expansile metastasis is seen in: RCC & follicular carcinoma thyroid**[Q] • **MC cause of osteoblastic & osteolytic secondaries in females: CA Breast**[Q] • **MC tumor metastasize to bone in females: CA Breast**[Q]

Annexure 26

NAMED OPERATIONS

Named Operations	Done for
• **Hadfield's** operation[Q]	**Duct ectasia**[Q]
• **Sistrunk** operation[Q]	**Thyroglossal cyst**[Q]
• **Hartley-Dunhill** procedure[Q]	**Subtotal thyroidectomy**[Q] (10-12 gm of thyroid remnant is left in the same lobe)
• **Puestow** procedure[Q] • **Duval** procedure[Q] • **Beger's** procedure[Q] • **Frey's** procedure[Q]	**Chronic Pancreatitis**[Q]
• **Whipple's** procedure[Q] • **Traverso-Longmire** procedure[Q]	**Periampullary carcinoma**[Q]
• **Kasai** procedure[Q]	**Extrahepatic biliary atresia**[Q]
• **Nissen's** fundoplication[Q]	**GERD**[Q]
• **Heller's** cardiomyotomy[Q]	**Achalasia cardia**[Q]
• **Ivor-Lewis** operation[Q] • **Orringer** transhiatal esophagectomy[Q] • **Mckeon** en-bloc esophagectomy[Q]	**Carcinoma esophagus**[Q]
• **Shoemaker** procedure[Q] • **Pouchet** procedure[Q] • **Kelling-Madlener** procedure[Q] • **Csendes** procedure[Q]	**Type IV gastric ulcer**[Q]
• **Ramstedt-Fredet** pyloromyotomy[Q]	**Infantile hypertrophic pyloric stenosis**[Q]
• **Bishop-Koop** operation[Q]	**Meconium ileus**[Q]
• **Bianchi** procedure[Q]	**Short bowel syndrome**[Q]
• **Ladd's** operation[Q]	**Malrotation of gut**[Q]
• **Swenson** operation[Q] • **Duhamel** operation[Q] • **Soave** operation[Q]	**Hirschsprung's disease**[Q]
• **Hartmann's** procedure[Q]	**Carcinoma sigmoid colon**[Q]
• **Kocher's** maneuver[Q]	**Mobilization of duodenum**[Q]
• **Extended Kocher's** maneuver[Q]	**Right sided medial visceral rotation**[Q]
• **Mattox** maneuver[Q]	**Left sided medial visceral rotation**[Q]
• **Cattell-Braasch** maneuver[Q]	**For extensive retroperitoneal exposure**[Q]
• **Mitrofanoff's** procedure[Q]	**Appendicovesicostomy**[Q]
• **Malone** procedure[Q]	**Appendicolostomy**[Q]
• **Milligan-Morgan** open hemorrhoidectomy[Q] • **Ferguson** closed hemorrhoidectomy[Q] • **Whitefield** submucosal hemorrhoidectomy[Q] • **Longo's** stapler hemorrhoidectomy[Q]	**Hemorrhoidectomy**[Q]
• **Well's** procedure[Q] • **Ripstein** procedure[Q] • **Frykman & Goldberg** procedure[Q]	**Abdominal rectopexy**[Q]
• **Delorme's** mucosectomy[Q] • **Thiersch** anal encirclement[Q] • **Altmier's** rectosigmoidectomy[Q]	**Perineal rectopexy**[Q]
• **Lord's** procedure[Q] • **Notara's** lateral sphincterostomy[Q]	**Fissure in ano**[Q]
• **Bascom** procedure[Q] • **Karydakis** procedure[Q]	**Pilonidal sinus**[Q]

Contd...

Contd...

Procedure	Condition
• **Bassini** repair, **Shouldice** repair[Q] • **McVay** repair[Q] • **Lichtenstein** repair[Q]	**Inguinal hernia**[Q]
• **Lockwood** operation[Q] • **Lothiessen** operation[Q] • **McEvedy** operation[Q] • **Henry** procedure[Q]	**Femoral hernia**[Q]
• **Dowd's** operation[Q]	**Lumbar hernia**[Q]
• **Mayo's** repair[Q]	**Umbilical hernia**[Q]
• **Rovsing's** operation[Q]	**Deroofing of cyst in ADPKD**[Q] (**Rovsing's sign**: Pain in right lower quadrant during palpation of left lower quadrant in **acute appendicitis**) (**Rovsing's syndrome**: Abdominal pain, nausea & vomiting on hyperextension of spine in **horse shoe kidney**)
• **Anderson Hynes dismembered pyeloplasty**[Q]	**PUJ obstruction**[Q]
• **Lich-Gregoir** technique[Q] • **Leadbetter-Politano** technique[Q]	**Methods of ureteric implantation in VUR**[Q]
• **Boari's** operation[Q]	**Lower ureteric reconstruction** with a strip of bladder wall
• **Frayer's suprapubic** prostatectomy[Q] • **Millin's retropubic** prostatectomy[Q] • **Young's perineal** prostatectomy[Q]	**Open prostatectomy for BPH**[Q]
• **Dennis-Brown** technique[Q] • **MAGPI**[Q] • **Mathiew** procedure[Q] • **Asopa or Duckett** technique[Q] • **Thiersch-Duplay or Bracka** technique[Q]	**Hypospadias**[Q]
• **Winter** shunt[Q] • **Al-Ghorab** shunt[Q] • **Quackel or Sacher** shunt[Q] • **Grayhack** shunt[Q] • **Barry** shunt[Q]	**Surgical management of ischemic priapism**[Q]
• **Nesbitt operation**[Q]	**Peyronie's disease**[Q]
• **Fowler-Stephens** orchiopexy[Q] • **Ladd & Gross** orchiopexy[Q] • **Ombridann's** orchiopexy[Q] • **Keetley-Torek** orchiopexy[Q]	**Undescended Testis**[Q]
• **Lord's plication of sac**[Q]	**Small hydrocele**[Q]
• **Jaboulay's eversion of sac**[Q]	**Medium sized hydrocele**[Q]
• **Palomo's** operation[Q]	**Varicocele**[Q]
• **Trendelenberg operation**[Q]	**Varicose vein**[Q]
• **Gilles, Neibulowitz & Kinmonth** procedure[Q]	**Reconstructive operation for lymphedema**[Q]
• **Kontoleons, Homans, Thompson & Charles** procedure[Q]	**Excisional operation for lymphedema**[Q]
• **Moh's micrographic surgery**[Q]	**BCC or SCC** involving **vital areas, cosmetic areas** or **recurrent tumors**[Q]
• **COMMANDO's** operation[Q]	**COM**bined **M**andibulectomy **A**nd **N**eck **D**issection **O**peration for **carcinoma tongue fixed to mandible** with **infiltration of floor of mouth**[Q].
• **Newman & Seabrocks'** operation[Q]	**Parotid fistula**[Q]
• **Millard rotation advancement technique**[Q] • **Thompson, Le Musurier & Tennison-Randall** operation[Q]	**Cleft lip repair**[Q]

Annexure 27

DIFFUSE LARGE B CELL LYMPHOMA (DLBL) IS MC TYPE OF LYMPHOMA IN

- **Primary CNS lymphoma**[Q]
  (in immunocompetent patients)
- **Orbital** lymphoma[Q]
- **Thyroid** lymphoma[Q]
- **Breast** lymphoma[Q]

- **Gastric** lymphoma[Q]
- **Small intestinal** lymphoma[Q]
- **Appendicular** lymphoma[Q]
- **Colorectal** lymphoma[Q]
- **Testicular** lymphoma[Q]

Annexure 28

TRIANGLES IN SURGERY

Calot's triangle	• Superiorly: **Cystic artery**[Q] • Medially: **Common hepatic duct**[Q] • Laterally: **Cystic duct**[Q]
Hepatocystic triangle	• Superiorly: **Inferior surface of liver**[Q] • Medially: **Common hepatic duct**[Q] • Laterally: **Cystic duct**[Q]
Femoral triangle	• Superiorly: **Inguinal ligament**[Q] • Medially: Medial border of **adductor longus** muscle[Q] • Laterally: Medial border of **sartorius** muscle[Q] (**Femoral artery pulsations** are felt at this site[Q])
Inferior triangle of Petit	• Inferiorly: **Iliac crest**[Q] • Medially: **Latissimus dorsi muscle**[Q] • Laterally: **External oblique muscle**[Q]
Superior triangle of Grynfelt	• Superiorly: **12th rib**[Q] • Medially: **Paraspinal muscles**[Q] • Laterally: **Internal oblique muscle**[Q]
Scalene triangle	• Anteriorly: **Scalenus anticus**[Q] • Posteriorly: **Scalenus medius**[Q] • Inferiorly: **First rib**[Q] (Trunk of **Brachial plexus & subclavian vessels** are **compressed** at Scalene triangle causing **thoracic outlet syndrome**[Q])
Sherren's triangle	• Bounded by lines joining **anterior superior iliac spine, pubic tubercle & umbilicus**[Q] • Area of **skin hyperaesthesia in acute appendicitis**[Q]
Simon's triangle	• Superiorly: **Inferior thyroid artery**[Q] • Laterally: **Common carotid artery**[Q] • Medially: **Esophagus**[Q] (**Simon's triangle** aids in **identification of recurrent laryngeal nerve**[Q])
Joll's triangle	• Laterally: **Upper pole** of thyroid gland & **superior thyroid vessels**[Q] • Superiorly: Attachment of **strap muscles & deep investing layer of fascia to hyoid**[Q] • Medially: **Midline**[Q] • Floor: **Cricothyroid muscle**[Q] (**External branch of superior laryngeal nerve** lies **in Joll's triangle**[Q])

Contd...

Contd...

Triangle of **Auscultation**	• Superiorly & medially: **Inferior portion of trapezius** • Inferiorly: **Upper border of latissimus dorsi** • Laterally: **Medial border of scapula** (Only part of back **not covered by muscles, respiratory sounds** are better heard)
Triangle of **Doom**	• Bounded **laterally** by the **gonadal vessels**[Q] • **Medially** by the **vas deferens**[Q] • **Apex** oriented superiorly at the **internal ring**[Q] (Contain **external iliac vessels**[Q], deep circumflex iliac vein, the femoral nerve & genital branch of the genitofemoral nerve)
Triangle of **Hesselbach**	• Laterally: **Epigastric artery**[Q] • Medially: **Lateral border** of **rectus abdominis**[Q] where it is attached to pubic crest • Inferiorly: **Inguinal ligament**[Q]

Triangle of **Pain**	• Medially: **Gonadal vessels**[Q]
	• Superiorly: **iliopubic tract**[Q]
	• Laterally: **Peritoneum**[Q]
	• This triangle **contains** from lateral to medial:
	  – **Lateral femoral cutaneous nerve**[Q] (**MC injured nerve**[Q])
	  – **Anterior femoral cutaneous**[Q]
	  – **Femoral branch** of the **genitofemoral nerve**[Q]
	  – **Femoral nerve**[Q]

Annexure 29

Condition	Most Commonly occurs on
Parathyroid insufficiency	2nd–5th day[Q]
Duodenal stump blowout	4th–7th day[Q]
Bowel anastomotic leak	7th day[Q]
Wound dehiscence	5th–8th day[Q]
T-tube cholangiogram	7th–10th day[Q]
Perforation in typhoid ulcer	3rd week[Q]

Condition	Location
Hemorrhoids	3, 7 & 11'O clock position[Q]
Vascular supply of bile duct	Co-axial 3'O clock & 9'O clock position[Q]
TUIP (Transurethral incision of prostate)	Incision at 5 & 7'O clock position[Q]
Fissure-in-ano	6'O clock position[Q]
Endoscopic sphincterotomy	11'O clock position[Q]
Optical internal urethrotomy	12'O clock position[Q]
MC position of appendix	12'O clock position[Q] (Retrocecal)

Annexure 30

Condition	MC Organism Responsible
Breast abscess Splenic abscess Acute pyelonephritis (hematogenous spread) Carbuncle Hand infections	• **Staphylococcus aureus**[Q]
Acute suppurative thyroiditis	• **Staphylococcus aureus**[Q] > **Streptococcus**[Q]
Pyogenic liver abscess	• **In Western countries: E. coli**[Q] • **In Asian countries: Klebsiella pneumoniae**[Q] • **In children with chronic granulomatous disease: Staphylococcus aureus**[Q]
Amoebic liver abscess	• **Entamoeba histolytica**[Q]
Hydatid cyst	• **Echinococcus granulosus**[Q]
Emphysematous cholecystitis	• **Clostridium welchiiQ (anaerobe) > E. coli**[Q] **(aerobe)**
Emphysematous pyelonephritis Acute pyelonephritis (ascending form) Chronic pyelonephritis Perinephric abscess UTI Acute & chronic bacterial prostatitis Prostatic abscess Infected pancreatic necrosis	• **E. coli**[Q]
Xanthogranulomatous pyelonephritis	• **Proteus**[Q]
Cholangitis	• **E. coli**[Q] > **Klebsiella**[Q]
Peptic ulcer MALT lymphoma	• **H. pylori**[Q]
Spontaneous bacterial peritonitis	• **In adults: E. coli**[Q] • **In children: Group 'A' Streptococci**[Q]
Secondary bacterial peritonitis	• **Bacteroides**[Q] **(anaerobe) > E. coli**[Q] **(aerobe)**
Peritonitis in CAPD	• **Staphylococcus epidermidis**[Q]
Acute mesenteric lymphadenitis	• **Yersinia enterocolitica**[Q]
Gastrointestinal tuberculosis Genitourinary tuberculosis	• **Mycobacterium tuberculosis**[Q]
Appendicular perforation	• **Bacteroides**[Q] **(anaerobe) > E. coli**[Q] **(aerobe)**
Anorectal abscess	• **E. coli**[Q] > **Bacteroides**[Q]
OPSI (Overwhelming post-splenectomy infection)	• **Streptococcus pneumoniae**[Q]
Struvite stone (Staghorn calculi)	• **Proteus**[Q]
Schistosomiasis	• **Schistosoma hematobium**[Q]
Acute epididymo-orchitis	• **Sexually active male <35 years: Chlamydia**[Q] • **Children, elderly males, homosexuals: E. coli**[Q]
Mycotic aneurysm	• **Staphylococcus aureus**[Q] **>Salmonella**[Q]
Lymphedema	• **Wuchereria bancrofti**[Q]
Burn sepsis	• **Pseudomonas**[Q]
Cellulitis	• **Streptococcus pyogenes**[Q]
Erysipelas	• **Beta-hemolytic group 'A' Streptococci**[Q]
Gas gangrene	• **Clostridium perfringens**[Q]
Chronic burrowing ulcer (Meleney gangrene)	• **Microaerophilic non-hemolytic Streptococci**[Q]

Annexure 31

Etiology	Type of Renal Calculus
• Laxative abuse	Ammonium urate[Q]
• Thiazide • Ileostomy	Uric acid[Q]
• Primary hyperparathyroidism • Crohn's disease • Short bowel syndrome • Excess intake of spinach, rhubarb, tea, chocolate & pepper	Calcium oxalate[Q]
• Ethylene glycol	Oxalate stone[Q]
• Inflammatory bowel disease	Calcium oxalate > Uric acid[Q]
• Allopurinol	Xanthine stone[Q]
• Renal tubular acidosis	Calcium phosphate[Q]

Image-based Questions

INSTRUMENTS

1. What is the name of given instrument?
- a. Kocher's thyroid dissector
- b. Doyen's retractor
- c. Joll's thyroid retractor
- d. Deaver's retractor

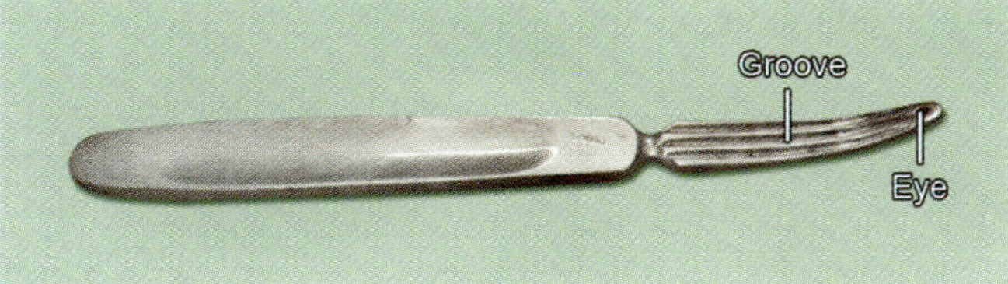

2. What is the name of given instrument?
- a. Aneurysm needle
- b. Veress needle
- c. Tracheal dilator
- d. Urethral dilator

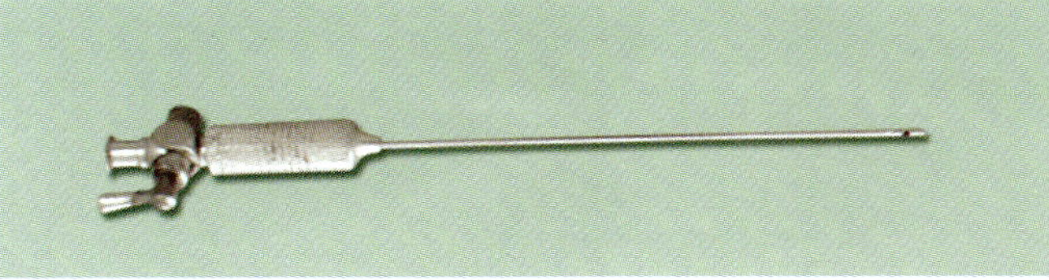

3. Which instrument is shown below? *(MCI June 2019)*
- a. Tongue depressor
- b. Doyen retractor
- c. Self-retaining retractor
- d. Langenbeck's retractor

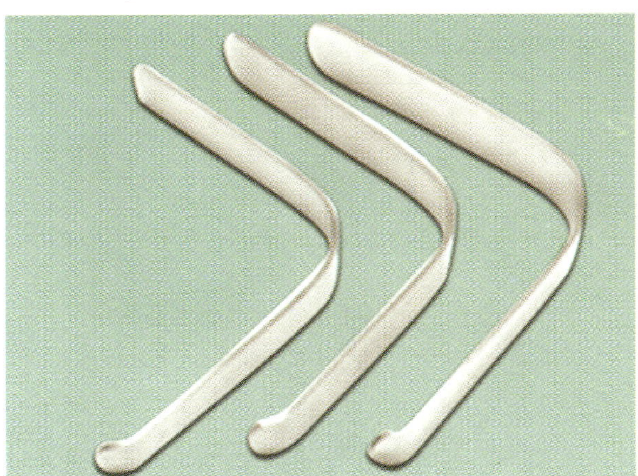

4. What is the name of given instrument?
- a. Doyen's towel clip
- b. Mayo's towel clip
- c. Moynihan's tetra towel clip
- d. Lanes tissue forceps

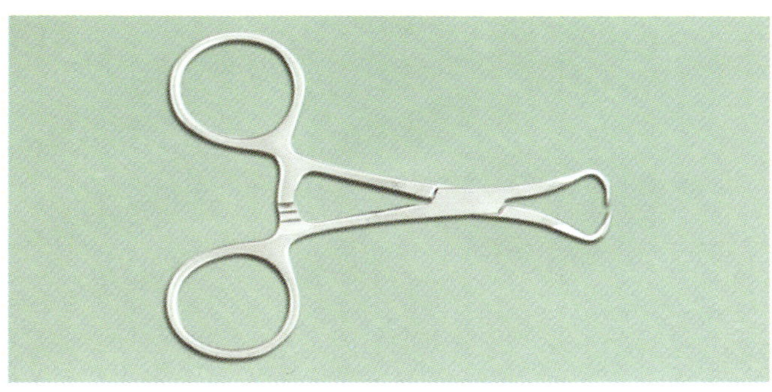

5. What is the name of given instrument?
- a. Doyen's towel clip
- b. Mayo's towel clip
- c. Moynihan's tetra towel clip
- d. Lanes tissue forceps

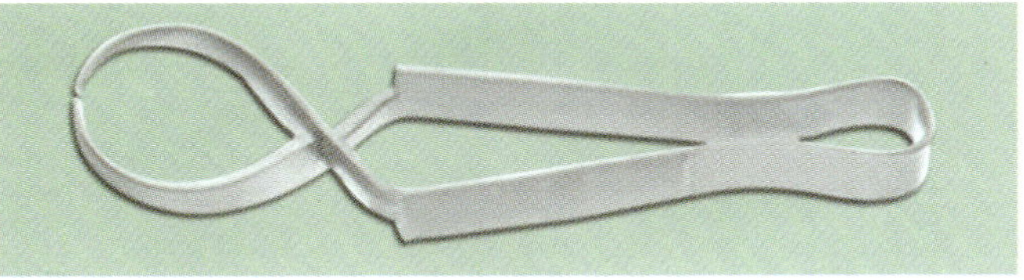

6. What is the name of given instrument?
- a. Doyen's towel clip
- b. Mayo's towel clip
- c. Moynihan's tetra towel clip
- d. Lanes tissue forceps

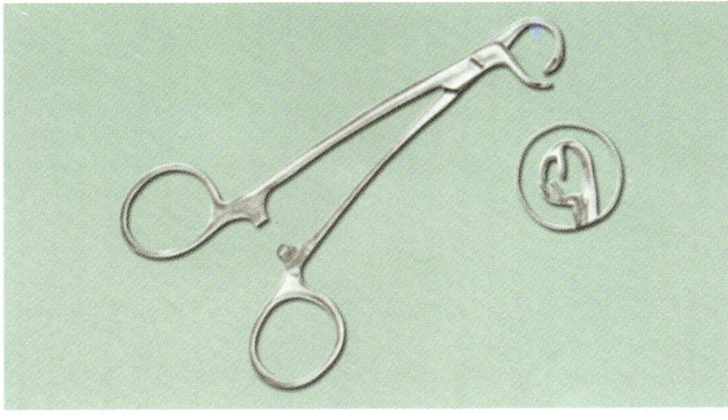

7. What is the name of given instrument?
- a. Doyen's towel clip
- b. Bone curette
- c. Aneurysm needle
- d. Doyen's coastal elevator

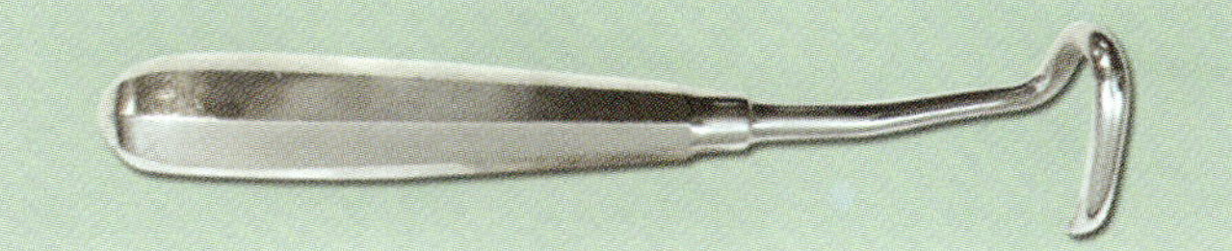

8. What is the use of given instrument?
   a.   Dissection in thyroid surgeries
   b.   Elevation of periosteum
   c.   Suturing
   d.   Used with blade for skin incision

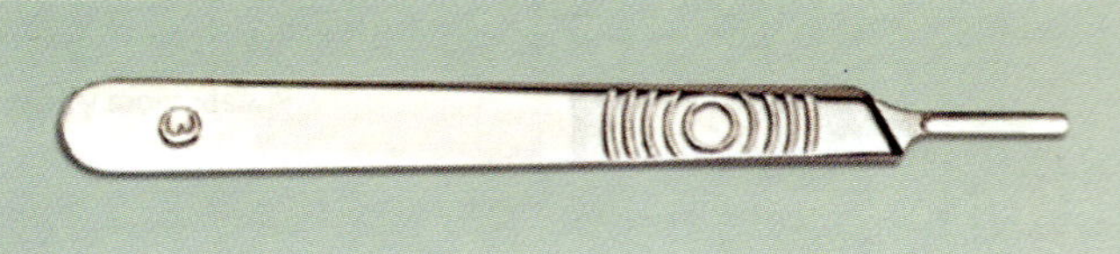

9. Identify the surgical blade used for incision and drainage:
(Recent Question 2019)
   a. 10   b. 11
   c. 15   d. 23

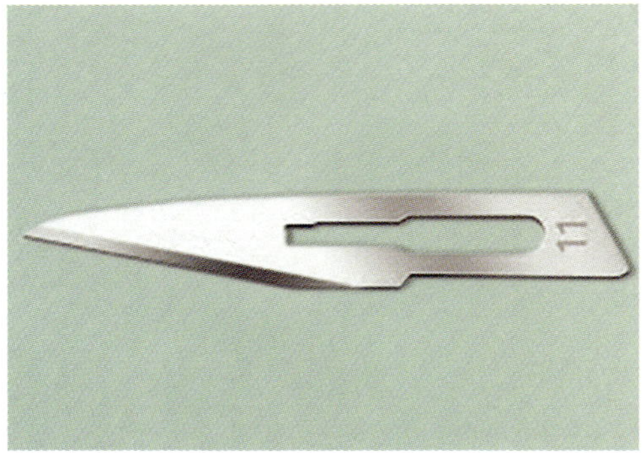

10. What is the use of instrument?   *(Recent Question 2017)*
   a.   Elevation of periosteum
   b.   Cutting the bone
   c.   Harvesting skin graft
   d.   Retraction of abdominal wall

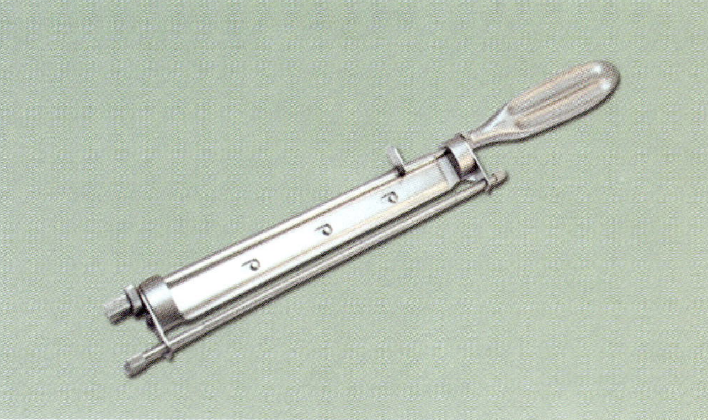

11. What is the name of given instrument?
   a.   Artery forceps   b.   Needle holder
   c.   Kocher's forceps   d.   Tissue forceps

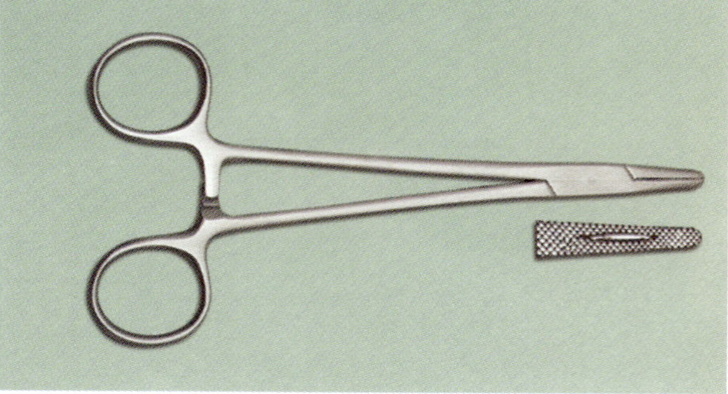

12. What is the name of given instrument?
   a.   Osteotome   b.   Bone cutter
   c.   Bone nibbler   d.   Rib shear

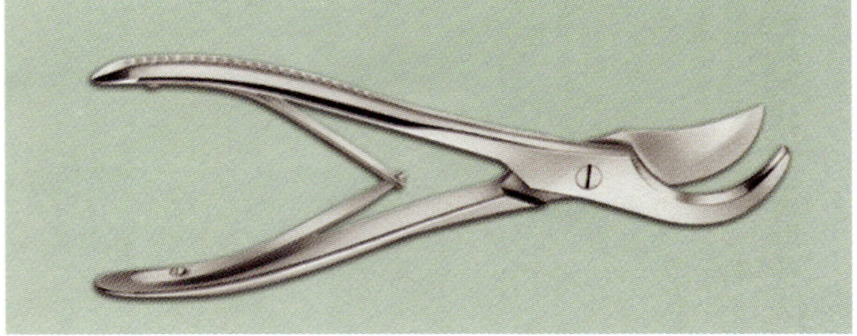

13. The given instrument is used for the diagnosis of:
(Recent Question 2018)
   a.   Hemorrhoids
   b.   Fissure-in-ano
   c.   Pilonidal sinus
   d.   All of the above

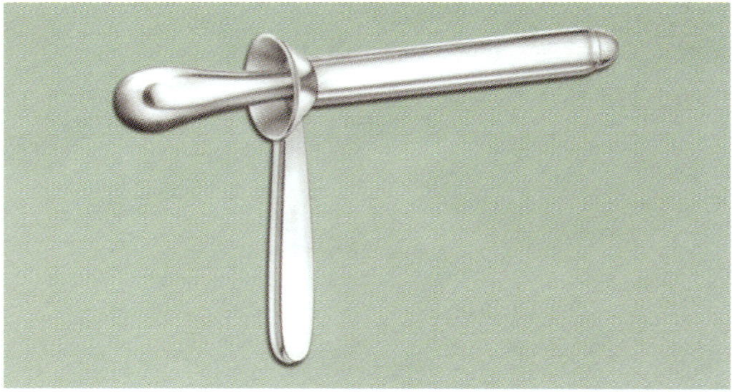

14. What is the name of given instrument?
   a.   Bone hook
   b.   Bone curette
   c.   Periosteal elevator
   d.   Kocher's dissector

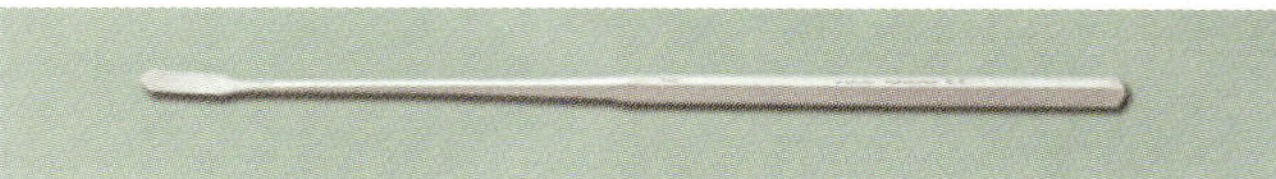

15. What is the name of given instrument?
   a.   Gigli saw
   b.   Mayo's vein stripper
   c.   Fogarty balloon catheter
   d.   Long intravenous catheter

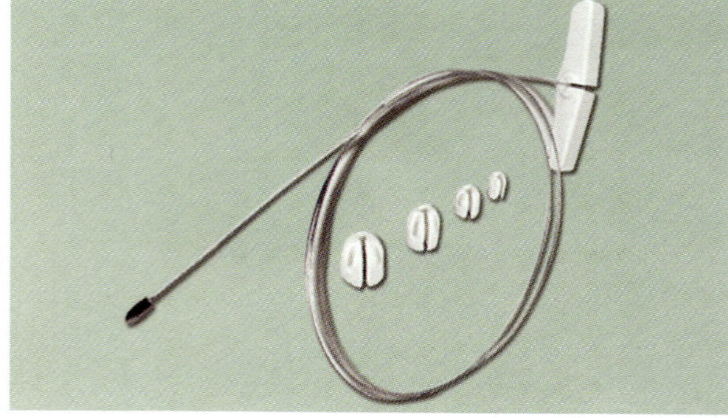

16. What is the name of given instrument?
   a.   Gigli saw
   b.   Mayo's vein stripper
   c.   Fogarty balloon catheter
   d.   Long intravenous catheter

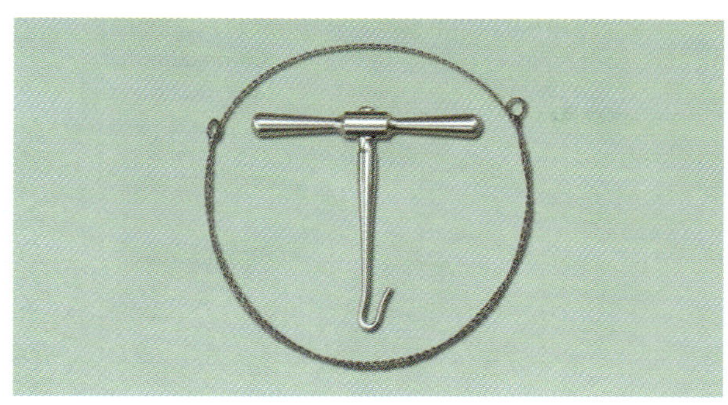

17. What is the name of given instrument?

(Recent Question 2016)

a. Aneurysm needle
b. Fistula probe
c. Veress needle
d. Bone hook

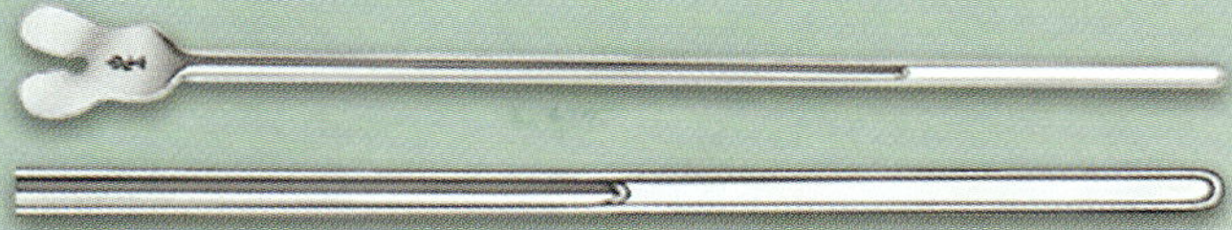

18. What is the name of given instrument?

a. Gallbladder trocar
b. Bone curette
c. Gallstone scoop
d. Laparoscopic trocar

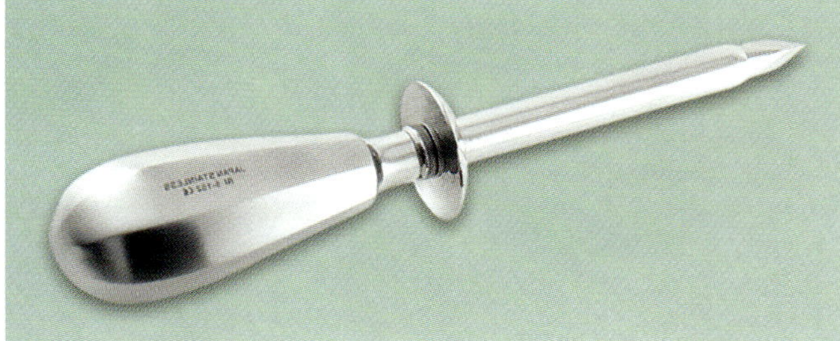

FORCEPS

19. What is the name of given instrument? *(Recent Question 2016)*

a. Ovum forceps
b. Sponge holding forceps
c. Cord holding forceps
d. Pile holding forceps

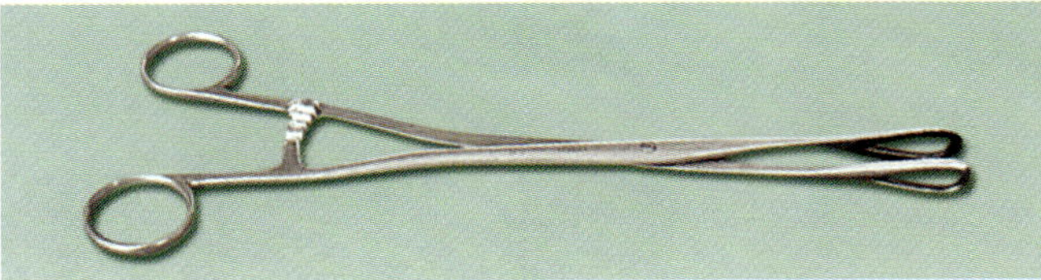

20. What is the name of given instrument?

a. Lister's sinus forceps
b. Kocher's hemostatic forceps
c. Babcock's tissue forceps
d. Lane's tissue forceps

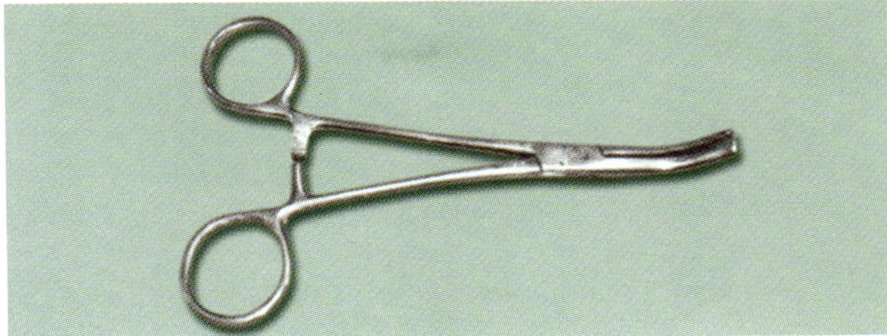

21. What is the name of given instrument?

a. Lister's sinus forceps
b. Kocher's hemostatic forceps
c. Babcock's tissue forceps
d. Lane's tissue forceps

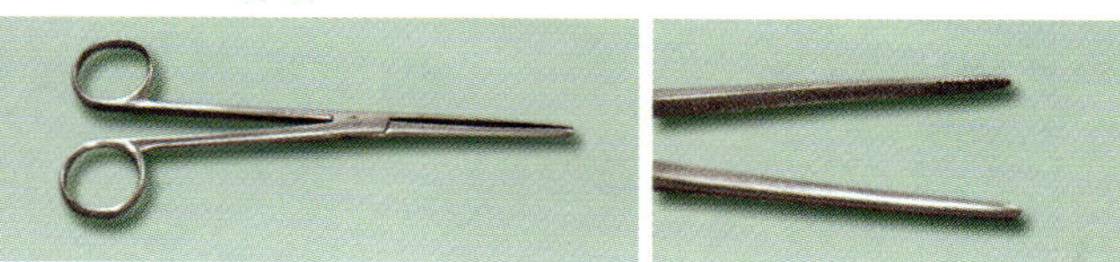

22. What are the uses of given instrument?

a. Used during laparotomy to retract skin margins
b. Used to hold neck of bladder during bladder neck resection
c. Used to hold skin flaps
d. All of the above

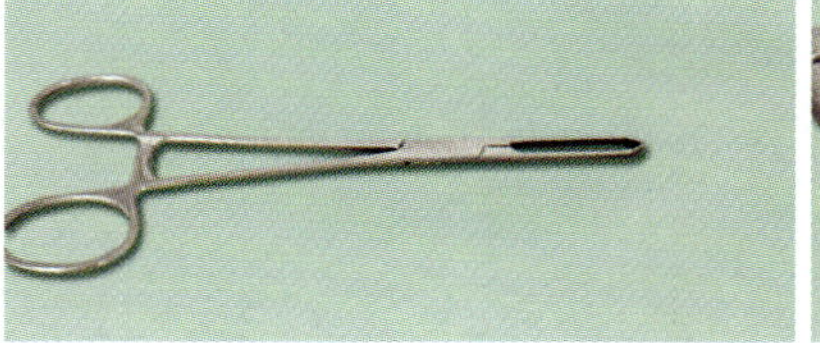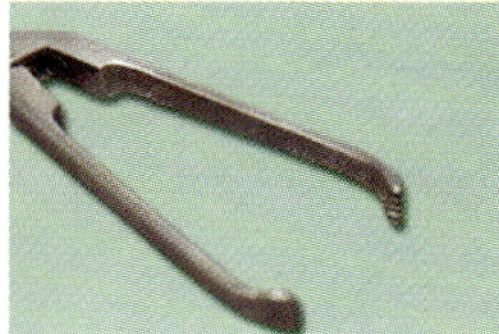

23. What is the name of given instrument? *(Recent Question 2017)*

a. Lister's sinus forceps
b. Kocher's hemostatic forceps
c. Babcock's tissue forceps
d. Lane's tissue forceps

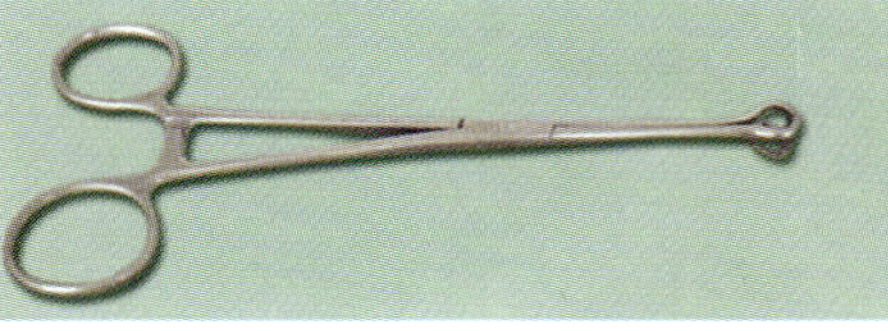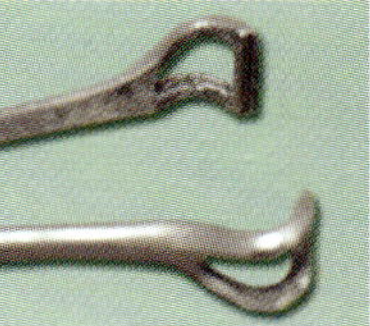

24. What is the name of given instrument?

a. Lister's sinus forceps
b. Kocher's hemostatic forceps
c. Babcock's tissue forceps
d. Lane's tissue forceps

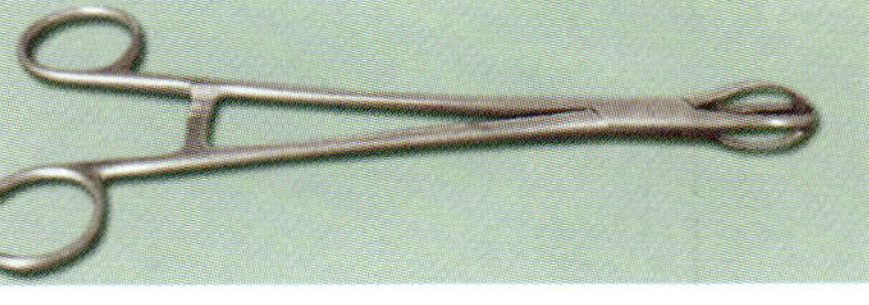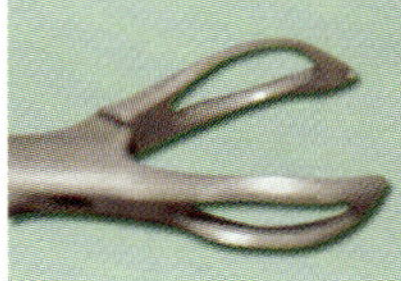

25. What are the uses of given instrument?

a. Used to hold the cut skin margins during suturing
b. Used to hold the linea alba or the rectus sheath during closure of abdominal incision
c. Used to hold the scalp during closure of scalp incision
d. All of the above

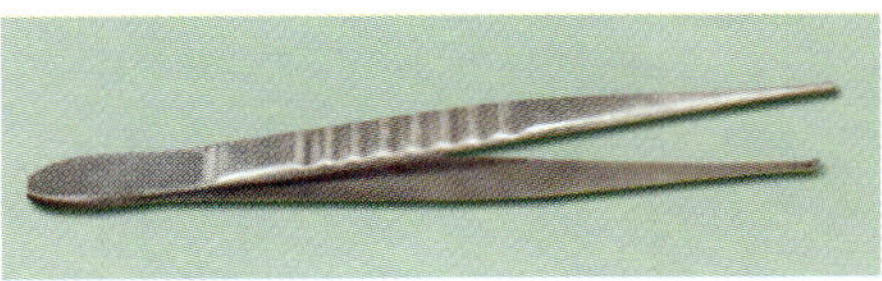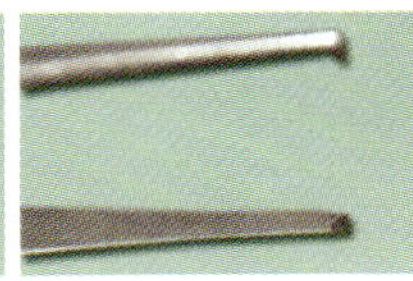

26. What is the name of given instrument?

a. Pyelolithotomy forceps
b. Sponge holding forceps
c. Desjardins forceps
d. Pile holding forceps

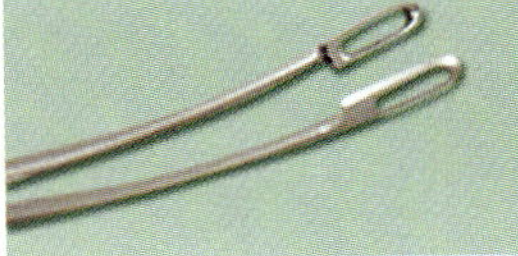

27. What is the name of given instrument?
a. Pyelolithotomy forceps   b. Sponge holding forceps
c. Sprapubic cystolithotomy forceps
d. Pile holding forceps

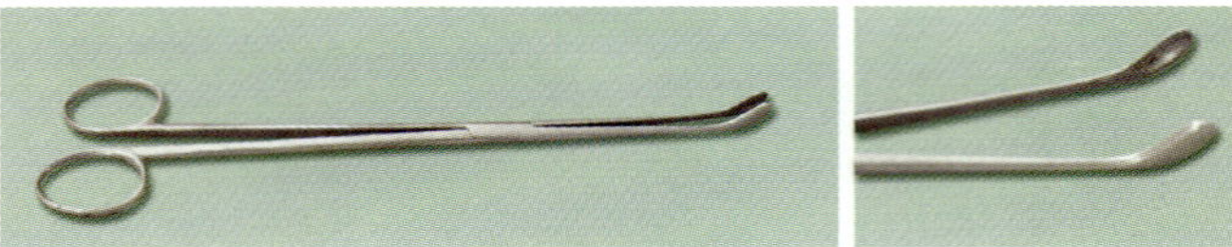

28. What is the name of given instrument?
a. Pyelolithotomy forceps   b. Sponge holding forceps
c. Sprapubic cystolithotomy forceps
d. Pile holding forceps

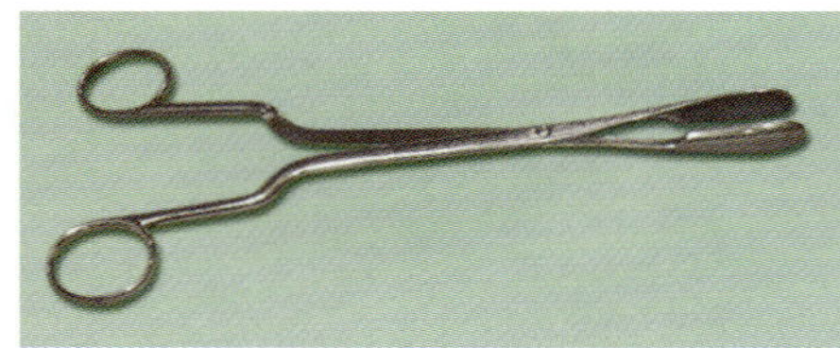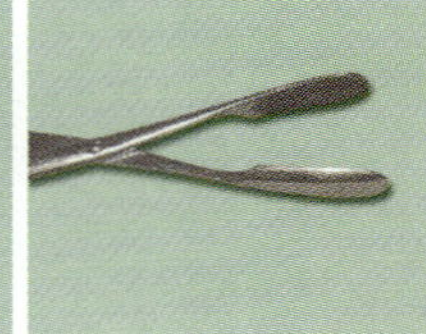

29. What is the use of given instrument?
a. Used for blunt dissections
b. Used to clean abscess cavity
c. Used to hold sponge during cleaning and draping
d. Used to pick sterilized instruments

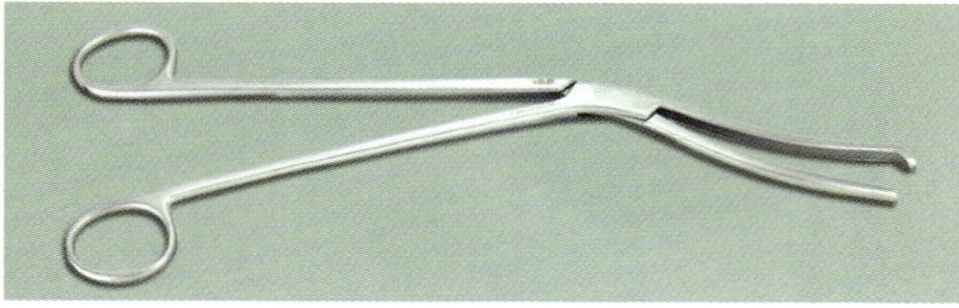

30. What is the name of given instrument?
a. Rampley's sponge holding forceps
b. Piles holding forceps
c. Duval lung holding forceps
d. Ovum forceps

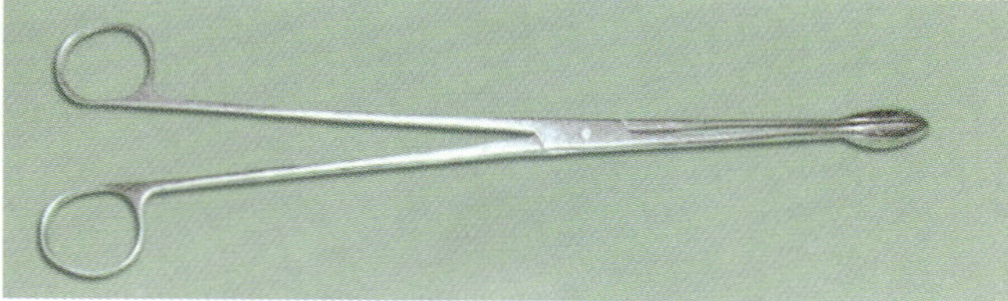

31. What is the name of given instrument?
a. Lister sinus forceps   b. Lanes tissue forceps
c. Russian tissue forceps   d. Kocher's forceps

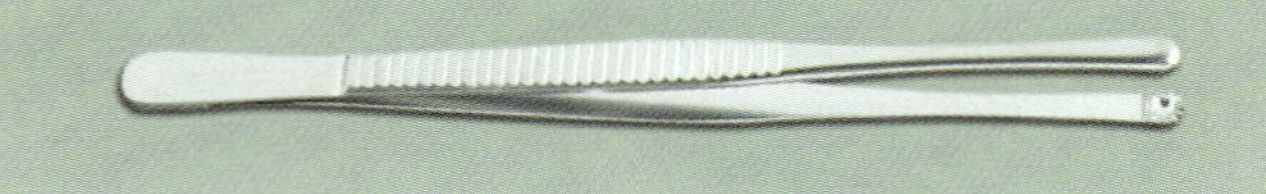

32. What is the name of given instrument?
a. Kocher's forceps   b. Right angle forceps
c. Lanes tissue forceps   d. Russian tissue forceps

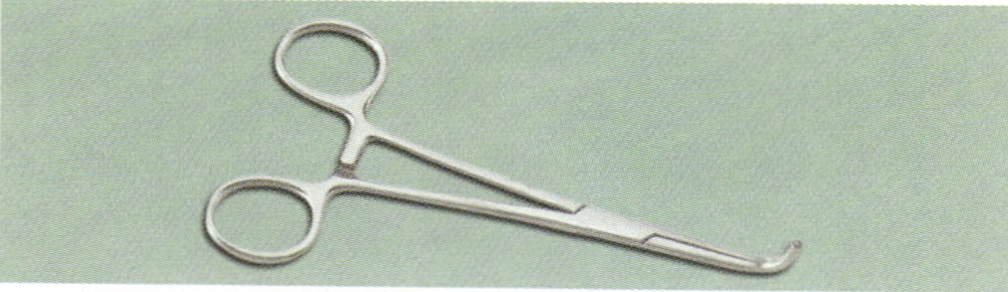

33. Which instrument is shown below?   *(MCI June 2019)*
a. Artery forceps   b. Kocher forceps
c. Allis forceps   d. Babcock forceps

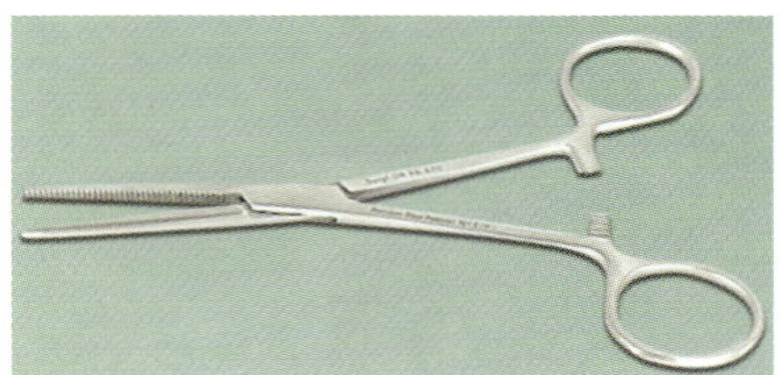

34. What is the name of given instrument?
a. Mosquito hemostatic forceps
b. Spencer Wells hemostatic forceps
c. Kocher's hemostatic forceps
d. Right angle forceps

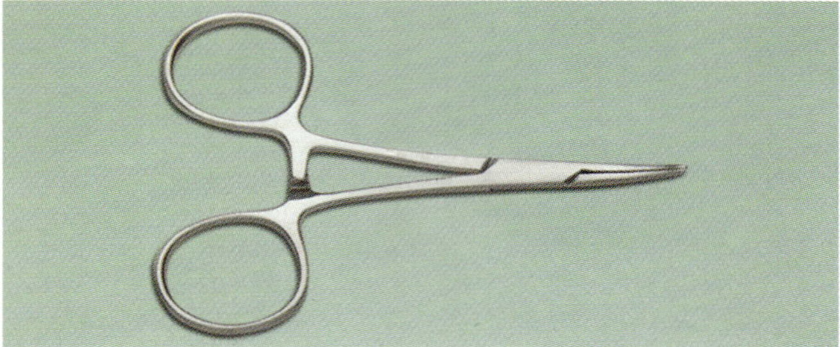

35. What is the name of given instrument?
a. Mosquito hemostatic forceps
b. Spencer Wells hemostatic forceps
c. Kocher's hemostatic forceps
d. Right angle forceps

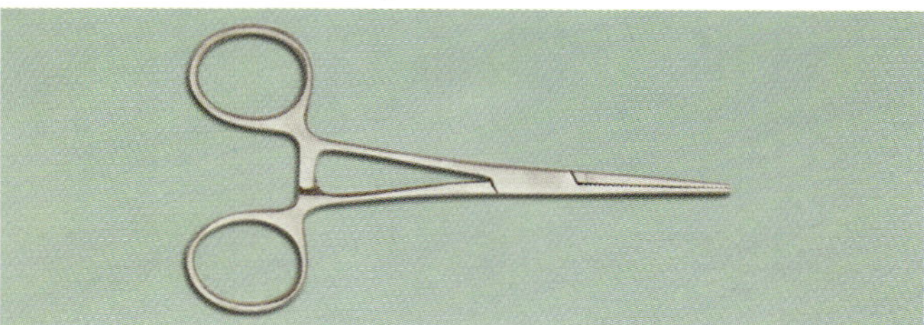

36. Identify the instruments shown here and choose the best combination: *(APPG 2016)*

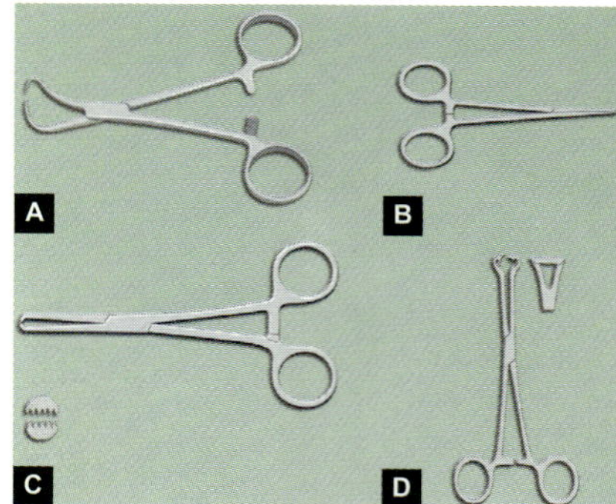

a. A = Dunhill's forceps. B = Halstead mosquito forceps.
C = Allis forceps. D = Crile's hemostatic forceps
b. A = Crile's hemostatic forceps
B = Allis intestinal forceps.
C = Schnidt tonsil forceps. D = Babcock intestinal forceps.
c. A = Backhaus towel clamp. B = Halstead mosquito forceps.
C = Allis forceps. D = Babcock intestinal forceps.
d. A = Backhaus towel clamp. B = Foerster sponge forceps.
C = Dunhill's forceps. D = DeBakey forceps.

RETRACTOR

37. What is the name of given instrument? *(Recent Question 2017)*
a. Morris retractor
b. Doyen's retractor
c. Czerney's retractor
d. Deaver's retractor

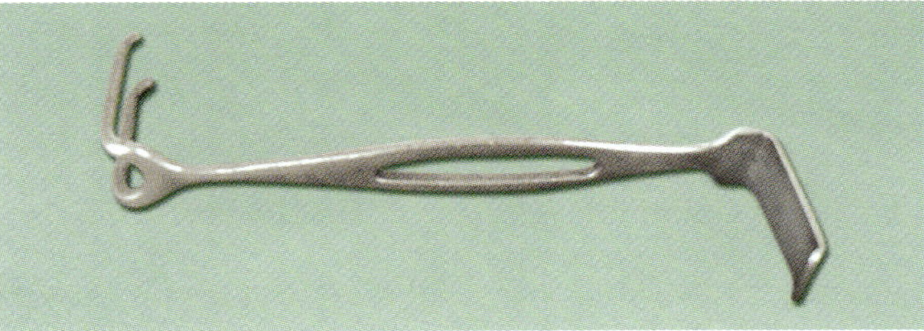

38. What is the name of given instrument?

(Recent Questions 2015)

a. Morris retractor
b. Doyen's retractor
c. Czerney's retractor
d. Deaver's retractor

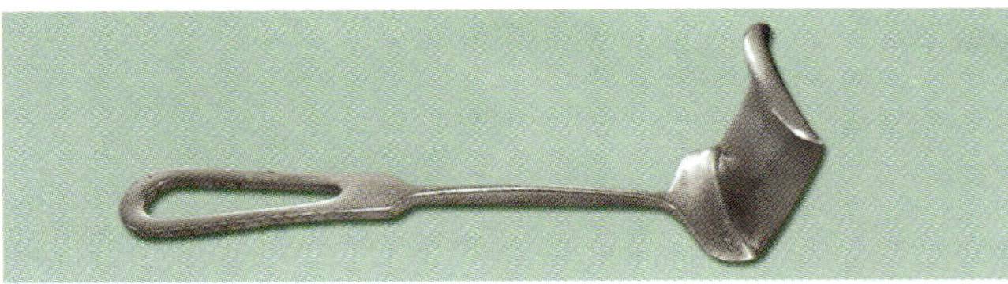

39. What are the uses of given instrument?
a. Used to retract skin flap for excision of sebaceous cyst
b. Used during venesection for retraction of skin
c. Used during tracheostomy for retraction of skin and thyroid isthmus
d. All of the above

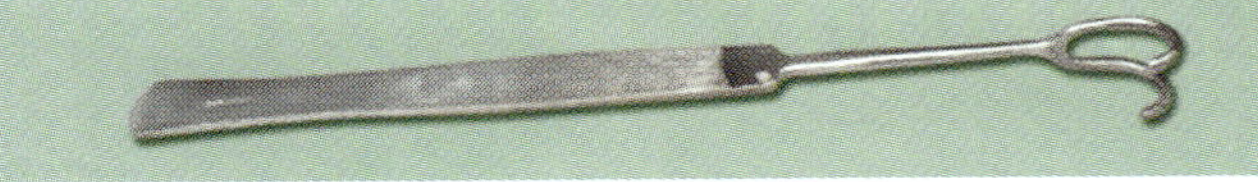

40. What is the name of given instrument?
a. Morris retractor b. Doyen's retractor
c. Volkman's retractor d. Deaver's retractor

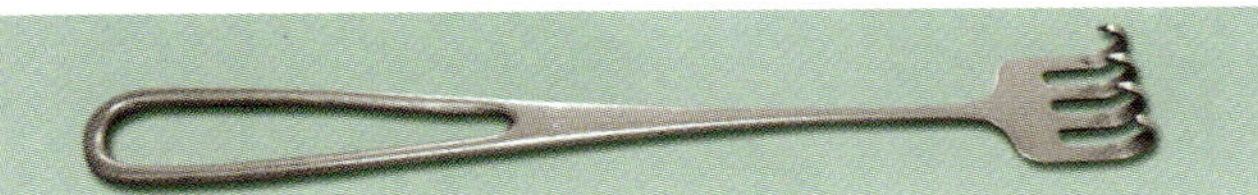

41. What is the name of given instrument? *(Recent Question 2017)*
a. Morris retractor b. Doyen's retractor
c. Volkman's retractor d. Deaver's retractor

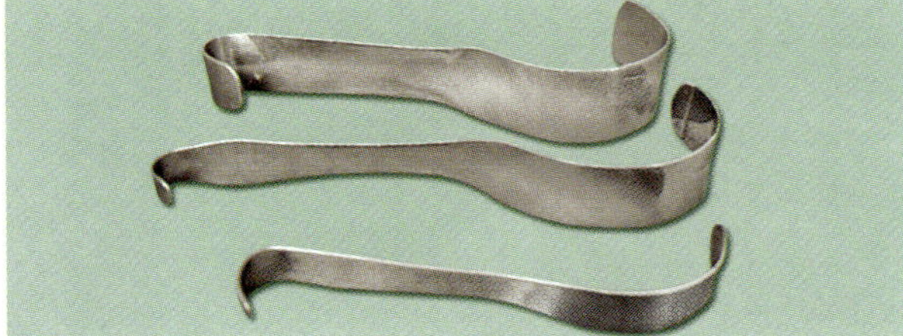

42. What is the name of given instrument?
a. Kocher's thyroid dissector
b. Doyen's retractor
c. Joll's thyroid retractor
d. Deaver's retractor

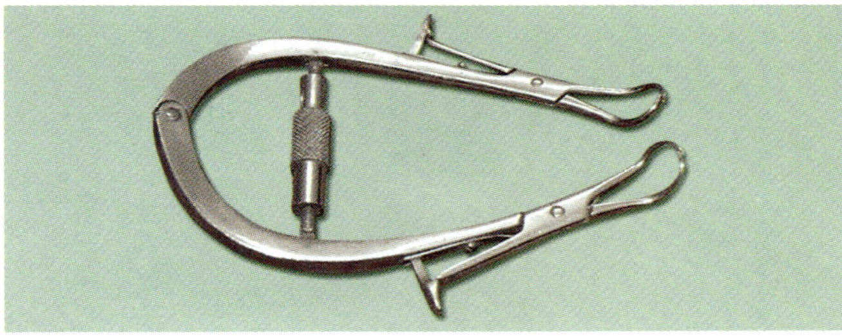

43. What is the name of given instrument?
a. Doyen's retractor *(Recent Question 2016)*
b. Doyen's intestinal occlusion clamp
c. Doyen's mouth gag
d. Joll's thyroid retractor

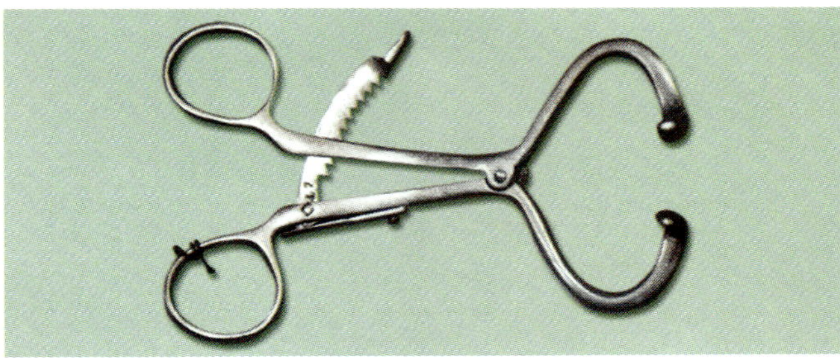

44. What is the name of given instrument?
a. Morris retractor
b. Volkman's retractor
c. Doyen's retractor
d. Balfours retractor

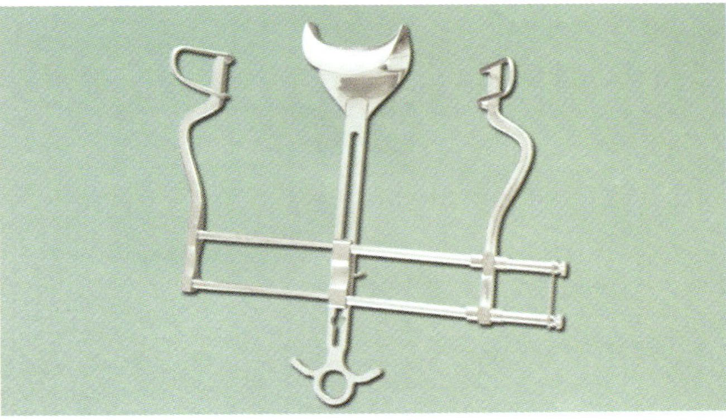

45. What is the name of given instrument?
a. Doyen's mouth gag
b. Beckman Weitlaner retractor
c. Cat's paw retractor
d. Bladder neck retractor

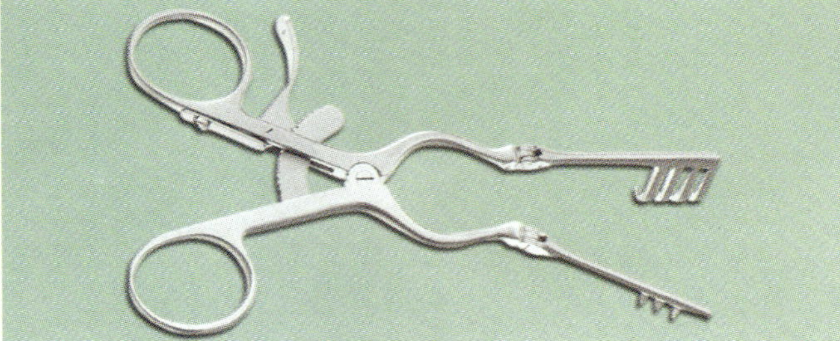

46. What is the name of given instrument?
a. Morris retractor
b. Farabeuf retractor
c. Doyen's retractor
d. Volkman's retractor

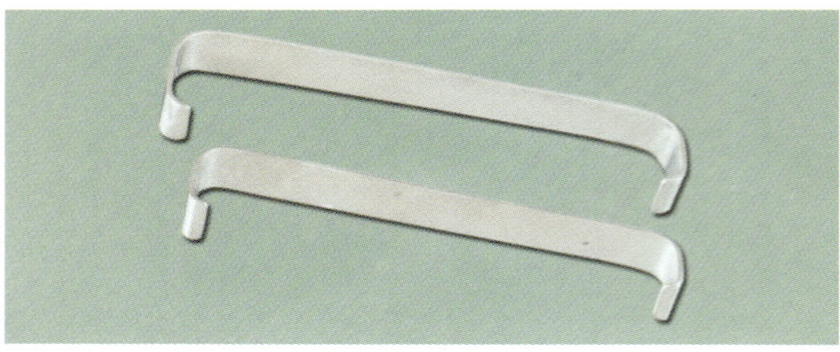

47. What is the name of given instrument?
a. Czerny's retractor
b. Morris retractor
c. Langenbeck's retractor
d. Doyen's retractor

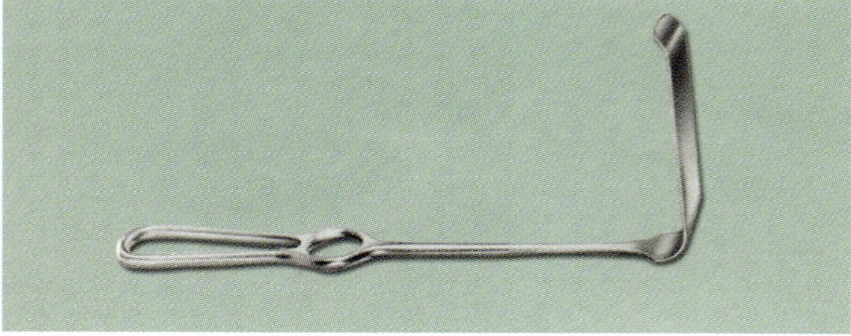

48. What is the name of this instrument?
a. Scapula retractor
b. Morris retractor
c. Kelly retractor
d. Doyen's retractor

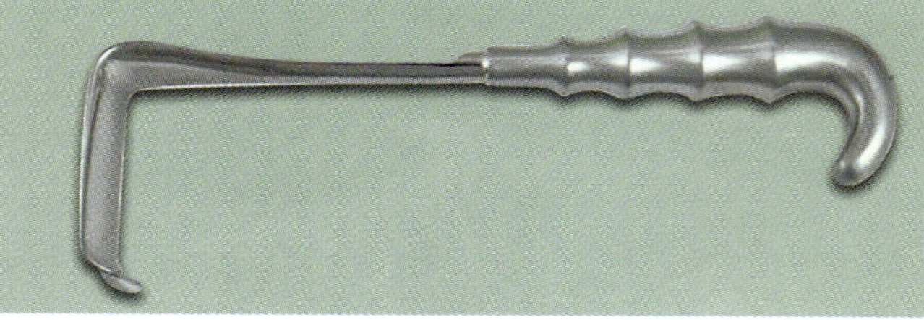

49. What is the name of this retractor?
a. Cat's paw retractor
b. Double hook retractor
c. Single hook retractor
d. Langenbeck's retractor

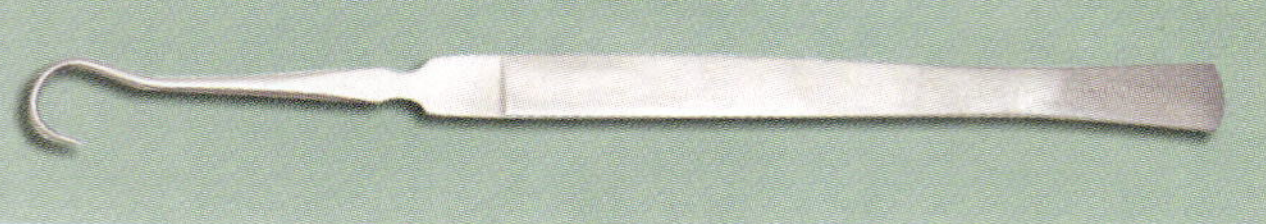

CLAMP

50. What is the name of given instrument?
a. Payr's crushing clamp
b. Doyen's intestinal occlusion clamp
c. Hemostatic clamp
d. Vascular clamp

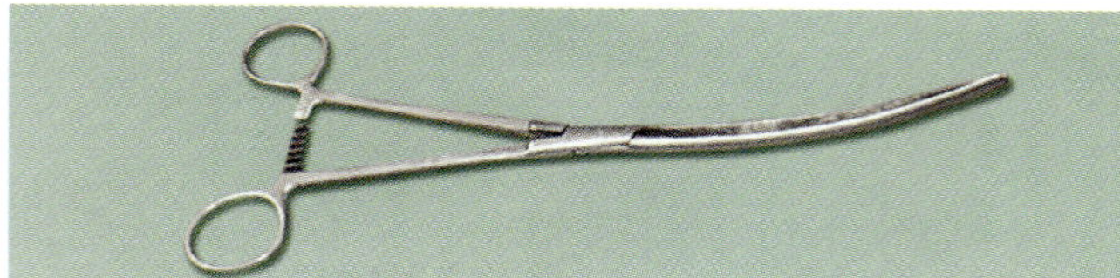

51. What is the name of given instrument?
a. Payr's crushing clamp
b. Doyen's intestinal occlusion clamp
c. Hemostatic clamp
d. Vascular clamp

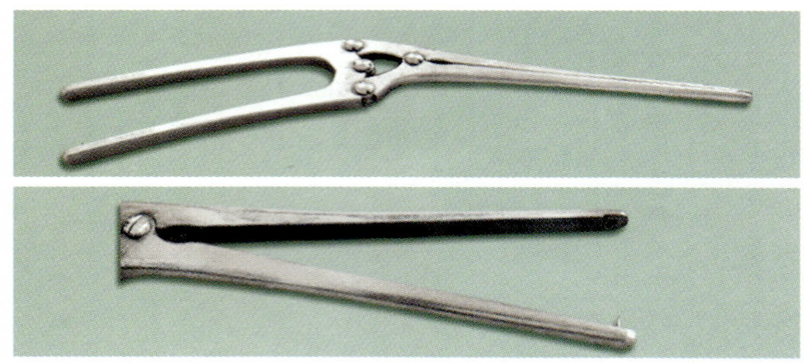

52. What is the name of given instrument?
a. Satinsky vascular clamp
b. Light bulldog clamp
c. Pott's bulldog clamp
d. Well's arterial clamp

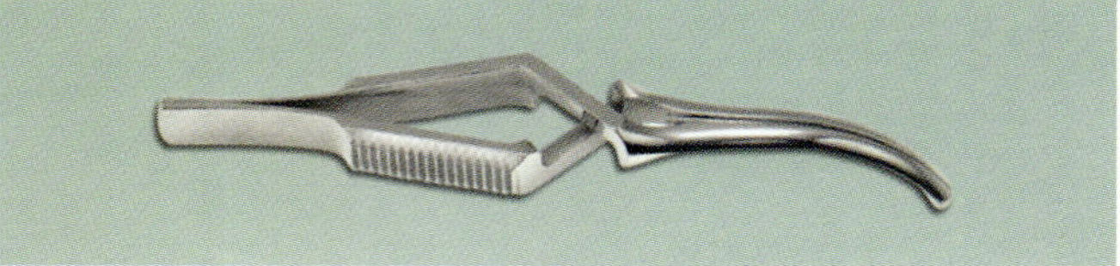

53. What is the name of given instrument?
a. Satinsky vascular clamp
b. Light bulldog clamp
c. Pott's bulldog clamp
d. Well's arterial clamp

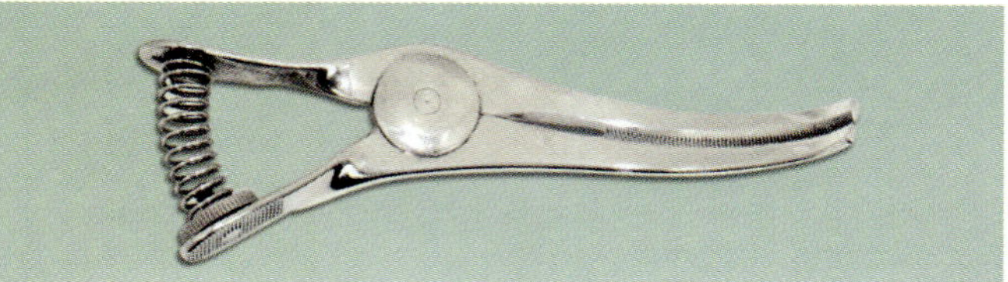

54. What is the name of given instrument?
a. Satinsky vascular clamp
b. Light bulldog clamp
c. Pott's bulldog clamp
d. Well's arterial clamp

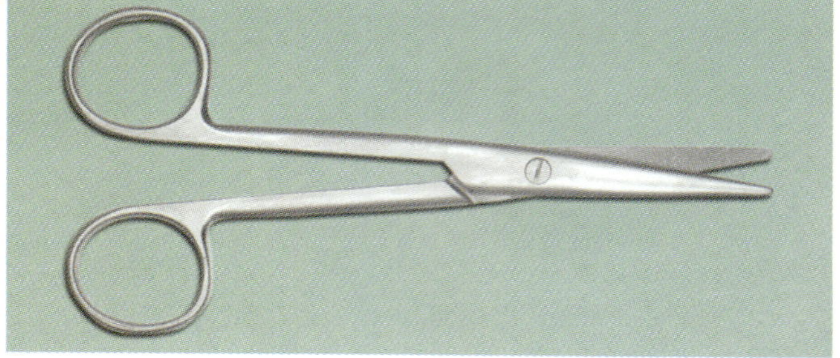

SCISSORS

55. What is the name of given instrument?
a. Mayo scissors
b. Metzenbaum scissors
c. Mcindoe scissors
d. None of the above

56. What is the name of given instrument?
a. Mayo scissors
b. Metzenbaum scissors
c. McIndoe scissors
d. None of the above

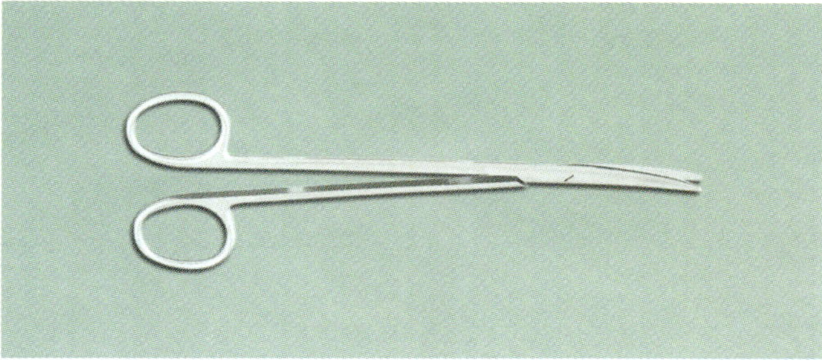

57. What is the name of given scissors?
a. Mayo's scissors
b. Metzenbaum scissors
c. Lister bandage scissors
d. Tenotomy scissors

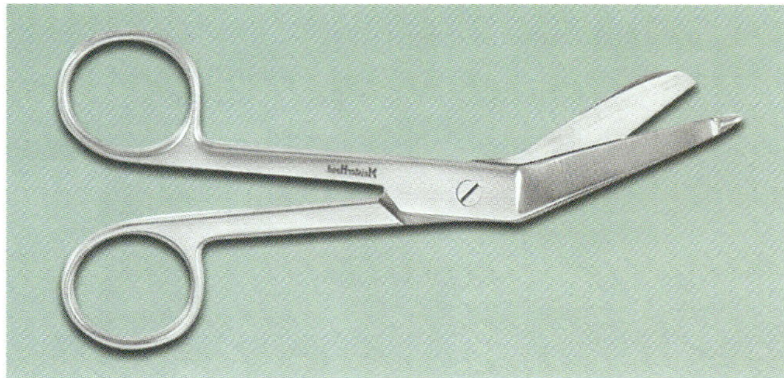

58. What is the name of given instrument?
a. Aneurysm needle
b. Cervical dilator
c. Tracheal dilator
d. Urethral dilator

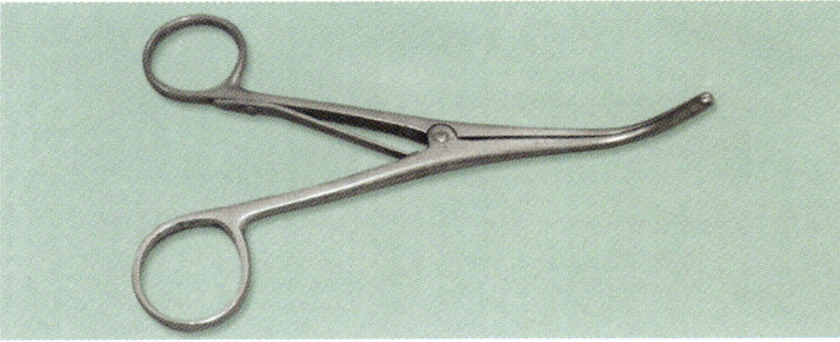

59. What is the name of given instrument?
a. Cervical dilator
b. Urethral dilator
c. Esophageal dilator
d. Anal dilator

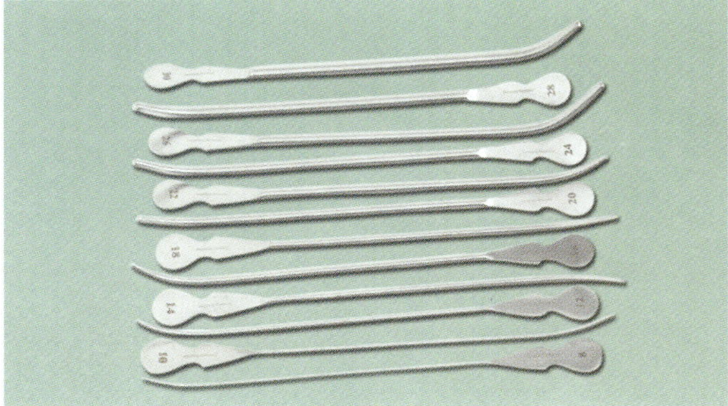

60. What is the name of given instrument?
a. Bile duct dilator
b. Ureteric dilator
c. Urethral dilator
d. Cervical dilator

SCOOP

61. What is the name of given instrument? *(Recent Question 2016)*
a. Volkmann scoop
b. Gallstone scoop
c. Bone curette
d. Biopsy scoop

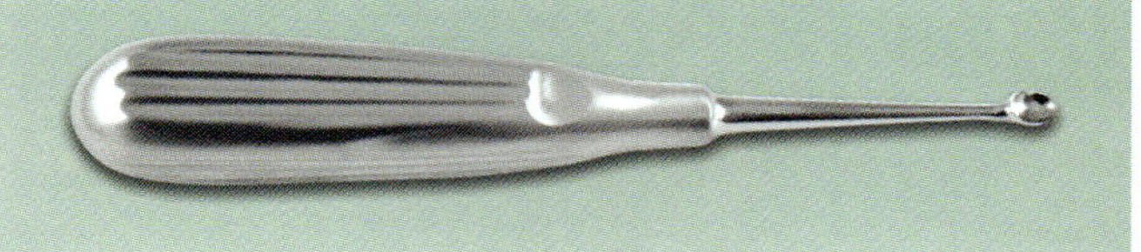

62. What is the name of given instrument?
a. Volkmann scoop
b. Gallstone scoop
c. Bone curette
d. Biopsy scoop

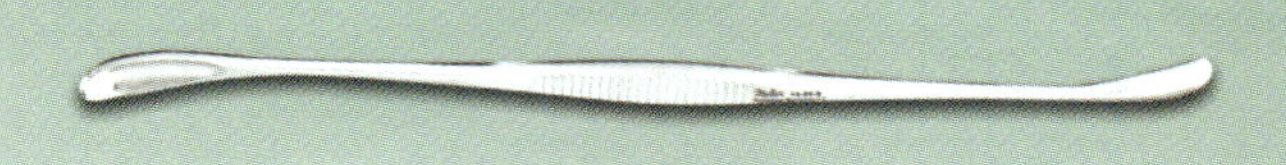

LAPAROSCOPIC INSTRUMENTS

63. What is the name of given instrument?
a. Ureteroscope
b. Cystoscope
c. Laparoscope
d. Sigmoidoscope

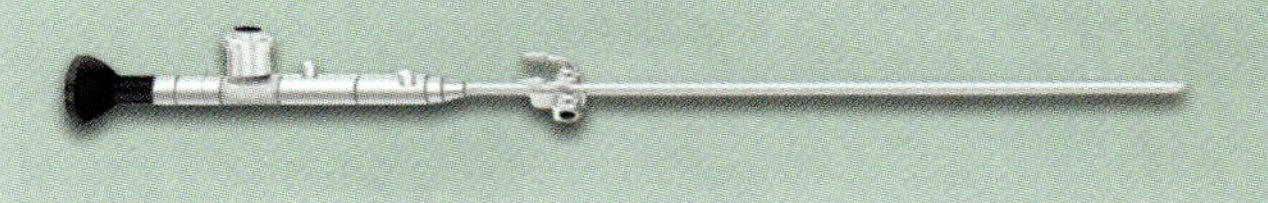

64. What is the name of given instrument?
a. Ureteroscope
b. Cystoscope
c. Laparoscope
d. Sigmoidoscope

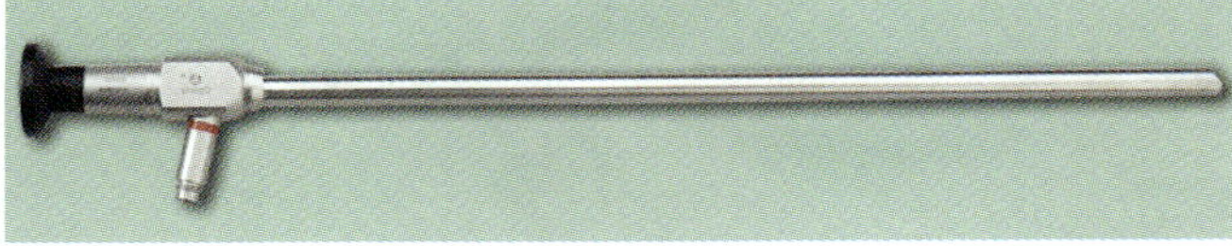

65. What is the name of given instrument?
a. Veress needle
b. Hasson cannula
c. Trocar
d. Laparoscope

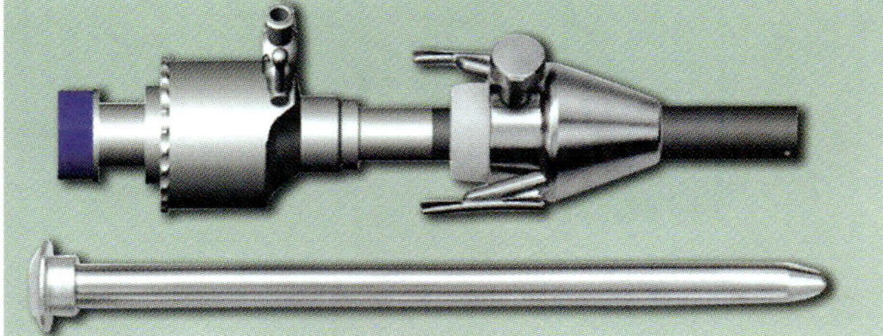

66. What is the name of given instrument?
a. Veress needle
b. Hasson cannula
c. Trocar
d. Laparoscope

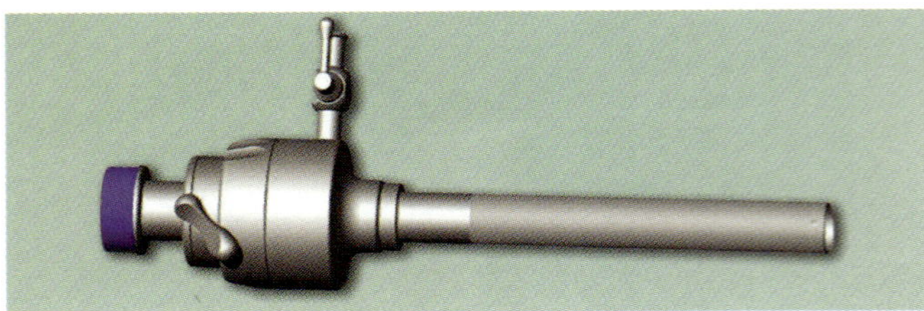

BIOPSY NEEDLE

67. What is the name of this needle? *(Recent Question 2016)*
a. Tru cut biopsy needle   b. Vim-Silverman needle
c. Menghini biopsy needle   d. Salah needle

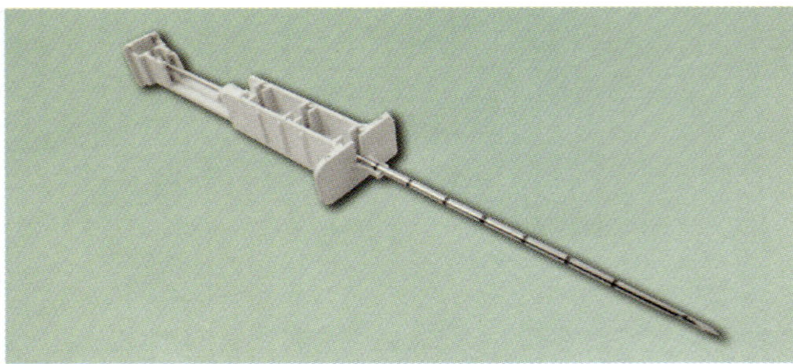

68. What is the name of this needle?
a. Tru cut biopsy needle   b. Vim-Silverman needle
c. Menghini biopsy needle   d. Salah needle

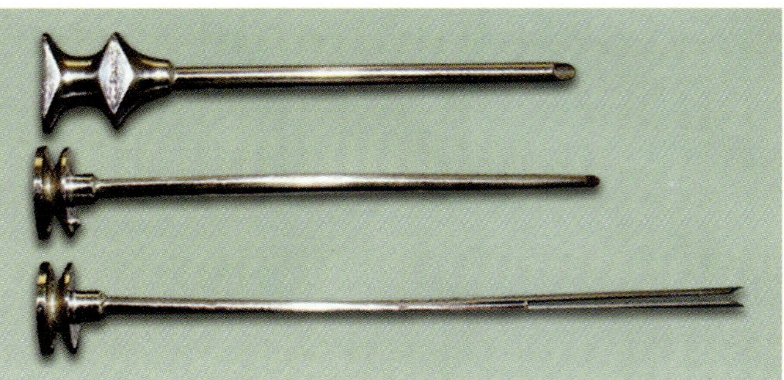

69. Identify the instrument shown below: *(AIIMS May 2016)*
a. Laparoscopic port trocar
b. Peritoneal dialysis catheter
c. Endoscopic ultrasound probe
d. DPL catheter

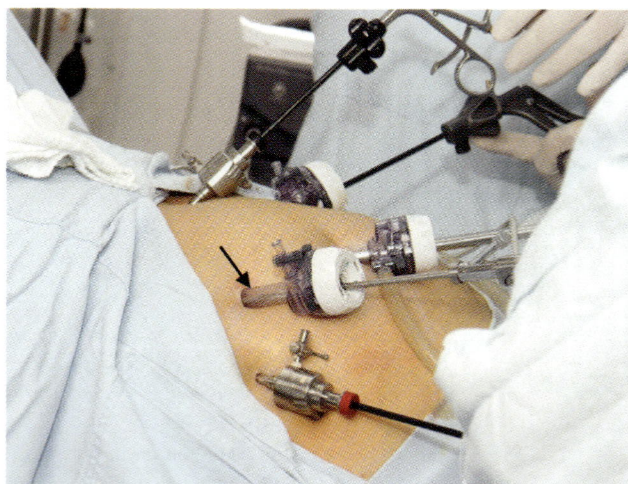

70. A 60 years old male came with bleeding per rectum and was diagnosed to have carcinoma colon. The patient underwent extended right hemicolectomy as shown below. Identify the instrument that the surgeon is using: *(AIIMS May 2016)*
a. Monopolar cautery
b. Ligasure vessel ligating system
c. Harmonic scalpel
d. Hyfrecator

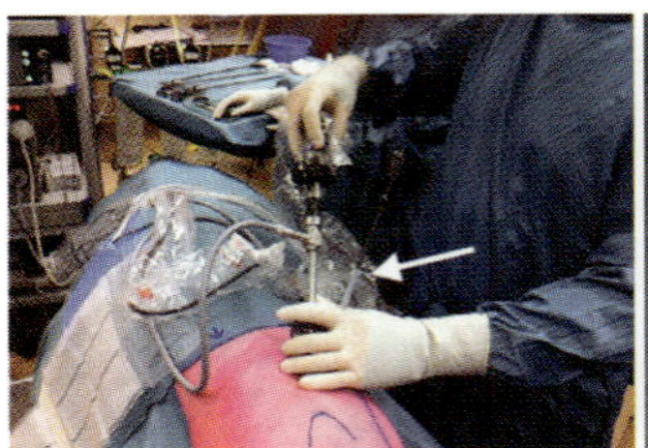
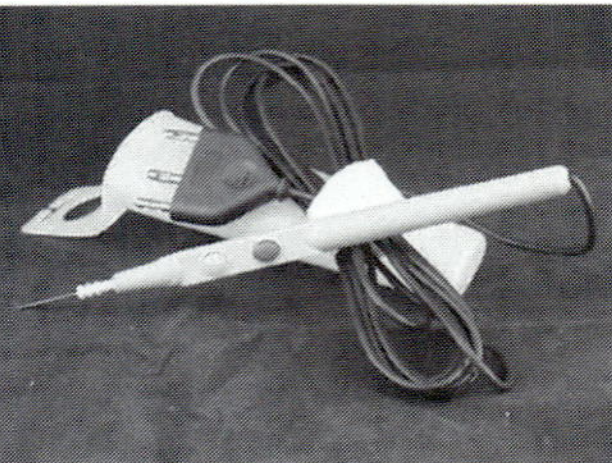

STAPLER

71. What is the name of given stapler?
a. Linear stapler   b. Intraluminal stapler
c. Skin stapler   d. Linear cutting stapler

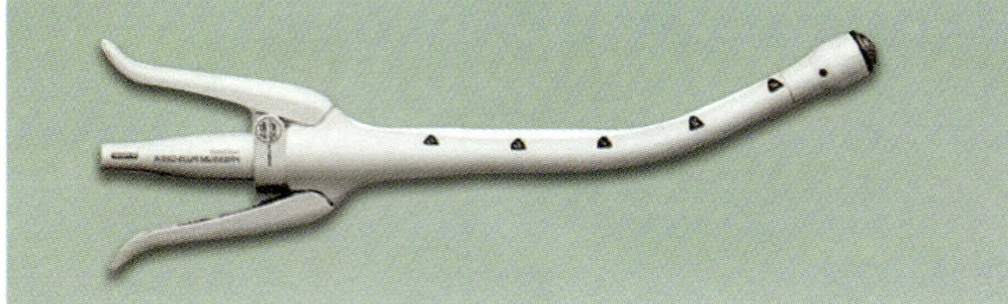

72. What is the name of given stapler?
a. Linear stapler
b. Intraluminal stapler
c. Skin stapler
d. Linear cutting stapler

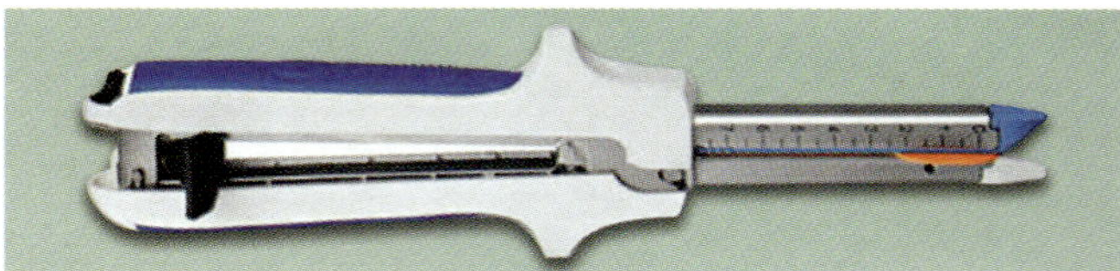

73. What is the name of given stapler?
a. Intraluminal stapler
b. Linear cutting stapler
c. Skin stapler
d. Linear stapler

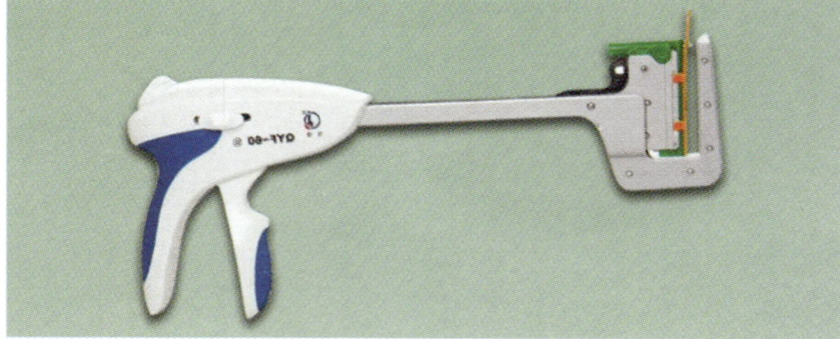

74. What is the name of given stapler?
a. Linear stapler
b. Intraluminal stapler
c. Skin stapler
d. Linear cutting stapler

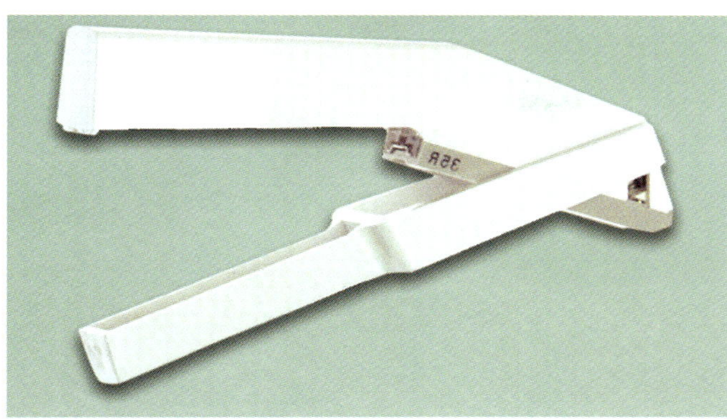

TUBES

75. What is the name of given tube?
- a. Kocher's T-tube
- b. Kehr's T-tube
- c. Lanz T-tube
- d. Mayo's T-tube

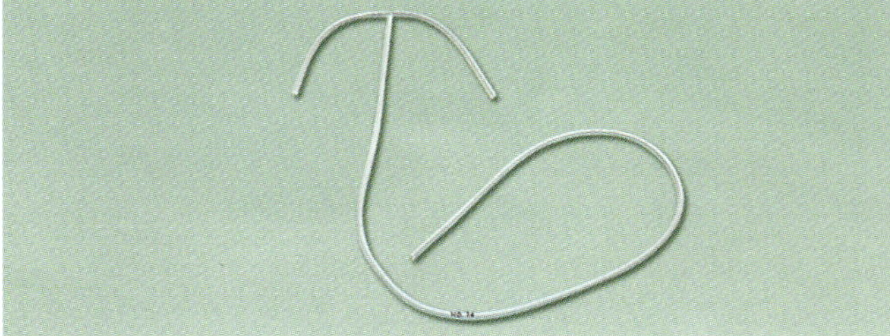

76. What is the name of given tube/catheter?
- a. Nelaton's catheter
- b. Fogarty catheter
- c. Sengstaken-Blakemore tube
- d. Bladder irrigation catheter

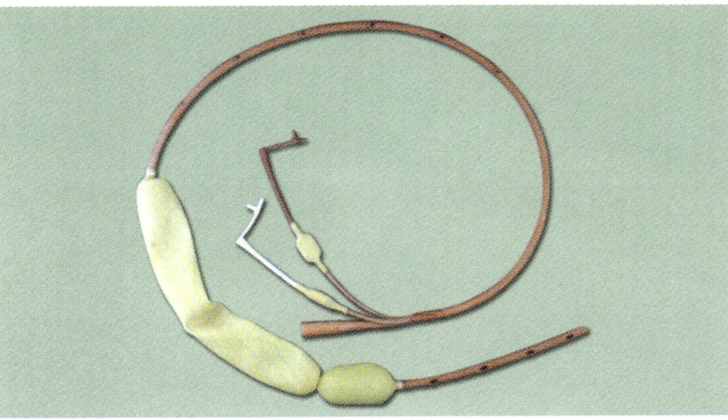

77. What is the name of given tube? *(Recent Question 2017)*
- a. Kehr's T-tube
- b. Flatus tube
- c. Ryle's tube
- d. Infant feeding tube

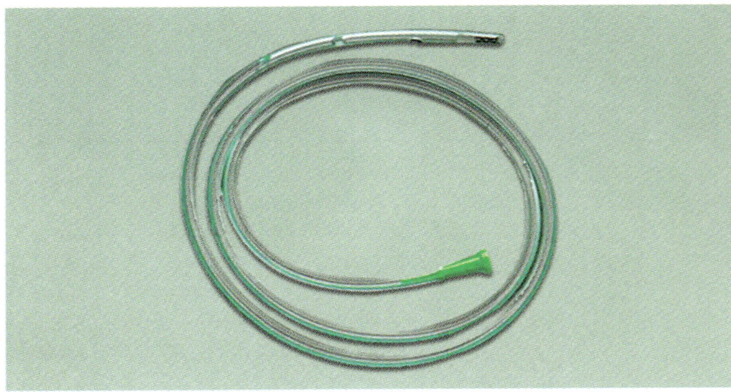

78. The correct procedure of inserting the following equipment in the image given below: *(AIIMS May 2018)*
- a. Supine with flexed neck
- b. Supine with extended neck
- c. Sitting with flexed neck
- d. Sitting with extended neck

79. What is the name of given tube? *(Recent Question 2017)*
- a. Kehr's T-tube
- b. Nelaton's catheter
- c. Ryle's tube
- d. Infant feeding tube

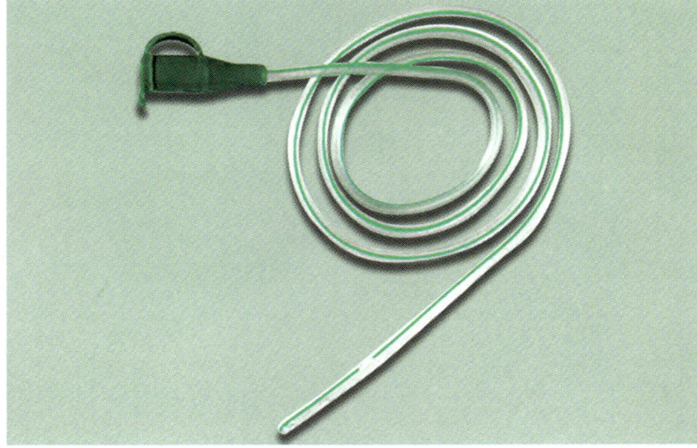

CATHETERS

80. What is the name of given catheter?
- a. Nelaton's catheter
- b. Fogarty catheter
- c. Infant feeding tube
- d. Ryle's tube

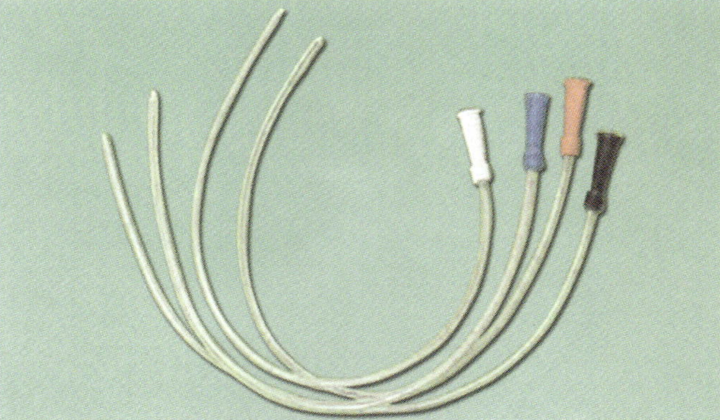

81. This tube/catheter is used in:
- a. Portocaval shunt
- b. Peritoneovenous shunt
- c. Mesocaval shunt
- d. Ventriculoperitoneal shunt

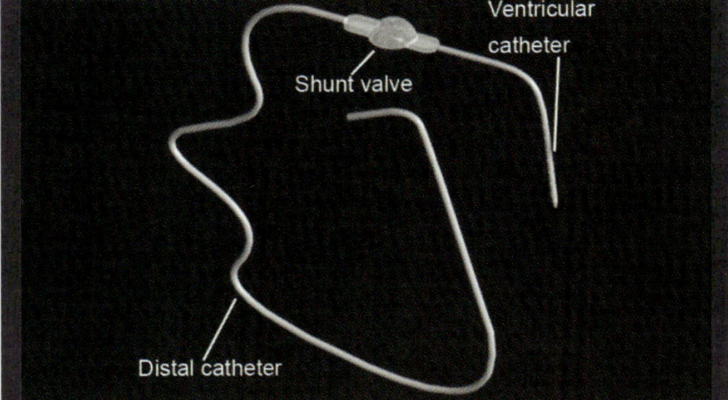

82. What is the name of given tube/catheter?
- a. Nelaton's catheter
- b. Fogarty catheter
- c. Sengstaken Blakemore tube
- d. Bladder irrigation catheter

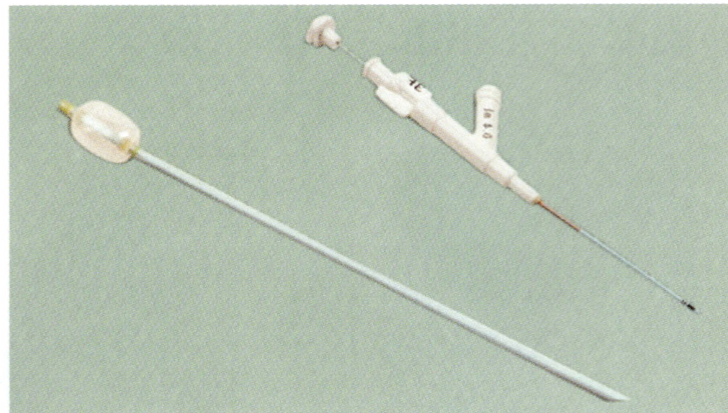

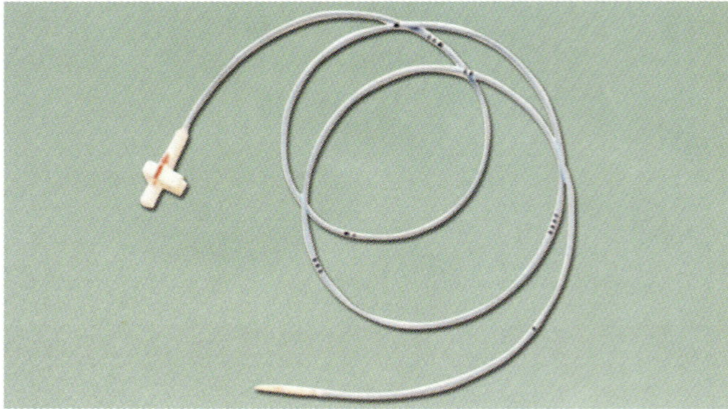

83. What is the name of given catheter?
a. Nelaton's catheter   b. Fogarty catheter
c. Foley's catheter   d. Malecot's catheter

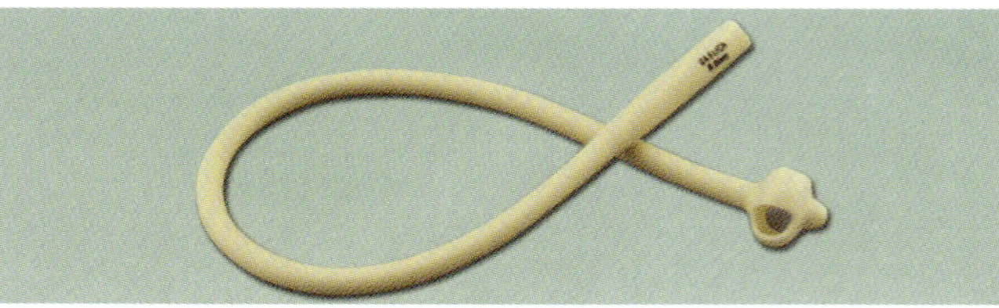

84. What is the name of given tube?
a. Foley's catheter   b. Red rubber catheter
c. Malecot's catheter   d. Nelaton's catheter

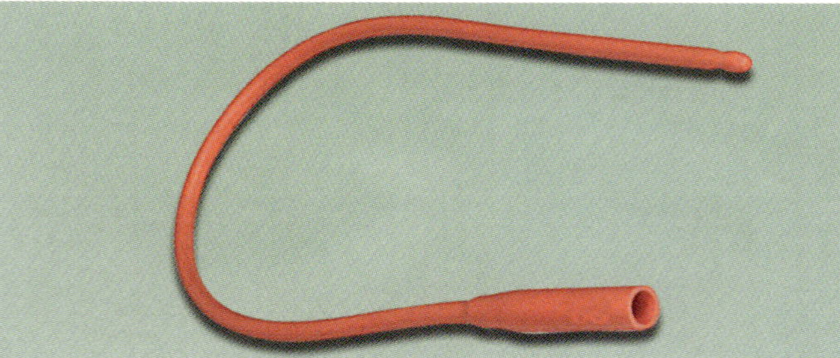

85. What is the name of given catheter?
a. Fogarty catheter   b. Central venous catheter
c. Bladder irrigation catheter   d. Nelaton's catheter

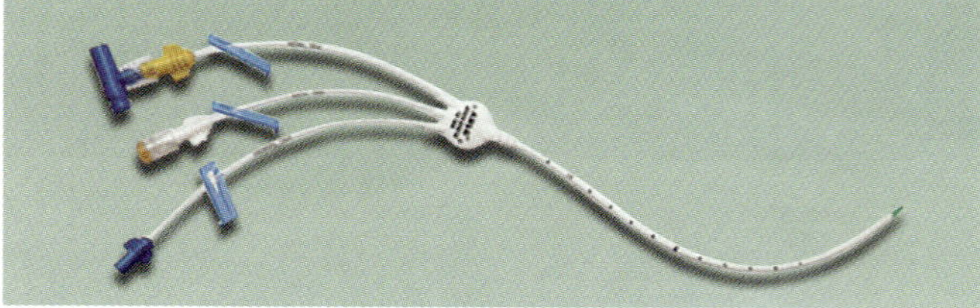

SUCTION AND DRAIN

86. What is the name of this drain?
a. Penrose drain   b. Jackson-Pratt drain
c. Romovac suction drain   d. Corrugated rubber drain

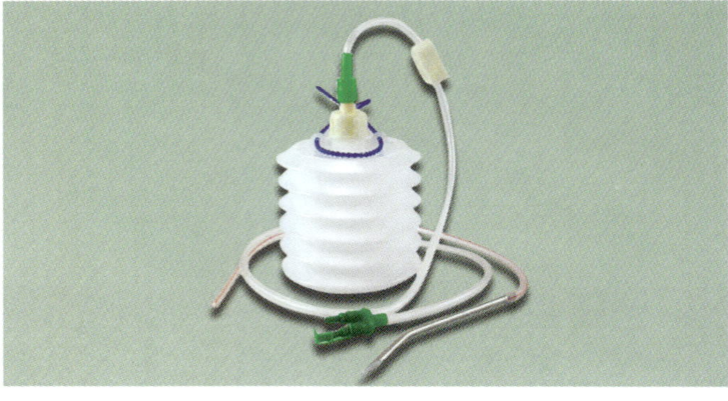

87. What is the name of given instrument?
a. Frazier suction tip   b. Poole suction tip
c. Adson suction tip   d. Yankauer suction tip

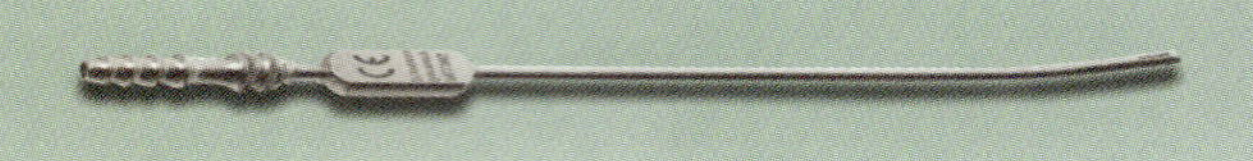

88. What is the name of given instrument?
a. Frazier suction tip   b. Poole suction tip
c. Adson suction tip   d. Yankauer suction tip

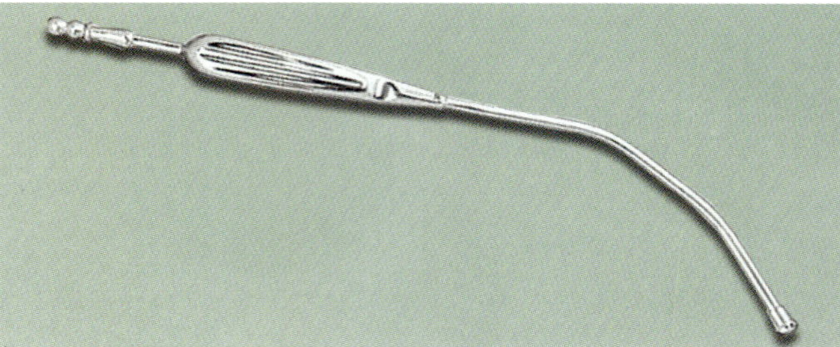

GASTROINTESTINAL SURGERY

89. Identify the labelled structures in the CT abdomen here:
(APPG 2016)

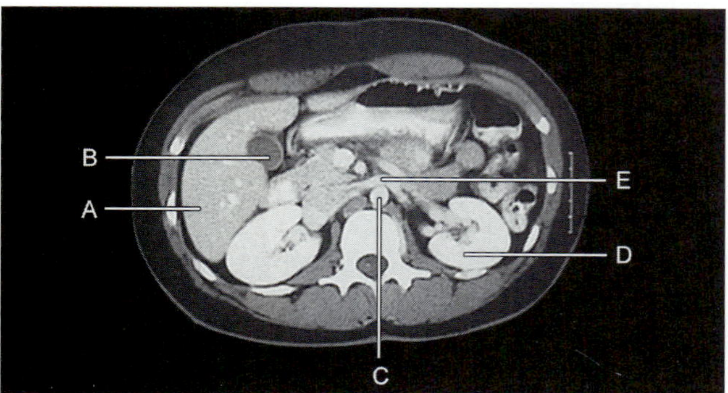

a. A = liver, B = inferior vena cava, C = head of pancreas, D = left kidney, E = transverse colon
b. A = right kidney, B = gallbladder, C = aorta, D = stomach E = pancreas
c. A = right kidney, B = inferior vena cava, C = head of pancreas, D = left psoas muscle, E = transverse colon
d. A = liver, B = gallbladder, C = aorta, D = left kidney, E = pancreas

Explanations

INSTRUMENTS

1. **Ans. a. Kocher's thyroid dissector** *(Ref: Jaypee Manual of Surgical Equipments/p 178)*

Kocher's Thyroid Dissector
• Used during thyroid surgeries, used **to dissect the superior thyroid pedicle**

2. **Ans. b. Veress needle** *(Ref: Jaypee Manual of Surgical Equipments/p 226)*

Veress Needle
• Used for **induction of pneumoperitoneum** during laparoscopic surgeries

3. **Ans. a. Tongue depressor**

4. **Ans. b. Mayo's towel clip** *(Ref: Jaypee Manual of Surgical Equipments/p 109)*

Mayo's Towel Clip
• **Curved blades** helps to **hold entire thickness of drapes firmly**
• **U**sed to **fix drapes, suction tubes, laparoscopic cables** and **diathermy wires** on OT table

5. **Ans. a. Doyen's towel clip** *(Ref: Jaypee Manual of Surgical Equipments/p 109)*

Doyen's Towel Clip
• **Short instrument** with **curved blades,** used to **fix the towels during draping**

6. **Ans. c. Moynihan's tetra towel clip** *(Ref: Jaypee Manual of Surgical Equipments/p 110)*

Moynihan's Tetra Towel Clip
• **Curved blades with four teeth** (two teeth in each blade)
• Used to **hold the cut edges of skin incision** to the four corners of draped towels to **isolate the operative field**

7. **Ans. d. Doyen's coastal elevator** *(Ref: Jaypee Manual of Surgical Equipments/p 223)*

Doyen Rib Raspatory (Doyen's Coastal Elevator)
• Used to **remove tissue** and **cartilage from the ribs**

8. **Ans. d. Used with blade for skin incision** *(Ref: Jaypee Manual of Surgical Equipments/p 127)*

Bard Parker Handle (BP Handle): Blades are held in position by BP Handle to give incisions

9. **Ans. b. 11**

Surgical Blade	Uses
10	• For skin incision (to open skin[Q])
11	• Arteriotomy[Q], incision & drainage[Q]
15	• Minor surgical procedures[Q], plastic & pediatric surgery[Q]
22	• Abdominal incisions[Q]
23	• For very thick skin[Q]

10. **Ans. c. Harvesting skin graft** *(Ref: Jaypee Manual of Surgical Equipments/p 247)*

Humby Knife
• A knife with a roller attached, **used for cutting skin grafts of varying thickness**
• The **distance** between the roller and blade of the knife **can be varied by means of a calibration device.**

11. Ans. b. Needle holder   *(Ref: Jaypee Manual of Surgical Equipments/p 136)*

Mayo Hegar Needle Holder
• Smaller distal blades with cross-serrations with a groove in middle • **Ratio of length of handle to blade is 4:1** • **Needle is placed** at junction of **proximal 2/3rd** and **distal 1/3rd of the blade** • **Used for suturing** skin and other organs

12. Ans. d. Rib shear   *(Ref: Jaypee Manual of Surgical Equipments/p 234)*

Rib Shear	
• Same as bone cutter but it has **one cutting blade**	• Used to **cut the ribs**

13. Ans. a. Hemorrhoids   *(Ref: Jaypee Manual of Surgical equipments/p189)*

14. Ans. c. Periosteal elevator   *(Ref: Jaypee Manual of Surgical Equipments/p 233)*

Periosteal Elevator
• Used to **elevate and dissect bone, tissue, nerves**, clean and scrape bone. • Used to **expose fracture sites** or bone in other procedures. • Used to **strip portions of the membrane (periosteum)** covering the exterior surface of a bone.

15. Ans. b. Mayo's vein stripper   *(Ref: Jaypee Manual of Surgical Equipments/p 175)*

Mayo's Vein Stripper: Used in the stripping of varicose veins

16. Ans. a. Gigli saw   *(Ref: Jaypee Manual of Surgical Equipments/p 235)*

Gigli's Saw: Used to **cut bones** in amputations

17. Ans. b. Fistula probe   *(Ref: Jaypee Manual of Surgical Equipments/p 190)*

Brodie's Fistula Probe
• **Winged blade, curved shaft** gradually tapered to **pointed tip with groove** along the curvature longitudinally • **Used to probe and treat fistula in ano; as a guide and protector to release tongue tie**

18. Ans. a. Gallbladder trocar   *(Ref: Scott-Conner & Dawson: Essential Operative Techniques and Anatomy/p 416)*

Gallbladder Trocar
• Gallbladder trocar is used to decompress the distended gallbladder during cholecystectomy

FORCEPS

19. Ans. b. Sponge holding forceps   *(Ref: Jaypee Manual of Surgical Equipments/p 108)*

Rampley's Sponge Holding Forceps
• Used for **cleansing the skin** with swab dipped in antiseptic solution during all operations • Used for **removing laminated membrane** and the **daughter cysts** during operation of hydatid cyst • Used to **hold the fundus** and Hartmann's pouch of gallbladder **during cholecystectomy** • Used to **swab an abscess cavity**

20. Ans. b. Kocher's hemostatic forceps   *(Ref: Jaypee Manual of Surgical Equipments/p 154)*

Kocher's Hemostatic Forceps
• Used during **appendectomy** to **crush the base** • Used to **hold perforating vessels** during **mastectomy** • Used during **subtotal thyroidectomy** • Used to **hold bleeding vessels** while operating on **palm** and **sole**

21. Ans. a. Lister's sinus forceps

Lister's Sinus Forceps
• Used for **incision and drainage** of abscess by **Hilton's method** • May be used to **hold a guaze swab to clean the abscess cavity**

22. Ans. d. All of the above   *(Ref: Jaypee Manual of Surgical Equipments/p 160)*

Allis Tissue Forceps

- Used during **laparotomy** to **retract skin margins**
- Used to **hold neck of bladder** during bladder neck resection
- Used to **hold skin flaps** while excising lipoma, sebaceous cyst or LN
- Used during thyroid operations, neck dissection to **hold the margins of skin** while raising skin flaps

23. Ans. c. Babcock's tissue forceps   *(Ref: Jaypee Manual of Surgical Equipments/p 160)*

Babcock's Tissue Forceps

- Used during **appendectomy**
- Used during **gastrectomy**, **gastrojejunostomy** to **hold the margins of stomach** while applying the occlusion clamps
- Used during small and large intestine resection anastomosis to **hold the margins of gut**
- Used to **hold the cut margins of bladder** during suprapubic cystolithotomy

24. Ans. d. Lane's tissue forceps   *(Ref: Jaypee Manual of Surgical Equipments/p 160)*

Lane's Tissue Forceps

- Used during **submandibular** or **parotid gland excision** to **hold the gland** during dissection from the adjacent structures
- During **mastectomy**, it may be used to **hold the breast** while dissecting it off from the pectoral fascia
- May be used to fix the draping sheets and suction tubes to the draping sheet

25. Ans. d. All of the above   *(Ref: Jaypee Manual of Surgical Equipments/p 146)*

Toothed Dissecting Forceps

- Used to **hold the cut skin margins** during **suturing**
- Used to **hold the linea alba** or the **rectus sheath** during closure of abdominal incision
- Used to **hold the scalp** during closure of scalp incision

26. Ans. c. Desjardins forceps   *(Ref: Jaypee Manual of Surgical Equipments/p 199)*

Desjardins Choledocholithotomy Forceps

- Used during **choledocholithotomy** for **stone removal**
- Used during **laparoscopic cholecystectomy** for **stone removal**
- May also be used during removal of kidney, ureteric or bladder stone

27. Ans. a. Pyelolithotomy forceps   *(Ref: Jaypee Manual of Surgical Equipments/p 199)*

Pyelolithotomy Forceps

- Used to **hold the stone** during **nephrolithotomy**, **pyelolithotomy** or **ureterolithotomy**

28. Ans. c. Suprapubic cystolithotomy forceps   *(Ref: Jaypee Manual of Surgical Equipments/p 195)*

Sprapubic Cystolithotomy Forceps

- Used for **suprapubic cystolithotomy**, to **hold and bring out the calculi** from urinary bladder

29. Ans. d. Used to pick sterilized instruments   *(Ref: Jaypee Manual of Surgical Equipments/p 107)*

Cheatle's Forceps

- Used to **pick sterile articles (instruments and drapes) to avoid touching the instruments** while transferring them from the tray to table

30. Ans. d. Ovum forceps   *(Ref: Jaypee Manual of Surgical Equipments/p 209)*

Ovum Forceps

- Used to **remove placental fragments, small endometrial polyps** from the uterus.
- Used to **remove gallstone from gallbladder during extraction** of gallbladder

31. Ans. c. Russian tissue forceps   *(Ref: Jaypee Manual of Surgical Equipments/p 161)*

Russian Tissue Forceps

- **Clubbed tip** in the blades with **serrated inner surface**
- Used to **hold skin while suturing**

32. Ans. b. Right angle forceps   *(Ref: Jaypee Manual of Surgical Equipments/p 159, 153)*

Right Angle Forceps (Meigster or Lahey)

- Used to **dissect pedicle, pass ligatures, to hold bleeding vessel in depth,** to dissect and pass **ligatures to cystic duct** and **cystic artery** in cholecystectomy

33. **Ans. a. Artery forceps**

34. **Ans. a. Mosquito hemostatic forceps**   *(Ref: Jaypee Manual of Surgical Equipments/p 152)*

Mosquito Hemostatic Forceps
• Used to hold fine bleeding vessels • Used to puncture the mesoappendix at an avascular site

35. **Ans. b. Spencer Wells hemostatic forceps**   *(Ref: Jaypee Manual of Surgical Equipments/p 152)*

Spencer-Wells Hemostatic Forceps
• Used to **hold the bleeding vessel** • Used to **split internal oblique** and **transversus abdominis during appendectomy** • Used to do **blunt dissection**

36. **Ans. c. A= Backhaus towel clamp. B = Halstead mosquito forceps. C = Allis forceps. D = Babcock intestinal forceps**

RETRACTOR

37. **Ans. c. Czerny's retractor**   *(Ref: Jaypee Manual of Surgical Equipments/p 140)*

Czerny's Retractor
• Used for **tissue retraction** in **appendectomy, thyroidectomy, mastectomy** and **inguinal hernia operation**

38. **Ans. a. Morris retractor**   *(Ref: Jaypee Manual of Surgical Equipments/p 141)*

Morris Retractor
• Used for tissue retraction **appendectomy, thyroidectomy, mastectomy** and **inguinal hernia operation**

39. **Ans. d. All of the above**   *(Ref: Jaypee Manual of Surgical Equipments/p 143)*

Double Hook Retractor
• Used to **retract skin flap for excision of sebaceous cyst** • Used during **venesection** for retraction of skin • Used during **tracheostomy** for retraction of skin and thyroid isthmus

40. **Ans. c. Volkman's retractor**   *(Ref: Jaypee Manual of Surgical Equipments/p 141)*

Cat's Paw or Volkman's Retractor
• Used for **retraction of skin flaps** or **fascia** for operation at the surface, e.g. excision of the sebaceous cyst, lipoma, dermoid.

41. **Ans. d. Deaver's retractor**   *(Ref: Jaypee Manual of Surgical Equipments/p 142)*

Deaver's Retractor
• Used during **cholecystectomy** for **retraction of right lobe of liver** • Used during **pancreaticojejunostomy** for **retraction of stomach** • Used during kidney operations to retract the abdominal wall

42. **Ans. c. Joll's thyroid retractor**   *(Ref: Jaypee Manual of Surgical Equipments/p 178)*

Joll's Thyroid Retractor
• **Self retaining** retractor used during thyroid operations to **retract skin flaps**

43. **Ans. c. Doyen's mouth gag**   *(Ref: Jaypee Manual of Surgical Equipments/p 304)*

Doyen's Mouth Gag
• Used to **open mouth during intraoral operations** like **glossectomy, cleft palate operation, excision of intraoral ranula**

44. **Ans. d. Balfours retractor**   *(Ref: Jaypee Manual of Surgical Equipments/p 144)*

Balfour Abdominal Retractor
• **Self-retaining retractor** used in **laparotomy procedures, cesarean sections** and **bowel resection.**

45. **Ans. b. Beckman Weitlaner retractor**   *(Ref: Jaypee Manual of Surgical Equipments/p 144)*

Beckman Weitlaner retractor: Used to **retract** or **hold back tissue** or **bone** for Surgical exposure

46. **Ans. b. Farabeuf retractor**   *(Ref: Jaypee Manual of Surgical Equipments/p 143)*

Farabeuf Double-Ended Retractor
• Versatile **handheld retractor** used in **dentistry, in wrist** and **hand procedures,** or in **hernia repair**

47. **Ans. c. Langenbeck's retractor**   *(Ref: Jaypee Manual of Surgical Equipments/p 140)*

Langenbeck's Retractor
• Retractor used in **hernia surgery** and **superficial surgeries to retract skin, fascia and muscles**

48. **Ans. c. Kelly retractor**   *(Ref: Jaypee Manual of Surgical Equipments/p 212)*

Kelly Retractor
• A **curved right-angled retractor,** used in **deep pelvic surgery** such as rectal dissection.

49. **Ans. c. Single hook retractor**   *(Ref: Jaypee Manual of Surgical equipments/p143)*

Single Hook Retractor
• Used for **superficial retraction** specially for **tough structures** like **skin, fascia of sole & palm**

CLAMP

50. **Ans. b. Doyen's intestinal occlusion clamp**   *(Ref: Jaypee Manual of Surgical Equipments/p 181)*

Doyen's straight intestinal occlusion clamp: Used for **gut resection** and **anastomosis**

51. **Ans. a. Payr's crushing clamp**   *(Ref: Jaypee Manual of Surgical Equipments/p 180)*

Payr's gastric crushing clamp: Used during **partial gastrectomies**

52. **Ans. b. Light bulldog clamp**   *(Ref: Jaypee Manual of Surgical Equipments/p 156)*

Light Bulldog Clamp
• It has **pinch cock action** to open and close with **fine transverse serrations** in the blade
• Used for **temporary occlusion of small peripheral blood vessels**
• Can be used as a **suture tag**

53. **Ans. c. Pott's bulldog clamp**   *(Ref: Jaypee Manual of Surgical Equipments/p 156)*

Pott's Bulldog Clamp
• **Paper clip like** instrument with serrations and **spring loaded handle** which permits a **secure grip** of the vessel
• Used for **temporary occlusion of small peripheral blood vessels**

54. **Ans. a. Satinsky vascular clamp**   *(Ref: Jaypee Manual of Surgical Equipments/p 226)*

Satinsky Vascular Clamp
• Used for **partial occlusion of blood vessel**
• Partially occlude the wall of a vessel over a distance; **blood flow to continue through the rest of the vessel.**

SCISSORS

55. **Ans. a. Mayo scissors**   *(Ref: Jaypee Manual of Surgical Equipments/p 137, 269)*

Mayo's Scissors: Used for **cutting tough tissues;** used for **cutting ligaments**

56. **Ans. b. Metzenbaum scissors**   *(Ref: Jaypee Manual of Surgical Equipments/p 137, 269)*

Metzenbaum Scissor: Used for **cutting delicate tissues like intestine, bladder** (viscera)

57. **Ans. c. Lister bandage scissors**   *(Ref: Jaypee Manual of Surgical Equipments/p 137, 269)*

Lister Bandage Scissors
• **Distal blades** are **bent at angle,** so that it is passed easily under the bandage
• **Flat blunt atraumatic tip** in the **lower blade**
• Used for **cutting bandages**

DILATOR

58. **Ans. c. Tracheal dilator**

Tracheal dilator: Used during **tracheostomy**

59. Ans. b. Urethral dilator   *(Ref: Jaypee Manual of Surgical Equipments/p 194)*

> **Urethral Dilator:** Used to **dilate urethra in urethral strictures** and **before cystoscopy**

60. Ans. a. Bile duct dilator

Bake Bile Duct Dilator

- Used in **choledocholithotomy**, after removing the stones from the bile duct
- Used to **sound the bile duct for any retained stone**
- Used to **check the patency of ampulla of Vater**

SCOOP

61. Ans. a. Volkmann scoop   *(Ref: Jaypee Manual of Surgical Equipments/p 235)*

Volkmann Scoop

- This instrument has a working end **similar to curette**
- Used for **debriding** the contents of an **abscess cavity, sinus or fistula** & **collection of cancellous bone grafts**

62. Ans. b. Gallstone scoop   *(Ref: Jaypee Manual of Surgical Equipments/p 173)*

Gallstone Scoop

- Flat and thin structure with **spoon like shape holder** on both sides
- Spoon like shape helps to **remove stones from gallbladder**

LAPAROSCOPIC INSTRUMENTS

63. Ans. b. Cystoscope   *(Ref: Jaypee Manual of Surgical Equipments/p 260)*

Cystoscope

- Lighted tube with a **telescopic lens** used to **examine inside of the bladder**

64. Ans. c. Laparoscope   *(Ref: Jaypee Manual of Surgical Equipments/p 260)*

Laparoscope

- **Laparoscopes** are based on **Hopkins optical** system which uses a **series of glass rods with lenses placed at appropriate intervals** along the shaft of instrument
- Provide **visualization** of Surgical field **with magnification**
- **Oblique viewing (30º) laparoscopes provide larger field of vision** than the end viewing (0º) laparoscopes

65. Ans. b. Hasson cannula   *(Ref: Jaypee Manual of Surgical Equipments/p 267)*

Hasson Cannula

- Used as alternative technique to **create pneumoperitoneum by open technique,** especially in patients with **upper abdominal surgeries** or **accompanying ileus**
- **Incidence of vessel injury is very less** with Hasson cannula

66. Ans. c. Trocar   *(Ref: Jaypee Manual of Surgical Equipments/p 267)*

Trocar

- **Trocars** are required **to access the peritoneal cavity during surgery** and for **maintaining pneumoperitoneum when instruments are exchanged**

BIOPSY NEEDLE

67. Ans. a. Tru cut biopsy needle   *(Ref: Jaypee Manual of Surgical Equipments/p 60)*

Tru Cut Biopsy Needle

- Tru cut biopsy needle consists of **cutting needle encased in a trocar.**
- Cutting needle slides into the trocar to a **preset depth.**
- Cutting needle is advanced rapidly into the organ tissue followed by trocar
- Needle and trocar are removed together and the **biopsy core** is **collected from the cutting needle.**

68. Ans. b. Vim-Silverman needle   *(Ref: Jaypee Manual of Surgical Equipments/p 60)*

Vim-Silverman Needle
• **Vim-Silverman needle** consists of **trocar, a fitting obturator** and a **cutting needle with prongs.**
• Trocar and fitting obturator are introduced together into organ tissue after which the obturator is removed and cutting needle with prongs is introduced through the trocar.
• **Biopsy core is collected between the prongs of cutting needle.**

69. Ans. a. Laparoscopic port trocar

The instrument marked in the laparoscopy image above is the port containing the trocar. It is used for creating pneumoperitoneum and inserting the instruments for the procedure.

70. Ans. a. Monopolar cautery   *(Ref: Sabiston 20/e p235-236)*

Monopolar Electrocautery	**Bipolar Electrocautery**	**LigaSure**	**Hyfrecators**

Surgical Devices and Energy Sources	
Monopolar Electrocautery	• Monopolar electrocautery is used for **cutting, blending, desiccation** and **fulguration.** • **Using a pencil instrument, active electrode is placed in the entry site** and can be **used to cut tissue and coagulate bleeding.** **Cutting:** • Cautery **activated** with a **constant waveform**[Q] • **Heat** is **generated relatively quickly** over the target with **minimal lateral thermal spread**[Q]. **Coagulation:** • Cautery activated with an **intermittent waveform**[Q] • **Less heat** is **generated** on a **slower frequency, with** the potential for **large lateral thermal spread**, resulting in **tissue dehydration** & **vessel thrombosis**[Q]. • **Blended waveform** have the **advantage of both cutting and coagulation** modes. • **Grounding pad** is placed securely on the patient **for monopolar cautery** device **to function properly** and **to prevent thermal burn injury** at the current reentry electrode site. • **MC used** because of **versatility and effectiveness**[Q].
Bipolar Electrocautery	• **Bipolar electrocautery** establishes a **short circuit between the tips of instrument** (forceps)[Q] • **Grounding pad** is **not required**[Q] • **Grasped tissue** between the **tips of instrument completes** the **circuit**[Q] • It provides **precise thermal coagulation** (generating **heat affects only the tissue within short circuit**)[Q] • **More effective than the monopolar instrument in coagulating vessels** due to **mechanical advantage of compression of tissue between the tips** of the instrument to the thermal coagulation[Q]. • Particularly useful for procedures in which **lateral thermal injury** or an **arcing phenomenon needs to be avoided**[Q].
LigaSure	• **LigaSure** is a **new electrothermal bipolar tissue sealing system**[Q] • Applied in **abdominal and pelvic surgery**, mostly **through laparoscopy**[Q]. • **Advantage:** It improves **vessel sealing** with **minimal lateral thermal spread**[Q].
Hyfrecators	• Hyfrecator functions by **sending electrical impulses into body with the use of a probe**[Q]. • It **works by emitting low-power high-frequency AC** (alternating current) **electrical pulses via a probe**, directly to the affected area of the body[Q]. • Hyfrecator is used for **removal of warts, pearly penile papules, desiccation of sebaceous gland disorders**, electrocautery of bleeding, **epilation,** destruction of small cosmetically **unwanted superficial veins**, destruction of skin cancers (**basal cell carcinoma**).

STAPLER

71. Ans. b. Intraluminal stapler   *(Ref: Berry & Kohn's Operating Room Technique by Nancymarie Phillips/p 335, 336, 551)*

Staplers used in Surgery	
• **Types of Stapler: Skin, Linear (cutting and stapling), Ligating and Intraluminal types.**	
Skin stapler	• Skin staplers are used to **approximate skin edges during skin closure.**
Linear stapler	• Linear staplers are used to **insert two straight, staggered evenly spaced, parallel rows of staples** into tissues. • Linear staplers are typically used to **staple tissue to be transected within the alimentary tract or thoracic cavity.**
Linear cutter	• Linear cutter is used to **staple and transect the tissue**, especially **in GI procedures.** • Linear cutters **deliver two double staple lines and contain a knife blade** that **passes between the two staple lines, dividing the tissue.**
Ligating clips	• Ligating clip is used to **occlude a single small structure (blood vessel or duct).**
Ligating cutter	• Ligating cutter ejects **two ligating clips side by side** and then **divides the tissue between the clips** with a single activation.
Intraluminal stapler	• Intraluminal (circular) staplers are **used to anastomose tubular structures** within the GIT. • This stapler **fires a double row of circular staples** and then **trims the lumen with a knife** located within the head of the stapler. • U**sed during resection and anastomoses** of the **distal colon or rectum**

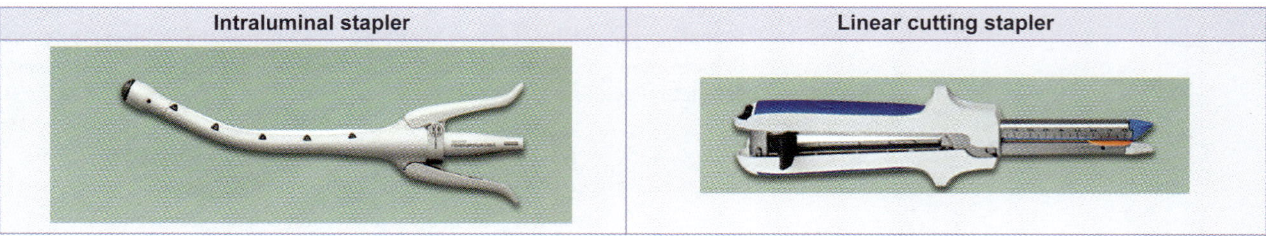

Intraluminal stapler

Linear cutting stapler

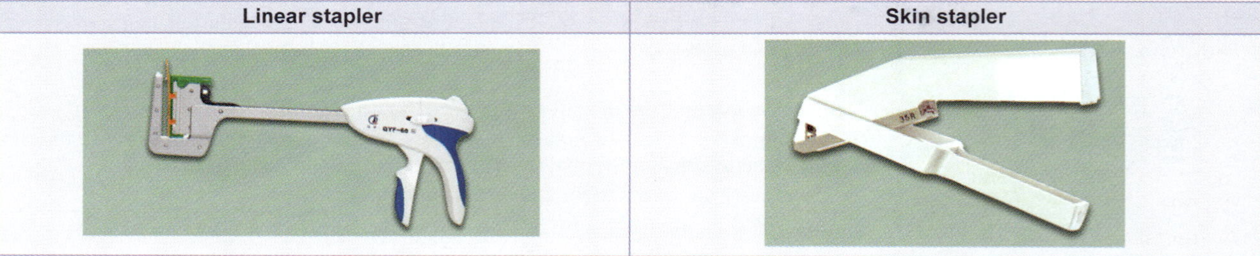

Linear stapler

Skin stapler

72. Ans. d. Linear cutting stapler   *(Ref: Berry & Kohn's Operating Room Technique by Nancymarie Phillips/p 335, 336, 551)*

73. Ans. d. Linear stapler   *(Ref: Berry & Kohn's Operating Room Technique by Nancymarie Phillips/p 335, 336, 551)*

74. Ans. c. Skin stapler   *(Ref: Berry & Kohn's Operating Room Technique by Nancymarie Phillips/p 335, 336, 551)*

TUBES

75. Ans. b. Kehr's T-tube   *(Ref: Jaypee Manual of Surgical Equipments/p 97)*

Kehr's T-tube
• Following choledochotomy, the bile duct is closed over a T-tube, as primary closure of bile duct is associated with higher incidence of leakage
• Used to drain bile duct following repair of bile duct injury. The T-tube acts as a stent and is usually kept for 4-6 weeks

76. Ans. c. Sengstaken Blakemore tube

Sengstaken Blakemore Tube
• The tube is passed down into esophagus & gastric balloon is inflated inside the stomach.
• **Traction** is applied to the tube so that **gastric balloon** will **compress the GE junction** & **reduce the blood flow to esophageal varices.**
• Used **only in emergencies** where **bleeding from presumed varices is impossible to control with medication alone**.
• **Endotracheal intubation** before the procedure is strongly advised to secure the airway **to prevent aspiration**

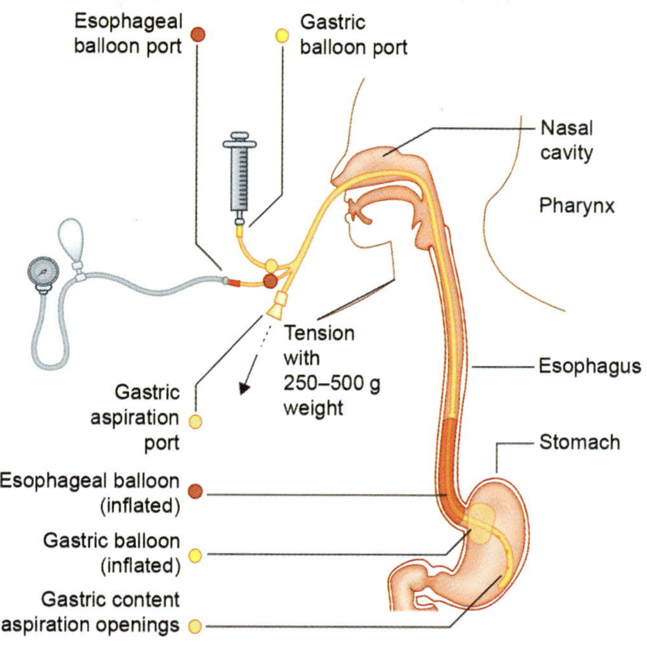

77. Ans. c. Ryle's tube *(Ref: Jaypee Manual of Surgical Equipments/p 96)*

Ryle's (Nasogastric) Tube
• To measure the required length of tube, measure from the tip of the patient's nose, to their ear, and then down to the xiphisternum.
• Markings of Ryle's tube (**GBPD**)

– **At 40 cm:** Indicates the level of <u>**GE**</u> **junction**[Q]	– **At 60 cm:** Indicates the level of **pylorus**[Q]
– **At 50 cm:** Indicates the level of <u>**body of stomach**</u>[Q]	– **At 65 cm:** Indicates the level of <u>**d**</u>**uodenum**[Q]

Indications of Ryle's Tube Insertion	
Diagnostic	**Therapeutic**
• **Saline load test** to confirm **gastric outlet obstruction** • To assess **free & total acid** in **peptic ulcers** • To diagnose **tracheoesophageal fistula** • In **Hollander's test** for completion of vagotomy	• **Decompression** in **intestinal obstruction, gastric outlet obstruction** • In **perforation peritonitis, upper GI bleed, abdominal surgeries** • **Enteral nutrition** in head injuries, comatose patients, maxillofacial injuries

78. Ans. c. Sitting with flexed neck

79. Ans. d. Infant feeding tube *(Ref: Jaypee Manual of Surgical Equipments/p 97)*

Infant Feeding Tube	
• **No markings** and **no shots** in Infant feeding tube	• Indications are similar to Ryle's tube in **infants & children**

CATHETERS

80. Ans. a. Nelaton catheter

Nelaton Catheter
• **Nelaton catheters** can be used for **one-time emptying of the bladder**, for instance **during/after surgery** or to **determine the amount of urine** in the bladder.

81. Ans. d. Ventriculoperitoneal shunt *(Ref: Bailey 27/e p655, 26/p-608)*

Ventriculoperitoneal Shunt
• **MC shunt for hydrocephalus: Ventriculoperitoneal shunt**
• It involves the **insertion of a catheter**[Q] **into the lateral ventricle** (usually **right frontal** or **occipital**)
• The catheter is then connected to a shunt valve under the scalp and finally to a distal catheter, which is tunneled subcutaneously down to the abdomen and inserted into the peritoneal cavity.
• If the CSF pressure exceeds the shunt valve pressure, then CSF will flow out of the distal catheter and be absorbed by the peritoneal lining.
• **Other options for distal catheter placement** include the **right atrium** via the deep facial and jugular vein (**ventriculoatrial shunt**) or the **pleural cavity** (**ventriculopleural shunt**).

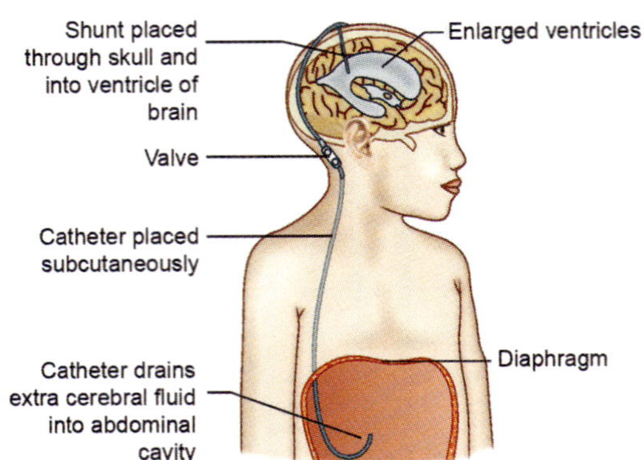

82. Ans. b. Fogarty catheter   *(Ref: Bailey 27/e p955)*

Fogarty Embolectomy Catheter

- Used to **remove fresh emboli from vessels**[Q]
- Consists of a hollow tube with an inflatable balloon attached to its tip.
- Inserted into the blood vessel through a clot. The balloon is then inflated to extract it from the vessel.

83. Ans. d. Malecot's catheter   *(Ref: Jaypee Manual of Surgical Equipments/p 96)*

Malecot's Catheter

- **Self retaining catheter** with an **umbrella or flower** at the **tip**
- **Used for draining urine** from the urinary bladder, when the urethra is damaged as in **suprapubic catheterization**; drainage of urine from the kidney by **percutaneous nephrostomy**
- Used for **drainage of fluid collections**, e.g. an abdominal abscess
- Used as **intercostal drain**

84. Ans. b. Red rubber catheter

Red Rubber Catheter

- **Non self retaining urinary catheter** with rounded and blunt tip
- Temporarily used to **drain urine from bladder** and **to estimate the residual urine**

85. Ans. b. Central venous catheter   *(Ref: Jaypee Manual of Surgical Equipments/p 105)*

Central Venous Catheter

- **Central venous catheters are used for fluid, medication and nutrition administration**[Q]
- **Used for monitoring pressure or volume changes to detect potential problems or evaluate patient improvement**[Q]

  - **Most preferred veins** for central venous catheterization **in operating room: Internal jugular vein**[Q]
  - **Most preferred veins** for central venous catheterization **outside operating room: Subclavian vein**[Q]
  - **Most preferred veins** for central venous catheterization **in acutely injured, critically ill** patients: **Femoral vein**[Q] (Relative ease of insertion)

SUCTION AND DRAIN

86. Ans. c. Romovac suction drain   *(Ref: Jaypee Manual of Surgical Equipments/p 98)*

Romovac Suction Drain

- Suction is created by pressing the suction corrugation
- Used for **mastectomy, thyroidectomy, flap and reconstructive surgeries**

87. Ans. c. Adson suction tip   *(Ref: Jaypee Manual of Surgical Equipments/p 101)*

Adson Suction Tip

- Angles with a vent or thumb rest to control suction
- **Fine suction tip** helps in **fine and meticulous surgeries** like **vascular, plastic or reconstructive surgeries**

88. Ans. d. Yankauer suction tip   *(Ref: Jaypee Manual of Surgical Equipments/p 101)*

Yankauer Suction Tip

- It has **large suction tip**
- Used in surgeries in which **large volume of fluid** has to be **sucked** (peritoneal cavity after lavage, in perforation peritonitis, hemoperitoneum)

GASTROINTESTINAL SURGERY

89. Ans. d. A = liver. B. = gallbladder. C. = aorta. D. = left kidney E. = pancreas

Endocrine Surgery

- Breast
- Thyroid
- Parathyroid and Adrenal Glands

Breast

■ NIPPLE DISCHARGE

Nipple Discharge

- Unilateral, spontaneous, serous or serosanguinous discharge from a single duct is usually caused by an intraductal papilloma[Q], or rarely by an intraductal cancer.
- Mostly the underlying cause is a duct papilloma or duct ectasia[Q], but since the chances of malignancy are high, it must be investigated further.
- Risk of malignancy increases if an underlying mass[Q] is present.[Q]

Causes of Nipple Discharge			
Colour	**Cause**		
Blood-stained	• **Duct papilloma[Q] (MC)**	• Intraductal carcinoma[Q]	• Duct ectasia[Q]
Serous	• **Fibrocystic disease[Q]**	• Duct ectasia[Q]	• Carcinoma[Q]
Black, green, paste like or grumous discharge	• Duct ectasia[Q]		

Investigations

- **Mammography:** Can show underlying suspicious lesions
- **Cytological examination:** (may identify malignant cells, but a negative finding does not rule out cancer)

Ductography

- **Primary indication: Nipple discharge[Q]** (particularly when the fluid contains **blood**)
- Radiopaque contrast media is injected into one or more of the major ducts and mammography is performed
- **Intraductal papillomas: Small filling defects[Q]** surrounded by contrast media
- **Cancers: Irregular masses** or as **multiple intraluminal filling defects[Q]**
- **Duct ectasia: Dilated cystic structure[Q]**

- **Ultrasound:** May show presence of an underlying mass or duct ectasia

Final Diagnosis

- Final diagnosis is made by **excising** the **involved duct (Microdochectomy)[Q]** and any **underlying mass** if present and subjecting then for a histopathological diagnosis.
- **Radical duct excision** (removal of all lactiferous ducts) is **not done[Q]**.

Treatment

- Firstly **exclude a carcinoma** by **occult blood test** and **cytology.**
- **Simple reassurance** may then be sufficient but, if the **discharge** is proving **intolerable**, an **operation to remove the affected duct** or **ducts** can be performed **(microdochectomy).**

■ CARCINOMA BREAST: RISK FACTORS

Risk Factors for Breast Cancer	
1. **Age**: Incidence **increases with age[Q]**	6. **Alcohol** and **high fat diet[Q]**
2. **Country of birth**: More common in **western countries[Q]**	7. **Personal history** of malignancy:
3. **Family history** and **genetic risk factors** (BRCA)[Q]	– Contralateral breast cancer[Q]
4. **Hyperestrogenemia:**	– **Ovarian** and **endometrial cancer[Q]**
– **Early menarche[Q], late menopause[Q]**	8. Previous **benign breast disease[Q]**
– **Nulliparity[Q]**	9. **High socioeconomic status[Q]**
– **Obesity[Q]**	10. **Radiation** exposure[Q]
5. **Late first** full term **pregnancy[Q]**	11. **Hormone replacement therapy[Q]**

- **Combined (estrogen + progesterone) HRT** is associated with **increased risk** of **CA breast.**[Q]
- **Only estrogen HRT** is **not associated** with increased **risk of CA breast**[Q].

> - **Smoking**[Q] and **OCPs**[Q] **does not** appear to **increase risk** of **breast cancer**
> - **Longer duration** of **breast feeding** has a **protective effect**[Q]

BRCA-1	BRCA-2
• Chromosome: **17**[Q]	• Chromosome: **13**[Q]
• **BRCA-1 associated** breast cancers:	• **BRCA-2 associated** cancers:
– Invasive **ductal carcinomas**	– Invasive ductal carcinomas
– **Poorly differentiated**[Q]	– **Well differentiated**[Q]
– **Hormone-receptor negative**[Q]	– **Hormone-receptor positive**[Q].
– **Early age** of onset	– **Early age** of onset
– **Bilateral**	– **Bilateral**
• Associated **ovarian, colon** and **prostate cancers**[Q].	• Associated **ovarian, colon, prostate, pancreas, gall-bladder, stomach** cancers and **melanoma**[Q].

CARCINOMA IN SITU

DUCTAL CARCINOMA IN SITU

- Although **DCIS** is **predominantly** seen in the **female breast**, it accounts for 5% of **male breast** cancers.
- DCIS carries a **high risk for progression** to an **invasive cancer**[Q].
- DCIS is **classified** on the basis of **nuclear grade & presence of necrosis**[Q].

Pathology

- Proliferation of epithelium that lines the minor ducts, resulting in **papillary growths within** the **duct lumina**.
- Papillary growths (**papillary growth pattern**) eventually coalesce & fill the duct lumina so that only scattered, rounded spaces remain between the clumps of atypical cancer cells, which show **hyperchromasia** and **loss of polarity (cribriform growth pattern)**.
- Eventually pleomorphic cancer cells with **frequent mitotic figures obliterate** the **lumina & distend** the **ducts (solid growth pattern)**.
- With continued growth, these cells outstrip their blood supply and become **necrotic (comedo growth pattern)**.

Histological Types of DCIS

- **Low Grade**: Cribriform, Papillary & Micropapillary[Q]
- **High Grade: Solid & Comedocarcinoma**[Q]

Diagnosis

- **Calcium deposition** occurs in the areas of necrosis and is a common feature seen on mammography[Q].
- **DCIS** most frequently **presents** as **mammographic calcifications**[Q].

Treatment

- **Non-palpable DCIS**: Section by **needle localisation** technique with **specimen mammography** to ensure that all visible evidence of cancer is excised
- **Low grade DCIS** (cribriform or papillary subtype <0.5 cm in diameter): **Lumpectomy** alone if margins are widely free of disease
- **DCIS with limited disease: Lumpectomy + Radiotherapy**[Q]
- **DCIS with Extensive disease** (>4 cm in diameter or disease in >1 quadrant): **Mastectomy**[Q]

	LCIS	DCIS
• Age (years)	• 44–47 (Early)	• **54–58 (Late)**[Q]
• Incidence	• 2–5% (Less common)	• **5–10% (More common)**[Q]
• Clinical signs	• None	• Mass, pain, nipple discharge
• Mammographic signs	• None	• **Microcalcifications**[Q]
• Premenopausal	• **2/3**[Q]	• 1/3
• Incidence of synchronous invasive carcinoma	• 5%	• **2–46%**[Q]
• Multicentricity	• **60–90%**[Q]	• 40–80%
• Bilaterality	• **50–70%**[Q]	• 10–20%
• Axillary metastasis	• 1%	• **1–2%**[Q]
• **Subsequent carcinomas:**		
– Incidence	• 25–35%	• **25–70%**[Q]
– Laterality	• **Bilateral**[Q]	• Ipsilateral
– Interval to diagnosis	• **15–20 years**[Q]	• 5–10 years
– Histologic type	• **Ductal**	• **Ductal**

LOBULAR CARCINOMA

- LCIS originates from the **terminal duct lobular units** and develops **only in** the **female breast**[Q].
- **LCIS is mostly multicentric & bilateral**
- Increased **risk of invasive carcinoma** is in the **both breasts**[Q].

Histopathology

- Characterized by **distention & distortion** of **terminal duct lobular units**[Q] by cancer cells
- **Cytoplasmic mucoid globules**[Q] are a distinctive cellular feature.
- **Histologic hallmark** of **invasive** lobular carcinoma is **tendency** of **tumor cells** to **invade** in **linear strands (Indian file pattern)**[Q]

Clinical Characteristics

- **Presenting symptom** in most cases is **breast mass with ill-defined margins**
- Usually presents as an **incidental finding**[Q], on breast biopsy performed for other indication.
- Average age at diagnosis: **44-47 years**; more common in **white women**[Q]
- **Invasive breast cancer** develops in **25-35%** of women with LCIS, **in either breast**, regardless of which breast harbored the initial focus of LCIS, and is **detected synchronously** with **LCIS** in **5%** of cases.
- In women with LCIS, up to **65%** of subsequent **invasive cancers** are ductal, not lobular, in origin.
- **Marker** of **increased risk** for **invasive breast cancer**[Q] rather than as an anatomic precursor.
- **Invasive lobular carcinoma: Different pattern** of metastases, propensity to **involve peritoneal surface & meninges**[Q], less likely to metastasize to lungs or bone.

Diagnosis

- **Calcifications** associated with LCIS typically **occur in adjacent tissues (neighborhood calcification)**[Q]
- **Neighborhood calcification** is a **unique feature** of **LCIS**[Q] and contributes to its diagnosis.

Treatment

- **Observation/Chemoprevention/Prophylactic bilateral mastectomy**[Q]

■ CARCINOMA BREAST

BREAST CANCER

- **MC cancer** in **women** in the **world**[Q] and **MC cancer** in **urban**[Q] women in India
- **MC type** is **adenocarcinoma**[Q] and most carcinoma arises from **terminal duct lobular unit**[Q]
- **MC type** of CA breast: **Invasive ductal** (schirrous) **carcinoma**[Q]
- **Least common type** of CA breast: **Papillary**[Q]

> - **Most malignant** type of CA breast: **Inflammatory breast cancer**[Q]
> - **Best prognosis** is seen in: **Tubular**[Q]
> - **MC site** of CA breast: Upper outer **quadrant**[Q] (left[Q] breast >right)
> - **Least common** site of CA breast: **Lower inner quadrant**[Q]   • **MC route of spread: Limphatic**
> - **MC site of metastasis is Bone**[Q] (**Osteolytic** deposits in **Lumbar vertebra >Femur >Thoracic vertebra >Rib >Skull**)

- **Metastatic disease (Malignant pleural effusion**[Q]**)** is the **principal cause of death** from **breast cancer**.
- **2nd MC cause** of **cancer related death in women**[Q] (MC is **CA lung** in both **males** and **females**)[Q]
- **Pathway of metastasis in breast cancer:** Cancer cells from breast → Posterior intercostal veins → Batson veretebral venous plexus → Intracranial dural venous sinus → Brain

Clinical Features

- **Early breast cancer** may be **asymptomatic**[Q]

Symptoms indicating possibility of **breast cancer**	
• **Change in size** or **shape** of breast[Q]	• **Single duct discharge,** particularly **blood stained**[Q]
• **Skin dimpling, nipple retraction**[Q]	• **Axillary node** enlargement[Q]

- **Peau-d-orange:** Due to **obstruction** of **subdermal lymphatics (lymphatic permeation** by **tumor cells**[Q]**)** leading to **cutaneous lymphatic edema**[Q]
- **Symptoms** indicating possibility of Metastasis:
  - Breathing difficulty, bone pain, symptoms of **hypercalcemia**[Q], abdominal distention, jaundice

> - **Multifocality: Second cancer** in the **same quadrant (within 4 cm)**
> - **Multicentricity: Second cancer** outside the quadrant of primary cancer (away at least 4 cm)
> - **Dimpling: Small depression** over skin of breast due to **infiltration of ligament of Cooper** by carcinoma[Q]
> - **Puckering: Small fold or wrinkle** of skin over the breast due to **infiltration of ligament of Cooper** by carcinoma[Q]
> - **Cancer en-cuirasse: Infiltration of breast skin** & chest wall with **multiple nodules & ulceration** by the carcinoma[Q]

Contd…

Contd…

Evaluation

Triple Assessment		
• **Clinical examination**[Q] • **Imaging (USG or mammography)**[Q] • **Tissue sampling (FNAC or true cut biopsy)**[Q]		
• **Confident diagnosis** by **triple assessment** in **99.9%**		

- **First investigation** for suspected case of breast cancer: **Mammography**[Q]   • **Best and diagnostic investigation: Biopsy**[Q]

■ CARCINOMA BREAST INVESTIGATIONS

INVESTIGATIONS IN CA BREAST

FNAC	True-cut (core-cut) Biopsy
• Size of needle: 22-26 Gauge[Q]	• Size of needle: 14-16 Gauge[Q]
• **FNA is easily performed**, but **requires a trained cytopathologist**[Q] for accurate specimen interpretation.	• Core cutting needle biopsy provides a **histologic specimen** suitable for **interpretation by any pathologist**[Q].
• **False-negative results**[Q] are **most common** in **fibrotic** or **well-differentiated tumors.**	• **ER, PR status** and **presence of HER-2 overexpression** can be **routinely determined**[Q] from core biopsy specimens,
• **FNA does not reliably distinguish invasive cancer from DCIS**[Q], potentially leading to the overtreatment of gross DCIS.	• **Diagnostic technique of choice** for patients who will **receive preoperative systemic therapy**[Q].

ULTRASONOGRAPHY IN BREAST DISEASE

- **Initial investigation** for palpable lesions in **women <35 years**[Q]
- **Young woman's breast** contains a **large proportion** of **glandular tissue** which appears as a **soft tissue density**[Q] and **lowers the sensitivity of mammogram**[Q].
- The **sensitivity of ultrasound** for **detecting DCIS** is **significantly lower than mammography**[Q] that is why USG is not a useful screening test for breast cancer.
- Ultrasonography is an important method of:
  - **Resolving equivocal mammographic findings**
  - Defining cystic masses
  - Demonstrating the echogenic qualities of specific solid abnormalities

• **Breast cysts**	• **Smooth margins** and echo-free center
• **Benign breast masses**	• **Smooth contours,** round or oval shapes, weak internal echoes **Well-defined anterior** and **posterior margins**[Q].
• **Breast cancer**	• **Irregular walls**[Q] but may have smooth margins with acoustic enhancement

MAMMOGRAPHY

- **Delivers** a radiation dose of **0.1 cGy**[Q] per study (**chest radiography** delivers **25%** of this dose)[Q].
- **Bremsstrahlung type of X-ray** is used in mammography.
- **No increased breast cancer risk**[Q] associated with the radiation dose delivered with screening mammography.
- Used to detect **unexpected breast cancer** in **asymptomatic women**.
- Two views of the breast are obtained, the **craniocaudal view** & **mediolateral oblique view.**

> - **MLO view** images the **greatest volume**[Q] of breast tissue, including **upper outer quadrant** & **axillary tail** of Spence
> - **CC view** provides better visualization of **medial aspect** of the breast & permits **greater breast compression**[Q]

- Mammography also is used to guide interventional procedures, including needle localization & needle biopsy.
- **Sensitivity** is much **reduced in younger** or **dense breasts**, considered **inappropriate** in patients **<35 years**[Q].

Mammographic Features Suggestive of Breast Cancer

- A **solid mass** with or without **stellate features**[Q]
- **Asymmetric thickening**[Q] of breast tissues
- **Clustered microcalcifications**[Q]

Advantages

- Around **33% reduction in mortality**[Q] for women after screening mammography.
- Starting at age **45 years**, **breast examinations** should be performed **yearly** and a **yearly mammogram** should be taken[Q].

Contd…

Contd…

Mammography	Benign	Malignant
Opacity	• **Smooth** margin • **Low density** • Homogeneous • **Thin halo**	• **Ill defined**[Q] margin, **irregular stellate, spiculated**[Q] margin, **comet tail**[Q] • **High density**[Q] • Heterogeneous • **Wide halo**[Q]
Calcification	• **Macrocalcification**[Q] (>0.5 mm in diameter)	• **Microcalcification**[Q] (<0.5 mm in diameter)
Breast Parenchyma	• Normal	• Architectural distortion[Q]
Nipple/areola	• Normal	• **± Retracted**
Skin	• Normal	• Thickened[Q]
Cooper ligaments	• Normal	• **Thickened**[Q], increased number
Subcutaneous retro mammary space	• Normal	• **Obliterated**[Q]

BIRADS (Breast Imaging Reporting and Data System)		
Category	**Definition**	**Likelihood of Malignancy**
0	**Incomplete assessment**, need **additional imaging** evaluation[Q]	Not applicable
1	**Negative, routine mammogram** in 1 year is recommended[Q]	0%
2	**Benign** findings, **routine mammogram** in 1 year is recommended[Q]	0%
3	**Probably benign** findings, short term **follow-up** suggested[Q]	>0 to ≤2%
4	**Suspicious** abnormality, **biopsy** should be considered[Q] (**4A-Low** suspicion; **4B-Moderate** suspicion; **4C-High** suspicion)	4A: >2-≤10% 4B: >10-≤50% 4C: >50-≤95%
5	**Highly suggestive** of malignancy, **appropriate action** should be taken[Q]	>95%
6	Known **biopsy-proven malignancy**	Not applicable

MRI

- Screening with **MRI** is **superior to mammography** in **detecting invasive breast cancer in younger women**[Q], where the **sensitivity of mammography is low** due to **presence of mammographically dense breast parenchyma**[Q]

Indications for Breast MRI
1. **Lobular carcinoma**[Q]: Difficult to detect and measure by conventional method because of multifocal and infiltrating
2. **Staging of primary breast cancer**[Q]
3. **Occult primary tumour** with malignant axillary lymphadenopathy and **normal mammogram** and **breast USG**[Q]
4. **Screen younger women** with **high familial risk** of breast cancer[Q]
5. Assessing the **integrity of breast implant**[Q]

Pattern of Calcification in Breast Diseases	
Carcinoma	**Microcalcification**, punctate, branching[Q]
Fibroadenoma	**Popcorn**[Q] (coarse, granular, crushed stone)
Fibrocystic disease	Powdery
Fat necrosis	Curvilinear

■ CLASSIFICATION OF BREAST CANCER

WHO Classification of Breast Cancer		
In-situ Carcinoma	**Invasive Carcinoma (MC)**	**Paget's Disease of Nipple**
• Ductal carcinoma in–situ • Lobular carcinoma in–situ	• Ductal carcinoma (**MC**) • Lobular carcinoma • **Tubular (Cribiform)** carcinoma • **Mucinous (Colloid)** carcinoma • **Medullary** carcinoma • **Papillary** carcinoma • Metaplastic carcinoma • Inflammatory carcinoma	

■ CARCINOMA BREAST STAGING

8th AJCC (2017) TNM Staging for Breast Cancer
T: Primary tumor
T1: Tumor ≤2 cm[Q]
T2: Tumor >2 cm & ≤5 cm[Q]
T3: Tumor >5 cm[Q]
T4a: Extension to **chest wall**, not including pectoralis muscle[Q] **T4b**: **Edema** (including peau d'orange) or **ulceration** of skin, or **satellite skin nodules** confined to the same breast[Q] **T4c**: Both **T4a & T4b**[Q] **T4d**: **Inflammatory carcinoma**[Q]

Note
• Invasion of dermis alone does not qualify as T4[Q]. • Chest wall includes ribs, intercostal muscles & serratus anterior but not the pectoral muscles[Q]. • Dimpling of the skin, nipple retraction, or other skin changes, except those in T4b & T4d, may occur in T1, T2 or T3 without affecting the classification[Q].

N: Regional lymph nodes
N1: Metastasis to **movable ipsilateral level I, II axillary LNs**[Q]
N2a: Metastasis in **ipsilateral level I, II axillary LNs fixed** or **matted**[Q] **N2b**: Metastasis only in **clinically apparent ipsilateral internal mammary LNs** and in the absence of clinically evident axillary LNs metastasis[Q]
N3a: Metastasis in **ipsilateral infraclavicular LNs**[Q] **N3b**: Metastasis in **ipsilateral internal mammary LNs** & **axillary LNs**[Q] **N3c**: Metastasis in **ipsilateral supraclavicular LNs**[Q]
M: Distant metastases
M0: No distant metastasis; M1: Distant metastasis

[*Note*: Clinically apparent is defined as detected by **imaging studies** (excluding lymphoscintigraphy) or by **clinical examination** or **grossly visible pathologically**[Q].]

Stage I	Stage IIA	Stage IIB	Stage IIIA	Stage IIIB	Stage IIIC	Stage IV
T1 N0M0	T0**N1** M0 **T1N1** M0 **T2** N0M0	**T2N1** M0 **T3** N0M0	T0 **N2** M0 **T1-2 N2** M0 **T3 N1-2** M0	**T4 N0-2** M0	AnyT **N3** M0	AnyT anyN **M1**

Special Conditions in Staging	
• **Positive LN** in **opposite axilla**	• **Metastasis**
• **Two mass** in same breast	• Staging according to **big mass**
• **Mass** in **both breasts**	• **Separate staging** for **both breasts**

■ CARCINOMA BREAST MANAGEMENT

BREAST CANCER TREATMENT

A. Early Invasive Breast Cancer (Stage I, IIA, IIB):
- **Mastectomy + Axillary LN status assessment**[Q] or
- **BCT + Axillary LN status assessment + RT**[Q]
- If sentinel LN can not be identified or found to harbor metastatic disease, axillary LN dissection (**Level I+II**) should be done

Indications of Adjuvant Chemotherapy
1. **LN positive**[Q]
2. **Tumor >1 cm**[Q]

3. **LN** negative, **>0.5 cm** with **adverse prognostic factors**:
    – **Blood vessel** or **lymph vessel** invasion[Q]
    – **High** nuclear or histologic **grade**[Q]
    – **Her-2-neu** over expression[Q]
    – **Negative hormone receptor** status[Q]

Contd…

Contd…

> • **Tamoxifen** should be given for **hormone receptor positive**, cancer >1 cm[Q]
> • **Trastazumab** should be given for **Her-2-neu positive** cancer[Q]

B. Locally Advanced Breast Cancer (Stage IIIA, IIIB, IIIC)[Q]:
- **Neoadjuvant chemotherapy** + **MRM** + **Adjuvant RT**[Q]
- **BCT** for IIIA with N1 with patients who achieve **good response** to **neoadjuvant chemotherapy**[Q]
- Systemic **chemotherapy** + **radiotherapy** are indicated in treatment of grossly involved internal mammary nodes (N3b)

C. Distant Metastases (Stage IV):
- **Prolong survival** and **improve quality** of life[Q]
- **Hormonal therapies** are **preferred** to cytotoxic therapy as it is associated with **minimal toxicity**[Q]

Indications of Hormonal Therapy	Indications of Systemic Chemotherapy
1. Hormone receptor positive (**ER/PR positive**)[Q]	1. Hormone receptor **negative**[Q]
2. **Bone** or **soft tissue metastases only**[Q]	2. Hormone **refractory**[Q] (after 3 endocrine regimens)
3. **Limited** or **asymptomatic** visceral metastases	3. **Symptomatic visceral metastases**[Q]

Local Regional Recurrence
• Who had **mastectomy**: **Resection** of local regional recurrence **with reconstruction + chemotherapy + hormonal therapy + RT** (if not received RT previously)[Q]
• Who had **lumpectomy**: Mastectomy with reconstruction + chemotherapy + hormonal therapy[Q]

INDICATIONS OF RADIOTHERAPY IN CARCINOMA BREAST

- **Locally Advanced Breast Cancer**[Q] (to decrease recurrence rate)
- **Margin** is **positive** after mastectomy[Q]
- After **breast conservation surgery**[Q]
- Metastases to **4** or **more lymph nodes**[Q]

■ CHEMOTHERAPY IN CARCINOMA BREAST

CHEMOTHERAPY IN CA BREAST

- **First-generation regimen** such as a 6-monthly cycle of **cyclophosphamide, methotrexate** and **5-fluorouracil (CMF)**[Q] will achieve a **25% reduction** in the **risk of relapse** over a 10- to 15-year period[Q].
- **CMF** is **no longer** considered **adequate adjuvant chemotherapy**[Q]
- Modern regimens include an **anthracycline (doxorubicin** or **epirubicin)** and **taxanes**.

> • Effect of **combining hormone** & **chemotherapy** is **additive** although **hormone therapy** is **started after completion** of **chemotherapy** to reduce side-effects.

- Most popular combinations were **CMF & CAF**[Q] (Cyclophosphamide, **Adriamycin [doxorubicin]**, and 5-fluorouracil.
- In the United States, a **combination** of **Adriamycin (doxorubicin)** and **cyclophosphamide (AC)** or **AC plus a taxane (docetaxel, paclitaxel)** are likely to be used as **polychemotherapy**[Q].
- For HER-2–positive breast cancer, adding **trastuzumab**[Q] to polychemotherapy is approved for use as a surgical adjuvant.
- **Anthracycline-containing combinations** are significantly **better than** no treatment, **single-agent treatment,** or **CMF**[Q].

New Drugs in CA Breast	
Ixabepilone	• Used for **antracycline & taxane resistant** breast cancer[Q]
Lapatinib	• Inhibitor of Her-2-neu & EGFR tyrosine kinase • Second line Her-2-neu therapy[Q]
Sunitinib	• Approved for **advanced renal cancer & refractory metastatic breast cancer**[Q]
Pertuzumab	• **Humanized monoclonal antibody** used for **metastatic Her-2-neu positive breast cancer**[Q]

■ HORMONE THERAPY IN CARCINOMA BREAST

Hormonal Therapy in Carcinoma Breast

1. **Ovarian suppression or ablation:**
  – Bilateral oophorectomy[Q]
  – Medically by LHRH agonist (**Goserelin, Leuperolide**)[Q]

2. **SERM: Tamoxifen** and **Raloxifene**[Q]

Contd…

Contd…

| |
| 3. **Aromatase Inhibitors:** |
| – **Non-steroidal: Letrozole** and **Anastrazole**[Q] |
| – **Steroidal: Exmestane**[Q] |
| 4. **Anti-estrogens: Fulvestrant**[Q] |
| 5. **Progestins:** Megesterol & Medroxyprogesterone acetate |

Aromatase Inhibitors
• **No increased risk** of **endometrial carcinoma**[Q]
• **Decreases bone mineral density** & increases risk of **fracture**[Q]
• **Used** in **postmenopausal patients**[Q]

Hormonal Therapy in Carcinoma Breast
• **Tamoxifen** is **DOC** in **premenopausal** patients[Q]
• **Aromatase inhibitors are DOC in postmenopausal patients**

TAMOXIFEN

- **Tamoxifen** is a **standard hormonal treatment** of breast cancer in both **premenopausal** & **postmenopausal women**[Q]
- Tamoxifen is **effective in Estrogen Receptor (ER) positive breast carcinoma** but some ER negative tumors also respond to tamoxifen[Q].

> - Tamoxifen is **approved for primary prophylaxis** of breast cancer in **high risk women**[Q]
> - It **reduces the recurrence rate** of breast cancer in **ipsilateral** as well **contralateral breast**[Q]
> - **Tamoxifen** is associated with **reduced risk of cancer** in the **contralateral breast**[Q].

- **Dose: 10 mg BD × 5-years**[Q]
- While tamoxifen blocks estrogen receptors on the breast, it stimulates these receptors in the uterus (because tamoxifen is a **partial against of ER**), may **lead** to **endometrial hyperplasia** & **endometrial cancer**[Q]

Tamoxifen
• **Potent antagonist** in **breast carcinoma cells, blood vessels** and at some peripheral sites[Q]
• **Partial agonist** in the **pi**tuitary, **b**one, **u**terus and **l**iver **(Pit Bul)**

- Tamoxifen causes **retinal deposits, decreased visual acuity** & **cataracts** in occasional patients[Q]
- Tamoxifen **increases** the **risk of thromboembolic events**[Q]

Adverse Effects of Tamoxifen	
• **Hot flushes**, nausea & vomiting **(MC)**[Q]	• **Thromboembolism**[Q]
• **Menstrual irregularities**[Q], vaginal bleeding, discharge, pruritus vulvae & dermatitis	• **Cataract**[Q]
	• Retinal deposits & decreased visual acuity
• **Endometrial cancer**[Q]	

■ LYMPH NODE METASTASIS IN CARCINOMA BREAST

LYMPHATIC METASTASIS IN CA BREAST

- **Lymphatic spread** in CA breast occurs **through subareolar lymphatic plexus of Sappey's** lymphatic plexus, **cutaneous lymphatics** & **inflammatory lymphatics**[Q].

> - **Lymphatic metastasis** occurs **primarily to the axillary (75%)**[Q] & **internal mammary lymph nodes**[Q].
> - **Tumors** in the **posterior one third** of breast are more likely to drain to the **internal mammary nodes**[Q].

- Involvement of LNs has both biological & chronological significance.
- It represents not only an evolutional event in the spread of the carcinoma but is also a **marker for** the **metastatic potential**[Q] of that tumour.
- Involvement of **supraclavicular nodes** and of **any contralateral lymph nodes** represents **advanced disease**[Q].
- LN metastasis is treated by **surgical dissection** or **radiotherapy**

Contd…

Contd…

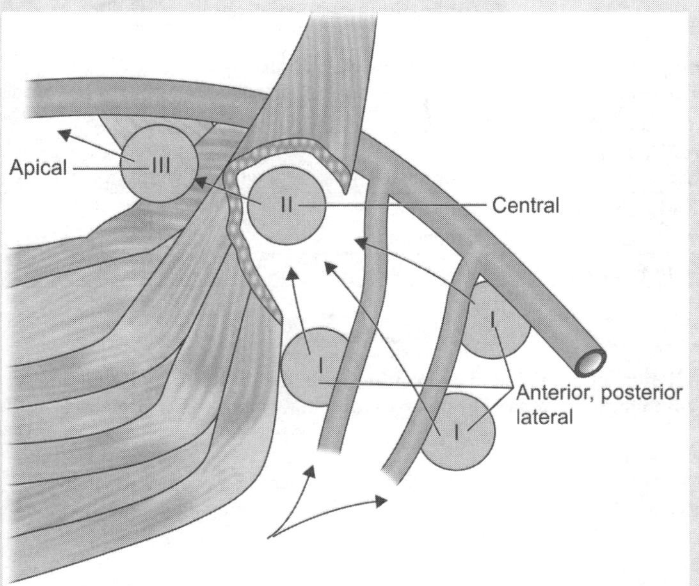

Axillary LN Levels in relation with Pectoralis minor		
Level	**Relation with Pectoralis minor**	**Axillary LNs Included**
I	Below or lateral	Anterior, posterior, lateral[Q]
II	Posterior (behind)	Central, Interpectoral[Q] (Rotter's nodes)
III	Medial or above	Apical[Q]

■ MASTECTOMY

Types of Mastectomy	
Simple or total mastectomy	Removal of **breast tissue, nipple-areola complex**, & **skin**[Q].
Extended simple mastectomy	Simple mastectomy + removal of **level I** axillary LNs.
Modified radical mastectomy	Removes all **breast tissue, nipple-areola complex, skin** and level **I & II** axillary LNs[Q].
Halsted's radical mastectomy	Removes all **breast tissue** and **skin, nipple areola complex, pectoralis major** and **minor** muscles and the level **I, II & III** axillary LNs[Q].

Variants of MRM	
Auschincloss Procedure	Removes all **breast tissue, nipple-areola complex, skin** and level **I & II** axillary LNs[Q].
Patey's Procedure	**Pectoralis minor** is **removed** to allow complete dissection of **level III** axillary LNs[Q]
Scanlon's Modification of Patey's Procedure	**Pectoralis minor** is **divided** instead of removing[Q]. Division of pectoralis minor allows **complete removal** of **level III** axillary LNs[Q]

■ COMPLICATIONS OF MASTECTOMY

Complications of Mastectomy

• **Seroma**
  – **MC complication**[Q], beneath skin flaps & axilla, occurs in **30%** cases
  – Catheter is retained until drainage is <30 mL/day

• **Wound Infection**   – Majority are due to **skin flap necrosis**

Contd…

Contd…

Complications of Mastectomy

• **Lymphedema**
  – Occurs less frequently with the standard axillary dissections.
  – Extensive LN dissection, radiation therapy, presence of positive LNs, obesity are predisposing factors[Q].

• **Injury to Long Thoracic (Motor) Nerve**
  – Seen in **10%** of all cases.
  – Result in a palsy of the Serratus anterior muscle (classical **winged scapula**)

• **Injury to Thoracodorsal Nerve**   – Leads to palsy of the latissimus dorsi muscle.
• **Redundant Axillary Fat Pad**

ANGIOSARCOMA

- Classified as **de novo**, as **postradiation**, or as arising in **association with postmastectomy lymphedema.**
- Stewart and Treves described **lymphangiosarcoma** of **upper extremity** in women with **ipsilateral lymphedema** after **radical mastectomy. (Stewart-Treves Syndrome)**[Q]
- Angiosarcoma is now the preferred name.
- **Average interval** between MRM or radical mastectomy and the development of an angiosarcoma is **10.5 years**[Q].
- **60% of women** developing this cancer have a **history of adjuvant radiation therapy**[Q].

Clinical Features

- **Acute worsening** of **edema**
- Appearance of **subcutaneous nodules** with propensity towards **hemorrhage and ulceration**

Radiation-induced Angiosarcoma	Angiosarcoma (in the absence of previous radiation therapy or surgery)
• **Reddish brown** to **purple raised rash** within the radiation portals and on the skin of the breast	• May form a **mass within** the **parenchyma of the breast**

Treatment

- **Preoperative chemotherapy** & **radiotherapy** followed by **surgical excision (radical amputation)**[Q]
- Associated with **poor prognosis**[Q]

■ BREAST CONSERVATIVE SURGERY

BREAST CONSERVATIVE SURGERY (BCT)

- Involves **resection** of **primary breast cancer** with a margin of normal appearing breast tissue, **adjuvant radiation therapy** with or without **assessment** of **axillary LN status**[Q].
- Surgical procedures employed: **wide local excision, lumpectomy, quadrantectomy**
- BCT is currently treatment for women with **DCIS, Stage I and Stage II invasive breast cancer**[Q].

Suitable Candidates for BCT

- Cancer is **solitary**, with no clinical or mammographic evidence of cancer elsewhere in the breast.
- Tumour can be **excised with tumor free surgical margins** without producing a cosmetically unacceptable breast.
- There are **no contraindications to radiation**
- Patients is **willing** & **motivated** for breast conservation

Contraindications for BCT

Absolute contraindications	Relative contraindications
1. **Pregnancy**[Q] is an absolute contraindication to the use of breast irradiation. 2. Women with **two** or **more primary tumors** in **separate quadrants** of the breast or with **diffuse malignant** appearing **micro calcifications**[Q]. 3. A **history** of prior **therapeutic irradiation**[Q] to the breast region that would require treatment to an excessively high total-radiation dose to a significant volume 4. **Persistent positive margins**[Q] after reasonable surgical attempts	1. History of **collagen vascular disorders**[Q] (**Scleroderma** and **active lupus erythematosus** but not the rheumatoid arthritis) 2. Presence of **multiple gross tumours** in the **same quadrant** and **indeterminate calcifications**[Q] 3. **Large tumour** in **small breast**[Q] 4. **Breast size, large pendulous breast**[Q] presents difficulty in delivering uniform radiation dose 5. **Centrally located tumour**[Q], for which removal of nipple-areola complex is required to obtain a tumour free margin

■ CARCINOMA BREAST PROGNOSTIC INDICATORS

> **Prognostic Factors in Carcinoma Breast**
>
> - **Most important prognostic factor** in CA breast: **Stage >Axillary LN status**[Q]
> - **In case of metastasis**, the **prognosis no more depends upon** the lymph node status[Q]
>
>> - In **breast carcinoma metastasis**, prognosis **best depends upon estrogen & progesterone receptor status**[Q] (ER & PR status)

> **Oncotype DX**
>
> - **Oncotype DX** is a **genomic test that predicts the likelihood of a cancer recurrence**, likelihood of benefit from chemotherapy, & likelihood of survival in patients with newly diagnosed breast cancer that **has not spread to LNs (node negative)** and is **hormone receptor-positive**.
> - Oncotype DX evaluates the **activity of 21 genes** from a sample of the patient's cancer **to determine the patient's Recurrence Score**.
> - **Recurrence Score** ranges from **0 to 100**, with a **higher score indicating a greater risk of recurrence**.
> - Oncotype DX diagnostic tests help individualize treatment planning for breast, colon and prostate cancer patients.

Oncotype DX may be used to guide chemotherapy decisions among certain women with:		
• Node-negative[Q]	• Hormone receptor-positive[Q]	• HER2-negative breast cancer[Q]

Name of Test	Brief Description	Scoring/Measurement	Tissue Needed
Oncotype DX	A genomic test that uses a **21-gene assay** to provide an **individual, quantitative assessment of the likelihood of disease recurrence**.	Recurrence Score, a number between **0 and 100** that **correlates to a specific likelihood of breast cancer recurrence within 10 years** of initial diagnosis	**Fixed-tissue blocks**
Mamma Print	A unique **70-gene assay** that has the ability to **identify which early-stage breast cancer patients** are **at risk of distant recurrence following surgery, independent of Estrogen Receptor status** and any **prior treatment**.	**Low risk or high risk**	**Paraffin embedded or fresh tissue**
PAM50	A **50-gene test** in development that is designed to be performed in local routine hospital pathology laboratories and has been optimized **to separate intrinsic disease subtypes that are used to generate a ROR score**.	**Risk of Recurrence (ROR) score**	**Fixed-tissue blocks**

■ GENE EXPRESSION PROFILING IN BREAST CANCER

- "**Gene expression profiling,** *which can measure the relative quantities of mRNA for essentially every gene, has* identified **five major patterns of gene expression** in the NST group: **luminal** A, **luminal** B, **normal**, **basal-like**, and **HER2 positive**. These molecular classes **correlate with prognosis** and **response to therapy,** and thus have taken on clinical importance."

Luminal Criteria	
Type	**Properties**
Luminal A (MC)	**ER & PR +ve, Her-2-neu –ve**[Q] **(MC type**[Q]; **Best prognosis**[Q]**)**
Luminal B	**ER, PR & Her-2-neu +ve** (Triple positive)[Q]
Normal breast-like	Well-differentiated, ER-positive
Basal cell type	**Triple negative, positive** for **myoepithelial markers**[Q] (basal keratins, P-cadherin, p63, or laminin)**, CK-5, 6 & 17, EGFR**
Her-2 type	**Her-2-neu +ve, ER & PR –ve**[Q] **(worst prognosis)**

■ TRIPLE-NEGATIVE BREAST CANCER (TNBC)

> **Triple-negative Breast Cancer (TNBC)**
>
> - **TNBC:** Breast cancer that **does not express** the genes for **ER, PR & Her-2-neu**[Q]
> - Accounts for **15–25%** of breast cancer cases.
> - More common in **premenopausal women**[Q]

Contd…

Contd...

Pathology

- **Germline mutations** of **BRCA1 & BRCA2 genes**[Q] are the causative factor
- Also known as **basal-like**[Q] (**75% of basal-type breast cancers are triple negative**)
- Some TNBC **overexpresses EGFR & transmembrane glycoprotein NMB**[Q] (GPNMB).

Treatment

- **Standard treatment: Surgery (Mastectomy/BCS) + Adjuvant chemotherapy + Radiotherapy**[Q]

> - **Didox (synthetic antioxidant)** in addition to chemotherapy **reduces drug resistance**[Q].
> - **Didox inhibits ribonucleotide reductase M2 (RRM2)**[Q]
> - **RRM2** contributes to **cells resistance of the chemotherapy** resulting in relapse[Q].

- **TNBCs** are very **susceptible to chemotherapy**[Q].
- **BRCA1-related TNBC** is particularly susceptible to **platinum-based agents & taxanes**[Q].

Prognosis

- **High risk of recurrence**[Q] after treatment

■ BREAST RECONSTRUCTION

Breast Reconstruction		
Autogenous	**Alloplastic**	**Combined**
• **TRAM flap (MC)**[Q] • **Lattisimus dorsi flap**[Q] • Gluteal flap • **Ruben's flap**[Q] • Thoracoepigastric flap • Lateral thigh flap	• **Silicone gel** implant[Q] • **Silicone implant** with **saline refill**[Q]	• **Lattisimus dorsi flap** with **implant**[Q] • **TRAM flap** with **implant**[Q]

- Placement of **implant in a submuscular plane** beneath **pectoralis major**[Q], **superior portion** of **rectus abdominis, & serratus anterior muscles** provides **better protection** against **implant extrusion**, as well as **decreased risk** for **capsular contracture & implant displacement**[Q]

Common Reconstructive Options after Mastectomy		
Type	**Advantages**	**Disadvantages**
Implant	**One stage** procedure, minimal prolongation, hospitalization, or recovery, low cost	**Poor symmetry**[Q] if skin removed or in large ptotic breasts. **Capsular contracture, leakage, rupture**[Q] possible.
Tissue expander	Short operative time, hospitalization, recovery not prolonged, low cost	**Multiple** physician **visits** post-op. **Poor symmetry** large or ptotic breasts. **Capsular contracture, leakage rupture**[Q] possible.
Latissimus dorsi flap	Short operative time, hospitalization, recovery not prolonged, low cost	**Donor site scar**[Q] Usually **requires an implant**[Q] Moderate prolongation hospitalization and recovery.
TRAM flap	Natural contour. Good match for large or ptotic breasts. Abdominoplasty.	**Donor site scar**[Q] **Fat necrosis, flap loss** possible. **Abdominal wall weakness** and **hernia**[Q]. Significant prolongation hospitalization plus recovery.

- **MC method** of **breast reconstruction**: Implants (silicon implants)[Q]
- **Surgical breast reconstruction** should **never done prior to RT**[Q].
- **Best flap** for breast reconstruction: **DIEP flap**[Q] (Deep inferior epigastric perforator flap) > **TRAM FLAP**[Q]

■ INFLAMMATORY BREAST CARCINOMA (MASTITIS CARCINOMATOSA)

- IBC (stage **IIIB**) accounts for **<3%** of breast cancers.
- Characterized by the skin changes of **brawny induration, erythema** with a raised edge, & **edema** (**rapid onset** peau d'orange) involving **>33%** of **skin** of breast[Q].

Pathology

- **Permeation** of **dermal lymph vessels** by **cancer cells** is seen in **skin biopsy** specimens[Q].
- There **may be** an associated **breast mass**[Q].

Contd...

Contd…

Clinical Features
- Characterized by skin changes of **brawny induration**, **erythema** with a raised edge, and **edema** (peau d'orange)[Q].
- IBC may be **mistaken for** a **bacterial infection**[Q] of the breast.
- More than **75%** of women present with **palpable axillary lymphadenopathy**[Q]
- **Distant metastases at diagnosis** in **25%** of white women with IBC.

Diagnosis
- IOC for diagnosis is **skin biopsy**[Q].

Treatment
- Multimodal approach (NACT + Mastectomy + RT ± Hormonal therapy)[Q]
- **Chest wall**, **supraclavicular**, **internal mammary** and **axillary** lymph node basins receive **adjuvant radiation therapy**.

> - Both **inflammatory breast cancer** & **Paget's disease may** or **may not** be **associated** with **breast mass**.

■ BREAST CANCER DURING PREGNANCY

BREAST CANCER DURING PREGNANCY

- Occurs in **1 of every 3000**[Q] pregnant women
- **MC non-gynecologic malignancy** associated with **pregnancy**[Q].
- **Ductal carcinoma** is **MC type,** accounting for **75–90%**[Q] of breast cancer in pregnancy.

Clinical Features
- Presents as **painless palpable mass**[Q] with or without nipple discharge
- **Axillary LN metastases** in up to **75%** patients
- Approx. **<25% nodules** developing during **pregnancy** and **lactation** will be **cancerous**[Q]
- **Present at a later stage** of disease because breast changes occurring in hormone-rich environment of pregnancy obscure early cancer

Diagnosis
- **USG** and **needle biopsy**[Q] are used for diagnosis
- **Mammography** is rarely indicated due to its **decreased sensitivity** during **pregnancy** and **lactation**

Treatment: Mainstay of therapy is surgical resection

• **Stage I and II**	• **Mastectomy with axillary dissection**[Q]
• **LABC**	• **NACT after 1st trimester + MRM in 2nd trimester + RT after delivery**[Q]

LABC in Pregnancy
• **MRM** can be performed during **first & second** trimester (increased risk of spontaneous abortion after first-trimester anesthesia), **chemotherapy after first trimester** and **radiotherapy after delivery**.
• **Chemotherapy** during **first trimester** carries a risk of **spontaneous abortion** and **12%** risk of **birth defects, given after first trimester.**
• No evidence of teratogenecity by chemotherapy during second and third trimester.

■ PAGET'S DISEASE OF NIPPLE

PAGET'S DISEASE OF NIPPLE

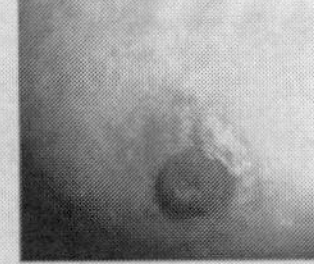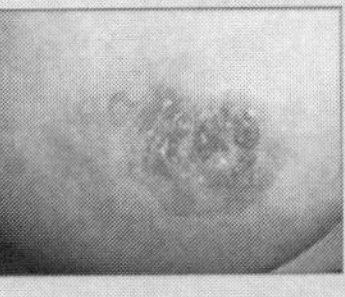

- **Chronic eczematous eruption** of **nipple** which may progress to an ulcerated weeping lesion.
- Differentiated by superficial spreading melanoma by **CEA positivity**[Q]

Histopathology
- Paget cell is **large**, pale staining with **round nuclei & large nucleoli**[Q]
- Paget cells **spread into lactiferous sinuses**[Q] under the nipple and upward to invade overlying epidermis of the nipple
- Paget cells **does not invade dermal basement membrane**[Q] (carcinoma in situ)

Clinical Features
- Most (**>97%**) patients with Paget's disease have an **underlying ductal carcinoma**[Q] (in situ or invasive)
- Paget's disease **may (54%)** or **may not (46%)** be accompanied by a **mass**[Q]
- **Invasive breast cancer coexists** with Paget's disease in **93%** of patients **with mass** and in **38%** of patients **without mass**[Q]

Diagnosis
- **Complete mammography** and **biopsy** is required to rule out occult multicentric disease
- **Biopsy** showing **Paget cell is diagnostic**[Q]

Treatment
- Most commonly utilized procedure is **simple mastectomy**[Q]
- Wide excision of nipple and areola to achieve clear ,margins + Radiotherapy + Axillary staging
- Lumpectomy + Radiotherapy + Axillary LN dissection

■ CARCINOMA OF MALE BREAST

CARCINOMA OF MALE BREAST

- Peak in **6th decade**[Q] of life, accounts for less than **1%** of all cases of breast cancer.
- MC Type: **Infiltrating ductal carcinoma**[Q].

> - Male breast cancer is **preceded by gynecomastia** in 20% of men[Q].
> - **Hormone receptor positive: 80%; Her-2-neu positive: 35%**

- **Lobular carcinoma** (both in-situ and invasive) is **rarely seen** due to **absence of lobules** in males.

Predisposing Factors
- Excess endogenous or exogenous **estrogen** (Testicular disease, **infertility, obesity, cirrhosis**)[Q]
- **Radiation** therapy, **Klinefelter's syndrome** and **testicular feminizing syndromes**[Q].
- **BRCA2 mutations**[Q]

> - **Gynecomastia is not a risk factor** for **carcinoma male breast**[Q].

Clinical Features
- **MC presentation is lump**[Q].
- Local pain, axillary adenopathy, nipple retraction, ulceration, bleeding, & discharge.

> - **Breast cancer** in **men** more commonly **involves** the **pectoralis major muscle**[Q] due to **scanty breast tissue.**

Diagnosis
- Evaluation includes **breast imaging** studies and diagnostic **needle** or **surgical biopsy**.

Treatment
- Treatment of male breast cancer is **surgical** (Most common procedure: **MRM**) [Q]
- **Adjuvant radiation therapy** is in **high risk cases** for local-regional recurrence.
- **Eighty per cent** of male breast cancers are **hormone receptor positive**, and adjuvant **tamoxifen** is considered.

Prognosis
- Stage >**Lymph node status** is the **best prognostic indicator**[Q] as in female breast carcinoma.
- **Stage by stage prognosis** is **same as female CA breast**[Q]

■ CYSTOSARCOMA PHYLLODES

PHYLLODES TUMORS

- Tumors of **mixed connective tissue** & **epithelium** (biphasic proliferation of **stroma** & mammary **epithelium**) [Q]
- Also known as **serocystic disease of Brodie**[Q]
- Classified as benign, borderline, or malignant.

Pathology
- Sharply demarcated from surrounding breast tissue, which is compressed & distorted.
- **Connective tissue** composes the **bulk** of these tumors, which have mixed gelatinous, solid & cystic areas.
- **Cystic areas** represent sites of **infarction** & **necrosis**.
- Gross cut tumor surface: **Classical leaf-like (phyllodes) appearance**[Q].
- Most **malignant phyllodes tumors** contain **liposarcomatous** or **rhabdomyosarcomatous elements** rather than fibrosarcomatous elements[Q].
- Evaluation of **number of mitoses** & **presence or absence of invasive foci** at the tumor margins may help to identify a **malignant tumor**[Q].

Clinical Features
- **Smooth, rounded,** usually **painless** multinodular lesions
- Average **age: 4th decade**.
- Large, mostly **massive size** but always **mobile over chest wall**[Q]
- **Bosselated surface** with **pressure necrosis of overlying skin**[Q]
- Diagnosis is suggested by **larger size**, a history of **rapid growth**[Q], and occurrence in **older patients**.
- **Differentiated from carcinoma by: No fixity to skin** and **pectoralis, no nipple retraction, no LN involvement**[Q]
- **MC site of metastasis: Lungs**

Diagnosis
- **Diagnosis** is best made by **biopsy**[Q]

Contd...

Contd…

Treatment

• Small phyllodes tumors	• Wide local excision[Q]
• Large phyllodes tumors	• Mastectomy[Q]
• Phyllodes tumor with **suspicious malignant elements**	• **Re-excision** of biopsy site **to ensure complete excision** of tumor with a **1 cm margin**

- **Axillary dissection** is **not recommended** because axillary LN metastases rarely occur[Q].

■ BENIGN DISORDERS OF BREAST

ABERRATIONS OF NORMAL DEVELOPMENT AND INVOLUTION

- ANDI classification encompasses all aspects of breast condition, including pathogenesis and degree of abnormality.

Early Reproductive Years
- **Fibroadenomas** in younger women aged **15–25 years**
- Nipple inversion is a disorder of development of the major ducts, which prevents normal protrusion of the nipple.
- Mammary duct fistulas arise when nipple inversion predisposes to major duct obstruction, leading to recurrent subareolar abscess and mammary duct fistula.

Later Reproductive Years
- **Cyclical mastalgia** and **nodularity** usually are associated with **premenstrual enlargement** of the breast and are regarded as normal.
- In epithelial hyperplasia of pregnancy, papillary projections sometimes give rise to bilateral bloody nipple discharge.

Involution
- **Macrocysts** are common, are often **subclinical,** and do not require specific treatment.
- **Sclerosing adenosis** is considered a disorder of both the proliferative and the involutional phases of the breast cycle.
- **Duct ectasia** (dilated ducts) and periductal mastitis are other important components.
- **Sixty per cent** of women **70 years** of age exhibit some degree of **epithelial hyperplasia**.
- **Atypical** proliferative diseases include **ductal** and **lobular hyperplasia**, both of which display **some features** of **carcinoma in situ**.
- Women with **atypical ductal** or **lobular hyperplasia** have a **fourfold increase** in **breast cancer risk**.

ANDI Classification of Benign Breast Disorders			
	Normal	**Disorder**	**Disease**
Early reproductive years (age 15–25 years)	Lobular development Stromal development Nipple eversion	**Fibroadenoma**[Q] Adolescent hypertrophy Nipple inversion	Giant fibroadenoma Gigantomastia Subareolar abscess Mammary duct fistula
Later reproductive years (age 25–40 years)	Cyclical changes of menstruation Epithelial hyperplasia of pregnancy	**Cyclical mastalgia**[Q] Nodularity Bloody nipple discharge	**Incapacitating mastalgia**[Q]
Involution (age 35–55 years)	Lobular involution Duct involution Dilatation Sclerosis Epithelial turnover	Macrocysts Sclerosing lesions Duct ectasia Nipple retraction **Epithelial hyperplasia**	Periductal mastitis **Epithelial hyperplasia with atypia**[Q]

FIBROADENOMA

- **MC benign tumor** of female breast[Q];
- **MC age group: 15–30 years**[Q];
- Known as **breast mouse**[Q]
- Etiology: **Increased sensitivity** of **focal areas** of breast tissue **to estrogen**[Q]

Pathology
- **Encapsulated** spherical lesion, composed of **fibrous** and **glandular tissue**[Q]
- Arise from interlobular stroma, stromal cells can be monoclonal or polyclonal

Clinical Feature
- **Painless,** slowly growing **solitary mobile lump** in the breast (**Breast mouse**)[Q]

Diagnosis
- **IOC is FNAC**[Q] (**Antler horn configuration**[Q] of ductal epidermal cells)
- Characteristic **popcorn calcification**[Q] on mammography

Treatment
- **No treatment**[Q] is necessary when diagnosis is confirmed.
- **Excision biopsy** is the treatment of choice for **suspicious lesion**[Q] and for cosmetic indications.

BREAST CYST

- Occur most commonly in the **last decade** of **reproductive life**[Q] as a result of a non-integrated involution of stroma and epithelium.

Clinical Features

- Often **multiple**, may be **bilateral**[Q] and can mimic malignancy.
- Typically **present suddenly** and cause great alarm; **prompt diagnosis** and **drainage** provides **immediate relief**[Q].

Diagnosis

- Diagnosis can be confirmed by **aspiration** and/or **ultrasound**[Q].

Treatment

- **Aspiration** for Solitary cyst: If they **resolve completely**, and if the fluid is **not blood-stained, no further treatment** is required (**30% will recur** and require **reaspiration**)[Q]
- **Core biopsy** or **local excision**[Q]: If there is a **residual lump** or if the fluid is **blood-stained, for histological diagnosis** (exclude cystadenocarcinoma, which is more common in elderly women)

GALACTORRHEA

- Secretion of **milk looking discharge** from **one** or **both breasts unrelated to pregnancy**[Q] is called galactorrhea.
- Physiological galactorrhea is the continued production of milk after lactation has ceased and menses resumed and is often caused by continued mechanical stimulation of the nipple.
- In both **men** and **women**[Q], galactorrhea may **vary in colour** and **consistency**.
- Galactorrhea is commonly **associated with prolactinoma**[Q].

Treatment

- Treatment is aimed at **normalizing prolactin level**[Q].
- **Bromocriptine**[Q] (dopamine agonist) is the **drug of choice**.
- **Surgery** is considered when there is **failure of medical therapy**[Q] (Trans-nasal trans-sphenoidal excision of **pituitary adenoma** is done[Q])

AMAZIA

- **Congenital absence** of the **breast**[Q] may occur on one or both sides.
- It is sometimes **associated with absence** of the **sternal portion** of the **pectoralis major** (Poland's syndrome)[Q].
- It is **more common in males**[Q].

MONDOR'S DISEASE

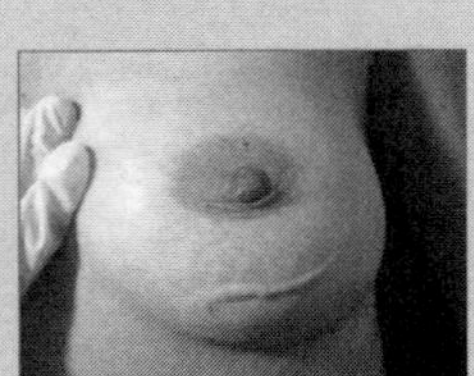

- A variant of **thrombophlebitis** involving the **superficial veins** of the **anterior chest wall**[Q] and breast.
- Also known as "**string phlebitis**," a thrombosed vein presenting as a **tender, cord-like structure**[Q].
- Frequently involved veins: **Lateral thoracic vein, thoracoepigastric vein**, superficial epigastric vein.
- **Benign, self-limited disorder.**

Clinical Features

- **Acute pain** in the **lateral aspect** of the **breast** or the **anterior chest wall**[Q].
- A **tender, firm cord** is found to follow the distribution of one of the major superficial veins.

Diagnosis

- When the diagnosis is **uncertain**, or when a **mass** is present near the tender cord, **biopsy** is indicated.

Treatment

- **NSAIDs** and application of **warm compresses**[Q] along the symptomatic vein with **restriction of motion** and **brassiere support** of the breast
- Usually **resolves** within **4–6 weeks**.
- When symptoms **persist** or are **refractory to therapy, excision** of the involved vein segment

DUCT PAPILLOMA

- Intraductal pailloma are true polyps of epithelium lined breast ducts.
- **Benign**[Q] lesions (**not pre-cancerous**)
- **Mostly solitary**[Q], located under the areola (within 4-5 cm of nipple orifice)
- Generally **<1 cm**, can grow up to 4–5 cm

Clinical Features

- **MC presentation: Bloody nipple discharge**[Q]
- **Intraductal papilloma** is **MC** cause of **bloody nipple discharge**[Q]

Diagnosis

- **Ductography: Small filling defects**[Q] surrounded by contrast media

Treatment

- **Microdochectomy:** Complete **excision** of the **involved duct** along with **tumor**[Q]

Duct Ectasia (Periductal Mastitis)

- **Dilatation** of the **breast ducts**, which is often associated **with periductal inflammation**.
- Pathogenesis is obscure, **more common** in **smokers**[Q].

Clinical Features

- **Nipple discharge** (of **any colour**), a **subareolar mass**, **abscess**, **mammary duct fistula** and/or **nipple retraction**[Q] are the most common symptoms.

Diagnosis

- **Ductography: Dilated cystic structure**[Q] in duct Ectasia
- In the case of a **mass** or **nipple retraction**, a **carcinoma** must be **excluded** by obtaining a **mammogram** and **negative cytology** or histology.

Treatment

- **Hadfield's operation**[Q]: Excision of all of the major ducts
- **Cessation of smoking**[Q] increases the chance of a long-term cure.

Breast Abscess

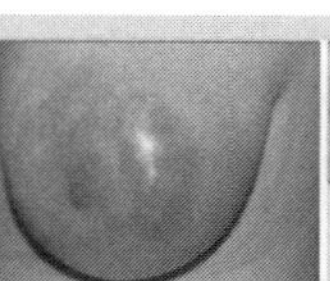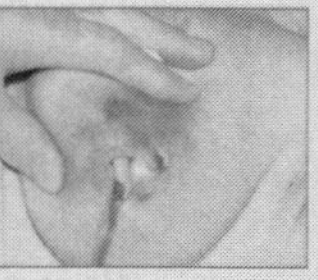

- Typically seen in **staphylococcal infections**[Q]
- Present with point **tenderness, erythema,** and **hyperthermia**
- **Related to lactation** and occur **within** the **first few weeks** of **breastfeeding**[Q].
- **S. aureus** are **transmitted** via **suckling neonate**[Q]

Staphylococcal infections **(MC)**	**Localized** and situated **deep** in the breast tissues
Streptococcal infections	**Diffuse superficial involvement**

Diagnosis

- Preoperative **ultrasonography** is effective in **delineating the required extent** of the drainage procedure

Treatment

- Local wound care, including application of warm compresses, & IV antibiotics.
- For **mastitis, first line antibiotics** are **dicloxacillin**[Q] or **Cloxacillin**[Q] (given for **10-14 days**).
- **Drainage procedure** is best accomplished via **circumareolar incisions** or incisions **paralleling Langer's lines**[Q].
- **Biopsy** of **abscess cavity wall** at the time of incision and drainage **to rule out** underlying or coexisting **breast cancer** with **necrotic tumor**[Q].

Multiple Choice Questions

■ NIPPLE DISCHARGE

1. **Blood stained nipple discharge is seen in:**
   (Recent Question 2017, DNB 2013, 2011, Orissa 2011, PGI June 2009, UPPG 2010, AIIMS Nov 2003, All India 2005)
   a. Breast abscess
   b. Fibroadenoma
   c. Ductal papilloma
   d. Fat necrosis of breast

2. **Green discharge is most commonly seen with:**
   (Recent Question 2016, Kerala PG 2015, WBPG 2015, AIIMS Nov 98)
   a. Duct papilloma
   b. Duct ectasia
   c. Retention cyst
   d. Fibroadenosis

3. **A 25 years old female complains of discharge of blood from a single duct in her breast. The most appropriate treatment is:**
   (All India 2008)
   a. Radical excision
   b. Microdochectomy
   c. Radical mastectomy
   d. Biopsy to rule out carcinoma

■ CARCINOMA BREAST INVESTIGATIONS

4. **Triple assessment for CA Breast includes:** *(Kerala PG 2015)*
   a. History, clinical examination and mammogram
   b. History, clinical examination and FNAC
   c. USG, mammogram and FNAC *(DNB 2010, All India 2009)*
   d. Clinical examination, mammogram and FNAC

5. **Breast triple assessment contains all except:**
   (MCI Dec 2018)
   a. Clinical examination
   b. Axillary sampling
   c. USG
   d. FNAC & Biopsy

6. **Best diagnostic method for breast lump is:** *(AIIMS June 95)*
   a. USG
   b. Mammogram
   c. Biopsy
   d. FNAC

7. **Investigation of choice for high risk breast cancer in female is:**
   a. MRI
   b. CT-PET *(DNB 2014)*
   c. Mammography
   d. USG

8. **Gold standard investigation for screening of breast carcinoma in patients with breast implant:**
   (Recent Question 2015)
   a. MRI
   b. USG
   c. Mammography
   d. CT Scan

9. **Best investigation to differentiate scar from recurrence after mastectomy done for carcinoma breast:** *(Recent Question 2016)*
   a. MRI
   b. CT
   c. PET scan
   d. Mammography

10. **All of the following are indications for MRI in breast carcinoma except:** *(Recent Question 2017)*
    a. Microcalcification
    b. High-risk cases
    c. Breast-implant patients
    d. Lobular carcinoma in situ

■ MAMMOGRAPHY

11. **Most sensitive imaging for ductal carcinoma in situ of breast is:** *(AIIMS Nov 2010)*
    a. Mammography
    b. MRI
    c. PET
    d. USG

12. **Dose of radiation per study in mammography:**
    a. 0.1cGy
    b. 0.2 *(Recent Question 2016)*
    c. 0.3
    d. 0.4

13. **BIRADS stands for:** *(AIIMS Nov 2012)*
    a. Breast Imaging Reporting and Data System
    b. Best Imaging Reporting and Data System
    c. Brain Imaging Reporting and Data System
    d. Best Imaging Reporting and Data System

14. **Popcorn calcification in mammography is seen in:**
    (Recent Question 2016, AIIMS June 2000)
    a. Fibroadenoma
    b. Fat necrosis
    c. Cystosarcoma phyllodes
    d. CA Breast

15. **What is the age of routine screening mammography?**
    a. 20 years
    b. 30 years *(DNB 2014)*
    c. 40 years
    d. 50 years

16. **BIRADS score 4 suggests:** *(Recent Question 2018)*
    a. Normal lesion
    b. Suspicion of malignancy
    c. Mostly benign
    d. Proven malignancy

17. **BIRADS score 5 is:** *(Recent Question 2015)*
    a. Negative
    b. Probably benign
    c. Suspicious abnormality
    d. Highly suggestive of malignancy

■ CARCINOMA BREAST RISK FACTORS

18. **Following condition has no increased risk of invasive breast carcinoma except:** *(MHCET 2016)*
    a. Hyperplasia atypical
    b. Sclerosing adenosis
    c. Apocrine metaplagia
    d. Duct ectasia

19. **Moderately increased risk for invasive breast carcinoma is associated with which of the following?**
    a. Sclerosing adenoma
    b. Apocrine metaplasia
    c. Duct ectasia *(DNB 2010, Kerala 2000)*
    d. Atypical ductal hyperplasia
    e. Fibro adenoma

20. **All of the following are predisposing factors for breast carcinoma except:** *(DNB 2008, MCI Sept 2008)*
    a. Family history of breast carcinoma
    b. First child at a younger age
    c. Early menarche and late menopause
    d. Nulliparous women

21. **BRCA-1 gene is located on which chromosome?**
    a. 11
    b. 13 *(MHCET 2016)*
    c. 17
    d. 22

22. **BRCA-2 gene is located on chromosome:**
    a. 17
    b. 13 *(Recent Question 2017)*
    c. 7
    d. 11

23. **All of the following are true about tumors associated with BRCA-1 except:** *(Recent Question 2017)*
    a. Hormone receptor positive
    b. Poorly differentiated
    c. Chromosome 17
    d. Early age onset

24. **All are risk factors for carcinoma breast except:**
    (Recent Question 2013)
    a. Early menarche
    b. Late menopause
    c. Ovarian cancer
    d. Early full term pregnancy

25. **% of malignancy in duct ectasia is:** *(Recent Question 2015)*
    a. No risk
    b. 15:1
    c. 7:1
    d. 10:1

26. **Premalignant lesion with high-risk for malignancy:**
    a. Atypical ductal hyperplasia *(Recent Question 2017)*
    b. Sclerosing adenosis
    c. Duct ectasia
    d. Papilloma

CARCINOMA BREAST

27. False about lobular carcinoma breast is: *(DNB 2008)*
a. Present as breast mass
b. Frequently bilateral
c. Poor prognosis
d. Multicentric

28. True about histology in infiltrating lobular breast carcinoma:
(JIPMER 2012, 2011)
a. Single file pattern
b. Pleomorphic cells in sheets
c. Cribiform pattern
d. Pin wheel pattern

29. Most common presentation of lobular carcinoma breast is:
a. Nipple discharge *(DNB 2012)*
b. Breast mass
c. Mammographic calcification
d. Nipple retraction

30. Histological variety of breast carcinoma with best prognosis is: *(DNB 2012, 2008, 2005, 2002)*
a. Medullary
b. Colloid
c. Lobular
d. Tubular

31. Breast cancer which is multicentric and bilateral?
(DPG 2008, AIIMS Feb 97, May 95, All India 96, PGI June 95)
a. Ductal carcinoma
b. Lobular carcinoma
c. Mucoid carcinoma
d. Colloid carcinoma

32. Single file pattern is seen breast cancer type: *(APPG 2004)*
a. Intraductal
b. Infiltrating lobular
c. Infiltrating ductular
d. None

33. Best prognosis amongst the following histological variants of breast carcinoma is seen with: *(All India 98)*
a. Intraductal
b. Colloid (Mucinous)
c. Lobular
d. Medullary

34. A 45-year-old female presented to your OPD with this lesion in the left breast. What is the most probable diagnosis?
a. DCIS
b. LCIS
c. Peau-d'orange
d. Paget's disease of nipple

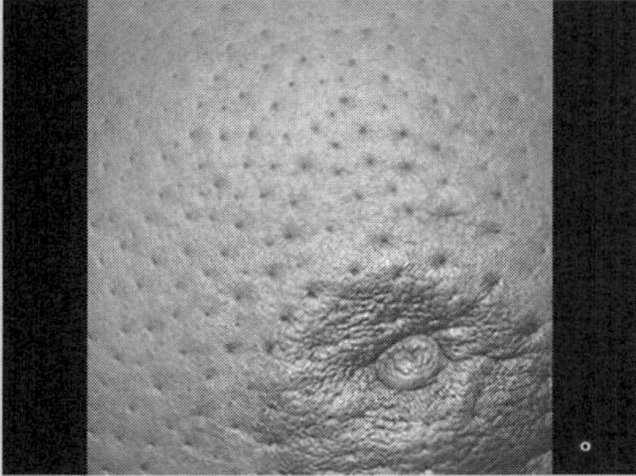

35. 'Peau-d-orange' appearance of the mammary skin is due to:
(DNB 2012, PGI June 95, Dec 95)
a. Intra-epithelial cancer
b. Sub-epidermal cancer
c. Lymphatic permeation
d. Vascular embolisation

36. Which is the most conspicuous sign in breast cancer?
A. Nipple retraction *(AIIMS Nov 2018)*
b. Peau-d'orange
c. Puckering
d. Both nipple retraction and puckering

37. Most common site of metastasis from breast carcinoma:
a. Thoracic vertebra
b. Pelvis *(DNB 2012)*
c. Femur
d. Lumbar vertebra

38. Carcinoma breast with high incidence of involving opposite breast is: *(Recent Question 2016, AIIMS Nov 94)*
a. Lobular carcinoma
b. Medullary carcinoma
c. Scirrhous adenocarcinoma
d. Atrophic scirrhous carcinoma

39. 'Peau-d-orange' is due to: *(DNB 2009, 2008, AIIMS Nov 93)*
a. Arterial obstruction *(AIIMS Nov 2015)*
b. Blockage of subdermal lymphatics
c. Invasion of skin with malignant cells
d. Secondary infection

40. Secondary deposits from carcinoma breast is commonest in:
(DNB 2010, 2001, All India 89)
a. Lung
b. Liver
c. Brain
d. Bone

41. Most common type of breast carcinoma: *(WBPG 2014, 2015)*
a. LCIS
b. DCIS
c. Phyllodes tumour
d. Invasive ductal carcinoma

42. Carcinoma breast is least commonly seen in:
a. Superior outer quadrant *(Recent Question 2013)*
b. Inferior outer quadrant
c. Subareolar
d. Lower inner quadrant

43. Nipple inversion occurs due to involvement of: *(DNB 2014)*
a. Cooper's ligament
b. Subareolar duct
c. Parenchyma of breast
d. Subdermal lymphatics

44. Van-Nuys classification does not include which of the following? *(Recent Question 2018)*
a. Patients age
b. Size of tumor
c. Presence of microcalcification
d. Her-2-neu receptor status

45. Dimpling in carcinoma breast is due to:
a. Edema *(Recent Question 2016)*
b. Contraction of Cooper's ligaments
c. Subdermal lymphangitis
d. Scarring

46. Most common site of metastases in carcinoma breast:
(Recent Question 2017)
a. Bone
b. Lung
c. Liver
d. Brain

CARCINOMA BREAST STAGING

47. In patients with breast cancer, chest wall involvement means involvement of any one of the following structures except: *(DPG 2010, AIIMS Nov 2005)*
a. Serratus anterior
b. Pectoralis major
c. Intercostal muscles
d. Ribs

48. Ipsilateral supraclavicular lymph nodes are positive in a patient of CA breast. Stage is:
(Recent Question 2013, AIIMS Nov 2008)
a. II
b. III B
c. III C
d. IV

49. TNM staging of breast carcinoma with positive bilateral supraclavicular lymph nodes is? *(DNB 2014)*
a. N3a
b. N3b
c. N3c
d. M1

CARCINOMA BREAST MANAGEMENT

50. True about modified radical mastectomy is: *(Punjab 2007)*
a. Pectoralis major is removed
b. Axillary lymph nodes are preserved
c. Pectoralis minor is divided
d. Internal mammary lymph nodes are removed

51. In a breast lump of 4 cm, no nodal metastasis is present. Which is the stage of breast cancer? *(MCI Nov 2017)*
a. Stage I
b. Stage II
c. Stage III
d. Stage IV

52. In Patey's modified mastectomy, which of the following is preserved? *(Recent Question 2014, MHSSMCET 2006)*
a. Intercostobrachial nerve
b. Pectoralis major
c. Pectoralis minor
d. Axillary fascia

53. Patey's mastectomy following are preserved except:
    (Recent Question 2014, MHSSMCET 2009)
    a. Teres major
    b. Teres minor
    c. Axillary vein
    d. Breast

54. Drug used in estrogen dependent breast cancer:
    (AIIMS May 2012)
    a. Tamoxifen
    b. Clomiphene citrate
    c. Estrogen
    d. Adriamycin

55. Superolateral boundary of axillary dissection is: *(DNB 2010)*
    a. Clavipectoral fascia
    b. Brachial plexus
    c. Axillary artery
    d. Axillary vein

56. Malti, a 45-year-female patient with a family history of breast carcinoma, showed diffuse microcalcification on mammography. Indraductal carcinoma is situ was seen on biopsy. Most appropriate management is:
    (Recenrt Question 2013, AIIMS June 2001)
    a. Quadrantectomy
    b. Radical mastectomy
    c. Simple mastectomy
    d. Chemotherapy

57. For CA breast best chemotherapeutic regimen:
    (AIIMS Sept 96, PGI June 96)
    a. Cyclophosphamide, methotrexate, 5-fluorouracil
    b. Methotrexate, cisplatin
    c. Cisplatin, adrimaycin, steroid
    d. Methotrexate, adriamycin, steroid

58. In breast conservation surgery, the healthy margin excised is typically:
    (DNB 2013)
    a. 1 cm
    b. 2 cm
    c. 3 cm
    d. 5 cm

59. In the breast conservation surgery, which of the following investigation is required:
    (DNB 2002)
    a. Serum calcium
    b. Total body scan
    c. Sentinel node biopsy
    d. Tumor markers

60. According to NSABP tamoxifen given in breast carcinoma for:
    a. 5 years
    b. 3 years   *(WBPG 2014)*
    c. 10 years
    d. Lifelong

61. In radical mastectomy, the structures preserved are all except:
    (Recent Question 2015)
    a. Axillary vein
    b. Cephalic vein
    c. Nerve to Serratus anterior
    d. Pectoralis minor

62. Treatment of choice for locally advanced breast cancer:
    a. Neoadjuvant chemotherapy followed by MRM followed by radiotherapy   *(Recent Question 2016)*
    b. Surgery alone
    c. Radiation alone
    d. Surgery followed by chemotherapy

63. Ixabepilone is used in: *(Recent Question 2017)*
    a. Melanoma
    b. Breast carcinoma
    c. Oat cell carcinoma
    d. Small cell carcinoma lung

64. Adjuvant therapy after mastectomy is needed in all of the following except:
    (Recent Question 2017)
    a. High risk, node positive
    b. Low risk, no node
    c. HR –ve
    d. Her-2-neu +ve

65. Level II axillary lymph node: *(Recent Question 2017)*
    a. Lateral to pectoralis major and minor
    b. Behind pectoralis minor
    c. Medial to pectoralis minor
    d. Superomedial to pectoralis major

66. Which of the following statements is not true about tamoxifen?
    (Recent Question 2019)
    a. It is used for visceral metastasis
    b. Tamoxifen is useful in post-menopausal and aromatase inhibitors in premenopausal patients
    c. Dose is 20 mg for 5 years
    d. It can cause endometrial carcinoma

■ CARCINOMA BREAST PROGNOSTIC INDICATORS

67. The most important prognostic factor of carcinoma breast is:
    (COMEDK 2010)
    a. Tumor size
    b. DNA content of tumour
    c. Histologic subtype
    d. Tumor grade

68. In case of CA breast most important prognostic factor is:
    a. Size of tumor   *(WB PG 2015, AIIMS Nov 96, Feb 97)*
    b. Lymph node status
    c. Presence of estrogen receptor
    d. Age of menopause

69. Molecular classification of breast cancer is based on:
    a. Serum hormone levels   *(AIIMS Nov 2014)*
    b. Expression of hormone receptors (ER/PR)
    c. In-vitro response to chemotherapeutic agents
    d. Gene expression profiling

70. Most common histo-immunological type of breast cancer:
    (Recent Question 2017)
    a. Luminal A
    b. Luminal B
    c. Basal cell type
    d. Her-2-neu type

71. Luminal A breast cancer shows following feature:
    (PGI May 2018)
    a. Low-grade tumor
    b. Her-2-neu amplification
    c. Good prognosis
    d. High-grade tumor
    e. ER-negative

72. Which patient has the better prognosis in breast cancer?
    a. Luminal A   *(MCI Dec 2019)*
    b. Luminal B
    c. Triple negative breast cancer
    d. Triple positive breast cancer

■ TRIPLE NEGATIVE BREAST CANCER

73. Which of the following is incorrect about triple negative breast cancer?   *(Recent Question 2016)*
    a. Does not express the genes for ER, PR and Her-2-neu
    b. More common in postmenopausal women
    c. Germline mutations of BRCA1 and BRCA2 genes increases the risk
    d. Very susceptible to chemotherapy

■ COMPLICATIONS OF MASTECTOMY

74. The tumour, which may occur in the residual breast or overlying skin following wide local excision and radiotherapy for mammary carcinoma is: *(Recent Question 2016, All India 2004)*
    a. Leiomyosarcoma
    b. Squamous cell carcinoma
    c. Basal cell carcinoma
    d. Angiosarcoma

75. Pain along medial aspect of arm in a post-mastectomy patient is due to:
    (DNB 2009, 2008)
    a. Phantom breast pain
    b. Intercostobrachial neuralgia
    c. Neuroma pain
    d. Other nerve injury pain

76. Winging of scapula is seen after mastectomy due to injury of:
    (Recent Question 2017)
    a. Musculocutaneous nerve
    b. Long thoracic nerve of Bell
    c. Intercostobrachial nerve
    d. Thoracodorsal nerve

77. Most common complication of mastectomy:
    a. Intercostobrachial nerve palsy   *(Recent Question 2017)*
    b. Long thoracic nerve palsy
    c. Thoracodorsal palsy
    d. Angiosarcoma

■ BREAST RECONSTRUCTION

78. **Reconstruction surgery in breast carcinoma, best myocuta-neous flap is:**   *(UPPG 2009)*
    a. Pectoralis minor   b. Pectoralis major
    c. Latissimus dorsi
    d. Transverse rectus abdominis

79. **Flap commonly used in breast reconstruction is:**
                                   (Recent Question 2014)
    a. Serratus anterior   b. TRAM
    c. Flap from arm   d. Delto pectoral flap

■ INFLAMMATORY CARCINOMA BREAST

80. **Most malignant type of carcinoma breast is:**
    a. Paget's disease   b. Anaplastic carcinoma
    c. Scirrhous carcinoma   *(Recent Question 2015)*
    d. Atrophic Scirrhous carcinoma
    e. Mastitis carcinomatosa

■ MALE BREAST CANCER

81. **True about breast carcinoma in men:** *(Recent Question 2016)*
    a. Estrogen receptor positive
    b. Associated with gynaecomastia
    c. Radiotherapy contraindicated due to close proximity to chest wall
    d. Seen in young males

82. **True abort male breast cancer:**   *(Recent Question 2014)*
    a. Invasive lobular carcinoma is most common type
    b. ER is negative
    c. Seen in young males
    d. BRCA-2 mutation is associated with increased risk

83. **Most common carcinoma breast in male is:**
                                   (Recent Question 2014)
    a. LCIS   b. DCIS
    c. Invasive ductal cancer   d. Invasive lobular cancer

■ CARCINOMA BREAST IN PREGNANCY

84. **True about breast cancer in pregnancy:**
    a. Occurs in 1 of every 3000 pregnant women
    b. MC non-gynecologic malignancy associated with preg-nancy
    c. Ductal carcinoma is MC type, accounting for 75-90% of breast cancer in pregnancy
    d. All of the above

■ MONDOR'S DISEASE

85. **Mondor's disease is:** *(MCI June 2018, Recent Question 2015, 2014)*
    a. Thrombophlebitis of the superficial veins of breast
    b. Carcinoma of the breast   *(DNB 2014, All India 96)*
    c. Premalignant condition of the breast
    d. Filariasis of the breast

86. **Mondor's disease is superficial thrombophlebitis of:**
                                   (COMEDK 2005)
    a. Axillary vein   b. Long saphenous vein
    c. Veins of the breast   d. Internal mammary vein

■ DUCTAL ANOMALIES

87. **Treatment of choice in duct papilloma of breast is:**
                     (Kerala PG 2015, All India 98, All India 96)
    a. Simple mastectomy   b. Microdochectomy
    c. Local wide excision   d. Chemotherapy

88. **Treatment for duct ectasia:**
    a. Hadfield's operation   *(Recent Question 2014, MAHE 2008)*
    b. Patey's mastectomy
    c. Modified radical mastectomy
    d. Radical mastectomy

89. **Slit shaped nipple is seen in:**   *(Recent Question 2015)*
    a. Duct ectasia   b. Duct papilloma
    c. Paget's disease   d. CA breast

90. **Using a small fine probe, single lactiferous duct is excised. What is the name of the procedure?**   *(Recent Question 2018)*
    a. Macrodochectomy   b. Microdochectomy
    c. Webster operation   d. Hadfield operation

91. **Sign seen in large duct papilloma is:**   *(DNB 2012)*
    a. Nipple discharge   b. Breast mass
    c. Skin excoriation   d. Lymph node involvement

■ CYSTOSARCOMA PHYLLODES

92. **Treatment of cystosarcoma phyllodes in a young woman:**
    a. Wide excision with a margin   *(JIPMER 2011)*
    b. Wide excision with chemotherapy
    c. Wide excision with radiotherapy
    d. MRM

93. **A 50 years old female presented with the given tumor in the OPD. The tumor was found to be malignant on biopsy. What is the best treatment option?**
    a. Breast conservation surgery
    b. Simple mastectomy
    c. Wide local excision
    d. Modified radical mastectomy

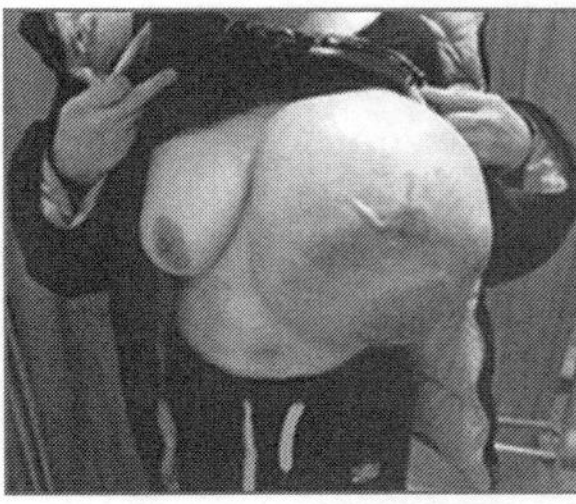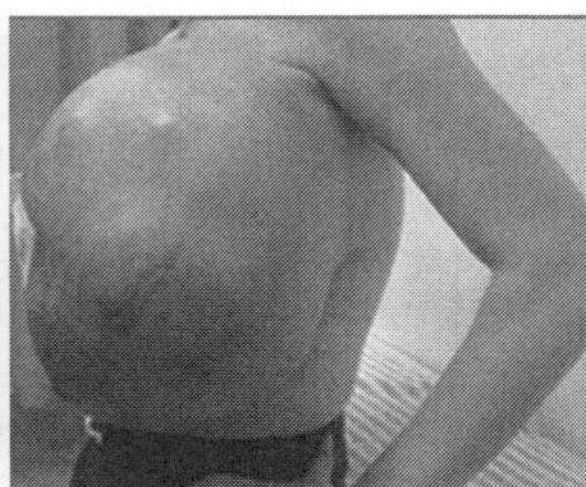

94. **Cystosarcoma phyllodes is treated by:**
                         (Recent Question 2015, AIIMS May 93)
    a. Simple mastectomy
    b. Radical mastectomy
    c. Modified radical mastectomy
    d. Antibiotic with conservative treatment

95. **True about cystosarcoma phyllodes is:**   *(DNB 2007)*
    a. Calcification   b. Cystic compondent
    c. Tendency to recur   d. All of the above

96. **Most common sarcoma of breast:**   *(Recent Question 2015)*
    a. Angiosarcoma   b. Phyllodes tumor
    c. Kaposi sarcoma   d. None

■ GYNECOMASTIA

97. **Gynecomastia may be seen in all of the following conditions except:**   *(All India 98)*
    a. Klinefelter's syndrome
    b. Cirrhosis of liver
    c. Cryptorchidism
    d. Sex-cord tumour of sertoli cells

98. **Gynaecomastia may be seen in patient with all except:**
                         (MCI Dec 2019, Recent Question 2016)
    a. Cimetidine therapy   b. Cirrhosis of liver
    c. Klinefelter's syndrome   d. Turner's syndrome

■ PAGET'S DISEASE OF NIPPLE

99. Paget's disease of breast, true statements are: *(PGI Nov 2009)*
   - a. Intraductal carcinoma
   - b. Mastectomy needed
   - c. Malignant
   - d. Bilateral

100. A 40-year-old female presented to your OPD with this lesion in the left breast. What is the most probable diagnosis?
   - a. DCIS
   - b. LCIS
   - c. Peau-d'orange
   - d. Paget's disease of nipple

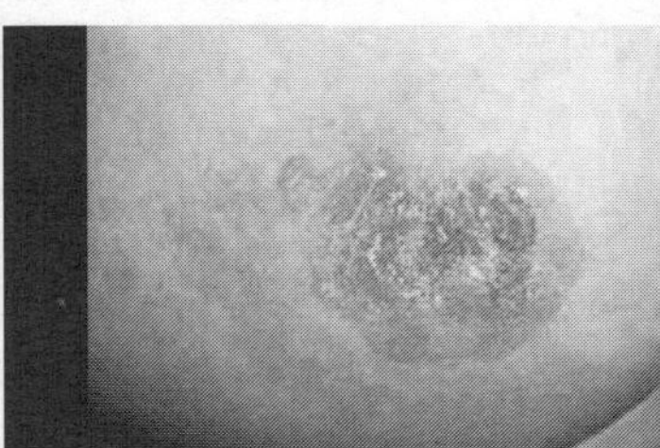 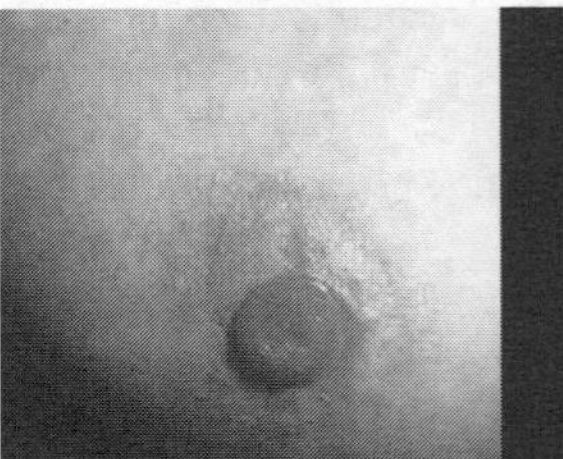

101. Primarily a disease of nipple and areola: *(DNB 2007)*
   - a. Duct papilloma
   - b. Paget's disease
   - c. Periductal mastitis
   - d. Fibroadenoma

102. Paget's disease of breast following are true except:
   - a. Treated by simple mastectomy *(Recent Question 2015)*
   - b. Represents underlying malignancy
   - c. Presents as eczema
   - d. Cytology diagnostic

103. All are true about Paget disease of breast except: *(DNB 2014)*
   - a. 1% associated with underlying invasive carcinoma of breast
   - b. Hormone receptor negative
   - c. Poor prognosis
   - d. Wedge or punch is biopsy taken from nipple for diagnosis

104. Correct description of Paget's disease of the breast:
   - a. Eczema of the skin of the nipple *(MCI Dec 2018)*
   - b. Eczema of the skin of areola
   - c. Mastitis carcinomatosis
   - d. Atrophic scirrhous carcinoma

105. Paget's disease of the nipple is: *(MCI June 2018)*
   - a. Infection
   - b. Dermatitis
   - c. Neoplasia
   - d. Hypopigmentation

■ BREAST ABSCESS

106. Which of the following is the first line drug for mastitis?
   (Recent Question 2019)
   - a. Cloxacillin
   - b. Cefazolin
   - c. Ampicillin
   - d. Metronidazole

107. A lady primigravida developed fluctuant painful mass of breast and fever after 14 days of delivery. Preferred treatment option is: *(Recent Question 2019)*
   - a. Stop lactation
   - b. Analgesics and continue breastfeeding
   - c. Antipyretic
   - d. Incision and drainage

■ MASTITIS AND BREAST ABSCESS

108. Acute mastitis commonly occurs during: *(DNB 2000)*
   - a. Pregnancy
   - b. Puberty
   - c. Lactation
   - d. Infancy

109. A lactating female presented with breast abscess. Most common organism responsible for her mastitis and abscess formation is: *(Recent Queston 2014, Punjab 2011)*
   - a. S. aureus
   - b. E. coli
   - c. Streptococci
   - d. Anaerobes

■ ANDI FIBROADENOMA AND FIBROADENOSIS

110. Fibroadenoma of the breast are:
   - a. Fixed mass
   - b. Diffuse mass
   - c. Multiple diffuse mass
   - d. Solitary mobile mass

111. A young female came to the surgery OPD with bilateral breast mass. On examination, mass was firm and mobile. What is the diagnosis on the basis of findings?
   - a. Breast cyst
   - b. Fibroadenoma
   - c. DCIS
   - d. LCIS

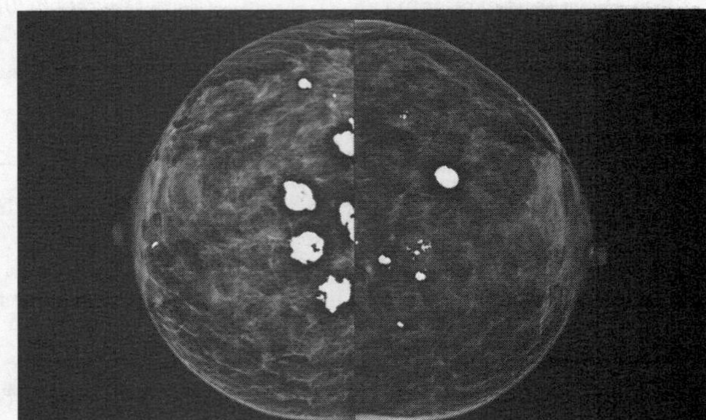

112. The following are suitable for simple mastectomy except:
   (Recent Question 2013)
   - a. Pagets disease
   - b. Fibroadenoma
   - c. Cystosarcoma phyllodes
   - d. None

113. Most common benign breast tumor: *(MCI Dec 2018)*
   - a. Fibroadenoma
   - b. Fibroadenosis
   - c. DCIS
   - d. Phyllodes tumor

114. Which of the following is not an indication for surgery in fibroadenoma? *(MCI Nov 2017)*
   - a. Patient's decision
   - b. Size more than 5 cm
   - c. Complex type
   - d. Recurrence

■ MISCELLANEOUS

115. Tylectomy literally means: *(DNB 91)*
   - a. Excision of a lump
   - b. Excision of LN
   - c. Excision of breast
   - d. Excision of skin

116. Most frequent site of accessory breast: *(Orissa 2011)*
   - a. Axilla
   - b. Groin
   - c. Buttock
   - d. Thigh

117. Zuska's disease common is smokers causes:
   (DNB 2012, 2007)
   - a. Acute mastitis
   - b. Chronic areolar abscess
   - c. Fibroadenosis
   - d. Acute abscess formation

118. Lymphatic from left upper quadrant of breast brain into all of the following group of lymphnodes except: *(DNB 2001)*
   - a. Anterior axillary
   - b. Central
   - c. Apical
   - d. Parasternal

119. In patients of breast pain, primrose oil is used for how many months? *(Recent Question 2017)*
   - a. 1
   - b. 2
   - c. 3
   - d. 4

■ SENTINEL LYMPH NODE BIOPSY

120. In sentinel node biopsy for breast cancer, the most commonly injured nerve is: *(AIIMS May 2013)*
   a. Lateral pectoral nerve
   b. Nerve to lattissimus dorsi
   c. Intercostobrachial nerve
   d. Long thoracic nerve (Nerve to serratus anterior)

121. Intraoperative sentinel lymph node detection in axilla is done by using: *(Recent Question 2013)*
   a. Mammography
   b. Isosulfan blue dye
   c. MRI
   d. CT

122. Sentinel lymph node biopsy in carcinoma breast is done if:
   a. LN palpable *(Recent Question 2013)*
   b. Breast mass but no lymph node palpable
   c. Breast lump with palpable axillary node
   d. Metastatic CA breast

123. Radioisotope used in sentinel lymph node biopsy in breast:
   a. Technetium iodine *(Recent Question 2017)*
   b. Technetium labeled colloid sulfur
   c. Tc99
   d. Iodine-131

124. Dye for sentinel lymph node biopsy is injected in which of the following site? *(MCI Dec 2018)*
   a. Axilla
   b. Tail of Spence
   c. Nipple
   d. Areola

Explanations

■ NIPPLE DISCHARGE

1. Ans. c. Ductal papilloma *(Ref: Schwartz 11/e p599, 10/e p554; Sabiston 20/e p824-826; Bailey 27/e p863)*

- MC cause of greenish discharge: Duct ectasia[Q]
- MC cause of blood-stained discharge: Duct papilloma[Q]

2. Ans. b. Duct ectasia   **3. Ans. b. Microdochectomy** *(Ref: Bailey 27/e p863; CSDT 12/e p299; Schwartz 11/e p552, 10/e p526)*

■ CARCINOMA BREAST INVESTIGATIONS

4. Ans. d. Clinical examination, Mammogram and FNAC *(Ref: Schwartz 11/e p567, 10/e p522-523; Sabiston 20/e p826-828; Bailey 27/e p863)*

- **Triple Assessment** includes a combination of **clinical assessment, radiological imaging** (USG/ Mammography) and **tissue sample analysis** (FNAC/Biopsy)[Q]
- The **positive predictive value** of Triple Assessment should **exceed 99.9%**[Q]

5. Ans. b. Axillary sampling *(Ref: Bailey 27/e p863)*

6. Ans. c. Biopsy *(Ref: Schwartz 11/e p575, 10/e p529-530; Sabiston 20/e p826-828; Bailey 27/e p862)*

CA BREAST

- First investigation for tissue sampling: FNAC[Q]
- Best and diagnostic investigation: Biopsy[Q]

7. Ans. a. MRI   **8. Ans. a. MRI**

9. Ans. c. PET scan   **10. Ans. a. Microcalcification** *(Ref: Schwartz 11/e p563, 10/e p527; Sabiston 20/e p828; Bailey 27/e p862)*

■ MAMMOGRAPHY

11. Ans. b. MRI *(Ref: Grainger 5/e p1190, 1188)*

- Screening with **MRI** is **superior to mammography** in **detecting invasive breast cancer in younger women**[Q], where the **sensitivity of mammography is low** due to **presence of mammographically dense breast parenchyma**[Q]

12. Ans. a. 0.1cGy   **13. Ans. a. Breast Imaging Reporting and Data System** *(Ref: Sabiston 20/e p831)*

14. Ans. a. Fibroadenoma *(Ref: Robbins 9/e p1069)*

Pattern of Calcification in Breast Diseases	
Carcinoma	**Microcalcification,** punctate, branching[Q]
Fibroadenoma	**Popcorn**[Q] (coarse, granular, crushed stone)
Fibrocystic disease	Powdery
Fat necrosis	Curvilinear

15. Ans. c. 40 years   **16. Ans. b. Suspicion of malignancy** *(Ref: Sabiston 20/e p831)*

17. Ans. d. Highly suggestive of malignancy

■ CARCINOMA BREAST RISK FACTORS

18. Ans. a. Hyperplasia atypical *(Ref: Schwartz 11/e p552, 10/e p508; Sabiston 20/e p832; Bailey 26/e p809)*

Cancer Risk Associated (with Benign Breast Disorders and In Situ Carcinoma of the Breast)	
Abnormality	**Relative Risk**
Nonproliferative lesions of the breast	No increased risk
Sclerosing adenosis	No increased risk
Intraductal papilloma	No increased risk
Florid hyperplasia	1.5 to 2-fold
Atypical lobular hyperplasia[Q]	**4–fold**
Atypical ductal hyperplasia[Q]	**4–fold**
Ductal involvement[Q] by cells of atypical ductal hyperplasia	**7–fold**
Lobular carcinoma in situ[Q]	**10–fold**
Ductal carcinoma in situ[Q]	**10–fold**

19. Ans. d. Atypical ductal hyperplasia

20. Ans. b. First child at a younger age

21. Ans. c. 17

22. Ans. b. 13 *(Ref: Schwartz 11/e p559, 10/e p515; Sabiston 20/e p832; Bailey 27/e p880)*

23. Ans. a. Hormone receptor positive *(Ref: Schwartz 11/e p559, 10/e p514; Sabiston 20/e p832; Bailey 27/e p880)*

24. Ans. d. Early full term pregnancy

25. Ans. a. No risk

26. Ans. a. Atypical ductal hyperplasia *(Ref: Schwartz 11/e p552, 10/e p508; Sabiston 20/e p831; Bailey 27/e p871)*

■ CARCINOMA BREAST

27. Ans. c. Poor prognosis

28. Ans. a. Single file pattern

29. Ans. b. Breast mass

30. Ans. d. Tubular

31. Ans. b. Lobular carcinoma

32. Ans. b. Infiltrating lobular

33. Ans. b. Colloid (Mucinous)

34. Ans. c. Peau-d'orange

35. Ans. c. Lymphatic permeation *(Ref: Bailey 27/e p873)*

PEAU-D-ORANGE

- Peau-d-orange is due to **cutaneous lymphatic edema**, where the infiltrated skin is tethered by sweat ducts, it can not swell, leading to an appearance like **orange skin[Q]**.
- Due to **obstruction** of **subdermal lymphatics** (**lymphatic permeation** by **tumor cells**)
- Seen in **advanced breast cancer** (may be seen in **chronic abscess**)

36. Ans. b. Peau-d'orange *(Ref: Schwartz 11/e p567, 10/e p518; Sabiston 20/e p860; Bailey 27/e p873)*

37. Ans. d. Lumbar vertebra *(Ref: Bailey 27/e p873)*

- Most common site of metastasis from breast carcinoma is lumbar vertebra.

Bailey says that "It is by this route (**spread by the bloodstream**) that **skeletal metastases** occur, although the initial spread may be via the lymphatic system. **In order of frequency** the **lumbar vertebrae, femur, thoracic vertebrae, rib and skull are affected** and these deposits are generally **osteolytic**."

38. Ans. a. Lobular carcinoma

39. Ans. b. Blockage of subdermal lymphatics

40. Ans. d. Bone

41. Ans. d. Invasive ductal carcinoma

42. Ans. d. Lower inner quadrant *(Ref: Bailey 27/e p874)*

- Upper inner (12–15%) • Upper outer (~ 50%) • Lower inner (3–5%) • Lower outer (6–10%) • Central/areolar (20%)

43. Ans. b. Subareolar duct *(Ref: Bailey 27/e p873)*

- Retraction of nipple is due to fibrosis in and around subareolar duct
- Retraction/dimpling of skin is due to involvement of cooper's ligament
- Peau-D-orange is due to blockage of subdermal lymphatics

44. Ans. d. Her-2-neu receptor status *(Ref: Sabiston 20/e p853; Bailey 27/e p872)*

45. Ans. c. Subdermal lymphangitis

46. Ans. a. Bone *(Ref: Schwartz 11/e p563, 10/e p543; Sabiston 20/e p838; Bailey 27/e p873)*

■ CARCINOMA BREAST STAGING

47. Ans. b. Pectoralis major *(Ref: Schwartz 11/e p576, 9/e p452; Sabiston 20/e p843)*

- **Chest wall involvement** means involvement of **ribs[Q], intercostal muscles[Q]** or **Serratus anterior[Q]** as **chest wall** is formed by these structures **not** the **pectoralis major.**

48. Ans. c. IIIC

49. Ans. d. M1

■ CARCINOMA BREAST MANAGEMENT

50. Ans. c. Pectoralis minor is divided *(Ref: Schwartz 11/e p592, 10/e p547-549; Sabiston 20/e p848-850; Bailey 27/e p876)*

51. Ans. b. Stage II *(Ref: Schwartz 11/e p576; Sabiston 20/e p843)*

52. Ans. b. Pectoralis major

53. Ans. d. Breast

54. Ans. a. Tamoxifen *(Ref: Schwartz 11/e p597, 10/e p552; Goodman and Gillman's 12/e p1179)*

55. Ans. d. Axillary vein *(Ref: Gray's 39/e p841)*

AXILLARY NODE CLEARANCE

- Axillary node clearance can be defined as clearing the axillary contents bounded by:
  - **Laterally:** Axillary skin
  - **Posteriorly:** Lattisimus dorsi, Teres major and Subscapularis
  - **Superiorly:** Lower border of **axillary vein**[Q]
  - **Anteriorly:** Pectoralis muscle   – **Medially:** Chest wall

56. Ans. c. Simple mastectomy   **57. Ans. a. Cyclophosphamide, methotrexate, 5-fluorouracil**

58. Ans. a. 1 cm *(Ref: Mastery of Surgery 5/e p525)*

BREAST CONSERVATION SURGERY

- The amount of breast tissue excised with the lesion may vary with the clinical situation, but is **typically 5 mm to 10 mm in all directions**.
- BCS may consist of **removal of tumor with 1 cm margin of normal tissue** (wide local excision) or a more extensive excision of a whole quadrant of breast (Quadrantectomy).

59. Ans. c. Sentinel node biopsy   60. Ans. a. 5 years

61. Ans. d. Pectoralis minor   62. Ans. a. Neoadjuvant chemotherapy followed by MRM followed by radiotherapy

63. Ans. b. Breast carcinoma *(Ref: Goodman Gilman 12/e p1709)*

"Ixabepilone is approved for breast cancer treatment." -Goodman Gilman 12/e p1709

64. Ans. b. Low risk, no node *(Ref: Schwartz 11/e p595, 583 10/e p550; Sabiston 20/e p853)*

65. Ans. b. Behind pectoralis minor *(Ref: Schwartz 11/e p546, 10/e p502; Sabiston 20/e p819)*

66. Ans. b. Tamoxifen is useful in post-menopausal and aromatase inhibitors in premenopausal patients *(Ref: Schwartz 11/e p597, 10/e p552; Sabiston 20/e p857; Bailey 27/e p878)*

■ CARCINOMA BREAST PROGNOSTIC INDICATORS

67. Ans. a. Tumor size *(Ref: Schwartz 11/e p579, 10/e p535-536; Bailey 27/e p875; Harrison 19/e p528)*

- The **most important** prognostic variables are provided by **tumor staging**[Q].
- The **size** of the tumor and status of the **axillary LN** provide resonably **accurate information** on the likelihood of **tumor relapse**[Q].

68. Ans. b. Lymph node status

PROGNOSIS IN MALE BREAST CANCER

- **Stage >Lymph node status** is the **best prognostic indicator**[Q] as in female breast carcinoma.

69. Ans. d. Gene expression profiling *(Ref: Harrison 19/e p526; Schwartz 11/e p580, 9/e p453; Sabiston 20/e p839)*
Molecular classification of breast cancer is based on gene expression profiling.

Gene expression profiling, *which can measure the relative quantities of mRNA for essentially every gene,* has identified **five major patterns of gene expression** in the NST group: **luminal A, luminal B, normal, basal-like,** and **HER2 positive.** These molecular classes **correlate with prognosis** and **response to therapy,** and thus have taken on clinical importance. *-Robbins 8/e p1084*

One of the most exciting aspects of breast cancer biology has been its recent subdivision into at least five subtypes based upon gene expression profiling. *-Harrison 19/e p526*

70. Ans. a. Luminal A *(Ref: Sabiston 20/e p840)*   **71. Ans. a. Low-grade tumor, c. Good prognosis** *(Ref: Sabiston 20/e p840)*

72. Ans. a. Luminal A *(Ref: Sabiston 20/e p840)*

■ TRIPLE NEGATIVE BREAST CANCER

73. Ans. b. More common in postmenopausal women *(Ref: Bailey 27/e p878; Schwartz 10/e p515)*

Triple-Negative Breast Cancer
• Tends to be **more aggressive**[Q] than other types of breast cancer.
• Tends to be **higher grade**[Q] than other types of breast cancer.
• Usually is a cell type called **"basal-like"**[Q]

■ COMPLICATIONS OF MASTECTOMY

74. Ans. d. Angiosarcoma *(Ref: Schwartz 11/e p593, 10/e p549; Sabiston 20/e p848; Bailey 27e p879)*

75. Ans. b. Intercostobrachial neuralgia *(Ref: Medical Care of Cancer Patients by Sai-Ching Jim Yeung, Carmen P. Escalanate, Robert F)*

76. Ans. b. Long thoracic nerve of Bell *(Ref: Schwartz 11/e p593, 590 10/e p548; Sabiston 20/e p848)*

77. Ans. a. Intercostobrachial nerve palsy *(Ref: Schwartz 11/e p590, 10/e p502)*

■ BREAST RECONSTRUCTION

78. Ans. d. Transverse rectus abdominis *(Ref: Schwartz 11/e p593; Sabiston 20/e p867; Bailey 26/e p816-817)*

79. Ans. b. TRAM *(Ref: Schwartz 11/e p593, 10/e p549-550; Sabiston 20e/ p867; Bailey 27/ep 879)*

■ INFLAMMATORY CARCINOMA BREAST

80. Ans. e. Mastitis carcinomatosa *(Ref: Schwartz 11/e p601, 10/e p555; Sabiston 20/e p860)*

- **MC type** of CA breast: **Invasive ductal carcinoma**[Q]
- **Most malignant** type of CA breast: **Inflammatory breast cancer**[Q]

■ MALE BREAST CANCER

81. Ans. a. Estrogen receptor positive, b. Associated with gynaecomastia *(Ref: Schwartz 11/e p600, 10/e p555; Sabiston 20/e p861; Bailey 27/e p862)*

82. Ans. d. BRCA-2 mutation is associated with increased risk   83. Ans. c. Invasive ductal cancer

■ CARCINOMA BREAST IN PREGNANCY

84. Ans. d. All of the above *(Ref: Schwartz 11/e p600, 10/e p554; Sabiston 20/e p2059-2060; Bailey 27/e p881)*

■ MONDOR'S DISEASE

85. Ans. a. Thrombophlebitis of the superficial veins of breast *(Ref: Schwartz 11/e p550, 10/e p507; Sabiston 19/e p1594; Bailey 27/e p867)*

86. Ans. c. Veins of the breast

■ DUCTAL ANOMALIES

87. Ans. b. Microdochectomy *(Ref: Bailey 27/e p865)*   88. Ans. a. Hadfield's operation *(Ref: Bailey 27/e p865)*

89. Ans. a. Duct ectasia   90. Ans. b. Microdochectomy *(Ref: Bailey 27/e p865)*

"Microdochectomy: A lacrimal probe or length of stiff nylon suture is inserted into the duct from which the discharge is emerging. A tennis racquet incision can be made to encompass the entire duct or a periareolar incision used and the nipple flap dissected to reach the duct. The duct is then excised." -Bailey 27/e p865

91. Ans. a. Nipple discharge

■ CYSTOSARCOMA PHYLLODES

92. Ans. a. Wide excision with a margin *(Ref: Schwartz 11/e p601, 10/e p555; Sabiston 20/e p841-842; Bailey 27/e p870)*

93. Ans. b. Simple mastectomy *(Ref: Schwartz 11/e p601, 10/e p555; Sabiston 20/e p841; Bailey 27/e p870)*

On the basis of clinical findings, patient is having malignant cystosarcoma phyllodes, which is best treated by simple mastectomy.

94. Ans. a. Simple mastectomy   95. Ans. d. All of the above   96. Ans. b. Phyllodes tumor

■ GYNECOMASTIA

97. Ans. c. Cryptorchidism *(Ref: Schwartz 11/e p549, 10/e p505-506; Sabiston 20/e p824; Bailey 27/e p882)*

98. Ans. d. Turner's syndrome

■ PAGET'S DISEASE OF NIPPLE

99. Ans. a. Intraductal carcinoma, b. Mastectomy needed, c. Malignant *(Ref: Schwartz 11/e p565, 10/e p506-521; Sabiston 20/e p860-861; Bailey 27/e p873)*

100. Ans. d. Paget's disease of nipple   101. Ans. b. Paget's disease

102. Ans. d. Cytology diagnostic   103. Ans. a. 1% associated with underlying invasive carcinoma of breast

104. Ans. a. Eczema of the skin of the nipple *(Ref: Schwartz 11/e p565; Sabiston 20/e p860-861; Bailey 27/e p873)*

105. Ans. c. Neoplasia *(Ref: Schwartz 11/e p565; Sabiston 20/e p860-861; Bailey 27/e p873)*

■ BREAST ABSCESS

106. Ans. a. Cloxacillin *(Ref: Sabiston 20/e p836; Bailey 27/e p866)*

107. Ans. d. Incision and drainage *(Ref: Schwartz 11/e p565, 10/e p506; Sabiston 20/e p836; Bailey 27/e p866)*

■ MASTITIS AND BREAST ABSCESS

108. Ans. c. Lactation *(Ref: Schwartz 11/e p550, 10/e p506; Sabiston 20/e p836; Bailey 27/e p866)*

> **NONEPIDEMIC (SPORADIC) PUERPERAL MASTITIS**
>
> - **Involvement** of the **interlobular connective tissue** of the breast by an infectious process.
> - The patient develops **nipple fissuring** and **milk stasis**, which initiate a **retrograde bacterial infection**[Q].
> - **Emptying of the breast** using breast suction pumps **shortens** the **duration** of symptoms[Q] and **reduces** the incidence of **recurrences.**
> - The addition of **antibiotic therapy**[Q] results in a satisfactory outcome in >95% of cases.

109. Ans. a. S. aureus *(Ref: Schwartz 11/e p550, 10/e p506; Sabiston 20/e p836; Bailey 27/e p866)*

■ ANDI FIBROADENOMA AND FIBROADENOSIS

110. Ans. d. Solitary mobile mass *(Ref: Bailey 27/e p870; Schwartz 11/e p554, 10/e p510; Sabiston 20/e p836)*

111. Ans. b. Fibroadenoma *(Ref: Schwartz 11/e p554, 10/e p510; Bailey 27/e p870)*

Pattern of Calcification in Breast Diseases	
Carcinoma	**Microcalcification**, punctate, branching[Q]
Fibroadenoma	**Popcorn**[Q] (coarse, granular, crushed stone)
Fibrocystic disease	Powdery
Fat necrosis	Curvilinear

112. Ans. b. Fibroadenoma   **113.** Ans. a. Fibroadenoma *(Ref: Bailey 27/e p868)*

114. Ans. a. Patient's decision *(Ref: Bailey 27/e p870; Schwartz 11/e p554; Sabiston 20/e p836)*

■ MISCELLANEOUS

115. Ans. a. Excision of a lump
- **Lumpectomy (Tylectomy):** Surgical procedure designed to remove a discrete lump

116. Ans. a. Axilla *(Ref: Bailey 27/e p865)*

117. Ans. b. Chronic areolar abscess *(Ref: Schwartz 11/e p550, 10/e p506)*

> **ZUSKA'S DISEASE (RECURRENT PERIDUCTAL MASTITIS)**
>
> - Condition of **recurrent retroareolar infections** and **abscesses**
> - **Smoking** has been implicated as a **risk factor**
> - Managed symptomatically by **antibiotics** with **incision** and **drainage**
> - **Prognosis**
> - The prognosis is favorable, with **5-** and **10-year** survival rates of **74** and **51%,** respectively.

118. Ans. d. Parasternal *(Ref: Bailey 27/e p873)*

119. Ans. c. 3 *(Ref: Bailey 27/e p869)*

> *"Treatment of mastalgia: Oil of evening primrose, in adequate doses given over 3 months, will help more than half of these women"*
> *-Bailey 27/e p869*

■ SENTINEL LYMPH NODE BIOPSY

120. Ans. c. Intercostobrachial nerve

121. Ans. b. Isosulfan blue dye *(Ref: Schwartz 11/e p590, 10/e p545)*

122. Ans. b. Breast mass but no lymph node palpable   *(Ref: Schwartz 11/e p590, 10/e 545)*

123. Ans. b. Technetium labeled colloid sulfur *(Ref: Schwartz 11/e p590, 10/e p545; Sabiston 20/e p850; Bailey 27/e p877)*

> *"Lymphatic mapping can be performed with a combination of ^{99m}Tc-labeled sulfur colloid and a vital blue dye, isosulfan blue (Lymphazurin), or with a single agent for localization of the sentinel node." -Sabiston 20/e p850*

124. Ans. d. Areola *(Ref: Schwartz 11/e p590; Sabiston 20/e p850; Bailey 27/e p877)*

Thyroid

THYROGLOSSAL CYST

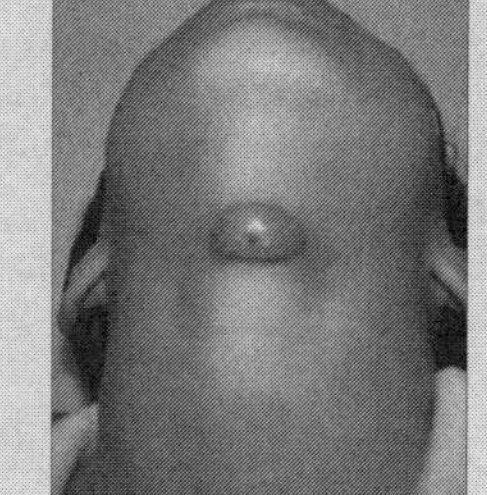

THYROGLOSSAL CYST

- **Cystic swelling** developed in the remnant of the **thyroglossal duct** or **tract**
- **Present** in **any part** of the **thyroglossal tract**[Q] (thyroglossal tract extends from foramen caecum to isthmus of thyroid)

Common Sites

- **Subhyoid (MC)**[Q]
- Region of the thyroid cartilages
- Suprahyoid
- Floor of mouth
- Beneath the foramen caecum

Clinical Features

- It is a **midline swelling**[Q], except in the region of thyroid cartilage, where thyroglossal tract is pushed to one side, usually to the left.
- Though it's a **congenital swelling**[Q] MC **age of presentation** is between **15 and 30 years**[Q].
- Cyst can be **moved sideways** but not vertically.
- Peculiar characteristic which helps in distinguishing thyroglossal cyst from other neck swelling
  - **Moves up with protrusion of tongue**[Q] as the thyroglossal tract is attached to the tongue.
  - **Moves with deglutition**[Q] so do all thyroid swellings, subhyoid bursitis.
- Cyst is lined by pseudostratified columnar epithelium and squamous epithelium with **heterotopic thyroid tissue** present in **20%** of cases.

Complications

- **Recurrent infections**[Q]
- Formation of **thyroglossal fistula**[Q]
- Carcinomatous change (**papillary carcinoma**[Q])

Treatment

- **Sistrunk operation: En-bloc cystectomy** and **excision** of **central hyoid bone**[Q] to minimize recurrence.

RETROSTERNAL GOITER

RETROSTERNAL (SUBSTERNAL/MEDIASTINAL/INTRATHORACIC GOITER)

- A goiter is said to be **retrosternal, substernal** or **mediastinal** if > 50% of **thyroid tissue** is **below** the **opening of thoracic cage**[Q].
- Usually arises from **lower pole** of a **nodular goiter**[Q].

Clinical Features

- **Often symptomless, discovered** on a routine **chest X-ray**[Q].
- **Can lead to tracheal deviation** and **scabbard trachea**[Q] (flattening of trachea caused by compression)

Severe Symptoms due to Mass Effect on the Trachea, Esophagus, Great Vessels and Nerves
1. **Dyspnea (MC symptom)** particularly at night, **cough** and **stridor**[Q]
2. Dysphagia
3. Enlargement of neck veins and superficial veins on the chest wall
4. Recurrent nerve palsy
5. **Pemberton's sign**[Q]: Symptoms of faintness with evidence of facial congestion and external jugular venous obstruction when the arms are raised above the head.

Treatment

- Virtually **all intrathoracic goiters** can be **removed via a cervical incision**[Q].

■ INVESTIGATIONS IN THYROID DISORDERS

THYROID SCAN

- Whereas ultrasound allows anatomic evaluation, **radionuclide scans** allow assessment of **thyroid function**[Q].
- [123]I and ^{131}I iodine scintigraphy is also used to evaluate the functional status of the gland.
- Advantages of scanning with ^{123}I include a **low dose of radiation** (30 mrad) and **short half-life**[Q].
- [131]I has a **longer half-life** (8 days) and **emits higher levels of β-radiation**[Q].
- [131]I is optimal for **imaging thyroid carcinoma**. It is the **screening modality of choice** for the **evaluation of distant metastasis**[Q].

Isotope	$t_{1/2}$
I^{132}	2.3 hours[Q]
I^{123}	13 hours[Q]
I^{131}	8 days[Q]

RADIOACTIVE IODINE (I^{131}) THERAPY

- I^{131} is an **effective agent** for **delivering high radiation doses** to thyroid tissue[Q]
- It emits mainly beta radiation (90%), which **penetrates** only **0.5 mm**[Q] of the **tissue** & allow therapeutic effects on thyroid **without any damage** to the surrounding structures, particularly **parathyroids**.

Mechanism of Action
- I^{131} emits **beta particles**[Q] and **γ-rays**.
- **Beta rays** are utilized for their **destructive effects** on **thyroid**[Q] cells.
- **X-rays** are useful for **tracer studies**.

Indications in Carcinoma Thyroid	Contraindications of I^{131} Therapy
1. **Distant metastasis**[Q] at diagnosis	1. **Childhood**[Q]
2. Incomplete tumor resection[Q]	2. **Pregnancy**[Q]
3. Patients at **high risk** for **mortality** or **recurrence**[Q]	3. **Lactation**[Q]

■ SOLITARY THYROID NODULE

SOLITARY THYROID NODULE

- **MC solitary thyroid nodule** is **benign colloid nodule**[Q], it accounts for **60%** cases of solitary thyroid nodule.
- **2nd MC cause** of solitary thyroid nodule is **follicular adenoma (30%)**[Q].

Management of Solitary Thyroid Nodule

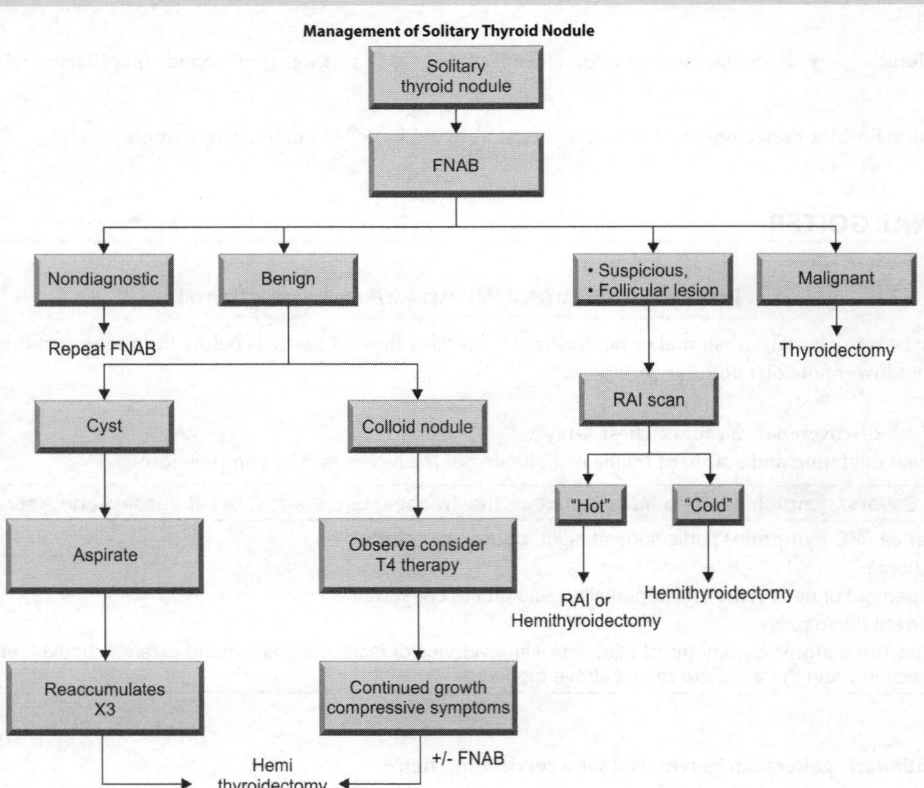

■ ACUTE (SUPPURATIVE) THYROIDITIS

ACUTE (SUPPURATIVE) THYROIDITIS

- Acute thyroiditis is rare and due to **suppurative infection** of the **thyroid**[Q].
- **More common** in **children** and often is **preceded by** an **upper respiratory tract infection** or **otitis media**[Q].

Etiology

- Thyroid gland is inherently resistant to infection due to its extensive blood & lymphatic supply, high iodide content, and fibrous capsule.

Infectious Agents Can Seed Thyroid
1. Via **hematogenous** or **lymphatic route**[Q]
2. Via direct **spread** from **persistent pyriform sinus fistulae** or **thyroglossal duct cysts**[Q]
3. As a result of **penetrating trauma**[Q]
4. Due to **immunosuppression**[Q]

- **MC organism** responsible: **Staph. aureus >Streptococcus**[Q]
- In **children & young adults**, **MC cause** is presence of a **pyriform sinus**[Q] (remnant of the **fourth branchial pouch** that connects the oropharynx with thyroid), such sinuses are predominantly **left-sided**[Q].
- **Long-standing goiter** and **degeneration** in **thyroid malignancy** are risk factors in **elderly**[Q]

Clinical Features

- **Thyroid pain**, often referred to the throat or ears, and a **small, tender goiter**[Q]
- **Fever, dysphagia** and **erythema** over the thyroid.
- Systemic symptoms of a **febrile illness** and **lymphadenopathy**[Q].

Diagnosis

- **ESR** and **WBC count** are usually **increased**, but **thyroid function** is **normal**.
- **FNA biopsy** shows infiltration by **polymorphonuclear leukocytes**.
- **Culture** of the sample can identify the organism.
- **Persistent pyriform sinus fistula** should be suspected in **children** with recurrent acute thyroiditis. A **barium swallow** demonstrates the anomalous tract with **80% sensitivity**[Q].

Treatment

- **Parenteral antibiotics** and **drainage** of **abscesses**[Q].
- Patients with **pyriform sinus fistulae** require **complete resection**[Q] of the sinus tract, including the area of the thyroid where the tract terminates, **to prevent recurrence**.

■ SUBACUTE THYROIDITIS

SUBACUTE /DE QUERVAIN'S/ GRANULOMATOUS/ VIRAL THYROIDITIS/GIANTCELL THYROIDITIS

- Also termed de Quervain's thyroiditis, granulomatous thyroiditis, or viral thyroiditis.
- Peak incidence: **30–50 years; women** are affected three times more frequently than men.
- Usually follows **upper respiratory tract infection**[Q]
- A **viral etiology** has been proposed
- **Strong association** with the **HLA-B35 haplotype**[Q]

The Disorder Classically Progresses through Four Stages
1. Initial **hyperthyroid phase**, due to release of thyroid hormone
2. **Euthyroid** phase
3. **Hypothyroidism**, occurs in about 20 to 30% of patients
4. **Resolution** and return to the **euthyroid state** in 90% of patients.

- In the **early stages** of the disease, TSH is **decreased**, and Tg, T4 , and T_3 levels are **elevated** due to the release of preformed thyroid hormone from destroyed follicles.
- **ESR** is typically **>100 mm/h**[Q].
- **RAIU** is **decreased**[Q]

Clinical Features

- **Painful** and **enlarged thyroid**, sometimes accompanied by fever.
- Features of **thyrotoxicosis** or **hypothyroidism**, depending on the phase of the illness.

Contd...

- Malaise and symptoms of an **upper respiratory tract infection** may **precede** the **thyroid-related features**[Q] by several weeks.
- The patient typically complains of a **sore throat** and **small exquisitely tender goiter**[Q]
- Pain is often referred to the jaw or ear.
- **Complete resolution** is the **usual outcome**[Q]
- Permanent hypothyroidism can occur, particularly in those with coincidental thyroid autoimmunity.

Laboratory Findings

- **ESR** is **markedly elevated**[Q]
- **Antithyroid antibodies** are **low** with T4, T3 and TSH levels depend on the stage of disease.

> - **RAIU** is **decreased** during the hyperthyroid stage (distinguishes from Grave's disease)
> - In doubt: **FNAC** (shows characteristic **giant multinucleated cells)**[Q]

Treatment

- Treatment is **primarily symptomatic**, as disease is **self-limited**[Q].
- **Aspirin** or other **NSAIDs** are sufficient to control symptoms in most cases.
- **Severe cases** with marked local or systemic symptoms may require **glucocorticoids.**
- **Short-term thyroid replacement** may be needed in the **hypothyroid phase**.
- **Thyroidectomy** is reserved for the **rare patients** who have a prolonged course **not responsive** to **medical measures.**

■ RIEDEL'S THYROIDITIS

RIEDEL'S THYROIDITIS

- A rare variant of thyroiditis also known as **Riedel's struma**[Q] or **invasive fibrous thyroiditis**
- Characterized by the **replacement of** all or part of the **thyroid parenchyma** by **fibrous tissue**
- Also **invades** into **adjacent tissues**[Q].
- **Etiology**: Primary **autoimmune etiology** (probably)

> **Riedel's Thyroiditis is Associated with**
>
> - **Mediastinal** and **retroperitoneal** fibrosis
> - **Periorbital** and **retro-orbital** fibrosis
> - **Sclerosing cholangitis**

Clinical Features

- Occurs predominantly in **women, 30–60 years**.
- Presents as a **painless, hard anterior neck mass**[Q], which progresses over weeks to years to produce **symptoms** of **compression**, including dysphagia, dyspnea, choking, and hoarseness.
- Patients may present with symptoms of **hypothyroidism** and **hypoparathyroidism**[Q] as the **gland** is **replaced** by **fibrous tissue**.
- Physical examination: **Hard, "woody" thyroid gland** with **fixation**[Q] to surrounding tissues.

Treatment

- **Surgery**[Q] is the **mainstay** of the treatment (decompress the trachea by **wedge excision of isthmus**)
- Some patients show dramatic improvement with **tamoxifen & corticosteroids.**

■ HASHIMOTO'S THYROIDITIS

HASHIMOTO'S THYROIDITIS

- First described by Hashimoto as **struma lymphomatosa**[Q], i.e. a transformation of thyroid tissue to lymphoid tissue.
- **MC inflammatory disorder** of the thyroid and **leading cause** of **hypothyroidism**[Q].

> - **Thyroid lymphoma**[Q] is a rare but **well-recognized complication**
> - **Papillary thyroid carcinoma**[Q] may be occasionally associated

- **Genetic association** has been noted with **HLA B8, DR3** and **DR5**[Q].
- More common in **women** (Male:female, 1:10), near menopause (**30-50 years**).

Etiopathogenesis

- **Autoimmune** disease
- Thought to be initiated by **activation of CD4+T (helper) lymphocytes** which further recruit cytotoxic CD8+T cells.

Contd...

Contd...

- Thyroid tissue is destroyed by **cytrotoxic T cells** and **autoantibodies**[Q].

Autoantibodies are Directed against
1. Thyroglobulin (Tg): 60%
2. **Thyroid peroxidase** (TPO): **95%**[Q]
3. TSH-R: 60%

- It is also thought to be **associated with:**
  - Increased intake of **iodine**
  - Drugs such as **interferon alpha, lithium, amiodarone**

Pathology

- **Gross examination: Mildly enlarged thyroid**[Q] with pale, gray-tan cut surface
- **Microscopic examination:**
  - Gland is **diffusely infiltrated** by **small lymphocytes** and **plasma cells**[Q]
  - Follicles are lined by **Hürthle** or **Askanazy cells**[Q] (characterized by abundant eosinophilic, granular cytoplasm).

Clinical Features

- **MC** presentation: **Minimally** or **moderately enlarged firm gland**[Q].
- On examination an **enlarged pyramidal lobe** is often palpable.
- Mild hyperthyroidism may be present initially (due to destruction of thyroid tissue).
- **Hypothyroidism** is inevitable and **usually permanent**[Q].

Laboratory Findings

- **Elevated TSH** and presence of thyroid **autoantibodies confirm** the **diagnosis**[Q].
- **Elevated TSH, reduced T4 and T3 levels**[Q].
- Presence to thyroid autoantibodies (particularly **TPO antibody**)[Q].
- In case of doubt, diagnosis is confirmed by **FNA biopsy.**

Management

- **Thyroid hormone replacement therapy** for overtly **hypothyroid** patients or in euthyroid patients to **shrink large goiters**[Q].
- **Surgery** may occasionally be indicated for **suspicion of malignancy** or for **goiters** causing **compressive symptoms** or cosmetic deformity.

■ PAINLESS OR SILENT THYROIDITIS

PAINLESS OR SILENT THYROIDITIS

- Painless thyroiditis, or "silent" thyroiditis, occurs in patients with **underlying autoimmune thyroid disease** and has a **clinical course similar to that of subacute thyroiditis.**
- Occurs in up to **5% of women 3–6 months after pregnancy** termed as **postpartum thyroiditis.**
- **Associated with presence of TPO antibodies antepartum**, three times **more common in women with type 1 DM.**

Clinical Features

- Characterised by **brief phase of thyrotoxicosis lasting 2–4 weeks, followed by hypothyroidism for 4–12 weeks, and then resolution.**

Diagnosis

- **Uptake of** ^{99m}**Tc pertechnetate or radioactive iodine is initially suppressed.**
- In addition to the **painless goiter**, silent thyroiditis can be **distinguished from subacute thyroiditis by a normal ESR & presence of TPO antibodies.**

Treatment

- Glucocorticoid treatment is not indicated for silent thyroiditis.
- **Severe thyrotoxic symptoms: Propranolol**
- **Thyroxine replacement** for hypothyroid phase but **should be withdrawn after 6–9 months, as recovery is the rule.**

■ GRAVE'S DISEASE (DIFFUSE TOXIC GOITER)

GRAVE'S DISEASE (DIFFUSE TOXIC GOITER)

- **MC cause** of **hyperthyroidism,** caused by **stimulatory autoantibodies** to **TSH-R**[Q].
- **Autoimmune disease** with strong **familial predisposition**[Q].
- More common in **females** with peak incidence between **40–60** years.
- Characterized by **thyrotoxicosis, diffuse goiter** & **extrathyroidal conditions**[Q] (ophthalmopathy, dermopathy, thyroid acropachy and gynecomastia).

Contd...

Contd…

Etiopathogenesis

- **Autoimmune process** with possible **triggers** (post-partum state, iodine excess, lithium therapy and bacterial or viral infections)
- Associated with **HLA-B8, HLA-DR3, HLA-DQA1*0501** and **CTLA-4**^{Q}
- **Thyroid stimulating antibodies**^{Q} **are hallmark** of Grave's disease

Clinical Features

- **Hyperthyroid symptoms**^{Q} (heat intolerance, increased sweating and thirst, weight loss despite adequate caloric intake)
- **Symptoms of adrenergic stimulation**^{Q} (palpitations, nervousness, fatigue, emotional lability, hyperkinesis and tremors)
- **MC GI symptom** is **increased frequency** of **bowel movements** and **diarrhea**^{Q}

> - **Female patients** often develop **amenorrhea, decreased fertility** and **increased** incidence of **miscarriage**^{Q}
> - **Children** experience **rapid growth** with **early bone maturation**^{Q}
> - **Older patients** present with **CVS complications (AF and CHF)**^{Q}

- Weight loss, facial flushing, warm and moist skin, tachycardia, cutaneous vasodilatation, **collapsing pulse** is seen on examination
- A **fine tremor, muscle wasting** and **proximal muscle** group **weakness** with **hyperactive tendon reflexes** often are present^Q

> - Overlying **bruit** or **thrill** at **upper pole**^{Q} due to **increased vascularity**
> - **Loud venous hum**^{Q} in supraclavicular space
> - **Ophthalmopathy** (orbital proptosis) occurs in **50%**, dermopathy in **1–2%.**^{Q}
> - Dermopathy is characterized by deposition of **glycosaminoglycans** leading to **thickened skin** in **pretibial region** and **dorsum of foot**^{Q} (pretibial myxedema).

- **Gynecomastia** is common in **young men**^{Q}
- Rare bony involvement leads to **subperiosteal bone formation** and **swelling in metacarpals**^{Q} (thyroid acropachy).

Diagnosis

- **Suppressed TSH** with or without an elevated free T4 or T3 level. **If eye signs are present,** other tests are generally not needed^Q.
- **In absence** of **eye signs, elevated RAIU** with **diffusely enlarged gland**^{Q} confirms the diagnosis.
- **Elevated TSH-R** or **thyroid-stimulating antibodies (TSAb)** are **diagnostic**^{Q} of Grave's disease and increased in about **90%** patients.
- **Anti-Tg** and **Anti-TPO antibodies** are **non-specific** and elevated in up to **75%** cases.
- **MRI of orbits** are useful in evaluating **Grave's ophthalmopathy.**

Treatment

- Treatment modalities: **Antithyroid drugs**, thyroid ablation with radioactive ^{131}I and **thyroidectomy**^{Q}.

■ TREATMENT OF GRAVE'S DISEASE

TREATMENT OF GRAVE'S DISEASE

- Treatment modalities are antithyroid drugs, thyroid ablation with radioactive ^{131}I, and thyroidectomy.

Antithyroid Drugs

- Administered in **preparation for RAI ablation** or **surgery**^{Q}.
- Drugs commonly used: **Propylthiouracil** and **methimazole**^{Q}.
- **Propylthiouracil** can cause **liver failure in pregnancy.**
- **Methimazole** is associated with **aplasia cutis & choanal atresia.**

> - **Antithyroid drug of choice in Graves: Methimazole**^{Q}
> - **Antithyroid drug of choice in pregnancy: Carbimazole**^{Q}
> - **Antithyroid drug of choice in thyroid storm: Propylthiouracil**^{Q}

- Most patients have **improved symptoms** in **2 weeks** and become **euthyroid** in about **6 weeks**^{Q}.
- **Catecholamine response** of thyrotoxicosis can be **alleviated** by **propranolol**^{Q}.

Radioactive Iodine Therapy (^{131}I)

- ^{131}I emits **beta (90%)** and **gamma rays**^{Q}

Indications of RAI Therapy
1. **Older patients** with **small** or **moderate-sized goiters**^{Q}
2. Patients **relapsed after medical** or **surgical therapy**^{Q}
3. **Antithyroid drugs** or **surgery** are **contraindicated**^{Q}

Contraindications of RAI	
Absolute Contraindications	**Relative Contraindications**
• **Pregnancy**^{Q}	• **Young patients** (children and adolescents)^Q
• **Lactation**^{Q}	• **Thyroid nodules**^{Q}
	• **Ophthalmopathy**^{Q}

Contd…

Contd…

Surgical Treatment

- **Surgery is recommended** when RAI is contraindicated[Q]
- **Treatment of choice: Total Thyroidectomy**

Indications of Surgery	
When RAI is Contraindicated	**Relative Indications**
• Confirmed **cancer** or **suspicious thyroid nodules**[Q] • **Young patients**[Q] • **Pregnancy and Lactation**[Q] • **Severe reactions** to antithyroid medications • **Large goiters** causing compressive symptoms • Reluctant to undergo RAI therapy	• **Smokers,** with **moderate to severe Grave's ophthalmopathy**[Q] • Patients desiring **rapid control of hyperthyroidism** with a chance of being euthyroid • **Poor compliance** to **antithyroid medications**.

■ TOXIC ADENOMA

TOXIC ADENOMA (PLUMMER'S DISEASE)

- Hyperthyroidism from a **single hyperfunctioning nodule**[Q] typically occurs in **younger patients**
- Increased thyroid hormone production occurs **independent of TSH control**[Q].
- Characterized by **somatic mutations** in the **TSH-R gene**[Q]

Clinical Features

- **Recent growth** of a **long-standing nodule** along with the symptoms of **hyperthyroidism**[Q].
- Hyperthyroidism from a **single hyperfunctioning nodule** typically occurs in **younger patients**
- Physical examination: **Solitary thyroid nodule** without palpable thyroid tissue on the contralateral side.
- Eye signs are not common, mainly **CVS dysfunction**
- **Rarely malignant**[Q].

Diagnosis

- **RAI scanning** shows a **"hot" nodule**[Q] with suppression the rest of the thyroid gland.

Treatment

- **Smaller nodules** may be managed with **antithyroid medications** and **RAI**[Q].
- **Most patients** are **euthyroid** after **radioiodine therapy**[Q] (radioiodine preferentially accumulates in hyperfunctioning nodules)
- Surgery (**Hemithyroidectomy**) is preferred in **young** patients with **larger nodules**[Q].

■ THYROTOXICOSIS

CVS FINDINGS IN THYROTOXICOSIS

- **MC cardiovascular manifestation** is **sinus tachycardia**[Q], often associated with **palpitations**, occasionally caused by **supraventricular tachycardia**[Q].
- **Exertional dyspnea**[Q]
- Hyperactive precordium with **loud first heart sound**, an accentuated pulmonic component of the second heart sound, and a **thirds heart sound**[Q].
- **Systolic ejection click**[Q]
- The high cardiac output produces a **bounding pulse**, **widened pulse pressure**[Q], and an **aortic systolic murmur** and can lead to worsening of angina or heart failure in the elderly or those with preexisting heart disease.
- **Atrial fibrillation** is more common in patients >50 years of age[Q].
- A systolic scratch, also known as **Means-Lerman scratch**[Q], is occasionally heard in 2nd left intercoastal space during expiration.
- **Systolic hypertension**

Cardiovascular Manifestations of Thyrotoxicosis	
Increased Atrial Irritability	**High Cardiac Output**
• **Sinus tachycardia (MC)** [Q] • Palpitations[Q] • Supraventricular tachycardia[Q] • Atrial fibrillations[Q]	• Bounding pulse • Wide pulse pressure[Q] • Hyperdynamic precordium[Q] • **Loud first heart sound**[Q], an accentuated pulmonic component of the second heart sound, and a **thirds heart sound**[Q]. • **Aortic systolic murmur**[Q] • **Means-Lerman scratch**[Q]

Contd…

Contd...

THYROID STORM (THYROTOXIC CRISIS)

- It is an **emergency** due to **decompensated hyperthyroidism**[Q].

Treatment

- **Non-selective beta blocker (Propranolol):**
  - **Most valuable measure** in **thyroid storm**[Q].
  - In thyroid storm most of the symptoms are because of adrenergic over activity due to **increased tissue sensitivity** to **catecholamines** in hyperthyroidism.
  - This **increased sensitivity** is due to **increased** number of **beta receptors**[Q].
- Quick relief is obtained by blocking **beta** receptors.
- **Propylthiouracil:**
  - **Antithyroid drug of choice** for **thyroid storm**[Q]
  - **Reduces hormone synthesis** as well as **peripheral conversion** of T_4 to T_3[Q]
  -
- **Corticosteroids (Hydrocortisone):**
  - **Inhibits** both **release of thyroid hormone** from the gland and **peripheral conversion** of T_4 to T_3[Q]
- **Iodides (Potassium iodide** or **ipanoic acid):**
  - Used to **inhibit** further **hormone release**[Q] from the gland.
- **Other Measures:**
  - **Diltiazem,** if **tachycardia** is not controlled by propranolol alone.
  - **Rehydration, anxiolytics, external cooling** and appropriate antibiotics

■ CARCINOMA THYROID

Type of Thyroid Carcinoma	Prevalence
Papillary (**MC**)	**80–90%**
Follicular	5–10%
Medullary	10%
Anaplastic	Rare
Lymphoma	1%

Well Differentiated Thyroid Cancer	
1. **Papillary** carcinoma of thyroid[Q]	2. **Follicular** carcinoma of thyroid[Q]
3. **Follicular variant** of **papillary** carcinoma thyroid[Q]	4. **Hurthle cell carcinoma** (variant of follicular carcinoma thyroid) [Q]

Carcinoma Thyroid		
Type	**Mode of spread**	**MC site of metastasis**
Papillary carcinoma	**Lymphatic**[Q] spread	Lungs
Follicular carcinoma	**Hematogenous**[Q] spread	Bones
Medullary carcinoma	Both **lymphatic** and **hematogenous**[Q] spread	Liver
Anaplastic carcinoma	**Direct invasion**[Q]	Lungs

Pulsating Secondaries	
1. **Follicular carcinoma thyroid**[Q]	2. **RCC**[Q]

Bone Metastasis in Carcinoma Thyroid	
Follicular carcinoma	**Osteolytic** metastasis (**Pulsating secondaries in flat bones**)[Q]
Medullary carcinoma	**Osteoblastic** metastasis[Q]

■ PAPILLARY CARCINOMA OF THYROID

PAPILLARY CARCINOMA OF THYROID

- Accounts for **80%** of all thyroid malignancies in **iodine-sufficient areas**[Q]
- **MC thyroid cancer** in **children** & **individuals** exposed to **external radiation**[Q].
- More often in **women, 30–40** years.

Contd...

Contd…

Pathology

- **Grossly: Hard** & **whitish remain flat** on sectioning with a blade with macroscopic **calcification, necrosis,** or **cystic changes**

> - **Multifocality**[Q] is **common** (up to **85%** of cases) on **microscopic examination.**
> - **Multifocality** is associated with an **increased risk** of **cervical nodal metastases**[Q], rarely **invade adjacent structures** such as the trachea, esophagus & RLNs.

- **Rarely encapsulated**[Q] (PCT are **seldom encapsulated**)
- **Other variants: Tall cell**[Q], **insular**[Q], columnar, diffuse sclerosing, clear cell, **trabecular,** and poorly differentiated types; account for about **1%**; associated with a **worse prognosis.**

Histological Characteristics of Papillary Carcinoma Thyroid

- **Papillary projections**[Q]: PTC contains branching papillae of cuboidal epithelial cells
- **Orphan Annie eye nuclei:**
  - The nuclei contain finely dispersed chromatin, which imparts an **optically clear** or **empty appearance**, giving rise to term **ground glass** or **Orphan Annie eye nuclei**[Q].
  - **Invaginations** of **cytoplasm** in cross-sections: **Intranuclear inclusions**[Q] (**pseudo-inclusion**) or **intranuclear grooves**[Q].
  - **Diagnosis** of PTC is **based on** these **nuclear characteristics**[Q] even in the absence of papillary structures.
- **Psammoma bodies**[Q]: **Microscopic, calcified deposits** representing clumps of sloughed cells

Clinical Features

- Most patients are **euthyroid** & present with a **slow-growing painless mass**[Q] in the neck.
- Dysphagia, dyspnea dysphonia are associated with locally advanced invasive disease.
- **Lymph node metastases** are **common**[Q], especially in **children young adults**, and may be the presenting complaint.

> - **"Lateral aberrant thyroid"** denotes a **cervical lymph node** that has been **invaded by metastatic cancer**[Q].

- **Distant metastases** are **uncommon** at initial presentation, but may ultimately develop in up to **20%** of patients.
- **MC sites of metastasis: Lungs**[Q] >bone >liver >brain.

Diagnosis

- **Diagnosis** is established by **FNAC** of the **thyroid mass** or **lymph node**[Q].
- Once thyroid cancer is diagnosed on FNAC, a **complete neck ultrasound** to evaluate the **contralateral lobe** and for **LN metastases** in the central & lateral neck compartments.

Treatment

- **Total** or **near-total thyroidectomy**[Q]
- During thyroidectomy, **enlarged central neck nodes** should be **removed**[Q].
- **Biopsy-proven lymph node metastases** detected clinically or by imaging in the lateral neck in patients with papillary carcinoma are managed with **modified radical neck dissection.**

Prognosis

- PTC have an **excellent prognosis** with a **>95% 10-year survival rate**[Q].

■ FOLLICULAR CARCINOMA THYROID

FOLLICULAR CARCINOMA OF THYROID

- FTC account for **10%** of **thyroid cancers**
- Occurs more commonly in **iodine-deficient areas**[Q].
- **More common** in **women** with mean age of **50 years**
- **Genes** implicated in FCT: p53[Q], PTEN[Q], Ras[Q], PAX8/PPAR1

Pathology

- Usually **solitary lesion** surrounded by **capsule**[Q].
- **Malignancy** is defined by the presence of **capsular** and **vascular invasion**[Q].
- **Tumor infiltration** and **invasion**, as well as **tumor thrombus** within the **middle thyroid** or jugular veins, may be apparent at operation.

Clinical Features

- Usually present as **solitary thyroid nodules**, occasionally with a history of **rapid size increase**, and **long-standing goiter**[Q].
- Preoperative clinical diagnosis of cancer is difficult unless distant metastases are present.
- Large follicular tumors (**>4 cm**) in **older men** are **more likely** to be **malignant**[Q].

> - **MC site** of **metastasis is bone** (Osteolytic metastasis with **pulsating secondaries in flat bones**)[Q]
> - **MC site of metastasis: Vertebra**[Q] >Ribs >Pelvis Bones >Skull

Contd…

Contd…

Diagnosis

- **FNAC** is **unable to distinguish benign** follicular lesions **from follicular carcinomas**[Q].
- **Intraoperative frozen-section** examination usually is **not helpful**, but should be **performed** when there is evidence of **capsular or vascular invasion**, or when **adjacent lymphadenopathy** is present.

Treatment

- **Follicular lesion: Hemithyroidectomy**[Q] (**80%** of these patients will have **benign** adenomas)
- **Thyroid cancer: Total thyroidectomy**[Q]
- **Prophylactic nodal dissection** is **unwarranted**[Q] because nodal involvement is infrequent.

Prognosis

- **Most important** prognostic factor: **Age** and **distant metastasis**.

Poor Long-term Prognosis	
• Age **>50 years**[Q]	• Marked **vascular invasion**[Q]
• Tumor size **>4 cm**[Q]	• **Extrathyroidal invasion**[Q]
• **Higher tumor grade**[Q]	• Distant **metastases**[Q]

■ MEDULLARY CARCINOMA THYROID

MEDULLARY CARCINOMA THYROID

- Neuroendocrine carcinoma **arising from parafollicular 'C' cells**[Q] of thyroid
- **Parafollicular 'C' cells** are derived from the **ultimobranchial bodies**[Q] & **secrete calcitonin**[Q]
- **'C' Cells** are concentrated **superolaterally** in thyroid lobes, from where MTC usually develops
- **Most MTCs** (75–80%) arise **sporadically**[Q]
- **Spread** is both **lymphatic** & **hematogenous**[Q]
- **MC site** of **metastasis: Liver**[Q]

Medullary Carcinoma Thyroid	
Sporadic: 80%[Q]	**Familial: 20%**[Q] (Non-MEN setting/ MEN-2A/MEN-2B)
• Originate in **one lobe**[Q] • Seen in **6th decade** • **RET protoncogene**[Q] mutation	• **Multicentric** and **bilateral**[Q] • Occur in **younger age**[Q] • Associoted with **C-cell hyperplasia**[Q] • **RET protoncogene**[Q] mutation

Clinical Features

Medullary Carcinoma Should Be Suspected
• **High level** of serum **Calcitonin**[Q] & **CEA**[Q]   • **Cervical lymph nodes** at time of presentation (**LN involvement**, thyroid and **blood borne metastases** occurs **early**)[Q]   • **Diarrhea**[Q] at the time of presentation.   • **Amyloid**[Q] in stroma histologically.   • **MEN setting**: Evidence of Pheochromocytoma/Hyperparathyroidism/Thyroid cancer in family.   • (Discovery of **medullary carcinoma thyroid** makes **family surveillance advisable**)[Q]

Diagnosis

- Diagnosed by **FNAC**[Q]
- **I**[131] scan is of **no use** as MTC is **TSH independent**[Q].
- **Tumor marker: Calcitonin** is raised in **almost all cases** of MTC
- **Calcitonin excess** in MTC is **not associated** with **hypocalcemia**

Treatment

- **Total thyroidectomy + Central LN dissection ± Ipsilateral MRND if tumor >1 cm**[Q]
- If **nodes** are **positive** on **ipsilateral side: Bilateral MRND**
- **Vandetanib (EGFR inhibitor)** is the only drug approved by US FDA for treatment of **advanced & progressive MTC**

Follow-up

- Level of **Calcitonin** falls after resection and is raises again in cases of recurrence, **used for follow up**[Q].

Prognosis

- MTC is **associated** with **poor prognosis**[Q].

■ ANAPLASTIC CARCINOMA

ANAPLASTIC CARCINOMA

- Accounts for **1%** of all thyroid malignancies
- **Mainly** affect **women in 7th and 8th decade**[Q]
- The typical patient has a **long-standing neck mass**, which **rapidly enlarges** and may be **painful**[Q].
- **Most aggressive** form of **thyroid cancer**[Q]

Pathology
- **Grossly: Firm & whitish** in appearance.
- Microscopically, sheets of cells with marked heterogeneity & characteristic **giant & multinucleated cells**[Q].

Clinical Features
- **Typical manifestation**: An **older patient** with **dysphagia, cervical tenderness** & a **painful, rapidly enlarging neck mass**[Q].
- **Superior vena cava syndrome** can also be part of the findings.
- The clinical situation **deteriorates rapidly** into **tracheal obstruction & rapid local invasion**[Q] of surrounding structures.
- Associated symptoms: **Dysphonia, dysphagia & dyspnea**

> - **Lymph nodes** usually are **palpable** at presentation.
> - **Evidence** of **metastatic spread** also may be present.
> - **MC site** of **metastasis: Lungs**[Q]

Diagnosis
- Confirmed by **FNAC** revealing characteristic **giant & multinucleated cells**[Q].
- **Incisional biopsy** occasionally is needed to **confirm** the **diagnosis**

Treatment
- **Thyroidectomy** for **resectable mass**[Q] (may lead to a small improvement in survival, especially in younger individuals)
- Combined **radiation & chemotherapy** in an adjuvant setting in patients with resectable disease has been associated with **prolonged survival**[Q].
- **Tracheostomy**[Q] to alleviate **airway obstruction**.

Prognosis
- **Most aggressive thyroid malignancies**[Q], with **<6 months** survival

■ METASTATIC TUMORS OF THYROID

METASTATIC TUMORS OF THYROID

- Rare, most cases are found in autopsy
- MC site of primary: **CA Breast**[Q] > CA Lung
- If thyroid metastases is detected pre-mortem, MC site of primary: **RCC**[Q] > CA Breast > CA Lung

■ THYROID LYMPHOMA

THYROID LYMPHOMA

- MC type is **NHL B cell**[Q] type, of **intermediate** grade.
- Majority of patients have thyroid disease plus **cervical** or **mediastinal lymph nodes**[Q].
- More common in **females**.
- Most thyroid lymphomas **develop in** patients with **Chronic Lymphocytic Thyroiditis**[Q]

Clinical Features
- **Lymphomas** are **rapidly growing tumours**, present with **rapidly enlarging neck mass** which is often **painless**.
- Patients may present with **acute respiratory distress & dysphagia**
- About **10–30%** present with symptoms relating to local invasion, including **hoarseness, dyspnoea** with stridor, or **dysphagia**.

> - **Painless**[Q] and associated with **fever**[Q]
> - Patients with thyroid lymphoma virtually **never have hyperthyroidism** but frequently have **hypothyroidism**[Q].
> - Hypothyroid patients have evidence of **autoimmune thyroiditis** or **Hashimoto's thyroiditis**[Q].

Diagnosis
- Diagnosis is confirmed by **core-needle biopsy**[Q].

Treatment: External Beam Radiotherapy + Chemotherapy[Q]
- Patients with **thyroid lymphoma** respond rapidly to chemotherapy (**CHOP**—cyclophosphamide, doxorubicin, vincristine, and prednisone) and associated with **improved survival**.
- Combined treatment with **radiotherapy & chemotherapy** often is recommended.
- To alleviate **pressure symptoms, surgical resection** (Thyroidectomy and nodal dissection) is recommended.

■ THYROIDECTOMY

STEPS OF THYROIDECTOMY

- A **Kocher transverse collar incision**, typically **4 to 5 cm** in length, is placed in or parallel to a **natural skin crease 1 cm below cricoid cartilage**.
- Subcutaneous tissues & platysma are incised sharply and subplatysmal **flaps are raised superiorly** to the level of **thyroid cartilage** and inferiorly to the **suprasternal notch**[Q]
- **Strap muscles** are **divided in the midline** along the entire length of mobilized flaps, & thyroid gland is exposed.
- **Middle thyroid veins** are ligated and **divided**[Q].

  - **Dissection plane** is kept as **close** to the **thyroid** as possible & **superior pole** vessels are individually identified, skeletonized, ligated, & divided low on the thyroid gland **to avoid injury** to **external branch** of **superior laryngeal nerve**[Q].

- RLNs can be most consistently identified at the **level of cricoid cartilage**.
- **Parathyroids** usually can be identified **within 1 cm of** the crossing of the **inferior thyroid artery** and **the RLN**[Q]

  - **Inferior thyroid vessels** are **dissected, skeletonized, ligated**, and **divided as close to the surface of thyroid gland as possible** to **minimize devascularization of the parathyroids** (extracapsular[Q] dissection) or **injury to the RLN**[Q].

- **RLN** is **most vulnerable to injury in** the vicinity of the **ligament of Berry**. Any **bleeding** in this area should be **controlled with gentle pressure** before carefully identifying the vessel & ligating it. Use of the **electrocautery should be avoided** in proximity to the RLN[Q].
- Once the ligament is divided, the thyroid can be separated from the underlying trachea by sharp dissection.

  - **Parathyroid glands** that have been **inadvertently removed** during the thyroidectomy should be resected, confirmed as parathyroid tissue by frozen section, **divided into 1-mm fragments**, and **reimplanted into** individual pockets in the **sternocleidomastoid**[Q] muscle. The sites should be **marked with silk sutures** and a **clip**[Q].

■ COMPLICATIONS OF THYROIDECTOMY

COMPLICATIONS OF THYROIDECTOMY

- **Hemorrhage**
  - Due to **slipping of ligature** on the **superior thyroid artery**[Q], bleeding from muscular artery
  - **Hematomas** may cause airway compromise and **must be evacuated immediately**[Q].
  - Hematomas may occur immediately or later on.
  - An **immediate bleed** occurs after or shortly before extubation when the patient lightens from anaesthesia and may **begin to cough**, causing a vessel to open.
- **Respiratory obstruction: Causes include**
  - Tension hematoma[Q]
  - Laryngeal edema (by anesthetic intubation): MC cause of respiratory obstruction[Q]
  - Bilateral recurrent laryngeal nerve paralysis[Q]
- **Recurrent laryngeal nerve paralysis**
  - May be unilateral or bilateral, transient or permanent.
  - Bilateral paralysis causes respiratory obstruction - Dyspnea, stridor.
- **Injury to other nerves**
  - **External branches of superior laryngeal nerve**[Q] (MC injured nerve during thyroid surgery: **External laryngeal nerve**[Q])
  - Cervical sympathetic trunk - may cause Horner's syndrome.
- **Parathyroid insufficiency**
  - Due to **removal of the parathyroid glands** or **infarction due to vascular injury**[Q].
  - **Vascular injury**[Q] is more important.
  - Cases usually present **2–5 days after operation**[Q] with symptoms of **hypocalcemia** (circumoral and fingertip numbness and tingling tetany, carpopedal spasm and laryngeal stridor)[Q]
  - Treatment with **oral calcium & vitamin D supplements**[Q]
  - **IV calcium gluconate**[Q] may be required in severe cases.
- **Thyroid insufficiency**
- **Thyrotoxic crisis**
  - Occurs if the thyrotoxic patient has been **inadequately prepared for thyroidectomy**[Q].

Multiple Choice Questions

■ PAPILLARY CARCINOMA

1. **Psammoma bodies may be seen in all of the following, except:** *(Recent Question 2016, All India 2011)*
   a. Follicular carcinoma of thyroid
   b. Papillary carcinoma of thyroid
   c. Meningioma
   d. Serous cystadenocarcinoma of ovary

2. **Most common thyroid malignancy is:** *(DNB 2012, MHPGMCET 2002)*
   a. Anaplastic carcinoma   b. Follicular carcinoma
   c. Medullary carcinoma   d. Papillary carcinoma

3. **Which thyroid malignancy is common after radiation exposure?** *(Recent Question 2016, MHSSMCET 2005)*
   a. Follicular   b. Papillary
   c. Medullary   d. Anaplastic

4. **Orphan Annie-eye nuclei seen in:** *(Orissa 2011)*
   a. Papillary carcinoma of thyroid
   b. Medullary carcinoma of thyroid
   c. Anaplastic carcinoma of thyroid
   d. Follicular carcinoma of thyroid

5. **Which of the following would be the best treatment for a 2 cm thyroid nodule in a 50 years old man with FNAC revealing it to be a papillary carcinoma?** *(All India 2009, Recent Question 2015)*
   a. Hemithyroidectomy
   b. Subtotal thyroidectomy with modified neck dissection
   c. Near total thyroidectomy with modified neck dissection
   d. Hemithyroidectomy with modified neck dissection

6. **True regarding papillary carcinoma of thyroid:**
   a. Undifferentiated carcinoma   *(MCI March 2006)*
   b. Blood-borne metastasis is commoner
   c. Excellent prognosis
   d. Capsulated

7. **Which type of thyroid carcinoma has the best prognosis?** *(DNB 2010, All India 96)*
   a. Papillary carcinoma   b. Anaplastic carcinoma
   c. Follicular carcinoma   d. Medullary carcinoma

8. **Occult thyroid malignancy with nodal metastasis is:** *(DNB 2005, 2001, AIIMS Sept 96)*
   a. Medullary carcinoma   b. Follicular carcinoma
   c. Papillary carcinoma   d. Anaplastic carcinoma

9. **A 21 years old woman has 3 cm node in the lower deep cervical chain on the left. The biopsy is interpreted as revealing normal thyroid tissue in a lymph node. The most likely diagnosis is:** *(DNB 2012, DPG 2009 Feb)*
   a. Subacute thyroiditis
   b. Metastatic carcinoma thyroid
   c. Hashimoto's disease   d. Lateral aberrant thyroid

10. **Most common type of carcinoma thyroid having least chances of hematogenous spread:** *(Recent Question 2015)*
    a. Follicular   b. Papillary
    c. Anaplastic   d. Medullary

11. **Orphan-Annie eye nuclei is seen in:** *(Recent Question 2017)*
    a. Papillary carcinoma thyroid
    b. Follicular carcinoma thyroid
    c. Medullary carcinoma thyroid
    d. Anaplastic carcinoma thyroid

12. **Psammoma bodies are seen in:** *(Recent Question 2017)*
    a. Papillary carcinoma thyroid
    b. Follicular carcinoma thyroid
    c. Medullary carcinoma thyroid
    d. Thyroid lymphoma

13. **A 27 years old woman presents with 26 weeks of gestation with a lesion, which is found to be papillary carcinoma of thyroid. Which is the best treatment for this patient?**
    a. Thyroid ablation using radioactive iodine
    b. Total thyroidectomy   *(MCI June 2019)*
    c. Observation   d. Hemi-thyroidectomy

■ FOLLICULAR CARCINOMA

14. **All of the following are true for follicular carcinoma of thyroid except:** *(COMEDK 2006)*
    a. Lymph node involvement rare
    b. Vascular involvement common
    c. Younger patients have good prognosis
    d. Diagnosis by FNAC

15. **Thyroid carcinoma with pulsating vascular skeletal metastasis is:** *(COMEDK 2007, All India 95)*
    a. Follicular   b. Anaplastic
    c. Medullary   d. Papillary

16. **FNAC is useful in all the following types of thyroid carcinoma except:** *(UPPG 2010, MCI March 2005, All India 95)*
    a. Papillary   b. Follicular
    c. Anaplastic   d. Medullary

17. **Most probable malignancy that develops in a case of long-standing goiter is:** *(MCI June 2018, Recent Question 2015, Kerala PG 2015, AIIMS Feb 97, Nov 2001)*
    a. Follicular carcinoma   b. Anaplastic carcinoma
    c. Papillary carcinoma   d. Medullary carcinoma

18. **Bone metastasis is common in which thyroid tumor:**
    a. Follicular   b. Papillary   *(AIIMS Nov 99)*
    c. Hurthle cell tumour   d. Anaplastic

19. **Metastasis from follicular carcinoma should be treated by:**
    a. Radioiodine   b. Surgery   *(MCI Sept 2006)*
    c. Thyroxine   d. Observation

20. **True regarding follicular carcinoma of thyroid:**
    a. Hematogemous spread   *(JIPMER 2014, 2013)*
    b. Commonly multifocal
    c. Readily diagnosed by face
    d. Most commonly carcinoma of thyroid

21. **FNAC cannot detect which of the following?** *(AIIMS Nov 2014)*
    a. Follicular carcinoma   b. Papillary carcinoma
    c. Colloid goiter   d. Hashimoto's thyroiditis

■ MEDULLARY CARCINOMA

22. **Screening method of medullary carcinoma thyroid is:**
    a. Serum calcitonin   b. Serum calcium
    c. Serum alkaline phosphate   *(All India 97, AIIMS Nov 95)*
    d. Serum acid phosphatase

23. **Treatment of medullary carcinoma thyroid:**
    a. Surgery and Radiotherapy   *(AIIMS May 2011)*
    b. Radiotherapy and Chemotherapy
    c. Surgery only
    d. Radioiodine ablation

24. Recommended age for prophylactic thyroidectomy for MEN-2 is: *(Recent Question 2015)*
    a. 5 years
    b. Before 1 year
    c. At the time of diagnosis
    d. Any time

25. A biopsy from a mass in front of the neck revealed parafollicular cells. How do you follow up? *(JIPMER Nov 2017)*
    a. Calcitonin
    b. T4
    c. Thyroxine
    d. Thyroglobulin

26. After thyroidectomy for medullary carcinoma of thyroid, which is important for determining recurrence of tumour?
    a. Thyroglobulin
    b. TSH   *(MCI Sept 2009)*
    c. CEA
    d. Thyroxine levels

27. The expression of the following oncogene is associated with a high incidence of medullary carcinoma of thyroid: *(AIIMS Nov 2005)*
    a. p53
    b. Her-2-neu
    c. Ret proto-oncogene
    d. Rb gene

28. Amyloid stroma is seen in which carcinoma thyroid: *(AIIMS June 2000)*
    a. Papillary carcinoma
    b. Medullary carcinoma
    c. Anaplastic carcinoma
    d. Follicular carcinoma

29. Serum calcitonin is a marker for: *(DNB 2003, All India 94)*
    a. Anaplastic carcinoma
    b. Papillary carcinoma
    c. Medullary carcinoma
    d. Follicular carcinoma

30. All are true regarding medullary carcinoma of thyroid except:
    a. It arises from 'C' cells   *(JIPMER 2014, 2013)*
    b. Secrete high levels of calcitonin
    c. It is dependent on TSH
    d. Most cases are familial

31. Which of the following does not take radioactive iodine?
    a. Medullary carcinoma thyroid   *(Recent Question 2017)*
    b. Papillary carcinoma thyroid
    c. Follicular carcinoma thyroid
    d. Hürthle cell carcinoma thyroid

32. Calcitonin is the marker for: *(Recent Question 2017)*
    a. Papillary carcinoma thyroid
    b. Follicular carcinoma thyroid
    c. Medullary carcinoma thyroid
    d. Anaplastic carcinoma thyroid

33. RET proto-oncogene is associated with development of:
    a. Medullary carcinoma thyroid   *(Recent Question 2018)*
    b. Astrocytoma
    c. Paraganglioma
    d. Hürthle cell tumor thyroid

■ ANAPLASTIC CARCINOMA

34. A patient with long standing multinodular goitre develops hoarseness of voice and swelling undergoes sudden increase in size. Likely diagnosis is: *(Recent Question 2014, All India 2001)*
    a. Follicular carcinoma
    b. Papillary carcinoma
    c. Medullary carcinoma
    d. Anaplastic carcinoma

35. Least common thyroid malignancy is: *(Recent Question 2015)*
    a. Papillary
    b. Follicular
    c. Medullary
    d. Anaplastic

■ THYROID METASTASIS

36. Metastasis in thyroid gland come most commonly from carcinoma of: *(PGI June 98)*
    a. Testis
    b. Prostate
    c. Breast
    d. Lungs

■ THYROID LYMPHOMA

37. All of the following are true about lymphoma of the thyroid except: *(All India 2007)*
    a. More common in females
    b. Slow growing
    c. Clinically confused with undifferentiated tumors
    d. May present with respiratory distress and dysphagia

■ CARCINOMA THYROID

38. The most common histologic type of thyroid cancer is: *(Recent Question 2015, All India 2008, 2004, AIIMS Nov 05, PGI Dec 2005)*
    a. Medullary type
    b. Follicular type
    c. Papillary type
    d. Anaplastic type

39. Which of the following is not a histological variant of thyroid neoplasm? *(All India 2007)*
    a. Follicular
    b. Merkel cell
    c. Insular
    d. Anaplastic

40. Thyroxine can be given in which thyroid carcinoma:
    a. Papillary
    b. Medullary *(MCI Sept 2009)*
    c. Anaplastic
    d. Undifferentiated

41. Which of the following is used in the treatment of well differentiated thyroid carcinoma: *(Recent Question 2013)*
    a. I^{131}
    b. 99m Tc
    c. 32P
    d. MIBG

■ SOLITARY THYROID NODULE

42. Initial preferred investigation for thyroid nodule is:
    a. FNAC
    b. Radionucleide test
    c. Thyroid function test
    d. USG   *(DPG 2008)*

43. Investigation of choice in discrete thyroid swelling is: *(Recent Question 2014)*
    a. Isotope scans
    b. Ultrasonography
    c. Autoantibody titres
    d. FNAC

44. A patient came with a small solitary nodule in right lobe of thyroid. FNAC shows follicular adenoma. The best surgery is: *(DNB 2002)*
    a. Enucleation
    b. Sub-total thyroidectomy
    c. Right hemithyroidectomy
    d. Near-total thyroidectomy

45. Which of the following is true about subtotal thyroidectomy?
    a. Removal of one lobe and isthmus   *(Recent Question 2018)*
    b. Removal of both lobes leaving behind 6-8 grams of tissue
    c. Removal of entire lobe with cervical lymph nodes
    d. Removal of one lobe with isthmus

46. Which is the investigation of choice to differentiate between benign and malignant thyroid nodule? *(DNB 2014)*
    a. USG
    b. FNAC
    c. Scintigraphy
    d. Biopsy

■ GOITER

47. The most common presentation of endemic goiter is: *(All India 96)*
    a. Hypothyroid
    b. Diffuse goiter
    c. Hyperthyroid
    d. Solitary nodule

48. Thoracic extension of cervical goitre is usually approached through: *(AIIMS May 2005)*
    a. Neck
    b. Chest
    c. Combined cervico-thoracic
    d. Thoracoscopic

49. Treatment of choice in cold nodule of thyroid: *(JIPMER 93)*
- a. Subtotal thyroidectomy
- b. Wait and watch
- c. I-131
- d. Hemithyroidectomy

■ RETROSTERNAL GOITER

50. Retrosternal goiter is characterized by: *(DPG 2005)*
- a. Stridor
- b. Always malignant
- c. Bilateral
- d. None of the above

51. Most commonly used approach for retrosternal goitre:
- a. Transthoracic via second intercostal space
- b. Transthoracic via fourth intercostal space
- c. Trans-sternal through anterior mediastinum
- d. Transcervical   *(Recent Question 2019)*

■ THYROTOXICOSIS

52. Thyroid storm after operation is due to: *(COMEDK 2007)*
- a. Inadequate control of hyperthyroidism
- b. Massive bleeding
- c. Recurrent laryngeal nerve injury
- d. Postoperative infection

53. Which of the following is the agent of choice for treating thyrotoxicosis during pregnancy? *(COMEDK 2010)*
- a. Carbimazole
- b. Propylthiouracil
- c. Methimazole
- d. Radioactive I-131

54. The drug of choice for hyperthyroidism in third trimester of pregnancy is: *(MCI Dec 2019)*
- a. Carbimazole
- b. Propylthiouracil
- c. Sodium iodide
- d. Radioactive iodine

55. All of the following are features of thyrotoxicosis, except:
- a. Diastolic murmur   *(Recent Question 2016)*
- b. Soft non-ejection systolic murmur
- c. Irregularly, irregular pulse
- d. Scratching sound in systole

56. Treatment of thyroid storm includes all, except:
(AIIMS Nov 2003)
- a. Propranolol
- b. Radioactive iodine
- c. Hydrocortisone
- d. Lugol's iodine

57. Difference between thyrotoxicosis and malignant hyperthermia is: *(AIIMS June 2001)*
- a. Hyperthermia
- b. Tachycardia
- c. Muscle rigidity
- d. Elevated serum CPK level

58. Thyroid storm after operation is due to: *(COMEDK 2007)*
- a. Inadequate control of hyperthyroidism
- b. Massive bleeding
- c. Recurrent laryngeal nerve injury
- d. Postoperative injection

59. All of the following conditions are associated with hyperthyroidism, except: *(All India 2011)*
- a. Hashimoto's thyroiditis
- b. Grave's disease
- c. Toxic multinodular goiter
- d. Struma ovary

60. Which of the following is a symptom of hypothyroidism?
(JIPMER 2014, 2007)
- a. Hyperactivity
- b. Palpitation
- c. Diarrhoea
- d. Hair loss

61. Reduction of size and vascularity prior to thyroidectomy is done by: *(Recent Question 2015)*
- a. Iodides
- b. Propylthiouracil
- c. Radioiodine
- d. Propranolol

62. Treatment of choice for recurrent thyrotoxicosis after surgery is: *(MCI June 2018)*
- a. Further surgery
- b. Radioiodine followed by surgery
- c. Radioiodine
- d. Observation & follow-up

■ GRAVE'S DISEASE

63. All of the following are features of Grave's disease except:
- a. More common in males
- b. Tremor   *(MCI Sept 2005)*
- c. Pretibial myxoedema
- d. Intolerance to heat

64. Pretibial myxedema is seen in: *(MHPGMET 2005)*
- a. Thyrotoxicosis
- b. Hypothyroidism
- c. Hyperparathyroidism
- d. All

65. Which of the following statements about Grave's disease is false? *(Recent Question 2018)*
- a. Results in hyperthyroidism
- b. Autoimmune disorder
- c. Common in male
- d. Referred as diffuse toxic goiter

■ HYPOTHYROIDISM

66. In case of hypothyroidism which investigation is most informative and most commonly used: *(AIIMS June 98)*
- a. Serum TSH level
- b. Serum T3, T4 level
- c. Serum calcitonin assay
- d. Serum TRH assay

■ POST THYROIDECTOMY COMPLICATIONS

67. During thyroidectomy, inferior thyroid artery is ligated at:
- a. Maximally away from the gland   *(MCI Sept 2005)*
- b. Close to the gland
- c. Half way from the gland
- d. None of the above

68. Complications of total thyroidectomy include all except:
(AIIMS May 2005)
- a. Hoarseness
- b. Airway obstruction
- c. Hemorrhage
- d. Hypercalcemia

69. Hypoparathyroidism following thyroid surgery occurs within: *(AIIMS Nov 2004, Nov 2003)*
- a. 24 hours
- b. 2–5 days
- c. 7–14 days
- d. 2–3 weeks

70. A post-thyroidectomy patient develops signs and symptoms of tetany. The management is: *(All India 2000)*
- a. IV calcium gluconate
- b. Bicarbonate
- c. Calcitonin
- d. Vitamin D

71. A patient presents with swelling in the neck following a thyroidectomy; what is the most likely resulting complication?
- a. Respiratory obstruction   *(All India 2001)*
- b. Recurrent laryngeal nerve palsy
- c. Hypovolemia
- d. Hypocalcemia

72. After thyroidectomy, patient developed stridor within 2 hours. All are likely cause of stridor except:
- a. Hypocalcemia   *(AIIMS Nov 2001, Nov 2000)*
- b. Recurrent laryngeal nerve palsy
- c. Laryngomalacia

73. Hemorrhage after thyroidectomy is due to:
(Recent Question 2014)
- a. External carotid artery
- b. Internal carotid artery
- c. Superior thyroid artery
- d. Inferior thyroid artery

■ THYROIDITIS

74. Thyroid biopsy of a patient showed the presence of Hurthle cells. Antibodies found in this condition are: *(Punjab 2011)*
- a. Anti-TPO
- b. Anti-mitochondrial
- c. Anti-RNP
- d. Anti-dsDNA

75. A patient with autoimmune thyroiditis present with hypothyroidism. Which of the following is true?
   a. Thyroid peroxidase antibodies   *(JIPMER 2011)*
   b. Painless enlargement of thyroid
   c. Common in men
   d. No malignant risk

76. Hashimoto's thyroiditis, all are true except: *(AIIMS May 2011)*
   a. Follicular destruction   b. Increase in lymphocytes
   c. Oncocytic metaplasia   d. Orphan Annie eye nuclei

77. The laboratory investigation of a patient shows ↓T4, and ↑TSH. Which of the following is the most likely diagnosis:
   (All India 2011)
   a. Grave's disease   b. Hashimoto's disease
   c. Pituitary failure   d. Hypothalamic failure

78. Which of the following conditions is associated with hypothyroidism?   *(All India 2011)*
   a. Hashimoto's thyroiditis
   b. Grave's disease
   c. Toxic multinodular goiter
   d. Struma ovary

79. Most common cause of thyroiditis is: *(All India 2000)*
   a. Reidel's thyroiditis
   b. Subacute thyroiditis
   c. Hashimoto's thyroiditis
   d. Viral thyroiditis

80. Not a feature of de-Quervain's disease: *(All India 2002)*
   a. Autoimmune in etiology
   b. ↑ ESR
   c. Tends to regress spontaneously
   d. Painful and associated with enlargement of thyroid

81. Which of the following is wrong about subacute thyroiditis?
   a. Usually presents with painful enlargement of thyroid gland   *(Orissa 2011)*
   b. There may be features of hyperthyroidism or hypothyroidism
   c. In the thyrotoxic phase radioiodine uptake is increased
   d. High ESR

82. In Hashimoto's disease serum antibodies are mainly against:
   (Recent Question 2016)
   a. Thyroid follicles   b. Thyroxine
   c. Thyroglobulins   d. Iodine

83. DeQvervain's thyroiditis is characterised by:
   a. Mononuclear cell infiltration   *(COMEDK 2014)*
   b. Histiocyte reaction
   c. Giant cell infiltration
   d. Eosinophilia

■ THYROGLOSSAL CYST AND FISTULA

84. A 10-year-old child presented with midline swelling in anterior position of neck. Most probable diagnosis is:
   a. Thyroglossal cyst   b. Thyroglossal fistula
   c. Cold abscess   d. Acute lymphadenitis

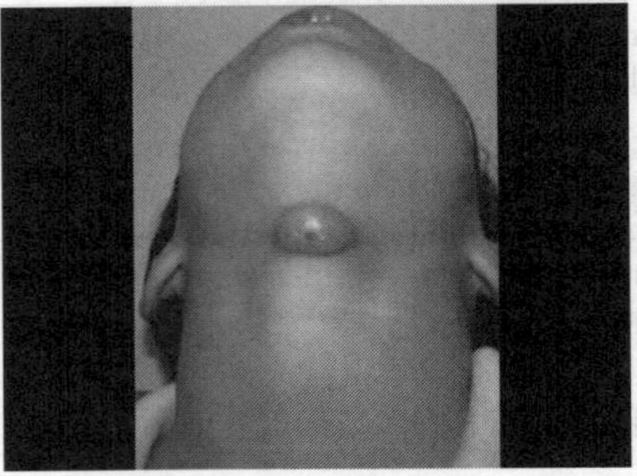

85. Sistrunk's operation is done in:
   (WBPG 2015, MHPGMCET 2008, 2006)
   a. Parotid tumor   b. Thyroglossal fistula
   c. Thyroglossal cyst   d. Branchial fistula

86. Most common site of thyroglossal cyst:
   (Recent Question 2013, DNB 2009, 2007, 2005, 2003, MHSSMCET 2005, AIIMS June 97)
   a. Suprahyoid   b. Hyoid
   c. Subhyoid   d. Intra-thyroid

87. Thyroglossal cyst may occasionally give rise to carcinoma:
   a. Papillary   b. Medullary
   c. Anaplastic   c. Follicular

88. Sistrunk's operation consists of: *(DPG 2009 March)*
   a. Excision of hyoid bone and cone of tongue muscle
   b. Excision of hyoid bone and the cyst
   c. Excision of central part of hyoid bone and cone of tongue muscles upto foramen caecum
   d. Excision of cyst only

■ MISCELLANEOUS

89. Pendred's syndrome is due to a defect in:
   (MCI June 2018, COMEDK 2007, 2008)
   a. Chromosome 7p   b. Chromosome 7q
   c. Chromosome 8p   d. Chromosome 8q

90. Reddish swelling in the region of foramen caecum:
   (DPG 2007)
   a. Lingual thyroid   b. Lingual tonsil
   c. Ranula   d. Thyroglossal cyst

Explanations

■ PAPILLARY CARCINOMA

1. **Ans. a. Follicular carcinoma of thyroid** *(Ref: Schwartz 11/e p1647, 10/e p1542; Sabiston 20/e p902; Bailey 27/e p818)*

Psammoma Bodies (PSM)	
1. **Papillary carcinoma thyroid**[Q]	2. **Papillary carcinoma (RCC)**[Q]
3. **Serous cystadenoma**[Q]	4. **Meningioma**[Q]

2. **Ans. d. Papillary carcinoma**
3. **Ans. b. Papillary**
4. **Ans. a. Papillary carcinoma of thyroid**
5. **Ans. c. Near total thyroidectomy with modified neck dissection**
6. **Ans. c. Excellent prognosis**
7. **Ans. a. Papillary carcinoma**
8. **Ans. c. Papillary carcinoma**
9. **Ans. d. Lateral aberrant thyroid**
10. **Ans. b. Papillary**
11. **Ans. a. Papillary carcinoma thyroid** *(Ref: Schwartz 11/e p1647, 10/e p1542; Sabiston 20/e p903)*
12. **Ans. a. Papillary carcinoma thyroid** *(Ref: Schwartz 11/e p1647, 10/e p1542; Sabiston 20/e p903)*
13. **Ans. b. Total thyroidectomy** *(Ref: Schwartz 11/e p1647; Sabiston 20/e p903)*

■ FOLLICULAR CARCINOMA

14. **Ans. d. Diagnosis by FNAC** *(Fef: Schwartz 11/e p1650, 10/e p1544, 1357; Sabiston 20/e p906; Bailey 27/e p818)*

LIMITATIONS OF FNAC IN THYROID DISEASES

1. **Not able** to **distinguish follicular adenoma** from **follicular carcinoma**[Q]
2. Not able to distinguish **Hurthle cell adenoma** from **Hurthle cell carcinoma**[Q]
3. **Useless** in **Reidel's thyroiditis**[Q] (Biopsy is preferred)[Q]
4. FNAC is **less reliable** in patients who have **history** of **head** and **neck irradiation** or **family history** of **thyroid cancer** due to higher likelihood of **multifocal lesions** and **occult cancer**[Q]

15. **Ans. a. Follicular**
16. **Ans. b. Follicular**
17. **Ans. a. Follicular carcinoma**
18. **Ans. a. Follicular**
19. **Ans. a. Radioiodine**
20. **Ans. a. Hematogenous spread**
21. **Ans. a. Follicular carcinoma**

■ MEDULLARY CARCINOMA

22. **Ans. a. Serum calcitonin** *(Ref: Schwartz 11/e p1655-1656, 10/e p1549-1550; Sabiston 20/e p909; Bailey 27/e p820; Harrison 20/e p2716)*
23. **Ans. c. Surgery only** *(Ref: Schwartz 11/e p1656, 10/e p1550; Sabiston 20/e p909; Bailey 27/e p820)*
24. **Ans. a. 5 years**
25. **Ans. a. Calcitonin** *(Ref: Schwartz 11/e p1656, 10/e p1549; Sabiston 20/e p909; Bailey 27/e p820)*
26. **Ans. c. CEA**
27. **Ans. c. Ret proto-oncogene**
28. **Ans. b. Medullary carcinoma**
29. **Ans. c. Medullary carcinoma**
30. **Ans. c. It is dependent on TSH**
31. **Ans. a. Medullary carcinoma thyroid** *(Ref: Schwartz 11/e p1656, 10/e p1550; Sabiston 20/e p909; Bailey 27/e p820)*
32. **Ans. c. Medullary carcinoma thyroid** *(Ref: Schwartz 11/e p1656, 10/e p1550; Sabiston 20/e p909; Bailey 27/e p820)*
33. **Ans. a. Medullary carcinoma thyroid** *(Ref: Schwartz 11/e p1656, 10/e p1541; Sabiston 20/e p909)*

■ ANAPLASTIC CARCINOMA

34. **Ans. d. Anaplastic carcinoma**
35. **Ans. d. Anaplastic**

■ THYROID METASTASIS

36. Ans. c. Breast *(Schwartz 11/e p1658, 10/e p1551)*

Metastatic Tumors of Thyroid

- Rare, most cases are found in autopsy
- MC site of primary: **CA Breast**[Q] > CA Lung
- If thyroid metastases is detected pre-mortem, MC site of primary: **RCC**[Q] >CA Breast > CA Lung

■ THYROID LYMPHOMA

37. Ans. b. Slow growing *(Ref: Schwartz 11/e p1657, 10/e p1551; Sabiston 20/e p910; Bailey 27/e p821; Harrison 19/e p2307)*

- Lymphomas of the thyroid gland are rapidly growing tumors and usually present with goiter that has grown significantly over a short period.

■ CARCINOMA THYROID

38. Ans. c. Papillary type

40. Ans. a. Papillary

39. Ans. b. Merkel cell

41. Ans. a. I^{131}

■ SOLITARY THYROID NODULE

42. Ans. c. Thyroid function test *(Ref: Sabiston 20/e p890; Harrison 20/e p2711)*

- **Initial investigation** done in **STN** is **thyroid function test** (TFT) [Q].
- **Investigation of choice** in **STN** for diagnosis is **FNAC**[Q].

Solitary Thyroid Nodule

- **Initial investigation** done in **STN** is **thyroid function test** (TFT) [Q].
- If **TFT** is **raised**, next investigation is **thyroid scan**, (For **hot nodules, RAI ablation** or **surgery** is done; For **warm or cold nodules, follow-up** or **surgery**) [Q]
- If **TFT** is **normal**, **USG** is **done** (**Aspiration** in **cystic lesions, FNAC** for **solid** or **heterogenous lesions**) [Q].
- **Investigation of choice** in **STN** for diagnosis is **FNAC**[Q].

43. Ans. d. FNAC

44. Ans. c. Right hemithyroidectomy

45. Ans. b. Removal of both lobes leaving behind 6-8 grams of tissue *(Ref: Sabiston 20/e p906; Bailey 27/e p814; Schwartz 11/e p1648, 10/e p1551)*

Surgery	Structure Removed
Hemithyroidectomy (Thyroid lobectomy)	Removal of **one lobe with isthmus**[Q]
Subtotal thyroidectomy	Removal of **both lobes leaving** behind 3-4 gms of tissue **in each lobe**[Q]
Near-total thyroidectomy	Leaving **<1 gm of tissue adjacent to RLN at ligament of Berry** on one side[Q]
Total thyroidectomy	Removal of **all visible thyroid tissue**[Q]
Hartley-Dunhill procedure	Removal of **one lobe with isthmus & second lobe partially (leaving 4-6 gms of thyroid tissue)**[Q]

46. Ans. b. FNAC

■ GOITER

47. Ans. b. Diffuse goiter *(Ref: Harrison 20/e p2711)*

Endemic Goiter

- Worldwide, **diffuse goiter** is most commonly caused by **iodine deficiency** and is termed **endemic goiter** when it affects **>5%**[Q] of the population.
- Endemic goiter occurs in **geographical areas** where the **soil, water** and **food** supply contains **low levels of iodine**[Q].
- The **lack of iodine** leads to decreased synthesis of thyroid hormones and a **compensatory increase in TSH** which in turn leads to **follicular cell hypertrophy** and **hyperplasia** and goitrous enlargement leading to **diffuse hyperplastic goiter**[Q].
- **Mostly, patients** are **euthyroid**[Q].

48. Ans. a. Neck *(Ref: Schwartz 11/e p1641, 10/e p1554)*

- Virtually **all intrathoracic goiters** can be **removed via a cervical incision**[Q].

49. Ans. d Hemithyroidectomy

■ RETROSTERNAL GOITER

50. Ans. a. Stridor

51. Ans. d. Transcervical *(Ref: Schwartz 11/e p1641, 10/e p1537; Sabiston 20/e p894; Bailey 27/e p810)*

■ THYROTOXICOSIS

52. Ans. a. **Inadequate control of hyperthyroidism** *(Ref: Schwartz 11/e p1638, 10/e p1534; Sabiston 20/e p920; Bailey 27/e p811, 758; Harrison 20/e p2712)*

53. Ans. a. **Carbimazole** *(Ref: Harrison 20/e p2706)*

54. Ans. a. **Carbimazole** *(Ref: Harrison 20/e p2706)*

55. Ans. a. **Diastolic murmur** *(Ref: Harrison 20/e p2704)*

56. Ans. b. **Radioactive iodine**

57. Ans. d. **Elevated serum CPK level**

- Both thyrotoxicosis and malignant hyperthermia may cause myopathy, but in hyperthyroidism serum CPK is often normal.

58. Ans. a. Inadequate control of hyperthyroidism

59. Ans. a. Hashimoto's thyroiditis

60. Ans. d. Hair loss

61. Ans. a. Iodides

62. Ans. c. Radioiodine

■ GRAVE'S DISEASE

63. Ans. a. **More common in males** *(Ref: Schwartz 11/e p1634, 10/e p1531-1533; Sabiston 20/e p892; Bailey 27/e p811; Harrison 20/e p2703)*

64. Ans. a. **Thyrotoxicosis**

65. Ans. c. **Common in male** *(Ref: Schwartz 11/e p1634, 10/e p; Sabiston 20/e p; Bailey 27/e p)*

■ HYPOTHYROIDISM

66. Ans. a. **Serum TSH level** *(Ref: Schwartz 11/e p1638, 10/e p1529; Sabiston 20/e p895; Bailey 27/e p802; Harrison 20/e p2701)*

- The **ultrasensitive TSH assay** has become the **most sensitive** and **specific test** for the **diagnosis of hyper- and hypothyroidism** and **for optimizing T$_4$ therapy**[Q].
- The **enhanced sensitivity** and **specificity of TSH assays** have **greatly improved laboratory assessment of thyroid function**[Q].

■ POST THYROIDECTOMY COMPLICATIONS

67. Ans. b. Close to the gland *(Schwartz 11/e p1658, 10/e p1551-1554; Sabiston 20/e p913; Bailey 27/e p813)*

- **Both superior** and **inferior thyroid vessels** should be **ligated close** to the **thyroid**[Q].
- Superiorly, **to avoid injury** to the **external branch** of the **superior laryngeal nerve**.
- Inferiorly, to **minimize devascularization of the parathyroids (extracapsular**[Q] **dissection)** or **injury to the RLN**[Q].

THYROIDECTOMY

- The **dissection plane** is kept as **close** to the **thyroid** as possible and the **superior pole vessels** are individually identified, skeletonized, ligated, and **divided low** on the **thyroid gland to avoid injury** to the **external branch** of the **superior laryngeal nerve**[Q]
- The **inferior thyroid vessels** are dissected, skeletonized, ligated, and **divided as close to the surface of the thyroid gland as possible** to **minimize devascularization of the parathyroids (extracapsular dissection)** or **injury to the RLN**[Q]. *-Schwartz 11/e p1658, 10/e p1553*

68. Ans. d. Hypercalcemia *(Ref: Schwartz 11/e p1662-1663, 10/e p1556; Sabiston 20/e p920; Bailey 27/e p815)*

69. Ans. b. 2–5 days

70. Ans. a. IV calcium gluconate

71. Ans. a. Respiratory obstruction

72. Ans. a. Hypocalcemia

73. Ans. c. Superior thyroid artery

■ THYROIDITIS

74. Ans. a. Anti-TPO *(Ref: Schwartz 11/e p1640, 10/e p1535; Sabiston 20/e p891; Bailey 27/e p821; Harrison 20/e p2699)*

75. Ans. a. Thyroid peroxidase antibodies

76. Ans. d. Orphan Annie eye nuclei

77. Ans. b. Hashimoto's disease

78. Ans. a. Hashimoto's thyroiditis

79. Ans. c. Hashimoto's thyroiditis

80. Ans. a. Autoimmune in etiology

81. Ans. c. In the thyrotoxic phase radioiodine uptake is increased

82. **Ans. c.** Thyroglobulins
83. **Ans. c.** Gaint cell infiltration

■ THYROGLOSSAL CYST AND FISTULA

84. **Ans. a.** Thyroglossal cyst *(Ref: Schwartz 11/e p1625, 10/e p1521; Sabiston 20/e p1861)*
85. **Ans. c.** Thyroglossal cyst   86. **Ans. c.** Subhyoid
87. **Ans. a.** Papillary
88. **Ans. c.** Excision of central part of hyoid bone and cone of tongue muscles up to foramen caecum

■ MISCELLANEOUS

89. **Ans. b.** Chromosome 7q *(Ref: Harrison 20/e p2693; Schwartz 10/e p1534)*

PENDRED'S SYNDROME

- Consists of **congenital sensorineural hearing loss + goitre**[Q]
- Due to defect in sulfate transport protein (chromosome 7q[Q]) to the thyroid gland and cochlea

Rafetoff Syndrome	**End organ resistance** to T4[Q]

90. **Ans. a.** Lingual thyroid *(Ref: Schwartz 11/e p1626, 10/e p1522)*
    Reddish swelling in the region of foramen caecum is Lingual thyroid.

LINGUAL THYROID

- Forms a **rounded swelling** at the **back of tongue** at the **foramen caecum**[Q]
- It may represent the **only thyroid tissue present**[Q]
- May cause dysphasia, impairment of speech, respiratory obstruction or hemorrhage
- **Medical treatment** options include administration of **exogenous thyroid hormone** to **suppress TSH** and **RAI ablation** followed by **hormone replacement**.
- **Surgical excision** is **rarely needed** but, if required, should be preceded by an evaluation of normal thyroid tissue in the neck to avoid inadvertently rendering the patient hypothyroid.

Parathyroid and Adrenal Glands

■ MULTIPLE ENDOCRINE NEOPLASIA

	MEN-1	MEN-2 (MEN-2A or Sipple syndrome)	MEN-3 (MEN-2B)	MEN-4 (MEN-X)
Components	• Parathyroid hyperplasia or adenoma[Q] • Pancreatic NET[Q] • Pituitary adenoma[Q] • Bronchial & thymic carcinoids[Q] • Adrenocortical tumors • Subcutaneous or visceral lipomas[Q] • Facial cutaneous angiofibromas[Q] • Collagenomas[Q]	• Medullary carcinoma thyroid[Q] • Pheochromocytoma[Q] • Parathyroid hyperplasia or adenoma[Q] • Hirschsprung's disease[Q] • Cutaneous lichen amyloidosis[Q]	• Medullary carcinoma thyroid[Q] • Pheochromocytoma[Q] • Intestinal ganglioneuroma[Q] • Mucosal neuromas[Q] • Megacolon[Q] • Marfanoid features[Q]	• Hyperparathyroidism • Pituitary adenoma • Pancreatic NET • Gonadal, adrenal, renal & thyroid tumors • (MEN-1 not having mutation of MEN1 gene is known as MEN-4)
Gene/Defect	MEN1 gene[Q]	RET oncogene (cysteine[Q] codon)	RET oncogene (tyrosine kinase[Q] domain)	Cyclin dependent kinase inhibitor (CDNKIB) gene
Chromosome	11	10[Q]	10[Q]	12
Transmission	Autosomal dominant[Q]	Autosomal dominant[Q]	Autosomal dominant[Q]	Autosomal dominant[Q]

MEN-1 (WERMER'S SYNDROME)

- Autosomal dominant[Q]
- **Defect:** MEN1 gene[Q] on chromosome **11**[Q] (encodes tumour suppressor protein, **menin**[Q])

Characteristic Features

Common Manifestations	Less Common Manifestations
• Parathyroid hyperplasia or adenoma[Q] • Pancreatic NET[Q] • Pituitary adenoma[Q]	• Bronchial and thymic carcinoids[Q] • Adrenocortical tumors • Subcutaneous or visceral lipomas[Q] • Facial cutaneous angiofibromas[Q] • Collagenomas[Q]

Parathyroid Gland

- **MC endocrine abnormality** (>98% of affected individuals) in MEN-1 is **multiglandular parathyroid tumors**[Q].
- **Hyperparathyroidism** is MC manifestation (**cardinal sign** of MEN-1 is **parathyroid adenoma** of **multicentricity**)[Q].
- **Parathyroid hyperplasia** is the MC cause of **hyperparathyroidism** in MEN-1.
- **Hypercalcemia** is **first biochemical abnormality**[Q] detected in MEN 1 and may precede the clinical onset of a pancreatic NET or pituitary neoplasm by several years.

Pancreatic Neuro-endocrine Tumors

- Pancreatic NET is **2nd MC manifestation**[Q].
- **Nonfunctioning** or that secrete **pancreatic polypeptide** are MC pancreatic NET in MEN-1[Q].
- MC **functional NET** in patients with MEN-1 is **gastrinoma**[Q] followed by insulinoma.
- MC increased pancreatic hormone: Pancreatic polypeptides >Gastrin >Insulin[Q]. (PGI)

Pituitary Adenoma

- **MC tumor:** Prolactinoma > Somatotrophinoma > Corticotrophinoma (**PSC**)

■ PRIMARY HYPERPARATHYROIDISM

PRIMARY HYPERPARATHYROIDISM

- PHPT arises from **increased PTH production**[Q] from abnormal parathyroid glands and results from a disturbance of normal feedback control exerted by serum calcium.
- More common in **women**[Q]

> - **Solitary adenoma**[Q] is the **MC cause** (in 80%)
> - **Parathyroid adenomas** are **most commonly located** in **inferior** parathyroid glands.

- Increased PTH production leads to **hypercalcemia** via:
  - **Increased GI absorption** of calcium
  - **Reduced renal calcium clearance**
  - **Increased** production of **vitamin D3**

Etiology

- Exposure to **low-dose therapeutic ionizing radiation** and **familial predisposition**[Q]
- Renal leak of calcium
- **Declining renal function** with age
- **Alteration in** the **sensitivity** of parathyroid glands to suppression by calcium
- **Lithium** therapy

Genetics

- **Most cases** of PHPT are **sporadic**

Clinical Features

- Patients with PHPT formerly presented with the **"classic" pentad** of symptoms:
  - **Kidney stones**[Q]
  - **Psychic moans**[Q]
  - **Painful bones**[Q]
  - **Fatigue overtones**[Q]
  - **Abdominal groans**[Q]
- Alteration in the "typical" patient with PHPT due to widespread use of automated blood analyzers.
- Patients are more likely to be minimally symptomatic or asymptomatic.
- Currently, **most patients** present with **weakness,** fatigue, **polydipsia, polyuria, nocturia, bone** and **joint pain, constipation**[Q], decreased appetite, nausea, heartburn, pruritus, depression, and memory loss.
- Renal **calculi** are typically composed of **calcium phosphate** or **oxalate**[Q].

Osteitis Fibrosa Cystica in Advanced PHPT
Pathognomonic radiologic findings on **X-rays** of **hands**, characterized by: • **Subperiosteal resorption**[Q] (most apparent on the **radial aspect**[Q] of **middle phalanx**[Q] of **2nd** and **3rd** fingers) • Bone cysts[Q] • **Tufting** of **distal phalanges**[Q]

Diagnosis

- **Elevated serum calcium** & **intact PTH** or two-site PTH levels, **without hypocalciuria** establishes the **diagnosis of PHPT** with virtual certainty[Q].
- **Decreased serum phosphate** (50%) & **elevated 24-hour urinary calcium** (60%) in **PHPT**[Q]

Localization

- ^{99m}**Tc-labeled sestamibi: Most widely used** & **accurate modality**[Q] (sensitivity >80% for detection of parathyroid adenomas)

Treatment

- **Parathyroidectomy** for patients having **"classic" symptoms** of PHPT or **<50 years**[Q]
- **SERM** and **bisphosphonates** are used to **lower serum calcium** and **increase BMD** in **PHPT.**

SECONDARY HYPERPARATHYROIDISM

- Secondary HPT **commonly occurs** in **chronic renal failure**[Q]
- May occur in hypocalcemia secondary to **inadequate calcium** or **vitamin D intake**, or **malabsorption**[Q].

Pathophysiology of HPT in Chronic Renal Failure

- Related to **hyperphosphatemia**[Q] (and resultant hypocalcemia)
- Deficiency of 1,25-dihydroxy vitamin D due to loss of renal tissue
- Low calcium intake
- Decreased calcium absorption
- Abnormal parathyroid cell response to extracellular calcium or vitamin D in vitro and in vivo.

Contd…

Contd…

Clinical Feature
- Patients generally are **hypocalcemic** or normocalcemic.

Treatment

> - **Low-phosphate diet, phosphate binders**, adequate intake of **calcium** and **1,25-dihydroxy vitamin D** and a high **calcium, low-aluminum dialysis bath**[Q].

- **Parathyroidectomy** should be considered if **PTH levels remain** high **despite optimal therapy**[Q].

■ TERTIARY HYPERPARATHYROIDISM

TERTIARY HYPERPARATHYROIDISM

- Development of autonomous parathyroid gland function, after long standing secondary hyperparathyroidism, most often in renal disease
- Cause problems similar to PHPT, such as pathologic fractures, bone pain, renal stones, peptic ulcer disease, pancreatitis, and mental status changes.
- **Operative intervention** is indicated in:
  - **Symptomatic disease**[Q]
  - If **autonomous PTH secretion** persists for **>1 year after** a successful **transplant**[Q].

Treatment
- **Subtotal** or **total parathyroidectomy** with **Autotransplantation + Upper thymectomy**[Q].

■ PARATHYROID CARCINOMA

PARATHYROID CARCINOMA

- Accounts for approximately **1%** of **PHPT** cases.

Clinical Features

Parathyroid Carcinoma is suspected preoperatively by	
Presence of **severe symptoms**[Q]	Serum **calcium levels > 14**[Q] mg/dL
Significantly **elevated PTH**[Q] levels (5 × normal)	

- **Palpable parathyroid**[Q] gland
  - **Local invasion**[Q] is most common; LN metastases in 15% & distant metastases in 33% at presentation.
  - **Intraoperatively:** Presence of a large, gray-white to gray-brown parathyroid **tumor adherent to** or **invasive into surrounding tissues**[Q] and enlarged LN.

Diagnosis
- **Histologic examination** that reveals **local tissue invasion, vascular or capsular invasion**[Q], trabecular or fibrous stroma, and frequent mitoses.

Treatments
- Parathyroid cancer: **Bilateral neck exploration + En-bloc excision** of **tumor** and ipsilateral **thyroid lobe** ± **MRND** in presence of LN metastases[Q]
- **Reoperation** for **locally recurrent** or **metastatic disease** to **control hypercalcemia**.
- **Cinacalcet**[Q] **(reduce PTH** levels by directly **binding** to **CASR cells** on parathyroid) is useful in **controlling hypercalcemia** in **refractory parathyroid carcinoma**.

■ INCIDENTALOMA

INCIDENTALOMA

- **Incidentally discovered adrenal masses** through imaging performed for unrelated/nonadrenal disease.
- Differential diagnosis includes both secreting & nonsecreting neoplasms.
- In patients with a **history of malignancy, metastatic disease** is the **most likely cause** of adrenal masses, particularly **when bilateral**[Q].
- In those **without a clear history of malignancy,** at least **80% of incidentalomas** will turn out to be **nonfunctioning cortical adenomas** or other **benign lesions** that **do not require surgical management**[Q].

Clinical Evaluation
- **Diagnostic work-up** of an incidentaloma is aimed at **identifying patients** that would **benefit from adrenalectomy**
- Workup for adrenal incidentaloma integrates **hormonal evaluation** with **size criteria**[Q].

Contd…

Contd...

- Evaluation begins with **history** taking, with a focus on **previous malignancy, hypertension**, and symptoms of **glucocorticoid** or **sex steroid excess**.
- **Biochemical investigations** for hormonally active tumors are followed by consideration of **size criteria**.
- Tumors **>6 cm** carry a **>25% risk for malignancy**[Q].

> - **CT-guided FNAC** is **rarely helpful**[Q] in the evaluation of adrenal masses and may be **hazardous**.
> - The **diagnosis** of **primary adrenal malignancy cannot be reliably based** on **cytologic criteria alone**[Q].

- **Use of FNAC** is generally confined to patients with a **history of extra-adrenal malignancy**[Q] in whom the clinician seeks to establish the diagnosis of **metastatic disease**[Q].
- **Pheochromocytoma must be excluded**[Q] before attempting such a procedure to avoid precipitating potentially fatal hypertensive crisis.

Treatments

- **Surgery** for **hormonally active tumors** and masses carrying **significant risk** for **malignancy**[Q].
- **Most incidentalomas** can be **removed laparoscopically**[Q], except for those displaying obvious malignant features on imaging.
- **Remove all incidentalomas** measuring **>5 cm** and to strongly consider removal of those measuring 3–5 cm, **follow up** with CT, every 6 months for **<3 cm**.

Indications of Surgery in Incidentaloma 3–5 cm	
1. **Suspicious** imaging characteristics (**heterogeneity, high attenuation**, or **irregular margins**)[Q] 2. **Young age**[Q]	3. **Few surgical risk factors**[Q] 4. **Interval tumor growth**[Q] 5. Patient preference

Adrenal Incidentalomas	
Tumor Types	**Percentage**
• **Presumed non-functional adenoma (MC)**	**82%**[Q]
• **Preclinical Cushing's**[Q]	5%
• **Pheochromocytoma**[Q]	5%
• **Adrenocortical carcinoma**	5%
• **Metastatic** carcinoma	2%
• Aldosterone producing adenoma	1%

■ ADRENOCORTICAL CARCINOMA

ADRENOCORTICAL CARCINOMA

- Adrenocortical carcinoma is a **rare tumor**
- **More than half** of adrenocortical carcinomas **are functional**[Q].
- **Cushing's syndrome**[Q] is **most commonly seen**, followed by virilization.

Pathology

- Microscopically: **Hyperchromatic cells** with and have **large nuclei**, prominent nucleoli.
- It is very difficult to distinguish benign adrenal adenomas from carcinomas by histologic examination alone.
- **Capsular** or **vascular invasion**[Q] is the **most reliable sign of cancer**.

Clinical Features

- Almost **all cases** occur in patients **40–50 years** of age
- **No gender predilection**
- **More than half** of adrenocortical carcinomas **are functional**.
- **Cushing's syndrome**[Q] is **most commonly seen**, followed by virilization.
- **Very large**[Q] at **initial evaluation** (mean tumor size, **9–12 cm**)
- Metastases to the lymph nodes, **liver**[Q], and lungs may be found.

Diagnosis

- **CT: Heterogeneous mass** with **irregular/indistinct borders, central necrosis**[Q], and invasion of adjacent structures.
- **Size** of adrenal mass is the **single most important criterion** to **diagnose malignancy**[Q]

Treatment

- **Radical open surgery: En-bloc resection** of **adjacent organs** or **regional lymphadenectomy**[Q] (or both).
- **Ketoconazole, aminoglutethimide** or **metyrapone (KAM)**: control **steroid hypersecretion**[Q].

Contd...

Contd…

Mitotane
• Principal chemotherapeutic agent, **derivative of** insecticide **DDT**[Q]
• Mitotane: Used as an **adjuvant to surgery** and as **primary therapy** in **unresectable** or **metastatic disease**[Q].
• Use is limited by **significant gastrointestinal** and **neurologic toxicity**[Q].

Prognosis

- Most **important predictor** of **survival: Adequacy of resection**[Q]

■ PHEOCHROMOCYTOMA

Section 1

Endocrine Surgery

PHEOCHROMOCYTOMA

- Tumors arise from **chromaffin cells**[Q] in adrenal medulla and elsewhere
- Peak incidence in **4th** and **5th** decade without any gender predilection
- **MC site of extra-adrenal tumor** is organ of **Zuckerkandl**[Q]
- **Extra-adrenal pheochromocytoma** is known as **paraganglioma**[Q].

Also Called 10% Tumor Because	
• 10% are **bilateral**[Q]	• 10% are **extra-adrenal**[Q]
• 10% are **malignant**[Q]	• 10% are **familial**[Q]
• 10% occur in **pediatric patients**[Q]	

Etiology and Risk Factors

- Either familial or sporadic. Familial can be syndromic or non-syndromic.

Syndromes Associated with **Pheochromocytoma (MVVS)**	
• **MEN-2A** and **MEN-2B**[Q]	• **Von-Recklinghausen syndrome**[Q] **(NF-1: MC)**
• **VHL syndrome**[Q]	• **Sturge-Weber syndrome**[Q]

- **Non-syndromic familial pheochromocytomas** are most commonly associated with **succinyl dehydrogenase D and B mutations**[Q].

Pathology

- Most are **unilateral & solitary**[Q]
- When pheochromocytoma develop in **MEN syndrome**, they are **rarely malignant**[Q]
- In contrast, patients with germline **SDHB mutation** appear to have **higher propensity** for **extra-adrenal** and **malignant tumors**[Q]
- Tumors are **not innervated**[Q], so catecholamines doesn't result from neural stimulation
- Tumors also secrete **endogenous opioids, adrenomedullin, erythropoetin, PTHrp, neuropeptide Y & chromogranin A**[Q].

> - **Most pheochromocytoma** produce both NA and Adr with **NA>Adr**[Q].
> - **Extra-Adrenal pheochromocytoma** secretes **NA exclusively**[Q] (Deficiency of enzyme PNMT-Phenylethanolamine-N-Methyltransferase).
> - Pheochromocytoma associated with **MEN** secretes **Adr alone**[Q].
> - Increased production of **dopamine and homovanillic acid** is usually seen in **malignant lesions**[Q].

Histologically Tumor Consists of

- Polygonal to spindle chromaffin cells clustered in small nests or alveoli (**Zelballen**) by a rich vascular network
- Nuclei are round with **salt & pepper chromatin**[Q]

> Criteria for **malignancy** are based **exclusively** on **presence of metastases**[Q] (because **capsular** or **vascular invasion** can be present in **benign tumors**)[Q]

Clinical Features

- Classic triad: **Headache + Diaphoresis+ Palpitation**[Q]
- **MC symptom** is **headache**[Q]
- **MC manifestation** is **hypertension**[Q] (remember hypertension is not a symptom)
- **Weight loss**[Q] due to increased energy expenditure

- **Cardiac manifestations:** Sinus tachycardia, sinus bradycardia, supraventricular arrhythmia and ventricular premature contractions
- **Carbohydrate intolerance** and increased hematocrit (**volume depletion**)

Diagnosis

Biochemical test:

- **Most sensitive screening test: Urinary catecholamines** and **VMA level**[Q]
- **Best test** for **diagnosis: Fractionated plasma metanephrines**[Q]

Contd…

Contd...

Pharmacological Test

- Positive response to **phentolamine** is reduction of BP of at least 35/25 mm Hg after 2 min. It is not diagnostic and biochemical confirmation is necessary.
- **Glucagon infusion** increases catecholamine release and causes **paroxysm of hypertension**[Q]

Imaging
- MRI is IOC for **adrenal**[Q], **extra adrenal pheochromocytoma**[Q] and in **pregnancy**[Q].
- MRI is **95% sensitive** and **100% specific** for pheochromocytoma[Q].
- CT scan should be performed **without contrast administration**[Q] to avoid hypertensive crisis.
- **MIBG scan** is useful for **extra-adrenal pheochromocytoma** but IOC is MRI[Q] even for extra adrenal pheochromocytoma.

> **Biopsy** is contraindicated as it **precipitates hypertensive crisis**[Q]

Treatment
- **Adrenalectomy is TOC**[Q].
- **Laparoscopic adrenalectomy** is preferred for **<5 cm tumors**[Q].
- **Pre-operatively alpha-blockers (phenoxybenzamine)**[Q] should be given.
- **Beta-blockers** are indicated **only if tachycardia develops** and should not be given until patient if **fully alpha blocked**[Q] to avoid hypertensive crisis due to unopposed alpha stimulation.

■ MALIGNANT PHEOCHROMOCYTOMA

MALIGNANT PHEOCHROMOCYTOMA

- Risk of malignancy increases with **size**[Q].
- Malignant tumors are more likely to express **p53, Bcl-2** and have **activated telomerase**[Q].

> - **Capsular** and **vascular invasion** may be seen in **benign lesions as well.**
> - **Malignancy** usually is **diagnosed** when there is evidence of **invasion** into **surrounding structures** or **distant metastasis**[Q].

- Increased production of **dopamine** and **homovanillic acid** is usually seen in **malignant lesions**[Q]
- **MC site of metastases is bone**[Q] > liver > lymph nodes.
- **Treatment: Resection** followed by **chemotherapy**[Q] **(cyclophosphamide + vincristine + dacarbazine)**

> **MDH:** Malignant pheochromocytoma secrete Dopamine **and HVA**[Q]

■ NEUROBLASTOMA

NEUROBLASTOMA

- Arise from **neural crest**[Q] and may originate anywhere along the distribution of sympathetic chain
- **MC tumor** diagnosed in **infants <1 year of age**[Q]
- **MC intra-abdominal malignancy** in **children**[Q]
- **Sporadic** in **majority** of cases

> - **MC site:** Adrenal (30%)[Q] > **Paravertebral reteroperitoneum**[Q] (28%) > **Posterior mediastinum**[Q] (15%) > **Pelvis (5%)** > **Cervical area**[Q]

- **Spontaneous regression** is unique behaviour especially in **stage 4S**[Q].

Pathology
- **Classic neuroblastomas:** Small, primitive-appearing cells with dark nuclei, scant cytoplasm
- **Mitotic activity**, nuclear breakdown (**"karyorrhexis"**)[Q], and **pleomorphism** may be prominent
- **Homer-Wright pseudorosettes**[Q] can be found
- Immunochemical detection of **neuron-specific enolase**[Q]

Clinical Features
- **MC presentation:** Fixed, lobular mass extending from the flank **toward the midline**[Q] of the abdomen
- **Most (80%) cases** present **before 4 years** and **peak incidence is 2 years**[Q] of age
- **Metastasis** is present in 60–70% of patients **at the time of diagnosis**[Q]

> - **Orbital metastasis** commonly present with **periorbital ecchymoses** and **proptosis** called as Raccoon eyes[Q].
> - Infants with **stage 4S** may display **cutaneous metastasis** called as **blueberry muffin lesions**[Q].
> - **Chronic watery diarrhea**[Q] (due to secretion of **VIP**) and **opsoclonus-myoclonus**[Q] (**dancing eyes, dancing feet**[Q]) are unusual paraneoplstic manifestations.

Contd...

Contd…

- **MC site** of **metastasis** in **older children** are **bones**[Q] (**Long bones–MC**, facial bones, skull particularly **sphenoid**), bone marrow and LN.
- In **infants** metastasis is confined to **liver** or **subcutaneous tissue**[Q].
- **Lung metastasis** are **rare**[Q] in **neuroblastoma**

Diagnosis

- Anemia, thrombocytopenia or **thrombocytosis** (more common)
- Increased LDH, ferritin, urinary catecholamines and neuron specific enolase
- **X-ray** or **CT: Stippled calcification**[Q] (MC abdominal tumor to demonstrate calcification prior to chemotherapy)

> - **Drooping Lily sign:** Neuroblastoma displaces **kidney inferolaterally**[Q]
> - **MRI**[Q] is **superior to CT** in assessing **vessel encasement**, vessel **patency**, **spinal cord compression** and **bone marrow involvement**.

- **MIBG scan** or **SRS** are used in the diagnosis of primary, residual and metastatic neuroblastoma.
- **MIBG** is one of the **single best studies** to document the **presence of metastatic**[Q] disease.

Treatment

- **Localized neuroblastoma: Excision**[Q]
- **Unresectable tumor: Biopsy**, initially treated by **chemotherapy** and **radiotherapy** followed by **surgical resection** of residual tumor[Q]
- **Disseminated disease: Chemotherapy**[Q] (Cyclophosphamide, vincristine, dacarbazine, doxorubicin, Cisplatin)

Prognosis

- **Shimada classification**[Q] describes prognosis based on the **degree of differentiation, mitosis-karyorrhexis index, presence** or **absence** of **Schwannian stroma**[Q].

International Neuroblastoma Staging System	
Stage	**Definition**
1	**Localized tumor** with **complete gross excision**, with or without microscopic residual disease; representative ipsilateral LNs negative for tumor microscopically (nodes attached to and removed with the primary tumor may be positive)
2A	Localized tumor with **incomplete gross excision**; representative ipsilateral nonadherent LNs negative for tumor microscopically
2B	Localized tumor with or without complete gross excision, with **ipsilateral nonadherent LNs**
3	**Unresectable unilateral tumor** with **contralateral regional LN involvement**; or midline tumor with **bilateral extension** by infiltration (unresectable) or by LN involvement
4	Any primary tumor with **dissemination** to **distant** LNs, bone, bone marrow, liver, skin, and/or other organs (except as defined for stage 4S)
4S	**Localized primary tumor** (as defined for stage 1, 2A, or 2B), with **dissemination limited to skin, liver**, and/or **bone marrow** (limited to infant **<1 year** of age)

Neuroblastoma Prognostic Factors

Favorable Prognosis	**Unfavorable Prognosis**
• Age **<1 year**[Q] • **Thoracic** primary lesion • **Shimada index** showing **well differentiated stromal rich** tumor[Q] • **Increased ratio** of VMA/HVA • **Normal** serum **ferritin** • **Hyperdiploid**[Q] or **near triploid**[Q] • **High level** of expression of **Trk-A gene**[Q]	• **N-myc amplification**[Q] (>10) • **Deletion** of **1p**[Q] (most characteristic cytogenetic abnormality) and **Gain** of **17q**[Q] • Expression of multidrug resistance protein • **Overexpression** of **telomerase**[Q] • **Increased** serum **ferritin** • Diploid[Q] • **Older patients** of **stages III** and **IV**[Q]

■ ESTHESIONEUROBLASTOMA

ESTHESIONEUROBLASTOMA (OLFACTORY NEUROBLASTOMA)

- Esthesioneuroblastoma is a **rare** unique tumor of **neural crest origin**[Q]
- Arises from the **basal neural cells** of the **olfactory mucosa** of the **cribiform plate**, upper nasal wall and superior turbinate[Q]
- Seen in **either sex** and most common in **3rd** and **4th** decade

Clinical Features

- Presents as a **unilateral polypoidal mass** in the **upper third** of the **nasal cavity** with symptoms of nasal obstruction, epistaxis and anosmia[Q]
- It is a **vascular tumor** that **bleeds profusely on biopsy**[Q]
- LN and systemic metastases can occur

Treatment

- Favored treatment is **surgical excision followed by radiation**[Q].

Multiple Choice Questions

■ MULTIPLE ENDOCRINE NEOPLASIA

1. **An infant is diagnosed with MEN-2B trait. Which the following will be best line of management?**
(Recent Question 2016, MHSSMCET 2007)
   a. Prophylactic surgery
   b. Clinical observation and follow up
   c. Regular FNAC
   d. All of the above

2. **Most common NET of pancreas seen in MEN-1:**
(Recent Question 2017)
   a. Gastrinoma
   b. Glucagonoma
   c. Insulinoma
   d. Somatostatinoma

3. **All of the following are true about MEN-I except:**
   a. Pituitary tumors   *(Recent Question 2017)*
   b. Parathyroid hyperplasia
   c. Medullary carcinoma
   d. Pancreatic endocrine tumors

4. **In MEN-2B prophylactic surgery in a child is indicated at:**
   a. 1 year   b. 3 years   *(Recent Question 2017)*
   c. 5 years   d. 10 years

■ PARATHYROID GLAND

5. **Treatment for parathyroid hyperplasia is:**   *(UPSC 2001)*
   a. Removal of all four glands
   b. Calcitonin
   c. Removal of 3½ glands
   d. Enlarged glands to be removed

6. **Parathyroid adenoma most commonly involves which of the following site:**   *(AIIMS June 2002)*
   a. Thyroid substance
   b. Superior parathyroid lobe
   c. Inferior parathyroid lobe
   d. In the mediastinum

7. **True about parathyroid carcinoma:**
   a. Parathyroid gland is palpable
   b. High calcium lebel
   c. Cinacalcet is used
   d. All of the above

8. **Commonest cause for hyperparathyroidism is:**
   a. Single adenoma
   b. Multiple adenomas
   c. Single gland hyperplasia
   d. Multiple gland hyperplasia

9. **Hypoparathyroidism occurs as a result of:**
   a. Idiopathic atrophy of parathyroids *(Recent Question 2015)*
   b. Following surgery
   c. Thyroiditis with secondary atrophy of parathyroids
   d. All of the above

10. **Hypocalcemia in immediate post-op period following excision of parathyroid adenoma is due to:**
   a. Stress   *(Recent Question 2015)*
   b. Increased uptake by bones
   c. Hypercalciuria
   d. Increased calcitonin

11. **Hyperparathyroidism is characterized by the following except:**   *(Recent Question 2016)*
   a. Generalized osteoporosis   b. Renal calculi
   c. Hypercalcemia   d. Osteosclerosis

12. **A patient has hypocalcaemia which was the result of a surgical complication. Which operation could it possibly have been?**   *(Recent Question 2015)*
   a. Nephrectomy   b. Thyroidectomy
   c. Gastrectomy   d. Vocal cord tumour biopsy

13. **A known patient with renal stone disease developed pathological fractures along with abdominal pain and certain psychiatric symptoms. He should be investigated for:**
(Recent Question 2016)
   a. Polycystic kidney   b. Renal tubular acidosis
   c. Hyperparathyroidism   d. Paget's disease of bone

14. **Which of the following is true about secondary hyperparathyroidism?**   *(Recent Question 2015)*
   a. Commonly occurs in CRF
   b. Related to hyperphophatemia
   c. Patients are generally hypocalcemic
   d. All of the above

15. **Parathyroid gland was implanted into forearm muscle. What is the type of transplantation?**   *(Recent Question 2016)*
   a. Orthotopic   b. Heterotopic
   c. Auxiliary   d. None

16. **Parathyroid autotransplantation is done in which of the following muscle?**   *(Recent Question 2019)*
   a. Brachioradialis   b. Biceps
   c. Triceps   d. Sartorius

17. **Which of the following is least sensitive for parathyroid imaging?**   *(Recent Question 2017)*
   a. USG   b. Sestamibi
   c. Sestamibi-SPECT   d. MRI

■ ADRENAL GLANDS

18. **During bilateral adrenalectomy, intra-operative dose of hydrocortisone should be given after:**   *(AIIMS Nov 2004)*
   a. Opening the abdomen
   b. Ligation of left adrenal vein
   c. Ligation of right adrenal vein
   d. Excision of both adrenal glands

19. **Parathyroid autotransplantation is done in which of the following muscle?**   *(Recent Question 2019)*
   a. Hyperparathyroidism
   b. Cushing's syndrome
   c. Zollinger-Ellison syndrome
   d. Adrenogenital syndrome

20. **Most common cause of Addison's disease in India:**
(AIIMS Nov 2011)
   a. Tuberculosis   b. Post-partum
   c. Autoimmune   d. HIV

21. **Indication for surgery in a case of adrenal incidentaloma:**
   a. Size >5 cm   *(MAHE 2008, 2007)*
   b. Bilateral adrenal metastasis
   c. Functional tumor
   d. All of the above

22. **True about adrenocortical carcinoma:** *(Recent Question 2016)*
    a. Rare tumor
    b. More than half are functional
    c. Most commonly associated with Cushing syndrome
    d. All of the above

23. **Which one of the following is not a CT feature of adrenal adenoma?** *(AIIMS Nov 2010)*
    a. Low attenuation
    b. Homogeneous density and well defined borders
    c. Enhances rapidly, contrast stays in it for relatively longer time and washes out late
    d. Calcification is rare

24. **Nonfunctional adrenal tumors are operated at what size:**
    a. >3 cm
    b. >5 cm *(MHSSMCET 2009)*
    c. >6 cm
    d. >10 cm

25. **Most prevalent incidentacoma is:** *(MHCET 2016)*
    a. Cushing's adenoma
    b. Pheochromocytoma
    c. Adrenocortical carcinoma
    d. Non-functioning adenoma

■ PHEOCHROMOCYTOMA

26. **Which one of the following clinical features is not seen in pheochromocytoma?** *(COMEDK 2011)*
    a. Hypertension
    b. Episodic palpitations
    c. Weight loss
    d. Diarrhea

27. **Episodic hypertension is a feature of:** *(JIPMER 2010)*
    a. Carcinoid tumor
    b. Insulinoma
    c. Pheochromocytoma
    d. Zollinger-Ellison syndrome

28. **All are true about pheochromocytoma except:**
    a. 90% are malignant *(All India 2011)*
    b. 95% occur in the abdomen
    c. They secrete catecholamines
    d. They arise from sympathetic ganglions

29. **Commonest symptom of pheochromocytoma is:** *(Recent Question 2015)*
    a. Palpitation
    b. Headache
    c. Sweating
    d. Dyspnea

30. **The most common site of ectopic pheochromo-cytoma is:**
    a. Organ of Zuckerkandl
    b. Bladder *(COMEDK 2008)*
    c. Filum terminale
    d. Celiac plexus

31. **Best way to localize extra-adrenal pheochromocytoma:** *(MCI June 2018)*
    a. X-ray
    b. Nucleotide scan
    c. VMA excretion
    d. Clinical examination

■ NEUROBLASTOMA

32. **All of the following are correct about neuroblastoma except:**
    a. Arises from adrenal cortex *(Recent Question 2017)*
    b. Can cause paraplegia
    c. May cause hypertension
    d. Secretes hormones

33. **Tumor arising from olfactory nasal mucosa is:**
    a. Nasal glioma *(All India 2012)*
    b. Adenoid cystic carcinoma
    c. Nasopharyngeal carcinoma
    d. Esthesioneuroblastoma

Explanations

■ MULTIPLE ENDOCRINE NEOPLASIA

1. **Ans. a. Prophylactic surgery** *(Ref: Schwartz 11/e p1677, 10/e p1550; Sabiston 20/e p1008)*

Prophylactic Thyroidectomy in RET Mutation Carriers	
MEN-2A	Before **5 years**[Q]
MEN-2B	Before **1 year**[Q]

2. **Ans. a. Gastrinoma** *(Ref: Sabiston 20/e p1000; Schwartz 11/e p1136, 10/e p1071; Bailey 27/e p857)*

3. **Ans. c. Medullary carcinoma** *(Ref: Sabiston 20/e p998; Schwartz 11/e p1677, 10/e p289; Bailey 27/e p857)*

4. **Ans. a. 1 year** *(Ref: Sabiston 20/e p1008; Schwartz 11/e p1677, 10/e p1550; Bailey 27/e p858)*

■ PARATHYROID GLAND

5. **Ans. c. Removal of 3½ glands** *(Ref: Harrison 20/e p2928; Schwartz 11/e p1671, 10/e p156; Sabiston 20/e p931)*

TREATMENT OF PRIMARY HYPERPARATHYROIDISM

- **Initial correction** of **hypercalcemia** (Rapid IV Normal saline with **furosemide**)[Q]
- **Neck exploration** is done and treatment is done accordingly

A **single parathyroid adenoma (85%)**[Q]	• **Resection**[Q]
Two adenomas (5%)	• **Resection**[Q]
Hyperplasia of all four glands (10-15%)	• **Resection** of **3½ glands**[Q] • **Resection** of **all four glands** with **autotransplantation** of a parathyroid gland in the forearm (**brachioradialis**) or **SCM muscle**[Q]

PARATHYROID AUTOTRANSPLANTATION

- Whenever **multiple parathyroids** are **resected**, it is preferable to **cryopreserve tissue**, so that it may be autotransplanted should the patient become hypoparathyroid[Q].
- Approx. **12–14 pieces** of 1 mm are transplanted into the **nondominant forearm** in belly of **brachioradialis**[Q] muscle

6. **Ans. c. Inferior parathyroid lobe** *(Ref: Harrison 20/e p2925)*
   - **Parathyroid adenomas** are **most commonly located** in **inferior**[Q] parathyroid glands.

7. **Ans. d. All of the above** *(Ref: Schwartz 11/e p1677, 10/e p1560; Sabiston 20/e p937; Bailey 27/e p835)*

8. **Ans. a. Single adenoma**

9. **Ans. b. Following surgery** *(Ref: Schwartz 11/e p1681, 10/e p1574; Sabiston 20/e p936; Bailey 27/e p825)*

PARATHYROID INSUFFICIENCY OR HYPOPARATHYROIDISM

- Mostly due to **removal of the parathyroid glands** or **infarction due to vascular injury**[Q].
- **Vascular injury**[Q] is more important.
- Cases usually present **2–5 days after operation**[Q] with symptoms of **hypocalcemia** (circumoral and fingertip numbness and tingling tetany, carpopedal spasm and laryngeal stridor)[Q]
- Treatment with **oral calcium** and **vitamin D supplements**[Q]
- **IV calcium gluconate**[Q] may be required in severe cases.

10. **Ans. b. Increased uptake by bones** *(Ref: Schwartz 11/e p1681, 10/e p73)*

> **HUNGRY BONE SYNDROME**
>
> - **Hypocalcemia** in **immediate postoperative period** following excision of parathyroid adenoma is due to **increased uptake by bones**[Q].
> - It is known as **Hungry Bone Syndrome**

11. **Ans. d. Osteosclerosis**

12. **Ans. b. Thyroidectomy**

13. **Ans. c. Hyperparathyroidism**

14. **Ans. d. All of the above** *(Ref: Schwartz 11/e p1679, 10/e p1572-1573; Sabiston 20/e p927-928; Bailey 27/e p833; Harrison 20/e p2933)*

15. **Ans. b. Heterotopic**

16. **Ans. a. Brachioradialis** *(Ref: Schwartz 11/e p1676, 10/e p1569; Sabiston 20/e p936; Bailey 27/e p830)*

> *"Total parathyroidectomy requires complete resection of all glands combined with immediate heterotopic transplantation of several 1- to 3-mm slices of fresh parathyroid tissue into individual pockets created in the brachioradialis muscle of the nondominant forearm." Sabiston 20/e p936*

17. **Ans. d. MRI** *(Ref: Sabiston 20/e p930; Schwartz 11/e p1672, 10/e p1565; Bailey 27/e p828)*

■ ADRENAL GLANDS

18. **Ans. d. Excision of both adrenal glands** *(Ref: Schwartz 11/e p1691, 10/e p1590-1590)*

> - Patients undergoing surgical treatment of endogenous hypercortisolism require glucocorticoid replacement.
> - Steroids are not given pre-operatively because these patients are already hypercortisolemic.
> - Instead **hydrocortisone** 100 mg IV is **given after** the **removal** of **second hyperplastic adrenal gland.**

19. **Ans. a. Hyperparathyroidism** *(Ref: Harrison 20/e p2923; Sabiston 20/e p925)*

20. **Ans. a. Tuberculosis** *(Ref: ASI 7/e p1073)*
    - **Most common cause** of **adrenal insufficiency (Addison's disease)** in **developing countries** is **Tuberculosis**[Q] followed by autoimmune disorders.

21. **Ans. d. All of the above** *(Ref: Schwartz 11/e p1697, 10/e p1589; Sabiston 20/e p985-987; Bailey 27/e p839; Harrison 20/e p2731)*

22. **Ans. d. All of the above** *(Ref: Schwartz 11/e p1696, 10/e p1588; Sabiston 20/e p979-980; Bailey 27/e p843; Harrison 20/e p2732)*

23. **Ans. c. Enhances rapidly, contrast stays in it for a relatively longer time and washes out late** *(Ref: Grainger Radiology 4/e p1388; Dahnert Wolfgang Radiology Review Manual 6/e p919)*

> - **Adrenal adenoma** on **contrast enhanced CT/MRI** show **rapid uptake** and relatively **rapid washout** of **contrast**[Q] material than do non adenomas.

CT Features of Adrenal Adenoma	
• Well defined /sharply defined[Q] • <5 cm in size[Q] • Low attenuation (<10 HU) due to lipid content[Q] • Mild homogenous enhancement	• Relatively rapid washout of contrast material (due to lack of large interstitial spaces) [Q] • Relatively rapid washout is characteristic of adenoma[Q]

24. **Ans. b. >5 cm**

25. **Ans. d. Non-functioning adenoma**

■ PHEOCHROMOCYTOMA

26. **Ans. d. Diarrhea** *(Ref: Schwartz 11/e p1693, 10/e p1586; Sabiston 20/e p980-985; Bailey 27/e p845; Harrison 20/e p2740)*

27. **Ans. c. Pheochromocytoma**

28. **Ans. a. 90% are malignant**

Management of Pheochromocytoma

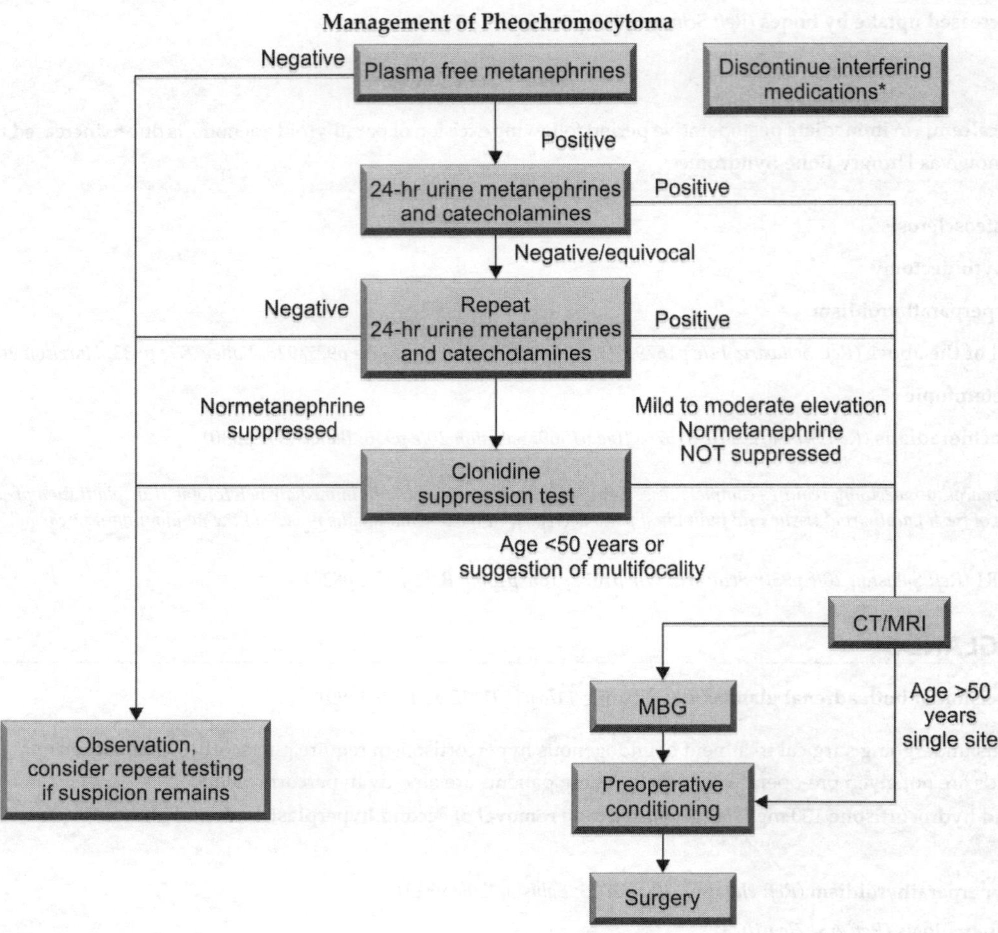

29. **Ans. b.** Headache

30. **Ans. a.** Organ of Zuckerkandl

31. **Ans. b.** Nucleotide scan *(Ref: Schwartz 11/e p1694, 10/e p1586; Sabiston 20/e p980; Harrison 20/e p2741)*

◼ NEUROBLASTOMA

32. **Ans. a.** Arises from adrenal cortex *(Ref: Sabiston 20/e p1887; Schwartz 11/e p1748, 10/e p1639; Bailey 27/e p847)*

33. **Ans. d.** Esthesioneuroblastoma *(Ref: Dhingra 5/e p217-218; Washington Manual of Surgical Pathology 2/e p45; Harrison 20/e p656)*

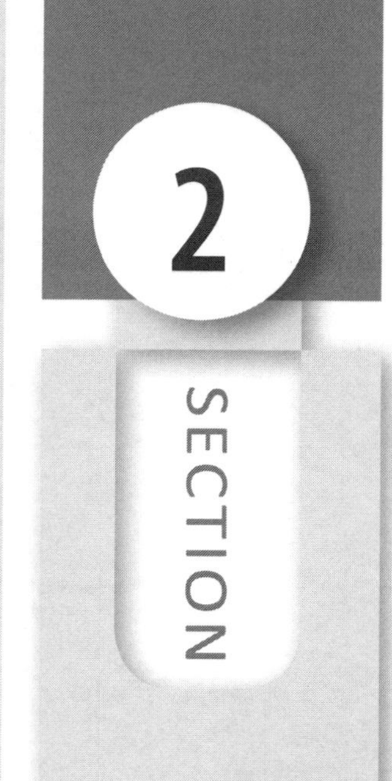

Hepatobiliary Pancreatic Surgery

- Liver
- Portal Hypertension
- Gallbladder
- Bile Duct
- Pancreas

Liver

■ PYOGENIC LIVER ABSCESS

<table>
<tr><td colspan="2" align="center">PYOGENIC LIVER ABSCESS</td></tr>
</table>

- Liver is **MC site** of **abdominal visceral abscess**[Q]
- PLA accounts for **majority** of hepatic abscesses[Q]

E. coli	MC in **western countries**[Q]
Klebsiella pneumoniae	MC in **Asian countries**[Q]
Staphylococcus	MC in **children**, suffering from **chronic granulomatous disease**[Q]

- **Multiple abscesses** occur in patients with a **biliary origin**[Q]
- **Solitary abscesses** are more likely than multiple abscesses to be **polymicrobial**.

Routes of Infection in PLA
• **Biliary tract (MC)**[Q]
• **Portal vein (2nd MC)**[Q]
• **Hepatic artery**[Q]
• **Direct extension**
• Penetrating or blunt trauma
• Cryptogenic

Clinical Features
- **MC presenting symptom** is **fever**[Q].
- **MC LFT abnormality** is an elevation of **ALP**[Q].
- **Classic presentation**: Fever, **jaundice (25%)**[Q], right upper quadrant pain & tenderness
- **Fever, chills**, & **abdominal pain** are the most common presenting symptoms
- Usually **single**, involve **right lobe**[Q]

Diagnosis
- **USG & CT** are the **main diagnostic modalities**[Q]
- **Diagnosis is confirmed** by **aspiration & culture**[Q]
- **CXR:** Elevated hemidiaphragm, right sided pleural effusion or atelectasis

Treatment
- **Percutaneous catheter drainage + IV antibiotics** has become the **treatment of choice**[Q].
- After 2 weeks of parenteral antibiotics, oral agents should be used for further 4 weeks.

■ AMOEBIC LIVER ABSCESS

<table>
<tr><td align="center">AMOEBIC LIVER ABSCESS</td></tr>
</table>

- Caused **by Entamoeba histolytica** whose cysts are acquired through the **feco-oral route**[Q]
- Trophozoites reach the liver through **portal venous system**[Q].

• **Solitary** and **more common** in **right lobe of liver**[Q].

- Majority of patients are **young men**

Pathogenesis
- MC form of invasive disease is **colitis**, frequently affects the **cecum & ascending colon**[Q]
- In colon: **Flask-shaped ulcers**[Q] (MC site: Cecum & ascending colon)[Q]
- **Synchronous hepatic abscess** is found in **one third** of patients with **active amebic colitis**.

Clinical Features
- **MC symptom** is abdominal pain[Q]
- **Typical clinical picture**: Patient of **20-40 yrs of age,** with history of travel to **endemic area**, presents with **fever**, chills, anorexia, **right upper quadrant pain**[Q].

Contd…

Contd...

- Results from an obligatory colonic infection, a **recent history** of **diarrhea** are **uncommon**[Q].

> - **Active colitis** and **amoebic liver abscess rarely occur simultaneously**, as a rule **colonic lesions** are **silent**[Q]
> - **Jaundice is rare**[Q]
> - **Raised PT is MC LFT abnormality**[Q].

Diagnosis

- **USG** and **CT** are the **main diagnostic modalities**[Q]

> - **Diagnosis** is **confirmed** by **serological tests**[Q] (**ELISA**) for antiamoebic antibodies.
> - **Cultures** of amoebic abscess are **usually sterile** or **negative**[Q].

- **CXR:** Elevated hemidiaphragm, right sided pleural effusion or atelectasis
- **ALA: Reddish-brown anchovy paste**[Q]; **more reliable characteristic** than color is the **odour** of the fluid.

Treatment

- **Metronidazole** (750 mg orally TDS × 10-14 days) is the **mainstay of treatment** and is **curative in** over **90%** of patients[Q], clinical improvement is seen within 3 days.
- **Luminal agents** include **iodoquinol, paromomycin & diloxanide furoate**[Q].
- Average time to **radiologic resolution** of abscess is **3-9 months**

Indications of Aspiration in ALA	
1. Diagnostic uncertainty[Q]	4. **High risk of rupture** (size **>5 cm**, **left lobe abscess**)[Q]
2. **Failure to respond** to therapy in 3-5 days[Q]	5. **Pregnancy**[Q] (Therapeutic trial with high dose
3. **Pyogenic superinfection**[Q]	Metronidazole is deemed inappropriate)

Complications

- Most frequent complications: Rupture into the **peritoneum (MC)**[Q], pleural cavity, or pericardium.
- **Size** of **abscess** appears to be the **most important risk factor** for rupture

■ HYDATID DISEASE

HYDATID DISEASE

- Hydatid disease is a **zoonosis**, occurs primarily in **sheep-grazing areas**[Q] of the world
- **Endemic in Mediterranean countries, Middle East, Far East, South America, Australia, New Zealand, & East Africa.**

> - **Humans** contract the **disease from dogs**, and there is **no human-to-human transmission**[Q].
> - Hydatid cyst is caused by **Echinococcus granulosus**[Q].
> - Other species affecting human beings: E. **multilocularis**, E. **vogelli**, E. **oligarthus**[Q]
> - **Malignant hydatidosis is caused by E. multilocularis**[Q]

Life-cycle

- **Dogs** are the **definitive host**[Q] of E. granulosus
- Eggs are passed (up to thousands of ova daily) and deposited with the dog's feces.

> - **Sheep**: Usual **intermediate host**[Q]
> - **Human: Accidental dead end intermediate host**[Q] without human to human transmission

- In the **human duodenum**, parasitic embryo releases an **oncosphere**, that **penetrate mucosa**, allowing access to **bloodstream**[Q].
- In the blood, **oncosphere** reaches **liver (MC)**[Q] or **lungs**, develops its **larval stage, hydatid cyst**.
- Organs most commonly involved are: **Liver >Lungs >Spleen >Kidney >Brain >Bone**[Q].

Hydatid Cyst
• Three weeks after infection, a visible hydatid cyst develops
• The cyst wall has two layers:
– **Ectocyst**: outer **gelatinous** membrane[Q]   – **Endocyst**: inner **germinal** membrane[Q]
• **Pericyst**: Fibrous capsule **derived from host tissues**, develops around the hydatid cyst.

- **Scoleces develop** into an **adult tapeworm** in **definitive host**[Q]
- Scoleces **differentiate into** a **new hydatid cyst** in **intermediate host**[Q]
- **Hydatid sand: Freed brood capsules** and **scoleces** in the hydatid fluid

Clinical Features

- **Equally common** in males & females, age of **45 years**.
- **Most** (75%) are **singular**, located in **right liver** (VII & VIII)[Q].
- **Mostly asymptomatic**[Q] until complications occur

> - **MC presenting symptoms**: Abdominal pain, dyspepsia & vomiting.
> - **MC sign: Hepatomegaly**[Q]

Contd…

- **Complications**: Rupture of the cyst into the **biliary tree (MC)**[Q] or **bronchial tree**, or free rupture into **peritoneal, pleural,** or **pericardial cavities**.
- **Intrabiliary rupture** is MC complication of hydatid liver cysts[Q]
- Free ruptures can result in disseminated echinococcosis and a potentially fatal anaphylactic reaction.

Diagnosis

- **USG** and **CT** are the **main diagnostic modalities**[Q]
  - **Daughter cyst** within the **large cyst (rosette appearance)** & **calcification** of **wall** are **highly suggestive** of **hydatid cyst**[Q].

> - **Diagnosis is confirmed** by **serological tests**[Q] (ELISA, Immunoblot, Arc-5, IHA) for antibodies.
> - **Ring like calcification** on **CECT** is seen in **hydatid cyst**[Q]

- In cases of **suspected biliary involvement (Jaundice)**, ERCP **(gold standard)**[Q] or PTC is necessary.

Treatment

- **Most cysts** are **treated surgically**[Q]
- **Conservative management** is appropriate in **elderly** patients with **small, asymptomatic, densely calcified cysts**[Q].
- **Treatment options**: PAIR, pericystectomy, marsupialization, leaving the cyst open, drainage of the cyst, omentoplasty, or partial hepatectomy to encompass the cyst.
- Currently, **PAIR** is the **preferred method** of **treatment**[Q] for **anatomically** & **surgically appropriate lesions**

> **Surgery remains the treatment of choice for cysts where**
> - **PAIR** is **not possible** or **cysts** are **refractory to PAIR**[Q]
> - For **complicated cysts** (communicating with biliary tract)[Q]

- **Radical (resection)** and **conservative (drainage & evacuation)** surgical approaches appear to be **equally effective** at controlling disease.
- **Pericystectomy** is the **preferred surgical approach**[Q] (complete cyst with surrounding fibrous tissue are removed)
- If surgical **cystectomy** is **not** technically **feasible**, then formal **liver resection** can be done.

> **Chemotherapy in Hydatid Disease**
> - Chemotherapy with **albendazole** or **mebendazole** is effective at **shrinking** the **cysts**
> - **Cyst disappearance** occurs in **fewer than 50%** of patients[Q].
> - **Preoperative treatment** may **decrease the risk for spillage**[Q] and is a reasonable and safe practice.
> - **Chemotherapy without definitive resection** or drainage is only considered **for:**
>   - **Widely disseminated disease**[Q]
>   - Patients with **poor surgical risk**[Q]

> **Treatment of E. multilocularis**
> - E. multilocularis cyst is **always multiloculated**[Q].
> - Treatment is **surgical resection**[Q].

■ PAIR

> **PAIR (Puncture, Aspiration of cyst content, Injection of scolicidal agent, and Reaspiration)**

- Currently, **PAIR** is **preferred method** of **treatment**[Q] for **anatomically** & **surgically appropriate lesions**
- The **efficacy of PAIR** in managing hydatid cysts is **>75%**.
- During PAIR, patient is given **prophylactic coverage of albendazole**

Scolicidal Agents

- **Hypertonic (20%) saline**[Q]: 100% scolicidal with contact time of 6 minutes
- 0.5% **cetrimide** with 0.05% **chlorhexidine**[Q]
- **Absolute alcohol**[Q]
- 10% **povidone iodine**[Q]

Contraindications of PAIR

- **Superficially located cysts**[Q]
- **Inaccessible** or **hazardous location**[Q] of cyst
- Cysts with **multiple internal septal**[Q] divisions (**honeycombing** pattern)
- **Dead** or **inactive cysts**[Q]
- Cysts **communicating with biliary tree**[Q]
- **Lung** or **brain cysts**[Q]

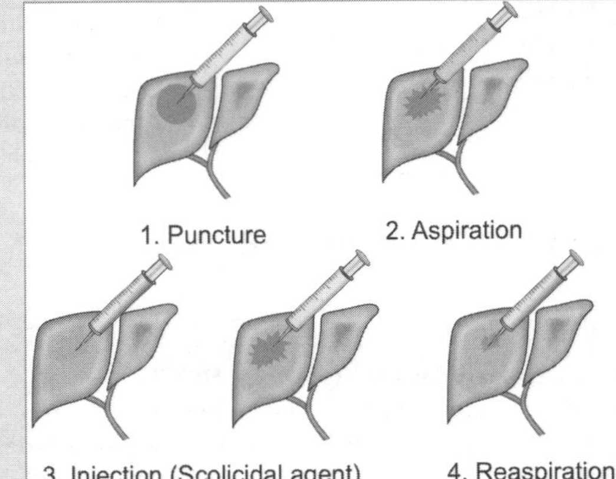

■ ACTINOMYCOSIS OF LIVER

ACTINOMYCOSIS OF LIVER

- Most commonly, Actinomyces **reaches liver through portal vein**[Q].
- **Liver** is gradually replaced by **multiple abscesses**, typical **honey comb liver**[Q]

Diagnosis

- Needle aspiration: **Actinomyces in pus**[Q]

Treatment

- Antibiotic **(Penicillin)** is the **DOC**[Q].

■ HEPATIC CYST

SIMPLE HEPATIC CYST

- Contain **serous fluid**, **do not communicate** with the biliary tree, and **do not have septations**[Q]
- **Single** in 50% cases[Q]

Treatment

- Nonsurgical treatment: **Aspiration** and **injection** of a **sclerosing agent** (most frequently **ethanol**)[Q].
- Surgical therapy: **Fenestration** or **unroofing** the **extrahepatic** portion of cyst[Q].

Complication

- **MC complication: Intracystic bleeding**[Q].

■ LIVER TUMORS

- **MC malignancy of liver: Metastasis**[Q]
- **MC primary malignancy of liver: HCC**[Q]
- **MC primary malignancy of liver in children: Hepatoblastoma**[Q]
- **MC benign tumor of liver: Hemangioma**[Q]

■ RISK FACTORS FOR HEPATOCELLULAR CARCINOMA

Conditions Associated with Hepatocellular Carcinoma					
1. Cirrhosis		**2. Metabolic diseases**		**3. Environmental**	
Condition	**Risk**	**Condition**	**Risk**	**Condition**	**Risk**
• HBV[Q]	High	• Hereditary **hemochromatosis**[Q]	High	• **Thorotrast**	Moderate
• HCV[Q]	High	• Hereditary **tyrosinemia**[Q]	High	• Androgenic **steroids**[Q]	Moderate
• **Alcohol**[Q]	High	• **Alpha-1 antitrypsin deficiency**	Moderate	• Cigarette **smoking**[Q]	Low to moderate
• Autoimmune chronic active hepatitis	High	• **Ataxia telangiectasia**[Q]	Moderate	• Aflatoxin[Q]	Moderate
• Cryptogenic cirrhosis	Moderate	• Types 1 & 3 glycogen storage disease	Moderate		
	Moderate	• **Galactosemia**[Q]	Moderate		
• Cirrhosis due to **NAFLD**[Q]		• **Citrullinemia**	Moderate		
		• Hereditary hemorrhagic telangiectasia	Moderate		
• **Primary biliary cirrhosis**[Q]	Low	• **Porphyria cutanea tarda**	Moderate		
		• **Wilson's disease**[Q]	Low		
		• Orotic aciduria	Moderate		
		• **Alagille's syndrome**[Q] (congenital cholestatic syndrome)	Moderate		

■ HEPATOCELLULAR CARCINOMA

HEPATOCELLULAR CARCINOMA

- **MC primary liver malignancy** is HCC[Q]
- HCC represents **MC solid organ cancers**[Q].
- **HCC: MC malignancy** responsible for **death in patients with cirrhosis**.

Contd…

Contd…

HEPATOCELLULAR CARCINOMA

- **MC primary liver malignancy** is **HCC**[Q]
- **HCC** represents **MC solid organ cancers**[Q].
- **HCC: MC malignancy** responsible for **death in patients with cirrhosis.**

> - More prevalent in **Asia** & **sub Saharan Africa**[Q] (high frequency of **chronic infection** with **HBV** & **HCV**[Q])
> - **100 folds increase** in risk in individuals with **HBV infection**[Q]

- More common in **males**, **60-90%** arise in **cirrhotic liver**[Q]
- **Post necrotic cirrhosis** has **highest risk**[Q] of developing into HCC
- **Alcoholic cirrhosis** & Primary biliary cirrhosis has **lower risk**[Q]

> - **Strong propensity** for **invasion of vascular channels**[Q]

Pathology
- **Gross Morphology:** Hanging, **pushing** & **invasive** tumors[Q].

Clinical Features
- **MC symptom** is **abdominal pain >weight loss**[Q]

> **Significant weight loss: 5% in 1 month or 10% in 6 months or 20% in 1 year**[Q]

- Usually presents at **late stage**[Q], symptoms at advanced stage are **vague**
- Non-specific symptoms (anorexia, weight loss) and **Hepatomegaly**[Q]

> **Paraneoplastic Syndromes in HCC**
> - **Hypercholesterolemia (MC)**[Q] **>hypoglycemia**[Q], erythrocytosis, hypercalcemia

- **Vascular bruit** (**25%**), GI bleed (10%), tumor rupture (2-5%), jaundice due to biliary obstruction (10%), paraneoplastic syndrome (<5%).

Tumor Markers
- Protein induced by Vitamin K Absence (**PIVKA**; Des-gamma-Carboxy Prothrombin); **glypican-3**; **AFP** fractions[Q]

> - Lectin fraction-3 of AFP (**AFP-L3**) is **highly specific to HCC** and also an indicator of **poorly-differentiated** histology and **unfavorable prognosis**[Q]
> - Serum **AFP** level is elevated above **20 ng/mL** in **>70%** of patients with HCC.

Diagnosis

> **Non-invasive Diagnostic Criteria for HCC**
> - **Focal lesion 1-2 cm: Two** imaging **techniques** with **arterial hypervascularization** & **venous washout**[Q].
> - **Focal lesion >2 cm: One** imaging **technique** with **arterial hypervascularization** & **venous washout**[Q].
> - Techniques to be considered: Dynamic CT & MRI.

- **Screening** is based on regular **ultrasound scanning** in **high risk population**[Q]
- **Biopsy** proof of HCC is **not required**[Q]

Treatment
- **Complete excision**[Q] by **partial hepatectomy** or by **total hepatectomy** and **transplant** is the only treatment modality with **curative** potential[Q].

> Remember: **Only 15-20% of HCC is resectable, because rest of the tumors have**
> - Multicentricity, Bilobar involvement[Q]
> - Portal vein invasion, Lymphatic metastasis[Q]

Okuda Staging System for HCC (BATA)[Q]		
Clinical parameter	Cut-off value	Points
Serum **B**ilirubin	<3 >3	0 1
Serum **A**lbumin	>3 <3	0 1
Tumor size	<50% >50%	0 1
Ascites	Absent Present	0 1
Stage I = 01; Stage II = 1–2 points; Stage III = 3–4 points.		

Cancer of the Liver Italian Program (CLIP)

- Components: **PACT** (Portal vein thrombosis, AFP levels, Child-Pugh stage, Tumor extension)[Q]
- CLIP system is applicable to **Hepatitis C-related** HCC cases[Q]

Chinese University Prognostic Index

- Components: **BA$_3$TS** (Bilirubin; A$_3$: Ascites, AFP, ALP; TNM stage; **Symptoms**)[Q]
- Applicable to **HBV** related HCC in **China**[Q].

Barcelona Clinic Liver Cancer Staging System

- It was developed to allow for the **indication** of the **best therapy** for **each stage of HCC**[Q] and is **best suited** for **treatment guidance** and to **select early-stage patients** who could benefit from **curative therapies**.
- It divides patients into four major groups (early, intermediate, advanced and end stage)
- It considers variables related to **tumor stage, liver functional status, physical status** and **cancer related symptoms**[Q].

Treatment Options for Hepatocellular Carcinoma	

1. Surgical:
  – Resection
  – Orthotopic liver transplantation
	4. Transarterial:
	  – Embolization
	  – Chemoembolization
	  – Radiotherapy

2. Ablative:
  – Ethanol injection
  – Acetic acid injection
  – Thermal ablation (**cryotherapy, radiofrequency ablation, microwave**)
	5. Systemic:
	  – Chemotherapy
	  – Hormonal
	  – Immunotherapy

3. Combination Transarterial and Ablative	**6. External-beam Radiation Therapy**

■ FIBROLAMELLAR HEPATOCELLULAR CARCINOMA

FIBROLAMELLAR HCC

- Occurs in **young adults without underlying cirrhosis**[Q]
- **Non-encapsulated** but well, circumscribed, so **high resectability rate**[Q]
- **Grows slowly** and & has **better prognosis**[Q]

Pathology

- **Well demarcated** & **non-encapsulated** and may have a **central fibrotic area**[Q].
- Composed of **large polygonal tumor cells** embedded in a **fibrous stroma** forming **lamellar structures**

> - **Calcification**[Q] differentiates FHCC from FNH in **35-55%** of **FHCC; heterogeneous enhancement**[Q] is also an important imaging finding.

Clinical Features

- Occurs in **younger patients**[Q] without a history of cirrhosis.

> - FHCC does not produce AFP[Q]
> - Associated with **elevated neurotensin**[Q] & Vitamin B$_{12}$ **binding globulin levels**[Q]

Treatment

- **Better prognosis** than HCC due to **high resectability rates, lack of chronic liver disease**, and a more **indolent course**[Q].
- Presence of **lymph node metastases** predicts a **worse outcome**[Q].

■ COLORECTAL LIVER METASTASIS

COLORECTAL LIVER METASTASIS

- About **20%** of these patients are candidates for a potentially **curative liver resection** with a **5-year survival rates** range from **25-58%**[Q].
- About **two-third** of cases **recur**, but in high-risk situations (**four** or **more** tumors, **extrahepatic** disease), recurrence rates are generally **80%** or higher[Q].
- Resections of **extrahepatic metastases** that appear to be associated with the **best outcome** are **limited lung metastases, locoregional recurrences** of the primary tumor, and **portal lymph nodes**.

■ HEPATOBLASTOMA

HEPATOBLASTOMA

- **MC primary hepatic tumor** of **childhood**, more common in **males**[Q].
- **Low birth weight** may represent a **risk factor**[Q].
- **Most cases** are sporadic, also associated with **Beckwith-Wiedemann syndrome** & **FAP**[Q]
- **Not associated** with **HBV** or **HCV infection** or any other **chronic viral hepatitis**[Q], cirrhosis or **inborn errors of metabolism**

Clinical Features

- **Median age** of presentation is **18 months**, and almost **all cases occur** before **3 years**[Q].
- **MC presenting sign** is an **asymptomatic abdominal mass**[Q].
- Mild **anemia & thrombocytosis**[Q] are commonly found at presentation.

  - Serum **AFP levels** are **elevated in 85-90%** of patients and can serve as a useful **marker for therapeutic response**[Q].

Diagnosis

- **CT scan** reveals a **vascular mass** that is often (50%) **speckled with calcification**[Q].
- To **confirm the diagnosis**, an **initial biopsy**[Q] is required.

Treatment

  - **For unresectable tumors**, the initial surgical procedure should include a **diagnostic biopsy** and **placement of a vascular access device for chemotherapy**[Q].
  - A **second laparotomy** is performed after **four cycles of chemotherapy**, if imaging studies show a good response, and the tumor appears resectable.

- **Neoadjuvant chemotherapy** (cisplatin, 5-fluorouracil, vincristine) followed by **resection**[Q]
- 50% of patients with **pulmonary metastases** can be **cured with resection**[Q] of the hepatic tumor and **chemotherapy** or resection of the pulmonary metastases[Q].

■ COURVOISIER'S LAW

COURVOISIER'S LAW

- In **obstruction** of the **CBD due to a stone, distention of gallbladder seldom occurs; the organ** usually **is shriveled**[Q].
- If there is no disease in the gallbladder and the **obstruction is due to cancer of ampulla, pancreas or bile duct**, then **gallbladder will be distended**[Q].

Exceptions to Courvoisier's Law

- **Double impaction of stones**[Q] (one in **cystic duct** & other in **CBD**).
- **Pancreatic calculus obstructing** the **ampulla of Vater**[Q]
- Oriental cholangiohepatitis[Q]
- **Mucocele** due to **stone** in the **cystic duct**[Q]

■ LIVER ANATOMY

Functional Anatomical Divisions of Liver

- **Functional anatomy of the liver is based on Couinaud's division of liver into eight (subsequently nine) functional segments**, based upon the distribution of **portal venous branches** & location of **hepatic veins** in the parenchyma (**Couinaud 1957**).

  - **Segment IX is a recent subdivision of segment I,** and describes that **part of segment that lies posterior to segment VIII**[Q].

- Liver is **divided into four portal sectors** by **four main branches of portal vein**. These are **right lateral, right medial, left medial & left lateral** (sometimes the term posterior is used in place of lateral & anterior in place of medial).
- **Three main hepatic veins lie between these sectors as intersectoral veins.** These **intersectoral planes** are also called **portal fissures (scissures). Fissures containing portal pedicles** are called **hepatic fissures.**
- **Each sector** is sub-divided **into segments (usually two)** based on their **supply by tertiary divisions of vascular biliary sheaths.**

Fissures of the liver:

- **Three major fissures**, not visible on the surface, run through the liver parenchyma and **harbor the three main hepatic veins (main, left & right portal fissures)**[Q].
- **Three minor fissures** are visible as **physical clefts of the liver surface (umbilical, venous & fissure of Gans)**[Q].

Sectors and segments of the liver:

- Sectors of liver are made up of between one & three segments: right lateral sector = segments VI & VII; right medial sector = segments V & VIII; left medial sector = segments III & IV (and part of I); left lateral sector = segment II.

  - **Segments are numbered in an ante-clockwise spiral centered on the portal vein** with the **liver viewed from beneath,** starting with segment I up to segment VI, and then back clockwise for the most cranial two segments VII & VIII.

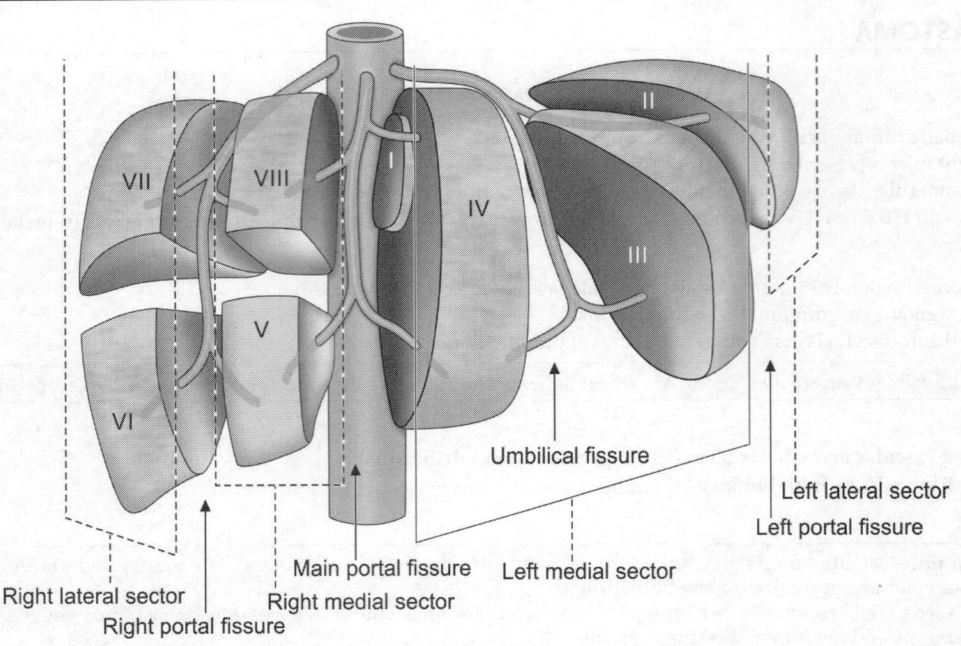

The fissures and sectors of the liver. (Right lateral = right posterior; right medial = right anterior)

Segmental Nomenclature			
I	Caudate lobe^Q	V	Right **anterior inferior** segment
II	Left **lateral superior** segment	VI	Right **posterior inferior** segment
III	Left **lateral inferior** segment	VII	Right **posterior superior** segment
IV	Left medial segment or **Quadrate lobe**^Q	VIII	Right **anterior superior** segment

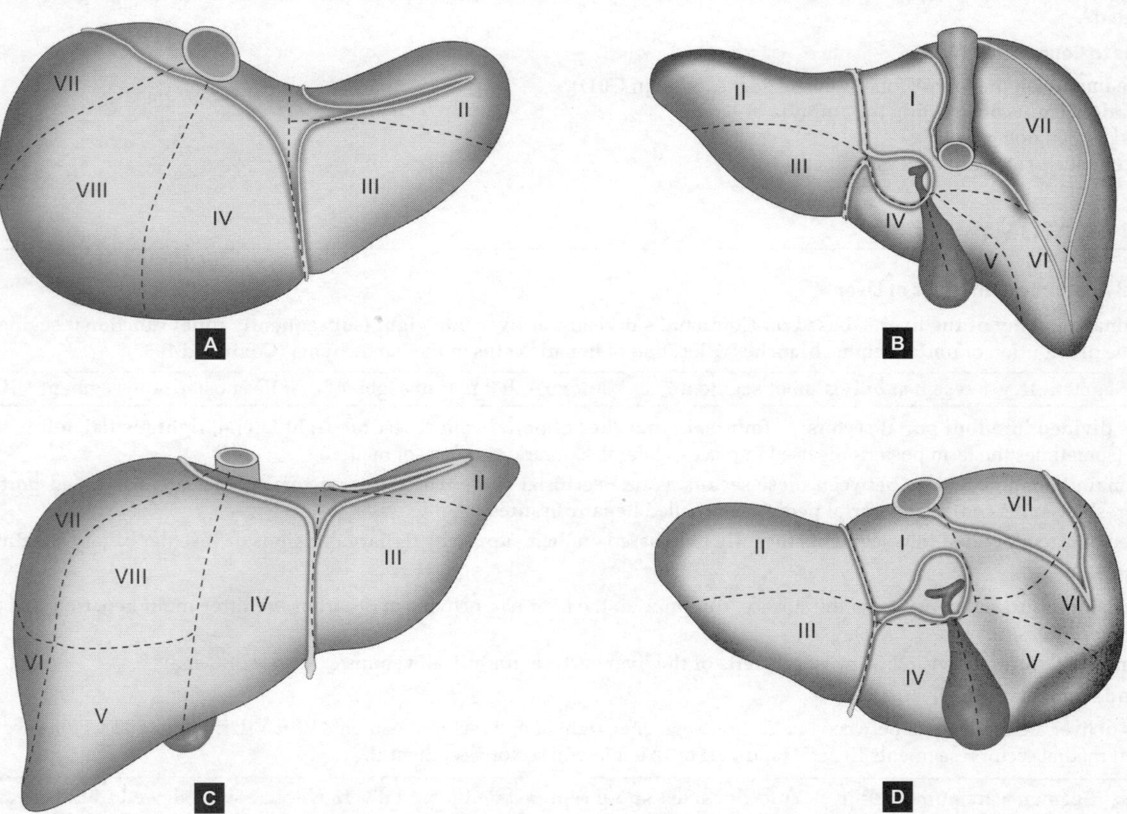

Segments of the liver (after Couinaud). (A) superior view; (B) posterior view; (C) anterior view; (D) inferior view.

■ LIVER ABSCESS

1. **Liver abscess ruptures most commonly in:** *(AIIMS GIS 2003)*
   a. Pleural cavity
   b. Peritoneal cavity
   c. Pericardial cavity
   d. Bronchus

2. **Commonest cause of pyogenic liver abscess:** *(AIIMS Sept 96)*
   a. Aspiration
   b. Hematogenous spread from a distant site
   c. Direct contact
   d. Lymphatic spread

3. **Anchovy sauce pus is a feature of:** *(All India 99)*
   a. Amebic liver abscess
   b. Lung abscess
   c. Splenic abscess
   d. Pancreatic abscess

4. **In pyogenic liver abscess commonest route of spread is:**
   (AIIMS Nov 98, AIIMS Nov 95)
   a. Hematogenous through portal vein
   b. Ascending infection through biliary tract
   c. Hepatic artery
   d. Local spread

5. **Flask shaped ulcers in colon is caused by:**
   (Recent Question 2019)
   a. Giardia lamblia
   b. Entamoeba histolytica
   c. H. pylori
   d. Enterobius vermicularis

6. **A 6 years old child is brought with high fever with rigors for 5-days with pain in the right hypochondrium. On examination the patient is anicteric and tenderness is noted in the right upper outer quadrant. What is the best investigation for this case?** *(MCI Dec 2018)*
   a. USG
   b. Serology
   c. LFT
   d. CECT

■ HYDATID CYST

7. **Water lily appearance in a chest radiograph suggests:**
   (COMEDK 2005, 2004)
   a. Metastasis
   b. Cavitating metastasis
   c. Aspergilloma
   d. Ruptured hydatid cyst

8. **Ultrasound was performed in a patient of hydatid cyst. What is the name of this sign?**
   a. Water lily sign
   b. Honeycomb sign
   c. Spoke wheel sign
   d. Triradiate sign

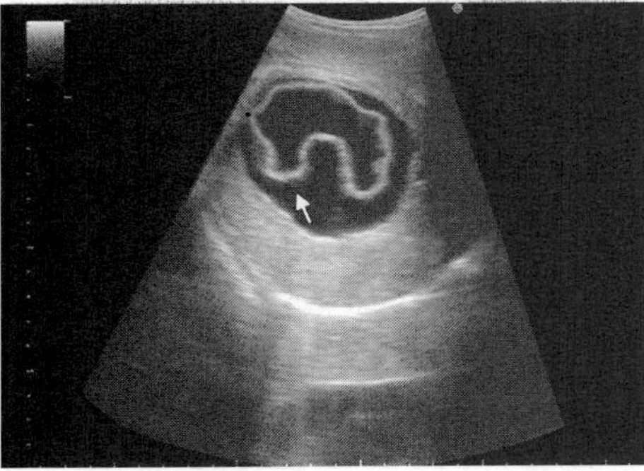

9. **A 40-year-old female presented with abdominal discomfort, dyspepsia and palpable abdominal mass. USG and CECT was performed. What is the diagnosis based on this ultrasound image?**
   a. Hydatid cyst
   b. Multiple HCC
   c. Liver secondaries
   d. Polycystic liver disease

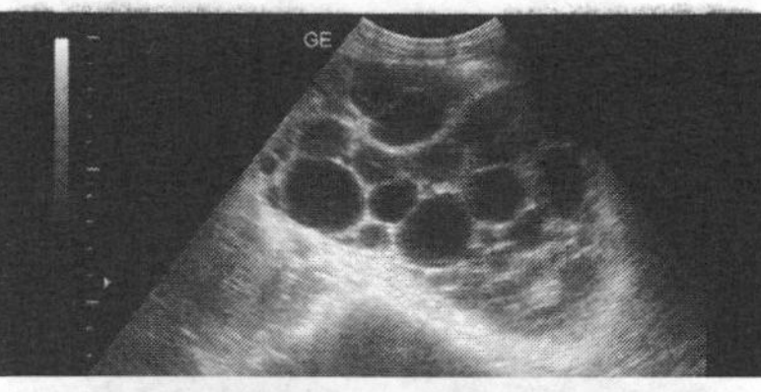

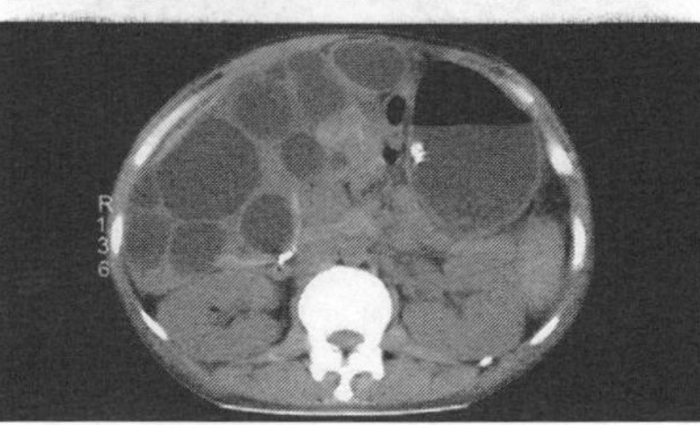

10. **A 40-year old male presents with a painless cystic liver enlargement of four years duration without fever or jaundice. The most likely diagnosis is:** *(UPSC 96)*
    a. Amoebic liver abscess
    b. Hepatoma
    c. Hydatid cyst of liver
    d. Choledochal cyst

11. **Ring like calcification on CECT is seen in:**
    (Recent Question 2016)
    a. HC
    b. FNH
    c. Liver metastasis
    d. Hydatid cyst

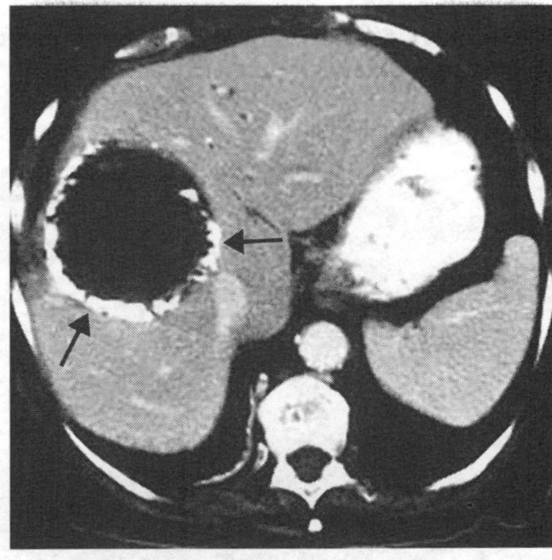

12. **Which of the following is true about hydatid cyst of liver?**
    a. Surgical management is done always
    b. Conservative treatment is effective
    c. Aspiration is safe *(Recent Question 2014, DPG 2007)*
    d. E. multilocularis is the most common cause

13. **Investigation of choice for hydatid disease is:**
    a. CT scan
    b. ELISA *(MCI Sept 2009)*
    c. Biopsy
    d. USG

14. **Malignant hydatidosis is caused by:** *(Recent Question 2016)*
    a. Echinococcus granulosus
    b. Echinococcus multilocularis
    c. Echinococcus vogelli
    d. Echinococcus oligarthus

15. **Malignant hydatid disease is caused by:**
    (Recent Question 2017)
    a. E. granulosus
    b. E. oligarthus
    c. E. vogelli
    d. E. multilocularis

16. **What is the name of this sign seen on CT chest?**
    (Recent Question 2017)

    a. Rising sun sign   b. Water lily sign
    c. Meniscus sign   d. Serpent sign

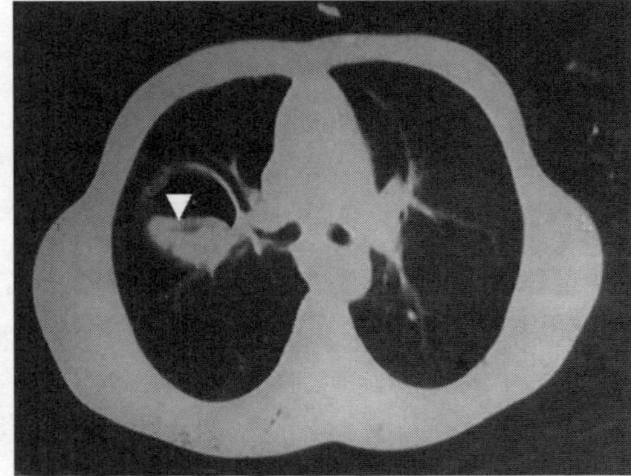

■ HEPATIC ADENOMA

17. **Most common liver tumor in those on OCPs:**
    (MHSSMCET 2007)

    a. HCC   b. Liver cell adenoma
    c. Bile duct adenoma   d. Focal nodular hyperplasia

18. **Which of the following liver tumors always merit surgery?**
    (DPG 2009 March)

    a. Hemangioma   b. Hepatic adenoma
    c. Focal nodular hyperplasia   d. Peliosis hepatis

■ FOCAL NODULAR HYPERPLASIA

19. **Radiographic image of a benign tumor is given below. What is the most probable diagnosis?**

    a. Hemangioma   b. Focal nodular hyperplasia
    c. Hepatic adenoma   d. Peliosis hepatis

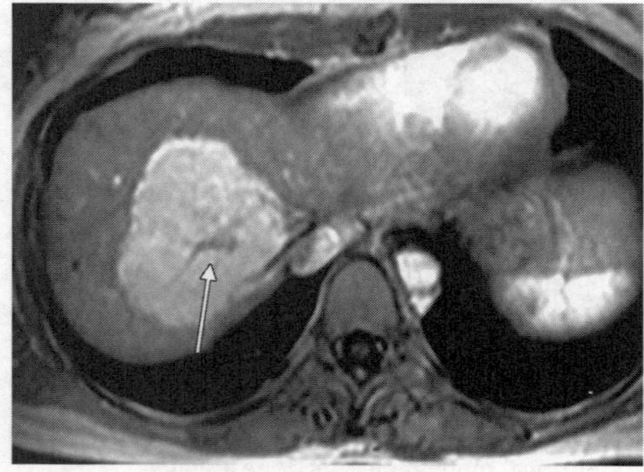

20. **Which one of the following hepatic lesions can be diagnosed with high accuracy by using nuclear imaging?**
    (AIIMS Nov 2004)

    a. Hepatocellular carcinoma   b. Hepatic adenoma
    c. Focal nodular hyperplasia   d. Hemangioma

■ HEMANGIOMA

21. **Most common benign tumor of liver is:**
    (DNB 2005, 2000, JIPMER GIS 2011)

    a. Hemangioma   b. Hepatic adenoma
    c. Hepatoma   d. Hamartoma

22. **Most common liver tumor in children:** *(Recent Question 2017)*

    a. Hemangioma   b. Non-parasitic cyst
    c. Adenoma   d. Focal nodular hyperplasia

■ HEPATIC CYST

23. **Solitary Hypoechoic lesion of the liver without septa or debris is most likely to be:** *(AIIMS Nov 2005)*

    a. Hydatid cyst   b. Caroli's disease
    c. Liver abscess   d. Simple cyst

24. **Treatment of choice for simple cyst of liver:**
    (JIPMER Nov 2017)

    a. Percutaneous drainage   b. Cysto-enterostomy
    c. Deroofing   d. Aspiration

■ POLYCYSTIC LIVER DISEASE

25. **Treatment of symptomatic polycystic liver disease is:**
    (DPG 2008)

    a. Deroofing of the cyst   b. Injection of sclerosant
    c. Hepatic resection   d. Liver transplantation

■ HEPATOCELLULAR CARCINOMA RISK FACTORS

26. **Which of the following most significantly increases the risk of HCC?** *(AIIMS May 2012)*
    a. HBV   b. HAV
    c. CMV   d. EBV

27. **True regarding HCC:** *(JIPMER 2010)*
    a. Non alcoholic steatohepatitis is a risk factor
    b. OCP's are a cause
    c. Focal nodular hyperplasia may turn malignant
    d. Chromosomal abnormalities are common

■ HEPATOCELLULAR CARCINOMA

28. **Okuda staging contains all except:** *(ILBS 2012)*
    a. Bilirubin   b. Tumor size
    c. Ascites   d. AFP

29. **Tumor marker for primary hepatocellular carcinoma are all except:** *(AIIMS May 2007)*
    a. Alpha-feto protein   b. Alpha-2 macroglobulin
    c. PIVKA-2   d. Neurotensin

30. **All of the following are modalities of therapy for hepatocellular carcinoma except:** *(AIIMS Nov 2005)*
    a. Radiofrequency ablation
    b. Transarterial catheter embolization
    c. Percutaneous acetic acid
    d. Nd-YAG laser ablation

31. **Which of the following liver tumour has a propensity to invade the portal or hepatic vein?** *(AIIMS June 2004)*
    a. Cavernous hemangioma   b. Hepatocellular carcinoma
    c. Focal nodular hyperplasia
    d. Hepatic adenoma

32. **Which of the following is not true about Milan's criteria?**
    a. Single tumor <5 cm in size   *(Recent Question 2017)*
    b. 3 nodules <3 cm in size
    c. >5 nodules   d. No extrahepatic disease

33. **AFP is a tumor marker for which of the following?**
    (MCI Dec 2018)

    a. HCC   b. RCC
    c. Oncocytoma   d. Chordoma

■ FIBROLAMELLAR HCC

34. **All of the following are true about fibrolamellar carcinoma of the liver except:** *(JIPMER 2012, All India 2001)*
    a. More common in females
    b. Better prognosis than HCC
    c. AFP levels always >1000 pg/ml
    d. Occur in younger individuals

35. Which of the following is having better prognosis?
    a. HCC   b. Cholangiocarcinoma
    c. Fibrolamellar variant of HCC
    d. Angiosarcoma

■ LIVER SECONDARIES

36. All of the following modalities can be used for in situ ablation of liver secondaries, except: *(All India 2006)*
    a. Ultrasonic waves   b. Cryotherapy
    c. Alcohol   d. Radiofrequency

37. Which of the following liver metastasis appear hypoechoic on ultrasound?   *(All India 2012)*
    a. Breast cancer   b. Colon cancer
    c. RCC   d. Mucinous adenocarcinoma

■ HEPATOBLASTOMA

38. All are true about hepatoblastoma except:
    a. Present in childhood   *(PGI SS June 2005)*
    b. Common in cirrhosis of liver due to HBV
    c. Chemosensitive
    d. Surgical resection is treatment of choice

39. AFP is raised in: *(KGMC 2011)*
    a. 100% of hepatoblastoma b. 90% of hepatoblastoma
    c. 100% of HCC   d. 90% of HCC

■ LIVER TRANSPLANTATION

40. Most common indication for liver transplantation in children is: *(JIPMER GIS 2011)*
    a. Biliary atresia   b. Indian childhood cirrhosis
    c. HCC   d. Hepatitis C infection

41. Auxiliary orthotopic liver transplant is indicated for:
    a. Metabolic liver disease   *(AIIMS May 2008)*
    b. As a standby procedure until finding a suitable donor
    c. Drug induced hepatic failure
    d. Acute fulminant liver failure for any cause

42. Liver after transplantation enlarges by: *(Recent Question 2015)*
    a. Increase in size of cell   b. Increase in number of cells
    c. Both of the above   d. None of the above

43. All are indications of liver transplantation except: *(Recent Question 2014)*
    a. Cholangiocarcinoma   b. Cirrhosis
    c. Biliary atresia   d. Fulminant hepatitis

■ HEPATIC RESECTION

44. Vascular inflow occlusion of the liver is by:
    a. Clamping the hepatic artery   *(DNB 2012)*
    b. Occluding the portal vein
    c. Clamping the hepatic veins
    d. The Pringle maneuver

45. Pringle maneuver may be required for treatment of:
    a. Injury to tail of pancreas
    b. Mesenteric ischemia
    c. Bleeding esophageal varices
    d. Liver laceration   *(APPG 2015, Recent Question 2014)*

■ HEPATIC REGENERATION

46. Following resection of 2/3rd of the liver, regeneration is complete within:
    a. 2-3 months   b. 8-10 weeks
    c. 4-6 months   d. 4-5 weeks

■ LIVER TRAUMA

47. A 17-years old boy is admitted to the hospital after a road traffic accident. Per abdomen examination is normal. After adequate resuscitation, his pulse rate is 80/min and BP is 110/70 mmHg. Abdominal CT reveals 1 cm deep laceration in the left lobe of the liver extending from the done more than half way through the parenchyma. Appropriate management at this time would be: *(DPG 2011, UPSC 2005)*
    a. Conservative management
    b. Abdominal exploration and packing of hepatic wounds
    c. Abdominal exploration and ligation of left hepatic artery
    d. Left hepatectomy

48. 'Beer-Claw' appearance on CECT abdomen is seen in: *(MHCET 2016)*
    a. Hepatic laceration   b. Pancreatic laceration
    c. HCC   d. RCC

■ LIVER ANATOMY

49. Which is not true regarding the basis of functional divisions of liver?   *(AIIMS May 2015)*
    a. Based on portal vein and hepatic vein
    b. Divided into 8 segments
    c. There are three major and three minor fissures
    d. 4 sectors

50. In Couinaud's classification, segment IV of liver is: *(AIIMS Nov 2007)*
    a. Caudate lobe   b. Quadrate lobe
    c. Right lobe   d. Left lobe

51. The Couinaud's segmental nomenclature is based on the position of the: *(All India 2004)*
    a. Hepatic veins and portal vein
    b. Hepatic veins and biliary ducts
    c. Portal vein and biliary ducts
    d. Portal vein and hepatic artery

■ LIVER FUNCTION TESTS AND JAUNDICE

52. Courvoisier's law is related to: *(Recent Question 2016)*
    a. Jaundice
    b. Ureteric calculi
    c. Portal hypertension
    d. The length of skin flap in skin grafting

53. Which of the following is an exception of Courvoisier's law?   *(Recent Question 2015)*
    a. Double impaction   b. Portal lymphadenopathy
    c. Periampullary Carcinoma d. None of above

Explanations

■ LIVER ABSCESS

1. **Ans. b.** Peritoneal cavity
2. **Ans. b.** Hematogenous spread from a distant site
   - Hematogenous spread is most common among the given options.
3. **Ans. a.** Amebic liver abscess
4. **Ans. b.** Ascending infection through biliary tract
5. **Ans. b.** Entamoeba histolytica *(Ref: Schwartz 11/e p1370, 10/e p1285; Bailey 27/e p58)*
6. **Ans. b.** Serology *(Ref: Bailey 27/e p1169)*

■ HYDATID CYST

7. **Ans. d.** Ruptured hydatid cyst *(Ref: Sabiston 20/e p1452-1455; Schwartz 11/e p1370, 10/e p1285-1286; Bailey 27/e p1169; Blumgart 6/e p1108; Shackelford 8/e p1425)*
8. **Ans. a.** Water lily sign *(Ref: Bailey 27/e p66)*
9. **Ans. a.** Hydatid cyst
10. **Ans. c.** Hydatid cyst of liver
11. **Ans. d.** Hydatid cyst *(Ref: Sabiston 20/e p1452)*
    - Ring like calcification on CECT is seen in hydatid cyst.
12. **Ans. c.** Aspiration is safe *(Ref: Bailey 27/e p1169)*
    - Aspiration is safe in Hydatid cyst of liver.
13. **Ans. b.** ELISA
14. **Ans. b.** Echinococcus multilocularis
15. **Ans. d.** E. multilocularis *(Ref: Sabiston 20/e 1452p; Schwartz 11/e p1371, 10/e p1286)*
16. **Ans. b.** Water lily sign *(Ref: Wolfgang 2/e p309)*

"The **water-lily sign** is seen in **hydatid cyst** when there is **detachment of the endocyst membrane** which results in **floating membranes within the pericyst** that mimic the **appearance of a water lily**. It is classically described on **plain radiographs** (mainly **chest X-ray**) when the **collapsed membranes are calcified** but may be seen on **ultrasound and CT**."

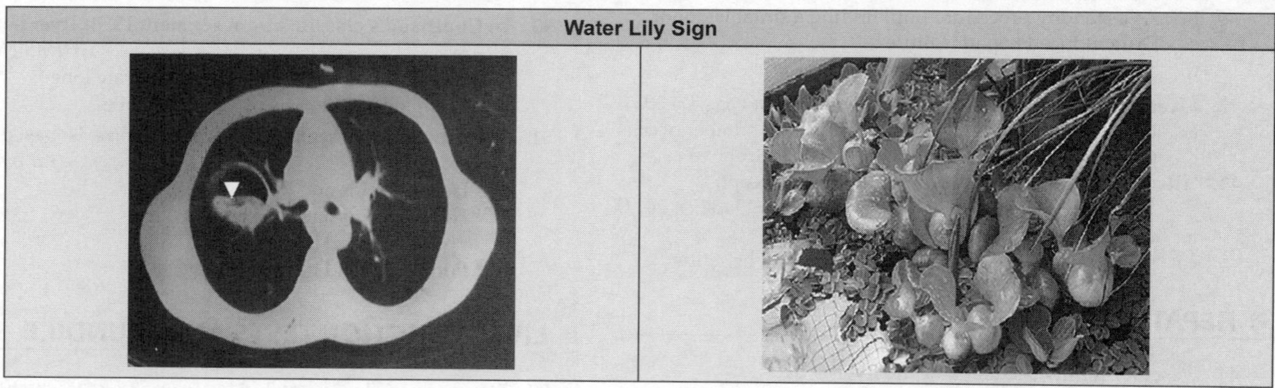

■ HEPATIC ADENOMA

17. **Ans. b.** Liver cell adenoma
18. **Ans. b.** Hepatic adenoma *(Ref: Bailey 27/e p1172; Taber's Medical Dictionary 19/e p1600)*

    Hepatic adenoma always merits surgery. As **no characteristic radiological features** to **differentiate** these lesions **from malignant tumor**. These tumors are thought **to have malignant potential** and **resection** is therefore the **treatment of choice**[Q].

■ FOCAL NODULAR HYPERPLASIA

19. **Ans. b.** Focal nodular hyperplasia *(Ref: Sabiston 20/e p1456; Schwartz 11/e p1376, 10/e p1291; Bailey 27/e p1172)*

    The given image shows central stellate scar, which is seen in focal nodular hyperplasia.

20. **Ans. c.** Focal Nodular Hyperplasia

■ HEMANGIOMA

21. **Ans. a.** Hemangioma
22. **Ans. a.** Hemangioma *(Ref: Sabiston 20/e p1456; Schwartz 11/e p1375, 10/e p1289; Bailey 27/e p1171)*

■ HEPATIC CYST

23. **Ans. d. Simple cyst** *(Ref: Sabiston 20/e p1469; Schwartz 11/e p1374, 10/e p1288-1289; Blumgart 6/e p530; Shackelford 8/e p1421)*

24. **Ans. c. Deroofing** *(Ref: Schwartz 10/e p1289; Sabiston 20/e p1469)*

■ POLYCYSTIC LIVER DISEASE

25. **Ans. a. Deroofing of the cyst** *(Ref: Sabiston 20/e p1469; Schwartz 11/e p1374, 10/e p1288-1289; Blumgart 6/e p1140; Shackelford 8/e p1424)*
Treatment of **symptomatic polycystic liver disease** is **deroofing** of the **cyst.**

■ HEPATOCELLULAR CARCINOMA: RISK FACTORS

26. **Ans. a. HBV**

27. **Ans. a. Non alcoholic steatohepatitis is a risk factor** *(Ref: Shackelford 8/e p1542)*
- **Cirrhosis due to NAFLD (Non-alcoholic fatty liver disease)** mainly **caused by obesity** is a **risk factor for HCC.**

■ HEPATOCELLULAR CARCINOMA

28. **Ans. d. AFP** *(Ref: Sabiston 20/e p1460; Blumgart 6/e p1335; Shackelford 8/e p1544)*   **29.** **Ans. b. Alpha-2 macroglobulin**

30. **Ans. d. Nd-YAG laser ablation** *(Ref: Sabiston 20/e p1461; Schwartz 11/e p1376, 10/e p1291, 1294-1296; Bailey 27/e p1174; Blumgart 6/e p1338; Shackelford 8/e p1547)*

TREATMENT OF HCC

- **Hepatic resection** as the **first-line treatment** for cirrhotic patients with small HCC and **preserved liver function** and reserve salvage **transplantation** for **recurrence** or **deterioration of liver function** after hepatic resection[Q]
- Only patients with **normal bilirubin** concentration and **absence of portal hypertension** should be considered for **resection[Q].**
- If not candidate for surgery offer **percutaneous ablation**; patients with more advanced disease (**large** or **multifocal HCC**) **without portal vein invasion** are candidates for **transarterial chemoembolization** if liver function is preserved (the sole palliative approach that has been shown to have a **positive impact** in **survival** is transarterial chemoembolization)[Q].

  - For **patients without cirrhosis** who develop HCC, **resection is the treatment of choice** [Q].
  - For those patients with **Child's class A cirrhosis** with **preserved liver function** and **no portal hypertension, resection also is considered** [Q].
  - If **resection** is **not possible** because of **poor liver function** and the **HCC meets the Milan criteria** (one nodule <5 cm, or two or three nodules all <3 cm, no gross vascular invasion or extrahepatic spread), liver transplantation is the **treatment of choice** [Q].

Milan Criteria (Mazzafero)		
• **One nodule <5 cm**	• **Two or three nodules all <3 cm**	• **No gross vascular invasion** or **extrahepatic spread**

31. **Ans. b. Hepatocellular carcinoma** *(Ref: Sabiston 20/e p1459; Schwartz 11/e p1376, 10/e p1291-1294-1296; Blumgart 6/e p1334; Shackelford 8/e p1547)*

HEPATOCELLULAR CARCINOMA

- **HCC derive its blood supply** from **hepatic artery**[Q].
- **HCC** is characterized by being **hyperdense** on the **arterial phase** of contrast imaging, meaning that they have **more arterial perfusion**[Q].
- **Arterial perfusion of HCC** also allows for **treatment** of the **lesions via embolization** of feeding artery[Q].
- **Characteristic of HCC: Propensity to invade** the **portal vein**[Q].
- **Risk of portal vein invasion** appears to **correlate with tumor size** & **differentiation**[Q].
- **Outcome** of patients with **portal venous invasion** is **worse** than that of patients whose tumor does not invade the portal vein.

32. **Ans. c. >5 modules** *(Ref: Shackelford 8/e p1551; Sabiston 20/e p645, Schwartz 11/e p1376, 1380, 10/e p1295; Bailey 27/e p1175)*
This is a **typical case of HCC**, remember **AFP is raised** in about **75% of Africans** and only **30% of patients in US** and **Europe.**

33. **Ans. a. HCC** *(Ref: Robbin's 9/e p337)*

■ FIBROLAMELLAR HCC

34. **Ans. c. AFP level always >1000 pg/mL**   **35.** **Ans. c. Fibrolamellar variant of HCC**

■ LIVER SECONDARIES

36. **Ans. a. Ultrasonic waves** *(Ref: Sabiston 20/e p1464-1465; Schwartz 11/e p1379, 10/e p1123; Bailey 27/e p1172; Blumgart 6/e p1665; Shackelford 8/e p1568)*
Ultrasonic waves are not described as a method of local ablative therapy for liver secondaries.

37. **Ans. a. Breast cancer** *(Ref: Focal Liver Lesions (Springer) 2006/266)*

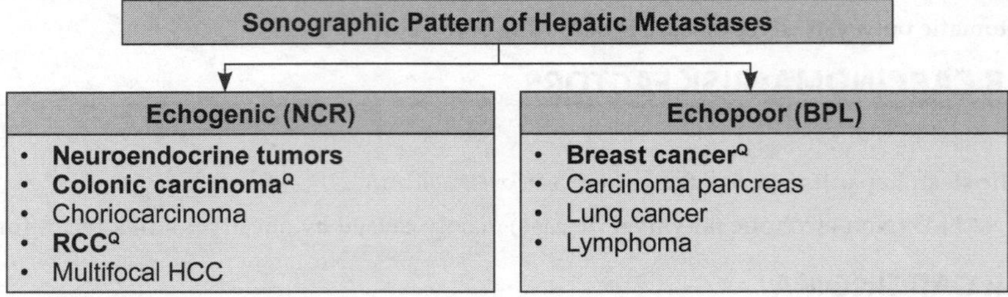

- **Metastases** from **breast cancer** are typically **hypoechoic (echopoor)**[Q] on **ultrasonography.**
- **Metastases** from **carcinoma colon** and **RCC** are typically **hyperechoic (echogenic)**[Q].
- **Metastases** from **mucinous adenocarcinoma** of **colon** are typically **calcified**[Q].

Sonographic Pattern of Hepatic Metastases

Echogenic (NCR)	Echopoor (BPL)
• **Neuroendocrine tumors** • **Colonic carcinoma**[Q] • Choriocarcinoma • **RCC**[Q] • Multifocal HCC	• **Breast cancer**[Q] • Carcinoma pancreas • Lung cancer • Lymphoma

■ HEPATOBLASTOMA

38. **Ans. b. Common in cirrhosis of liver due to HBV**   **39.** **Ans. b. 90% of hepatoblastoma**

■ LIVER TRANSPLANTATION

40. **Ans. a. Biliary atresia** *(Ref: Sabiston 20/e p637-638; Schwartz 11/e p1380, 10/e p1277; Bailey 27/e p1554; Blumgart 6/e p661; Shackelford 8/e p1365)*

41. **Ans. a. > d. Metabolic liver disease >Acute fulminant liver failure for any cause** *(Ref: Blumgart 6/e p 1779)*
APOLT is **used in acute fulminant liver failure** mainly **caused by metabolic liver diseases**, not in liver failure from any cause.

INDICATIONS OF AUXILIARY PARTIAL ORTHOTOPIC LIVER TRANSPLANTATION (APOLT)

1. **Reversible fulminant hepatic failure**[Q]**Small-for-size grafts**[Q]
2. **Non-cirrhotic metabolic liver disease**[Q]**ABO-incompatibility**[Q]

AUXILIARY PARTIAL ORTHOTOPIC LIVER TRANSPLANTATION (APOLT)

- **In fulminant hepatic failure, APOLT** provides **temporary support** until the **native liver** recovers and then immunosuppression can be withdrawn.
- **APOLT** can **compensate** for **enzyme deficiency** in **non-cirrhotic metabolic liver disease (most commonly Criggler-Najjar syndrome)** without complete removal of native liver.
- Transplants of **ABO-incompatible grafts** are often unavoidable due to **limited number of potential donor** candidates. A **high incidence** of **early graft failure** with a high rate of **biliary** and **vascular complications** in ABO-incompatible liver transplantation is reported. The **remnant liver** could **sustain a patient's life** if the anticipated **graft failure** occurred in an ABO-incompatible case.
- In **small-for-size graft**, the **remnant liver** is expected to **support** the function of **implanted graft** during the **early post-op period**. The graft liver expands its function in proportion to volume growth. After the graft liver has grown sufficiently, it can be expected to meet the hepatic functional demands of the recipient.

42. **Ans. b. Increase in number of cells**   **43.** **Ans. a. Cholangiocarcinoma**

■ HEPATIC RESECTION

44. **Ans. d. The Pringle maneuver** *(Ref: Sabiston 20/e p439; Blumgart 6/e p1581; Shackelford 8/e p1417)*

PRINGLE MANEUVER (TOTAL INFLOW OCCLUSION)

- **Total clamping** of the **hepatic pedicle,** by placing an **atraumatic clamp** across the **foramen of Winslow**[Q].
- **Appropriate-sized vascular clamp** or **loop snare** easily **controls hemorrhage** from either the **portal vein** or the **hepatic arteries**[Q].
- Inflow occlusion durations of up to **30 minutes** can be **tolerated safely** in **cirrhotic livers** and possibly up to **60 minutes** in **early disease.**
- If prolonged occlusion is required, intermittent clamping can be used with **repeated clampings** of **10-20 minutes** duration, each followed by **5 minutes declamping.**

45. **Ans. d. Liver Laceration**

■ HEPATIC REGENERATION

47. **Ans. c. 4-6 months**

LIVER REGENERATION

- Following **resection of 2/3ʳᵈ of the liver, regeneration** is **complete within 5-6 months.**

■ LIVER TRAUMA

47. **Ans. a. Conservative management** *(Ref: Sabiston 20/e p437-439; Schwartz 11/e p225, 10/e p173-174, 1642; Bailey 27/e p1161; Blumgart 6/e p1890-1891; Shackelford 8/e p1448)*

   In stable patients, conservative management is preferred option.

48. **Ans. a. Hepatic laceration**

■ LIVER ANATOMY

49. **Ans. b. Divided into 8 segments** *(Ref: Gray's 40/e p1165, 1166,1178; Sabiston 20/e p1421-1423; Blumgart 6/e p37; Shackelford 8/e p1250)*

   All of the given options are true. If we have to choose one answer, most preferred option is 'liver is divided into 8 segments', because sometimes segment IX is described. Segment IX is a recent subdivision of segment I, and describes that part of the segment that lies posterior to segment VIII.

   "Current understanding of the functional anatomy of the liver is based on Couinaud's division of the liver into eight (subsequently nine) functional segments, based upon the distribution of portal venous branches and the location of the hepatic veins in the parenchyma (Couinaud 1957)."-Gray's 40/e p1165

   "Segment IX is a recent subdivision of segment I, and describes that part of the segment that lies posterior to segment VIII." -Gray's 40/e p1166

50. **Ans. b. Quadrate lobe**

51. **Ans. a. Hepatic veins and portal vein**

■ LIVER FUNCTION TESTS AND JAUNDICE

52. **Ans. a. Jaundice** *(Ref: Saiston 20/e p1544)*

53. **Ans. a. Double impaction**

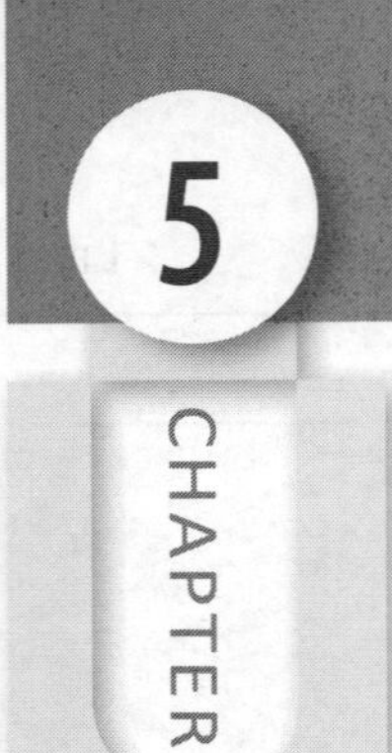

Portal Hypertension

■ ETIOLOGY OF PORTAL HYPERTENSION

Etiology of Portal Hypertension		
Presinusoidal	**Sinusoidal**	**Postsinusoidal**
Extrahepatic or sinistral: • Splenic vein thrombosis[Q] • Splenomegaly[Q] • Splenic arteriovenous fistula[Q]	**Intrahepatic: Cirrhosis** due to- • **HBV, HCV, Alcohol**[Q] • Metabolic abnormality • Autoimmune hepatitis • Primary biliary cirrhosis & **PSC**	**Intrahepatic:** • Veno-occlusive disease[Q]
Intrahepatic: • **Schistosomiasis**[Q] • Congenital hepatic fibrosis • Nodular regenerative hyperplasia • Idiopathic portal fibrosis • **Myeloproliferative disorder**[Q] • **Sarcoid** and **GVHD**		**Posthepatic** • **Budd-Chiari syndrome**[Q] • **Congestive heart failure** • IVC web[Q] • **Constrictive pericarditis**[Q]

- **MC cause** of **intrahepatic presinusoidal** portal hypertension: **Schistosomiasis**[Q]
- **MC cause** of **sinusoidal** portal hypertension: **Cirrhosis**[Q]

■ PORTAL HYPERTENSION

Portal Pressure

- Normal portal vein pressure: **5–10 mm Hg**[Q]
- Normal portal vein pressure: **10–15 cm saline**[Q]
- **Variceal formation** occurs when portal pressure is **>10 mm Hg**[Q].
- **Variceal bleeding** occurs when portal pressure is **>12 mm Hg**[Q].

Portal Hypertension

- **Definition:** Portal pressure **>10 mm Hg**[Q]
- **MC cause** of portal hypertension in **United States: Cirrhosis**[Q].
- Consequence of **both increased portal vascular resistance & increased portal flow**[Q].
- Portal hypertension results in **splenomegaly** with enlarged, tortuous, & even aneurysmal splenic vessels.

- **Cruveilhier-Baumgarten murmur**[Q]: Audible **venous hum** in **caput medusa**

- **Hyperdynamic portal venous circulation** seems to be **related to severity of liver failure**[Q].
- **Upper GI bleeding** is caused by **portal hypertension** in about **90%** of instances.
- Most bleeding episodes occur during the **first 1 to 2 years** after **identification of varices**[Q].
- **Colour Doppler** is **investigation of choice** for evaluation of **PHT**.

- About **one third** of **deaths** in patients with known esophageal varices are due to **upper GI bleed**[Q]
- A **larger proportion** dies as a result of **liver failure**[Q].

- **MC causes** of **death** in **cirrhosis** patients: Hepatic failure[Q]
- **2nd MC causes** of **death** in **cirrhosis** patients: **variceal hemorrhage**[Q]

■ CHILD-TURCOTTE-PUGH (CTP) SCORING SYSTEM

CHILD-TURCOTTE-PUGH (CTP) SCORING SYSTEM

- **CTP score** is a measure to **assess hepatic function**[Q] in many liver diseases.
- It was **initially devised to classify patients** into **risk groups** prior to **undergoing porto-systemic shunt surgeries**[Q].
- It is used to **assess prognosis in cirrhosis**[Q] and many liver diseases.

Child-Turcotte-Pugh (CTP) Score			
Variable	1 Point	2 Points	3 Points
Serum albumin (g/dL)	>3.5	**2.8–3.5**[Q]	<2.8
Bilirubin (mg/dL)	<2	2–3[Q]	>3
Prothrombin time (sec above normal) or **INR**	<4 <1.7	**4–6**[Q] **1.7–2.3**[Q]	>6 >2.3
Ascites	None	**Controlled**[Q]	Uncontrolled
Encephalopathy	None	**Controlled**[Q]	Uncontrolled

Class A	**5–6** points[Q]
Class B	**7–9** points[Q]
Class C	**10–15** points[Q]

- **Major surgeries** can be done **only in Class A**[Q]
- **Only minor surgical procedures** can be performed in **Class B**[Q]
- **No surgical intervention** should be done in **Class C (Best treatment** is **liver transplantation)**[Q].

■ LEFT SIDED PORTAL HYPERTENSION

LEFT SIDED PORTAL HYPERTENSION

- Portal hypertension **due to isolated splenic vein thrombosis**[Q] is known as left sided portal hypertension or **sinistral hypertension**[Q].
- **Pressure** in **portal vein** and **SMV** are **normal**[Q]
- There is **gastrosplenic venous hypertension** leading to **formation of gastric varices**[Q]

Causes

- **Pancreatitis (MC)**[Q] leading to splenic vein thrombosis
- Neoplasm
- Trauma

Treatment

- **Splenectomy** is the **treatment of choice**[Q].

■ ESOPHAGEAL VARICES

ESOPHAGEAL VARICES

- **Most significant clinical finding** associated with **PHT** is development of **GE varices**[Q].
- **Major blood supply** to GE varices is **anterior branch** of **left gastric** or **coronary vein**[Q].
- **Variceal bleeding** is **leading cause** of **morbidity & mortality** associated with **PHT**[Q]

Prevention of Variceal Bleeding

- Current measures aimed at preventing variceal bleeding include:
  - Improvement of liver function (**abstention from alcohol**)[Q]
  - **Avoidance** of aspirin & **NSAIDs**[Q]
  - Administration of **propranolol** or **nadolol (nonselective beta blockers)**[Q]

- **Beta blockers reduce** the **index variceal bleed** by 45% and reduce **bleeding mortality** by 50%[Q].

Contd...

Section 2

Hepatobiliary Pancreatic Surgery

Contd...

- **Prophylactic endoscopic variceal ligation (EVL)** is associated with a **lower incidence** of **first variceal bleed**[Q].
- **EVL** is recommended for **medium to large varices**, performed **every 1 to 2 weeks**[Q] until obliteration, followed by endoscopy 1 to 3 months later and surveillance endoscopy every 6 months to monitor for recurrence of varices.

Management of Acute Variceal Bleeding

- Patients should be **admitted to** an ICU for **resuscitation** and management[Q].
- **Blood resuscitation** should be performed to a **hemoglobin level of 8 g/dL**[Q].
- **Over-replacement** of packed **red blood cells** and the overzealous administration of **saline** can lead to both **rebleeding** and **increased mortality**[Q].
- Administration of **FFP** and **platelets** in patients with **severe coagulopathy**[Q].

> - Use of **short-term prophylactic antibiotics** has been shown both to **decrease** the **rate of bacterial infections** and to **increase survival**[Q].
> - **Ceftriaxone 1 g/day IV** is often given[Q].

Pharmacologic therapy for Variceal Hemorrhage
• Pharmacologic therapy can be initiated as soon as the diagnosis of variceal bleeding is made.
• **Vasopressin**, is the **most potent vasoconstrictor**, its use is **limited by** its large number of **side effects**, and it should be administered for **only a short period** to prevent ischemic complications[Q].
• **Somatostatin** and **octreotide** also cause **splanchnic vasoconstriction**[Q].
• **Octreotide** is the **preferred pharmacologic agent** for **initial management** of acute variceal bleeding[Q].

- In addition to pharmacologic therapy **endoscopy** should be carried out **as soon as possible** and EVL should be performed.
- Combination of **pharmacologic and EVL therapy improve** initial **control of bleeding** and **increase the 5-day hemostasis rate**[Q].
- **Shunt therapy (surgical shunts** or **TIPS)** has been shown to **control refractory variceal bleeding** in >90% of treated individuals[Q].
- **Shunt surgery** is considered only in patients with **preserved hepatic function (CTP** class **A)**[Q]
- **TIPS** is used in patients with **decompensated liver disease (CTP** class **B** or **C)**[Q].

Sengstaken-Blakemore Tube
• Balloon tamponade using will **control refractory variceal bleeding** in >80% of patients[Q].
• Its **application** is **limited** due to complications (**aspiration** and **esophageal perforation**)[Q]
• Use of a Sengstaken-Blakemore tube should be **limited** to **short-term therapy (<24 hours)** in those patients awaiting definitive care[Q].

■ BALLOON TAMPONADE

BALLOON TAMPONADE

- Sengstaken and Blakemore designed a **triple-lumen**[Q] (esophageal balloon, gastric balloon, & gastric aspiration) tube.
- Airway should be protected by placement of an **endotracheal tube**[Q].
- Use of **water** or **oily contrast** media to inflate the balloon is **contraindicated**[Q].
- In the case of Sengstaken–Blakemore tube, the **gastric balloon** is inflated with **50 mL of air**[Q] and **after proper positioning**, the gastric balloon inflated with **250 mL** of air and plugged snug against the GE junction.

> - If bleeding does not stop promptly, the **gastric balloon** may be inflated to at least a volume of **300 mL**, or the **esophageal balloon** may be inflated to a pressure of **40 mm Hg**[Q].

Complication

- **MC complication** of balloon tamponade is **aspiration**[Q] pneumonia.

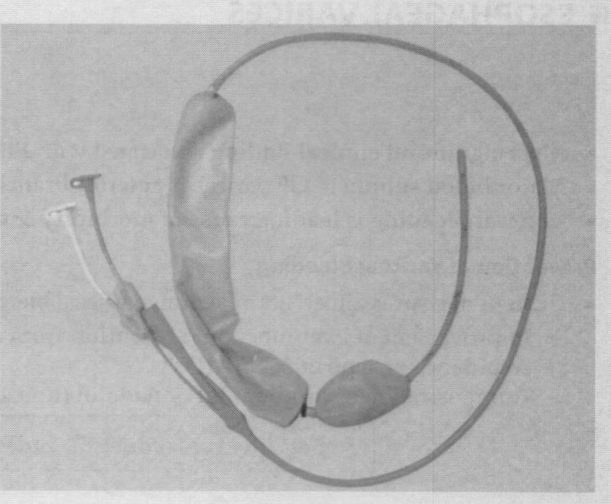

■ TRANSJUGULAR INTRAHEPATIC PORTAL-SYSTEMIC SHUNT (TIPSS)

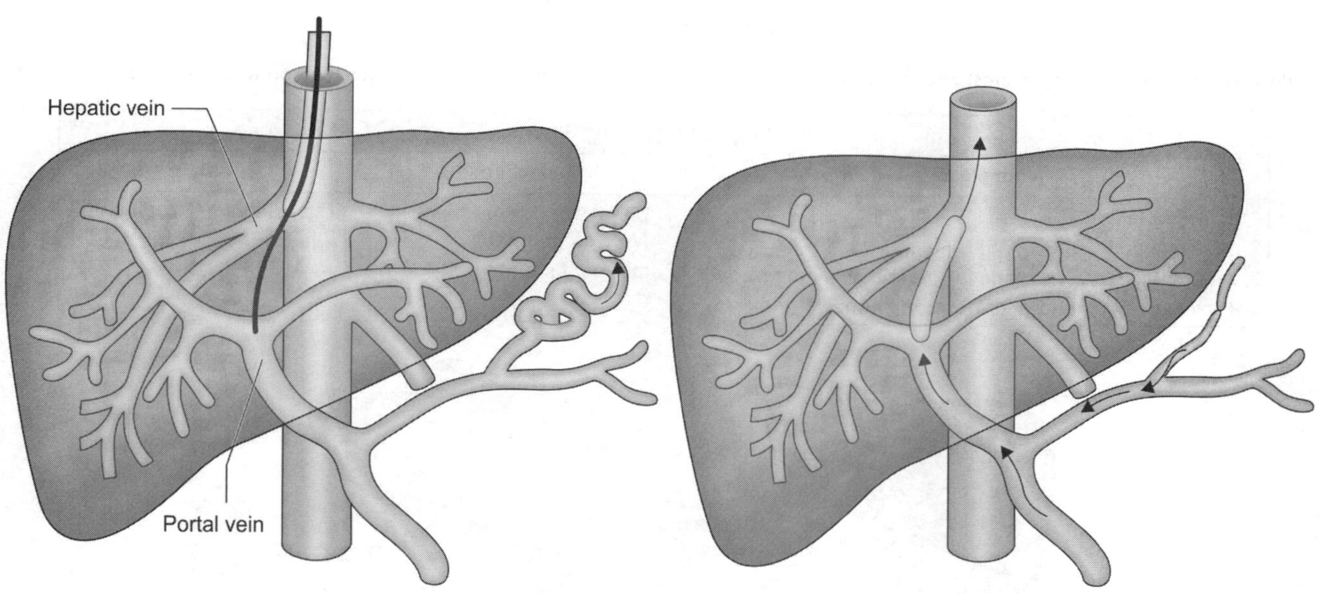

Transjugular intrahepatic portosystemic shunt (TIPS)

TRANSJUGULAR INTRAHEPATIC PORTAL-SYSTEMIC SHUNT (TIPSS)

- TIPSS is a **non-selective shunt**, created between **portal** and **hepatic vein**[Q]
- TIPSS is **portahepatic** or **intrahepatic shunt**[Q]

Technique of Placement

- Initial venous access is through the **right internal jugular vein** because this is the **shortest** and **most direct path** to catheterize the hepatic veins[Q].
- **Right hepatic vein** is MC used because it is the **largest hepatic vein** and usually has the **most favourable orientation**[Q].
- Portal vein is cannulated by **Rosch needle**.

Stent

- **VIATORR** is a **stent-graft**[Q] specifically designed for TIPSS.

Indications of TIPSS	
1. **Prevention of rebleeding** from varices (**MC**)[Q]	5. Refractory hepatic hydrothorax[Q]
2. **Acute variceal bleeding**[Q]	6. Budd-Chiari syndrome[Q]
3. **Refractory ascites**[Q]	7. Hepatic veno-occlusive disease[Q]
4. **Hepatorenal syndrome**[Q]	8. Portal hypertensive gastropathy[Q]

Contraindications of TIPSS	
Absolute	**Relative**
1. **Right-sided heart failure**[Q]	1. Portal vein thrombosis[Q]
2. **Polycystic liver disease**[Q]	2. Hypervascular liver tumors[Q]
3. **Pulmonary hypertension**[Q]	3. Encephalopathy[Q]
4. **Hepatopulmonary syndrome**[Q]	

Complications

- **Encephalopathy (10–20%)**[Q]:
- **Stenosis** or **thrombosis (5–15%)**[Q]:
  - **Shunt stenosis** is usually secondary to **neointimal hyperplasia** and is **more common than thrombosis**[Q].

Surveillance

- **Doppler duplex ultrasonography** at 24 hours, 1 month, 3 months, and 6 months after the initial TIPS procedure.

■ PORTOSYSTEMIC SHUNTS

PORTOSYSTEMIC SHUNTS

- **Portosystemic shunts** are the **most effective** means of **preventing recurrent hemorrhage**[Q] in patients with portal hypertension.

Types of Portosystemic Shunts

Nonselective	Selective	Partial
1. **Eck fistula**[Q] 2. Side-to-side PCS (**SSPCS**)[Q] 3. Interposition graft (**portacaval, mesocaval, mesorenal**)[Q] 4. Proximal splenorenal shunt (**Linton shunt**[Q])	1. **Distal** splenorenal shunt (**Warren shunt**[Q]) 2. **Inokuchi shunt**[Q]	1. Diameter of shunt **<10 mm**[Q]

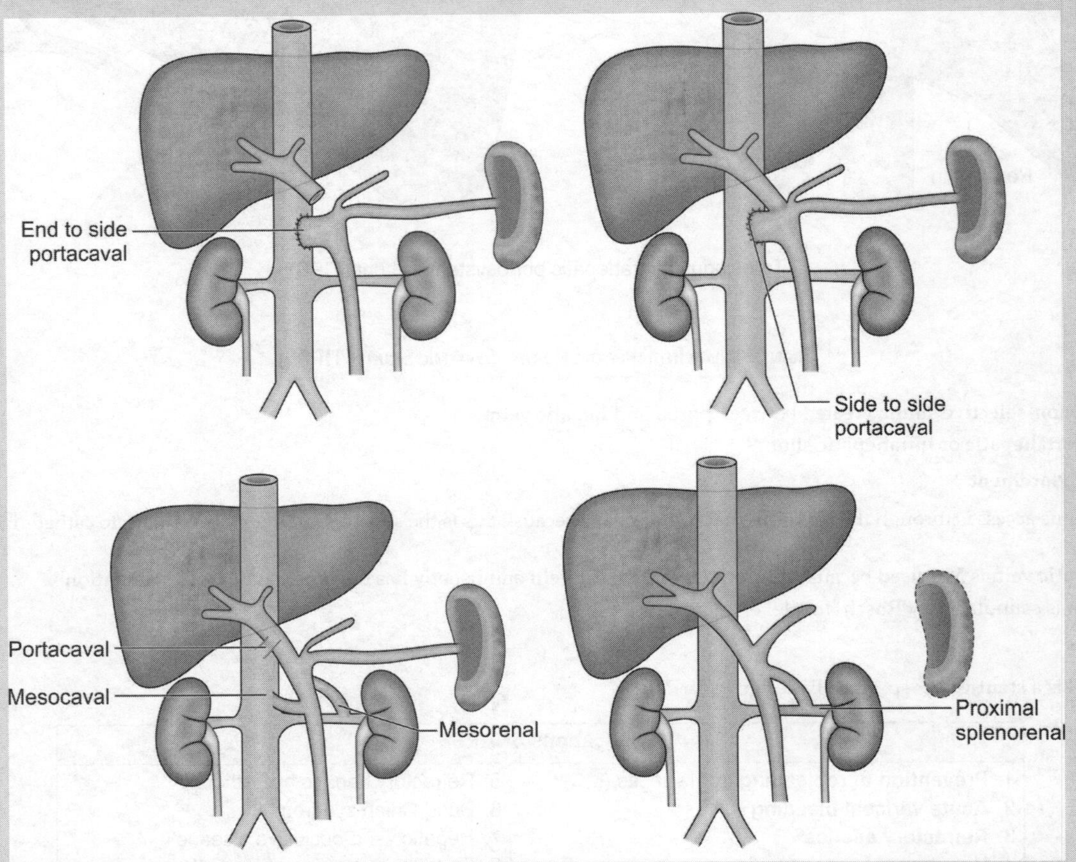

Non-selective shunts

- In the current era, indications for a **nonselective shunt** would include an **emergency shunt** for **variceal hemorrhage**, an **elective shunt** in the presence of **significant ascites** and treatment of **Budd-Chiari syndrome**[Q].
- Patients in whom a **future liver transplant** is required should be treated with a **shunt** in which **dissection** is **performed outside** of the **porta hepatis**.
- Choice (TIPS or shunt) is based on the predicted time to transplantation:
  - **TIPS** if transplant is **delayed <1 year**[Q]
  - **Portosystemic shunt** if transplant is **delayed >1 year**[Q].
- Patients who live in **remote locations** and those who **fail endoscopic** and **drug therapy** receive a **selective shunt**.
- **MC causes** of **death in:**
  - **Medically treated** patients: Rebleeding[Q]
  - **Shunted** patients: Accelerated hepatic failure[Q]
- **Rex shunt** is an **internal jugular vein graft (mesenteric-left portal vein bypass)**[Q] used in **EHPVO**[Q].
- **Eck's Fistula** is an **end-to-side portacaval shunt**[Q].

■ PERITONEOVENOUS SHUNT

PERITONEOVENOUS SHUNT

- **Le-Veen shunt** is designed for the **relief of ascites due to chronic liver disease**[Q].
- One end of silastic tube is inserted into the ascites within the peritoneal cavity other end is tunneled subcutaneously to the neck, where it is **inserted under direct vision into the internal jugular vein and fed into the SVC**[Q].

Mechanism of Action

- Owing to a one-way valve within the tubing, peritoneal fluid is drawn from the abdomen and drained to the circulation due to the **lower pressure in the SVC** in comparison with the abdomen during the respiratory cycle[Q].

> - In an attempt to prevent the high occlusion rate, a further development was the **insertion of a chamber placed over the costal margin to allow digital pressure and evacuation of any debris within the peritoneovenous shunt (Denver shunt)**[Q].

■ ENCEPHALOPATHY

ENCEPHALOPATHY

- Cerebral toxins include ammonia, mercaptans and GABA. **Severity** of encephalopathy **does not correlate** with blood **ammonia** levels.

> - **MC cause** is **azotemia**[Q]; most episodes are **acute**[Q]
> - **MC setting** for the development of encephalopathy is in patients with **cirrhosis** who undergo a **procedural shunt**[Q].

- **Only drugs with proven effectiveness:**
  - **Neomycin**[Q]: A poorly absorbed antibiotic that **suppresses urease containing bacteria**
  - **Lactulose**[Q]: A nonabsorbable disaccharide that **acidifies colonic contents** and also has **cathartic effects**
- **Unproven therapies** include the enteral or parenteral administration of **branch chain amino acids** and the drug **flumazenil**, a selective antagonist of benzodiazepine receptor.

Factors Precipitating Hepatic Encephalopathy			
Nitrogenous causes		**Non-nitrogenous causes**	
• Uremia/**Azotemia (MC)**[Q]	• **Hypokalemia**[Q]	• **Sedative**, benzodiazepines	• Hypothyroidism
• GI **bleeding**[Q]	• **Constipation**[Q]	• **Barbiturates**[Q]	• Anemia
• Dehydration	• Excessive dietary **protein**[Q]	• **Hypoxia**[Q]	
• Metabolic **alkalosis**[Q]	• **Infection**[Q]	• **Hypoglycemia**[Q]	

■ NONCIRRHOTIC PORTAL HYPERTENSION

NONCIRRHOTIC PORTAL HYPERTENSION

- **Noncirrhotic portal hypertension** encompasses two distinct pathological condition that present with similar clinical features.
  - **Non cirrhotic portal fibrosis (NCPF)**   – **Extra-Hepatic Portal Venous Obstruction (EHPVO)**
- Distinction between the two conditions should ideally be made by further investigations as the similarly in presentation makes clinical criteria unreliable.

NCPF	EHPVO

• NCPF presents in **young adults**[Q]
• Most commonly during the **2nd & 3rd decade**[Q]
	• EHPVO may present in two age groups:
	  – **Children: 1st and 2nd** decade due to congenital malformations[Q]
	  – **Adults: 4th and 5th** decade due to thrombotic event[Q]

Clinical Presentation: • Gradual onset of symptoms • **Splenomegaly** is about **4 times more common** in **NCPF** than EHPV[Q]	**Clinical Presentation:** • **Gradual onset** in **children**, where the cause is **congenital malformation**[Q] • **Acute onset** in adults where the cause is a **thrombotic event**[Q] • Splenomegaly is 4 times less common in patients with EHPV[Q]

■ MELD SCORE AND PELD SCORE

MODEL FOR END-STAGE LIVER DISEASE (MELD) SCORE

- **MELD score** is used to **assess** the **severity of chronic liver disease**[Q]
- It was **initially developed** to **predict death within 3 months** of surgery in patients that had **undergone TIPS.**[Q]
- It is calculated by using **3 variables (CBI)**: S. Creatinine, S. Bilirubin, INR[Q]

  - MELD score is **currently used** by United Network for Organ Sharing (UNOS) for **prioritizing allocation of liver transplant**[Q].

- It is **6–40 point** scale
- **Relative risk of mortality** increases by **14% for each 1point increase in MELD score.**
- **MELD score = 3.8log(e) (S. bilirubin mg/dL) + 11.2Log(e) (INR) + 9.6Log(e) (S. creatinine mg/dL)**

PEDIATRIC END-STAGE LIVER DISEASE (PELD) SCORE

- **PELD score** utilizes following variables (**NABIA**)[Q]:
  1. Nutritional status[Q]   2. Age[Q]   3. Bilirubin[Q]   4. INR[Q]   5. Albumin[Q]

MELD score (CBI)	Creatinine, Bilirubin, INR[Q]
PELD score (NABIA)	Nutritional status, Age, Bilirubin, INR, Albumin[Q]

Multiple Choice Questions

■ PORTAL HYPERTENSION

1. **Normal portal vein pressure is:**
   (Recent Question 2016, COMEDK 2008)
   a. < 3 mm Hg   b. 3–5 mm Hg
   c. 5–10 mm Hg   d. 10–12 mm Hg

2. **Left sided portal hypertension is best treated by:**
   (Recent Question 2016, AIIMS June 2001)
   a. Splenectomy   b. Portocaval shunt
   c. Lieno-renal shunt   d. Spleno-renal shunt

3. **Child-Pugh criteria does not include:**   *(Punjab 2010)*
   a. Encephalopathy   b. ALT
   c. Ascites   d. Albumin

4. **MELD score doesn't include:**
   (Recent Question 2017, AIIMS GIS Dec 2011, Dec 2006)
   a. INR   b. S. bilirubin
   c. S. creatinine   d. Blood urea

5. **Child's Criteria is used in:**   *(DNB 2005, 2001, 2000)*
   a. Pancreatitis   b. Cirrhosis
   c. Multiple myeloma   d. AIDS

6. **Child-Pugh score is used for:**   *(Recent Question 2017)*
   a. Hepatic encephalopathy   b. Uremic encephalopathy
   c. Chronic liver disease   d. Head injury

7. **All of the following are true in case of chronic liver disease except:**   *(Recent Question 2019)*
   a. MELD score is used frequently to see whom needs liver transplant early
   b. MELD score includes serum albumin, creatinine, and INR
   c. Child Pugh score includes PT-INR, albumin and bilirubin
   d. Child Pugh score has class A, B, C

■ ESOPHAGEAL VARICES

8. **What is the most probable diagnosis on the basis of given endoscopy image?**   *(Recent Question 2016)*
   a. GAVE   b. Schatzki ring
   c. Barrett's esophagus   d. Esophageal varices

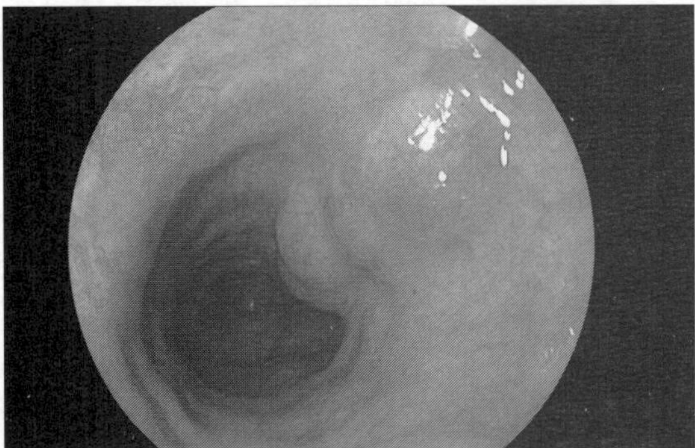

9. **Best test for esophageal varices is:**   *(UPPG 2009)*
   a. CT-scan   b. Gastro-esophagoscopy
   c. Tomography   d. Ultrasound

10. **Which of the following agents is recommended for medical treatment of variceal bleed?**   *(All India 2011)*
    a. Octreotide   b. Desmopressin
    c. Vasopressin   d. Nitroglycerine

■ GASTRIC VARICES

11. **Most common cause of gastric varices is:** *(AIIMS GIS Dec 2011)*
    a. Splenic vein thrombosis
    b. Splenectomy
    c. Cirrhosis
    d. Mesenteric thrombosis

■ TIPS

12. **TIPS means creating anastomosis between which of the following?** *(WB PG 2015, MHSSMCET 2009, Karnataka 2006)*
    a. Portal vein and hepatic artery
    b. Portal vein and IVC
    c. Portal vein and hepatic vein
    d. Hepatic vein and hepatic artery

13. **Early complication of TIPS procedure:**
    a. Shunt stenosis and blockage   *(JIPMER Nov 2017)*
    b. Capsular haemorrhage
    c. Metabolic encephalopathy
    d. Recurrent variceal bleed

■ SURGICAL SHUNTS

14. **What is the type of this shunt?**

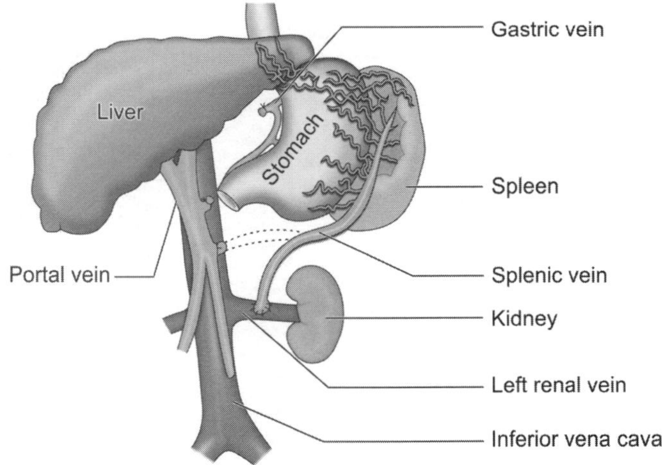

    a. Non-selective shunt   b. Selective shunt
    c. Partial shunt   d. None of the above

15. **Denver shunt is used in:**   *(DNB 2012)*
    a. Ascites   b. Dialysis
    c. Raised ICT   d. Raised IOP

16. **The Le-Veen shunt in ascites is done between peritoneum and:**   *(Recent Question 2016, AIIMS Nov 2014)*
    a. Cisterna chyli   b. Renal pelvis
    c. Superior vena cava   d. Gallbladder

17. **Which of the following is a selective shunt?**
    a. Proximal splenorenal shunt   *(Recent Question 2017)*
    b. Warren shunt
    c. Side-to-side portocaval shunt
    d. Mesocaval shunt

■ EXTRA-HEPATIC PORTAL VENOUS OBSTRUCTION

18. A 12-year-old boy presents with hematemesis, melena and mild splenomegaly. There is no obvious jaundice or ascites. The most likely diagnosis is: *(All India 2011)*
    a. EHPVO
    b. NCPF
    c. Cirrhosis
    d. Malaria with DIC

19. Treatment of choice for extrahepatic portal thrombosis:
    a. Mesocaval shunt *(MHSSMCET 2009)*
    b. Porto caval shunt
    c. Mesorenal shunt
    d. Splenorenal shunt

■ NONCIRRHOTIC PORTAL FIBROSIS

20. Which of the following is the most common presenting symptom of non-cirrhotic portal hypertension?
    a. Chronic liver disease *(All India 2006)*
    b. Ascites
    c. Upper gastrointestinal bleeding
    d. Encephalopathy

■ BUDD-CHIARI SYNDROME

21. The obstruction of two or more major hepatic veins is seen in: *(MHCET 2016)*
    a. Budd-Chiari syndrome   b. Reye's syndrome
    c. Rotor syndrome   d. Crigler-Najjar syndrome

22. Classical triad of Budd-Chiari syndrome:
    a. Fever, jaundice, abdominal pain *(Recent Question 2016)*
    b. Fever, ascites, jaundice
    c. Hepatomegaly, abdominal pain, ascites
    d. Abdominal pain, jaundice, hepatomegaly

23. Most commonly performed hepatobiliary shunt in Budd-Chiari syndrome: *(Recent Question 2016)*
    a. Rex shunt   b. Lienorenal shunt
    c. Mesocaval shunt
    d. Side to side portocaval shunt

■ VENO-OCCLUSIVE DISEASE

24. Veno-occlusive disease is seen in all except: *(AIIMS GIS Dec 2011)*
    a. Bone marrow transplant   b. Bush teas
    c. Mushroom poisoning   d. Cytosine arabinoside

Explanations

■ PORTAL HYPERTENSION

1. **Ans. c. 5–10 mm Hg** *(Ref: Sabiston 20/e p1436-1437; Schwartz 11/e p1366, 10/e p1280-1281; Harrison 20/e p2410)*

2. **Ans. a. Splenectomy**

3. **Ans. b. ALT**

4. **Ans. d. Blood urea** *(Ref: Sabiston 20/e p640; Schwartz 11/e p13365, 10/e p1280; Harrison 20/e p2416)*

MELD score (CBI)	Creatinine, Bilirubin, INR[Q]
PELD score (NABIA)	Nutritional status, Age, Bilirubin, INR, Albumin[Q]

5. **Ans. b. Cirrhosis**

6. **Ans. c. Chronic liver disease** *(Ref: Sabiston 20/e p1436; Schwartz 11/e p1366, 10/e p1280; Bailey 27/e p1156)*

7. **Ans. b. MELD score includes serum albumin, creatinine, and INR**

■ ESOPHAGEAL VARICES

8. **Ans. d. Esophageal varices** *(Ref: Sabiston 20/e p1437; Schwartz 11/e p1366, 10/e p1281; Bailey 27/e p1126; Harrison 20/e p2411)*

9. **Ans. b. Gastro-esophagoscopy**

10. **Ans. a. Octreotide** *(Ref: Harrison 20/e p2411)*

- **Somatostatin** and/or its analog **octreotide** are the **agents of choice** for **medical management** of **variceal bleed[Q].**
- **Octreotide** and **Somatostatin** have been found to be effective in **achieving hemostasis** and **preventing early rebleeding[Q].**
- **Terlipressin** is released in sustained and slow manner. It does not share several systemic side effects of vasopressin and **may be used** to **control variceal bleeding[Q].**

Drugs used in Portal Hypertension	
Drugs Decreasing portal blood flow	**Drugs decreasing intrahepatic resistance**
• Non-selective beta blockers • Vasopressin and **Terlipressin** • Somatostatin and **Octreotide (DOC)[Q]**	• Nitrates • Alpha1-blockers (Prazosin) • Angiotensin receptor blockers

■ GASTRIC VARICES

11. **Ans. c. Cirrhosis** *(Ref: Sabiston 20/e p1232; Schwartz 11/e p1367, 10/e p1088)*

- **MC cause** of **gastric varices: Cirrhosis[Q]**
- **MC cause** of **isolated gastric varices: Splenic vein thrombosis[Q]**

■ TIPS

12. **Ans. c. Portal vein and hepatic vein**

13. **Ans. c. Metabolic encephalopathy** *(Ref: Schwartz 11/e p1367, 10/e p1282; Sabiston 20/e p1440; Bailey 27/e p1164)*

■ SURGICAL SHUNTS

14. **Ans. b. Selective shunt** *(Ref: Sabiston 20/e p1442; Schwartz 11/e p1368, 10/e p1283)*

The given shunt is distal splenorenal shunt, which is a selective shunt.

15. **Ans. a. Ascites** *(Ref: Textbook of Hepatology by Erwin Kuntz/317)*

16. **Ans. c. Superior vena cava** *(Ref: Bailey 26/e p1077; Textbook of Hepatology by Erwin Kuntz/317)*

The Le-Veen shunt in ascites is done between peritoneum and superior vena cava.

"The Le-Veen shunt is designed for the relief of ascites due to chronic liver disease. One end of the silastic tube is inserted into the ascites within the peritoneal cavity and the other end is tunneled subcutaneously to the neck, where it is inserted under direct vision into the internal jugular vein and fed into the SVC."- Bailey 26/e p1077

17. **Ans. b. Warren shunt** *(Ref: Sabiston 20/e p1442; Schwartz 11/e p1368, 10/e p1283)*

■ EXTRA-HEPATIC PORTAL VENOUS OBSTRUCTION

18. **Ans. a.** EHPVO *(Ref: Blumgart 6/e p1216)*

19. **Ans. a. > d.** Mesocaval shunt > Splenorenal shunt

- Since obstruction is in the portal vein, to bypass the obstruction the shunt should be preferably **Rex shunt (mesenterico-left portal shunt)**[Q] or a **mesocaval shunt**.
- Splenorenal shunt is also done in EHPVO but in **50%** of patients of **EHPVO, splenic vein is thrombosed**, not available for **splenorenal shunt**[Q].

■ NONCIRRHOTIC PORTAL FIBROSIS

20. **Ans. c.** Upper gastrointestinal bleeding *(R p1216)*

■ BUDD-CHIARI SYNDROME

21. **Ans. a.** Budd-Chiari syndrome

22. **Ans. c.** Hepatomegaly, abdominal pain, ascites

23. **Ans. d.** Side to side portocaval shunt

■ VENO-OCCLUSIVE DISEASE

24. **Ans. c.** Mushroom poisoning

Gallbladder

■ GALLSTONES: PATHOGENESIS

PATHOGENESIS OF CHOLESTEROL GALLSTONES

- **Cholesterol** is **insoluble** in **water** (**water** is major constituent of bile, **85-95%**)[Q].
- **Bile acid** & **phospholipids** in bile keep cholesterol in solution by the formation of **micelles**[Q].
- An **excess of cholesterol** relative to bile acids & phospholipids allows cholesterol to form crystals and such bile is called **lithogenic** or **supersaturated bile**[Q].

Factors Responsible for Formation of Gallstones		
Lithogenic bile	Nucleation	Stasis or GB hypomotility

• **Increased Biliary Cholesterol:**
  – **Obesity**[Q]
  – Cholesterol rich diet[Q]
  – **Clofibrate** therapy[Q]
• **Decreased Bile Acids:**
  – Primary biliary cirrhosis
  – **OCPs**[Q]
  – Mutation of **CYP7A1** gene[Q]
  – **Impaired enterohepatic circulation** of bile acids: **Ileal disease** or **resection, cholestyramine** or **colestipol** (bile acid sequestrants)[Q]
• **Decreased Biliary Lecithin**:
  – **MDR-3** gene **mutation**[Q] leads to defective lecithin secretion in bile
	• Cholesterol monohydrate crystal agglomerate to become macroscopic crystal by nucleation
	• **Pro-nucleating Factors**:
	  – **Mucin**[Q]
	  – Non-mucin glycoprotein[Q]
	  – Infection[Q]
	• **Anti-nucleating Factors**:
	  – Apolipoprotein A-I & A-II[Q]
	• **Excess** of **pro-nucleating factors** or **deficiency** of **anti-nucleating factors** results in formation of gallstones
		• Prolonged **TPN**[Q]
		• Prolonged **fasting**[Q]
		• **Pregnancy**[Q]
		• **Octreotide**[Q]
		• **OCPs**[Q]
		• Massive **burns**[Q]

- **Cholesterol gallstones** are made up of **crystalline cholesterol monohydrate**[Q].

Pigmented Stones	
Black Stones	Brown Stones

• **Black stones** are composed of **insoluble bilirubin pigment polymer**[Q] mixed with **calcium phosphate** & calcium **bicarbonate**[Q].
• **Predisposing Factors:**
  – **Hemolytic disorders**[Q] (Hereditary spherocytosis, sickle cell anemia)
  – Mechanical **prosthetic heart valves**[Q]
  – **Cirrhosis**
  – **Gilbert's syndrome**[Q]
  – **Cystic fibrosis**[Q]
  – Ileal disease or resection
	• **Brown pigment** stones contain **calcium bilirubinate**, calcium **palmitate** & calcium **stearate** as well as cholesterol[Q].
	• Typically found in **Asia**[Q]
	• **Rare** in **GB**[Q]
	• **Formed** in **bile duct**[Q]
	• **Related** to the **bile stasis and infection:**
	  – Gram negative bacteria (**E. coli** & **Klebsiella**)[Q] secretes **beta-glucuronidase**[Q], which **deconjugate** soluble **conjugated bilirubin**
	  – **Free unconjugated bilirubin precipitates** & combines **with calcium** and **bile** to form **brown pigment stones**.
	  – Stones form whenever static foreign bodies are present in the bile duct (**stents** or parasites such as **Clonorchis sinensis** & **Ascaris lumbricoides**)[Q]

■ GALLSTONES INVESTIGATIONS

- Ultrasonography
- Initial imaging modality of choice in obstructive jaundice[Q]
- It is **operator dependent** and may be **suboptimal due to excessive body fat** and **intraluminal bowel gas[Q]**.

USG can demonstrate		
• **Biliary calculi[Q]** • **Thickness** of GB wall[Q]	• **Size** of **GB and CBD[Q]**	• Presence of **inflammation[Q]** around GB • Occasionally, **presence of stones within** the **biliary tree[Q]**.

- It may even show a **carcinoma** of the **pancreas occluding** the **CBD[Q]**.

USG in obstructive jaundice
• **Initial imaging modality** of **choice** in **obstructive jaundice[Q]**
• It **can identify intra-** and **extrahepatic biliary dilatation[Q]**
• Identify the **level of obstruction[Q]**
• **Cause of the obstruction[Q]** may also be identified
• (**Gallstones** in the gallbladder, common hepatic or **CBD stones** or lesions in the wall of the duct suggestive of a **cholangiocarcinoma** or enlargement of the pancreatic head indicative of a **pancreatic carcinoma**) [Q]

- **Iopanoic acid** is used in **oral cholecystography[Q]**.
- **Biligraffin** is used in **IV cholangiography[Q]**.

RADIOISOTOPE SCANNING

- **Technetium-99m labelled derivatives** of **iminodiacetic acid** (HIDA, IODIDA) are, when injected intravenously, **selectively taken up** by the **reticuloendothelial cells** of the liver and **excreted into bile[Q]**.

HIDA Scan
• Allows **visualization** of the **biliary tree** and **gallbladder[Q]**
• Presence of **inflammation[Q]** around GB
• Occasionally, **presence of stones within** the **biliary tree[Q]**.
• **GB is visualized within 30 min** of **isotope injection** in **90%** of normal individuals and within 1 hour in the remainder.
• The **bowel** is usually **seen within 1 hour** in the majority of patients.
• **Nonvisualization** of the **GB** is suggestive of **acute cholecystitis[Q]**.
• If the patient has **contracted gallbladder**, as often occurs in **chronic cholecystitis**, **GB visualization** may be **reduced** or **delayed[Q]**.

- **Biliary scintigraphy** may also be **helpful in diagnosing bile leaks** and **iatrogenic biliary obstruction[Q]**.
- **Scintigraphy can confirm** the **presence & quantify the leak[Q]**.

■ ACUTE CHOLECYSTITIS

ACUTE CHOLECYSTITIS

- Acute cholecystitis is **related to gallstones** in **90–95%[Q]** of cases.
- **Characteristic triad: RUQ pain + Fever + Leukocytosis[Q]**

Clinical Features

- **RUQ pain** of **much longer duration** than biliary colic, is the **MC symptom[Q]**
- Other common symptoms: Fever, nausea, and vomiting.
- **Physical examination**: RUQ **tenderness** and **guarding** are usually present **inferior to** the **right costal margin**, distinguishing the episode from simple biliary colic.
- A **mass** (gallbladder & adherent omentum) is occasionally palpable[Q]
- **Murphy's sign[Q]: Inspiratory arrest** with **deep palpation** in the **RUQ** in acute cholecystitis (also known as **Naunyn's sign**)
- **Boa's sign[Q]:** Hyperesthesia below right scapula in acute cholecystitis.

• A **mild leukocytosis** is **usually present** (12,000–14,000 cells/mm³).
• Mild elevations in serum bilirubin (>4 mg/dL), ALP, transaminases, & amylase may be present.

Diagnosis

• **USG: IOC** for diagnosing **acute cholecystitis[Q]** (sensitivity 85%, specificity 95%).
• **HIDA scan: Gold standard[Q]** for diagnosing **acute cholecystitis**

Contd...

Contd...

Treatment

- **IV fluids, antibiotics**, and **analgesia** should be initiated[Q].
- **Cholecystectomy** is the **definitive treatment**[Q] for patients with acute cholecystitis.

> - **Early cholecystectomy** performed **within 2 to 3 days (within 72 hours)** [Q] of presentation **is preferred over interval** or **delayed cholecystectomy** that is performed 6 to 10 weeks after initial medical therapy.
> - **Laparoscopic cholecystectomy** is the **preferred approach** to patients with **acute cholecystitis**[Q].

■ MEDICAL THERAPY FOR GALLSTONES

MEDICAL THERAPY FOR GALLSTONES

- Medical therapy for gallstones utilizes bile acids: **Chenodeoxycholic acid (CDCA) & Ursodeoxycholic acid (UDCA)**[Q]

Mechanism of Action

- They **inhibit HMG-CoA reductase**[Q], rate limiting enzyme for cholesterol synthesis, thus **decreases cholesterol saturation of bile**[Q]
- They cause **dispersion** of **cholesterol from** the **stones** by **physicochemical means**[Q]

Prerequisites for Medical Treatment	Drawbacks of Medical Treatment
• **Radioluscent (cholesterol)** stones[Q] • **Stones <10 mm** in diameter[Q] • **Functioning GB**[Q] • **Non-acute symptoms**[Q]	• **Low rates** of **complete resolution**[Q] • **High recurrence** rate[Q] • **Not cost-effective** (expensive drug has to be taken for up to 2 years)[Q] • **Need** of **maintenance therapy** to prevent recurrence[Q]

■ GALLSTONE ILEUS

GALLSTONE ILEUS

- Passage of **stone** through a **spontaneous biliary-enteric fistula** leading to a **mechanical bowel obstruction**[Q]
- **MC site** of fistula: Between the **gallbladder** and **duodenum**[Q]
- **2nd MC site**: Between **gallbladder** and **transverse colon**[Q].

Clinical Features

> - **Rigler's triad**[Q]: Classic plain abdominal film triad of **small bowel obstruction, pneumobilia, & ectopic gallstone** is considered pathognomonic[Q].

- **Most cholecystoduodenal fistula** does **not result in Gallstone ileus**[Q].
- Occurs **most commonly** in the **elderly (>70 years)**[Q]
- **Nausea, vomiting, and abdominal pain, signs** & symptoms of intestinal obstruction
- A history of **gallstone-related symptoms** may be present in only 50% of patients.
- **Pain** may be **episodic** and **recurrent** as the impacted stone temporarily obstructs the bowel lumen and then dislodges and moves distally, known as **tumbling obstruction**[Q].
- **MC site** of **obstruction** is ileum[Q] (60%); **jejunum** (15%); **stomach** (15%) colon (5% > sigmoid colon); & duodenum (5%).

Diagnosis

- **Abdominal X-ray**: Evidence of an **intestinal obstruction** with **pneumobilia** or a **calcified stone**[Q] distant from the gallbladder.

Treatment

- It is a **surgical emergency**[Q] without a period of waiting in the hope that stone will pass
- In case of **obstruction in the ileum calculus** can be **manipulated proximally** to a **healthy jejunum**[Q] where a **safe enterotomy** and stone removal may be executed.
- **Stable patients**: Takedown of the **biliary-enteric fistula** and **cholecystectomy**[Q] during the same procedure is warranted because recurrent cholecystitis and cholangitis are common.

> - **Unstable patients** or a **significant inflammation** in RUQ: Unstable to withstand a prolonged **operative procedure**, the fistula can be addressed at a second laparotomy[Q].

■ MUCOCELE

- Mucocele (Hydrops)
- **Hydrops** or **mucocele** result from **prolonged obstruction** of the **cystic duct**, usually by a **large solitary calculus**[Q].
- **Obstructed GB lumen** is progressively **distended** by **mucus** (mucocele) or by a **clear transudate (hydrops)** produced by mucosal epithelial cells[Q].
- Clinical Features
- A **visible, easily palpable, nontender gallbladder**[Q] sometimes extending from the RUQ into the right iliac fossa may be found on physical examination.
- The patient with hydrops of the gallbladder **frequently remains asymptomatic**[Q], although chronic RUQ pain may also occur.
- Treatment
- **Early cholecystectomy**[Q], because empyema, perforation, or gangrene may complicate the condition.

GALLBLADDER EMPYEMA

- GB empyema results from **progression of acute cholecystitis** with **persistent cystic duct obstruction** to **superinfection**[Q] of the stagnant bile with a pus-forming bacterial organism.

Clinical Features
- Clinical picture resembles that of **cholangitis** with **high fever; severe RUQ pain**; marked **leukocytosis**; and often, **prostration**[Q].
- Empyema carries a **high risk of gram-negative sepsis** and/or **perforation**[Q].

Treatment
- **Emergency surgical intervention** with **antibiotic coverage** is required as soon as the diagnosis is suspected.

■ PROPHYLACTIC CHOLECYSTECTOMY

Indications of Prophylactic Cholecystectomy	
• **Cardiac transplant** recipients[Q]	• **Family history** of **GB cancer** and asymptomatic stones[Q]
• **Lung transplant** recipients[Q]	• Cholelithiasis encountered during **elective abdominal procedures**[Q]
• Chronic **TPN** requirement[Q]	
• Recipients of **biliopancreatic diversion**[Q] (bariatric patient)	• **Nonfunctioning** GB[Q]
• Children with **hemoglobinopathy**[Q] (sickle cell, thalassemia and spherocytosis)	• **Typhoid carrier** with positive bile culture[Q]
• Asymptomatic gallstone ≥3 cm[Q]	• **Trauma** to GB[Q]
• **Stone** associated with the **polyp**	• **Porcelain GB**

■ ACALCULOUS CHOLECYSTITIS

ACALCULOUS CHOLECYSTITIS

- Acute **inflammation of gallbladder without stones**[Q]
- **More fulminant course**[Q] than the acute calculous cholecystitis. **More commonly progresses** to gangrene, empyema, or perforation[Q].

Predisposing Factors
- **Burns**[Q]
- **Long-term TPN**[Q]
- **Elderly** and **critically ill patients** after **trauma**[Q]
- Major operations **(abdominal aneurysm repair & cardiopulmonary bypass**[Q])

Etiopathogenesis
- Exact etiology is not clear

- **GB stasis & ischemia**[Q] have been implicated as causative factors.

Clinical Features
- **Similar** to **acute calculous cholecystitis**[Q].
- Patients may present with only **unexplained fever, leucocytosis** and **hyperamylasemia & RUQ tenderness**[Q].

Diagnosis
- **Ultrasonography** is the **diagnostic test of choice**[Q], especially because it can be done at the bed side.
- **Cholescintigraphy** demonstrates **absent gallbladder filling**

Treatment
- **Emergency cholecystectomy**[Q] for **stable**[Q] patients
- **Open cholecystectomy**[Q] is often the **preferred approach**.

Percutaneous Cholecystostomy
• If patients are **unfit for surgery**, percutaneous, ultrasound guided, or **CT guided cholecystostomy** is the **treatment of choice**[Q].
• About **90% patients improve** with **percutaneous cholecystostomy**.

■ XANTHOGRANULOMATOUS CHOLECYSTITIS

XANTHOGRANULOMATOUS CHOLECYSTITIS

- **XGC:** Inflammatory disease characterized by a **focal or diffuse destructive inflammatory process** with **lipid-laden macrophages**[Q]

Clinical Features

- Similar to acute cholecystitis

Diagnosis

- **Thickening** of GB wall is **most common radiological finding**, sometimes presence of **hypoattenuated bands**[Q].

Treatment

- Surgical treatment **(Laparoscopic cholecystectomy)** remains **the most** effective and **feasible option for XGC**

■ EMPHYSEMATOUS CHOLECYSTITIS

EMPHYSEMATOUS CHOLECYSTITIS

- Thought to begin with acute cholecystitis (calculous or acalculous), followed by ischemia or gangrene of GB wall and **infection** by **gas producing organisms**[Q].
- Occur most frequently in **elderly men** and patients with **diabetes mellitus**[Q].

Causative organisms of Emphysematous Cholecystitis
• **Anaerobes: Cl. welchii or Cl. perfringens (MC)** [Q]
• **Aerobes: E. coli**[Q]

Clinical Features

- Clinical manifestations are essentially indistinguishable from those of nongaseous cholecystitis.

Diagnosis

- **Diagnosis** is usually made on **abdominal X-ray**[Q]
- **Abdominal X-ray** findings: **Gas within the GB lumen**, dissecting within GB wall to form a **gaseous ring** or in **pericholecystic tissues**[Q].
- **IOC for diagnosis: CT scan**[Q]

Treatment

- **Prompt surgical drainage** coupled with appropriate **antibiotics** is mandatory[Q].
- **Cholecystectomy** is **best treatment** of complicated acute cholecystitis[Q].
- **Unstable patients: Percutaneous cholecystostomy** under **LA**[Q] can be performed to drain GB.

■ MIRIZZI'S SYNDROME (FUNCTIONAL HEPATIC SYNDROME)

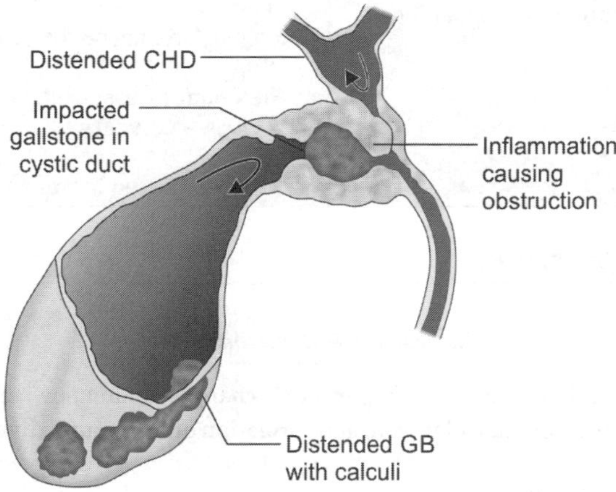

MIRIZZI'S SYNDROME (FUNCTIONAL HEPATIC SYNDROME)

- It is defined as **obstruction** of the **common hepatic duct** or **CBD** by **external compression** or by **erosion** of stone in the **Hartmann pouch** or **cystic duct**[Q].
- **External compression** has been classified as **type 1** whereas **erosion** as **type 2** Mirizzi syndrome by **McSherry**[Q].
- **Csendes** subclassified type 2 into three categories based on the percentage of the wall of CBD eroded by offending calculus.

Contd...

Contd...

Csendes Classification of Mirizzi's Syndrome	
Type I	**Obstruction** of common duct by **external compression only** (no erosion)[Q]
Type II	Erosion of **less than one-third** circumference of common duct[Q]
Type III	Erosion of **up to two-third** circumference of common duct[Q]
Type IV	**Total/near total** circumferential destruction of common duct[Q]
Type V	**Erosion of GB in common duct** with **cholecystoenteric fistula**

Treatment

Type I	**Partial cholecystectomy**[Q]
Type II & Type III	**Partial cholecystectomy** leaving behind a cuff of gallbladder for reconstruction of bile duct (**choledochoplasty**) with **T-tube drainage**[Q]
Type IV & V	Bilioenteric anastomosis[Q]

- **Stenosis** of the **biliary tree** often **resolves spontaneously** in the **postoperative period**, and **choledochotomy** is **seldom indicated**[Q].

■ STRAWBERRY GALLBLADDER (CHOLESTEROLOSIS)

STRAWBERRY GALLBLADDER (CHOLESTEROLOSIS)

- **Acquired**[Q] histologic abnormality of GB epithelium
- Associated with **excessive accumulation** of lipid (**cholesterols esters & triglyceride**)[Q] within epithelial macrophage of GB wall.
- **Cholesterol stones** are found in **half** of the **cases**[Q].

Pathology
- **Gross Appearance:** Mucosa has **pale, yellow streaks** running longitudinally giving rise to the term **strawberry gallbladder**[Q] (although the mucosa is usually bile stained rather than red).
- **Diffuse form** ("strawberry gallbladder"): GB mucosa is **brick red** and speckled with **bright yellow flecks** of lipid[Q].
- **Localized form: Solitary** or multiple "**cholesterol polyps**" studding the gallbladder wall[Q].

Treatment
- **Cholecystectomy** is indicated in **symptomatic cholesterolosis** or when **cholelithiasis** is present[Q].

■ GALLBLADDER POLYPS

Polypoid Lesions of the Gallbladder	
Cholesterol polyps	**Adenomatous polyp**

• **Cholesterol polyps** are the **most common**[Q]
• Usually **<10 mm** in size[Q]
• Have a characteristic echogenic **pedunculated**[Q] appearance on USG
• **Multiple (30% of cases)**[Q]
	• Adenomatous polyp has **malignant potential**[Q].
	• Adenoma may be **difficult to distinguish from adenocarcinoma** of GB
	• Main differentiating feature is a **lack of transmural invasion** on USG[Q]
	• **Risk factors** associated with **malignancy:**
	  – **Age > 60 years**[Q] – Coexistence of **gallstones**[Q]
	  – Documented **increase in size**[Q] – **Size > 10 mm**[Q]

■ GALLBLADDER ADENOMYOMATOSIS

GALLBLADDER ADENOMYOMATOSIS

- **Adenomyomatosis** is a benign condition characterized by **hyperplastic changes**[Q] of unknown etiology involving the GB wall.
- It causes **overgrowth of mucosa, thickening of muscular wall,** and **formation of intramural diverticula** or sinus tracts termed as **Aschoff-Rokitansky sinuses**[Q].
- These **sinuses** may contain **cholesterol crystals**[Q].

Diagnosis

> - **USG:** The presence of cholesterol crystals in these sinuses can result in "**diamond ring sign**"[Q], "**V-shaped**"[Q], or "**comet-tail" artifacts**[Q] on USG.

Treatment
- **Cholecystectomy** is indicated in **symptomatic adenomyomatosis** or when **cholelithiasis** is present[Q].

■ RISK FACTORS FOR CARCINOMA GALLBLADDER

Risk Factors for Carcinoma Gallbladder	
• Gallstones >3 cm[Q] • **Porcelain gallbladder**[Q] • Anomalous pancreaticobiliary junction[Q] • **Choledochal cysts**[Q]	• **Adenomatous** polyps[Q] • **Primary sclerosing cholangitis**[Q] • Obesity[Q] • **Salmonella typhi infection**[Q]

■ PORCELAIN GALLBLADDER

PORCELAIN GALLBLADDER

- Porcelain GB is characterized by **extensive calcium encrustation** of GB wall[Q].
- The term porcelain gallbladder has been used to emphasize the **blue discoloration** & **brittle consistency** of GB wall at surgery[Q].

Pathology

- **Calcium salt deposition** within the wall of a **chronically inflamed gallbladder**[Q]

Clinical Features

- Most porcelain GB (**90%**) are **associated** with **gallstones**[Q].
- Mean **age** of patients is **54 years**.
- Patients are usually **asymptomatic** and the condition is usually **found incidentally** on **plain abdominal radiographs,** sonograms or CT images.
- **Incidence of CA GB: 6%**

Diagnosis

- In porcelain GB, **plain radiographic findings** are usually **straight forward**[Q].
- **CT scan** is **diagnostic** in cases of **doubt**

Treatment

- **Cholecystectomy** in **all patients**[Q] with porcelain GB (high incidence of development carcinoma GB).

■ CARCINOMA GALLBLADDER

CARCINOMA GALLBLADDER

- **Highest incidence** of CA GB in **India** and **Pakistan**[Q]
- More common in **women** of **6th** & **7th** decade[Q]
- **Cholelithiasis** is seen in **75–98%** of all patients with CA GB[Q].
- **Incidence** of CA GB **in** a population of **patients with gallstones** is from **0.3–3%**[Q].
- CA GB is an **aggressive malignancy** with **poor prognosis**[Q]
- **Nevin classification**[Q] is used for **CA GB staging**.
- **MC gene mutation** in **CA GB: p53> K-ras>BRAF**[Q]
- **MC mode** of CA GB **spread: Direct invasion**[Q] into the adjacent organs.

Pathology

- **MC Site: Fundus (60%)**[Q] >Body (30%) >Neck (10%)
- **Histological types:**
  - **Diffuse Infiltrative: MC type**[Q]
  - **Nodular** or **mass forming**
  - **Papillary:** Exhibits **polypoid** or cauliflower appearance and have **best prognosis**[Q].
- **Adenocarcinoma**[Q] is the MC histologic subtype of CA GB.
- In CA GB: **Direct hepatic invasion in 59%**[Q] , **LN metastasis in 45%**, **perineural invasion in 42%** cases.

Clinical Features

- Most commonly presents with **RUQ pain** often **mimicking cholecystitis** and cholelithiasis[Q].
- **Weight loss, jaundice,** and an **abdominal mass** are less common presenting symptoms.
- **Chronic cholecystitis** with a **recent change** in **quality** or **frequency** of the **painful episodes** in 40% patients[Q]
- Malignant biliary obstruction with jaundice, weight loss, and RUQ pain.

Diagnosis

- **USG** is **first diagnostic modality**[Q] used in evaluation of patients with **RUQ pain**.

  - **USG:** A **heterogeneous mass replacing** the **GB lumen** and an **irregular gallbladder wall**[Q]
  - **CT scan:** Mass replacing the **gallbladder (MC finding)**; focal or diffuse gallbladder **wall thickening;** and an **intraluminal polypoidal mass.**[Q]

Contd...

Contd...

- **Unresectable** or **incurable CA GB**: Percutaneous biopsy or FNAC for **confirmatory tissue diagnosis.**[Q]

Tumor Markers

- **Best tumor marker** for CA GB is **CA19-9**[Q]
- **CEA >4 ng/mL** is associated with **93% specificity** but **50% sensitivity.**

■ TNM CLASSIFICATION OF CARCINOMA GALLBLADDER

8th AJCC (2017) TNM Classification of Carcinoma Gallbladder	
T1a	**Lamina propria** invasion[Q]
T1b	**Muscular invasion**[Q]
T2	Invade the **perimuscular connective tissue**[Q] **T2a:** Invade the **perimuscular connective tissue** on the **peritoneal side** with **no extension to serosa**[Q] **T2b:** Invade the **perimuscular connective tissue** on the **hepatic side** with **no extension into the liver**[Q]
T3	**Serosal perforation** and/or **direct invasion of the liver** (regardless of extent) and/or invasion of any other **single extrahepatic organ**[Q].
T4	Tumor invades the main **portal vein, hepatic artery** or **two** or **more extrahepatic organ**[Q]
N1	Metastasis to **1-3 regional nodes**[Q]
N2	Metastasis to **4 or more regional nodes**[Q]
M1	Distant metastasis

Stage IA	Stage IB	Stage IIA	Stage IIB	Stage IIIA	Stage IIIB	Stage IVA	Stage IVB
T1a N0M0	T1b N0M0	T2a N0M0	T2b N0M0	T3 N0M0	T1-3 N1M0	T4 N0-1M0	Tany **N2**M0 Tany Nany **M1**

■ TREATMENT OF CARCINOMA GALLBLADDER

Treatment of Carcinoma Gallbladder

- Gallbladder cancer: Incidental pathological finding after Laparoscopic cholecystectomy
- **T1a** with **negative cystic duct margin**: No further therapy[Q]
- **T1a** with **positive cystic duct margin**: **Reresection** of **cystic duct** or **CBD** to negative margin[Q]

> - **T1b, T2, T3** tumor with no evidence of metastasis: Reresection, **extended cholecystectomy** (possible CBD or extended hepatic resection)[Q]

- **T4**: **Extended cholecystectomy** with **extended right hepatectomy**[Q]
- **N2** or **M1** disease: **Clinical trial** (chemoradiation or chemotherapy) in good performance status[Q]
- Laparoscopic **trocar site scars** are **excised for staging purpose** to identify **M1** disease than for any potential therapeutic benefit[Q].

Preoperatively diagnosed CA GB

- **T2, T3**: Extended cholecystectomy[Q]
- **T4 N0**: Extended cholecystectomy with **extended right hepatectomy**[Q]
- **N1** or **hilar invasion**: Extended cholecystectomy with **CBD resection**[Q]
- **N2 or M1**: **Clinical trial** (chemoradiation or chemotherapy) in good performance status, **palliative care** in poor performance status[Q]

Surgical Technique

- For patients suspected of having resectable gallbladder cancer, begin **surgical exploration with laparoscopy**, in the absence of disseminated disease, proceed with open laparotomy.

> - **Extended cholecystectomy** consists of **cholecystectomy with en bloc resection** of segments **IVB** and **V**; including **lymphadenectomy** of the **cystic duct, pericholedochal, periportal,** and **posterior pancreaticoduodenal** and **local interaortocaval** lymph nodes.

- During a **standard cholecystectomy** the **serosa** of the gallbladder is **typically opened** and the avascular subserosal layer is used as the surgical plane of dissection.
- In case of **suspected carcinoma** the **plane of dissection** is along the **cystic plate** of the liver to avoid violation of the gallbladder subserosa.
- Only **15%** of patients develop **loco-regional recurrence** while most **(85%)** had **recurrence** involving a **distant site.**

Unresectable Carcinoma Gallbladder

- Goal of palliation is to relieve jaundice, pain, bowel obstruction and prolongation of life.
- **Gemcitabine** plus **cisplatin (reference regimen)** is used for **palliation** of **unresectable disease**[Q].

■ GALLBLADDER: ANATOMY AND PHYSIOLOGY

GALLBLADDER: ANATOMY AND PHYSIOLOGY

- It is lined by a single, highly-folded, **tall columnar epithelium**
- The **mucus** originates in **tubuloalveolar glands**[Q] found in mucosa lining the infundibulum & **neck**, but are **absent** from the **body & fundus**.
- It is **covered by** the **serosa** except where it is embedded in the liver

> - GB lacks a muscularis mucosa & submucosa[Q].

- Normal capacity of the gallbladder is **30–50 mL**[Q].
- Mucosa contain **crypt of Luschka**[Q].

Cystic Duct
• **Cystic duct** measures **2–4 cm** in length & contains prominent **concentric folds** known as **spiral valves of Heister**[Q].
• Cystic duct frequently exhibits a **tortuous** or **serpentine course**[Q].
• Diameter of the cystic duct ranges from **1–5 mm**.
• Mucosa of the **cystic** duct is arranged in **spiral folds** known as **valves of Heister**[Q] surrounded by a sphincteric structure called **sphincter of Lutkans**[Q].

- **Cystic artery** is nearly **found within** the **Hepatocystic triangle**[Q], the area bound by the cystic duct, common hepatic duct and the liver margin.
- GB mucosa has the **greatest absorptive capacity**[Q] per unit of any structure in the body.
- **Hartmann's pouch** is an **acquired diverticulum**[Q] of the infundibulum or **neck** of the gallbladder.

Functions of Gallbladder
• Reservoir of bile
• **Concentration of bile 5-10 times**[Q]
• Secretion of **mucus, 20 mL/ day** by **tubuloalveolar glands**
• **Acidification of bile**

■ GALLSTONES: PATHOGENESIS

1. Cholesterol gallstones are made up of: *(Recent Question 2019)*
   a. Crystalline cholesterol monohydrate
   b. Crystalline cholesterol dihydrate
   c. Amorphous cholesterol monohydrate
   d. Amorphous cholesterol dihydrate

2. True statement about gallstones are all except:
   (AIIMS Nov 99)
   a. Lithogenic bile is required for stone formation
   b. May be associated with carcinoma gallbladder
   c. Associated with diabetes mellitus
   d. More common in males between 30–40 years of age

3. All are component of Saint's triad except: *(AIIMS Nov 95)*
   a. Renal stones   b. Hiatus hernia
   c. Diverticulosis of colon   d. Gallstones

4. Commonest type of gallstone is: *(DNB 2011)*
   a. Cholesterol stone   b. Pigment
   c. Mixed   d. All are equally common

5. Percentage of gallstones which are radiopaque:
   (NEET 2013, JIPMER 86)
   a. 10%   b. 20%
   c. 30%   d. 40%

6. Which of the following statement is correct about gallstones?
   a. 1-Cholesterol, 2-Black, 3-Brown
   b. 1-Cholesterol, 2- Brown, 3- Black
   c. 1- Brown, 2-Black, 3- Cholesterol
   d. 1- Black, 2- Brown, 3- Cholesterol

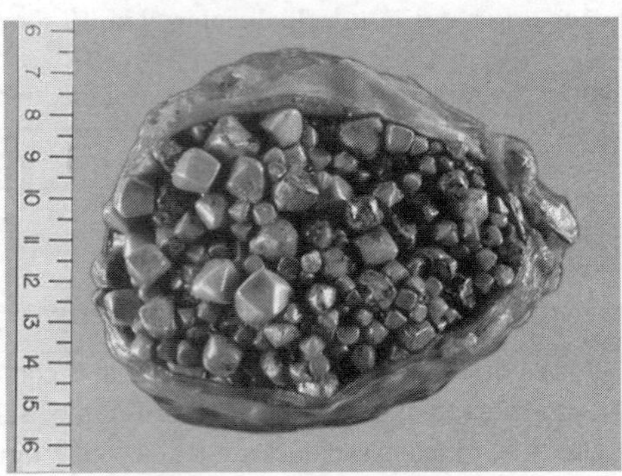

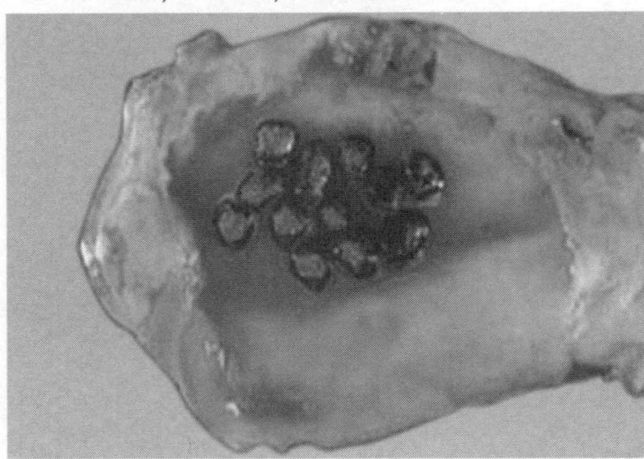

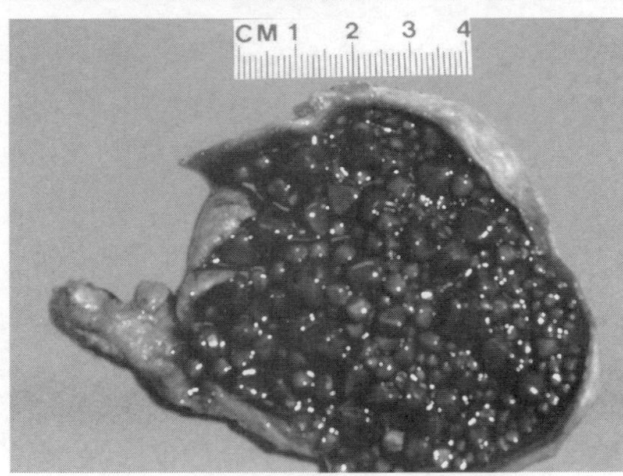

7. Gallstones do not contain: *(Recent Question 2014)*
   a. Oxalate   b. Cholesterol
   c. Phosphate   d. Carbonate

8. True color of cholesterol stone is: *(DNB 2012)*
   a. Black   b. Brown
   c. Dark yellow   d. Pale yellow

9. Most common type of gallstone in India is: *(MCI March 2009)*
   a. Cholesterol   b. Pigment
   c. Mixed   d. Both a and c

10. Calculous cholecystitis is associated with all of the following except: *(MCI March 2005)*
    a. Oral contraceptives   b. Estrogen
    c. Obesity   d. Diabetes

11. 80% of gallstones contain: *(Recent Question 2015)*
    a. Bile pigments   b. Cholesterol
    c. Calcium salts   d. Phospholipids

■ GALLSTONES: INVESTIGATIONS

12. Investigation of choice in acute cholecystitis: *(PGI Dec 2005)*
    a. OCG   b. HIDA scan
    c. USG   d. CT

13. Mercedes Benz sign or Seagull sign is seen in:
    (Recent Quetion 2015 MHSSMCET 2006)
    a. Gallstones   b. Renal stones
    c. CBD stones   d. Hydatid cyst

14. Initial investigation of choice for biliary obstruction:
    a. CT Abdomen   b. ERCP   *(JIPMER 2013)*
    c. MRCP   d. USG

15. Investigation of choice in suspected gallbladder stone is:
    (Recent Question 2017, UPPG 2010, MCI March 2010)
    a. Ultrasound   b. X-ray
    c. Barium study   d. Oral cholecystography

16. Investigation for assessing proper functioning of biliary system: *(MCI March 2007)*
    a. USG   b. CT scan
    c. HIDA scan   d. All of the above

■ GALLSTONES COMPLICATIONS AND TREATMENT

17. Not a complication of gallstones: *(JIPMER 2010)*
    a. Mucocele   b. Diverticulosis
    c. Acute cholangitis
    d. Empyema of the gallbladder

18. Which of the following is a contraindication for medical management of gallstones? *(Karnataka 2012)*
    a. Radiopaque stones
    b. Radioluscent stones
    c. Normal functioning gallbladder
    d. Small stones

■ GALLSTONE ILEUS

19. In gallstone ileus, obstruction is seen at:
    (Recent Question 2014, AIIMS GIS Dec 2009)
    a. Jejunum
    b. Proximal ileum
    c. Distal ileum
    d. Colon

20. The treatment of gallstone ileus is: *(PGI June 99, UPSC 2008)*
    a. Cholecystectomy alone
    b. Removal of obstruction
    c. Cholecystectomy, closure of fistula and removal of stone by enterotomy
    d. Cholecystectomy with closure of fistula

■ MUCOCELE

21. The treatment of choice for a mucocele of gallbladder is:
    a. Aspiration of mucous *(AIIMS June 2004)*
    b. Cholecystectomy
    c. Cholecystostomy
    d. Antibiotics and observation

22. Which of the following is false about mucocele of gallbladder? *(Recent Question 2015)*
    a. Complication of gallstones
    b. Treatment is early cholecystectomy
    c. Obstruction at neck of gallbladder
    d. Gallbladder is never palpable

■ CHOLECYSTITIS AND CHOLECYSTECTOMY

23. The technique of laparoscopic cholecystectomy was first described by? *(AIIMS May 2011)*
    a. Erich Muhe
    b. Phillip Moure
    c. Kurt Semm
    d. Eddie Reddick

24. Which of the following is the absolute contraindication for laparoscopic cholecystectomy?
    a. Clotting factor deficiency *(NEET 2013, MHSSMCET 2005)*
    b. Perforation peritonitis
    c. Empyema of the gallbladder
    d. Adhesions

25. Contraindications of laparoscopic cholecystectomy is:
    a. Coagulopathy *(Recent Question 2015, DNB 2011)*
    b. Obstructive pulmonary disease
    c. End stage liver disease
    d. All of the above

26. A patient underwent laparoscopic cholecystectomy and was discharged on the same day. On postoperative day 3, he presented to the hospital with fever. Ultrasonography showed a 5 × 5 cm collection in the right subdiaphragmatic region. What will be the management? *(AIIMS May 2017)*
    a. Observe with antibiotic cover
    b. Re-explore the wound with T-tube insertion
    c. Pigtail insertion and drainage
    d. ERCP and proceed

27. Referred pain to inferior angle of right scapula in acute cholecystitis is known as: *(Recent Question 2017)*
    a. Murphy's sign
    b. Naunyn's sign
    c. Boa's sign
    d. Cullen's sign

28. A 32-year-old man presented with fever and pain in upper right hypochondrium after food intake. Investigation of choice for the diagnosis is: *(MCI Dec 2019)*
    a. CECT
    b. Ultrasound
    c. MRI
    d. HRCT

■ ACALCULOUS CHOLECYSTITIS

29. Acalculous cholecystitis can be seen in all except:
    (Punjab 2008, AIIMS Nov 2005)
    a. Dengue hemorrhagic fever
    b. Malaria
    c. Leptospirosis
    d. Enteric fever

30. All of the following are causes of acalculous cholecystitis except: *(Recent Question 2013)*
    a. Bile duct stricture
    b. Schistostoma
    c. Prolonged TPN
    d. Major operations

■ XANTHOGRANULOMATOUS CHOLECYSTITIS

31. All of the following statements about Xanthogranulomatous inflammation are true except: *(NEET Pattern)*
    a. Foam cells are seen
    b. Yellow nodules are seen
    c. Multinucleated giant cells are seen
    d. Associated with tuberculosis

■ EMPHYSEMATOUS CHOLECYSTITIS

32. Acute emphysematous cholecystitis is caused by:
    a. Pseudomonas aeuroginosa *(JIPMER 2012, 2010)*
    b. Staphylococcus
    c. Clostridium perfringens
    d. Streptococcus pyogenes

33. All of the following are correct regarding emphysematous cholecystitis except: *(NEET Pattern, DNB 2010)*
    a. More common in males
    b. More common in diabetics
    c. In many cases the gallbladder does not contain stone
    d. It is caused most commonly by Pseudomonas

■ MIRIZZI'S SYNDROME

34. Mirizzi syndrome is: *(Recent Question 2015, 2014, DNB 2011)*
    a. GB stone compressing common hepatic duct
    b. GB carcinoma invading IVC
    c. GB stone causing cholecystitis
    d. Pancreatic carcinoma

■ STRAWBERRY GALLBLADDER

35. Cholesterolosis is: *(Karnataka 94)*
    a. Disease of defective metabolism of choline
    b. Concerned with epithelial tumors of brain
    c. Diffuse deposition of cholesterol in mucosa of gallbladder
    d. Disease concerned with obstructive jaundice

36. Gross appearance of gallbladder specimen is suggestive of:
    a. Emphysematous cholecystitis
    b. Xanthogranulomatous cholecystitis
    c. Gallbladder cholesterolosis
    d. Adenomyomatosis

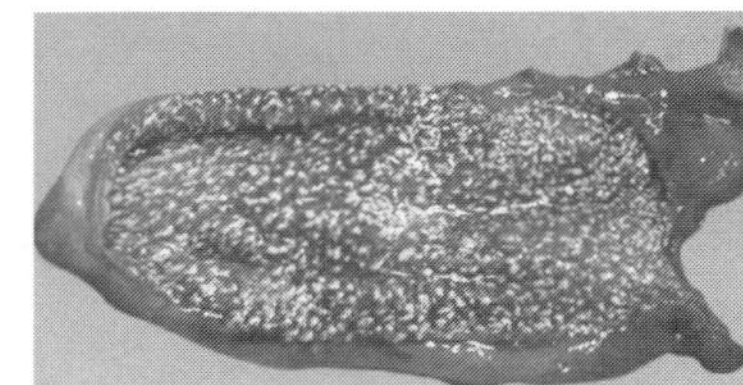

■ GALLBLADDER POLYP AND ADENOMYOMATOSIS

37. Risk factors for malignant change in an asymptomatic patient with a gallbladder polyp on ultrasound include all of the following, except: *(AIIMS May 2011, All India 2009)*
    a. Age > 60 years
    b. Rapid increase in size of polyp
    c. Size of polyp > 5 mm
    d. Associated gallstones

38. Identify the diagnosis of the given gross specimen:
    (AIIMS Nov 2017)

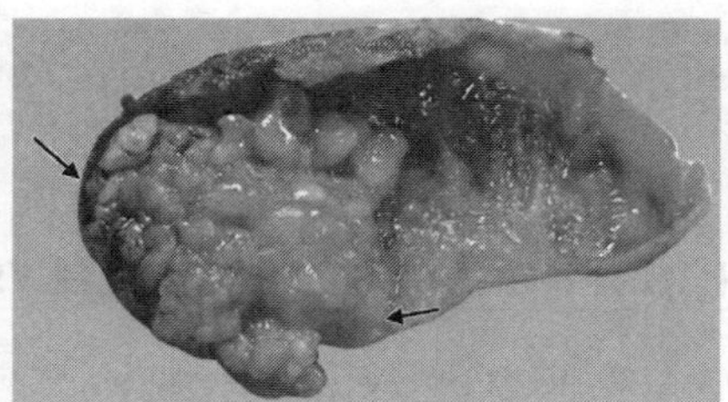

    a. Cancer gallbladder   b. Cholesterolosis
    c. Strawberry gallbladder d. Polyps in gallbladder

39. On abdominal ultrasound gallbladder shows diffuse wall thickening with hyperechoic nodules at neck and comet tail artifacts. The most likely diagnosis will be:
    a. Adenomyomatosis   *(AIIMS May 2011)*
    b. Adenocarcinoma of gallbladder
    c. Xanthogranulomatous cholecystitis
    d. Cholesterol crystals

40. This incidental finding on ultrasound abdomen is suggestive of:
    a. Gallbladder stone
    b. Gallbladder polyp
    c. Adenomyomatosis
    d. Xanthogranulomatous cholecystitis

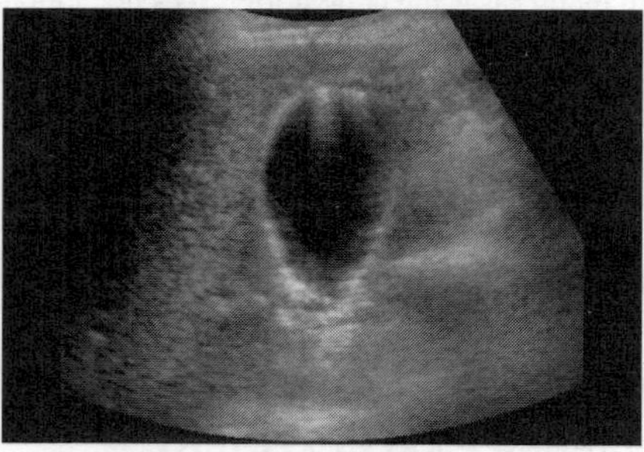

■ CARCINOMA GALLBLADDER PREDISPOSING FACTORS

41. Organism associated with fish consumption and also causes carcinoma gallbladder: *(AIIMS Nov 2012, AIIMS Nov 2010)*
    a. Gnathostoma
    b. Anglostrongyloidosis cantonensis
    c. Clonorchis sinensis
    d. H. dimunata

42. All of the following are risk factors for carcinoma gallbladder, except: *(AIIMS June 2004)*
    a. Typhoid carriers
    b. Adenomatous gallbladder polyps
    c. Choledochal cyst
    d. Oral contraceptives

43. All of the following are the risk factors for carcinoma gallbladder except: *(Recent Question 2017)*
    a. Primary sclerosing cholangitis
    b. Porcelain gallbladder
    c. Multiple 2 cm gallstones
    d. Choledochal cyst

44. All of the following are true about porcelain gallbladder except: *(Kerala PG 2015)*
    a. May be seen on plain X-ray
    b. More commonly diagnosed on CT
    c. It is an indication for cholecystectomy
    d. Always denotes benign etiology

45. Incidental finding in a female patient of age 56 years who underwent the CECT abdomen is suggestive of:
    a. Carcinoma gallbladder   b. Gallbladder polyp
    c. Porcelain gallbladder   d. Gallstone

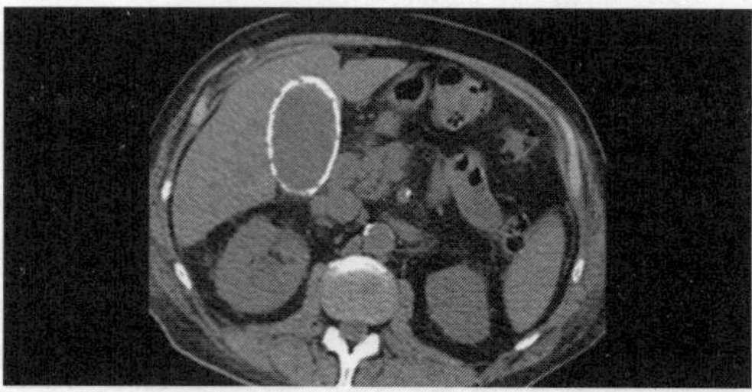

■ CARCINOMA GALLBLADDER

46. Commonest type of carcinoma gallbladder with gallstones is: *(AIIMS Nov 95)*
    a. Adenocarcinoma   b. Anaplastic carcinoma
    c. Squamous cell carcinoma d. Transitional cell carcinoma

47. Commonest association seen in carcinoma gallbladder: *(AIIMS 91)*
    a. Peritoneal deposits   b. Duodenal infiltration
    c. Secondaries to liver   d. Cystic node involvement

48. Most common type of cancer gallbladder in a patient with gallstone: *(APPG 2005)*
    a. Adenocarcinoma   b. Squamous carcinoma
    c. Sarcoma   d. None

49. Most appropriate treatment option for the carcinoma gallbladder with invasion of perimuscular connective tissue, diagnosed after laparoscopic cholecystectomy:
    (Recent Question 2017)
    a. Resection of segment IVb & V of liver with nodal clearance
    b. Resection of segment IVb & V of liver with nodal clearance with port site excision
    c. Wedge excision of liver with lymphadenectomy
    d. Wedge excision of liver with lymphadenectomy and port-site excision

Explanations

■ GALLSTONES: PATHOGENESIS

1. **Ans. a. Crystalline cholesterol monohydrate** *(Ref: Robbins 9/e p876; Sleisenger & Fordtran 9/e p1098)*

   "There are two general classes of gallstones: cholesterol stones, containing more than 50% of crystalline cholesterol monohydrate, and pigment stones composed predominantly of bilirubin calcium salts." (Robbins 9/e p876)

2. **Ans. d. More common in males between 30–40 years of age**   3. **Ans. a. Renal stones**

4. **Ans. c. Mixed** *(Ref: Bailey 27/e p1198)*

Mixed Gallstones

   - **Most common gallstones**, account for **90% calculi**[Q]

5. **Ans. a. 10%**

   - Most (90%) gallstones are radioluscent[Q].   - Most (90%) kidney stones are radiopaque[Q].

6. **Ans. d. 1- Black, 2- Brown, 3- Cholesterol** *(Ref: Sabiston 20/e p1491-1492; Schwartz 11/e p1403, 10/e p1318-1319; Bailey 27/e p1198)*

7. **Ans. a. Oxalate**   8. **Ans. d. Pale yellow**

9. **Ans. b. Pigment** *(Ref: Bailey 27/e p1198)*

   - In the **USA** and **Europe, 80%** are **cholesterol** or **mixed stones**, whereas in **Asia, 80%** are **pigment stones**[Q].
     - **MC gallstone: Mixed (90%)**[Q]
     - **MC gallstones in USA** and **Europe: Cholesterol stones**[Q] **(Mixed**, if given in the option)
     - **MC gallstones in India (Asia): Pigment stones (80%)**[Q]

10. **Ans. d. Diabetes**

Classification of Gallstones			
	Cholesterol	**Black pigment**	**Brown pigment**
Location	Gallbladder and bile duct	Gallbladder and bile duct	**Bile ducts**[Q]
Major constituent	Cholesterol	Bilirubin pigment **polymer**[Q]	**Calcium bilirubinate**[Q]
Consistency	Crystalline with nucleus	**Hard**[Q]	**Soft, friable**[Q]
% Radiopaque	15%	**60%**[Q]	**0%**[Q]

11. **Ans. b. Cholesterol**

■ GALLSTONES: INVESTIGATIONS

12. **Ans. c. USG** *(Ref: Sabiston 20/e p1493; Schwartz 11/e p1404, 10/e p1319; Bailey 27/e p1199; Shackelford 8/e p1269-1270)*

   - **IOC** for **acute cholecystitis: USG**[Q]   - **Gold standard** for **diagnosis of acute cholecystitis: HIDA scan**[Q]
     - **USG is IOC** for **acute calculous cholecystitis, chronic cholecystitis** and **cholelithiasis**[Q].

13. **Ans. a. Gallstones** *(Ref: Bailey 27/e p1199)*   14. **Ans. d. USG**   15. **Ans. a. Ultrasound**

16. **Ans. c. HIDA scan** *(Ref: Sabiston 20/e p1488; Schwartz 11/e p1399, 10/e p1320; Bailey 27/e p1199; Blumgart 5/e p254-270; Shackelford 7/e p1306)*

■ GALLSTONES COMPLICATIONS AND TREATMENT

17. **Ans. b. Diverticulosis** *(Ref: Sabiston 20/e p1492-1493; Bailey 27/e p1199; Blumgart 6/e p554)*

Effects and Complications of Gallstones			
In gallbladder		**In Bile duct**	**In Intestine**
- Silent stones	- Empyema	- Obstructive jaundice	- **Gallstone ileus**
- Acute cholecystitis	- Perforation	- Cholangitis	
- Chronic cholecystitis	- Gangrene	- **Acute pancreatitis**	
- Mucocele	- Carcinoma		

18. **Ans. a. Radiopaque stones**

■ GALLSTONE ILEUS

19. Ans. c. Distal ileum (*Ref: Sabiston 20/e p1506-1507; Blumgart 6/e p563; Shackelford 8/e p844*)   **20.   Ans. b. Removal of obstruction**

■ MUCOCELE

21. Ans. b. Cholecystectomy (*Ref: Bailey 27/e p1199; Harrison 20/e p2428*)

22. Ans. d. Gallbladder is never palpable

■ CHOLECYSTITIS AND CHOLECYSTECTOMY

23. Ans. a. Erich Muhe (*Ref: Blumgart 6/e p6,551*)

HISTORY OF LAPAROSCOPIC CHOLECYSTECTOMY

- Dr. **Kurt Semm**, the **father of "pelviscopy,"** performed the **first laparoscopic appendectomy** in **1980[Q]**.
- **Eric Muhe[Q]** performed the **first laparoscopic cholecystectomy** in **1982**. He used a **modified operating laparoscope** placed at the umbilicus after establishing pneumoperitoneum.
- In 1987, **Phillipe Mouret** performed the **first video laparoscopic cholecystectomy** by using a **camera attached to the laparoscope[Q]**.

24. Ans. a. Clotting factor deficiency (*Ref: Blumgart 6/e p575*)

Contraindications to Laparoscopic Cholecystectomy

Absolute	Relative
• **Unable** to **tolerate general anesthesia[Q]** • **Refractory coagulopathy[Q]** • Suspicion of **carcinoma[Q]**	• Previous **upper abdominal surgery[Q]** • **Cholangitis[Q]** • **Diffuse peritonitis[Q]** • **Cirrhosis** or **portal hypertension[Q]** • Chronic obstructive pulmonary disease • **Cholecystenteric fistula[Q]** • **Morbid obesity[Q]** • **Pregnancy[Q]**

Indications of Open Cholecystectomy

• Poor pulmonary or cardiac reserve[Q] • Cirrhosis and portal hypertension[Q] • Combined procedure	• Suspected or known gallbladder cancer[Q] • Third-trimester pregnancy[Q]

25. Ans. d. All of the above

26. Ans. c. Pigtail insertion and drainage (*Ref: Sabiston 20/e p1506; Schwartz 11/e p1417, 10/e p1332; Bailey 27/e p1203*)

27. Ans. c. Boa's sign   **28.   Ans. b. Ultrasound** (*Ref: Bailey 27/e p1199*)

■ ACALCULOUS CHOLECYSTITIS

29. Ans. b. Malaria

- Both malaria and dengue are uncommon causes of acalculous cholecystitis.
- **Malaria[Q]** seems to be more common between the two.

30. Ans. b. Schistostoma

■ XANTHOGRANULOMATOUS CHOLECYSTITIS

31. Ans. d. Associated with tuberculosis (*Ref: www.medscape.com/viewarticle/449665*)

■ EMPHYSEMATOUS CHOLECYSTITIS

32. Ans. c. Clostridium perfringens (*Ref: Sabiston 20/e p1493; Blumgart 6/e p562*)

33. Ans. d. It is caused most commonly by Pseudomonas

■ MIRIZZI'S SYNDROME

34. Ans. a. GB stone compressing common hepatic duct

■ STRAWBERRY GALLBLADDER

35. Ans. c. Diffuse deposition of cholesterol in mucosa of gallbladder (*Ref: Bailey 27/e p1201*)

36. Ans. c. Gallbladder cholesterolosis (*Ref: Bailey 27/e p1201*)

■ GALLBLADDER POLYP AND ADENOMYOMATOSIS

37. **Ans. c.** Size of polyp > 5 mm
38. **Ans. d.** Polyps in gallbladder *(Ref: Sabiston 20/e p1511; Bailey 27/e p1210)*
39. **Ans. a.** Adenomyomatosis *(Ref: Sabiston 19/e p1505; Bailey 27/e p1201)*
40. **Ans. c.** Adenomyomatosis *(Ref: Sabiston 20/e p1511)*
    - The presence of cholesterol crystals in these sinuses in adenomyomatosis can result in **"diamond ring sign"**[Q], **"V-shaped"**[Q], or **"comet-tail" artifacts**[Q] on USG.

■ CARCINOMA GALLBLADDER PREDISPOSING FACTORS

41. **Ans. c.** Clonorchis sinensis *(Ref: www.ncbi.nlm.gov/pubmed/3993073)*

CLONORCHIS SINENSIS

- Clonorchis sinensis is a **liver fluke, acquired** by **ingestion of raw** or inadequately cooked **freshwater fishes**[Q].
- In human body, it **lives within bile ducts** and causes **inflammatory reaction** leading to **cholangiohepatitis** and **biliary obstruction**[Q].
- It is a well known **risk factor** for **cholangiocarcinoma**[Q].
- It is a **rare**, but **mentioned risk factor** for **carcinoma gallbladder**[Q].

42. **Ans. d.** Oral contraceptives
43. **Ans. c.** Multiple 2 cm gallstones *(Ref: Sabiston 20/e p1512; Schwartz 11/e p1421, 10/e p1334; Bailey 27/e p1210)*
44. **Ans. d.** Always denotes benign etiology
45. **Ans. c.** Porcelain gallbladder *(Ref: Sabiston 20/e p1512; Schwartz 11/e p1401-1402, 10/e p1317; Bailey 27/e p1190)*

■ CARCINOMA GALLBLADDER

46. **Ans. a.** Adenocarcinoma
47. **Ans. c.** Secondaries to liver

- Metastasis in Carcinoma Gallbladder
- **Direct hepatic invasion** in **59%**[Q], **LN metastasis** in **45%**, **perineural invasion** in **42%** cases.

48. **Ans. a.** Adenocarcinoma
49. **Ans. b.** Resection of segment IVb & V of liver with nodal clearance with port site excision *(Ref: Sabiston 20/e p1514; Schwartz 11/e p1422, 10/e p1335; Bailey 27/e p1211)*

Bile Duct

■ CHOLEDOCHAL CYST

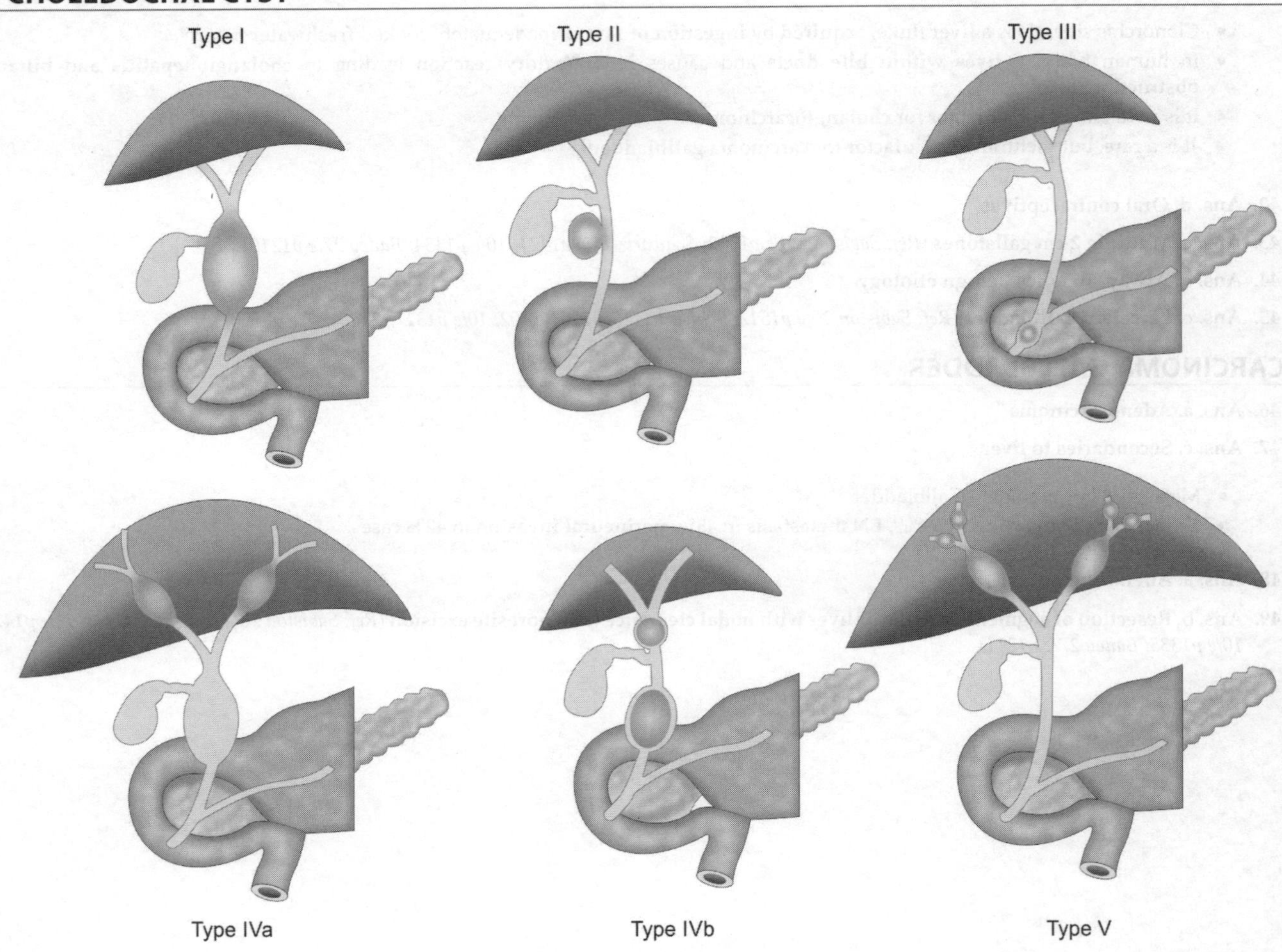

Todani modification of Alonso-Lej classification

Choledochal Cyst

- Cystic dilation of biliary ducts, more common in **females**[Q]

Etiology

- Most widely accepted hypothesis: **Abnormal pancreaticobiliary ductal junction (APBDJ)**[Q]
- **APBDJ** results in **reflux of pancreatic fluid** into distal common hepatic duct and results in mucosal injury, chronic inflammation, and **weakening of bile duct wall**[Q].

Classification

- MC choledochal cyst: **Type I > Type IV > Type III (143)**[Q]

Contd...

Contd...

Todani Modification of Alonso-Lej Classification[Q]	

Type I (MC)	• Dilation of extrahepatic biliary tree
	  – Type Ia: **cystic dilation**[Q] **(MC type)**
	  – Type Ib: **focal segmental dilation**[Q]
	  – Type Ic: **fusiform dilation**[Q]

Type II	• **Diverticular dilation**[Q] of extrahepatic biliary tree
Type III	• Cystic dilation of intraduodenal portion of common bile duct **(choledochocele)**[Q]
Type IVA	• Dilation of the **extrahepatic & intrahepatic biliary tree**[Q]
Type IVB	• Dilation of multiple sections of **extrahepatic bile ducts**[Q]
Type V	• Dilation confined to intrahepatic bile ducts **(Caroli's disease**[Q]**)**
Type VI	• **Cystic dilatation of cystic duct**[Q] (not included in Todani's modification)

Clinical Features

- **Classic triad: Pain, jaundice (intermittent)** & abdominal **mass (10%)**[Q].

> - **MC symptom** in **Infants: Jaundice** (in 80%)[Q]
> - **MC symptom** in patients **>2 years** of age: **Abdominal pain**[Q]

- In **children**, the major clinical symptoms are recurrent **abdominal pain (81.8%),** nausea & vomiting (65.5%), mild jaundice (43.6%), an abdominal mass (29.0%), and fever (29.0%).
- In **adults, abdominal pain** (87%) and **jaundice** (42%) are present frequently. Less common clinical findings include nausea (29%), cholangitis (26%), pancreatitis (23%), and an **abdominal mass (13%).**

Diagnosis

- **IOC** for **choledochal cyst: MRCP** (non-invasive)
- **ERCP:** More useful in defining the distal ductal anatomy and the presence of APBDJ
- **PTC:** Useful in defining the proximal ductal anatomy and the presence of intrahepatic disease.

Treatment of Choledochal Cyst	
Type I	• **Roux-en-Y hepaticojejunostomy**[Q]
Type II	• **Excision** with **T-tube repair**[Q] • **Roux-en-Y hepaticojejunostomy**[Q]
Type III	• **Endoscopic sphincterotomy** and cyst unroofing[Q]
Type IVA	• **Hepatic resection** for **localized** disease[Q] • **Liver transplantation** for **diffuse** disease[Q]
Type IVB	• Transduodenal sphincteroplasty and **Roux-en-Y hepaticojejunostomy**[Q]
Type V	• **Hepatic resection** for **localized disease**[Q] • **Liver transplantation** for **diffuse disease**[Q]

Complications of Choledochal Cyst	
• Recurrent cholangitis[Q] • Pancreatitis[Q] • Gallstones[Q]	• Cirrhosis with portal hypertension • Portal vein thrombosis • Malignancy[Q]

■ CHOLEDOCHOLITHIASIS

CHOLEDOCHOLITHIASIS

- **CBD stones** are classified by **point of origin**
- Found in **6–12%** of patients with GB stones[Q]
- **Retained stones** discovered **within 2 years** of cholecystectomy[Q]
- **Recurrent stones** detected **>2 years** following cholecystectomy[Q]

Primary CBD stone	Secondary CBD stone
• **Formed** within the **biliary tract**[Q]	• **Formed** initially in the **GB**[Q]
• Associated with biliary **Stasis and infection**[Q]	• **Migrate through** the **cystic duct** into CBD[Q]
• More commonly seen in **Asian**[Q] populations	• Most common bile duct stones in **Western countries**[Q]
• **Soft, friable, light-brown stones** or **sludge** in the CBD	• Usually **cholesterol stones**[Q]

Contd...

Contd...

Clinical Features

- CBD stones may be **silent** and are often **discovered incidentally**[Q]. In these patients, biliary obstruction is transient, and laboratory tests may be normal.
- Clinical features suspicious for **biliary obstruction** due to **CBD stones** include **biliary colic, jaundice, clay colored stools,** and **darkening of the urine**[Q].
- **Fever** and **chills** may be present in patients with choledocholithiasis and **cholangitis**.
- Serum **bilirubin** (>3.0 mg/dL), **aminotransferases**, and **ALP** are commonly elevated in patients with biliary obstruction but are **neither sensitive nor specific** for the presence of common duct stones.

Diagnosis

- USG: **First test**, can document **GB stones** and estimate the **CBD diameter**[Q]
- A **dilated bile duct** (>8 mm in diameter) in a patient with **gallstones, jaundice** and **biliary pain** is **highly suggestive** of choledocholithiasis.
- MRCP: Provides excellent anatomic detail, with **sensitivity** and **specificity** of 95% and 98%, respectively, for **CBD stones**[Q].

> - **ERCP: Diagnostic and therapeutic test of choice for patients with suspected CBD stones**[Q].

Treatment

- Treatment options are **ERCP, laparoscopic** or **open CBD Exploration.**

■ CHOLANGITIS

Cholangitis

- **Ascending bacterial infection**[Q] of the biliary ductal system with obstruction
- **MC cause** of acute cholangitis is **choledocholithiasis**[Q]
- **MC organisms** present in the bile in patients with cholangitis: **E. coli**[Q], **Klebsiella pneumoniae**[Q], Streptococcus faecalis, & Bacteroides fragilis.

Etiology

- **Choledocholithiasis (MC)**[Q]
- Biliary-enteric anastomotic strictures
- Benign strictures
- Cholangiocarcinoma and periampullary cancer

Clinical Features

- Characterized by **Charcot's triad**[Q]: **Abdominal pain + jaundice + fever**
- Cholangitis may be either **self-limited** or **toxic with severe illness**, including **jaundice, fever, abdominal pain, mental status changes,** and **hypotension (Reynold's pentad)**[Q].

> - **Fever & chills** are the **MC presentation** (due to **cholangiovenous & cholangiolymphatic reflux**)[Q]

- **Fever** is the **most consistent sign**, generally **intermittent, spiking** and associated **with shaking chills**[Q].

Diagnosis

- **Leukocytosis, hyperbilirubinemia**, and **raised ALP** and **transaminases**[Q]
- **Positive blood culture** is **more common** in **partial obstruction**[Q] than with complete obstruction

> - **Cholangiography** (If ERCP is not available, PTC should be performed) is **mandatory** as a **diagnostic** and **potentially therapeutic intervention**[Q].

Treatment

- **Initial treatment: IV antibiotics & aggressive hydration**[Q]
- **Septic shock** with **toxic cholangitis: ICU monitoring** and **vasopressors** to support blood pressure.
- **Most patients** will **respond to these measures** alone.
- **Urgent biliary decompression** will be necessary in 15% cases[Q].
- Biliary decompression may be performed endoscopically or by a percutaneous transhepatic route based on the level of the obstruction.
- Methods of Biliary Decompression

ERCP with Sphincterotomy and Stone Extraction	Percutaneous Transhepatic Cholangiography (PTC)	Surgical Decompression
- **Procedure of choice**[Q] - Early endoscopy is **diagnostic & therapeutic**[Q] - Permits biliary decompression by **sphincterotomy & stone extraction**[Q] - If stone can't be removed, a **nasobiliary catheter** or stent is inserted to decompress biliary tract[Q]	**PTC is performed if:** - **ERCP** has **failed** or not **available**[Q] - **Proximal** or hilar obstruction[Q] - **Stricture** of **biliary enteric anastomosis**[Q]	- Surgical decompression is indicated when **neither ERCP nor PTC** is **possible**[Q]. - Consists of CBD **decompression** with a **T-tube**[Q]

Contd...

Contd...

Elective Definitive Treatment in Stabilized Patients

- **Cholecystectomy** with **choledochotomy** and **CBD exploration**[Q]
- **T-tube** is left in place for **cholangiography** and **removal** of any **retained stone**[Q]
- **T-tube cholangiogram** is done on **7th-10th day post-operatively**[Q]
- **Remove** the T-tube if **cholangiogram** is **normal**[Q]
- If **residual stone** is discovered **on** the post-operative **cholangiogram**, T-tube should be **left in place** for **4-6 weeks** for the tract to mature[Q].
- The **stones** are **removed percutaneously** through the **matured tract** by **Burhenne's technique**[Q].

■ ERCP

ERCP

- Endoscopic clearance of CBD stones can **avoid** the **need for an open operation**[Q] if expertise in laparoscopic common bile duct exploration is not available.

Indications of preoperative ERCP

• Patients with **worsening cholangitis**[Q]	• **Biliary pancreatitis**[Q]
• **Ampullary stone impaction**[Q]	• **Cirrhosis**[Q]

Contraindications of Endoscopic sphincterotomy

- CBD diameter **>2 cm**[Q]
- Long suprasphincteric **stricture, >15 mm**[Q]
- **Peri-vaterian diverticulum**[Q]
- **Duodenal wall** and **head** of the pancreas **severely inflamed**[Q]

■ BILE DUCT INJURY

BILE DUCT INJURY

- **Most benign strictures** follow **iatrogenic bile duct injury**[Q]
- **Most commonly** during **laparoscopic cholecystectomy**[Q]
- **Incidence** of bile duct injury during **open** cholecystectomy is **0.1–0.2%**[Q]
- **Incidence** of bile duct injury during **laparoscopic** cholecystectomy is **0.3–0.85%**[Q]

■ BISMUTH CLASSIFICATION OF BILE DUCT STRICTURES

Bismuth Classification of Bile Duct Strictures	
Type 1	**Low** common hepatic duct stricture; hepatic duct **stump >2 cm**[Q]
Type 2	Mid common hepatic duct **stump < 2 cm**[Q]
Type 3	**High** stricture **(hilar)**, no hepatic duct stump; **confluence intact**[Q]
Type 4	**Destruction of** the hilar **confluence**; right and left hepatic ducts separated[Q]
Type 5	Involvement of **aberrant right sectoral hepatic duct** alone **with or without** a concomitant **hepatic duct stricture**[Q]

■ STRASBERG CLASSIFICATION OF LAPAROSCOPIC BILIARY INJURIES

Strasberg Classification of Laparoscopic Biliary Injuries	
Type A	• **Bile leaks** from **minor ducts** still in continuity with the CBD[Q] • Includes **leakage from cystic duct** stump and from a **subvesical duct of Luschka**[Q] • **MC causes of biliary leaks** seen after laparoscopic cholecystectomy[Q]
Type B	• **Occlusion** of a part of the biliary tree, almost always an **aberrant right sectoral duct**[Q]
Type C	• **Transection without ligation** of an aberrant right sectoral duct[Q]
Type D	• A **lateral injury** to an **extrahepatic duct**[Q]
Type E	• Includes biliary strictures, divided into **E1 to E5** as classified by **Bismuth**

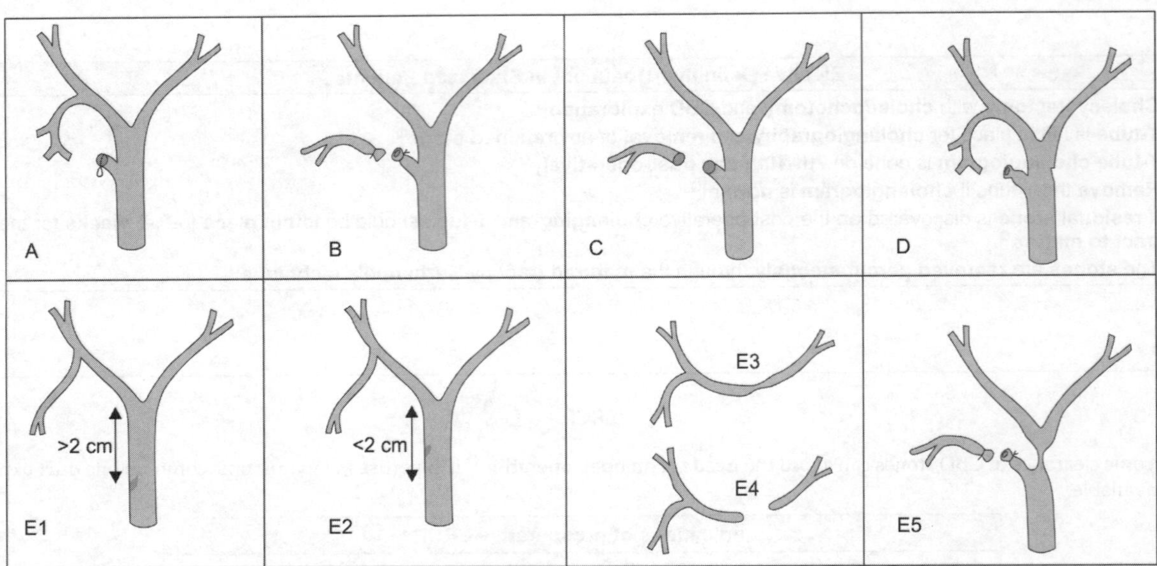

Strasberg classification of postoperative bile duct strictures

■ MANAGEMENT OF THE BILE DUCT INJURY RECOGNIZED AFTER CHOLECYSTECTOMY

Management of the Bile Duct Injury Recognized after Cholecystectomy

- Patients with a **bile leak** will **present early**[Q]
- Patients with **postoperative biliary strictures** alone often present with jaundice or cholangitis **months to years** after the initial injury[Q].

Intraoperative Considerations
- Management of postoperative biliary strictures following ductal injury depends on the degree **of injury**, the presence of **stricture-induced complications**, and the **operative risk** of the patient.

Planning of the following specific goals	
• **Control** the **infection** (abscess or cholangitis)[Q]	• **Drain the biloma**[Q]
• Complete the **cholangiography**[Q]	
• Provide definitive therapy with **controlled reconstruction** or **stenting**[Q]	

■ BILIARY ATRESIA

Biliary Atresia

- Characterized by **progressive obliteration** of the **extrahepatic** and **intrahepatic** bile ducts[Q].
- **Etiology** is **unknown; incidence 1 in 12,000 live births**[Q].
- Presently, there is **no medical therapy** to **reverse** the **obliterative process**[Q]

> - Patients who are **not offered surgical treatment** uniformly develop biliary cirrhosis, portal hypertension, and **death** by **2 years of age**[Q].

- **MC indication** for **pediatric liver transplantation**[Q]

Pathology
- **Bile duct proliferation, severe cholestasis** with **plugging**, and **inflammatory cell infiltrate** are the **pathologic hallmarks** of this disease[Q].
- Over time, these changes **progress to fibrosis with end-stage cirrhosis**[Q].
- Positive for neural cell adhesion molecule (**CD56**) staining

Classification

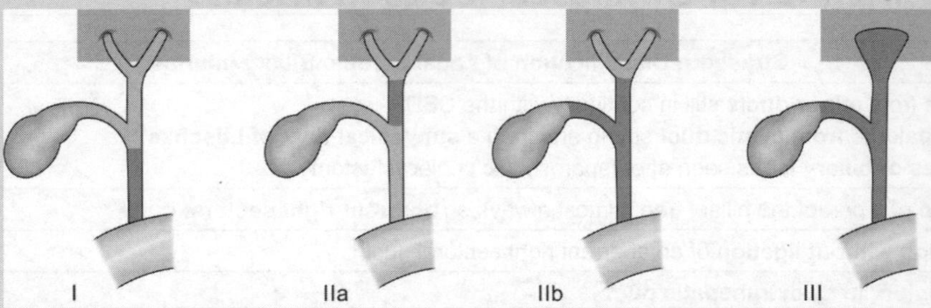

Contd...

Contd...

Kasai Classification of Biliary Atresia	
• Type I	• **CBD** is **obliterated**, proximal bile ducts are patent[Q]
• Type IIa	• **Atresia of** common hepatic duct **(CHD)** with patent cystic duct & CBD[Q]
• Type IIb	• **Obliteration of CHD, cystic duct & CBD**[Q]
• Type III	• **Atresia of CBD, cystic duct & hepatic ducts up to porta hepatis**[Q] **(MC type,** responsible for **> 90% cases**[Q])

Clinical Features

- Infants with biliary atresia present with **jaundice at birth** or **shortly thereafter**[Q].
- Infants with biliary atresia characteristically have **acholic, pale gray stools**, secondary to obstructed bile flow.
- With passage of time, **progressive failure to thrive** and, if untreated, develop **stigmata of liver failure** and **portal hypertension** (splenomegaly and esophageal varices)
- **Associated malformations in 25%: Polysplenia, malrotation, preduodenal portal vein,** and **intrahepatic vena cava**[Q].

Diagnosis

- USG of the liver and GB is important in the evaluation of the infant with cholestasis.

> - **USG: GB is shrunken** and **CBD** is **not visible**[Q]. A **triangle cord sign**[Q] found on ultrasound has a **predictive accuracy of 95%,** the **gallbladder ghost triad**[Q] in which the **gallbladder** is **short** (<1.9 cm) and **irregular** and **lacks an echogenic inner lining** also got good sensitivity.

- **Next diagnostic step:** Percutaneous **liver biopsy**[Q] if the hepatic synthetic function is normal (diagnostic accuracy 90%).
- **Hepatobiliary scintigraphy:** In cases in which the **USG** and **biopsy** findings are **inconclusive (absent excretion into the intestine)**[Q]

> - **Gold standard for diagnosing biliary atresia: Intraoperative cholangiography**[Q] *(Blumgart 6/e p658)*
> - Although **percutaneous liver biopsy** is **highly accurate,** there are **no histologic findings** that are **pathognomonic for BA**

Treatment

- **Exploratory laparotomy:** If the needle biopsy or abdominal ultrasound is consistent with BA
- **Intra-operative cholecystocholangiography: To confirm** the **diagnosis,** demonstration of the **fibrotic biliary remnant** and definition of **absent proximal** and **distal bile duct patency**[Q]

> - Treatment of choice: **Kasai hepatoportoenterostomy**[Q] (Roux-en-Y hepaticojejunostomy)

Postoperative Management

- **Ursodeoxycholic acid** (facilitate bile flow) + **Methylprednisolone** (anti-inflammatory agent) + **TMP-SMX** (antimicrobial prophylaxis)[Q]

> - **Cholangitis** is the **MC** postoperative **complication**[Q].

Prognosis

- About **30%** of infants undergoing hepatoportoenterostomy **before 60 days** of age will have a **long-term successful outcome** and **not require liver transplantation**[Q].
- **Liver transplantation** in the patients who develop **progressive hepatic fibrosis** with resultant **portal hypertension** and progressive cholestasis[Q].
- **Serum bilirubin** at **3 months** after surgery seems to be **strongly predictive of long-term survival**[Q].

■ PRIMARY SCLEROSING CHOLANGITIS

PRIMARY SCLEROSING CHOLANGITIS

- PSC is a **cholestatic liver disease** characterized by **fibrotic strictures** involving **intrahepatic & extrahepatic biliary tree**[Q] in the absence of a known precipitating cause.
- More common in HLA **B8/DR3**[Q]

> - **Incidence** of UC in PSC ranges from **75–80%**[Q].
> - **PSC** is **present** in **5.5%** of patients with **chronic UC**[Q].

- Patients with PSC are at **increased risk** for developing **cholangiocarcinoma**[Q].
- **Smoking** is **protective** in UC & **PSC**[Q].

Pathology

- **Cholangiocytes**[Q], epithelial cells that lines the bile duct are **target cell** of injury in PSC.
- Histologic finding of **"onion skin appearance"**[Q] is **pathognomic** of PSC, but seen in **<10%** cases.

Contd...

Section 2 — Hepatobiliary Pancreatic Surgery

Contd...

> - Involvement of **large intrahepatic** and **extrahepatic duct**[Q] distinguishes PSC from PBC.
> - **Absence of the smallest intrahepatic ducts** leading to a **reduction in the branching** of biliary tree (give rise to **pruned-tree appearance**[Q] on direct cholangiography).

Clinical Features

- More common in **males**[Q], mean age at presentation is **40–45 years**[Q]
- About **75% of patients** are **symptomatic**[Q] at presentation with evidence of cholestatic liver disease such as **jaundice, pruritus,** and **fatigue**[Q].
- Symptoms of bacterial cholangitis are uncommon.
- Condition is characterized by **relapses & remissions**[Q], with quiescent periods.

Diagnosis

- **Asymptomatic elevation** of GGT is the **earliest finding**[Q], ALP and bile acids are also increased.
- **Normal ALP does not always rule out** diagnosis of **PSC**[Q].
- **Cholangiography confirms** the **diagnosis of PSC** with evidence of **diffuse multifocal strictures** found in both **intrahepatic & extrahepatic bile ducts**[Q].

ERCP Findings in PSC
• **ERCP** is the **gold standard**[Q] for diagnosis of PSC.
• Typical cholangiographic findings of PSC: **Multifocal stricturing & beading**[Q] throughout the biliary tree
• **Beaded** or **pruned tree appearance**[Q]
• **Pseudodiverticula**[Q]

Treatment

- Treatment of choice: Liver transplantation
- Medical therapy for PSC include **high dose UDCA**[Q] (25–30 mg/kg/day).

■ PRIMARY BILIARY CIRRHOSIS

PRIMARY BILIARY CIRRHOSIS

- Believed to be an **autoimmune etiology**, leading to **progressive destruction** of **intrahepatic bile ducts**[Q]
- More common in **females**[Q]

Pathology

- **Florid duct lesion** is characterized by **lymphocytic** or **granulomatous bile duct infiltration**[Q].
- In the setting of **positive AMA**, florid duct lesion is **essentially diagnostic**[Q].

Clinical Features

- Most patients are **asymptomatic, pruritus** is the **commonest & earliest symptom**[Q].
- **Pruritus precedes jaundice in PBC**[Q], **Pruritus is most bothersome in evening**[Q].
- **Jaundice, fatigue, melanosis**[Q] (gradual darkening of exposed areas of skin), deficiency of fat soluble vitamins due to malabsorption.
- **Xanthomas & xanthelesmas**[Q] due to protracted elevation of serum lipids.

Laboratory Findings

- **Increased ALP, hyperlipidemia & positive antimitochondrial antibody**[Q].

Diagnosis

- **Diagnosis** can be **made by AMA**[Q].
- **IOC for diagnosis: Biopsy**[Q]

Treatment

- **Cholestyramine** is **mainstay** of treatment of **pruritus**[Q].
- **Ursodeoxycholic acid** is associated with **significant delay** to time of transplantation[Q].
- **Transplantation in PBC** may also be indicated for **intolerable lethargy** or **intractable pruritus**[Q].

■ RISK FACTORS FOR CHOLANGIOCARCINOMA

Risk Factors for Cholangiocarcinoma	
• **Choledochal cyst**[Q]	• RPC or **hepatolithiasis**[Q]
• **Primary sclerosing cholangitis**[Q]	• **Biliary enteric anastomosis**[Q]
• **Ulcerative colitis**[Q]	• **HBV, HIV, HCV**[Q]
• **Choledocholithiasis**[Q]	• **Radon**
• **Clonorchis sinensis & Opisthorchis viverrini**[Q]	• Asbestos, Nitrosamines, Dioxin **(AND)**[Q]
• **Cirrhosis**[Q]	• Diabetes, Obesity, OCPs, Smoking, Thorotrast, Isoniazid **(DOSTI)**[Q]

■ CHOLANGIOCARCINOMA

CHOLANGIOCARCINOMA

- Tumors arising from bile duct epithelium
- **MC type** is **adenocarcinoma**[Q]
- Differentiated by anatomic site of origin: **Intrahepatic** (10%), **hilar (65%)**[Q] and **distal** (25%).
- Hilar cholangiocarcinoma is also known as **Klatskin tumor**[Q]
- **MC gene mutation: K-ras >p16 (KRAP-16)**[Q]
- MC Type: Sclerosing

Clinical Features

- **Painless jaundice (70–90%)** is **MC symptom**[Q] of cholangiocarcinoma, followed by **pruritus** (66%), **abdominal pain**, **weight loss** (30–50%), **fever** (20%).
- **Distant metastasis** occurs in **one third**[Q] of patients.
- **MC site** of metastasis: **Lung** or **mediastinum**, liver and peritoneum.
- **Tumor markers: CA19-9**[Q], **CEA.**
- **Raised CA19-9** is a **poor prognostic factor**[Q] in cholangiocarcinoma.

Diagnosis

- **IOC for diagnosis: MRI+MRCP**

Treatment

Perihilar cholangiocarcinoma	**CBD resection + Lymphadenectomy + Hepatic resection**[Q]
Intrahepatic cholangiocarcinoma	**Hepatic resection**[Q]
Distal cholangiocarcinoma	Pancreaticoduodenectomy **(Whipple's procedure)**[Q]

Palliation

- **Chemotherapy: Gemcitabine + Cisplatin**[Q] is the reference regimen

■ HEMOBILIA

HEMOBILIA

- Bleeding into the biliary tract from an **abnormal arterial source** to **intrahepatic biliary tract** fistula
- **Arterial hemobilia** is the **MC source**[Q]

Etiology

- **Trauma:**
  - **Iatrogenic trauma (PTC)** is the **MC cause**[Q]
  - **Blunt trauma** is more common cause than penetrating trauma
- Gallstones
- Vascular pathology: Aneurysm, angiodysplasia, hemangioma
- Uncommon causes: Malignancy, parasitic infestation, liver abscess, cholangitis

Clinical Features

- Characterized by **Quinck's triad (Sandblom's**[Q] **triad): GI hemorrhage + biliary colic + jaundice**[Q].
- **Presentation: Melena (90%)**[Q], **hematemesis** (60%), **biliary colic** (70%), and **jaundice** (60%).
- Tendency for **delayed presentations** (up to weeks) and **recurrent brisk** but **limited bleeding** over months and even years[Q].

Diagnosis

- **Endoscopy: First investigation**[Q] to be done (visualize bleeding from the ampulla of Vater)
- **Angiography: Investigation of choice**[Q] (reveal the source of bleeding in 90%)
- **Transarterial embolization** is **curative** in **major hemobilia**[Q]

Treatment

- Treatment is focused on **stopping bleeding** and **relieving biliary obstruction**[Q].
- Most cases of **minor hemobilia** can be **managed conservatively**[Q] with correction of coagulopathy, adequate biliary drainage and close observation.

> - **First line therapy** for **major hemobilia: Transarterial embolization (TAE)**[Q]
> - **TAE** is **curative** in **major hemobilia** (success rates of 80-100%)[Q]
> - **Surgery:** When **conservative therapy** and **TAE** have **failed.**

■ BILE DUCT: ANATOMY AND PHYSIOLOGY

BILE DUCT: ANATOMY AND PHYSIOLOGY

Anatomy

- It lies in front of the portal vein and to the **right of** the **hepatic artery**[Q].
- Common hepatic duct is **1–4 cm** in **length** and has a **diameter** of approx. **4 mm**[Q].
- CBD is about **7–11 cm** in length & **5–10 mm** in diameter[Q].
- A **fibroareolar tissue** containing **scant smooth muscle** surround the mucosa (a **distinct muscle layer** is **absent**)[Q].
- Most important **arteries** to the supraduodenal bile duct run parallel to the duct at the **3 & 9 o' clock**[Q] positions.

> - Approximately **60%** of the blood supply to the supraduodenal bile duct originates **inferiorly** from the **pancreaticoduodenal** and **retroduodenal arteries**[Q].
> - Whereas **38%** of the blood supply originate **superiorly** from the **right hepatic artery** and **cystic duct artery**[Q].
> - **Mnemonic: Neeche se PR (Pancreaticoduodenal artery, Retroduodenal artery) upar se CR (Cystic artery, Right hepatic artery)**

Multiple Choice Questions

■ CHOLEDOCHAL CYST

1. Caroli's disease is: *(AIIMS GIS Dec 2006)*
   a. Type I choledochal cyst
   b. Type III choledochal cyst
   c. Type IV choledochal cyst
   d. Type V choledochal cyst

2. A 10-year-female presents with pain in the right hypochondrium, fever, jaundice and a palpable mass in the right hypochondrium. The probable diagnosis is: *(COMEDK 2011)*
   a. Hepatitis
   b. Hepatoma
   c. Choledochal cyst
   d. Mucocele gallbladder

3. A 10 years old female presented with recurrent attacks of cholangitis. CECT was done, the diagnosis on the basis of CECT is: *(Recent Question 2017)*
   a. Type 1 choledochal cyst
   b. Type 3 choledochal cyst
   c. Type 4 choledochal cyst
   d. Type 5 choledochal cyst

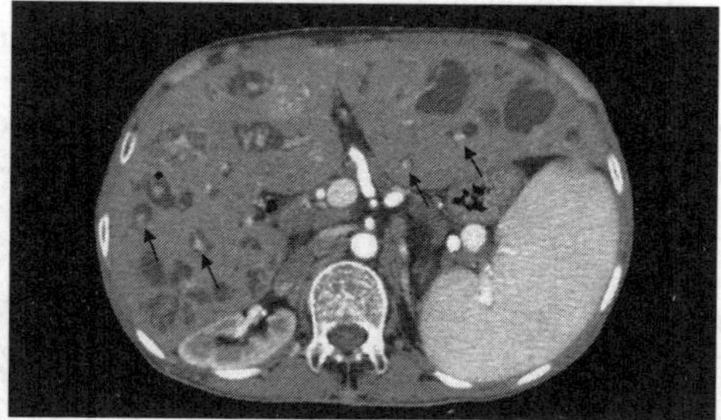

4. Central dot sign is seen in:
   (Recent Question 2016, AIIMS May 2011, Nov 2008, ILBS 2012)
   a. Primary sclerosing cholangitis
   b. Liver Hamartoma
   c. Caroli's disease
   d. Polycystic liver disease

5. Clinical features of choledochal cyst in adult are:
   a. Pain, lump and intermittent jaundice *(UPSC 2004)*
   b. Pain, fever and intermittent jaundice
   c. Pain, lump and progressive jaundice
   d. Pain, fever and progressive jaundice

6. Choledochal cyst develops due to: *(DNB 2006)*
   a. Stenosis of sphincter
   b. Dysfunction of long circular fibre
   c. Congenital
   d. Iatrogenic

7. All of the following are true about choledochal disease except: *(Recent Question 2017)*
   a. Type IV is Caroli's disease
   b. Type I is most common
   c. Type III is also called choledochocele
   d. Type II is diverticular disease

8. Choledochocele is which type of choledochal cyst?
   a. II
   b. III *(Recent Question 2017)*
   c. IV
   d. V

9. Both intra and extrahepatic choledochal cyst is seen in:
   a. II
   b. III *(Recent Question 2017)*
   c. IV
   d. V

■ CHOLEDOCHOLITHIASIS AND CHOLANGITIS

10. The procedure of choice for elective removal of CBD stones for most patients is: *(COMEDK 2006)*
    a. Open choledocholithotomy
    b. Endoscopic papillotomy
    c. Laparoscopic choledocholithotomy
    d. Percutaneous choledocholithotomy

11. The Reynold's pentad of fever, jaundice, right upper quadrant pain, septic shock and mental status change is typical of: *(COMEDK 2008)*
    a. Cholangitis
    b. Hepatitis
    c. Cholecystitis
    d. Pancreatitis

12. Charcot's triad:
    (Recent Question 2014, JIPMER 2010, All India 96, 95)
    a. Fever, abdominal pain, jaundice
    b. Fever, vomiting, jaundice
    c. Fever, jaundice, abdominal distension
    d. Fever, diarrhea, jaundice

13. Triad of abdominal pain, fever and jaundice is known as:
    (MCI Dec 2019)
    a. Charcot's triad
    b. Saint's triad
    c. Virchow triad
    d. Renault's triad

14. Sphincterotomy of sphincter of Oddi is performed at:
    (DNB 2006)
    a. 3 O'clock position
    b. 6 O'clock position
    c. 9 O'clock position
    d. 11 O'clock position

15. Most common cause of cholangitis: *(AIIMS June 94)*
    a. Viral infection
    b. CBD stone
    c. Surgery
    d. Amebic infection

16. The treatment of choice for an 8 mm retained common bile duct (CBD) stone is: *(DNB 2011, AIIMS May 2005, Nov 2003)*
    a. Laparoscopic CBD exploration
    b. Percutaneous stone extraction
    c. Endoscopic stone extraction
    d. Extracorporeal shock wave lithotripsy

17. Ramu presents with recurrent attacks of cholelithiasis, USG examination shows a dilated CBD of 1 cm. The next line of management is: *(AIIMS June 2001)*
    a. ERCP
    b. PTC
    c. Cholecystostomy
    d. Intravenous cholangiogram

18. Most common surgical cause of obstructive jaundice:
    (AIIMS Nov 94, AIIMS Nov 96, All India 98, 2000)
    a. Periampullary carcinoma
    b. Carcinoma gallbladder
    c. Carcinoma head of pancreas
    d. CBD stones

19. Common bile duct stones will manifest all except:
    (MCI March 2008, All India 89)
    a. Distended gallbladder
    b. Jaundice
    c. Itching
    d. Clay colored stools

20. In cholangitis, the organism mostly responsible is:
    (Recent Questions 2016)
    a. E. coli
    b. Streptococcus
    c. E. histolytica
    d. Clostridium

21. **All of the following are seen with bile duct stone except:**
    a. Obstructive jaundice   *(MCI March 2008)*
    b. Distended and palpable gallbladder
    c. Pruritus
    d. Clay colored stools

■ CHOLEDOCHOTOMY AND CBD EXPLORATION

22. **Choledochotomy is indicated in all of the following except in patients with:**   *(COMEDK 2010)*
    a. Palpable CBD stones
    b. History of jaundice or cholangitis
    c. Abnormal alkaline phosphatase
    d. Abnormal gamma glutamyl transferase

23. **After exploration of common bile duct, the T-tube is removed on which of the following days?**   *(Karnataka 96)*
    a. 3rd postoperative day
    b. 4th postoperative day
    c. 12th postoperative day
    d. 6th postoperative day

24. **Cholangiography via T-tube done after how many days of cholecystectomy:**   *(TN 99)*
    a. 1–5 days   b. 5–9 days
    c. 10–14 days   d. 15–20 days

25. **Most common complication of common bile duct exploration:**
    a. Retained stone   *(DPG 2008)*
    b. Pancreatitis
    c. Stricture of common bile duct
    d. T-tube displacement

■ BILE DUCT INJURY AND BILIARY STRICTURES

26. **Biliary stricture developing after laparoscopic cholecystectomy usually occurs at which part of common bile duct?**   *(Punjab 2008, All India 2006)*
    a. Upper   b. Middle
    c. Lower   d. All with equal frequency

27. **According to Bismuth Strasberg classification of bile duct injury, causing occlusion of a branch of biliary tree would be which type?**   *(MHSSMCET 2010)*
    a. Type A   b. Type B
    c. Type C   d. Type D

28. **Strasburg's class 'B' bile injury means:**   *(MHSSMCET 2010)*
    a. Bile leak from a minor duct
    b. Occlusion of a branch of biliary tree
    c. Injury of bile duct not in communication with CBD
    d. Circumferential injury to major bile ducts

29. **The initial investigation of choice for a post cholecystectomy biliary stricture is:**   *(AIIMS May 2005)*
    a. Ultrasound scan of the abdomen
    b. Endoscopic cholangiography
    c. Computed tomography
    d. Magnetic resonance cholangiography

30. **Most common cause of biliary stricture is:**   *(AIIMS June 94)*
    a. CBD stone   b. Trauma
    c. Asiatic cholangitis   d. Congenital

■ BILIARY FISTULA

31. **Most common cause of gallbladder fistula is:**   *(DPG 2008)*
    a. Liver abscess aspiration
    b. Laparoscopic surgery
    c. Gallstones   d. Trauma

32. **Which does not contribute to enterobiliary fistula?**
    a. Gastric ulcer   b. Duodenal ulcer
    c. Carcinoma gallbladder   d. Gallstones   *(Punjab 2008)*

■ BILIARY ATRESIA

33. **The gold standard for the definitive diagnosis of the extrahepatic biliary atresia is:**
    a. Per-operative cholangiography
    b. Hepatobiliary scintigraphy
    c. Alkaline phosphatase level
    d. Liver biopsy   *(Recent Question 2016, AIIMS, Nov 2002)*

34. **Kasai's procedure is the treatment of choice for:**
       (Recent Question 2017, Recent Question 2013, Orissa 2011)
    a. Congenital hypertrophic pyloric stenosis
    b. Duodenal atresia
    c. Biliary atresia   d. Hirschprung's disease

■ PRIMARY SCLEROSING CHOLANGITIS

35. **A 50-year-old male presents with pain upper abdomen, pruritus, jaundice and weight loss, elevated ANA, the likely diagnosis is:**   *(COMEDK 2011)*
    a. Primary sclerosing cholangitis
    b. Klatskin tumor
    c. Secondary sclerosing cholangitis
    d. Choledocholithiasis

36. **A 45-year-old male presented with recurrent attacks of cholangitis. MRCP and ERCP findings are given below. What is the most probable diagnosis?**

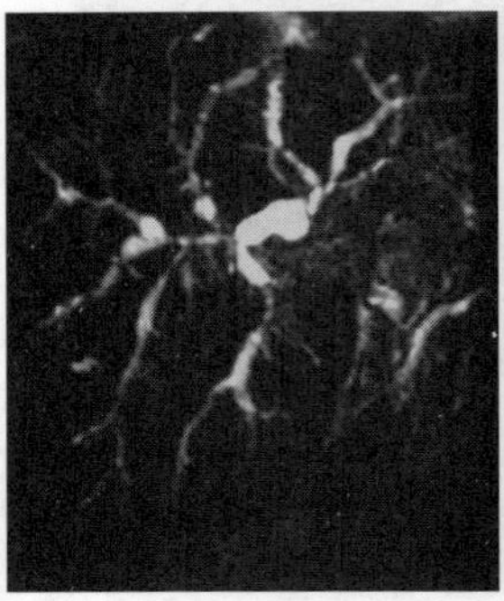 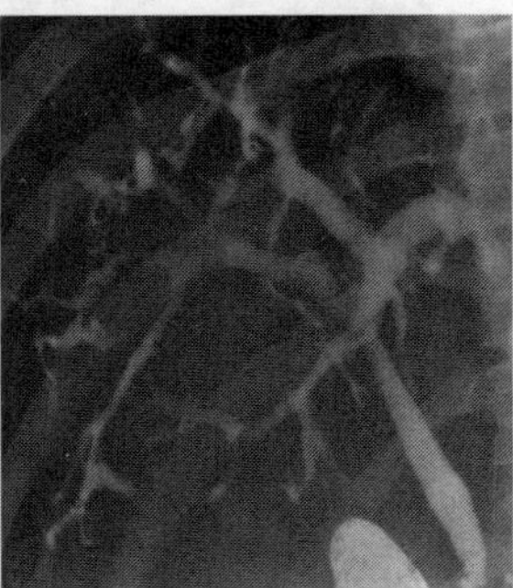

    a. Primary biliary cirrhosis
    b. Primary sclerosing cholangitis
    c. Oriental cholangiohepatitis
    d. Caroli's disease

37. **Primary sclerosing cholangitis is likely to be associated with:**
    a. Adenocarcinoma of pancreas   *(JIPMER 2012, 2011)*
    b. Cholangiocarcinoma
    c. Hepatocellular carcinoma
    d. Adenocarcinoma of gallbladder

38. **"Onion skin" fibrosis of bile duct is seen in:**
    a. Primary biliary cirrhosis   *(COMEDK 2009)*
    b. Primary sclerosing cholangitis
    c. Extrahepatic biliary fibrosis
    d. Congenital hepatic fibrosis

39. **True regarding primary sclerosing cholangitis associated with ulcerative colitis are all of the following except:**
       (MCI March 2007)
    a. Biliary cirrhosis is a known complication
    b. Increased risk of hilar cholangiocarcinoma
    c. May have raised levels of alkaline phoshphatase
    d. Primary sclerosing cholangitis resolves after total colectomy

■ PRIMARY BILIARY CIRRHOSIS

40. **Pruritus precedes jaundice in:**   *(ILBS 2011)*
    a. Primary biliary cirrhosis
    b. Secondary biliary cirrhosis

c. Primary sclerosing cholangitis
d. CBD stone

41. **The earliest symptom in primary biliary cirrhosis is:**
    (COMEDK 2008, 2007)
    a. Jaundice
    b. Pruritus
    c. Melanosis
    d. Vomiting

42. **Commonest presentation of primary biliary cirrhosis:**
    a. Pruritus
    b. Pain   *(All India 98)*
    c. Jaundice
    d. Fever

■ CHOLANGIOCARCINOMA PREDISPOSING FACTORS

43. **Not a predisposing factor for cholangiocarcinoma:**
    (Punjab 2007)
    a. Asiatic cholangio-hepatitis
    b. Cholelithiasis
    c. Ulcerative colitis
    d. Choledochal cyst

44. **Cholangiocarcinoma has been associated with infection by:**
    a. Paragonimus westermani
    b. Clonorchis sinensis
    c. Loa Loa   *(Recent Question 2016, 2015, COMEDK 2004)*
    d. Schistosoma haematobium

45. **All of the following are known predisposing factors for cholangiocarcinoma except:**
    a. CBD stones   *(Recnet Question 2016, All India 97)*
    b. Clonorchis sinensis
    c. Ulcerative colitis
    d. Primary sclerosing cholangitis

■ CHOLANGIOCARCINOMA

46. **Klatskin tumor is:**   *(JIPMER 2010)*
    a. Merkel cell carcinoma of skin
    b. Primitive neuroectodermal tumor of chest wall
    c. Common hepatic duct tumor
    d. Adenocarcinoma of anal canal

47. **Most common site of cholangiocarcinoma:**
    (AIIMS Nov 2011, May 2011, Nov 2008)
    a. Distal biliary duct
    b. Hilum
    c. Intrahepatic duct
    d. Multifocal

48. **ERCP is indicated for the following except:**
    a. Distal CBD tumor
    b. Hepatic porta tumor
    c. Proximal cholangiocarcinoma
    d. Gallstone pancreatitis   *(Recent Question 2013)*

49. **According to Bismuth classification, type IV cholangiocarcinoma involves:**   *(Recent Question 2015)*
    a. Common hepatic duct
    b. Bifurcation only
    c. Bifurcation and bilateral secondary intrahepatic ducts
    d. Bifurcation and unilateral secondary intrahepatic ducts

50. **Most common site of metastasis in cholangiocarcinoma:**
    (Recent Question 2016)
    a. Liver
    b. Bones
    c. Lung
    d. Pancreas

■ HEMOBILIA

51. **Most common cause of hemobilia:**
    (DNB 2005, 2000, AIIMS GIS 2003)
    a. Trauma
    b. Iatrogenic
    c. Parasites
    d. Tumors

52. **Not true of hemobilia:**
    (DNB 2010, Punjab 2009, ComedK 2007)
    a. GI bleeding
    b. Fever
    c. Jaundice
    d. Colicky RUQ pain

53. **True regarding hemobilia:**   *(DPG 2007)*
    a. Triad of jaundice, pain, melena
    b. MC cause- rupture of portal vein into biliary system
    c. MR angiography is the IOC
    d. None of the above

Explanations

■ CHOLEDOCHAL CYST

1. **Ans. d. Type V choledochal cyst** *(Ref: Sabiston 20/e p 1511; Schwartz 11/e p1417, 1374, 10/e p1289, 1630; Bailey 27/e p1197; Blumgart 6/e p762; Shackelford 8/e p1374)*

CAROLI'S DISEASE (TYPE V CHOLEDOCHAL CYST)

- Congenital malformation, consists of multiple **sacular dilatations** limited to the **intrahepatic**[Q] bile ducts (segmental bile ducts).
- **About half** the cases are **associated with congenital hepatic fibrosis**[Q] (affect **interlobular** bile ducts).
- Cyst with congenital hepatic fibrosis is known as **Grumbach's disease**[Q].

Clinical Features

- Symptoms include **cholangitis (64%)**[Q], portal hypertension (22%), and abdominal pain (18%)
- More common in **male**s
- Frequent episodes of **cholangitis** indicates **poor prognosis**[Q].

Diagnosis

- **CT findings**: Portal vein radicals can be seen after enhancement within dilated intra-hepatic bile ducts (**central dot sign**)[Q].

Treatment

- **Hepatic resection** for **localized disease**[Q]
- **Liver transplantation** for **diffuse disease**[Q].

2. **Ans. c. Choledochal cyst**

3. **Ans. d. Type 5 choledochal cyst** *(Ref: Sabiston 20/e p15; Schwartz 11/e p1374, 10/e p1289; Bailey 27/e p1168; Blumgart 6/e p762; Shackelford 8/e p1374)*
   - Central dot sign is seen in **Caroli's disease (Type V Choledochal cyst)**.

4. **Ans. c. Caroli's disease**

5. **Ans. a. Pain, lump and intermittent jaundice**

CHOLEDOCHAL CYST

- **Classic triad: Pain, jaundice (intermittent)** and abdominal **mass (10%)**[Q].

6. **Ans. c. Congenital**

7. **Ans. a. Type IV is Caroli's disease** *(Ref: Sabiston 20/e p1510; Schwartz 11/e p1374, 10/e p1289; Bailey 27/e p1168)*

8. **Ans. b. III** *(Ref: Sabiston 20/e p1510; Schwartz 11/e p1417, 10/e p1330; Bailey 27/e p1198)*

9. **Ans. c. IV** *(Ref: Sabiston 20/e p1510; Schwartz 11/e p1417, 10/e p1330; Bailey 27/e p1198)*

■ CHOLEDOCHOLITHIASIS AND CHOLANGITIS

10. **Ans. b. Endoscopic papillotomy** *(Ref: Sabiston 20/e p1494-1496; Schwartz 11/e p1407, 10/e p1321-1322; Bailey 27/e p1205)*

- **ERCP: Diagnostic** and **therapeutic test of choice** for patients with suspected **CBD stones**[Q].`

11. **Ans. a. Cholangitis** *(Ref: Sabiston 20/e p1507; Schwartz 11/e p1407, 10/e p1322-1323; Bailey 27/e p1205)*

12. **Ans. a. Fever, abdominal pain, jaundice**

- **Charcot's triad**[Q]: **Abdominal pain + jaundice + fever**[Q]
- **Reynold's pentad**[Q]: **Charcot's triad + altered mental status + shock (hypotension)**[Q]

13. **Ans. a. Charcot's triad** *(Ref: Bailey 27/e p1168)*

14. **Ans. d. 11 O'clock position** *(Ref: Sabiston 20/e p1496; Schwartz 11/e p1407, 10/e p1327)*

TRANSDUODENAL SPHINCTEROPLASTY

- This **cut is made superiorly** (at the **11 o'clock position**)[Q] for 4 to 5 mm.
- The **sphincter** is **incised at** the **11–O'clock position to avoid injury to the pancreatic duct**[Q].

15. **Ans. b. CBD stone**

16. **Ans. c. Endoscopic stone extraction**

17. **Ans. a.** ERCP

18. **Ans. d.** CBD stones

19. **Ans. a.** Distended gallbladder

20. **Ans. a.** E. coli

21. **Ans. b.** Distended and palpable gallbladder

■ CHOLEDOCHOTOMY AND CBD EXPLORATION

22. **Ans. d.** Abnormal gamma glutamyl transferase

23. **Ans. c.** 12th postoperative day

24. **Ans. b.** 5–9 days

25. **Ans. a.** Retained stone *(Ref: Sabiston 20/e p1496)*

Most common complication of common bile duct exploration retained stone.

- **Clearance** of all **common bile duct stones** is achieved **in 75–95%** of patients with **laparoscopic CBD exploration**[Q].
- The rate of **retained CBD stone** is <5%.
- MC complication of **laparoscopic CBD exploration**[Q] is **retained stone**.

■ BILE DUCT INJURY AND BILIARY STRICTURES

26. **Ans. a.** Upper *(Ref: Sabiston 20/e p1502)*

- **Most common duct injuries** occur **during attempted dissection** of the **cystic duct** when the **CBD is mistaken for cystic duct**[Q].
- These injuries involve **transection** of the **upper part** of the **CBD**[Q] and excision of a variable portion of the CBD proximal to first transection, including cystic duct-common duct junction.

THE STEWART-WAY CLASSIFICATION OF LAPAROSCOPIC BILE DUCT INJURY

- The **Stewart-Way classification** is based primarily on the **anatomic pattern** and **mechanism** of a particular injury and the presence of associated **vascular injury**.

Class	Criteria
	The Stewart-Way classification of laparoscopic bile duct injury
I.	**CBD mistaken** for **cystic duct** but **recognized**; cholangiogram incision of cystic duct extended into CBD
II.	**Lateral damage** to **common hepatic duct** from cautery or clips placed on duct; associated bleeding, poor visibility
III.	**CBD mistaken** for **cystic duct, not recognized**; CBD, CHD, RHD, LHD transected or resected
IV.	**RHD mistaken** for **cystic duct, RHA mistaken** for **cystic artery**, RHD and RHA transected; lateral damage to the RHD from cautery or clips placed on ducts

27. **Ans. b.** Type B

28. **Ans. b.** Occlusion of a branch of biliary tree

29. **Ans. c.** Computed tomography *(Ref: Blumgart 6/e p701)*

CT is **probably the best initial study**, the results of which **help direct further investigations**.

30. **Ans. b.** Trauma

- MC cause of **benign biliary stricture** is **laparoscopic cholecystectomy (operative trauma)**[Q].

■ BILIARY FISTULA

31. **Ans. c.** Gallstones *(Ref: Blumgart 6/e p682; Shackelford 8/e p1309)*

32. **Ans. a.** Gastric ulcer *(Ref: Blumgart 6/e p685)*

■ BILIARY ATRESIA

33. **Ans. a.** Per-operative cholangiography *(Ref: Blumgart 6/e p658)*

*"Despite these advancements in noninvasive imaging of hepatobiliary anatomy, **intraoperative cholangiography remains the gold standard for diagnosing biliary atresia**. Although endoscopic retrograde **cholangiopancreatography (ERCP) may be possible, equipment and expertise in performing ERCP in infants is limited**. Preoperative liver biopsy has become an increasingly safe and used method to help exclude other causes of neonatal jaundice. **Although percutaneous liver biopsy is highly accurate, there are no histologic findings that are pathognomonic for BA. Findings suggestive of BA** include portal or bridging fibrosis, bile duct proliferation, inflammation, or giant cell hepatitis, some of which may not be evident on samples taken from very young infants, thereby necessitating repeat biopsy at a later date."- Blumgart 6/e p658*

34. **Ans. c.** Biliary atresia

■ PRIMARY SCLEROSING CHOLANGITIS

35. Ans. a. Primary sclerosing cholangitis
36. Ans. b. Primary sclerosing cholangitis *(Ref: Sabiston 20/e p1508-1509; Schwartz 11/e p1417, 10/e p1292; Bailey 27/e p1206)*

> *In the MRCP and ERCP image, there is presence of multiple strictures involving both intrahepatic and extrahepatic bile duct and history of repeated attacks of cholangitis is highly suggestive of primary sclerosing cholangitis.*

37. Ans. b. Cholangiocarcinoma
38. Ans. b. Primary sclerosing cholangitis
39. Ans. d. Primary sclerosing cholangitis resolves after total colectomy

■ PRIMARY BILIARY CIRRHOSIS

40. Ans. a. Primary biliary cirrhosis *(Ref: Sabiston 20/e p639; Blumgart 6/e p1155; Shackelford 8/e p1406)*
41. Ans. b. Pruritus
42. Ans. a. Pruritus

■ CHOLANGIOCARCINOMA PREDISPOSING FACTORS

43. Ans. b. Cholelithiasis

> • **Choledocholithiasis, not the cholelithiasis** is a risk factor for **cholangiocarcinoma**[Q].

44. Ans. b. Clonorchis sinensis
45. Ans. None

■ CHOLANGIOCARCINOMA

46. Ans. c. Common hepatic duct tumor
47. Ans. b. Hilum
48. Ans. c. Proximal cholangiocarcinoma
49. Ans. c. Bifurcation and bilateral secondary intrahepatic ducts
50. Ans. a. Liver

■ HEMOBILIA

51. Ans. b. Iatrogenic *(Ref: Sabiston 20/e p1472-1474; Blumgart 6/e p1915; Shackelford 8/e p1275)*
52. Ans. b. Fever
53. Ans. a. Triad of jaundice, pain, melena

Pancreas

PANCREAS DIVISUM

PANCREAS DIVISUM

- **MC congenital anomaly** of pancreas[Q]
- It occurs when the ductal systems of the **dorsal** & **ventral pancreatic duct fail to fuse**[Q] during the second month of gestation.

Diagnosis

- **IOC** for diagnosis of **pancreas divisum: MRCP**[Q]
- **Gold standard** investigation for diagnosis: **ERCP**[Q]

Treatment

- Operative **dorsal duct sphincterotomy, with or without sphincteroplasty**[Q], is the preferred surgical treatment.

ANNULAR PANCREAS

ANNULAR PANCREAS

- **Circumferential** or near-circumferential **band of pancreas tissue** surrounding the **2nd** part of **duodenum**[Q]
- It is of **ventral pancreas origin** and is usually **proximal to ampulla**[Q].

> - **Duodenal stenosis** or **atresia** is present at the site of annulus in **40%**[Q]
> - **Down's syndrome**[Q] (trisomy 21) is present in **15-25%**.

- Intestinal malrotation, tracheoesophageal fistula, & congenital heart defects, Meckel's diverticulum and imperforate anus are also not uncommon.

Diagnosis

- **Definitive diagnosis** is made by ERCP.

Treatment

- Treatment of choice: **Duodenoduodenostomy**[Q] >Duodenojejunostomy.
- **Duodenoduodenostomy** has **replaced duodenojejunostomy** as the **treatment of choice** because it has a **lower incidence** of **postoperative complications**, particularly **obstruction** & **blind-loop syndromes**[Q].

ETIOLOGY OF ACUTE PANCREATITIS

Causes of Acute Pancreatitis	
Common Causes	**Uncommon Causes**
• **Gallstones** including microlithiasis **(MC)**[Q] • **Alcohol (2nd MC)**[Q] • **Hypertriglyceridemia**[Q] • **ERCP**[Q] • Blunt abdominal trauma • Postoperative • Drugs • Sphincter of Oddi dysfunction **Rare Causes:** • Infections (**CMV, Coxsackie, Mumps, Echovirus, (CME)** parasites)[Q] • Autoimmune (Sjogren syndrome)	• Vascular causes and vasculitis (ischemic-hypoperfusion states after cardiac surgery) • Connective tissue disorders • **TTP**[Q] • **CA pancreas**[Q] • **Hypercalcemia (Hyperparathyroidism)**[Q] • Periampullary diverticulum • **Pancreas divisum**[Q] • Hereditary pancreatitis • **Cystic fibrosis**[Q] • Renal failure

Drugs Associated with Pancreatitis		
Definite Cause (MAD CAT PET TV FM)		**Probable Cause (PILAAS)**
• 6-**M**ercaptopurine[Q]	• **E**strogens[Q]	• **P**henformin
• **A**zathioprine[Q]	• **T**rimethoprim-sulfamethoxazole[Q]	• **P**rocainamide
• **D**ideoxyinosine		• **I**soniazid
• **C**ytosine arabinoside	• **T**hiazide[Q]	• **L**-Asparaginase[Q]
• 5-**A**minosalicylate[Q]	• **V**alproic acid[Q]	• **A**cetaminophen[Q]
• **T**etracycline	• **F**urosemide	• **A**lpha-Methyl-dopa
• **P**entamidine[Q]	• **M**etronidazole[Q]	• **S**ulindac

■ ACUTE PANCREATITIS

ACUTE PANCREATITIS

- **AP is mild & self-limited** in most patients[Q]
- **Rapidly progressive inflammatory response** associated with prolonged length of hospital stay and significant morbidity & mortality occur in **10-20%**[Q] of patients
- **Mortality rate: Mild** pancreatitis <1%; **Severe** pancreatitis **10-30%**[Q].

> - **MC cause of death** in this group of patients is **multiorgan dysfunction syndrome**[Q].
> - **First sign of Multi-system organ failure** in AP commonly is **impaired lung function** caused by **ARDS**[Q].

- Mortality in the **first 2 weeks (early phase)**: Due to **multiorgan dysfunction**[Q]
- Mortality **after 2 weeks (late period)**: Caused by **septic complications**[Q]

Clinical Features
- **Cardinal symptom: Epigastric** and/or periumbilical **pain** that **radiates to the back, relieved by sitting** & **leaning forward**[Q].
- Up to **90%** of patients have **nausea** and/or **vomiting** that typically does not relieve the pain.
- Dehydration, poor skin turgor, tachycardia, hypotension, & dry mucous membranes are commonly seen in patients with AP.
- **Severe pancreatitis:** Significant abdominal distention, associated with generalized rebound tenderness and abdominal rigidity.

> - **Flank (Grey Turner)**[Q], **periumbilical (Cullen's sign)**[Q] & **inguinal ecchymosis (Fox sign)**[Q] are indicative of **retroperitoneal bleeding** associated with **severe pancreatitis.**

- Associated with **left sided pleural effusion**[Q]

Diagnosis
- Cornerstone of the diagnosis of AP: **Clinical findings + elevation of pancreatic enzyme** levels in the plasma[Q].

Pancreatic Enzymes
• A **threefold or higher** elevation of **amylase & lipase** levels **confirms** the **diagnosis**[Q].
• **Amylase's** serum **half-life** is **shorter** as compared with lipase.
• Lipase is also a **more specific marker of AP**[Q] because serum amylase levels can be elevated in peptic ulcer disease, mesenteric ischemia, salpingitis, and macroamylasemia.

- **X-ray Abdomen:** Localized ileus of **duodenum** and **proximal jejunum** (sentinel loop)[Q] or that of **transverse colon** up to **its mid point** (colon cut off sign)[Q].
- **IOC for acute pancreatitis: CECT**[Q] (Should be performed **after 72 hours of acute pancreatitis**[Q])

Treatment
- **Cornerstone of the treatment: Aggressive fluid resuscitation**[Q] (Fluid of choice: RL[Q]) with **supplementary oxygen**
- **Narcotics** are usually preferred, especially **Buprenorphine >morphine**[Q] as analgesics.

In Acute Pancreatitis	
• **NSAIDs of choice**	• **Metamizole**[Q]
• **Opiate of choice**	• **Buprenorphine**[Q]

- **Nutritional support: Enteral nutrition**[Q] is associated with less infectious complications and reduces the need for pancreatic surgery as compared to TPN.
- **Enteral nutrition** is **started within 24 hours** via NG tube.
- **TPN** can be given if patient is in **shock** & having **severe pancreatitis**.
- **Prophylactic antibiotic** should **not be given**[Q].

> - **ERCP:** Beneficial for patients with **severe acute biliary pancreatitis & cholangitis**[Q]
> - **Laparoscopic cholecystectomy:** Indicated for **all patients with mild acute biliary pancreatitis**[Q] with the **exception** of **older** patients and those with **poor performance status**[Q]

■ ASSESSMENT OF SEVERITY OF ACUTE PANCREATITIS

ASSESSMENT OF SEVERITY OF ACUTE PANCREATITIS

- **Severe pancreatitis** is diagnosed if **three or more**[Q] of the **Ranson's criteria** are fulfilled.
- Main disadvantage is that it does not predict the severity of disease at the time of the admission because six parameters are only assessed after 48 hours of admission.
- An **APACHE II score** of ≥8[Q] defines **severe pancreatitis**. The main advantage is that it can be used on admission and repeated at any time.
- A **CRP level ≥130 mg/mL**[Q] defines **severe pancreatitis**.

Tools for Predicting Severity in Acute Pancreatitis Ready for Clinical Use		
On Admission	**At 24 Hours**	**At 48 Hours**
• APACHE-II Score ≥8[Q] • **IL-6** • **Urea >60 mmol/L**	• Polymorphonuclear **elastase** • Urinary **trypsinogen 2** • Urinary **trypsinogen** activation peptide	• Ranson/Glasgow score ≥ 3[Q] • CRP ≥130[Q] mg/mL

Ranson's Prognostic Criteria for Non-Gallstone Pancreatitis	
At Admission	**During Initial 48 Hours**
• Age >55 years[Q] • WBC >**16,000**[Q] cells/mm³ • Blood glucose >**200**[Q] mg/dL • Serum LDH >**350**[Q] IU/L • AST >**250**[Q] U/L	• Hematocrit fall >**10**[Q] percentage points • BUN elevation >**5**[Q] mg/ dL • Serum calcium fall to <**8**[Q] mg/ dL • Arterial PO_2 <**60**[Q] mm Hg • Base deficit >**4**[Q] mEq/L • Estimated fluid sequestration >**6**[Q] **Litres**

ACUTE PHYSIOLOGY AND CHRONIC HEALTH EVALUATION (APACHE)-II SCORING SYSTEM

- **APACHE-II scoring system** incorporates 12[Q] physiological and laboratory parameters as well as age and comorbid conditions to estimate severity of any disease process.

The 12 physiologic variables are BT ↑ HR at CWG SHOP-2		
1. Mean arterial **Blood pressure**[Q]	5. **Creatinine**	9. **Hematocrit**
2. **Temperature**	6. **WBC count**[Q]	10. **Oxygenation**
3. **Heart rate**	7. **Glasgow Coma Scale**[Q]	11. Arterial **pH**[Q]
4. **Respiratory rate**	8. **Sodium**	12. Serum potassium

- **Score ≥8** signifies **severe, acute pancreatitis**[Q]

Computed Tomography Severity Index (CTSI) for Acute Pancreatitis

- CTSI (CT severity index scoring system) = Balthazar grade score + necrosis score
- **Highest attainable score = 10**[Q]

Pancreatic Inflammation		Pancreatic Necrosis	
Normal pancreas	0	None	0
Focal or **diffuse** pancreatic **enlargement**	1	≤ 30%	2
Intrinsic pancreatic alterations with **peripancreatic fat inflammatory** changes	2	30–50%	4
Single fluid collection/or phlegmon	3	>50%	6
Two or **more** fluid collections or **gas**, in or adjacent to the pancreas	4		

- **CTSI score:**
  - 0-3: Mortality 3%, morbidity 8%   – 4-6: Mortality 6%, morbidity 35%   – 7-10: Mortality 17%, morbidity 92%

BISAP score: Bedside Index for Severity of Acute Pancreatitis

- **BUN > 25 mg/dL**   • **Impaired mental status**   • SIRS ≥ 2 of 4 present   • **Age > 60 years**   • **Pleural effusion**`
  (Score **0–2**: Mortality < **2%**; Score **3–5**: Mortality > **15%**)

Quick Sequential Organ Failure Assessment (SOFA) Score	
qSOFA (Quick SOFA) Criteria	**Points**
• **Respiratory rate ≥22/min**[Q]	1
• Change in **mental status**[Q]	1
• **Systolic BP ≤100 mm Hg**[Q]	1

■ COMPLICATIONS OF ACUTE PANCREATITIS

Local Complications of Acute Pancreatitis				
	Acute (<4 weeks, No defined wall)		Chronic (>4 weeks, Defined wall)	
Content	No Infection	Infection	No Infection	Infection
Fluid	**Acute pancreatic fluid collection[Q] (APFC)**	Infected APFC	**Pseudocyst[Q]**	Infected pseudocyst
Solid ± Fluid	**Acute necrotic collection[Q] (ANC)**	Infected ANC	**Walled off necrosis[Q] (WON)**	Infected WON

Vascular Complications of Acute Pancreatitis

- Acute pancreatitis is **rarely associated with arterial vascular complications**.
- **MC vessel affected: Splenic artery**[Q]
- **Other vessels: Superior mesenteric, cystic, and gastroduodenal arteries**[Q]

> **Vascular Thrombosis**
> - Pancreatic inflammation can produce **vascular thrombosis**
> - **MC affected vessel: Splenic vein**[Q]
> - Imaging demonstrates **splenomegaly, gastric varices**, and **splenic vein occlusion**
> - **Thrombolytics** have been described in the **acute early phase. Most patients** can be managed with **conservative treatment**
> - **Recurrent episodes** of **upper GI bleeding** caused by venous hypertension should be **treated with splenectomy**[Q]

Pathogenesis

- It has been proposed that **pancreatic elastase damages** the **vessels**, leading to **pseudoaneurysm formation**.

Clinical Features

- **Spontaneous rupture**[Q] results in massive bleeding.
- Clinical manifestations include sudden onset of **abdominal pain, tachycardia**, and **hypotension**.

Treatment

- If possible, **arterial embolization** should be attempted **to control the bleeding**[Q].
- **Refractory cases** require **ligation of** the **affected vessel**.

> - **MC affected vessel** in **acute pancreatitis: Splenic artery (pseudoaneusysm formation)**[Q]
> - **MC affected vessel** leading to **vascular thrombosis** caused by acute pancreatitis: **Splenic vein**[Q]

■ PSEUDOPANCREATIC CYST

Pseudopancreatic Cyst

- A chronic collection of pancreatic fluid surrounded by a **nonepithelialized wall of granulation tissue & fibrosis**[Q]
- Pseudocysts account **75% of cystic lesions**[Q] of the **pancreas**.
- **MC complication** of **chronic pancreatitis**[Q]

> - Located anywhere from the **mediastinum** to the **scrotum**[Q]
> - **MC site of pseudocyst: Lesser sac**[Q]
> - **Traumatic pseudocysts** tend to occur **anterior to** the **body**[Q] of the gland
> - **Chronic pancreatitis pseudocysts** are commonly located **within the substance** of the gland

- **Incidence of Pseudocysts:**
  - **Acute pancreatitis: 10-20%** of patients[Q]
  - **Chronic pancreatitis: 20-40%** of patients
- **Multiple in 17%**[Q] cases
- **Alcohol is MC cause** of **pancreatitis related pseudocysts**[Q].

Pathophysiology

- **Pancreatic duct leak** with extravasation of pancreatic juice results in a pancreatic fluid collection (PFC).
- **Acute pseudocyst:** Over a period of **3 to 4 weeks**[Q], the PFC is sealed by an inflammatory reaction that leads to development of a wall of acute granulation tissue without much fibrosis.
- Acute pseudocysts may **resolve spontaneously** in up to **50% of cases**, over a course of **6 weeks** or longer[Q].
- **Pseudocysts >6 cm resolve less frequently** than smaller ones but may regress over a period of weeks to months[Q].

Clinical Features

- Pseudocysts usually cause symptoms of pain, fullness, or early satiety.

> - **Abdominal pain is MC symptom**[Q], occurs in up to 90% of patients
> - Other common symptoms include **early satiety, nausea & vomiting** (50% to 70%), **weight loss** (20% to 50%), **jaundice** (10%), and low-grade fever (10%)[Q]

Contd...

Contd...

- **Physical examination**: Upper abdominal tenderness in the majority of patients, and **25-45%** will have a **palpable abdominal mass**[Q].

Pseudocyst Complications (Shackelford 7th/1159)	
• **Infection (MC)[Q]: 14%**	• Duodenal obstruction
• Pain due to expansion	• Rupture
• Hemorrhage: up to 10%	• Abscess

Diagnosis
- **Elevated serum amylase & lipase**[Q] concentrations may occur in **half** of these patients.
- **Persistently elevated amylase** after resolution of atitis should prompt investigation for a pseudocyst.
- **IOC for diagnosis of pseudocyst. CECT**

Treatment
- Pseudocyst **5 cm** in diameter and **<6 weeks** old should be **observed**[Q], as they tend to **resolve spontaneously**[Q].
- **Pseudocyst >5 cm** diameter is an indications for **drainage**[Q]

- **Cystojejunostomy** has a **slightly lower recurrence rate**, but it is associated with significantly **more blood loss** and operative time

Clinical Pancreatic Syndromes and Associated Genetic Mutations	
• **Hereditary Pancreatitis**	• **PRSS1**[Q] (Cationic trypsinogen) gene
• **Idiopathic chronic Pancreatitis**	• **CFTR**[Q]
• **Tropical calcific Pancreatitis**	• **SPINK1 (PTSI)**[Q]

■ CHRONIC PANCREATITIS

CHRONIC PANCREATITIS

- Characterized by **persistent inflammation & irreversible fibrosis** associated with **atrophy** of pancreatic parenchyma[Q].
- Associated with **chronic pain** and **endocrine & exocrine insufficiency**[Q]

  > - In most cases of chronic pancreatitis, **exocrine insufficiency precedes endocrine insufficiency** by **many years**[Q]

- Approximately **90%** of **beta cell mass must be lost** before clinical **diabetes** develops.
- Classification of various causes of chronic pancreatitis based on the **TIGAR-O system**[Q] (TIGAR-O consist of toxic-metabolic, idiopathic, genetic, autoimmune, recurrent severe, obstructive).

Etiology
- **Heavy alcohol consumption** is MC cause of CP **(70-80%)**[Q]
- **Smoking increases** the **risk**[Q] of alcohol-induced CP.
- **Other causes**: Chronic duct obstruction, trauma, pancreas divisum, cystic dystrophy of the duodenal wall, **hyperparathyroidism, hypertriglyceridemia, autoimmune pancreatitis, tropical pancreatitis, & hereditary pancreatitis** (account for <10% of all cases)

Pathology
- Clinical Features
- **Classic triad**: DM + Pancreatic calcification + Steatorrhea **(DPS)**
- **Abdominal pain** is the primary manifestation and **MC symptom** of CP[Q].
- **Intensity, frequency, & duration** of pain gradually **increase with worsening disease**[Q].
- Pancreatic **inflammation** and **fibrosis** decrease the number & function of acinar cells.

  > - At least **90%** of the **gland** needs to be **dysfunctional** before **steatorrhea, diarrhea**, and other symptoms of **malabsorption** develop[Q]
  > - **Exocrine insufficiency** occurs in **80-90%** of patients with **long-standing CP**[Q]

- **Diabetes** is developed in **40-80%** of patients, typically occurs **many years after** the onset of **abdominal pain** and **pancreatic exocrine insufficiency**[Q].

Diagnosis
- **X-ray abdomen**: Diffuse pancreatic calcification is seen in **30-40%** cases of CP[Q]
- **IOC for diagnosis: MRCP**

  > - **ERCP**: Considered the **gold standard** for the diagnosis of CP, the advent of **secretin MRCP** and **EUS** have **significantly decreased its role** as a **diagnostic test**[Q]

- **Steatorrhea**: If the **stool fat** content **exceeds 7 gm/day**[Q]

Contd...

Section 2
Hepatobiliary Pancreatic Surgery

Contd...

Treatment

- Patients should be strongly encouraged to stop drinking and smoking.
- **NSAIDs** are the first line of treatment, patients with severe pain should be treated with potent long-acting **narcotics**[Q].
- **Pancreatic enzyme replacement**[Q] in patients with pancreatic exocrine insufficiency.
- **ERCP**: Primary modality for **treating symptomatic pancreatic duct obstruction** with **dilation** and **polyethylene stent placement**[Q].
- **Endoscopic stone extraction** should be considered for patients with **pain** and **pancreatic duct dilation secondary to stones**[Q].

■ SURGICAL PROCEDURES IN CHRONIC PANCREATITIS

PROCEDURES IN CHRONIC PANCREATITIS

Surgical Procedures in Chronic Pancreatitis	
Drainage Procedure	**Resection Procedure**
• **Puestow Procedure**[Q] (Longitudinal Pancreaticojejunostomy): **Resection of tail** followed by a longitudinal pancreaticojejunostomy[Q]	• **Beger's Procedure** (Duodenal Preserving Pancreatic Head Resection **DPPHR**[Q]) • **Frey's Procedure** (Local Resection of the Head of the Pancreas Combined with Longitudinal Pancreaticojejunostomy **LR-LPJ**)[Q]

SURGICAL PROCEDURES IN CHRONIC PANCREATITIS

- **Ideal procedure**: DPPHR[Q] (Beger's)
- **In** presence of **portal vein thrombosis**: Frey's[Q]

■ SEROUS CYSTADENOMA OF PANCREAS

- Serous Cystadenoma of Pancreas
- **Mucsite**: Head of pancreas; Affect **women** almost **exclusively**[Q]
- Most are **benign** and have **no malignant potential**[Q]
- Pathology
- SCNs are **large**[Q], well-circumscribed masses (**microcystic**)
- Typically have **small cyst**[Q] filled with clear fluid with **spongelike** or **honeycomb appearance**[Q].

Clinical Features

- Most are **asymptomatic**[Q]
- Patients commonly present with **vague abdominal pain**[Q] and less frequently with weight loss & obstructive jaundice.

Diagnosis

- Aspiration from cyst yields **non-viscous fluid** with **low CEA** & **low amylase** levels[Q].

  - **Central calcification** gives rise to a characteristic **central sunburst**[Q], **radial,** or **stellate scar pattern** on **CT scan**[Q] (10-20%)

Treatment

- SCN is benign, **resection** is indicated when **diagnosis** is **in doubt** or when they become **symptomatic**[Q], size > 4 cm

■ MUCINOUS CYSTADENOMA OF PANCREAS

MUCINOUS CYSTADENOMA OF PANCREAS

- **MCN: MC cystic neoplasm**[Q] of pancreas
- Frequently seen in **young women**, mean age **5th decade**[Q]; MC site: **body** & **tail** of pancreas

Pathology

- MCNs contain **mucin-producing epithelium**[Q], **macrocystic**
- Histology: Presence of **mucin-rich cells** and **ovarian-like stroma**[Q]
- **Estrogen** & **progesterone staining** are **positive** in **most cases**[Q]

Clinical Features

- Up to **50%** of patients present with **vague abdominal pain**.
- A **history of pancreatitis** may be found in up to **20%** of patients, which explains the common misdiagnosis of pseudocyst.

Contd...

Diagnosis

- **CT scan**: Presence of a **solitary cyst** with **fine septations** & **rim of calcification**[Q]

  - Presence of **eggshell calcification**, **larger** tumor **size**, or a **mural nodule** on cross-sectional imaging is **suggestive of malignancy**[Q]
  - **Cyst fluid analyses**: **Mucin-rich** aspirate, **high CEA** & **low amylase** levels[Q]

Treatment

- **Surgical excision is indicated** for all mucinous cystic neoplams[Q]
- **Pancreatic resection** is the **standard treatment** for MCNs[Q].

■ INTRADUCTAL PAPILLARY MUCINOUS NEOPLASM (IPMN)

INTRADUCTAL PAPILLARY MUCINOUS NEOPLASM

- **IPMN** is also known as **mucin-secreting carcinoma**[Q], villous adenoma of the duct of Wirsung
- Seen in **6th** to **7th** decade of life; **Equal sex distribution**[Q]
- More common in **head** & **uncinate process**[Q] of the pancreas

Types of IPMN

- **Side branch IPMN:** Involves dilation of the pancreatic duct side **branches**
- **Main duct IPMN:** Abnormal cystic dilation of the **main pancreatic duct**
- **Mixed-type IPMN:** **Side branch** IPMN that has extended to **involve** the **main pancreatic duct**

Clinical Features

- Present with **abdominal pain** or **recurrent pancreatitis**, (caused by obstruction of pancreatic duct by **thick mucin**[Q]).
- Some patients (5-10%) have **steatorrhea, diabetes**, & **weight loss** secondary to pancreatic insufficiency.

  - **Predictors of malignancy: Jaundice, elevated** serum **ALP, mural nodules, diabetes**, & main pancreatic **duct diameter ≥ 7 mm**[Q]

Diagnosis

- **Endoscopy: Mucus extruding** through a large, **fish-mouth** like papillary orifice is **virtually diagnostic of IPMN**[Q]
- **CT scans: Dilated main pancreatic duct**, cysts of varying sizes, and possibly **mural nodules**[Q]
- **Aspirated fluid: Mucinous** content with **elevated CEA** & **amylase** level[Q]

Treatment

- **Partial pancreatectomy:** For **main duct, symptomatic**, and **large branch-type IPMNs (>3 cm)**, or IPMNs with an **invasive component**[Q]
- **Observation:** For **asymptomatic small (< 3 cm) branch duct IPMNs** without **associated nodularity**.

■ RISK FACTORS FOR PANCREATIC CARCINOMA

RISK FACTORS FOR PANCREATIC CARCINOMA

- There is **association** between risk of **pancreatic cancer, H. pylori** colonization, & **ABO** blood groups[Q].
- Older age, African American race, low socioeconomic status, Ashkenazic jewish heritage are associated with increased risk of pancreatic cancer.
- **Host etiologic factors** associated with increased risk of pancreatic cancer include history of **diabetes mellitus, chronic cirrhosis** and **pancreatitis**, a **high fat** or **cholesterol diet**, and **prior cholecystectomy**[Q].

Risk Factors for Pancreatic Carcinoma		
• **Established**	• **Tobacco**[Q]	• **Inherited susceptibility**[Q]
• **Associated**	• **Chronic pancreatitis**[Q]	• **Diabetes mellitus** type 2[Q] • **Obesity**[Q]
• **Possible**	• **Physical inactivity**[Q]	• Certain pesticides • High carbohydrate/sugar intake

Genetic Mutation in Pancreatic Cancer (KRAP-16: K-ras >p16))	
Gene	**Pancreatic Cancer %**
• p16[Q]	• 82
• K-ras[Q]	• 95-100 (MC)
• p53[Q]	• 75
• DPC4	• 55
• BRCA2	• 7

Predisposing Conditions for Familial Pancreatic Cancer (H₃-AFP)	
• Hereditary pancreatitis[Q] • HNPCC[Q] • Hereditary Breast Cancer associated with the BRCA2 mutation[Q]	• Ataxia Telangiectasia[Q] • FAMMM (Familial atypical multiple mole melanoma) syndrome[Q] • Peutz-Jegher syndrome[Q] (Highest risk)

■ CARCINOMA PANCREAS

CARCINOMA PANCREAS

- **MC type** is **pancreatic ductal adenocarcinoma (PDAC)**[Q]; MC site: Head (75%) > Body (15%) >Tail (10%)[Q]
- More common in **Men, African Americans**, mean age at diagnosis is **72 years**[Q]

> • **K-ras2** oncogene is **activated** (by point mutation) in >95% of pancreatic cancers (**MC gene mutation**)[Q]

Clinical Features

- **MC symptom** for patients with PDACs in the periampullary region is **jaundice**[Q].
- **Pain** typically arising in epigastrium & radiating to the back.
- **Weight loss** affecting more than 50% of individuals.
- For tumors of **body** & **tail** of pancreas, **pain** & **weight loss** become more common at presentation.
- A **palpable distended gallbladder** in **1/3rd of patients** with periampullary PDAC (**Courvoisier Law**)[Q]
- With widespread disease, a left supraclavicular node (**Virchow's node**)[Q] may be palpable. Periumbilical lymphadenopathy may be palpable (**Sister Mary Joseph's node**)[Q].
- In cases of **peritoneal dissemination**, perirectal tumor involvement may be palpable via DRE, referred to as **Blumer's shelf**[Q].

Presenting Symptoms of Periampullary Tumors	
• **Jaundice (75%)**[Q]	• Pruritus (11%)
• **Weight loss (51%)**[Q]	• Fever (3%)
• **Abdominal pain (39%)**	• Gastrointestinal bleeding (1%)
• Nausea/vomiting (13%)	

- **MC site of metastasis in CA pancreas: Liver**[Q]

Diagnosis

- Tumor markers: **CA19-9 (most sensitive)**[Q] & **CEA**.
- **MDCT** is **investigation of choice** for the evaluation of **lesions arising** in the **pancreas**[Q].

> • **ERCP:** Reserved for cases requiring **therapeutic** or **palliative intervention**[Q]
> • **Double duct sign** on ERCP is highly suggestive of **pancreatic head cancer**[Q]

- **EUS:** For identifying lesions <2 cm[Q] that do not appear on CT scans
- **Tissue diagnosis** is **not necessary prior to** routine **resection**[Q].

Treatment

- **Surgical resection** remains the **only potentially curative treatment** of pancreas cancer.

• Tumors of **head** of pancreas	• **Pylorus preserving pancreaticoduodenectomy or Longmire-Traverso procedure** is preferred[Q]
• Tumors of **body & tail** of pancreas	• **Distal pancreatectomy** and **en-bloc splenectomy**[Q]

- **MC complication** of pancreaticoduodenectomy is delayed gastric emptying[Q]
- **MC cause** of **death** following **pancreaticoduodenectomy** is **cardiopulmonary complications**[Q].
- **Most important predictor** of **post-operative survival** is R0 resection.
- **Most important margin** in **pancreaticoduodenectomy** is retroperitoneal or uncinate margin[Q].

Palliative Therapy for Pancreatic Cancer	
• Biliary obstruction	• **ERCP** with **metal stent placement (Best)**[Q] • Roux-en-Y hepaticojejunostomy
• Gastric outlet obstruction	• **Endoscopic stenting (Preferred)**[Q] • Double bypass (Roux-en-Y hepaticojejunostomy + gastrojejunostomy)
• Pain	• **NSAIDs** or **opiates**[Q] • **Celiac nerve block**[Q]

Contd...

Contd...

Chemotherapy
- **Gemcitabine**[Q] is currently the standard of care for patients with **metastatic pancreatic cancer**.

Prognosis
- **Five-year** survival **after curative resection** (pancreaticoduodenectomy) approaches **15-20%**[Q]
- Overall, 5 year survival rate **with pancreatic cancer** is 5%[Q].

Median Survival in Carcinoma Pancreas	
• **Resectable** disease (stage **I** and **II**)	• **15-20** months[Q]
• **Locally advanced** disease (stage **III**)	• **6-10** months[Q]
• **Metastatic** disease (stage **IV**)	• **3-6** months[Q]

■ TNM CLASSIFICATION OF PANCREATIC CANCER

8th AJCC (2017) TNM Classification of Pancreatic Cancer	
Tis	Carcinoma in situ
T1	Tumor limited to pancreas **upto 2 cm** in greatest dimension
	T1a: Tumor ≤0.5 cm in greatest dimension
	T1b: Tumor >0.5 cm but ≤1 cm in greatest dimension
	T1c: Tumor >1 cm but ≤2 cm in greatest dimension
T2	Tumor limited to pancreas **>2-4 cm** in greatest dimension
T3	Tumor **>4 cm** in greatest dimension
T4	Tumor involves **celiac axis**, **superior mesenteric artery** and/or **common hepatic artery**
N1	Metastasis in **1-3** regional LN
N2	Metastasis in **4 or more** regional LN
M1	Distant metastasis

Stage 0	Stage IA	Stage IB	Stage IIA	Stage IIB	Stage III	Stage IV
Tis N0 M0	**T1** N0 M0	**T2** N0 M0	**T3** N0 M0	**T1-T3 N1** M0	**T1-T3 N2** M0 **T4** AnyN M0	Any T AnyN **M1**

■ CARCINOMA PANCREAS: TREATMENT

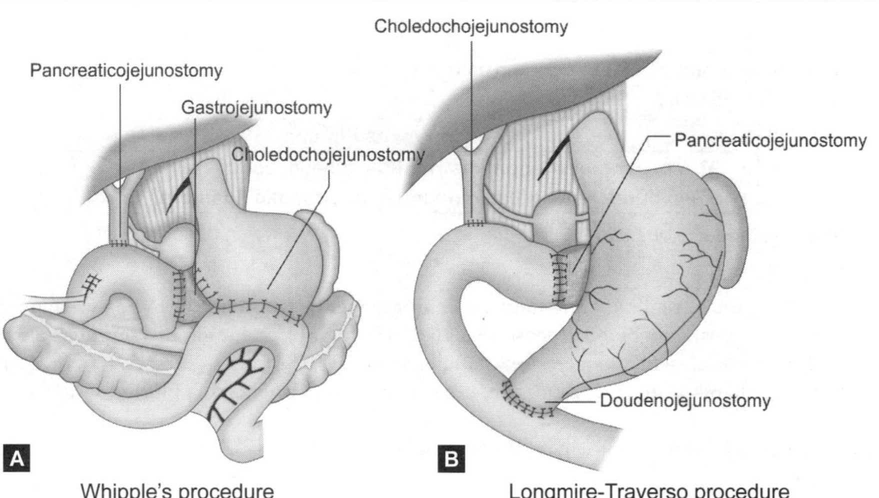

Whipple's procedure   Longmire-Traverso procedure

WHIPPLE'S PROCEDURE (PANCREATICODUODENECTOMY)

- It consists of complete **removal of the pancreatic and hepatoduodenal ligament lymph nodes**, the **duodenum** with a **short segment of the proximal jejunum** and the **distal half to two-thirds of the stomach** with the **right half of the greater omentum**.

Whipple's Procedure Involves Resection of	
• Distal stomach[Q]	• Duodenum[Q]
• Gallbladder[Q]	• Proximal jejunum[Q]
• CBD[Q]	• Regional lymphatics
• Head of pancreas[Q]	

Contd...

Contd...

Restoration of GI Continuity Requires
• Pancreaticojejunostomy[Q]
• Hepaticojejunostomy[Q]
• Gastrojejunostomy[Q]

- **Pylorus Preserving Pancreaticoduodenectomy (PPPD)** or **Longmire-Traverso procedure** is the **preferred surgery** for **carcinoma head** of pancreas[Q].
- The **Whipple procedure** is now **reserved for situations** in which the **entire duodenum has to be removed** (e.g. **in FAP**) or where the **tumour encroaches** on the **1st part** of **duodenum** or the **distal stomach** and a **PPPD would not achieve a clear resection margin**[Q].
- Pylorus Preserving Pancreaticoduodenectomy or Longmire-Traverso Procedure
- To retain a functioning pylorus, the entire stomach and 2cm of first part of duodenum & their neurovascular supply are preserved[Q].

■ NEURO ENDOCRINE TUMORS (NET) OF PANCREAS

NET OF PANCREAS

- **MC NET** of Pancreas: **Non-functional** (Mostly malignant) >**Insulinoma**[Q]
- **MC benign NET** of Pancreas: **Insulinoma**[Q]
- **MC malignant functional NET** of Pancreas: **Gastrinoma**[Q]

LOCALIZATION OF NET OF PANCREAS

- **Somatostatin receptors** are present in >**90% of gastrinomas**; in contrast, pancreatic adenocarcinomas do not possess somatostatin receptors. They are **also present in** a significant portion of **glucagonomas** and **nonfunctioning endocrine tumors**[Q].
- The **sensitivity for SRS** is **over 80%** for **all pancreatic NET excluding insulinomas**[Q]
- **SRS** has an **overall sensitivity** of **80% to 100%** and **specificity >90%** for **gastrinomas**[Q].
- **SRS** is also **useful for detecting hepatic metastases** from **noninsulinoma endocrine tumors**

■ INSULINOMA

INSULINOMA

- Insulinoma is **MC functioning tumor** of the **endocrine pancreas**[Q]
- The average age at diagnosis is **45 years**.

Location of Insulinoma
• **97%** in **pancreas** (**equal distribution** in head, body, & tail)[Q]
• **3%** in **duodenum, splenic hilum,** or **gastrocolic ligament**[Q]

- **Typically small**, with an average size of **1.0 to 1.5 cm**.

Clinical Features

- **Diagnostic hallmark is Whipple's triad**[Q]: Fasting-induced **neuroglyopenic symptoms** of hypoglycemia (diaphoresis, shaking, mental confusion, obtundation, & seizures), **low blood glucose** levels (40 to 50 mg/dL), and **relief of symptoms** after administration of glucose.
- **Sympathetic overactivity**[Q] in response to hypoglycemia: Fatigue, weakness, fearfulness, hunger, tremor, diaphoresis, & tachycardia.
- **CNS disturbance**: Apathy, irritability, anxiety, confusion, excitement, loss of orientation, blurred vision, delirium, stupor, coma, and/or seizures.
- **Significant weight gain**: Patients eat frequently to prevent hypoglycemia.
- It is a **painless condition**.

Diagnosis

- **Gold standard test** for the **diagnosis** of insulinoma is the **72-hour fasting**[Q] test
- An **insulin-to-glucose** ratio > **0.4** is consistent with insulinoma[Q]

- **CECT** or **MRI: Hyperattenuating** as compared with surrounding pancreatic tissue because of **rich vascular supply**[Q]

Localization

- **Angiography** will detect approximately **70%** of **insulinomas >5 mm**, showing a characteristic **vascular blush**[Q]

- **Portal venous sampling** for insulin with or without **arterial stimulation** with **calcium** is the **best pre-operative method** of **localization**[Q]
- **EUS** with **intra-operative palpation** is **best localization technique** for **Insulinoma**[Q]

Contd...

Contd...

Treatment

- **Diazoxide** decreases beta cell release of insulin, used to prevent or attenuate symptoms of hypoglycemia prior to surgical intervention once the diagnosis is made[Q].
- Insulinomas are well suited for **laparoscopic resection** or **enucleations**[Q].

• **Insulinoma** of **head** of pancreas	• **Enucleation** is **TOC**[Q]
• **Insulinoma** of **body** or **tail** of pancreas	• **Distal pancreatectomy** is **TOC**[Q]

■ GASTRINOMA/ZOLLINGER-ELLISON SYNDROME

ZOLLINGER-ELLISON SYNDROME

- Gastrinoma is **MC functioning malignant**[Q] pancreatic endocrine tumor.
- **More common** in **men**, mean age **50 years**[Q]
- ZES occur in **two forms: Sporadic (75%) & MEN-1 association (25%)**[Q]
- Those associated with **MEN-1** are almost always **multiple, early onset,** more common in **duodenum**[Q]

> • **MC site** of Gastrinoma: **Duodenum > Pancreas**[Q]

- **All gastrinomas** also produce **chromagranin A**[Q]

> • **Gastrinoma** → increased gastrin secretion → marked gastric **acid hypersecretion** → Peptic ulcer

Location

- **MC site** is duodenum followed by **Pancreas**[Q]
- In **Duodenum, MC in 1st part**[Q] (71%) >2nd part (21%) >3rd part (8%)
- About **70-90%** of gastrinomas are located **within the Passaro's triangle**[Q].

Boundaries of Passaro's Triangle
• **Junction of cystic duct** and **CBD**[Q]
• **Junction of 2nd & 3rd part of duodenum**[Q]
• **Junction of neck & body of pancreas**

Clinical Features

- Gastric acid hypersecretion causes **peptic ulcer disease** often **refractory severe diarrhea**
- **MC presenting symptoms** are **abdominal pain**[Q] (70-100%), **diarrhea** (50-70%) & **GERD** (30-35%).

> • **Unique characteristic** of acid-induced diarrhea: **Halted by nasogastric aspiration** of gastric secretions[Q]

- Most patients have peptic ulcers (**MC are duodenal ulcers**)[Q]
- **MC cause of death** in ZES: **Liver metastasis**[Q]

Diagnosis

- **Hypergastrinemia** with **increased secretion of gastric acid** confirms the diagnosis
- Elevated gastrin alone is not sufficient to diagnose ZES (**Basal gastric acid hypersecretion** must be demonstrated).

Zollinger-Ellison Syndrome
• 100% patients will have a fasting serum gastrin level >100 pg/mL
• **BAO >15 mEq/hr** in most patients and **>5 mEq/hr** in patients with **prior surgery** to decrease gastric acid secretion
• Levels **>1000 pg/mL** are **diagnostic**[Q]

- **Elevated serum gastrin level** with a **pH <2** in the gastric aspirate is **almost diagnostic** of ZES[Q].

Provocative Test in Gastrinoma

- If the **diagnosis is in doubt**, the **provocative tests** are highly useful.
- **Secretin provocation test** is **best.**

> • **Secretin Provocation Test**: An increase of **>200 pg/mL** in the **gastrin value** after administration of secretin is **diagnostic**[Q]

Localization

- SRS is **imaging test of choice** for **localizing** both **primary & metastatic gastrinomas**[Q].

Contd...

Contd...

Treatment

- **Acid secretion** is controlled by **PPIs**[Q]

  - **ZES in MEN-1:** **Hyperparathyroidism** should be **treated first** because it can complicate the management of their gastrinoma, **neck exploration** should be performed **before resection** of **gastrinoma**[Q].

- **Distal pancreatectomy:** Gastrinoma involving **body** or **tail**[Q] of pancreas
- **Pancreaticoduodenectomy:** Gastrinoma involving **head**[Q] of pancreas

■ GLUCAGONOMA

GLUCAGONOMA (HYPERGLYCEMIC CUTANEOUS SYNDROME)

- Compared with other pancreatic NET, they tend to be **larger**[Q], averaging **5-10 cm**[Q] in **size** at the time of diagnosis.
- More common in **females**; 70% are **malignant**[Q].
- **MC site: Body** and **tail**[Q] of pancreas.

Clinical Features

- **Classic presentation** of the 4Ds: **Diabetes, dermatitis, DVT,** and **depression**[Q].

  - **Necrolytic erythema migrans** are **MC manifestations** of the disease, seen in **2/3rd** of **patients**[Q].
  - **Necrolytic erythema migrans:** The characteristic rash occur in **areas of friction; rash is migratory, red,** and **scaling,** associated with **intense pruritus**[Q]

- **Parenteral administration** of **amino acids** was found to result in the **disappearance** of the **skin lesions**[Q]

Diagnosis

- **Fasting glucagon** level >50 pmol/L is considered **diagnostic**[Q].
- **Glucagonomas,** are **usually larger** and **easily localized** by **CT**[Q].
- **SRS** can be performed **if CT is not informative.**

Treatment

- **Resection** is the **treatment of choice** for, **glucagonomas,** and remains the **only curative option**[Q].

■ VIPomas (VERNER-MORRISON SYNDROME)

VIPomas (VERNER-MORRISON SYNDROME)

- Also known as WDHA syndrome (**watery** diarrhea, hypokalemia, achlorhydria) or **pancreatic cholera**[Q]
- Usually **solitary**; MC site is **tail of pancreas**[Q]
- **Two-thirds** are **malignant**[Q].

Clinical Features

- **Diagnostic triad: Secretary diarrhea + High** levels of circulating **VIP + Pancreatic tumor**[Q].
- **Profuse, watery, iso-osmotic secretary diarrhea** is **MC presenting symptom** and may exceed a volume of 3 to 5 liters/day.

  - Characterized by: **Hypokalemia, hypercalcemia,** hypochlorhydria & **hyperglycemia**[Q].

Diagnosis

- **Constant features** are **diarrhea, hypovolemia, hypokalemia** and **acidosis,** variable features are **achlorhydria** or hypochlorhydria, **hyperglycemia** and **flushing with rash**[Q].
- **VIPomas,** are **usually larger** & **easily localized** by **CT**[Q].

Treatment

- **Aggressive preoperative hydration** and **correction of electrolyte abnormalities** & acid-base disturbances[Q].
- **Octreotide** is commonly used preperatively **to reduce diarrhea volume** and facilitate fluid & electrolyte replacement.
- **Resection** is the **treatment of choice for VIPomas,** and remains the **only curative option**[Q].

■ PANCREATIC TRAUMA

PANCREATIC TRAUMA

- Pancreatic injuries are uncommon.
- **Penetrating injuries** into the abdomen are the **MC injuries** seen in **adults**[Q].
- Isolated pancreatic injuries are not common.

Contd...

- Up to 90% of patients present with associated hepatic, gastric, splenic, renal, colonic, or vascular lesions.
- **MC associated injury** is to a **hollow viscus** (38%)[Q]; followed by the liver (19%); and spleen (11%).

Pancreatic Trauma in Children
• **MC mechanism** in **children** is **abdominal blunt trauma**[Q].
• Direct compression of the epigastrium against the vertebral column and a blunt object (**handlebar**) is typically seen after **bicycle injuries**[Q].
• **MC segment** of the pancreas affected is the **body**[Q].

Pancreatic Organ Injury Scale		
Grade		Type of Injury
I	Hematoma	**Minor contusion** without duct injury
	Laceration	**Superficial laceration** without duct injury
II	Hematoma	**Major Contusion** without duct injury or tissue loss
	Laceration	**Major Laceration** without duct injury or tissue loss
III	Laceration	**Distal transaction** or **parenchymal injury with duct injury**
IV	Laceration	**Proximal transaction** or parenchymal injury **involving ampulla**
V	Laceration	**Massive disruption** of pancreatic **head**

Diagnosis

- **CT scan: Investigation of choice** to evaluate patients with **abdominal trauma**[Q].
- **CT findings**: Peripancreatic hematomas, free fluid in the lesser sack, or abnormal thickening of Gerota's fascia suggest pancreatic injury.

• **ERCP: Most reliable test** to demonstrate **pancreatic duct integrity**[Q]

- **Isolated pancreatic amylase** level measurement is **not recommended** because up to 40% of patients with pancreatic duct transected have normal serum amylase levels. **Serial quantification levels**[Q] increase the sensitivity of the assay.

Treatment

- Definitive treatment is based on surgical findings.
- **Major pancreatic resections** in **stable patients** with **isolated pancreatic injury**[Q].
- **Damage control surgery** is indicated for **complex injuries** or **unstable patients**[Q].
- **Most** (up to 75%) of **deaths occur within** the **48 to 72 hours** after trauma, and most are related to **hypovolemic shock**[Q].

Complication

- A **persistent drain output** or **pancreatic fistula** is the MC complication after **pancreatic trauma**[Q].

Grading	Treatment of Pancreatic Injuries
• **Grade I**	• **Observation alone**[Q]
• **Grade II**	• **Debridement, drainage, possible repair**[Q]
• **Grade III**	• **Distal resection, possible Roux-en-Y drainage**[Q]
• **Grades IV and V**	• **Damage control**[Q], hemostasis/drainage • Resection and possible **Roux-en-Y drainage**[Q] • **Triple-tube decompression**[Q] • **Pyloric exclusion technique** • **Duodenal diverticularization**[Q] • Pancreaticoduodenectomy

■ ACUTE PANCREATITIS: ETIOLOGY AND RISK FACTORS

1. Which of the following is the most common non-alcoholic cause of acute pancreatitis? *(COMEDK 2008, 2007)*
   a. Thiazides
   b. Hypercalcemia
   c. Hyperlipidemia
   d. Gallstones

2. The commonest cause of acute pancreatitis is: *(COMEDK 2008)*
   a. Biliary calculi
   b. Alcohol abuse
   c. Infective
   d. Idiopathic

3. Most common complication after ERCP is: *(AIIMS May 2007)*
   a. Acute pancreatitis
   b. Acute cholangitis
   c. Acute cholecystitis
   d. Duodenal perforation

4. Which of the following is not an etiological factor for pancreatitis? *(AIIMS May 2014)*
   a. Abdominal trauma
   b. Hyperlipidemia
   c. Islet cell hyperplasia
   d. Germline mutations in the cationic trypsinogen gene

5. Which of the following drug causes acute pancreatitis? *(Recent Question 2017)*
   a. L-Asparaginase
   b. Metronidazole
   c. Ciprofloxacin
   d. Penicillin

■ ACUTE PANCREATITIS: CLINICAL FEATURES, DIAGNOSIS AND TREATMENT

6. Which of the following is most diagnostic investigation for acute pancreatitis? *(MHPGMCET 2003)*
   a. Serum amylase
   b. Serum lipase
   c. Serum P-isoamylase
   d. Serum LDH

7. Which of the following is not a feature of acute pancreatitis? *(DNB 2011, Orissa 2011)*
   a. Hyperbilirubinemia
   b. Hypercalcemia
   c. Hyperglycemia
   d. Increased serum LDH level

8. Which one is not the bad prognostic sign for pancreatitis? *(AIIMS June 2000)*
   a. TLC >16,000/μL
   b. Calcium <8 mmol/L
   c. Glucose >200 mg%
   d. Prothrombin >2 times the control

9. Destruction of fat in acute pancreatitis is due to: *(MHCET 2016)*
   a. Lipase and trypsin
   b. Secretin
   c. Lipase and elastase
   d. Cholecystokinin and trypsin

10. Gasless abdomen in X-ray is a sign of: *(Recent Question 2019)*
    a. Acute pancreatitis
    b. Necrotizing enterocolitis
    c. Ulcerative colitis
    d. Intussusception

11. Which of the following is not a component of APACHE score? *(DNB 2012)*
    a. Serum potassium
    b. Serum sodium
    c. Serum calcium
    d. Creatinine

12. Acute pancreatitis causes all except: *(DNB 2007)*
    a. Pleural effusion
    b. Pseudocyst
    c. Gallbladder stone
    d. Pancreatic necrosis

13. Most common causes of death due to acute pancreatitis:
    a. Shock
    b. Infection *(DNB 2001)*
    c. Hypocalcemia
    d. Diabetes

14. Which of the following does not correlate with severity of acute pancreatitis? *(AIIMS Nov 2011, GB Pant 2010)*
    a. Serum glucose
    b. Serum amylase
    c. Serum calcium
    d. AST

15. Which of the following is not associated with Pancreatitis? *(JIPMER 2014, 2011)*
    a. Raised serum amylase
    b. Raised serum lipase
    c. Hypocalcemia
    d. Hypoglycemia

16. Balthazar scoring system is used for: *(DNB 2014)*
    a. Acute pancreatitis
    b. Acute appendicitis
    c. Acute cholecystitis
    d. Cholangitis

17. Ideal fluid of choice in a 35 years old man presenting with acute pancreatitis: *(Recent Question 2018)*
    a. Isotonic crystalloid by IV line
    b. Hypertonic saline by IV line
    c. Hypotonic saline by central line
    d. Vasopressin

■ ACUTE PANCREATITIS: COMPLICATIONS

18. Grey Turner's sign (flank discoloration) is seen in: *(MCI June 2018, COMEDK 2008)*
    a. Acute pyelonephritis
    b. Acute cholecystitis
    c. Acute pancreatitis
    d. Acute peritonitis

19. When to do surgery in pancreatic ascites? *(JIPMER May 2018)*
    a. Symptomatic
    b. Recurrent ascites following abdominal drainage
    c. Not responding to medical therapy
    d. Leak from the stented duct

20. Cullen's sign: *(UPPG 2007)*
    a. Bluish discoloration of the flanks
    b. Bluish discoloration around umbilicus
    c. Migratory thrombophlebitis
    d. Subcutaneous fat necrosis

21. Cullen's sign is seen in: *(Bihar PG 2014, Kerala 94)*
    a. Acute cholecystitis
    b. Acute pancreatitis
    c. Acute hemorrhagic pancreatitis
    d. Blunt injury abdomen

22. Hemorrhagic pancreatitis, bluish discoloration of flank: *(Recent Question 2013)*
    a. Grey Turner sign
    b. Cullen sign
    c. Trousseau sign
    d. None

■ CHRONIC PANCREATITIS: ETIOLOGY, CLINICAL FEATURES AND DIAGNOSIS

23. All are seen in chronic calcific pancreatitis except: *(Kerala 96)*
    a. Diabetes mellitus
    b. Fat malabsorption
    c. Hypercalcemia
    d. Recurrent abdominal pain
    e. Increased incidence of pancreatic carcinoma

24. "Chain of lakes" appearance seen in:
    a. Acute pancreatitis   *(MHCET 2016, UPPG 2007, 2005)*
    b. Chronic pancreatitis
    c. Carcinoma pancreas
    d. Strawberry gallbladder

25. Chronic calcific pancreatitis is associated with all of the following except: *(MCI Sept 2005)*
    a. Hypercalcemia   b. Diabetes mellitus
    c. Malabsorption of fat
    d. Diabetes associated complications are uncommon

26. Most common cause of chronic pancreatitis:
    (Recent Question 2018)
    a. Gallstones   b. Alcohol
    c. Hereditary   d. ERCP

27. All of the following are true about tropical pancreatitis except: *(Recent Question 2017)*
    a. Caused by tapioca ingestion
    b. Dilatation of pancreatic ducts with large stones with fibrosis
    c. Increase the risk of pancreatic cancer
    d. Treatment is mainly surgical

28. Gold standard investigation for chronic pancreatitis:
    a. MRI   b. ERCP   *(DNB 2014)*
    c. Pancreatic function tests   d. Fecal fat estimation

■ CHRONIC PANCREATITIS: TREATMENT AND COMPLICATIONS

29. Patient with chronic pancreatitis gives chain of lakes appearance in ERCP examination. Management is:
    a. Total pancreatectomy   *(AIIMS Nov 2000)*
    b. Sphincteroplasty
    c. Side to side pancreaticojejunostomy
    d. Resecting the tail of pancreas and performing a pancreatojejunostomy

30. Pain relief in chronic pancreatitis can be obtained by destruction of: *(Recent Question 2016)*
    a. Celiac ganglia   b. Vagus nerve
    c. Anterolateral column of spinal cord
    d. None of the above

31. Complication of chronic pancreatitis include all except:
    (Recent Question 2013)
    a. Renal artery stenosis   b. Pseudocyst
    c. Splenic vein stenosis   d. Fistulae

32. All of the following are true about chronic pancreatitis is except: *(DNB 2014)*
    a. Damage to exocrine part with damage to endocrine part
    b. Can lead to malignancy
    c. Whipple's procedure can be done
    d. Gallbladder stone is the most common cause

33. Most common complication of both acute and chronic pancreatitis: *(Recent Question 2017)*
    a. Portal vein thrombosis   b. Pancreatic abscess
    c. Pseudocyst   d. Pancreatic necrosis

■ PSEUDOPANCREATIC CYST

34. A chronic alcoholic presented with repeated episodes of nonbilious vomiting after meals. On the basis of CECT findings, what is the diagnosis?   *(Recent Question 2016)*
    a. Gastric outlet obstruction b. Pseudocyst
    c. Carcinoma pancreas   d. Chronic pancreatitis

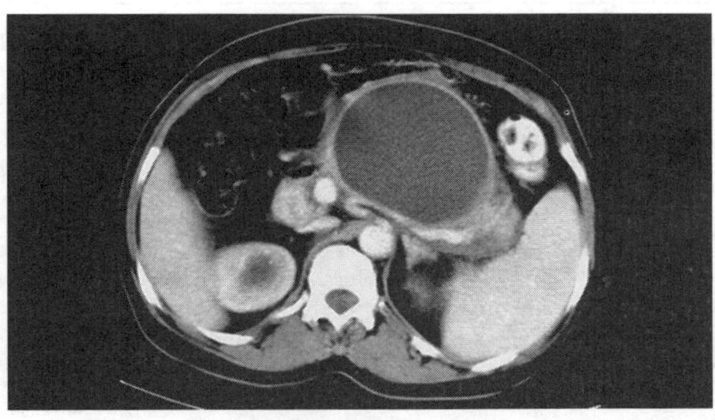

35. Most common complication of pseudocyst:
    (DNB 2003, PGI SS Dec 2009)
    a. Infection   b. Rupture
    c. Hemorrhage   d. Compression

36. Major complication of cysto-gastrostomy for pseudopancreatic cyst is: *(DPG 2011, COMEDK 2005)*
    a. Infection   b. Obstruction
    c. Fistula   d. Hemorrhage

37. Treatment of choice for asymptomatic pseudocyst pancreas is: *(DNB 2010)*
    a. Marsupialization   b. Conservative
    c. Drainage   d. Cystogastrostomy

38. All are features of pseudopancreatic cyst, except:
    a. Follows acute pancreatitis   *(All India 97)*
    b. Lined by false epithelium
    c. May regress spontaneously
    d. Treatment of choice is percutaneous aspiration

■ CYSTIC NEOPLASMS OF PANCREAS

39. Increased amylase, mucin and CEA is seen in: *(ILBS 2012)*
    a. IPMN
    b. Mucinous cystadenoma
    c. Serous cystadenoma
    d. Solid pseudopaillary tumor

40. Not true about mucinous cystadenoma pancreas:
    a. Microcystic adenoma   *(AIIMS May 2011)*
    b. Lined by columnar epithelium
    c. Premalignant
    d. Focus of ovarian stroma in it

41. A 60-year-old female present with history of recurrent abdominal pain. Imaging shows multiple small cystic lesions like bunch of grapes in the head of pancreas with a grossly dilated main pancreatic duct. The most likely diagnosis is:
    a. SCN   b. MCN   *(All India 2012)*
    c. IPMN   d. Pancreatic pseudocyst

42. All of the following are true about mucinous cystic neoplasm except: *(Recent Question 2017)*
    a. Less amylase in fluid
    b. Enucleation is performed
    c. Estrogens receptors are positive
    d. More common in females

■ CARCINOMA PANCREAS: ETIOLOGY AND RISK FACTORS

43. Earliest genetic change in carcinoma pancreas: *(ILBS 2012)*
    a. Her-2-neu   b. p53
    c. p16   d. DCC

44. **Not a risk factor for carcinoma pancreas:**   *(ILBS 2012)*
    a. Acute pancreatitis   b. Diabetes
    c. Smoking   d. Obesity

45. **Most common mutation in pancreatic adenocarcinoma:**
    a. K-ras   b. p16   *(GB PANT 2010)*
    c. p53   d. BRAF

46. **Which of the following does not predispose to CA pancreas?**
    (Recent Question 2017, AIIMS GIS May 2008)
    a. Familial breast cancer
    b. HNPCC
    c. PJS
    d. Cronkhite-Canada syndrome

47. **Maximum risk of carcinoma pancreas is seen in which of these?**   *(AIIMS May 2017)*
    a. Hereditary atypical multiple mole melanoma syndrome
    b. Hereditary pancreatitis
    c. Peutz-Jegher's syndrome
    d. Familial adenomatous polyposis

48. **First gene mutated in pancreatic adenocarcinoma is:**
    (Recent Question 2017)
    a. K-ras   b. p53
    c. p16   d. BRAF

■ CARCINOMA PANCREAS: CLINICAL FEATURES AND DIAGNOSIS

49. **Most common symptom of CA head of pancreas:**
    (ILBS 2012, AIIMS GIS Dec 2011, Dec 2006)
    a. Weight loss   b. Pain
    c. Jaundice   d. Anorexia

50. **In carcinoma head of pancreas, nausea and vomiting is due to:**   *(JIPMER May 2018)*
    a. External compression of duodenum
    b. Portal vein infiltration
    c. Proliferation infiltration of tumor into duodenum
    d. Chemotherapy related

51. **Diagnostic investigation in carcinoma pancreas:**   *(ILBS 2012)*
    a. MDCT   b. PET scan
    c. ERCP   d. MRCP

52. **According to AJCC 8th edition, staging of 2 cm size pancreatic cancer if it involves portal vein in:**   *(JIPMER May 2018)*
    a. T1   b. T2
    c. T3   d. T4

53. **Most appropriate initial method of investigation for carcinoma head of pancreas:**   *(Recent Question 2018)*
    a. Laparoscopic guided biopsy
    b. MRI guided biopsy
    c. CECT guided biopsy
    d. EUS guided transgastric biopsy

54. **Inverted "3" sign seen in:**   *(PGI Dec 97)*
    a. Ampullary carcinoma   b. Insulinoma
    c. CA head pancreas   d. CA stomach

55. **Most common tumor of pancreas is:**   *(UPPG 2007)*
    a. Adenocarcinoma
    b. Squamous cell carcinoma
    c. Adeno-squamous cell carcinoma
    d. Ductal adenocarcinoma

56. **The commonest pancreatic tumor is:**   *(Recent Question 2016)*
    a. Ductal adenocarcinoma   b. Cystadenoma
    c. Insulinoma   d. Non islet cell tumor

57. **Most sensitive investigation of pancreatic carcinoma is:**   *(Recent Question 2016)*
    a. Angiography   b. ERCP
    c. Ultrasound   d. CT scan

58. **Most appropriate initial method of investigation for carcinoma head of pancreas:**   *(Recent Question 2018)*
    a. EUS guided transgastric biopsy
    b. CECT guided biopsy
    c. MRI guided biopsy
    d. Laparoscopic biopsy

59. **Double duct sign is seen in:**   *(Recent Question 2017)*
    a. Periampullary carcinoma
    b. Chronic pancreatitis
    c. HCC
    d. Carcinoma gallbladder

60. **Most common site for carcinoma pancreas is:**   *(Recent Question 2013)*
    a. Head   b. Body
    c. Tail   d. Neck

■ CARCINOMA PANCREAS: TREATMENT AND PROGNOSIS

61. **A patient with obstructive jaundice due to pancreatic cancer might have all of the following clinical findings except:**
    a. A palpable gallbladder   *(COMEDK 2004)*
    b. Pain is early in the course of the disease
    c. Pulmonary metastasis
    d. Thrombocytopenia

62. **Which of the following drugs has been found to increase the survival in locally advanced pancreatic cancer?**
    (COMEDK 2006)
    a. Doxorubicin   b. Streptozocin
    c. Gemcitabine   d. Paclitaxel

63. **Components of Whipple's operation are following except:**
    (MHSSMCET 2009)
    a. Gastrojejunostomy   b. Duodenojejunostomy
    c. Choledochojejunostomy   d. Pancreaticoduodenostomy

64. **All are resected in Whipple's operation except:**
    (AIIMS Nov 98, AIIMS Feb 97, All India 96)
    a. Duodenum   b. Head of pancreas
    c. Portal vein   d. Common bile duct

65. **False about CA pancreas:**   *(KGMC 2011)*
    a. Most common site is head and uncinate process
    b. Pain suggests unresectability
    c. Two third patients present with diabetes
    d. Acute pancreatitis never occurs in CA pancreas

66. **Which of the following is not a contraindication for resection of head of pancreas:**   *(Recent Question 2015)*
    a. Liver metastasis
    b. Ascites
    c. Peritoneal seedings
    d. Involvement of major artery

67. **Which of the following is not resected in pylorus preserving pancreaticoduodenectomy?**   *(Recent Question 2016)*
    a. Pyloric antrum   b. CBD
    c. Duodenum   d. Gallbladder

68. **Most common complication after Whipple's procedure:**
    (Recent Question 2017)
    a. Delayed gastric emptying   b. Pancreatic fistula
    c. Wound infection   d. Anastomotic leak

69. **Median survival in carcinoma pancreas after surgery and adjuvant therapy:** *(Recent Question 2017)*
   a. 12 months
   b. 22 months
   c. 32 months
   d. 44 months

70. **Order of anastomosis in Whipple's procedure:**
   (Recent Question 2016, JIPMER SS 2016)
   a. Pancreaticojejunostomy, gastrojejunostomy, hepaticojejunostomy,
   b. Hepaticojejunostomy, pancreaticojejunostomy, gastrojejunostomy
   c. Gastrojejunostomy, pancreaticojejunostomy, hepaticojejunostomy,
   d. Pancreaticojejunostomy, hepaticojejunostomy, gastrojejunostomy

■ INSULINOMA

71. **Localization in insulinoma is best with:** *(COMEDK 2011)*
   a. Contrast CT
   b. Magnetic Resonance Imaging
   c. Somatostatin Receptor Scintigraphy
   d. Selective arteriography

72. **A 55-year-old male presents with tachycardia, sweating, palpitation, giddiness. Most probable diagnosis:**
   a. Insulinoma *(JIPMER 2011)*
   b. Zollinger-Ellison syndrome
   c. Carcinoma pancreas
   d. Carcinoid

73. **Gold standard test for insulinoma:** *(AIIMS May 2011)*
   a. 72-hours fasting test
   b. Plasma insulin levels
   c. C-peptide levels
   d. Low glucose levels < 30 mg/dL

74. **Which of the following is the most common endocrine tumor of pancreas?** *(AIIMS June 2004, PGI June 2006)*
   a. Insulinoma
   b. Gastrinoma
   c. VIPoma
   d. Glucagonoma

75. **Insulinoma is most commonly located in which part of the pancreas?** *(AIIMS June 2002)*
   a. Head
   b. Body
   c. Tail
   d. Equally distributed

76. **Whipples triad is seen in:**
   (APPG 2015, WBPG 2012, DNB 2011, AIIMS Feb 97)
   a. Insulinoma
   b. Somatostatinoma
   c. Glucagonoma
   d. CA pancreas

77. **Most common site of insulinoma:** *(Recent Question 2017)*
   a. Head
   b. Body
   c. Tail
   d. Equally distributed in head, body and tail

■ ZOLLINGER-ELLISON SYNDROME

78. **MC site of gastrinoma:** *(GB Pant 2011)*
   a. Duodenum
   b. Pancreas
   c. Stomach
   d. Colon

79. **All are true about gastrinoma except:** *(GB Pant 2011)*
   a. Abnormal peptic ulcer location
   b. Diarrhea
   c. Decreased BAO and MAO
   d. Best treatment is omeprazole

80. **Localization of gastrinoma is best done by:** *(GB Pant 2011)*
   a. USG
   b. CT
   c. MRI
   d. SRS

81. **Which of the following is correct with Zollinger-Ellison syndrome?** *(MCI Nov 2017)*
   a. Associated with MEN1
   b. Most common site is stomach
   c. Best test for diagnosis is pentagastrin test
   d. Metastasis to adjacent gut

82. **All are true about Zollinger-Ellison syndrome except:**
   (DNB 2007, AIIMS GIS Dec 2011)
   a. Recurrent ulceration after acid reducing surgery
   b. Raised gastrin levels in all cases
   c. Decreased BAO/MAO
   d. Diarrhea

83. **Treatment of Zollinger-Ellison syndrome:**
   a. Total gastrectomy with removal of tumor
   b. Partial gastrectomy *(DNB 2004, All India 88)*
   c. Excision of tumor alone
   d. H_2 receptor antagonist

84. **The investigation of choice to detect gastrinoma < 5 mm size is:** *(COMEDK 2014)*
   a. Endoscopic ultrasound
   b. Octreotide scan
   c. CT scan
   d. Portal venous sampling

85. **What is the name of this triangle?** *(Recent Question 2019)*

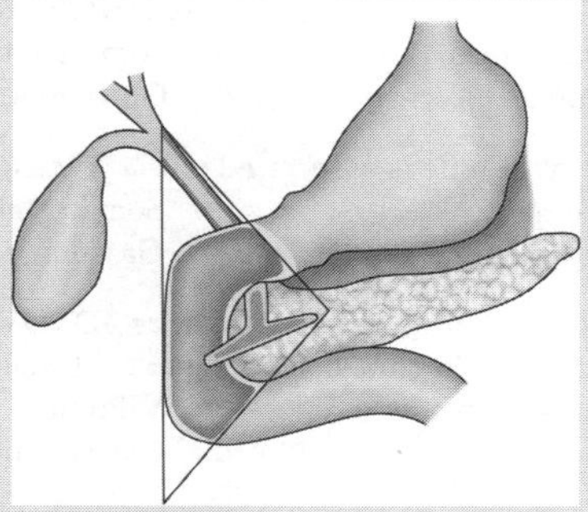

   a. Gastrinoma triangle
   b. Calot's triangle
   c. Doom's triangle
   d. Cholecystohepatic triangle

86. **Not a boundary of gastrinoma triangle:** *(DNB 2011, DPG 2007)*
   a. Junction of 2nd and 3rd part of duodenum
   b. Junction of 3rd and 4th part of duodenum
   c. Junction of head with body of pancreas
   d. Junction of cystic duct with common bile duct

87. **Which of the following is not true for Zollinger-Ellison syndrome?** *(DNB 2002, MCI June 2018, Sept 2008)*
   a. Recurrence after operation
   b. Reduced BAO: MAO ratio
   c. Gastrin producing tumour
   d. Diarrhea may be a presenting features

88. **Diarrhoea with non-healing Gastric ulcer with PPI is due to:**
   a. MEN 1 syndrome *(DNB 2014)*
   b. Zollinger-Ellison syndrome
   c. H. pylori infection
   d. VIPoma

89. **Which of the following does not form the boundary of gastrinoma triangle?** *(Recent Question 2017)*
   a. Pylorus
   b. Junction of neck and body of pancreas
   c. Cystic duct and CBD junction
   d. Junction of 2nd and 3rd part of duodenum

90. **A patient presented with pain in left hypochondrium, vomiting, diarrhea, melena and weight loss. Most probable diagnosis is:** *(Recent Question 2015)*
   a. Cholangitis
   b. Enterocolitis
   c. Zollinger-Ellison syndrome
   d. Amoebiasis

91. **A 30-year-old patient is having weakness due to secretory diarrhea. Endoscopy shows large duodenal ulcer. Probable diagnosis is:** *(MCI Dec 2019)*
   a. Gastrinoma
   b. Primitive neuroectodermal tumour
   c. Carcinoid syndrome
   d. Autoimmune gastritis

■ ENDOCRINE TUMORS OF PANCREAS

92. **Most common endocrine tumor of pancreas is:**
    (AIIMS GIS Dec 2006)
    a. Insulinoma
    b. Gastrinoma
    c. Somatostinoma
    d. VIPoma

93. **Best investigation for neuroendocrine tumors of pancreas:**
    a. Portal venous sampling   *(AIIMS GIS Dec 2006)*
    b. CECT
    c. EUS
    d. SRS

94. **Necrolytic migratory erythema is seen in:**
    (Recnet Question 2016, AIIMS GIS May 2011)
    a. Glucagonoma
    b. Somatostinoma
    c. VIPoma
    d. Insulinoma

95. **The triad of diabetes, gallstones and steatorrhoea is associated with which one of the following tumors?**
    (COMEDK 2014, 2009, 2007)
    a. Gastrinomas
    b. Somaststationomas
    c. VIPomas
    d. Glucagonomas

96. **WDHA syndrome is associated with:** *(Recent Question 2017)*
    a. VIPoma
    b. Somatostinoma
    c. Glucagonoma
    d. Gastrinoma

97. **Which of the following is known as 4D (DVT, Depression, Dermatitis & Diarrhoea) syndrome:** *(Recent Question 2017)*
    a. Glucagonoma
    b. VIPoma
    c. Somatostinoma
    d. Gastrinoma

■ PANCREAS DIVISUM

98. **Pancreas divisum:**   *(AIIMS GIS May 2008)*
    a. Most common congenital anomaly
    b. Most are symptomatic
    c. Failure of fusion of dorsal and ventral pancreas
    d. Dorsal duct dilation at lesser papilla is curative

■ ANNULAR PANCREAS

99. **Treatment of choice for annular pancreas:**
    (NEET Pattern, MHSSMCET 2006)
    a. Duodenojejunostomy   b. Distal pancreatectomy
    c. Proximal pancreatectomy   d. Duodenoduodenostomy

100. **Treatment of choice for annular pancreas is:** *(All India 2010)*
    a. Division of pancreas
    b. Duodenoduodenostomy
    c. Doudenojejunostomy
    d. Roux-en-Y loop

■ PANCREATIC TRAUMA

101. **Which of the following is true about pancreatic injury?**
    a. Most cases are iatrogenic   *(Recent Question 2015)*
    b. Blunt trauma is the most common cause
    c. Urine amylase is diagnostic
    d. HRCT is investigation of choice

102. **Regarding injury to pancreas, which is not true?**
    (AIIMS Nov 94)
    a. Majority of postoperative complications are due to missed duct injury
    b. Fracture is common at the junction of head and body
    c. Commonly associated with vascular injury
    d. Peritoneal lavage is good for making the diagnosis

■ PANCREATIC TRANSPLANTATION

103. **The advantage of bladder drainage over enteric drainage after pancreatic transplantation is better monitoring of:**
    (All India 2009)
    a. HBA IC levels
    b. Amylase levels
    c. Glucose levels
    d. Electrolyte levels

■ MISCELLANEOUS

104. **Open sphincteroplasty is done at:**   *(MHSSMCET 2009)*
    a. 12 O' clock position
    b. 11 O' clock position
    c. 6 O' clock position
    d. 2 O' clock position

105. **Investigation of choice to visualise pancreas is:** *(DNB 2006)*
    a. MRI
    b. CT Scan
    c. USG abdomen
    d. ERCP

Explanations

■ ACUTE PANCREATITIS: ETIOLOGY AND RISK FACTORS

1. **Ans. d. Gallstones** *(Ref: Sabiston 20/e p1525-1526; Schwartz 11/e p1440, 10/e p1351-1360; Bailey 27/e p1222; Blumgart 6/e p883; Shackelford 8/e p1128; Harrison 20/e p2438)*

2. **Ans. a. Biliary calculi**

3. **Ans. a. Acute pancreatitis** *(Ref: Sabiston 20/e p1526; Bailey 27/e p1222; Blumgart 6/e p889; Shackelford 8/e p1076)*

COMPLICATIONS OF ERCP

- **Complications:** Pancreatitis, hemorrhage, cholangitis and **perforation.**
- **MC complication** is **acute pancreatitis (5%)**[Q]
- **Hemorrhage** requires **surgical intervention most commonly, sphincterotomy** usually is **converted into** formal surgical **sphincteroplasty,** which includes the bleeding artery[Q].
- **Cholangitis** is confined to patients in whom **CBD clearance** has **not** been **achieved**, and measures should be directed at providing **adequate bile drainage** and administering **parenteral antibiotics. Emergency surgery** for cholangitis carries high risk, but is indicated in **patients** who do **not improve within 24 hours**[Q].
- **Perforation** may be **asymptomatic** and noticed only as **retroperitoneal gas** or **extravasation of** radiographic **contrast** material, but **even in symptomatic patient, conservative treatment** is often effective with spontaneous resolution and avoidance of potentially difficult surgery[Q].

4. **Ans. c. Islet cell hyperplasia**

5. **Ans. b. Metronidazole** *(Ref: Sabiston 20/e p1526; Schwartz 11/e p1440, 10/e p1353; Bailey 27/e p1222)*

■ ACUTE PANCREATITIS: CLINICAL FEATURES, DIAGNOSIS AND TREATMENT

6. **Ans. b. Serum lipase**
7. **Ans. b. Hypercalcemia**
8. **Ans. d. Prothrombin >2 times the control**
9. **Ans. a. Lipase and trypsin**

10. **Ans. a. Acute pancreatitis** *(Ref: Sabiston 20/e p1527; Schwartz 11/e p1444, 10/e p1351-1360; Bailey 26/e p1128, 1135, 1138)*

Radiological Appearance		
Acute Pancreatitis	**Chronic Pancreatitis**	**CA Pancreas**
• **Renal halo** sign[Q] • **Gasless abdomen**[Q] • **Ground glass appearance**[Q] • **Colon cut off** sign[Q] • **Sentinel loop**[Q]	• **Chain** of **lakes appearance**[Q] • **String** of **pearl appearance**[Q] • **Beaded appearance**[Q] • Numerous **irregular calcifications**[Q] are pathognomonic (on X-ray)	• **Double contour** of medial border of duodenal C loop • **Double duct sign**[Q] • **Dilated / widening** of **duodenal C loop**[Q] • **Mucosal irregularity**[Q] • **Scrambled egg appearance** • **Inverted / reverse 3 sign** of **Frostberg**[Q]: Seeing CA head of pancreas • **Rose thorning** of **medial wall** of **2**nd part of duodenum[Q]

11. **Ans. c. Serum calcium**
12. **Ans. c. Gallbladder stone**
13. **Ans. b. Infection**
14. **Ans. b. Serum amylase**
15. **Ans. d. Hypoglycemia**
16. **Ans. a. Acute pancreatitis**

17. **Ans. a. Isotonic crystalloid by IV line** *(Ref: Sabiston 20/e p1528; Schwartz 11/e p1446, 10/e p1358; Bailey 27/e p1225)*

"While there are proponents for aggressive fluid therapy and for specific resuscitation goals, it is probably best to resuscitate with a balanced crystalloid and to restore normal blood volume, blood pressure, and urine output. On the basis of recent data it appears that lactated Ringer's solution may be superior to normal saline in reducing the systemic inflammatory response."
—*Schwartz 11/e p1446, 10/e p1358*

■ ACUTE PANCREATITIS: COMPLICATIONS

18. **Ans. c. Acute pancreatitis**

19. **Ans. d. Leak from the stented duct** *(Ref: Schwartz 11/e p1447, 10/e p1378; Sabiston 20/e p1531; Bailey 27/e p1228)*

20. **Ans. b. Bluish discoloration around umbilicus**

21. **Ans. c. Acute hemorrhagic pancreatitis**
22. **Ans. a. Grey Turner sign**

■ CHRONIC PANCREATITIS: ETIOLOGY, CLINICAL FEATURES AND DIAGNOSIS

23. **Ans. c. Hypercalcemia** (*Ref: Sabiston 20/e p1532; Schwartz 11/e p1452, 10/e p1360, 1366-1367; Bailey 27/e p1230; Harrison 20/e p2445*)

24. **Ans. b. Chronic pancreatitis**　　　　　　25. **Ans. a. Hypercalcemia**

26. **Ans. b. Alcohol** (*Ref: Sabiston 20/e p1531; Schwartz 11/e p1451, 10/e p1362; Bailey 27/e p1230*)

27. **Ans. d. Treatment is mainly surgical** (*Ref: Sabiston 20/e p1532; Schwartz 11/e p1468, 1470, 10/e p1366; Bailey 27/e p1230*)

28. **Ans. b. ERCP**

■ CHRONIC PANCREATITIS: TREATMENT AND COMPLICATIONS

29. **Ans. c. Side to side pancreaticojejunostomy**

30. **Ans. a. Celiac ganglia** (*Ref: Sabiston 20/e p1534; Schwartz 11/e p1469, 10/e p1380; Bailey 27/e p1231*)

CHRONIC PANCREATITIS

- **Pain from** the **pancreas** is carried in **sympathetic fibers** that traverse the **celiac ganglia,** reach the sympathetic chain through the splanchnic nerves, and then ascend to the cortex
- **Celiac plexus nerve blocks**[Q] performed either **percutaneously** or **endoscopically** have been employed to **abolish this pain** with inconsistent results

31. **Ans. a. Renal artery stenosis**　　　　32. **Ans. d. Gallbladder stone is the most common cause**

33. **Ans. c. Pseudocyst** (*Ref: Sabiston 20/e p1530*)

■ PSEUDOPANCREATIC CYST

34. **Ans. b. Pseudocyst**　　　　　　35. **Ans. a. Infection**

36. **Ans. d. Hemorrhage** (*Ref: CSDT 11/e p638*)

- Serious post-op hemorrhage from cyst occurs from cystogastrostomy[Q].

37. **Ans. b. Conservative**　　　　38. **Ans. d. Treatment of choice is percutaneous aspiration**

■ CYSTIC NEOPLASMS OF PANCREAS

39. **Ans. a. IPMN** (*Ref: Sabiston 20/e p1538-1539; Schwartz 11/e p1502, 9/e p1234; Blumgart 6/e p960; Shackelford 8/e p1162*)

40. **Ans. a. Microcystic adenoma** (*Ref: Sabiston 20/e p1537; Schwartz 11/e p1500-1501, 10/e p 1410-1413*)

- **Mucinous cystadenoma** is **macrocystic,** not the microcystic adenoma.

41. **Ans. c. Intraductal papillary mucinous neoplasm (IPMN)**

42. **Ans. b. Enucleation is performed** (*Ref: Sabiston 20/e p1537; Schwartz 11/e p1500-1505, 10/e p1410; Bailey 27/e p1234*)

■ CARCINOMA PANCREAS: ETIOLOGY AND RISK FACTORS

43. **Ans. a. Her-2-neu** (*Ref: Sabiston 20/e p1541-1542; Schwartz 11/e p1485, 10/e p1395; Bailey 27/e p1234*)

- **K-ras mutations** and **HER2/neu over expression** are the **earliest changes** to occur in **pancreatic carcinoma**[Q]

44. **Ans. a. Acute pancreatitis** (*Ref: Sabiston 20/e p1541-1542; Schwartz 11/e p1484, 10/e p1395; Bailey 27/e p1234*)

45. **Ans. a. K-ras** (*Ref: Sabiston 20/e p1542; Schwartz 11/e p1485, 10/e p1395; Bailey 27/e p1234*)

46. **Ans. d. Cronkhite-Canada syndrome**　　　　47. **Ans. c. Peutz-Jegher's syndrome** (*Ref: Sabiston 20/e p1542*)

48. **Ans. a. K-ras** (*Ref: Sabiston 20/e p1543; Schwartz 11/e p1485, 10/e p1395; Bailey 27/e p1234*)

■ CARCINOMA PANCREAS: CLINICAL FEATURES AND DIAGNOSIS

49. **Ans. c. Jaundice** (*Ref: Sabiston 20/e p1544; Schwartz 11/e p1485, 10/e p 1394; Bailey 27/e p1234; Blumgart 6/e p979; Shackelford 8/e p1138*)

50. **Ans. a. External compression of duodenum** (*Ref: Schwartz 11/e p1485, 10/e p1395; Sabiston 20/e p1544; Bailey 27/e p1234*)

51. **Ans. a. MDCT**

- **Diagnostic investigation** in **carcinoma pancreas** is **MDCT**[Q]
- **MDCT** is **investigation of choice** for the evaluation of **lesions arising** in the **pancreas**[Q]
- **IOC** for **diagnosis, staging** and **follow-up** in **CA pancreas: MDCT**[Q]

52. **Ans. a. T1**

53. **Ans. d. EUS guided transgastric biopsy** (*Ref: Schwartz 11/e p1487-1488, 10/e p1397-1399; Sabiston 20/e p1544; Bailey 27/e p1235*)

- *"EUS is useful if CT fails to demonstrate a tumour, if tissue diagnosis is required prior to surgery* (e.g. a mass has developed on a background of chronic pancreatitis and a distinction needs to be made between inflammation and neoplasia), *if vascular invasion needs to be confirmed, or in separating cystic tumours from pseudocysts. Transduodenal or transgastric FNA or Trucut biopsy performed under EUS guidance avoids spillage of tumour cells into the peritoneal cavity. Percutaneous transperitoneal biopsy of potentially resectable pancreatic tumours should be avoided as far as possible. Histological confirmation of malignancy is desirable but not essential, particularly if the imaging clearly demonstrates a resectable tumour. The lack of a tissue diagnosis should not delay appropriate surgical therapy. In patients judged to have unresectable disease, tissue diagnosis should be obtained prior to starting palliative therapy."* -Bailey 27/e p1235

54. Ans. c. CA head of pancreas   **55.** Ans. d. Ductal adenocarcinoma

56. Ans. a. Ductal adenocarcinoma

57. Ans. d. CT scan *(Ref: CSDT 11/e p645; Schwartz 11/e p1487, 10/e p1398)*

- **Investigation of choice** for carcinoma pancreas: **MDCT**[Q]
- Currently **CT** is probably the single **most versatile** and **cost effective** tool **for diagnosis of pancreatic cancer**

58. Ans. a. EUS guided transgastric biopsy *(Ref: Sabiston 20/e p1544; Schwartz 11/e p1487-1488, 10/e p1399; Bailey 27/e p1235)*

59. Ans. a. Periampullary carcinoma *(Ref: Shackelford 7/e p1183)*   **60.** Ans. a. Head

■ CARCINOMA PANCREAS: TREATMENT AND PROGNOSIS

61. Ans. b. Pain is early in the course of the disease *(Ref: Sabiston 20/e p1544)*

Carcinoma Pancreas
• Symptoms include **unexplained episodes of pancreatitis**[Q], **painless jaundice**, nausea, vomiting, steatorrhea, and **unexplained weight loss**   • With **further spread beyond the pancreas**, these patients may **note upper abdominal** or **back pain** when **peripancreatic nerve plexuses** are **involved** and **ascites** when **peritoneal carcinomatosis** or **portal vein occlusion** develops[Q]

62. Ans. c. Gemcitabine *(Ref: Bailey 27/e p1237; Blumgart 6/e p1040; Shackelford 8/e p 1146)*

- **Gemcitabine**[Q] is currently the standard of care for patients with **metastatic pancreatic cancer**.

63. Ans. b. Duodenojejunostomy *(Ref: Sabiston 20/e p1546; Bailey 27/e p1237; Shackelford 8/e p1185)*
- **Duodenojejunostomy** is done **in PPPD**, not in Whipple's procedure.
- **Gastrojejunostomy** is done **in Whipple's procedure**.

64. Ans. c. Portal vein

65. Ans. d. Acute pancreatitis never occurs in CA pancreas *(Ref: Sabiston 20/e p1544)*

- Clinical Features of Carcinoma Pancreas
- **MC site** is **head and uncinate process**[Q]
- Patients with lesions that occur near the bile duct, such as those near the **ampulla, head** of the pancreas, and **uncinate process**, are much more likely to have **obstructive jaundice**[Q].
- Those with **lesions in the body or tail of the pancreas** are more likely to complain of **pain**.
- **Pain** suggests **unresectability**[Q] in carcinoma pancreas
- **Two third (65%)** patients present with **diabetes in carcinoma pancreas**[Q]
- Patients may also have **acute pancreatitis secondary to obstruction of the pancreatic duct**[Q].
- **Elderly patients with acute pancreatitis** but **without a history of alcohol use** or **gallbladder stones** should be **screened for a neoplasm**[Q].

66. Ans. b. Ascites   **67.** Ans. a. Pyloric antrum

68. Ans. a. Delayed gastric emptying *(Ref: Sabiston 20/e p1548; Schwartz 11/e p1497, 10/e p1406; Bailey 27/e p1236)*

69. Ans. b. 22 months *(Ref: Sabiston 20/e p1547)*

"After surgical resection and adjuvant therapy for pancreatic cancer, the median survival is approximately 22 months, with 5-year survival of 15% to 20%. Most patients experience relapse of disease in the form of metastatic disease (85%) and, less commonly, local recurrence (40%). In the absence of surgical resection, those with locally advanced disease who receive palliative chemotherapy may survive 10 to 12 months, whereas those with metastases rarely survive beyond 6 months." -Sabiston 20/e p1547

70. Ans. d. Pancreaticojejunostomy, hepaticojejunostomy, gastrojejunostomy

■ INSULINOMA

71. Ans. d. Selective arteriography

- **Portal venous sampling** for insulin with or without **arterial stimulation** with **calcium** is the **best pre-operative method** of **localization**[Q].
- **EUS** with **intra-operative palpation** is **best localization technique** for Insulinoma[Q].

72. Ans. a. Insulinoma   **73.** Ans. a. 72-hours fasting test

74. Ans. a. Insulinoma

NET OF PANCREAS

- **MC NET of Pancreas: Non-functional** (Mostly malignant) >**Insulinoma**[Q]
- **MC benign NET of Pancreas: Insulinoma**[Q]
- **MC malignant functional NET of Pancreas: Gastrinoma**[Q]

75. Ans. d. Equally distributed   76. Ans. a. Insulinoma

77. Ans. d. Equally distributed in head, body and tail *(Ref: Sabiston 20/e p952; Schwartz 10/e p1391; Bailey 27/e p849)*

■ ZOLLINGER-ELLISON SYNDROME

78. Ans. a. Duodenum *(Ref: Sabiston 20/e p954; Schwartz 11/e p1481, 10/e p1071-1073; Bailey 27/e p850; Blumgart 6/e p999; Shackelford 8/e p702)*

79. Ans. c. Decreased BAO and MAO

- **Basal acid output is increased in Gastrinoma**[Q].

80. Ans. d. SRS   81. Ans. a. Associated with MEN1 *(Ref: Sabiston 20/e p954; Schwartz 11/e p1481; Bailey 27/e p850)*

82. Ans. c. Decreased BAO/MAO   83. Ans. d. H_2 receptor antagonist   84. Ans. a. Endoscopic ultrasound

85. Ans. a. Gastrinoma triangle *(Ref: Schwartz 11/e p1482, 10/e p1392; Sabiston 20/e p954; Bailey 27/e p1141)*

86. Ans. b. Junction of 3rd and 4th part of duodenum   87. Ans. b. Reduced BAO: MAO ratio

88. Ans. b. Zollinger-Ellison syndrome   89. Ans. a. Pylorus *(Ref: Sabiston 20/e p1210; Schwartz 11/e p1481, 10/e p1392; Bailey 27/e p851)*

90. Ans. c. Zollinger-Ellison syndrome

91. Ans. a. Gastrinoma *(Ref: Sabiston 20/e p954; Schwartz 11/e p1481; Bailey 27/e p850)*

■ ENDOCRINE TUMORS OF PANCREAS

92. Ans. a. Insulinoma   93. Ans. d. SRS *(Ref: Sabiston 20/e p947)*   94. Ans. a. Glucagonoma

95. Ans. b. Somaststationomas   96. Ans. a. VIPoma *(Ref: Sabiston 20/e p965; Schwartz 11/e p1482, 10/e p1392; Bailey 27/e p849)*

97. Ans. a. Glucagonoma *(Ref: Sabiston 20/e p957; Schwartz 11/e p1483, 10/e p1393; Bailey 27/e p849)*

■ PANCREAS DIVISUM

98. Ans. a. Most common congenital anomaly *(Ref: Sabiston 20/e p1522; Schwartz 11/e p1432, 10/e p1365-1366; Bailey 27/e p1219; Blumgart 6/e p861; Shackelford 8/e p1127)*

■ ANNULAR PANCREAS

99. Ans. d. Duodenoduodenostomy *(Ref: Blumgart 6/e p860)*   100. Ans. b. Duodenoduodenostomy

■ PANCREATIC TRAUMA

101. Ans. d. HRCT is investigation of choice

102. Ans. b. Fracture is common at the junction of head and body, d. Peritoneal lavage is good for making the diagnosis

■ PANCREATIC TRANSPLANTATION

103. Ans. b. Amylase levels *(Ref: Sabiston 20/e p644-665; Schwartz 11/e p375-377, 10/e p340-344; Bailey 27/e p1553; Blumgart 6/e p1881; Shackelford 8/e p1230)*

- Bailey 25/e p1425: '**Urinary drainage** of the pancreas has the **advantage** that **urinary amylase levels can be used to monitor graft rejection**'[Q]

■ MISCELLANEOUS

104. Ans. b. 11 O' clock position *(Ref: Sabiston 20/e p1396; Schwartz 11/e p1447, 10/e p1327)*

TRANSDUODENAL SPHINCTEROPLASTY

- This **cut is made superiorly** (at the **11' O clock position**)[Q] **for 4 to 5 mm.**
- The **sphincter** is **incised** at the **11' O clock position** to **avoid injury to the pancreatic duct**[Q].

105. Ans. b. CT scan *(Ref: Sutton 7/e p796)*

- **CT is the mainstay of pancreatic imaging**, able to demonstrate **focal masses within the gland calcifications, duct dilatation, cysts, abscesses** and associated abnormalities in upper abdominal organs (hepatic metastases), lymph nodes and peri-pancreatic vascular structures.
- **CT is a useful tool for guiding percutaneous pancreatic biopsy and cyst aspiration** or **drainage.**

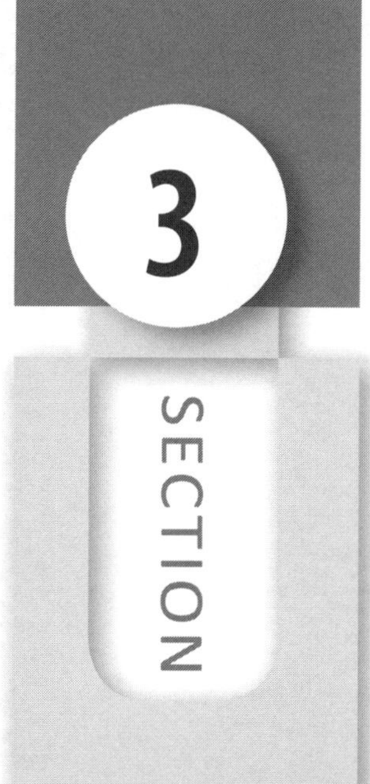

Gastrointestinal Surgery

- Esophagus
- Stomach and Duodenum
- Peritoneum
- Intestinal Obstruction
- Small Intestine
- Large Intestine
- Ileostomy and Colostomy
- Inflammatory Bowel Disease
- Vermiform Appendix
- Rectum and Anal Canal
- Hernia and Abdominal Wall
- Spleen

Esophagus

■ CONGENITAL DIAPHRAGMATIC HERNIA (BOCHDALEK HERNIA OR POSTEROLATERAL HERNIA)

CONGENITAL DIAPHRAGMATIC HERNIA (BOCHDALEK HERNIA OR POSTEROLATERAL HERNIA)

- **CDH** term is used for **Bochdalek hernia**[Q]
  - **Incidence 1 in 2000 to 5000**[Q] live births.
  - **Most CDH defects** are on the **left side** (80%); up to 20% on **right side**[Q].
- **Bag & Mask ventilation** is **contraindicated** in **CDH**[Q].

Pathogenesis

- Result from **failure of normal closure** of the **pleuroperitoneal canal**[Q] in the developing embryo.
  - **Main factors** affecting morbidity and mortality: **Pulmonary hypoplasia** & **pulmonary hypertension**[Q].

Clinical Features

- Classic triad: **Respiratory distress + Dextrocardia + Scaphoid abdomen**[Q]
- **MC** presentation is **respiratory distress** due to severe hypoxemia.
- **Anteroposterior diameter** of the **chest** may be **large**, & **abdomen** may be **scaphoid**[Q].

Diagnosis

- **Diagnosis** is made at the time of a **prenatal ultrasound** during pregnancy.
- **Postnatal diagnosis** by a **plain chest radiograph** demonstrates the **gastric air bubble** or **loops of bowel** within the **chest**[Q].
- **Pneumothorax** always occurs on **contralateral** to the **side of CDH**[Q].

Treatment

- **Physiologic stress** associated with **early repair** probably **adds more insult** and that **survival is not improved**[Q] when compared with delayed repair.
- A variable period of time (**24–72 hours**) to allow **for stabilization** before **surgical repair**[Q].
  - The **viscera** are **reduced** into the abdominal cavity, & **posterolateral defect** in diaphragm is **closed** using **interrupted, nonabsorbable sutures**[Q].
- In **most cases (80%–90%)**, a **hernia sac** is **not present**. If **identified**, it is **excised** at the time of repair[Q].
- Advantage of a **prosthetic patch** is that a **tension-free repair** can be frequently obtained in **large defects**[Q].

■ MORGAGNI HERNIAS (RETROSTERNAL HERNIAS OR LARREY'S HERNIA[Q])

MORGAGNI HERNIAS (RETROSTERNAL HERNIAS OR LARREY'S HERNIA[Q])

- **Congenital hernia** of **anteromedial, retrosternal diaphragm**
- Occur in the **triangular space** between the muscle fibers that make up the diaphragm
- They extend from the **xiphisternum** and **costal margin** to the central tendon of diaphragm.
  - **Ninety percent** are **right sided**[Q] because the pericardium itself prevents left-sided hernias
  - **Superior epigastric vessels** may **pass through Morgagni space**[Q]
  - **Most commonly involved viscus is transverse colon**[Q]

Clinical Feature

- Patients are **usually asymptomatic**[Q]

Diagnosis

- **Anterior mediastinal masses** are found incidentally on **chest radiographs**[Q].

Contd…

Contd…

Treatment

- **Prompt surgical repair** after diagnosis is prudent **to avoid incarceration** or **strangulation** of abdominal organs.
- A **transabdominal route**[Q] is the preferred choice.
- **Prosthetic mesh** is generally required **to repair the defect**[Q].

■ HIATUS HERNIA

Types of Hiatal hernia	
Type I	**Sliding** hiatal hernia (**MC**)[Q]
Type II	**True** paraesophageal hernia[Q]
Type III	**Mixed** paraesophageal hernia (**I and II**)[Q]
Type IV	Paraesophageal hernia containing other **intra abdominal organs**[Q]

TYPES OF HIATAL HERNIA

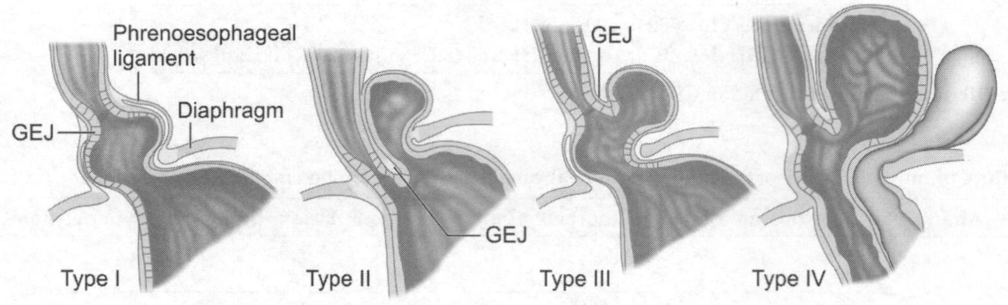

PATHOPHYSIOLOGY OF HIATUS HERNIA

Type I Hernia or Sliding HH

- Characterized by **upward displacement** of **GE junction** into the **posterior mediastinum**[Q].
- The **stomach** remains in its **usual longitudinal alignment**[Q].
- **Majority** of patients with HH are **asymptomatic**[Q]
- The **prevalence** and **size** of the sliding HH **correlate with** increasing **severity of reflux disease**[Q].

Type II Hernia

- **True PEH:** Defined by a **normally positioned intra abdominal GE junction** with **upward herniation** of the **stomach**[Q] alongside it.
- A PEH develops when there is a **defect**, possibly **congenital**, in the **hiatus anterior** to the esophagus.
- **Persistent posterior fixation** of the **GE junction** is the essential difference between a PEH and a sliding HH.

Type III Hernia

- **Mixed hernia:** Characterized by **displacement** of **both** the **GE junction** and a **large portion** of the **stomach** cephalad into the posterior mediastinum[Q].
- **Starts** as a **sliding HH**, and over time as the **hiatus enlarges**, and more of **fundus** and **body** of the stomach **herniate** into the chest.

Type IV Hernia

- Esophageal hiatus has dilated to such an extent that the **hernia sac** also **contains** other organs such as the **spleen, colon**, or **small bowel**[Q].
- Bowel obstruction and **complications**[Q] due to altered anatomy.

■ FACTORS AFFECTING LES PRESSURE

Lower Esophageal Sphincter (LES) Pressure	
Decreased by	**Increased by**
• **P**rostaglandin E1 and E2, **P**rogesterone[Q] • **M**orphine and **M**eperidine[Q] • **T**heophylline[Q] • **B**arbiturates, **D**iazepam[Q], **D**opamine • **CCB, A**tropine, **N**itrates[Q] • **C**hocolate, **C**offee[Q] • **A**lcohol, **P**ippermint[Q] • **S**moking, **F**at[Q]	• **B**ombesin, **A**ngiotensin II[Q] • **PP, S**ubstance P, **M**otilin[Q] • **G**astrin[Q] • **A**ntacids[Q] • **C**holinergics[Q] • **D**omeperidone • **M**etoclopramide[Q] • **P**rostaglandin $F_{2\alpha}$

- **PMT BD CAN decrease LES pressure**: Prostaglandin E1 and E2, Progesterone, Morphine and Meperidine, Theophylline, Barbiturates, Diazepam, Dopamine, CCB, Atropine, Nitrates
- **CAPS Fat decrease LES pressure**: Chocolate, Coffee, Alcohol, Pippermint, Smoking, Fat.
- **PSM BAG increase LES pressure**: PP, Substance P, Motilin, Bombesin, Angiotensin II, Gastrin

■ GASTROESOPHAGEAL REFLUX DISEASE (GERD)

GASTROESOPHAGEAL REFLUX DISEASE (GERD)

- **Classical triad** of symptoms is **retrosternal burning pain, epigastric pain & regurgitation**[Q].
- **GERD** is associated with **complications** such as **esophageal ulcerations** (5%), **peptic strictures** (4–20%), & **Barrett's esophagus** (8–20%).

Pathophysiology

- LES has the **primary role** of **preventing reflux** into the esophagus.

Factors Contributing to the High-pressure Zone in the Lower Esophagus
• **Intrinsic musculature**[Q] of the distal esophagus which are in a state of tonic contraction
• **Sling fibers** of the **cardia**[Q] which are at the same anatomic depth of the circular muscle fibers of the esophagus but are oriented in a different direction
• **Diaphragm**[Q]: during inspiration the anteroposterior diameter of the **crural opening** is decreased, compressing the esophagus and increasing the measured pressure at the LES
• **Transmitted pressure**[Q] of the abdominal cavity

- **GERD** is **often associated with** a **hiatal hernia** (MC type is **type I** or **sliding** hernia[Q]).

Clinical Features

- **Classical triad** of symptoms is **retrosternal burning pain, epigastric pain** and **regurgitation**.
- **MC presentation** of GERD: **Long-standing history** of **heartburn** and a **shorter history of regurgitation**[Q].

• **Symptoms of GERD: Heartburn** (80%)[Q], **Regurgitation** (54%), Abdominal pain (29%), **Cough** (27%), Dysphagia for solids (23%), Belching (15%), Bloating (15%), Aspiration (14%), Wheezing (7%).

Diagnosis

- **Endoscopy: Exclude other diseases**, especially a tumor, and to **document** the presence of **peptic esophageal injury**. An **essential step in** the **evaluation of GERD**, who are being **considered for operative intervention**[Q].

• **Manometry:** For **information about** the **function of** the **esophageal body** and **LES**[Q]

24-hour pH Monitoring

• **Gold standard** for **diagnosing** and **quantifying acid reflux** is the **24-hour pH test**[Q].
• **DeMeester score**[Q]: An overall score is obtained with the use of a formula that assigns a **weight to each item** according to its capacity **to cause esophageal injury.**
• **DeMeester score** needs to be **<14.7**[Q].

- **Esophagogram:** For evaluation of **symptoms of GERD** when an **operation is contemplated** or when the **symptoms do not respond as expected. Presence** and **size** of a **hiatal hernia** may be **characterized**[Q].

Treatment

- **Lifestyle modifications:** Cessation of smoking, **decreased caffeine intake**, and **avoidance** of **large meals** before lying down[Q]
- **Medical Management: Double dose of PPI** is the **initial approach**[Q]
- Compared with H$_2$ blockers, **PPIs** are **more effective** at **healing** esophageal **ulceration** secondary to acid exposure.

Indications of Surgical Therapy
• **Severe esophageal injury (ulcer, stricture**, or **Barrett's mucosa)**[Q]
• **Incomplete resolution** of **symptoms** or **relapses** while on medical therapy
• **Long duration** of **symptoms**[Q]
• **Symptoms** persist **at a young age**[Q]

- **Antireflux surgery:** Laparoscopic Nissen fundoplication is gold standard for GERD[Q].

■ TYPES OF FUNDOPLICATION

Type of Fundoplication	Degree of Wrap
Watson	• **90-degree anterior** fundoplication[Q]
Dor	• **180-degree anterior** fundoplication[Q]
Toupet	• 180-degree **posterior** fundoplication subsequently modified to a **270-degree wrap**[Q]
Belsey Mark IV	• **270-degree anterior** fundoplication[Q]
Nissen	• **360-degree** fundoplication[Q]

■ ACHALASIA CARDIA

ACHALASIA CARDIA

- MC motility disorder of esophagus[Q]
- MC hypomotility disorder of esophagus[Q]
- **Achalasia** means "**failure to relax**[Q]" (**sphincter** remains in a **constant state of tone** with periods of relaxation)
- Both the **muscle** of **esophagus** & **LES** are **affected**[Q].
- **Prevailing theory: Destruction** of the nerves to **LES** is **primary pathology** & **degeneration** of **neuromuscular function** of **body of esophagus** is **secondary**[Q].
- **Premalignant condition** leading to **squamous cell carcinoma**

> - **Triple A-syndrome** or **Allgrove disease**[Q]: Achalasia, Alacrima and ACTH-resistant Adrenal insufficiency.

Pathogenesis

> - **Progressive inflammation** & **selective loss** of **inhibitory myenteric neurons** in **Auerbach's plexus** of esophagus that normally secrete VIP & nitric oxide[Q].

- This results in **failure of relaxation of LES** and **aperistalsis of esophageal body** with subsequent **functional obstruction** at the level of **GE junction** & **gradual dilatation** of esophagus[Q].

Clinical Features

- **Classic triad** of symptoms consists of **dysphagia, regurgitation**, and **weight loss**.
- Heartburn, postprandial choking, & nocturnal coughing are seen commonly.

> - **Men** & **women** are **equally affected**, with **no ethnic predisposition** to the disease[Q].

- **Regurgitation** of undigested, foul-smelling foods is common, and with **progressive disease, aspiration** can become life-threatening[Q].
- **Pneumonia, lung abscess**, & bronchiectasis often result from **long-standing achalasia**.

Diagnosis

- **Barium swallow:**

> - **Dilated esophagus** with a **distal narrowing**[Q]
> - "**Bird's beak**", "**Pencil-tip**" or "**Rat's tail**" appearance[Q]

- **Hurst phenomenon: Thin stream of barium flows beyond bird beak due to increased esophageal pressure**[Q]
- Massive esophageal dilation, tortuosity, and a **sigmoidal esophagus (megaesophagus)** in **advanced stage**[Q]

> - **Mecholyl test** is **positive in Achalasia**[Q]
> - **CCK test** is **positive in Achalasia**[Q]

- **Manometry** is **gold standard test** for diagnosis.
  - **Absence** of **body peristalsis** & **poor LES relaxation** is **mandatory**[Q] for diagnosis.

Treatment

- **Early stage:** Sublingual **nitroglycerin, nitrates**, or **calcium channel blockers**[Q] may offer hours of relief of chest pressure before or after a meal.
- **Bougie dilation**[Q] up to 54 French may offer several months of relief but requires repeated dilations to be sustainable.
- **Botulinum toxin:**
  - Injection of **botulinum toxin (Botox)** directly into the LES **blocks acetylcholine release**, preventing smooth muscle contraction, and effectively **relaxes** the LES[Q].

> - **Laparoscopic Heller myotomy** is now the **operation of choice**[Q].
> - **Extent of Heller's myotomy: 2 cm above GE junction to 1 cm below**[Q], over stomach.

- **Partial antireflux procedure (Toupet** or **Dor fundoplication)**[Q] will restore a barrier to reflux and decrease postoperative symptoms.
- **Esophagectomy** is considered **megaesophagus, sigmoid esophagus, failure of more than one myotomy**, or an **undilatable reflux stricture**[Q].

■ DIFFUSE ESOPHAGEAL SPASM

DIFFUSE ESOPHAGEAL SPASM

- **Esophageal contractions** are **repetitive, simultaneous**, and of **high amplitude**[Q].
- Basic pathology **motor abnormality** of **esophageal body** is most notable in **lower two thirds** of esophagus.
- More common in **women** and is often found in patients with multiple complaints[Q].

Clinical Features

- Clinical presentation: **Chest pain** and **dysphagia**[Q] (may be related to eating or exertion and may mimic angina)
- Complain of a squeezing pressure in the chest that may radiate to the jaw, arms, and upper back.

Contd…

Contd…

Diagnosis

- **Barium swallow:**
    - **Corkscrew** or **rosary-bead** esophagus, **segmental spasm** or **pseudodiverticulosis** appearance[Q]
- **Manometry** is **gold standard test** for diagnosis[Q].
    - Classic manometry findings: **Simultaneous, multipeaked contractions** of **high amplitude** (>120 mm Hg) or **long duration** (>2.5 sec).

Treatment

- **Mainstay of treatment** for DES is **nonsurgical**, and **pharmacologic** (Nitrates, calcium channel blockers) or **endoscopic intervention** (Bougie dilation) is preferred[Q].
- **Indications of surgery** (**long esophagomyotomy**):
    - **Incapacitating chest pain** or **dysphagia** who have **failed medical** and **endoscopic therapy**[Q]
    - Presence of a **pulsion diverticulum** of the thoracic esophagus

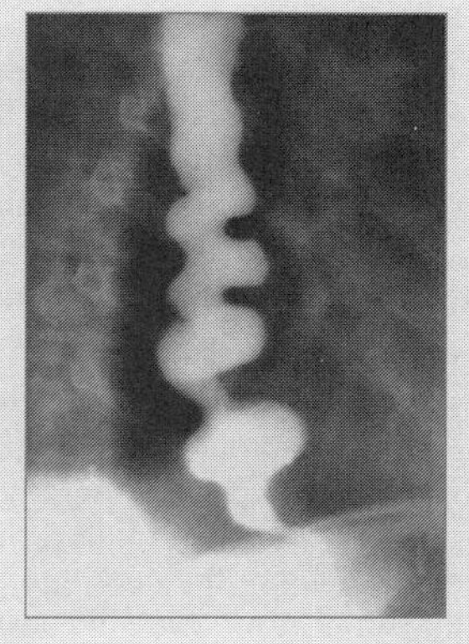

■ NUTCRACKER ESOPHAGUS

NUTCRACKER ESOPHAGUS

- **Hypermotility disorder** also known as **supersqueeze esophagus**[Q].
- Esophagus with **hypertensive peristalsis** or **high-amplitude peristaltic contractions**.
- **Most common and most painful** esophageal **hypermotility disorder**[Q].
- Associated with **hypertrophic musculature** resulting in high-amplitude contractions of the esophagus

Clinical Feature

- **Chest pain** and **dysphagia** are typical symptoms.

Diagnosis

- 10c for diagnosis: Manometry
- On manometry, **amplitude >180 mm Hg** and **duration of contraction >6 seconds**

Treatment

- Treatment is **medical** (**Calcium channel blockers, nitrates, and antispasmodics**)[Q]

■ HYPERTENSIVE LES

HYPERTENSIVE LES

- The **LES pressure** is **above normal**, motility of esophageal body may be **hyperperistaltic** or **normal**.

Clinical Feature

- Patients with **hypertensive LES** present with **chest pain** or **dysphagia**[Q].

Diagnosis

- Diagnosis is made by **manometry**.
    - **Elevated LES pressure** (>26 mm Hg) and **normal relaxation** of the LES.
    - Esophageal body may be **hyperperistaltic** or **normal**.

Treatment

- **Botox injections** alleviate symptoms temporarily, and **hydrostatic balloon dilation** may provide long-term symptomatic relief.
- **Surgery** in patients who **fail interventional treatments** and those with **significant symptoms**.
- A **laparoscopic modified Heller esophagomyotomy** is the **operation of choice**.

■ ZENKER'S OR PHARYNGOESOPHAGEAL DIVERTICULA

ZENKER'S OR PHARYNGOESOPHAGEAL DIVERTICULA

- **Mucosal outpouching** (**pulsion diverticulum**) occurring **through** the triangular bare area (**Killian's triangle**)[Q], between the **upper oblique fibers** (**thyropharyngeus muscle**) and **lower horizontal fibers** (**cricopharyngeus muscle**) of the **inferior constrictor muscle**[Q]
- It is **not a true esophageal diverticula**[Q]
- MC esophageal diverticula[Q]

Contd…

Contd…

Pathology

- **Neuromuscular incordination**[Q] in this region
- May be due to **different nerve supply** of the **two parts of inferior constrictor muscle**[Q]
    - **Thyropharyngeus (oblique fibers)** supplied by **pharyngeal plexus**
    - **Cricopharyngeus (horizontal fibers)** by **recurrent laryngeal nerve**

Clinical Features

- Usually seen in patients over **50 years**[Q]
- MC symptom is **dysphagia**[Q]
- **Undigested food** is **regurgitated into the mouth**, especially when the patient is in **recumbent position**[Q]
- Swelling of the neck, gurgling noise after eating, halitosis, and a sour metallic taste in the mouth are common symptoms
- **Cervical webs** are seen **associated in 50%**[Q] of patients.

Diagnosis

- **Barium swallow** is **diagnostic**

Complications

- **Pneumonia** and **lung abscess** due to **aspiration**[Q] **(MC)**
- Perforation, Bleeding   •   Carcinoma

Management

- Surgical therapy **(Cricopharyngeal myotomy + Diverticulopexy)** is **treatment of choice**[Q]

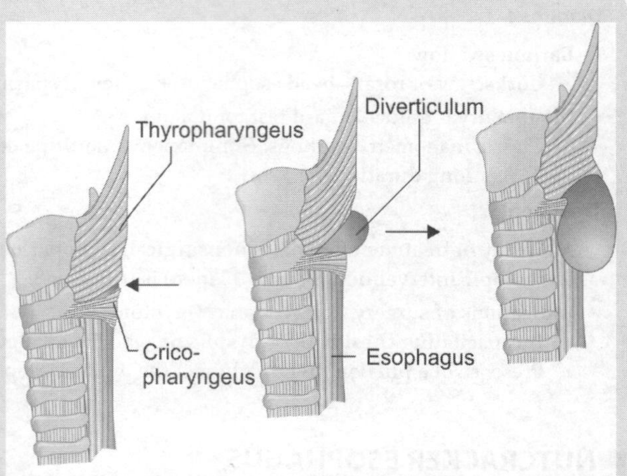

Treatment Options for Zenker's Diverticula
• **Cricopharyngeal myotomy**- a myotomy alone is sufficient for small diverticula
• **Myotomy with excision of sac**- done for large (>4 cm) diverticula
• **Diverticulopexy**

• **Diverticulo-esophagostomy** using a linear cutting staple gun
  – Septum between esophagus diverticula is divided
  – Also known as **Dohlman procedure**[Q]

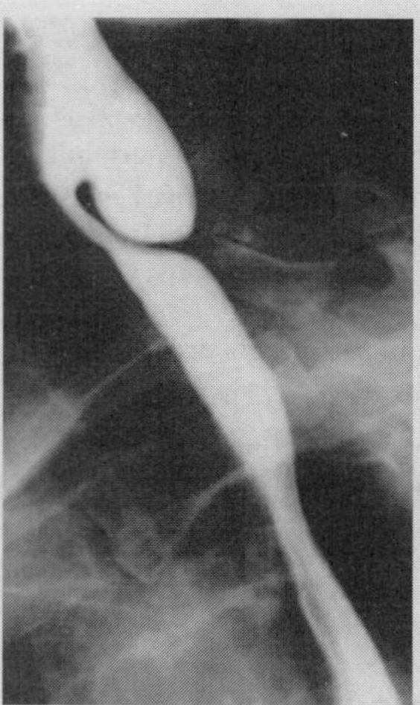

■ MIDESOPHAGEAL OR TRACTION DIVERTICULA

MIDESOPHAGEAL OR TRACTION DIVERTICULA

- **Inflammation** of **lymph nodes** exerts **traction** on wall of the esophagus leading to formation of a **true diverticulum** in the midesophagus.

> • Caused by **inflamed mediastinal lymph nodes** from **tuberculosis, histoplasmosis**[Q] and resultant fibrosing mediastinitis.

- Typically present on **right**.

Clinical Features

- **Most patients** are **asymptomatic**, incidentally found during a workup for some other complaint.
- **Dysphagia, chest pain**, and **regurgitation** can be present and are usually indicative of an **underlying primary motility disorder**.

Diagnosis

- **Investigation of choice** is **barium swallow**[Q] (lateral views to determine side)
- **CT scan** is helpful to identify any **mediastinal lymphadenopathy** and may help to **lateralize the sac**.
- **Manometry** in **all patients**, symptomatic or not, **to identify** a **primary motor disorder**.

Treatment

- In **asymptomatic patients** who have inflamed mediastinal lymph nodes from **tuberculosis** or **histoplasmosis**: ATT or **antifungal agents**[Q]
- **Diverticulopexy** for **symptomatic** or **2 cm or larger** diverticulum
- **Esophagomyotomy** in **severe chest pain** or **dysphagia** and a documented **motor abnormality**[Q]

■ BARRETT'S ESOPHAGUS

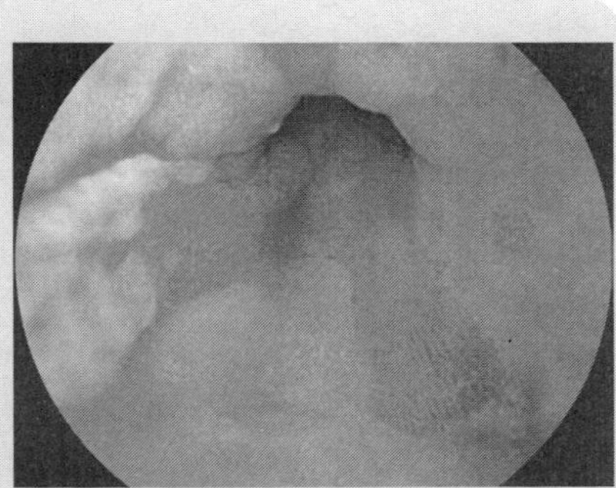

BARRETT'S ESOPHAGUS

- **Distal squamous mucosa** is **replaced by metaplastic specialized (intestinalized columnar) epithelium**, e.g. **goblet cells**, as a response to **chronic injury**; may regress after treatment[Q]
- Also called **columnar lined esophagus**[Q]
- **Metaplasia** of esophageal **squamous epithelium into columnar** in **distal**[Q] esophagus
- **MC type** of columnar epithelium is **intestinal epithelium (Intestinal metaplasia**[Q]**)**

Etiology

- Usually due to **chronic GERD**[Q]
- **Columnar epithelium of Barrett's** may be **more resistant to acid, pepsin & bile**[Q]
- Often associated with **sliding hiatal hernia**[Q]

Clinical Features

- Higher incidence in **whites, males & obese**
- **Symptoms: long history of heartburn** & other reflux symptoms; more massive reflux with more numerous and longer episodes than most reflux patients
- Major risk factor for **esophageal adenocarcinoma**[Q]

Diagnosis

- Characteristic **endoscopic appearance plus characteristic histologic findings**[Q]
- **8 random biopsies recommended**
- Report should include type of epithelium present and **presence/absence of dysplasia, grade of dysplasia**, & **extent of dysplasia**[Q]

> - **Barrett's esophagus** requires **both endoscopically visible segment of columnar lining** of distal esophagus and **intestinal metaplasia** showing goblet cells on biopsy[Q]

Endoscopy

- **Red velvety GI type mucosa** between **pale squamous mucosa** of lower esophagus & **lush pink gastric mucosa**[Q]
- May have **tongues extending up from GE junction** or a broad band displacing GE junction proximally

Positive Stains

- **Goblet cells contain acid mucin, usually sialomucin**[Q] (**Alcian blue+ at pH 2.5**, although stain generally not needed or recommended), **columnar cells contain neutral mucins (PAS+)**; intestinal metaplastic cells are often CK7+/CK20-; also **CDX2+.**
- **Guanylyl cyclase C+, Hep+**
- In routine practice, **only H&E is used for diagnosis**

Treatment

- **Antireflux therapy**[Q]
- **Endoscopy every 1-2 years to detect dysplasia or early adenocarcinoma** with **4 quadrant biopsies using jumbo forceps at intervals of 2 cm** or less throughout the length of the Barrett's segment **plus any suspicious lesions**[Q].

■ PREDISPOSING FACTORS FOR CARCINOMA ESOPHAGUS

Predisposing Factors for Carcinoma Esophagus	
Squamous Cell Carcinoma	**Adenocarcinoma**
<ul><li>**Alcohol**[Q]</li><li>**Smoking**[Q]</li><li>**Ingested carcinogens**:<ul><li>**Nitrates**[Q], nitrites, **nitrosamines**[Q]</li><li>**Smoked opiates**[Q]</li><li>**Fungal toxins** in pickled vegetables</li></ul></li><li>**Mucosal damage**:<ul><li>Chronic **Achalasia**[Q]</li><li>**Lye (caustic) ingestion**</li><li>**Long term ingestion** of **hot liquids**</li><li>**Radiation induced strictures**[Q]</li></ul></li><li>**Plummer-vinson syndrome**[Q]</li><li>**Tylosis palmaris et plantaris**[Q]: Congenital **Hyperkeratosis**[Q] and **pitting** of **palms** and **soles**[Q]</li><li>**Human papilloma virus**[Q]</li><li>**Esophageal diverticula**[Q]</li><li>**Bulimia**[Q]</li><li>**Deficiency**: Vitamin **A, zinc, molybdenum**</li></ul>	<ul><li>**GERD** (leading to **Barrett's esophagus**[Q])</li><li>**Obesity**[Q]</li><li>**Scleroderma**[Q]</li></ul><blockquote>**Scleroderma: Smooth muscle atrophy** in **lower 2/3rd** of esophagus → **Incompetent LES → GERD → Stricture**</blockquote><ul><li>Diet deficient in fruits and vegetables</li><li>Diet **high** in **animal protein** and **cholesterol**[Q]</li></ul>

■ CARCINOMA ESOPHAGUS

CARCINOMA ESOPHAGUS

- MC esophageal cancer worldwide: **Squamous cell carcinoma**[Q]
- MC esophageal cancer in United States (Western countries): **Adenocarcinoma**[Q]
- More common in **males**[Q]
- MC site of CA esophagus: Middle 1/3rd (Overall)[Q]
- Chemotherapy regimen: Epirubicin + Cisplatin[Q] + 5-FU (ECF)

Clinical Features

- Early-stage cancers: Asymptomatic or mimic symptoms of GERD.

> • MC symptom: Dysphagia >Weight loss[Q]

- **Most patients** with esophageal cancer **present with dysphagia** and **weight loss**, symptoms that usually indicate advanced disease.
- Choking, coughing, and aspiration from a tracheoesophageal fistula (In advanced cases)[Q]
- Hoarseness and vocal cord paralysis from direct invasion into the recurrent laryngeal nerve (In advanced cases)[Q]
- MC site of metastasis: Liver[Q] >lung >bone
- Paraneoplastic manifestation associated with adenocarcinoma: Motor Neuropathy[Q]

Diagnosis

- Barium swallow: First investigation done[Q] in suspected case of CA esophagus (classic finding of an apple core lesion[Q])

> • **Endoscopy** with biopsy: Investigation of choice for **diagnosis** of CA esophagus[Q].
> • **Endoscopic Ultrasound:** Investigation of choice for **staging** of CA esophagus, best for T staging and LN metastasis[Q].

- CECT (abdomen and chest): Assess the length of the tumor, thickness of the esophagus and stomach, **regional LN status** and **metastasis to liver** and **lungs**[Q].

Treatment of CA Esophagus	
High-grade dysplasia (Tis) or T1a	• Endoscopic Mucosal Resection[Q]
Localized Esophageal Cancer	• **T1**: Vagal sparing or transhiatal or **minimal invasive esophagectomy** with limited LN dissection[Q] • **T2** and **T3**: Neo-adjuvant chemoradiation + Surgery[Q] • **Cervical SCC** or **Non-ideal candidate** for resection: **Definitive chemoradiation**[Q]
Locally Advanced Cancer	• **Chemoradiation**[Q] (± Surgical resection in T4a)
Metastatic Disease	• **Definitive chemoradiation**[Q] (for involved distant LN or metastatic disease)
Malignant TEF	• **Coated SEMS**[Q] (self-expanding metallic stents)

- Postoperative chemoradiation is reserved for GE junction tumors[Q]
- Extent of Resection: An in-situ **margin of 10 cm**[Q] should be the goal

Prognosis

Long-term Survival Following Esophagectomy Depends on		
• **Depth** of **tumor** invasion (T)[Q]	• **Number** of **involved lymph nodes** (N)[Q]	• **Location**[Q] of the tumor in the esophagus

■ TNM CLASSIFICATION OF CARCINOMA OF THE ESOPHAGUS

8th AJCC (2017) TNM Classification of Carcinoma of the Esophagus	
Tis: Carcinoma-in-situ/ High-grade dysplasia	**N1**: Metastasis in **1-2** regional LNs[Q]
T1a: Tumor invades **lamina propria or muscularis mucosa**[Q] **T1b**: Tumor invades **submucosa**[Q]	**N2**: Metastasis in **3-6** regional LNs[Q]
T2: Tumor invades **muscularis propria**[Q]	**N3**: Metastasis in **7 or more** regional LNs[Q]
T3: Tumor invades **adventitia**[Q]	**M1**: Distant metastasis[Q]
T4a: Tumor invades **pleura, pericardium, azygous vein, diaphragm or peritoneum**[Q] **T4b**: Tumor invades other adjacent structures such as **aorta, vertebral body or trachea**[Q]	

■ TYPES OF ESOPHAGECTOMY

Types of Esophagectomy	
Ivor-Lewis	• Transthoracic esophagectomy[Q] • **Double incision: Midline laparotomy** followed by **right sided thoracotomy**[Q] • Done **for tumors** of middle 1/3rd of **esophagus**[Q]
Orringer	• Transhiatal esophagectomy[Q] • **Double incision: Midline laparotomy** followed by **Cervical incision**[Q] • **MC procedure done** for carcinoma esophagus[Q]
McKeon	• En-bloc esophagectomy[Q] • Three incisions: **Right sided thoracotomy**, followed by **midline**[Q] laparotomy, followed by **cervical incision**[Q] • Associated with **maximum morbidity** and **mortality**[Q]

■ REPLACEMENT CONDUITS AFTER ESOPHAGECTOMY

REPLACEMENT CONDUITS AFTER ESOPHAGECTOMY

- **Best conduit** after esophagectomy (overall): **Stomach**[Q]
- **Conduit of choice** after esophagectomy in **CA esophagus**: **Stomach**[Q]
- **Conduit of choice** after esophagectomy in **benign disorders (caustic injuries, acid-peptic disease), unhealthy stomach**: Colon[Q]
- **Conduit of choice** for **short segment replacement**: Jejunum[Q]

Routes of Replacement of Esophagus
• **Posterior mediastinum**[Q] through the bed of the resected esophagus
• **Anterior mediastinal** in the **retrosternal**[Q] position
• **Lateral traspleural** placement behind the lung root[Q]
• Antethoracic or presternal **subcutaneous route**[Q]

- **Gastric conduit** is based on **right gastric and right gastroepiploic vessels**[Q]
- **Left colon** is based on **left colic artery** (Branch of IMA), placed in **isoperistaltic** direction.
- **Posterior mediastinal route** is **preferred (shortest route)**[Q]

■ LEIOMYOMA

LEIOMYOMA

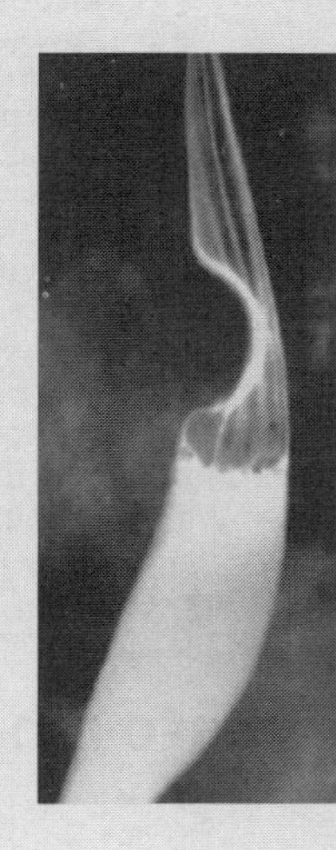

- Leiomyoma is **MC benign esophageal tumor**[Q].
- The average age **4th-5th** decades, more common in **males**[Q].
- Originate in **smooth muscle, 90%** are located in **lower two thirds** of the esophagus.
- Usually **solitary** and typically **oval**.[Q]
- They remain **intramural**, having the **bulk** of their mass **protruding toward** the **outer wall**
- The **overlying mucosa** is **freely movable** and **normal** in appearance[Q].

Clinical Features

- Many leiomyomas are **asymptomatic. Dysphagia** and **pain** are **MC symptoms**[Q].
- Location and size tend not to correlate consistently with symptoms

Diagnosis

• **Barium swallow** is **IOC** for leiomyoma (**classical, smooth, contoured, punched-out defect**)[Q]

- **Endoscopy**: Freely movable mass, which bulges into the lumen,
- **Should not be biopsied** because of an **increased chance** of **mucosal perforation** at the time of surgical **enucleation**[Q].

Treatment

- **Enucleation** is **TOC** for leiomyoma[Q].

■ DYSPHAGIA LUSORIA

DYSPHAGIA LUSORIA

- It is a **disorder of swallowing** caused **due to vascular anomalies**[Q] (**congenital abnormalities**)[Q]
- **Vascular rings** and **pulmonary slings** occur as a result of **developmental abnormalities** of the great vessels that cause **compression of the esophagus**[Q].

• **MC anomaly** is **right subclavian artery** arising from **descending aorta** and **travels behind** the **esophagus** to complete its course to the right upper extremity, may cause **significant posterior compression**[Q] of the esophagus.

Clinical Features

- Both vascular rings and pulmonary artery slings cause **dysphagia**.
- **Recurrent respiratory infections** and **difficulty in breathing** are also common symptoms.

Diagnosis

- **Barium swallow: Extrinsic anterior** or **posterior compression** of the esophagus.
- **Angiography** or **HRCT**: Identify the **anomalous anatomy**[Q].

Treatment

- In **symptomatic patients**, both vascular rings and pulmonary artery slings are **repaired**.
- Results: **Dysphagia resolves** nearly **100% of the time**[Q].

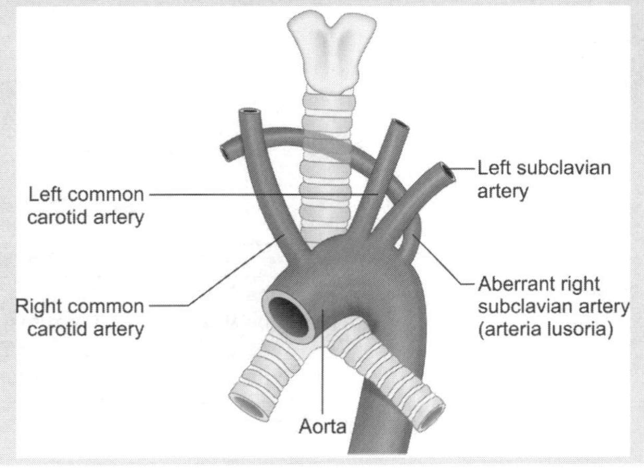

■ BOERHAAVE SYNDROME

BOERHAAVE SYNDROME

- **Spontaneous rupture** usually occurs on **left posterolateral side** of **distal esophagus** into **left pleural cavity** or just above the **gastroesophageal junction**.
- These patients are typically **male** (85%), **40 to 60 years** of age, who have a history of **recent emesis**[Q].

Clinical Features

> - **Mackler's triad**[Q] of **thoracic pain, vomiting,** and **cervical subcutaneous emphysema** is seen in spontaneous esophageal perforation.

- Thoracic perforations cause **substernal** and **epigastric pain**[Q].
- **Mediastinal emphysema** & **pleural effusions** are common, but early cervical subcutaneous emphysema is noted in only 20% or less of patients.
- **Fever & sepsis** develop with increasing contamination and inflammation of the mediastinum and pleural cavities.
- Patients with an **abdominal perforation** have **epigastric abdominal pain** that is also often referred to the **back** and **left shoulder**[Q].

Diagnosis

- **Chest X-ray: Hydropneumothorax**[Q]
- The **diagnosis** is **confirmed with** a **contrast esophagogram**[Q]. This technique will demonstrate extravasation in 90% of patients.

> - **Gastrografin (water soluble)** is **preferred**[Q] to prevent extravasation of barium into the mediastinum or pleura. **If no leak** is seen, a **barium study** should follow.

- **Chest CT: Mediastinal air** and **fluid** at the site of perforation.
- **Endoscopy:** If the **esophagogram** is **negative** or if **operative intervention** is planned.

Treatment

- Appropriate **resuscitation**, secured **airway**, **IV fluids** and **broad-spectrum antibiotics** are started immediately, and the patient is monitored in an ICU.

Within 24 Hours	After 24 Hours
• **Golden period** for **primary closure** of an esophageal perforation is within the **first 24 hours**[Q]. • Within 24 hours of perforation, **inflammation** is generally **minimal**, and **primary surgical repair** is recommended[Q]. • Mortality rate: **8-20%**	• **Debridement** of devitalized tissue + **Esophageal diversion** or **resection** + Creation of an **esophagostomy** + **Wide drainage** + **feeding jejunostomy**[Q] • Mortality rate: **>50%**[Q]

■ TRACHEO-ESOPHAGEAL FISTULA

TRACHEOESOPHAGEAL FISTULA

- TEF is an **abnormal communication** (fistula) between the **esophagus** and **trachea**[Q].
- TEF is usually **associated with esophageal atresia**, however it **may also exist without atresia**[Q].
- **MC anomaly** associated with TEF is **CVS (VSD)**[Q].

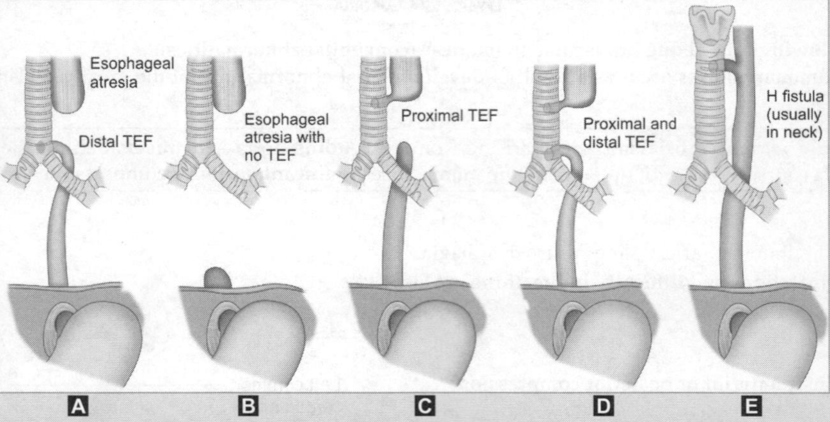

Classification of TEF
• **Type A:** Atresia only (6%)
• **Type B:** Atresia with proximal TEF (2%)
• **Type C: Atresia with distal TEF (85%): Most common**[Q]
• **Type D:** Atresia with both proximal and distal TEF (rare)
• **Type E:** TEF only (1%)

Contd…

Contd…

Clinical Features

- The diagnosis of EA is entertained in an **infant with excessive salivation** along with **coughing** or **choking during** the **first oral feeding**.
- A **maternal history** of **polyhydramnios** is often present.
- The newborn baby with atresia **regurgitates all of its first** and **subsequent feeds**[Q].
- **Saliva pours continuously** from its mouth[Q].
- Repeated episodes of **coughing, choking** and **cyanosis**[Q] occur on feeding in TEF.

Associated Anomalies

• **MC anomaly** associated with TEF is **CVS** (**VSD**).
• Esophageal atresia may occur as part of **VACTERL**[Q] group of anomalies:
  – **V**: Vertebral body segmentation defects[Q]
  – **A**: Anal atresia[Q]
  – **C**: **Cardiovascular** (PDA, **VSD**)[Q]
  – **TE**: Tracheoesophageal fistula[Q]
  – **R**: Renal (unilateral renal agenesis)[Q]
  – **L**: Limb anomalies (radial ray hypoplasia)[Q]

Diagnosis

- The **inability to pass** a NG **into** the **stomach** is a **cardinal feature** for the **diagnosis of EA**.
- If gas is present in the GIT below the **diaphragm**, an **associated TEF is confirmed**
- **Inability to pass a NG tube** with **absent radiographic evidence** for **gastrointestinal gas** is **virtually diagnostic** of an **isolated EA without TEF**.
- For **H-type: Tracheobronchoscopy + Endoscopy** should be performed

Treatment

- **Surgical repair** with **tension free esophageal anastomosis**

Outcome

- The mortality in TEF is **directly related to the associated anomalies**, particularly **cardiac defects** and **chromosomal abnormalities**[Q].

■ SCHATZKI'S RINGS

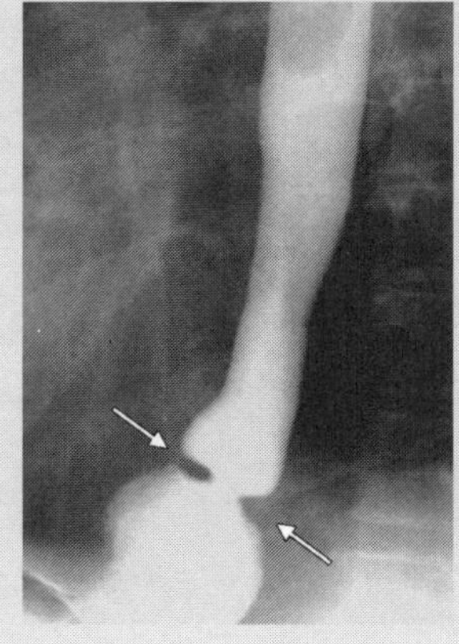

Schatzki's Rings

- Consists of a **concentric symmetric narrowing** representing an area of **restricted distensibility** of the **lower esophagus**[Q].

> • **Lying** precisely at the **squamocolumnar mucosal GEJ**, involves **mucosa** and **submucosa**[Q]

- It consists of **esophageal mucosa above** and **gastric mucosa below**.
- It is **often accompanied** by a **small hiatal hernia**

Clinical Features

- **Most patients** with Schatzki's rings present with **dysphagia**.
- The **dysphagia** is usually to **solid foods only** and comes on **abruptly** with nearly complete obstruction.

> • **Episodic aphagia: Intermittent obstruction** of the nondistensible ring by **large pieces of meat**[Q].

Diagnosis

- Diagnosis of a Schatzki's ring is made with a **barium swallow**[Q].
- **Schtazki ring: Type 'B' ring is located at GE junction**[Q]

Treatment

- Asymptomatic patients **incidentally found** to have a Schatzki's ring **require no treatment**.
- Best form of treatment of a **symptomatic Schatzki's ring** without reflux: **Esophageal dilation** for relief of the obstructive symptoms.
- Ring with **proven reflux** and mechanically defective sphincter: **Antireflux procedure**
- **Surgical excision** is **not indicated**, can cause **devastating esophageal strictures**.

■ ANATOMY AND PHYSIOLOGY OF ESOPHAGUS

ANATOMY AND PHYSIOLOGY OF ESOPHAGUS

- Narrowest tube of GIT; Narrowest region of esophagus: Cricopharynx (15 mm diameter)
- Extent: C6-T11[Q]; Length: 25-30 cm[Q]
- Cervical esophagus begins as a **midline structure** that **deviates slightly** to **left**[Q] of trachea as it passes through the neck into thoracic inlet.
- At the level of **carina**, it **deviates to right** to accommodate the arch of aorta.
- It then winds its way back under the left main-stem bronchus and **remains slightly deviated to left** as it **enters the diaphragm** through the esophageal hiatus[Q].
- **Immediately before entering** the abdomen, esophagus is pushed anteriorly by **descending thoracic aorta**[Q].

> - **Only Auerbach plexus** is present in **esophagus (Meissner's plexus is absent)**[Q].
> - **Lymphatic channels** in the **lamina propria** are the anatomic features **unique** to the esophagus[Q].

- Dense submucosal lymphatic plexus facilitates **early dissemination** of esophageal **malignancies**. In submucosa elastic fibers & collagen combine to make this the **strongest esophageal layer**. Submucosal glands of **mixed type** are the **characteristic** of the esophagus[Q].

> - **Lacks** a **serosal layer**[Q]; **Strongest Cayer: submucosa**[Q]
> - **Lining:** Lined by **stratified, non-keratinized squamous epithelium**[Q]

- Muscles:
    - Upper cervical region- Stratified muscle[Q]
    - Middle- Gradual transition from stratified to smooth muscle[Q]
    - Lower- Smooth muscle[Q]

Upper Esophageal Sphincter	Lower Esophageal Sphincter
• **Length: 4-5 cm**[Q] • **Pressure: 60 mm Hg**[Q] • Comprises **three skeletal muscle groups**: Distal portion of **inferior** pharyngeal **constrictor**, cricopharyngeus and circular muscle of **proximal esophagus**[Q]	• **Length: 5 cm**[Q] • **Abdominal length: 2 cm**[Q] • **Pressure: 6-26 mm Hg**[Q]

Multiple Choice Questions

■ CONGENITAL DIAPHRAGMATIC HERNIA

1. **All are true about Bochdalek hernia except:** *(GB Pant 2011)*
   a. Posterolateral
   b. Left side
   c. Present in second decade
   d. Congenital

2. **Most common organ that herniates in Morgagni's hernia:**
   a. Spleen
   b. Liver *(MHSSMCET 2009)*
   c. Stomach
   d. Transverse colon

3. **Which of the following is contraindication for Bag and mask ventilation?** *(AIIMS June 2000)*
   a. Septicemia
   b. Tracheoesophageal fistula
   c. Meconium aspiration
   d. Diaphragmatic hernia

4. **Not true about Bochdalek hernia:**
   a. Seen on right side *(Recent Question 2015, AIIMS Nov 97)*
   b. Associated with hypoplasia of lung
   c. Associated with hiatus hernia
   d. Pericardial cyst is a differential diagnosis

5. **Most common site of Morgagni hernia:** *(AIIMS Nov 2006)*
   a. Right anterior
   b. Right posterior
   c. Left anterior
   d. Left posterior

6. **Most common content of Morgagni foramen:** *(Recent Question 2017)*
   a. Stomach
   b. Small intestine
   c. Transverse colon
   d. Spleen

7. **Most common diaphragmatic hernia in a newborn infant:** *(Recent Question 2017)*
   a. Bochdalek
   b. Morgagni
   c. Paraesophageal type I
   d. Paraesophageal type III

■ HIATUS HERNIA

8. **The most common complication seen in hiatus hernia is:** *(DNB, 2011, All India 2005)*
   a. Esophagitis
   b. Aspiration pneumonitis
   c. Volvulus
   d. Esophageal stricture

9. **For hiatal hernia, investigation of choice is:**
   a. Barium meal follow through *(DPG 2006, DPG 2005)*
   b. Barium meal upper GI
   c. Barium meal upper GI in Trendelenburg position
   d. Barium meal double contrast

10. **Fundoplication is used in treatment of:** *(DNB 2012, MHPGMCET 2002)*
    a. Hiatus hernia
    b. Achalasia cardia
    c. CHPS
    d. CA esophagus

11. **Retrocardiac lucency with air fluid level is seen in:**
    a. Hiatus hernia *(Recent Question 2013)*
    b. Distal end esophageal obstruction
    c. Eventration of diaphragm
    d. None

■ REFLUX ESOPHAGITIS

12. **LES pressure is decreased by all except:** *(GB Pant 2011)*
    a. Alcohol
    b. Protein
    c. Fat
    d. Peppermint

13. **The lower esophageal sphincter tone (pressure) is increased by:** *(COMEDK 2005)*
    a. Glucagon
    b. Gastrin
    c. Emptying of the stomach
    d. Chocolate

14. **The gold standard for diagnosis of gastroesophageal reflux disease (GERD) is:**
    (Recent Question 2017, MHCET 2016, JIPMER 2014, Orissa 2011, COMEDK 2008, 2007, PGI June 1998)
    a. Barium swallow
    b. Endoscopy
    c. 24-hours pH monitoring
    d. Esophageal manometry

15. **Which of the following is the earliest indicator of pathological gastroesophageal reflux in infants (GERD)?** *(All India 2011)*
    a. Respiratory symptoms
    b. Postprandial regurgitation
    c. Upper GI bleed
    d. Stricture esophagus

16. **Best test to diagnose gastroesophageal reflux disease and quantify acid output is:** *(AIIMS May 2011, Nov 2008)*
    a. Esophagogram
    b. Endoscopy
    c. Manometry
    d. 24-hours pH monitoring

17. **Most important pathophysiological cause of GERD is:**
    a. Hiatus hernia *(AIIMS May 2012)*
    b. Transient LES relaxation
    c. LES hypotension
    d. Inadequate esophageal clearance

18. **Most common cause of esophagitis is:** *(AIIMS May 2009)*
    a. Alcohol
    b. Smoking
    c. Spicy and hot food
    d. Esophageal reflux

■ ACHALASIA CARDIA

19. **All of the following are true about achalasia cardia except:** *(Recent Question 2017)*
    a. Achalasia means absence of relaxation
    b. Heller's myotomy is the treatment choice
    c. It is premalignant condition
    d. Caused by selective loss of stimulatory myenteric neurons

20. **A female patient has dysphagia, intermittent epigastric pain. On endoscopy, esophagus was dilated above and narrow at the bottom. Treatment is:** *(AIIMS May 2012)*
    a. PPI
    b. Esophagectomy
    c. Dilatation
    d. Heller's cardiomyotomy

21. **Hellers operation is done for:**
    (Recent Question 2018, Recent Question 2016, 2014, DNB 2013, 2012)
    a. Achalasia cardia
    b. Hiatus hernia
    c. Diaphragmatic
    d. Reflux esophagitis

22. **A young patient presents with history of dysphagia more to liquid than solids. The first investigation you will do is:** *(AIIMS June 2003)*
    a. Barium swallow
    b. Esophagoscopy
    c. Ultrasound of the chest
    d. CT scan of the chest

23. **Treatment for achalasia associated with high rate of recurrence:** *(All India 2002)*
    a. Pneumatic dilatation
    b. Laparoscopic myotomy
    c. Open surgical myotomy
    d. Botulinum toxin

24. Bird's beak appearance is seen in:
    (Recent Question 2017, Recent Question 2015, J and K 2001)
    a. Volvulus
    b. Intussusception
    c. Achalasia
    d. Ulcerative colitis

■ ESOPHAGEAL MOTILITY DISORDERS

25. Corkscrew esophagus is seen in which of the following conditions? *(Recent Question 2017, Recent Question 2015, Bihar PG 2014, NEET 2013, DNB 2008, 2005, 2001)*
    a. Carcinoma esophagus
    b. Scleroderma
    c. Achalasia cardia
    d. Diffuse esophageal spasm

26. This characteristic appearance is seen on barium swallow in:
    (Recent Question 2016)
    a. Achalasia cardia
    b. Nutcrackers esophagus
    c. Diffuse esophageal spasm
    d. Hypertensive LES

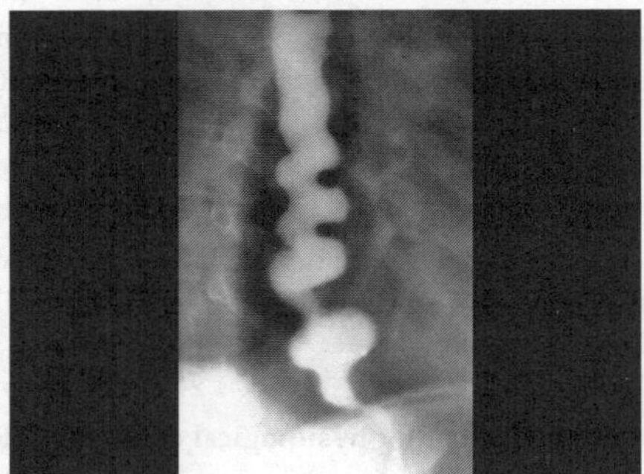

27. Most common motility disorder leading to dysphagia:
    (JIPMER 2010)
    a. Nut cracker esophagus
    b. Esophageal web
    c. Diffuse esophageal spasm
    d. Achalasia cardia

■ ZENKER'S DIVERTICULUM

28. Best investigation for Zenker's diverticulum is:
    (Recent Question 2014, AIIMS Nov 2011, AIIMS GIS Dec 2010)
    a. Barium swallow
    b. Endoscopy
    c. CECT
    d. EUS

29. What is the location of Killian dehiscence? *(MCI June 2019)*
    a. Below superior constrictor
    b. Below inferior constrictor
    c. Below cricopharyngeal muscle
    d. Below upper 1/3rd of smooth muscle of esophagus

30. True statement about Zenker's diverticulum:
    a. Congenital *(NEET Pattern, GB Pant 2011)*
    b. Feeling of obstruction in esophagus
    c. Traction diverticulum
    d. Not present with recurrent aspiration pneumonitis

31. A 50-year-old male Raju, presents with occasional dysphagia for solids, regurgitation of food and foul smelling breath. Probable diagnosis is: *(Recent Question 2016, AIIMS June 99)*
    a. Achalasia cardia
    b. Zenker's diverticulum
    c. CA esophagus
    d. Diabetic gastroparesis

32. Commonest complication of Zenker's diverticulum is:
    (AIIMS Nov 96)
    a. Dysphonia
    b. Gastroesophageal reflux
    c. Lung abscess
    d. Perforation

33. Dohlman's procedure is used in: *(Recent Question 2013)*
    a. Rectal prolapsed
    b. Esophageal achalasia
    c. CA esophagus
    d. Zenker's diverticulum

34. Dohlman surgery in Zenker's diverticulum is:
    a. Endoscopic stapling of septum *(Recent Question 2019)*
    b. Endoscopic suturing of pouch
    c. Resection of pouch
    d. Laser excision

■ ESOPHAGEAL DIVERTICULA

35. Which of the following is a true diverticulum of esophagus?
    (AIIMS Nov 2016)
    a. Zenker's diverticulum
    b. Meckel's diverticulum
    c. Epiphrenic diverticulum
    d. Parabronchial diverticulum

■ PLUMMER–VINSON SYNDROME

36. In Plummer–Vinson syndrome, obstruction is due to:
    (DPG 2006)
    a. Esophageal dysmotility
    b. Esophageal stenosis
    c. Postcricoid webs
    d. None of the above

37. All are features of Plummer-Vinson syndrome except:
    (COMEDK 2008)
    a. Esophageal web
    b. Iron deficiency
    c. Achalasia cardia
    d. Dysphagia

■ BARRETT'S ESOPHAGUS

38. All of the following are correct about Barrett's esophagus except: *(Recent Question 2019)*
    a. Predisposes to adenocarcinoma
    b. Columnar to squamous metaplasia
    c. Associated with GERD
    d. Acquired condition

39. Barrett's esophagus is diagnosed by:
    (AIIMS May 2012, Nov 2007, DNB 2008)
    a. Squamous metaplasia
    b. Intestinal metaplasia
    c. Squamous dysplasia
    d. Intestinal dysplasia

40. What is the most probable diagnosis on the basis of given endoscopy image? *(Recent Question 2016)*
    a. GAVE
    b. Schatzki ring
    c. Barrett's esophagus
    d. Esophageal varices

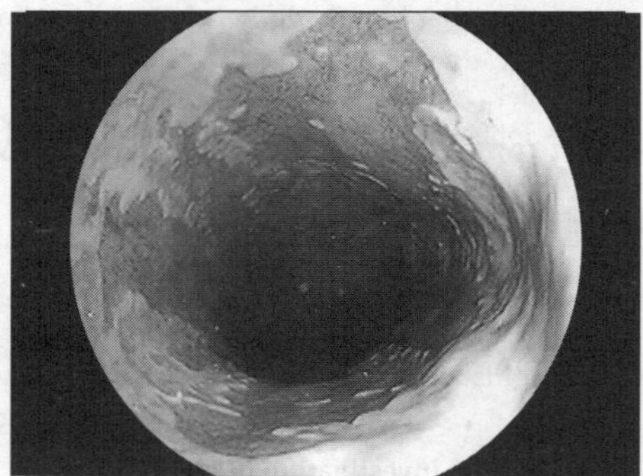

■ CARCINOMA ESOPHAGUS PREDISPOSING FACTORS

41. All are the predisposing factors for carcinoma esophagus except: *(COMEDK 2011)*
    a. Achalasia
    b. Paterson Brown Kelly Syndrome
    c. Zenker's diverticulum
    d. Ectodermal dysplasia

42. The adenocarcinoma of esophagus develops in:
    (Recent Question 2017, Bihar PG 2014, COMEDK 2014, All India 2002, 98)
    a. Barrett's esophagus
    b. Long standing achalasia
    c. Corrosive stricture
    d. Alcohol abuse

43. Not a predisposing factor for carcinoma esophagus:
    (AIIMS May 2009)
    a. Diverticula
    b. Human papilloma virus
    c. Mediastinal fibrosis
    d. Caustic ingestion

44. **Risk factor for adenocarcinoma of esophagus:** *(KGMC 2011)*
    a. Barrett's esophagus b. Corrosive injury
    c. Achalasia cardia d. All of the above

45. **Risk factors of carcinoma esophagus are all except:**
    (MCI Dec 2019)
    a. GERD b. Betel chewing
    c. Caustic injury d. Spicy food

■ CA ESOPHAGUS CLINICAL FEATURES, DIAGNOSIS AND TREATMENT

46. **T-staging of esophagus is best done by:**
    (AIIMS GIS Dec 2011, DNB 2002)
    a. EUS b. CT
    c. MRI d. PET

47. **Which of the following is not done in carcinoma esophagus?**
    (MCI Dec 2018)
    a. Biopsy b. 24-hours pH monitoring
    c. CT chest d. PET Scan

48. **Barium esophagogram findings in carcinoma esophagus are all except:** *(UPPG 2009)*
    a. Rat-tail deformity b. Pencil tip appearance
    c. Apple-core appearance d. Filling defect

49. **A 60-year-old chronic smoker presented with progressive dysphagia. Barium swallow was done, what is the name of sign?** *(Recent Question 2017)*
    a. Bird beak appearance b. Pencil tip appearance
    c. Apple core appearance d. Rat tail appearance

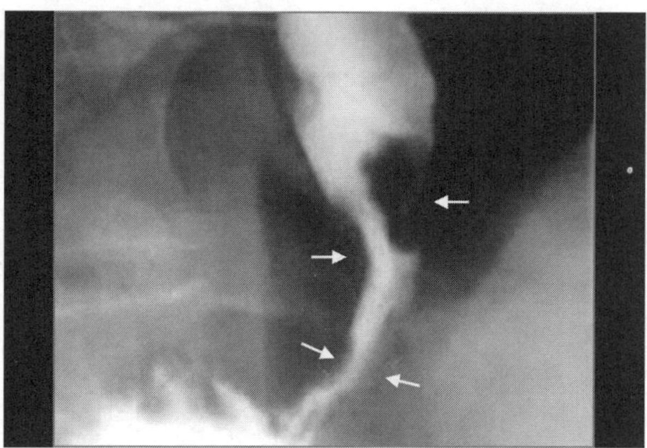

50. **MC site of CA esophagus is:**
    (MCI Nov 2017, Recent Question 2015, AIIMS Feb 2007)
    a. Middle 1/3rd b. Upper 1/3rd
    c. Lower 1/3rd d. Lower end of esophagus

51. **The commonest site of carcinoma esophagus in India is:**
    (AIIMS Nov 2003)
    a. Upper 1/3rd b. Middle 1/3rd
    c. Lower 1/3rd d. GE junction

52. **Treatment of choice for CA esophagus:** *(PGI SS Dec 2009)*
    a. Esophagectomy b. External radiotherapy
    c. Internal radiotherapy d. Chemotherapy

53. **Stage of CA esophagus is best decided by:** *(PGI SS June 2009)*
    a. Depth of tumor b. Size of tumor
    c. Histopathological grade d. Age of the patient

54. **Treatment of advanced esophageal cancer is:** *(DNB 2006)*
    a. Chemoradiation only
    b. Curative en-bloc resection
    c. Chemoradiation followed by curative enbloc resection
    d. Chemoradiation followed by palliative enbloc resection

55. **False statements about carcinoma esophagus are all of the following except:** *(MCI March 2009)*
    a. Most common in lower third
    b. Histologically, adenocarcinoma only
    c. Unrelated to tobacco chewing
    d. It is more common in females

56. **In Esophageal cancer prognosis is best determined by:**
    (AIIMS May 2015)
    a. Cellular differentiation b. Age of patient
    c. T stage d. Length of involvement

■ ESOPHAGECTOMY

57. **Conduit in gastric pull up is based on:**
    (AIIMS GIS Dec 2011, May 2008)
    a. Right gastric and right gastroepiploic artery
    b. Right gastric and left gastroepiploic artery
    c. Left gastric and right gastroepiploic artery
    d. Left gastric and left gastroepiploic artery

58. **Which is the best substitute for esophagus?**
    (MHSSMCET 2005, MP 99, All India 96, PGI Dec 95)
    a. Stomach b. Jejunum
    c. Left sided colon d. Right sided colon

59. **Ivor Lewis operation is the treatment of choice for cancer involving .... esophagus:** *(MHSSMCET 2009)*
    a. Upper 1/3rd b. Middle 1/3rd
    c. Lower 1/3rd d. Entire esophagus

60. **Which of the following surgical approach was first described by Orringer for the management of carcinoma esophagus?**
    (J amd K 2005)
    a. Transhiatal b. Thoracoscopic
    c. Left thoracoabdominal d. Right thoracoabdominal

61. **The ideal replacement for the esophagus after esophagectomy is:** *(COMEDK 2010)*
    a. Stomach b. Jejunum
    c. Colon d. Synthetic stent

■ LEIOMYOMA

62. **Commonest benign tumor of the esophagus:**
    (JIPMER 2014, DPG 2009 Feb)
    a. Leiomyoma b. Papilloma
    c. Adenoma d. Hemangioma

63. **This characteristic appearance is seen on barium swallow in:**
    (Recent Question 2017)
    a. Achalasia cardia b. Carcinoma esophagus
    c. Leiomyoma d. Diffuse esophageal spasm

■ DYSPHAGIA

64. **Odynophagia occurs in:** *(AIIMS GIS Dec 2011, PGI June 96)*
    a. Achalasia b. Herpes esophagitis
    c. Monilial esophagitis d. Barrett's esophagus

65. A 40-year-old female patient presented with dysphagia to both liquids and solids and regurgitation for 3 months. The dysphagia was non-progressive. What is the most likely diagnosis?   *(AIIMS May 2006)*
    a. Carcinoma of the esophagus
    b. Lower esophageal mucosal ring
    c. Achalasia cardia
    d. Reflux esophagitis with esophageal stricture

■ DYSPHAGIA LUSORIA

66. Dysphagia lusoria is due to:
                    (Recent Question 2016, 2014, AIIMS Nov 2003)
    a. Esophageal diverticulum
    b. Aneurysm of aorta   c. Esophageal web
    d. Compression by aberrant blood vessel

67. All are true about dysphagia lusoria except: *(DPG 2008)*
    a. Right aortic arch
    b. Vascular ring
    c. Due to aberrant subclavian artery causing pressure on esophagus
    d. Acquired in later life

■ ESOPHAGEAL PERFORATION AND INJURY

68. Mackler's triad includes: *(PGI Nov 2009)*
    a. Vomiting   b. Subcutaneous emphysema
    c. Lower thoracic pain   d. Peripheral cyanosis
    e. Pleural effusion

69. Which is most common site for iatrogenic esophageal perforation? *(Recent Question 2017, Recent Question 2014, DNB 2013, 2012, AIIMS Nov 97)*
    a. Abdominal portion   b. Cervical portion
    c. Above arch of aorta   d. Below arch of aorta

70. Commonest cause of esophageal perforation is:
    a. Acid ingestion   b. Hyperemesis
    c. Instrumentation   d. Carcinoma infiltrating

71. In majority of patients with esophageal leaks in thoracic cavity of less than 12 hours duration, the treatment of choice is:
    a. Primary closure, drainage and antibiotics   *(UPSC 97)*
    b. Early esophagogastrostomy
    c. Exclusion and diversion of continuity
    d. Total esophagectomy and gastric pull up

72. In esophageal perforation all are seen except: *(UPPG 2000)*
    a. Pain   b. Bradycardia
    c. Fever   d. Hypotension

73. Boerhaave's syndrome is due to:
                    (Recent Question 2016, DNB 2012, UPPG 2007)
    a. Drug induced esophagus perforation
    b. Corrosive injury
    c. Spontaneous perforation
    d. Gastroesophageal reflux disease

74. Most common site a spontaneous rupture of esophagus is:
    a. Cricopharyngeal junction   *(Recent Question 2017, DNB 2009)*
    b. Cardioesophageal junction
    c. Mid esophagus
    d. After the crossing of arch of aorta

75. Investigation of choice for esophageal rupture is?
    a. Dynamic MRI   *(DNB 2014)*
    b. Rigid esophagoscopy
    c. Barium contrast swallow
    d. Water soluble low molecular weight contrast swallow

76. Which of the following is true about Boerhaave's syndrome?
    a. May present with peritonitis   *(Recent Question 2017)*
    b. Forceful vomiting against open glottis
    c. Upper third esophagus location
    d. Most patients are managed by conservative management

77. A 28-years-old alcoholic patient walks to hospital with the complaints of binge vomiting, chest pain, fever and pneumomediastinum. The most probable diagnosis is:
                                      (MCI Dec 2019)
    a. Boerhaave's syndrome   b. Tension pneumothorax
    c. Peptic ulcer perforation d. Mallory-Weiss tear

■ TRACHEOESOPHAGEAL FISTULA

78. Esophageal atresia is most commonly associated with:
    a. Respiratory anomalies   b. Anorectal malformations
    c. Genitourinary   d. CVS   *(KGMC 2011)*

79. Which is the first investigation to be done in case of neonate presenting with frothiness in mouth and dyspnoea?
                                      (MCI June 2019)
    a. Bronchoscopy with injection of methylene blue
    b. NG tube insertion and CXR to check position of tube
    c. CT chest   d. Endoscopy

80. The most common type of tracheoesophageal fistula is:
    (Recent Question 2017, Recent Question 2014, MAHE 2008, 2007)
    a. Esophageal atresia without tracheoesophageal fistula
    b. Esophageal atresia with proximal tracheoesophageal fistula
    c. Esophageal atresia with distal tracheoesophageal fistula
    d. Esophageal atresia with proximal and distal tracheo-esophageal fistula

■ ESOPHAGEAL RINGS AND WEBS

81. Schatzki's ring is: *(PGI Dec 98)*
    a. Mucosal ring at squamocolumnar junction
    b. Muscular ring   c. Dysphagia is the symptom
    d. Inflammatory stricture

82. What is the diagnosis based on the given barium swallow findings?

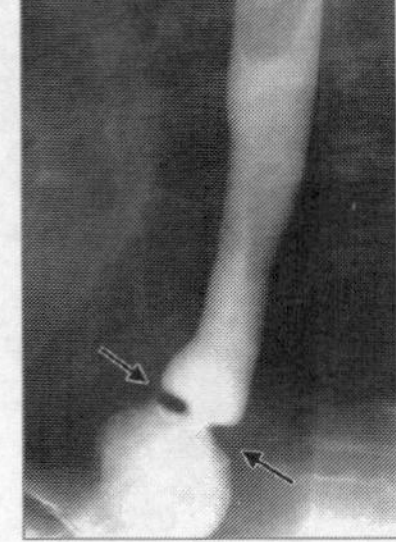

    a. Esophageal web   b. Carcinoma esophagus
    c. Schatzki ring   d. Leiomyoma

83. Schatzki ring is seen at: *(UPPG 2009)*
    a. Mid-esophagus   b. Lower-esophagus
    c. Junction of lower esophagus
    d. None

84. Schatzki ring: *(DNB 2007, MHSSMCET 2007)*
    a. Can be treated by PPI alone
    b. Occurs at GE junction
    c. Type A ring   d. Type C ring

85. What is the most probable diagnosis on the basis of given endoscopy image?   *(Recent Question 2016)*
    a. GAVE   b. Schatzki ring
    c. Barrett's esophagus   d. Esophageal varices

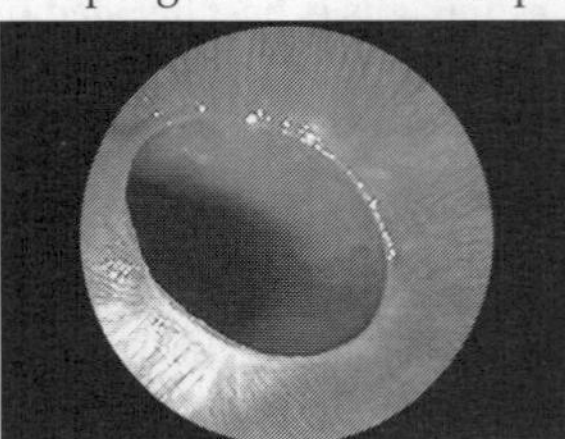

■ FOREIGN BODY

86. A foreign body usually gets arrested in which part of esophagus? *(DNB 2003)*
   a. Cardiac part of the esophagus
   b. In the middle third of the esophagus
   c. Below the cricopharynx
   d. Above the cricopharynx

87. A child was brought by his mother to the emergency with history of accidental swallowing of coin. Chest X-ray is given below. What is the location of foreign body in this child?
   (Recent Question 2016)
   a. Esophagus   b. Trachea
   c. Bronchus   d. None of the above

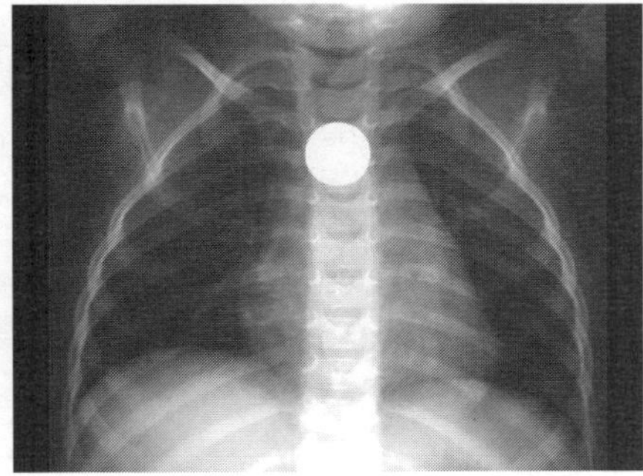

■ ESOPHAGUS: ANATOMY AND PHYSIOLOGY

88. Non-progressive contraction of esophagus are:
   (AIIMS May 2011, All India 2009)
   a. Primary   b. Secondary
   c. Tertiary   d. Quaternary

89. Distance between upper incisors and gastroesophageal junction is: *(DPG 97)*
   a. 25 cm   b. 30 cm
   c. 40 cm   d. 60 cm

90. Normal LES pressure: *(Recent Question 2017)*
   a. 6–26 mm Hg   b. 30–50 mm Hg
   c. 50–60 mm Hg   d. 60–70 mm Hg

91. Dysphagia in esophagus means which invasion?
   (Recent Question 2017)
   a. Mucosal   b. Submucosal
   c. Transmural d. Node

■ DIAPHRAGM

92. Diagnosis of traumatic rupture of diaphragm is made by:
   a. Laparoscopy *(PGI June 2007)*
   b. Chest X-ray
   c. Diagnostic peritoneal lavage
   d. CT

93. Which of the following incisions is taken for diaphragmatic surgery? *(AIIMS May 2014)*
   a. Transverse   b. Circumferential
   c. Vertical   d. Radial

■ MISCELLANEOUS

94. 'Pencil tip' deformity is seen in: *(PGI June 95)*
   a. Carcinoma esophagus   b. Achalasia cardia
   c. Barrett's esophagus   d. None of the above

95. Hamman's sign is seen with: *(MHPGMCET 2006)*
   a. Acute pericarditis   b. Aortic dissection
   c. Tracheal compression   d. Esophageal perforation

96. Feline esophagus is: *(Recent Question 2018)*
   a. Eosinophilic esophagitis
   b. GERD
   c. Radiation esophagitis
   d. Chemotherapy induced esophagitis

97. Serpiginous ulcers in lower esophagus are seen in:
   (Recent Question 2019)

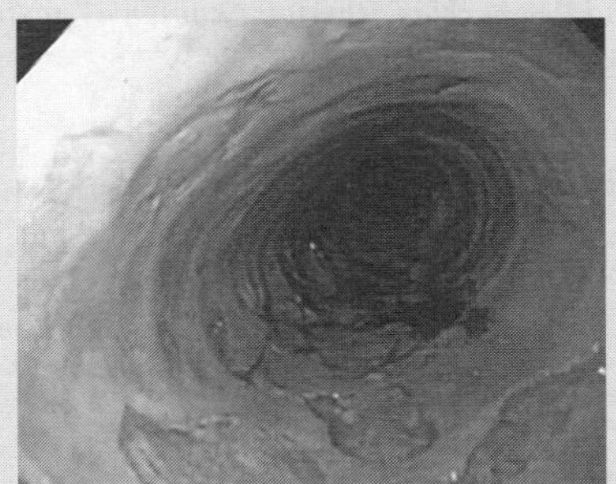

   a. CMV esophagitis   b. Candida esophagitis
   c. Corrosive esophagitis d. Pill induced esophagitis

98. Small punched out lesions on endoscopy in lower esophagus in the immunocompromised patients is seen in:
   (Recent Question 2019)

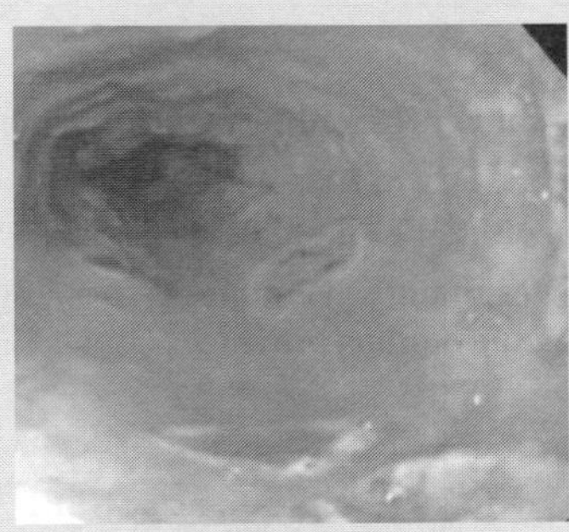

   a. CMV esophagitis   b. Candida esophagitis
   c. Corrosive esophagitis d. Herpes simplex esophagitis

Explanations

■ CONGENITAL DIAPHRAGMATIC HERNIA

1. Ans. c. Present in second decade

2. Ans. d. Transverse colon *(Ref: Sabiston 20/e p1863-1864; Schwartz 11/e p1712, 9/e p1416-1418; Bailey 27/e p938)*

3. Ans. d. Diaphragmatic hernia   4.   Ans. a. Seen on right side

5. Ans. a. Right anterior

6. Ans. c. Transverse colon *(Ref: Sabiston 20/e p1863; Bailey 27/e p938)*

> *"The foramen of Morgagni: A hernia in the anterior part of the diaphragm with a defect between the sternal and costal attachments. The most commonly involved viscus is the transverse colon."*-Bailey 27/e p938

7. Ans. a. Bochdalek *(Ref: Shackelford 7/e p506; Sabiston 20/e p1863; Schwartz 11/e p1712, 10/e p1604)*

> *"Bochdalek hernias otherwise known as posterolateral hernias, make up 85% of congenital hernias. They occur on the left side 80% of the time."*- Shackelford 7/e p506

■ HIATUS HERNIA

8. Ans. a. Esophagitis

9. Ans. c. Barium meal upper GI in Trendelenburg position *(Ref: Bailey 27/e p1084)*

> ### BARIUM STUDIES IN HIATAL HERNIA
>
> - **To facilitate visualization** of the **hernia**, the **patient** may **be placed** in a **Trendelenburg position during** studies of **barium swallowing**^{Q}.

10. Ans. a. Hiatus hernia   11.   Ans. a. Hiatus hernia

■ REFLUX ESOPHAGITIS

12. Ans. b. Protein *(Ref: Shackelford 7/e p56)*   13.   Ans. b. Gastrin

14. Ans. c. 24-hours pH monitoring *(Ref: Sabiston 20/e p1043-1048; Schwartz 11/e p1032, 10/e p964-980; Bailey 27/e p1077; Shackelford 7/e p174-180, 215-237)*

15. Ans. a. Respiratory symptoms *(Ref: Nelson 20/e p1791)*

   Recurrent respiratory symptoms (Wheezing, stridor, chronic cough, apnea, aspiration) are the **earliest indicators** of pathological reflux **among the options provided.**

> ### GERD IN INFANTS
>
> - **Most frequent complications** of **GERD** in **infants** are **failure to thrive** and **recurrent pulmonary symptoms**^{Q}.
> - **Regurgitation alone does not indicate pathological reflux.**
> - Presence of **upper GI bleed** is an **uncommon marker** for pathological reflux or esophagitis.
> - Presence of **stricture esophagus** is an **uncommon** and **late complication** of untreated pathological GERD.
> - **Recurrent pulmonary symptoms** are **frequent** and **early indicators** of **pathological GERD**^{Q}.

16. Ans. d. 24-hours pH monitoring

17. Ans. b. Transient LES relaxation *(Ref: Harrison 19/e p1906)*

   - Harrison says **"Transient LES relaxations account for** at least **90%** of **reflux** in **normal subjects** or **GERD patients** without hiatus hernia^Q."

18. Ans. d. Esophageal reflux

■ ACHALASIA CARDIA

19. Ans. d. Caused by selective loss of stimulatory myenteric neurons *(Ref: Sabiston 20/e p1017; Schwartz 11/e p1060, 10/e p990; Bailey 27/e p1095-1097)*

20. Ans. d. Heller's cardiomyotomy   21.   Ans. a. Achalasia cardia

22. **Ans. a.** Barium swallow   23. **Ans. d.** Botulinum toxin   25. **Ans. a.** Volvulus, **c.** Achalasia

■ ESOPHAGEAL MOTILITY DISORDERS

26. **Ans. d.** Diffuse esophagus spasm *(Ref: Sabiston 20/e p1015-1016; Schwartz 11/e p1060, 10/e p992; Bailey 27/e p1099; Shackelford 7/e p142-143)*

27. **Ans. c.** Diffuse esophageal spasm *(Ref: Sabiston 20/e p1015-1016; Schwartz 11/e p1060, 10/e p992; Bailey 27/e p1099; Shackelford 7/e p142-143)*

> • **Corkscrew** or **rosary-bead** esophagus, **segmental spasm** or **pseudodiverticulosis** appearance[Q] **is characteristic of diffuse esophageal spasm.**

28. **Ans. d.** Achalasia cardia

■ ZENKER'S DIVERTICULUM

29. **Ans. a.** Barium swallow *(Ref: Sabiston 20/e p1019-1020; Schwartz 11/e p1053, 10/e p989; Bailey 27/e p1101; Shackelford 7/e p336-346)*

24. **Ans. b.** Below inferior constrictor *(Ref: Bailey 27/e p1101)*

30. **Ans. b.** Feeling of obstruction in esophagus   31. **Ans. b.** Zenker's diverticulum

32. **Ans. c.** Lung abscess   33. **Ans. d.** Zenker's diverticulum

34. **Ans. a.** Endoscopic stapling of septum *(Ref: Sabiston 20/e p1020)*

> • *"An alternative to open surgical repair is the endoscopic* **Dohlman procedure,** *which has become more popular.* **Endoscopic division of the common wall between the esophagus and diverticulum using a laser, electrocautery, or stapler device has been similarly successful. Because of the configuration of the inline stapling device,** *this approach has been advocated for larger diverticula."*
> *-Sabiston 20/e p1020*

■ ESOPHAGEAL DIVERTICULA

35. **Ans. d.** Parabronchial diverticulum

■ PLUMMER–VINSON SYNDROME

36. **Ans. c.** Postcricoid webs   37. **Ans. c.** Achalasia cardia

■ BARRETT'S ESOPHAGUS

38. **Ans. b.** Columnar to squamous metaplasia *(Ref: Schwartz 11/e p1035, 10/e p967; Sabiston 20/e p1050; Bailey 27/e p1081)*

39. **Ans. b.** Intestinal metaplasia

40. **Ans. c.** Barrett's esophagus *(Ref: Sabiston 20/e p1050; Schwartz 11/e p1035, 10/e p967; Bailey 27/e p1081; Shackelford 7/e p285, 294)*

■ CARCINOMA ESOPHAGUS PREDISPOSING FACTORS

41. **Ans. d.** Ectodermal dysplasia *(Ref: Sabiston 20/e p1027-1028; Schwartz 11/e p1068, 10/e p1003-1014; Bailey 27/e p1085; Shackelford 7/e p375-380)*

42. **Ans. a.** Barrett's esophagus   43. **Ans. c.** Mediastinal fibrosis

44. **Ans. a.** Barrett's esophagus

45. **Ans. b.** Betel chewing *(Ref: Sabiston 20/e p1027-1028; Schwartz 11/e p1068; Bailey 27/e p1085)*

■ CA ESOPHAGUS CLINICAL FEATURES, DIAGNOSIS AND TREATMENT

46. **Ans. a.** EUS *(Ref: Shackelford 7/e p397)*

47. **Ans. b.** 24-hours pH monitoring *(Ref: Bailey 27/e p1085, 1089, 1091)*

48. **Ans. b.** Pencil tip appearance *(Ref: Surgical radiology Clinical Cases by Prabhakar Fajiah (2007)/113)*

Features of CA Esophagus on Barium Swallow	
• **Mucosal irregularity** and **shouldering**[Q]	• **Annular stricture**[Q]
• **Narrowing**[Q] of the lumen	• **Sharp** and **clear cut edge** of **filling defect**[Q]
• **Irregular "rat-tail" filling defect**[Q] of the distal esophagus with **shouldered edge**[Q]	• **Proximal dilatation**[Q] of the esophagus

> • **"Bird's beak"** , **"Pencil-tip"** or **"Rat's tail"** appearance is seen in **Achalasia**[Q].

49. **Ans. c.** Apple core appearance *(Ref: Sabiston 20/e p1028)*
> • Barium swallow: First investigation done[Q] in suspected case of Carcinoma esophagus (classic finding of an apple core lesion[Q]).

50. Ans. a. Middle 1/3rd

51. Ans. b. Middle 1/3rd

52. Ans. a. Esophagectomy

53. Ans. a. Depth of tumor

54. Ans. d. Chemoradiation followed by palliative enbloc resection

55. Ans. None

56. Ans. c. T stage

■ ESOPHAGECTOMY

57. Ans. a. **Right gastric and right gastroepiploic artery** *(Ref: Sabiston 20/e p1035-1036; Bailey 27/e p1092; Shackelford 7/e p518-520)*

58. Ans. a. **Stomach**

59. Ans. b. **Middle 1/3rd** *(Ref: Sabiston 20/e p1035-1036; Schwartz 11/e p1076, 10/e p1009; Bailey 27/e p1092; Shackelford 7/e p427-430)*

TUMOR MARGIN FOR CURATIVE EXCISION

- In GI malignancies (stomach[Q], small intestine[Q], colon[Q] and proximal rectum[Q]), tumor margin for curative excision is 5cm[Q] except:
  - Esophagus: 10 cm[Q]
  - Distal rectum: 2 cm[Q]

60. Ans. a. **Transhiatal**

61. Ans. a. **Stomach**

■ LEIOMYOMA

62. Ans. a. **Leiomyoma** *(Ref: Sabiston 20/e p1032; Schwartz 11/e p1081, 10/e p1216; Bailey 27/e p1084; Shackelford 7/e p465-469)*

63. Ans. c. **Leiomyoma** *(Ref: Sabiston 20/e p1032; Schwartz 11/e p1081, 10/e p1017; Bailey 27/e p1085)*

- **Barium swallow** is **IOC** for leiomyoma (**classical, smooth, contoured, punched-out defect**)[Q]

■ DYSPHAGIA

64. Ans. b. **Herpes esophagitis, c. Monilial esophagitis** *(Ref: Harrison 19/e p1901, 1909; Bailey 27/e p1103)*

If **odynophagia** is present, **candidial (monilial)** or **herpes esophagitis** or **pill induced esophagitis** should be suspected.

ODYNOPHAGIA

- Odynophagia means **painful swallowing** seen in **inflammatory lesions** of food passage (i.e. **oral cavity, pharynx** and **esophagus**)
- **Causes:**
  - **Candidial (monilial)** esophagitis[Q]
  - **Herpes** esophagitis[Q]
  - **Pill induced** esophagitis[Q]

65. Ans. c. **Achalasia cardia**

Presence of dysphagia to both solids and liquids suggests the diagnosis of achalasia.

■ DYSPHAGIA LUSORIA

66. Ans. d. **Compression by aberrant blood vessel** *(Ref: Sabiston 20/e p1581; Bailey 27/e p1105)*

67. Ans. d. **Acquired in later life** *(Ref: Sabiston 20/e p1581)*

Dysphagia lusoria is a **disorder of swallowing** caused **due to vascular anomalies**[Q] (**developmental** or **congenital abnormalities**).

■ ESOPHAGEAL PERFORATION AND INJURY

68. Ans. a. **Vomiting, b. Subcutaneous emphysema, c. Lower thoracic pain** *(Ref: Sabiston 20/e p1025-1026; Schwartz 11/e p1083, 10/e p1018; Bailey 27/e p1073; Shackelford 7/e p478-484)*

69. Ans. b. **Cervical portion** *(Ref: Sabiston 20/e p1025-1026; Schwartz 11/e p1083, 10/e p1018; Bailey 27/e p1073; Shackelford 7/e p478-479)*

Esophageal Perforation	
Iatrogenic	**Spontaneous**
• **Most common type**[Q] • Caused by **endoscopy**[Q] • **MC site** is **cervical esophagus (cricopharyngeal area)**[Q]	• Esophageal rupture after vomiting • **MC site: left posterolateral side** of the **distal esophagus**[Q]

70. Ans. c. **Instrumentation**

71. Ans. a. **Primary closure, drainage and antibiotics**

OPERATIVE REPAIR OF ESOPHAGEAL PERFORATION

- The principles of repair comprise a **clear exposure of** the **perforation** and **debridement** of devitalized tissue, followed by a **primary closure**.
- **Following debridement** of devitalized tissue, **primary mucosal repair** should then be **performed with interrupted, absorbable suture**, taking care to minimize esophageal stricturing while obtaining adequate suture purchase on vital tissue.
- The **muscular layer** is then reapproximated with an **interrupted** or **running suture**[Q].

> - **Subsequent coverage** with a **vascular pedicle**, such as an **intercostal muscle flap**, and **pleural, pericardial**, or **omental pedicle allows further buttressing** of a repair and is **recommended whenever feasible**[Q].
> - **Gastric fundus** may also be **suitable tissue reinforcement** especially **for** the distal **perforation**[Q].

- Depending on the site of perforation, any of the antireflux procedures (**Belsey Mark IV, Nissen, Dor, Toupet**) may be used to **buttress the repair**.

72. **Ans. b.** Bradycardia

73. **Ans. c.** Spontaneous perforation

74. **Ans. b.** Cardioesophageal junction

75. **Ans. d.** Water soluble low molecular weight contrast swallow

76. **Ans. a.** May present with peritonitis *(Ref: Sabiston 20/e p1025; Schwartz 11/e p1083, 10/e p1018; Bailey 27/e p1072)*

77. **Ans. a.** Boerhaave's syndrome *(Ref: Bailey 27/e p1072, 1073)*

■ TRACHEOESOPHAGEAL FISTULA

78. **Ans. d.** CVS *(Ref: Sabiston 20/e p1866-1868; Schwartz 11/e p1717, 10/e p608-609; Bailey 27/e p133; Shackelford 7/e p509-515)*

79. **Ans. b.** NG tube insertion and CXR to check position of tube *(Ref: Sabiston 20/e p1866-1868; Schwartz 11/e p1717; Bailey 27/e p133)*

80. **Ans. c.** Esophageal atresia with distal tracheoesophageal fistula

■ ESOPHAGEAL RINGS AND WEBS

81. **Ans. a.** Mucosal ring at squamocolumnar junction, **c.** Dysphagia is the symptom *(Ref: Sabiston 20/e p1026-1027; Schwartz 11/e p1049, 10/e p984; Bailey 27/e p1102; Shackelford 7/e p89-90)*

82. **Ans. c.** Schatzki ring *(Ref: Sabiston 20/e p1027; Schwartz 11/e p1049, 10/e p984; Bailey 27/e p1102)*

83. **Ans. b.** Lower esophagus

84. **Ans. b.** Occurs at GE junction *(Ref: Gastroenterol Hepatol (NY); 2010 November 6 (11): 701-704)*

Types of Esophageal Ring on Barium Examination	
Type A	Located **few cm proximal to GE junction**
Type B	**Schatzki's ring: MC esophageal ring** found on esophagogram, **at GE junction**[Q]
Type C	Located at **most distal portion of esophagus**, formed by diaphragmatic crural pressure

85. **Ans. b.** Schatzki ring *(Ref: Sabiston 20/e p1026; Schwartz 11/e p1049, 10/e p984; Bailey 27/e p1102; Shackelford 7/e p89-90)*

■ FOREIGN BODY

86. **Ans. d.** Above the cricopharynx *(Ref: Schwartz 9/e p2378; Dhingra 4/e p64)*

The first constriction where the esophagus commences is at the **cricopharyngeal sphincter**: This is the **narrowest portion of the esophagus** and is the **most common site of foreign body**.

87. **Ans. a.** Esophagus

"Coins in the esophagus are round in appearance on the frontal view whereas coins in the trachea are usually seen on end and are linear in shape."

Foreign Body	
• Coins account for 70% of pediatric ingested foreign bodies • Coins will typically become 'stuck' at the level of the cricopharyngeus muscle.	

Coin	Chest X-ray Anteroposterior (AP) View
In trachea	• Visualized in the **sagittal plane**[Q] (acquired while entering through vocal cords)
In esophagus	• Visualized in **coronal orientation**[Q]

■ ESOPHAGUS: ANATOMY AND PHYSIOLOGY

88. **Ans. c. Tertiary** *(Ref: Sabiston 20/e p1014-1015)*

TERTIARY CONTRACTIONS OF ESOPHAGUS

- Tertiary contractions are **simultaneous, non progressive, non peristaltic waves** that can occur **throughout the esophagus**[Q]
- Tertiary contractions represent **uncoordinated contractions** of the **smooth muscles** that are **responsible for** the **'Cork Screw' appearance** of **esophageal spasm** on Barium swallow
- Tertiary contractions do not have a physiological function and may be **observed in** the **elderly** and in patients with **esophageal motility disorders**[Q]

89. **Ans. c. 40 cm**

Esophageal Constrictions			
No.	Distance from incisor teeth	Bony level	Anatomical Landmark
1	15 cm[Q]	C6	Pharyngoesophageal junction (At beginning[Q])
2	25 cm[Q]		Aortic arch, left bronchus[Q]
3	40 cm[Q]	T10	Pierces diaphragm[Q]

BALD: Beginning, Aortic arch, Left Bronchus, Diaphragm[Q]

90. **Ans. a. 6–26 mm Hg** *(Ref: Sabiston 20/e p1016; Bailey 27/e p1068)*

"The normal LOS is 3–4 cm long and has a pressure of 10–25 mm Hg."-Bailey 27/e p1068

91. **Ans. c. Transmural** *(Ref: Schwartz 11/e p1009, 10/e p1004)*

■ DIAPHRAGM

92. **Ans. a. Laparoscopy** *(Ref: Sabiston 20/e p432; Schwartz 11/e p224-225, 10/e p202-203; Bailey 27/e p365)*

93. **Ans. b. Circumferential** *(Ref: Sabiston and Spencer's Surgery of Chest 8/e p chapter 7)*

Circumferential incision is generally taken for diaphragmatic surgery.

DIAPHRAGMATIC INCISIONS

- **Diaphragmatic incisions** can be divided into three groups: **circumferential, central tendon,** and **radial.**
1. **Circumferential incisions:**
   - Circumferential incisions in the periphery result in little loss of function.
   - Must be at least 5 cm lateral to the edge of the central tendon to avoid the posterolateral and anterolateral branches of the phrenic nerve.
   - **Difficult to correctly realign after a long operation.**
   - Placement of surgical clips on each side of the muscular incision can greatly facilitate the correct spatial orientation on closing.
2. **Incisions in the central tendon:**
   - Do not interrupt any major branch of the nerve itself.
   - **Provide excellent visualization of the abdomen from the thorax,** and vice versa.
   - **Easy to open and to close.**

3. **Transverse radial incision:**
   - Made from the midaxillary line centrally
   - **Relatively safe**
   - **May result in segmental diaphragmatic paralysis** if the incision transects the crural or posterolateral branches of the phrenic nerve.

■ MISCELLANEOUS

94. **Ans. b. Achalasia cardia**

95. **Ans. d. Esophageal perforation** *(Ref: Harrison 19/e p1720)*

HAMMAN'S SIGN OR HAMMAN'S CRUNCH

- A **crunching, rasping sound, synchronous with heartbeat, heard over the precordium** and sometimes at a distance from the chest in spontaneous mediastinal emphysema[Q].
- **Hamman's sign** may be present in **acute Mediastinitis** (as in **esophageal perforation**) [Q].

96. Ans. a. Eosinophilic esophagitis *(Ref: Schwartz 11/e p1051, 10/e p986)*

> *"Eosinophilic esophagitis (EE): A barium swallow should be the first test obtained in the patient with dysphagia. EE has a characteristic finding often called the "ringed esophagus" or the "feline esophagus," as the esophageal rings are felt to look like the stripes on a housecat. The endoscopic appearance of EE is also characteristic, and also appears as a series of rings." -Schwartz 11/e p1051, 10/e p986*

97. Ans. a. CMV esophagitis *(Ref: Harrison 20/e p2218)*

> *"CMV esophagitis occurs primarily in immunocompromised patients, particularly organ transplant recipients. CMV is usually activated from a latent stage. Endoscopically, CMV lesions appear as serpiginous ulcers in an otherwise normal mucosa, particularly in the distal esophagus." -Harrison 20/e p2218*

Causes of esophagitis			
Severe reflux esophagitis with **mucosal ulceration & friability**	**Cytomegalovirus esophagitis**	**Herpes simplex virus esophagitis** with **target-type shallow ulcerations**	**Candida esophagitis** with **white plaques adherent to esophageal mucosa**

98. Ans. d. Herpes simplex esophagitis *(Ref: Harrison 20/e p2218)*

> *"Herpes simplex virus type 1 or 2 may cause esophagitis. Vesicles on the nose and lips may coexist and are suggestive of a herpetic etiology. Varicella-zoster virus can also cause esophagitis in children with chickenpox or adults with zoster. The characteristic endoscopic findings are vesicles and small, punched-out ulcerations." -Harrison 20/e p2218*

Stomach and Duodenum

■ HELICOBACTER PYLORI

HELICOBACTER PYLORI

- First successful culture of organism was done by **Marshall and Warren**[Q], who named it Campylobacter pyloridis.

  - Around **90%** of **duodenal ulcers** and **75%** of **gastric ulcer** are associated with **H. pylori infection**[Q].
  - **Gastric antrum** is **MC site of colonization**[Q].

- It can live only in **gastric epithelium**, because only gastric epithelium expresses specific adherence receptors in vivo that can be recognized by organism.

  - Also found in **heterotopic gastric mucosa** in **proximal esophagus, Barrett's esophagus**, gastric metaplasia in the **duodenum**, **Meckel's diverticulum**, and heterotopic gastric mucosa in the **rectum**[Q].

- Mechanisms by which **H. pylori** promote ulcer formation include **stimulation** of **gastrin** release, **inhibition** of **somatostatin** release, interruption of inhibitory vagal reflexes and **inhibition** of gastroduodenal **bicarbonate** secretion[Q].
- **After eradication** of the organism, ulcer **recurrence is rare**[Q].

Characteristic Features
- **Spiral shaped, gram (-)ve rod, motile** with **lophotrichous flagella**[Q]
- The sole source is human gastric mucosa

  - Biochemical reactions: **Catalase, oxidase and urease positive**[Q]

- Grows well when incubated at **37°C in microaerophilic conditions**[Q].
- Media used include **Skirrow's medium, chocolate medium**[Q].

Pathogenesis
- Grows optimally at **pH 6.0-7.0**[Q] and would be killed at pH within the gastric lumen.
- But it survives as it is found deep in mucus layer near epithelial surface, without invading mucosa where physiologic pH is present. It produces **potent urease**, which **provides ammonia to buffer acid**[Q].
- Major diseases associated H. pylori virulence factors are **vacuolating cytotoxin (Vac A)**[Q], and group of genes called **CagPal**[Q].

  - **H. pylori colonization decreases somatostatin** producing cells →↑ Gastrin →↑Acid → Gastric metaplasia in duodenum → Ulceration[Q].

Clinical Manifestations
- **90% of duodenal ulcer and 75% of gastric ulcer**[Q] are related to H. pylori
- **Increase risk of gastric adenocarcinoma, gastric MALT lymphoma**[Q].
- Extra-gastrointestinal pathologies that are linked include **ischemic heart disease** and **cerebrovascular disease**[Q].

  - **CAG-A positive strain** is **protective for adenocarcinoma** esophagus but **can lead to SCC** of esophagus[Q].

Diagnosis
- **Histologic visualization** of H. pylori is the **gold standard** of **diagnostic test**[Q] (special stains used are **silver, Giemsa, Genta or Warthin starry stain**)[Q].

  - The **method of choice to diagnose** if endoscope is employed is **rapid urease test**[Q].
  - **Serology** is the test of choice for **initial diagnosis** when endoscopy is not required.
  - After treatment, **Urea breath test** is the method of choice but should be performed **after 4 weeks** of therapy[Q].

Accuracy of Diagnostic Methods
- **Chronic inflammation** on a gastric mucosal **biopsy** specimen is **100% sensitive** test[Q].
- **Rapid Urease test** on a gastric mucosal biopsy specimen is **100% specific** test[Q].

■ PEPTIC ULCER

Gastric Ulcer	Duodenal Ulcer
Etiology: – Atrophic gastritis – **H. pylori (75%)**[Q] – **Smoking, Alcohol**[Q] – **Lower socioeconomic status**[Q] – Altered mucosal barrier function (**NSAIDs**)[Q] – There is either **normochlorhydria** or **achlorhydria**[Q] – **Cirrhosis**[Q]	**Etiology:** – **Stress, anxiety**: '**hurry, worry, curry**'[Q] – **H. pylori (90%)**[Q] – **NSAIDs, steroids**[Q] – Blood group **O+ve**[Q] – **Endocrine: Zollinger-Ellison syndrome, MEN-1, Cushing's syndrome, hyperparathyroidism**[Q] – **Alcohol, smoking, vitamin deficiency**[Q] – **Chronic pancreatitis, Cirrhosis**[Q]
MC Site: – **Lesser curvature** along the **incisura angularis (Type 1)**[Q]	**MC site:** – **1st part** of **duodenum** (**overall MC site** for **peptic ulcer**)[Q]
Clinical features: – **Equal** in both sexes – **Pain in** the **epigastrium after** taking **food**[Q]; relieved by vomiting – Pain is uncommon during night – **Hematemesis** common – Appetite good, but **hesitant to eat** as eating leads to pain that results in **loss of weight**[Q]	**Clinical features:** – More common in **males**[Q] – **Pain** in early morning, decreases after food (**hunger pain**[Q]) – Pain **common during night**[Q] – **Melena** common – **Appetite good**, eats more frequently and there is **weight gain**[Q]
Features on Barium meal: – **Niche** on **lesser curve** with **notch** on **greater curve**[Q] – Regular/round margin of ulcer create **spoke wheel pattern**[Q] – **Overhanging mucosa** at the margins of a benign gastric ulcer projects inwards, towards the ulcer: **Hampton's line**[Q] – **Converging mucosal folds** at the **base of the ulcer**[Q]	**Features on Barium meal:** – **Deformed** or **absent duodenal cap** (because of spasm)[Q] – Appearance of **trifoliate duodenum** due to **secondary duodenal diverticula**[Q]
Complications: – **Perforation**: MC complication of **gastric ulcer** (Into **lesser sac**)[Q] – **Hour glass contracture:** Exclusively in women due to **cicatricial contracture** of **lesser curve ulcer**[Q] – **Tea pot stomach (hand bag stomach):** Cicatrisation and **shortening of the lesser curvature**[Q] – **Malignant transformation**[Q]	**Complications:** – **Bleeding: MC complication,** on **posterior wall, gastroduodenal artery**[Q] is most commonly involved – **Perforation**: More on **anterior wall,** if posterior, into pancreas – **Gastric outlet obstruction** due to **pyloric stenosis**- least common[Q] – Duodenal ulcers are **benign (No malignant transformation)**[Q]

■ TYPES OF GASTRIC ULCER

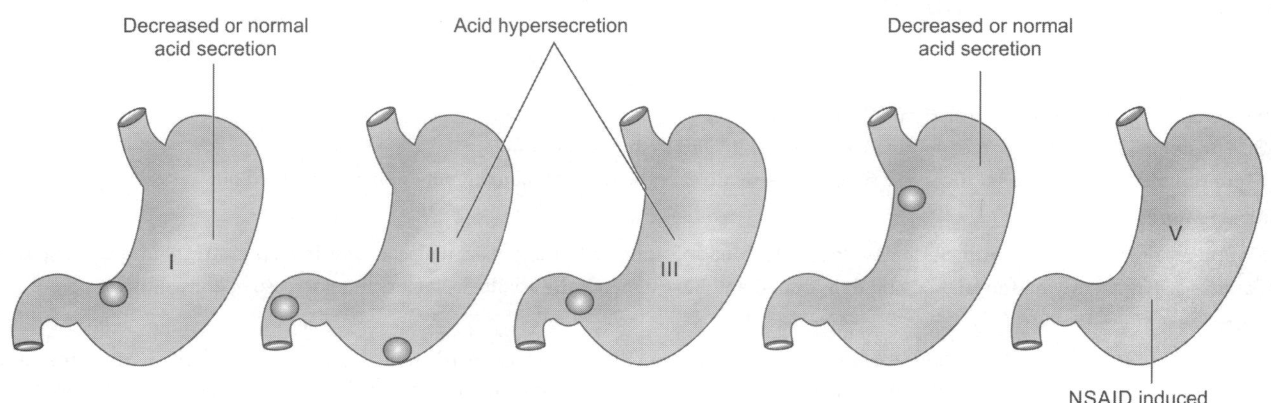

Modified Johnson's Classification of Gastric Ulcer		
Type	**Location**	**Acid Secretion**
I	Lesser curvature, near incisura angularis (**MC**)[Q]	Low
II	Body of the **stomach** and **duodenum**[Q]	**High**[Q]
III	**Prepyloric**[Q] (within 2-3 cm of the pylorus)	**High**[Q]
IV	**High** on the **lesser curve**, near **GE junction**[Q]	Low
V	Anywhere, induced by medication (NSAIDs)	Low

Gastric Ulcer	
Benign Ulcer	**Malignant Ulcer**
• Generally at **lesser curvature**[Q]	• At **greater curvature**[Q]
• **Smooth radiating folds**[Q] with **Hampton line and collar**[Q]	• Interrupted **nodular, clubbed folds** with **Lasman Kirklin complex**[Q] (malignant ulcer with no mass)
• **Overhanging margins**[Q] showing regeneration	• **Eccentric** with **heaped up** and **everted margins**[Q]
• **Mucosal rugae projects outwards** from the **margins of ulcer**[Q]	• **Mucosal rugae stop far** of the ulcer[Q]
• **Penetrating sign** (ulcer crater projects into stomach wall rather than into a mass in a stomach wall).	• **Carman's meniscus sign** (meniscoid appearance of trapped barium in ulcer bed)
• Huge base[Q]	• Necrotic base[Q]
• Preserved peristalsis[Q]	• No peristalsis[Q]
• Heals within 8-10 weeks[Q]	• No healing[Q]

◼ COMPLICATIONS OF PEPTIC ULCER

Complications of Peptic Ulcer
• **Intractability** (Non-healing)
• **Bleeding: MC complication** of peptic ulcer[Q]
• **Perforation: MC complication** of gastric ulcer[Q]
• **Gastric outlet obstruction** (Rare)

Duodenal Ulcer	
Complications	*Treatment*
Intractable	Highly selective vagotomy[Q]
Bleeding	**Truncal vagotomy** with **pyloroplasty**[Q] and oversewing of bleeding vessel
Perforated	**Omental patch repair** (with **Truncal vagotomy** in **stable** patients[Q])
Obstruction	(Rule out malignancy) • **Truncal vagotomy** with **antrectomy** is **ideal procedure**[Q] • **Truncal vagotomy** with **gastrojejunostomy** in cases of **inflammation** and **scarring** of duodenal bulb[Q]

◼ GASTRIC OUTLET OBSTRUCTION

GASTRIC OUTLET OBSTRUCTION

- **MC cause** of **gastric outlet obstruction: CA stomach**[Q]
- **Site of stenosis** or **obstruction** in **peptic ulcer disease: 1ˢᵗ part** of the **duodenum**[Q]
- **More common** with **duodenal ulcer** and **type III gastric ulcer** and requires that malignancy should be ruled out.

Clinical Features

- Symptoms of gastric retention, including **early satiety**, **bloating**, indigestion, anorexia, nausea, **vomiting**, epigastric pain, and **weight loss**.
- Patients are frequently **malnourished** and **dehydrated** and have a **metabolic alkalosis**, factors that increase operative risk.

Diagnosis

- A **saline load test** is helpful, it is performed by emptying the stomach with a nasogastric tube and instilling **750 mL** of saline, the patient is placed in **sitting position**, and **30 minutes** later the nasogastric tube is aspirated, normally **< 400 mL** should remain in the stomach, and 90% of subjects have a residue of less than 200 mL.
- The finding of **> 400 mL** residual saline is consistent with a **diagnosis** of **gastric outlet obstruction**.

Treatment

- **Surgery** is generally indicated if the obstruction fails to resolve despite **48–72 hours** of adequate **IV fluid replenishment**, **antisecretory therapy** and **nasogastric decompression**[Q].

• **Truncal vagotomy** and **antrectomy**[Q] is the **ideal procedure**.

- The **inflammation** and **scarring** at **duodenal bulb** or **previous proximal duodenal surgeries** prevents safe performance of an antrectomy, in this setting **truncal vagotomy** with **drainage (Gastrojejunostomy)** is the preferred approach[Q].

■ TYPES OF VAGOTOMY

Types of Vagotomy		
Highly Selective Vagotomy	*Vagotomy and Drainage*	*Vagotomy and Antrectomy*
• **Procedure of choice** for **chronic** or **intractable** duodenal **ulcers**[Q] • **Nerves of Latarjet supplying** the **antrum** are **preserved**[Q] (and hence gastric motility) • **Drainage procedure** is **not required**[Q] • **Lowest mortality rate** and **side effects**[Q] • **Minimal chances** of **dumping syndrome** and **gastric atony**[Q] • Relatively **high recurrence**[Q]	• **TV** is performed by **division** of **left** and **right vagus nerves above** the **hepatic** and **celiac branches**[Q] just above the GE junction. • **MC operation performed** for **duodenal ulcer**[Q] • **Intermediate morbidity** and **recurrence rate**[Q]	• **Procedure of choice** for **recurrent** duodenal **ulcers**[Q] • **Lowest recurrence** rate[Q] • **High mortality and morbidity**[Q]

■ OPERATIONS FOR GASTRIC ULCER

Operations for Gastric Ulcer	
Billroth-I Gastrectomy	*Billroth-II Gastrectomy*
• **Gastroduodenostomy**[Q] • Performed when there is a **sufficient portion** of **upper duodenum remaining**[Q] • **Remaining portion of stomach** is **reattached to the duodenum**[Q]	• **Loop gastrojejunostomy**[Q] • Performed if the **stomach cannot be reattached** to **duodenum**[Q] • **Remaining portion of duodenum** is **sealed off**, a **hole is cut into** the **jejunum** & **stomach is reattached**[Q] at this hole.

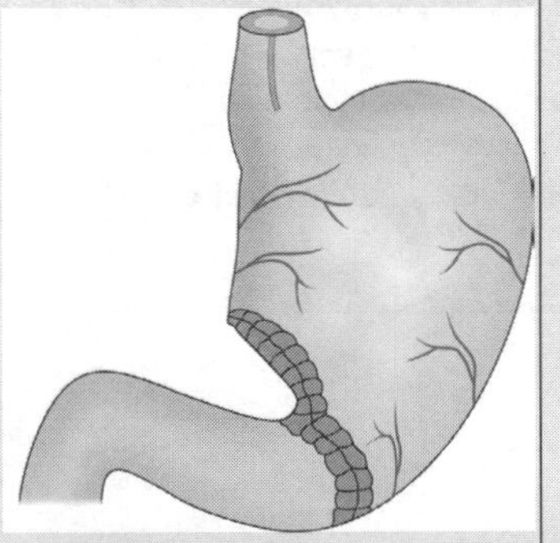

50 to 60 cm

Billroth I (Gastroduodenal) anastomosis

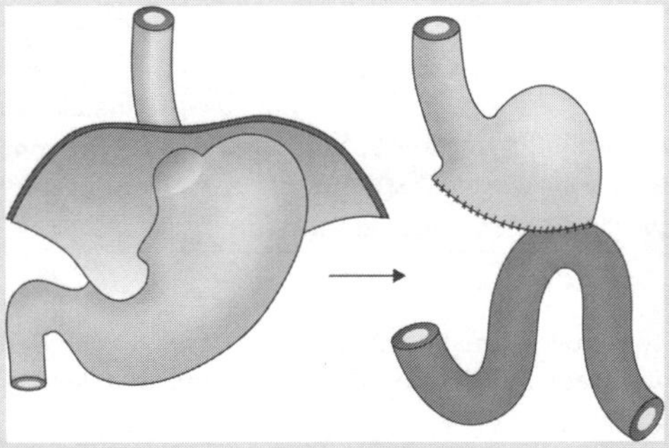

Billroth II Gastrectomy (Loop Gastrojejunostomy)

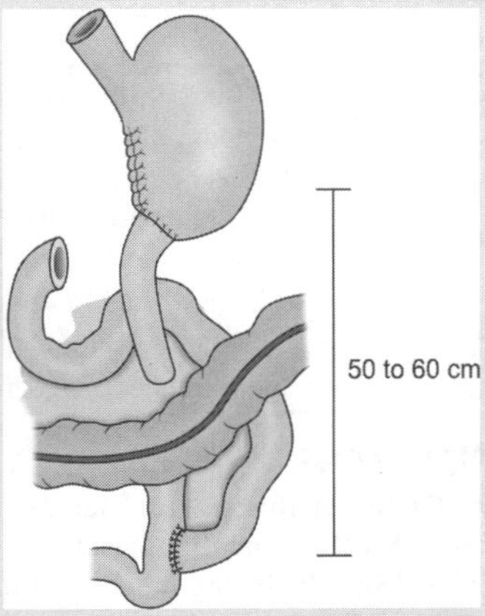

Roux-en-Y Gastrojejunostomy

Elective Gastric Ulcer Operations	
Type	**Procedure**
Type **I**	• **Distal gastrectomy** with Billroth I or II reconstruction[Q]
Type II and **III**	• **Truncal vagotomy** plus **antrectomy**[Q]
Type **IV**	• **Schoemaker** procedure[Q] • **Pouchet** procedure[Q] • **Kelling-Madlener** procedure (For **unstable** patients[Q]) • **Csendes** procedure (For **stable** patients[Q])

■ COMPLICATIONS AFTER GASTRECTOMY

Postgastrectomy/Vagotomy Syndrome		
Secondary to Gastric Resection	**Secondary to Gastric Reconstruction**	**Postvagotomy Syndrome**
• **Dumping syndrome**[Q] • Metabolic disturbances[Q]	• **Afferent loop** syndrome[Q] • **Efferent loop** obstruction[Q] • **Alkaline reflux gastritis**[Q] • **Retained antrum**[Q] syndrome	• Postvagotomy **diarrhea**[Q] • Postvagotomy **gastric atony**[Q] • **Incomplete vagal transection**[Q]

Metabolic Complications after Gastrectomy

- **Metabolic complications** are **more common** and **serious after partial gastrectomy**[Q] than after vagotomy.
- **More common** in **Billroth II**[Q] >Billroth I procedure
- **Severity** is **directly related** to the **extent of gastric resection**[Q].
- **MC metabolic defect** appearing **after gastrectomy: Anemia**[Q]

Anemia

- **MC metabolic defect** appearing **after gastrectomy**: Anemia[Q]
- **Iron deficiency anemia (IDA)** is more common than vitamin B_{12} deficiency anemia[Q].

■ DUMPING SYNDROME

Dumping Syndrome

- Dumping syndrome refers to a constellation of **post-prandial symptoms** occurring due to **accelerated emptying** (dumping) of **hyperosmolar stomach contents** into the small bowel.
- It is usually seen in operation which destroys the pyloric sphincter (i.e **gastrectomy, antrectomy** and **drainage procedures**)[Q].
- It also affects a small percentage of patients with highly selective vagotomy due to loss of receptive relaxation of stomach.

Dumping Syndrome	
Early Dumping	**Late Dumping**
• It occurs **immediately after meals** (after **15-30 minutes**)[Q] • Dumping of **hyperosmolar contents** into **small bowel**[Q] results in rapid fluid influx from the circulation into gastrointestinal tract. This leads to **acute intestinal distention** and peripheral & splanchnic vasodilatation[Q]. • This gives rise to **vasomotor** & **abdominal symptoms**: Epigastric fullness, sweating, light headedness, tachycardia, diarrhea. • Symptoms can be **ameliorated by lying down** & **saline infusion**[Q].	• It is seen **2-3 hrs after meal**[Q] • Occurs due to **reactive hypoglycemia**[Q]. • Carbohydrate load in small bowel → Increased plasma glucose → Increased insulin secretion → Hypoglycemia • Symptoms are **relieved by administration of sugar**[Q].

Management
- **Dietary management**: Diet therapy is done to reduce jejunal osmolality.
  - **Multiple small meals**, food **low in carbohydrate** and **rich in fat** and **proteins** are taken[Q].
  - **Liquids during meals** should be **avoided**[Q].
- **Somatostatin analogues (octreotide):**
- Diet therapy is usually successful but if it fails, the patient is started on octreotide.
- **Surgery:**
  - Surgery is **rarely required**[Q] as most of the patients improve with time, dietary management and Octreotide.

■ UPPER GI BLEED

Risk Stratification Systems for Upper GI Bleeds

- Help to **identify the patients at higher risk of major bleeding or death** (facilitate patient triage)
- Commonly used scoring systems:
  - **Rockall score** (takes account of **endoscopic findings; most useful**[Q])
  - **Blatchford score** (used during **initial assessment, does not require endoscopic data**[Q])

Commonly Used Risk Stratification Systems for Upper GI Bleeds	
Blatchford Score (PUSH + Melena/Syncope + Cardiac/Hepatic Dysfunction)	**Rockall & Baylor Score** (CASDE)
• **P**ulse[Q] • Blood **U**rea nitrogen[Q] • **S**ystolic BP[Q] • **H**emoglobin[Q] • Presence of **M**elena[Q], **S**yncope[Q], **H**epatic[Q] or **C**ardiac dysfunction[Q]	• **C**omorbid disease[Q] (cardiac, hepatic, renal, or disseminated cancer) • **A**ge[Q] (<60 years, 60-79 years, >80 years) • **S**hock[Q] (systolic BP <100 mm Hg, HR >100 beats/min) • **D**iagnosis at the time of endoscopy[Q] (Mallory-Weiss tears, nonmalignant lesions, or malignant lesions) • **E**ndoscopic stigmata of recent bleed[Q]

Bleed Risk Classification
• To **predict risk** of **rebleeding & mortality** in **upper GI bleed** • Predicts **risk on initial presentation** based on **five criteria:** 1. Ongoing **Bleeding**[Q] 2. **Low systolic BP**[Q] (<100 mm Hg) 3. **Elevated PT**[Q] (>1.2 times the control value) 4. **Erratic mental status**[Q] 5. Unstable comorbid **Disease**[Q]

■ THE FORREST CLASSIFICATION

The Forrest Classification (For Endoscopic Findings and Rebleeding Risk)		
Grade	Description	Rebleeding Risk
Ia	Active, **pulsatile** bleeding[Q]	**High**
Ib	**Oozing**[Q], non-pulsatile bleeding	High
IIa	Non-bleeding **visible vessel**[Q]	**High**
IIb	Adherent **clot**[Q]	Intermediate
IIc	**Black dot**[Q]	Low
III	**Clean base**[Q]	Low

- •**High rebleeding** risk: I & IIa[Q]
- **Intermediate risk**: IIb[Q]
- **Low risk**: IIc & III[Q]

■ MALLORY WEISS SYNDROME

MALLORY WEISS SYNDROME

- Mallory-Weiss tears are related to **forceful vomiting, retching, coughing,** or **straining**[Q]
- **Forceful contraction** of **abdominal wall** against an **unrelaxed cardia**, resulting in **mucosal laceration** of **proximal cardia**[Q] as a result of the increase in intragastric pressure.

> • Results in **disruption** of **gastric mucosa** high on the **lesser curve** at **cardia** (just below GE junction)[Q]

- Tear is **partial thickness**, extending through the **mucosa and submucosa**[Q]

Clinical Features

- Classically, seen in **alcoholic patients**[Q] after a period of **intense retching** and **vomiting** after binge drinking.
- Cause of up to **15%** of all **severe upper GI bleeds**[Q]

> • **Arterial bleeding** (usually from **left gastric artery**[Q]), usually **painless** and are **rarely**[Q] associated with **massive bleeding**.

Diagnosis

- Usually diagnosed by **history**
- **Endoscopy** is used to **confirm the diagnosis**[Q].

Treatment

- **Supportive therapy** is often all that is necessary because **90%** of **bleeding episodes** are **self-limited**, and the **mucosa** often **heals within 72 hours**[Q].

Persistent Bleeding in Mallory Weiss Syndrome is managed by
• **Endoscopic electrocoagulation**[Q] or endoscopic therapy with injection • **Angiographic embolization**[Q] • Surgery consists of laparotomy and **high gastrotomy** with **oversewing of the linear tear**[Q], if above maneuvers fails.

Remember: A **Sengstaken-Blakemore tube** will **not stop bleeding** in Mallory-Weiss syndrome, as the **bleeding is arterial** and the pressure in the balloon is not sufficient to overcome the arterial pressure and is **contraindicated**[Q].

Gastrointestinal Surgery

Section 3

■ DIEULAFOY'S GASTRIC LESION

DIEULAFOY'S GASTRIC LESION

- Caused by an **abnormally large (1–3 mm)**[Q], **tortuous artery** coursing through the **submucosa**
- Occurs **6–10 cm** from the **GE junction**, generally in **'fundus'** near the **cardia** along **lesser curvature**[Q].

> - **Erosion** of **superficial mucosa** overlying the artery occur **secondary to pulsations** of **large submucosal vessel**[Q] arteriole

- **Artery** is exposed to **gastric contents**, leading to **further erosion** & **bleeding** occurs[Q].
- **Mucosal defect** is **2–5 mm** in size

Clinical Features

- More common in **men** (2:1) with **peak incidence** in **5th decade**[Q].
- Associated with **sudden** onset of **massive, painless, recurrent hematemesis** with **hypotension**
- **Recurrent bleeding** with **spontaneous cessation** is common[Q].

Diagnosis

- **Endoscopy** is the **diagnostic modality of choice**, correctly identifying the lesion in 80% of patients.

> - **Repeated endoscopies** may be needed to correctly identify the lesion because of **intermittent nature** of the **bleeding**[Q]

- **Angiography** showing a **tortous ectatic artery** in the distribution of the **left gastric artery** with accompanied **contrast extravasation** in the setting of acute bleeding.

Treatment

- **Initial attempts** at **endoscopic control** are **often successful**[Q].
- **Application of thermal** or **sclerosant therapy** is **effective in 80–100% of cases.**[Q]
- **In cases that fail endoscopic therapy, angiographic coil embolization** can be successful[Q].
- **Gastric wedge resection** to include the offending vessel is reserved **when other modalities have failed**[Q].

■ WATERMELON STOMACH (GASTRIC ANTRAL VASCULAR ECTASIA)

WATERMELON STOMACH (GASTRIC ANTRAL VASCULAR ECTASIA)

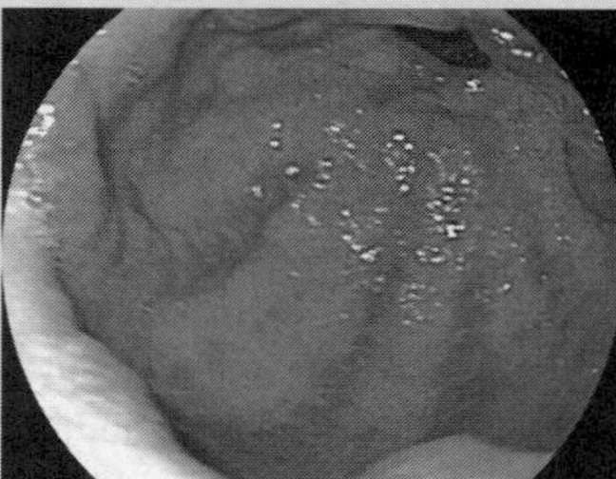

- A rare entity characterized by presence of both **inflammatory** and **vascular components** in **mucosa**[Q].

Pathology

- **Dilated mucosal blood vessels** in the lamina propria, often containing **thrombi,** with **no evidence of vascular malformation** on angiographic and morphologic examination[Q].
- **Mucosal fibromuscular hyperplasia** and **hyalinization** are often present[Q].
- Predominantly affects the **distal portion (Antrum)**[Q] of the stomach

Clinical Features

- Patients are generally **elderly women** with **chronic bleeding**[Q].
- Most have an **associated autoimmune connective tissue** disorders, and at least **25%** have **chronic liver disease**[Q].
- Patients typically have **iron deficiency anemia** & **chronic blood loss** requiring transfusions[Q].

Diagnosis

- Diagnosis is based on **typical endoscopic** and **biopsy appearance** of mucosa[Q].

> - Gross endoscopic examination reveals **prominent longitudinal folds** with **parallel striking red stripes** atop the mucosal folds of the **distal stomach**, much like the **rind of a watermelon**[Q].

Treatment

- Lesions are treated by **endoscopic cautery**[Q].
- In patients with **portal hypertension, TIPS** should be considered first[Q].

■ RISK FACTORS FOR CARCINOMA STOMACH

Factors Associated with Increased Risk of Developing Stomach Cancer	
Nutritional	**Medical**
• **Low fat** or **protein** consumption[Q]	• **Prior gastric surgery**[Q]
• **Salted** meat[Q]	• **H. pylori**[Q] infection
• **High nitrate** consumption[Q]	• **Epstein-Barr** virus[Q]
• High **complex-carbohydrate** consumption[Q]	• **Gastric atrophy** and **gastritis**[Q]
	• **Adenomatous polyps**[Q]
	• **Male** gender[Q]

Contd...

Contd…

Social		Occupational	
• **Low** social class[Q]		• Rubber workers[Q]	
		• Coal workers[Q]	
Environmental		**Genetic factors**	
• Poor food preparation (**smoked, salted**)[Q]		• Blood group 'A'[Q]	
• **Lack of refrigeration**[Q]		• **Pernicious anemia**[Q]	
• Poor drinking water (**well water**)[Q]		• Family history	
• **Smoking**[Q]		• **Hereditary nonpolyposis colon cancer**[Q]	
		• **Li-Fraumeni syndrome**[Q]	

- **Decreased risk of carcinoma stomach: Aspirin**, Diet (high fresh fruit and vegetable intake), Vitamin A and C, calcium, selenium, zinc and iron[Q].
- **Alcohol** is **not a risk factor** for **CA stomach**[Q].

■ CLASSIFICATION SYSTEM FOR CARCINOMA STOMACH

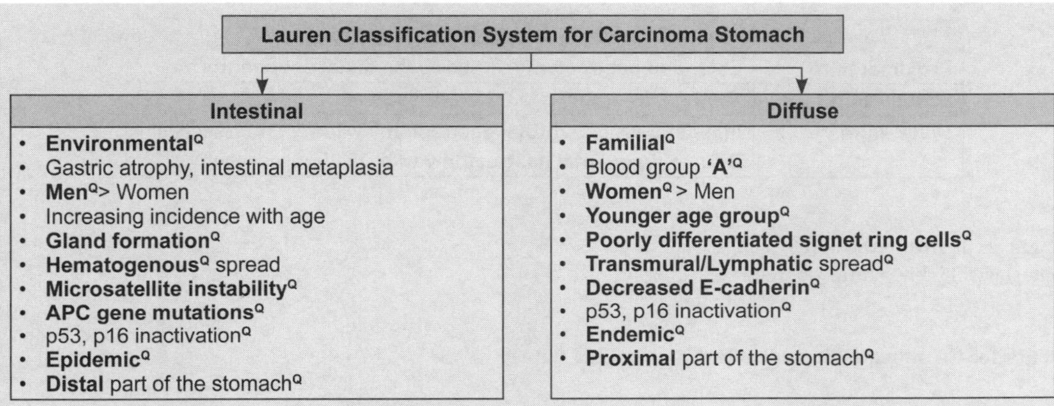

Bormann Classification (Based on macroscopic appearance)	
Type I	**Polyploid** or **fungating**[Q] cancers
Type II	Fungating & ulcerated with surrounded by **elevated borders**[Q]
Type III	Ulcerated lesions **infiltrating** the **gastric wall**[Q]
Type IV	Infiltrates diffusely (**Linitis plastica**)[Q]
Type V	Unable to be classified

■ CARCINOMA STOMACH

CARCINOMA STOMACH

- Incidence of **gastric cancer**, especially **distal cancer** is **decreasing**[Q]; Distribution: **Distal (40%) > Middle (30%) = Proximal (30%)**
- Incidence of **GE junction tumors** are **increasing**[Q]
- Approximately **90%** of all tumors of the stomach are **malignant**, the vast majority of which are **gastric adenocarcinoma**[Q].

> • **MC genetic abnormalities: p53** and **COX-2 gene**[Q] (SPC: Stomach, **p53** and **COX-2 gene**)

- **Tumor Markers: CEA, CA 19-9, CA-125, CA 72-4** & **beta-hCG**

Clinical Features

- **MC Symptoms: Abdominal pain (62-91%)**[Q] > **weight loss (22-61%)**.
- Typically, pain is constant, nonradiating, & unrelieved by food ingestion.
- **Proximal tumors** involving the gastroesophageal junction often present with **dysphagia**, whereas **distal antral tumors** may present as **gastric outlet obstruction**[Q].

> • **Diffuse mural involvement by tumor**, as occurs in **linnitis plastica**, leads to **decreased distensibility** of the stomach and complaints of **early satiety**[Q].

- **Ascitis, jaundice** or **palpable mass** indicate **incurable disease**[Q].
- **Transverse colon** is a potential site for **malignant fistulization** & **obstruction** from gastric primary tumor.

Contd…

Contd…

> • Patients may present with a palpable abdominal mass, a palpable **supraclavicular (Virchow's)** or **periumbilical (Sister Mary Joseph's)** lymph node, **left axilla (Irish nodes) peritoneal metastasis palpable** by rectal examination (**Blummer's shelf**), or a palpable ovarian mass (**Krukenberg's tumor**)[Q] via **retrograde lymphatics**[Q] most commonly.

- Paraneoplastic syndromes include thrombophlebitis (**Trousseau's syndrome**), neuropathies, nephrotic syndrome, & DIC.

Lymph Node Metastasis

- **Proximal stomach & GE junction tumors:** Higher propensity of spread to nodes in the **mediastinum & pericardial region**[Q].
- Tumors in the **body of stomach:** Highest likelihood of spreading to **nodes along** the **greater & lesser curvature, near** the location of **primary tumor** mass[Q].
- Tumors in the **distal stomach:** High likelihood of spread to the **periduodenal, peripancreatic, & porta hepatis** nodes[Q].

Diagnosis

- **Endoscopy with biopsy** is the **best method**[Q] to diagnose gastric cancer
- **IOC for staging of early gastric cancer:** EUS
- **Best investigation** for preoperative staging: **CECT**[Q]

Treatment of Carcinoma Stomach according to site	
Proximal-third	**Extended gastrectomy**, including the **distal esophagus**[Q]
Middle-third	**Total gastrectomy** and **D2** LN dissection[Q].
Distal-third	**Intestinal-type: Subtotal gastrectomy** with **D2** LN dissection[Q]
	Diffuse-type: Total gastrectomy with **D2** LN dissection[Q]

Recurrence

- **Most recurrences** occur **within** the **first 3 years**[Q].
- **MC site of metastasis: Liver**[Q] > lung > bone.

Prognosis

- **Prognostic factors** for **CA stomach: Depth**[Q] of **invasion** and **LN status**[Q]

LYMPH NODE STATIONS

1. Right cardiac; **2.** Left cardiac; **3.** Lesser curvature; **4.** Greater curvature; **5.** Suprapyloric; **6.** Infrapyloric **7.** Left gastric; **8.** Common hepatic; **9. Celiac; 10.** Splenic hilus; **11. Splenic artery; 12. Hepatoduodenal ligament**; **13.** Retropancreatic; **14.** Mesenteric root; **15.** Transverse mesocolon; **16.** Paraaortic

■ TNM CLASSIFICATION OF CARCINOMA OF THE STOMACH

8th AJCC (2017) TNM Classification of Carcinoma of the Stomach	
Tis: Carcinoma in situ: intraepithelial tumor without invasion of the lamina propria, high grade dysplasia	**N1:** Metastasis in **1-2** regional LNs[Q]
T1a: Tumor invades **lamina propria or muscularis mucosa**[Q]	**N2:** Metastasis in **3-6** regional LNs[Q]
T1b: Tumor invades **submucosa**[Q]	**N3a:** Metastasis in **7-15** regional LNs[Q]
T2: Tumor invades **muscularis propria**[Q]	**N3b:** Metastasis in **16 or more** regional LNs[Q]
T3: Tumor penetrates **subserosal connective tissue** without invasion of visceral peritoneum or adjacent structures[Q]	
T4a: Tumor invades **serosa (visceral peritoneum)**[Q]	**M1:** Distant metastasis
T4b: Tumor invades **adjacent structures**[Q]	

Stage Grouping								
Stage	**IA**	**IB**	**IIA**	**IIB**	**IIIA**	**IIIB**	**IIIC**	**IV**
	T1N0	T1N1	T1N2	T1N3a	T2N3a	T1-2N3b	T3-4aN3b	Any T, Any N, **M1**
		T2N0	T2N1	T2N2	T3N2	T3-4aN3a	T4bN3a-3b	
			T3N0	T3N1	T4aN1-2	T4bN1-2		
				T4aN0	T4bN0			

◼ LEATHER BOTTLE STOMACH (LINITIS PLASTICA)

LEATHER BOTTLE STOMACH (LINITIS PLASTICA)

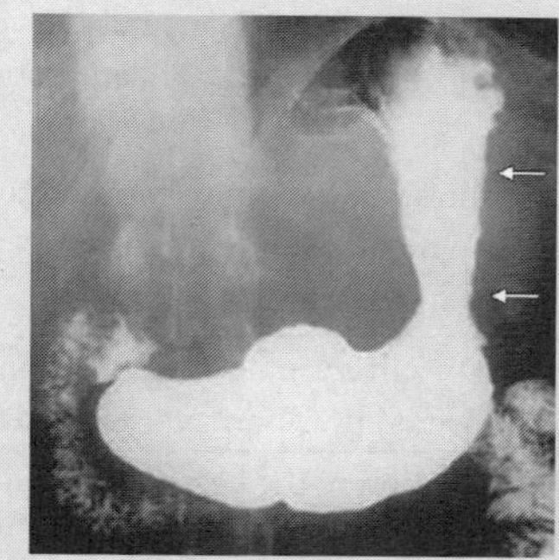
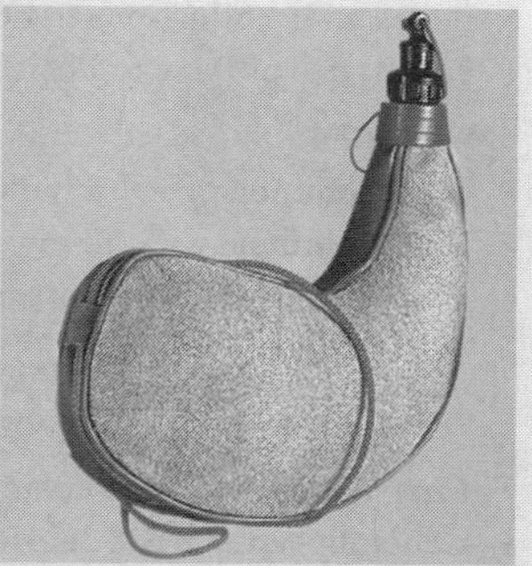

- Pyloric antrum is **MC site** affected in **localized variety**[Q]
- Stomach is **massively thickened** (feels like **leather**)[Q]

Pathology

- Caused by **proliferation of fibrous tissue** mainly in **submucosa**[Q]
- Characterized by **Mother of pearl appearance**
- Mucosa appears normal

Clinical Features

- **Early satiety** due to **reduced stomach capacity**[Q]
- **LN metastasis** is common[Q]

Treatment

- Treated by **radical gastrectomy**[Q]

Prognosis

- Associated with **poor prognosis**[Q]

◼ GASTROINTESTINAL STROMAL TUMOR

GASTROINTESTINAL STROMAL TUMOR

- GISTs: **MC mesenchymal tumor** of the **GI tract**[Q]
- MC primary site for GIST: **Stomach** (60–70%) > **small bowel** (20–25%) > **colorectum & esophagus** (5% each)[Q].

> - Most GISTs are **positive for CD-117** (95%), **BCL-2** (80%), **CD-34** (70%)[Q].

- **Types: Spindle cell** (70%) and **Epitheloid** (30%)[Q]

Pathology

- Arise from the **muscularis propria** and most likely originate from the **cells of Cajal**[Q]
- Expression of the receptor tyrosine kinase **KIT** (**CD 117**), 5% express platelet derived growth factor receptor alpha (**PDGFRA**)[Q].
- **PDGFRA mutations** in GIST appear to confer a **very favorable prognosis** with **low risk of recurrence**[Q].
- New tumor markers of GIST: **DOG-1** (discovered on GIST-1) & **protein kinase C-theta**

Clinical features

- Patients usually present after the fourth decade, with the mean age of **60 years** at diagnosis.
- **MC presentations** of gastric GISTs: **GI bleeding** and **pain** or dyspepsia.

Carney triad
Association of **extra-adrenal paragangliomas, pulmonary chondromas & multifocal GIST**[Q].

Diagnosis

> - **CT: IOC** for evaluation of **primary tumor & accurate staging**[Q]
> - **PET-CT: Gold standard** for recurrent GIST[Q]

Treatment

- **Bleeding** manifestation is the **MC indication** for **surgery**[Q].
- GIST should be treated with **segmental resection**[Q] (margins of **1cm**)

> - **LN metastasis** are **uncommon, regional lymphadenectomy** is **not recommended**[Q]
> - **Intraoperative incisional biopsy** prior to resection should be **avoided**, because it risks **tumor spillage**[Q]

- **Imatinib**[Q] (selective inhibitor of **type 3** tyrosine kinase KIT), is approved for use in **CD117-positive unresectable** and **metastatic GISTs**.

> - Functional imaging of GIST with **18FDG-PET** scanning represents a useful diagnostic modality for **early-response assessment** with **imatinib therapy**[Q].
> - **Sunitinib**[Q] is used in **imatinib-refractory disease**.
> - **Regorafenib**[Q]: Third line therapy in the **patients failing imatinib & sunitinib therapy**[Q].

Prognosis

- **Tumor size** is a **predominant factor for survival** in surgical series for primary GIST.
- **MC sites** of **disease failure** after complete resection: **Liver**[Q], **omentum** or **peritoneal cavity**.

■ BEZOARS

BEZOARS

- Bezoars are **collections** of **nondigestible materials**, usually of vegetable origin (phytobezoar) but also of hair (trichobezoar).
- **Four types of Bezoar:** Phytobezoars, Trichobezoars, Pharmacobezoar and Lactobezoar

Phytobezoar

- **Most common type**[Q], a high concentration of tannin, exposed to gastric acid form a coagulum leading to bezoar formation
- **Most commonly** found in patients who have undergone **surgery** of the **stomach** and have **impaired gastric emptying**[Q].
- **Diabetics** with **autonomic neuropathy**[Q] are also at risk.

  > - **Symptoms: Early satiety**, nausea, **pain, vomiting**, and **weight loss** with palpable **large mass**[Q]
  > - **Diagnosis** confirmed by a **barium examination** or **endoscopy**[Q].

- **Enzymatic therapy** to attempt dissolution of the bezoar. **Papain** and **cellulase** have been used with some success.
- Generally, **enzymatic débridement** is followed by **aggressive Ewald tube lavage** or **endoscopic fragmentation**[Q]. Failure of these therapies would necessitate surgical removal.

Trichobezoar

- Concretions of hair, generally found in **long-haired girls** or **women** who often deny eating their own hair (**trichophagy**)[Q].
- Typically **black** regardless of the color of the hair ingested because of enzymatic oxidation of gastric acid

  > - **Most common** type in **Children**[Q]
  > - **Trichobezoars** are **most likely** to **require surgical management**[Q]
  > - **Rapunzel Syndrome:** Gastric trichobezoars with a long **extension** of hairs that trails **into the duodenum.**

- **Symptoms: Pain** from **gastric ulceration** and fullness from **gastric outlet obstruction** with occasional **gastric perforation** and **small bowel obstruction**[Q].
- **Larger trichobezoars** require **surgical removal**[Q].
- The trichophagy requires **psychiatric care**[Q] because recurrent bezoar formation is common.

■ STRESS GASTRITIS (STRESS ULCERATIONS)

STRESS GASTRITIS (STRESS ULCERATIONS/ STRESS EROSIVE GASTRITIS/ HEMORRHAGIC GASTRITIS)

- Characterized by **multiple, superficial** (nonulcerating) **erosions** that **begin in** the **proximal or acid-secreting portion** of the stomach and **progress distally**[Q].
- **Almost always** seen in the **fundus**[Q] & **rarely** in **distal stomach**.

  > - **Cushing's ulcer:** Occur in the setting of central nervous system disease (**Head trauma**)[Q]
  > - **Curling's ulcer:** as a result of **thermal burn injury** involving > 35% of BSA[Q]

- **Increased acid secretion in Cushing's ulcer** but **not in Curling's ulcer**[Q]

Pathophysiology

Risk factors or Predisposing clinical conditions		
• **ARDS**[Q]	• **Hepatic dysfunction**[Q]	• **Hypotension**[Q]
• **Multiple trauma**[Q]	• **Oliguric renal failure**[Q]	• **Prolonged** surgical procedures[Q]
• Major burn **> 35%** of BSA[Q]	• Large **transfusion**[Q] requirements	• **Sepsis**[Q]

Clinical Features

- More than **50%** of patients develop their **stress gastritis within 1–2 days** after a traumatic event.
- Only clinical sign may be **painless upper GI bleeding** that may be delayed at onset.
- **Bleeding** is usually **slow** and **intermittent**[Q]

Diagnosis

- **Endoscopy** is required to **confirm the diagnosis**[Q] and to differentiate stress gastritis from other sources of GI hemorrhage.

Treatment

- **Definitive fluid resuscitation** with **correction** of any **coagulation abnormalities** and **treatment of the underlying sepsis**[Q]
- **Intraluminal gastric pH** should be maintained >5.0 with **antisecretory agents**.
- **Most of** the **superficial erosions** are not actively bleeding **do not require ligature unless** a **blood vessel** is seen at its **base**[Q].

  > - Operation is completed by **closing the anterior gastrotomy** and performing a **truncal vagotomy & pyloroplasty**[Q] to reduce acid secretion.

■ GASTRIC VOLVULUS

GASTRIC VOLVULUS

- **Organoaxial (two thirds)**: Torsion occurs along the stomach's **longitudinal axis**[Q]
- **Mesenteroaxial (one third)**: Torsion occurs along the **vertical axis**[Q]

Primary Gastric Volvulus	Secondary Gastric Volvulus
• Seen in association with **congenital asplenia & wandering spleen**[Q] • Usually **mesenteroaxial**[Q] • **Partial (<180 degree) & recurrent**[Q] • Not associated with a diaphragmatic defect	• Occur secondary to some anatomic abnormality, (**Most commonly diaphragmatic hernia**)[Q] • Usually **organoaxial**[Q] • **Paraesophageal hiatal hernia** is the most common cause in **adults** & **congenital diaphragmatic hernia** (Bochdalek hernia) in **children**[Q]

Clinical Features

- **Organoaxial gastric volvulus** occurs **acutely** & is associated with a diaphragmatic defect
- **Mesenteroaxial volvulus** is **partial** (< 180 degrees), **recurrent**, and not associated with a diaphragmatic defect.
- Major symptoms at presentation are **abdominal pain** that is acute in onset, distention, vomiting, & **upper GI hemorrhage**[Q].

> - **Borchardt's triad**: (Epigastric pain + Inability to vomit + Inability to pass a nasogastric tube) is characteristic feature of gastric volvulus[Q].

Diagnosis

- **X-ray abdomen**: Gas-filled viscus in the **chest** or upper abdomen[Q].
- **Diagnosis** can be **confirmed** by **barium** contrast study or **endoscopy**[Q].

Treatment

- **Acute volvulus**: It is a **surgical emergency. Stomach** is **reduced & uncoiled. Diaphragmatic defect** is **repaired** with consideration given to a fundoplication in the setting of a paraesophageal hernia[Q].
- In **strangulation** (5–28%), **compromised segment** of stomach is **resected**[Q].
- **Spontaneous volvulus,** without an associated diaphragmatic defect, is treated by **detorsion & fixation** of the stomach by gastropexy or tube gastrostomy[Q].

■ INFANTILE HYPERTROPHIC PYLORIC STENOSIS

INFANTILE HYPERTROPHIC PYLORIC STENOSIS

- In HPS, **hypertrophy** of **circular muscle**[Q] of **pylorus** results in constriction & obstruction of gastric outlet.
- **Acquired condition**
- **Incidence** of **1 in 3000 to 4000**[Q] live births.
- **Most common between** the ages of **3–6 weeks**[Q].
- **Associated anomalies** in **6–20%** cases: Esophageal atresia, Hirschprung's disease, ARM & malrotation

Etiology

- **Ethnic origin** is important because **highest incidence** is found among **whites of Scandinavian**[Q] decent and **lowest risk** among **African Americans** and **Chinese.**

> | • **Males** outnumber females by a ratio of **4:1**[Q] | • **First-born males**[Q] are frequently encountered. |

- **Higher risk** for developing HPS in **offspring of parents**[Q] with **this condition**

Clinical Presentation

- Infant is **normal at birth, symptomatic between** the ages of **3–6 weeks**[Q]
- Infants with HPS typically present with **projectile nonbilious vomiting**[Q].

> - **Visible gastric peristalsis** may be seen as a wave of contraction **from the left upper quadrant** to the **epigastrium**[Q].

- The infants usually **feed vigorously** between episodes of vomiting.
- Typical electrolyte abnormality: **Hypochloremic, hypokalemic, metabolic alkalosis** with **paradoxical aciduria**[Q].

Diagnosis

- **Palpation of the** pyloric tumor or **olive** in the **epigastrium**[Q] or right upper quadrant by a skilled examiner is **pathognomonic** for the diagnosis of HPS[Q].
- If the olive is palpated, **no additional diagnostic testing** is necessary[Q].

> - When the olive **cannot be palpated**, the diagnosis of HPS can be made with an **ultrasound exam** or fluoroscopic UGI series.
> - Absence of radiation exposure and cost make the **ultrasound** the **usual preferred study**[Q].

Contd…

Contd…

- **Diagnostic Sonographic measurements**:
  - **Pyloric wall thickness** of at least **4 mm**[Q]   – Transverse diameter **>13 mm**   – **Channel length** of at least **17 mm**[Q]
- **Barium Meal**:
  - **String sign**[Q]: indicating a narrowed elongated pyloric canal that does not relax is seen (**most specific sign**)
  - **Shoulder sign**[Q]: caused by hypertrophied muscle indenting the antrum
  - **Double-track sign**[Q]: caused by redundant mucosa

Treatment

- Pyloric stenosis is **never a surgical emergency** although dehydration and electrolyte abnormalities may present a **medical emergency**[Q]
- **Fluid resuscitation** and **correction of electrolyte abnormalities**[Q] and metabolic alkalosis is essential before surgery.
  - It is important that the underlying metabolic alkalosis is **slowly corrected** with **normal saline**.
  - Treatment of HPS is by a **Ramstedt-Fredet pyloromyotomy** (**cutting across** the **abnormal pyloric musculature**[Q] while preserving the underlying mucosa).

■ DUODENAL ATRESIA

DUODENAL ATRESIA

- Occurs as a **result of failure of vacuolization** of the **duodenum** from its solid cord stage.

Anatomic variants of Duodenal Atresia
Type I → **Mucosal web** with intact muscular wall (**windsock deformity**)
Type II → Two ends separated by a **fibrous cord**
Type III → **Complete separation with a gap** within the duodenum.

Clinical Features

- In most cases, the **duodenal obstruction** is **distal to the ampulla of Vater**, and infants present with **bilious emesis** in the **neonatal period**[Q].

Diagnosis

- **X-ray abdomen**: Double-bubble sign (air-filled stomach and **duodenal bulb**[Q]).

> - **Diagnosis is confirmed**, if there is **no distal air**[Q].
> - **If distal air** is present, an **upper GI contrast study** is **performed rapidly**, not only **to confirm the diagnosis of duodenal atresia** but also to **exclude midgut volvulus**[Q].

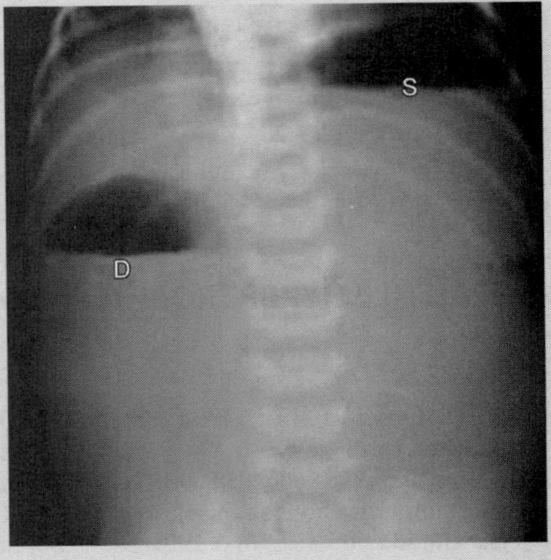

Treatment

- **Diamond-shaped duodenoduodenostomy** is the **treatment of choice**[Q].
- **5 'D's of duodenal atresia**: **D**A, **D**own's syndrome, **D**istal to ampulla, **D**ouble bubble sign, **D**uodenoduodenostomy

■ H. PYLORI

1. **H. pylori has been implicated in all, except:** *(Orissa 2011)*
   a. Gastric ulcer
   b. Gastric carcinoma
   c. Gastric lymphoma
   d. Gastric leiomyoma

2. **Which of the following is a common gastric lesion associated with H. pylori and undergoes regression following eradication of the infection?** *(MHPGMCET 2009)*
   a. Inflammatory polyp
   b. Metaplastic polyp
   c. Fundic gland
   d. True adenomas

3. **Eradication of helicobacter pylori has been proved to be beneficial in which of the following disorders of the stomach?** *(COMEDK 2006)*
   a. Low grade MALT lymphoma
   b. Erosive gastritis
   c. Carcinoma stomach
   d. Gastroesophageal disease

4. **H. pylori infection is associated with development of which malignancy:** *(DPG 2011)*
   a. MALTomas
   b. Atherosclerosis
   c. Sarcoma
   d. Gastrointestinal stromal tumor (GIST)

■ PEPTIC ULCER ETIOLOGY AND CLINICAL FEATURES

5. **Peptic ulcer is associated with all except one:**
   a. Cirrhosis *(AIIMS Feb 97)*
   b. Zollinger Ellison syndrome
   c. Primary hyperparathyroidism
   d. Pernicious anemia

6. **The causative agent for duodenal ulcer is:** *(MCI Dec 2019)*
   a. Shigella
   b. E. coli
   c. H. pylori
   d. Lactobacilli

7. **Which one is not associated with peptic ulcer?**
   a. Smoking cigarette *(AIIMS Nov 95)*
   b. Zollinger-Ellison's syndrome
   c. Plummer-Vinson syndrome
   d. Cirrhosis

8. **Commonest site of peptic ulcer is:** *(All India 99)*
   a. 1st part of duodenum
   b. 2nd part of duodenum
   c. Distal 1/3rd of stomach
   d. Pylorus of the stomach

9. **The most common site of a benign (peptic) gastric ulcer is:**
   a. Upper third of lesser curvature *(AIIMS June 2004)*
   b. Greater curvature
   c. Pyloric antrum
   d. Lesser curvature near incisura angularis

10. **Burning epigastric pain is due to:** *(AIIMS June 2004)*
    a. Vomitting
    b. Reflux esophagitis
    c. Duodenal ulcer
    d. Gastric ulcer

11. **Prepyloric or channel ulcer in the stomach is termed as:** *(Recent Question 2016, COMEDK 2008)*
    a. Type 1
    b. Type 2
    c. Type 3
    d. Type 4

12. **Gastric ulcer type III is located at:** *(Recent Question 2017)*
    a. Lesser curvature
    b. Body
    c. Prepyloric region
    d. GE junction

13. **Most common location for chronic gastric ulcer:** *(Recent Question 2018)*
    a. Antrum
    b. Fundus
    c. Greater curve
    d. Lesser curve

■ PEPTIC ULCER COMPLICATIONS

14. **Which of the following vessel is most commonly involved in hemorrhage from duodenal ulcer?**
    a. IVC *(Recent Question 2016, 2014, All India 2012)*
    b. Gastroduodenal artery
    c. SMA
    d. Inferior pancreatico duodenal artery

15. **Most common complication of chronic gastric ulcer is:**
    a. Tea pot stomach *(AIIMS June 93)*
    b. Scirrhous carcinoma (Adenocarcinoma)
    c. Perforation
    d. Massive hematemesis

16. **In gastric outlet obstruction in a peptic ulcer patient, the site of obstruction is most likely to be:** *(All India 2002, AIIMS June 93)*
    a. Antrum
    b. Duodenum
    c. Pylorus
    d. Pyloric canal

17. **Percentage of patients with perforated peptic ulcer who show free gas under the diaphragm:** *(UPPG 2009)*
    a. 100%
    b. 75%
    c. 50%
    d. 90%

18. **Posterior perforation of peptic ulcer drain into:** *(DNB 2009)*
    a. Omental bursa
    b. Greater sac
    c. Foramen of Winslow
    d. Paracolic gutter

19. **The vessel which needs to be ligated in a patient with a bleeding peptic ulcer is:** *(APPG 2015)*
    a. Gastroduodenal artery
    b. Superior pancreatico-duodenal artery
    c. Left gastric artery
    d. Left gastroepiploic artery

20. **In last decade, duodenal ulcer and its morbidity is reduced due to:** *(Recent Question 2015)*
    a. Lifestyle modification
    b. Eradication of H. pylori
    c. Proton pump inhibitors
    d. None of the above

■ PEPTIC ULCER DIAGNOSIS AND TREATMENT

21. **PPI's for peptic ulcer disease should be taken:** *(JIPMER 2011)*
    a. Before breakfast
    b. After breakfast
    c. After lunch
    d. After dinner

22. **Stump of stomach and duodenum is present in:** *(MHSSMCET 2006)*
    a. Billroth-I operation
    b. Billroth-II operation
    c. Whipple's operation
    d. Truncal vagotomy

23. **Barium meal characteristic feature of malignant gastric ulcer is:** *(JIPMER Nov 2017)*
    a. Hampton line
    b. Carman's meniscus sign
    c. Ulcer cap
    d. Ulcer crater

24. A patient who has undergone partial gastrectomy presents with neurological symptoms. Most probable diagnosis:
(JIPMER 2011)
   a. Folic acid deficiency
   b. Thiamine deficiency
   c. Vitamin B_{12} deficiency
   d. Iron deficiency

25. In a highly selective vagotomy, the vagal supply is severed to:
   a. Proximal two-thirds of stomach *(COMEDK 2008)*
   b. Antrum
   c. Pylorus
   d. Whole of stomach

26. Surgery of choice for chronic duodenal ulcer is:
   a. Vagotomy + antrectomy
   b. Total gastrectomy *(Recent Question 2014, AIIMS June 93)*
   c. Truncal vagotomy + pyloroplasty
   d. Highly selective vagotomy

27. Lowest recurrence rate in duodenal ulcer treatment is seen with: *(MHCET 2016, Recent Question 2014, AIIMS Nov 94, All India 2002)*
   a. Highly selective vagotomy
   b. Truncal vagotomy
   c. Truncal vagotomy and antrectomy
   d. Truncal vagotomy and pyloroplasty

28. Maximal reduction in gastric acidity is achieved by:
(Recent Question 2014, UPCS 97)
   a. Truncal vagotomy and pyloroplasty
   b. Truncal vagotomy and antrectomy
   c. Partial gastrectomy
   d. Highly selective vagotomy

29. Perforated peptic ulcer is treated by: *(SGPGI 2005)*
   a. Vagotomy + Pyloroplasty
   b. Vagotomy + Antrectomy
   c. Vagotomy + repair of perforation
   d. Graham's repair

30. The most commonly practiced operative procedure for a perforated duodenal ulcer is:
(Recent Question 2014, Karnataka 2005)
   a. Vagotomy and pyloroplasty
   b. Vagotomy and antrectomy
   c. Vagotomy and perforation closure
   d. Graham's omentum patch repair

GASTRECTOMY AND COMPLICATIONS

31. A patient of partial gastrectomy presents with neurological symptoms. Most probable diagnosis is: *(JIPMER 2011)*
   a. Folic acid deficiency
   b. Thiamine deficiency
   c. Vitamin B_{12} deficiency
   d. Iron deficiency

32. Dumping syndrome is due to: *(Recent Question 2017, Recent Question 2015, All India 99)*
   a. Diarrhea
   b. Presence of hypertonic content in small intestine
   c. Vagotomy
   d. Reduced gastric capacity

33. Which is not true about dumping syndrome? *(DNB 2014)*
   a. Post vagotomy
   b. Small frequent meals is beneficial
   c. Starch is beneficial
   d. Clinical features include diarrhea and bloating

34. A patient underwent gastrectomy. After eating, within 20 minutes patient started developing sweating, diarrhoea. What could be the cause? *(MCI Dec 2019)*
   a. Hyperglycemia
   b. Early dumping syndrome
   c. Late dumping syndrome
   d. Hypoglycemia

35. Duodenal blow out following Billroth gastrectomy most commonly occurs on which day:
(Recent Question 2015, AIIMS June 93)
   a. 2nd day
   b. 4th day
   c. 6th day
   d. 12th day

36. Anemia is greater in which of the following gastric resection:
   a. Billroth-II
   b. Billroth-I
   c. Both of the above are equal *(Recent Question 2016)*
   d. Neither of the above

37. Gastrojejunostomy is an example of:
   a. Clean contaminated wound *(DNB 2001, JIPMER 2008)*
   b. Clean uncontaminated wound
   c. Unclean uncontaminated wound
   d. Unclean contaminated wound

38. Which is a clean surgery: *(Recent Question 2013)*
   a. Hernia surgery
   b. Gastric surgery
   c. Cholecystectomy
   d. Rectal surgery

39. The first gastrectomy was performed in 1881 by:
   a. Miculikz
   b. Wolfer *(Bihar PG 2016)*
   c. Billroth
   d. Moynihan

UPPER GI BLEED

40. In Forrest classification, high-risk of bleeding is associated with all except: *(KGMC 2011)*
   a. Visible vessel
   b. Visible pulsatile bleeding
   c. Adherent clot
   d. Visible oozing from vessel

41. Investigation of choice for UGI bleed:
(WBPG 2012, PGI SS 2004, June 97)
   a. Endoscopy
   b. Angiography
   c. CT
   d. Barium studies

42. A 42-year-old company executive presents with sudden upper GI bleed (5 litres) of bright red blood, with no significant previous history. The diagnosis is: *(All India 2000)*
   a. Esophageal varices
   b. Duodenal ulcer
   c. Gastritis
   d. Gastric erosion

43. Following resuscitation, a patient with bleeding esophageal varices should be treated initially with: *(AIIMS Nov 2004)*
   a. Sclerotherapy
   b. Sengstaken Blackmore tube
   c. Propranolol
   d. Surgery

44. The most sensitive test to detect GI bleeding is:
   a. Selective angiography *(Recent Question 2016)*
   b. Radiolabelled erythrocyte scanning
   c. I-131 fibrinogen studies
   d. Stool for occult blood

45. In the Forrest classification for bleeding peptic ulcer with a visible vessel of pigmented protuberance is classified as:
(Recent Question 2016, COMEDK 2006)
   a. FI
   b. FII a
   c. FII b
   d. FII c

46. Most common cause of upper gastrointestinal tract bleeding is: *(Recent Question 2015, 2014, 2013)*
   a. Esophageal varices
   b. Peptic ulcer
   c. Gastritis
   d. Mallory weiss tear

47. Among the following, the least common cause of acute upper GI bleeding is: *(APPG 2015)*
   a. Vascular ectasia
   b. Mallory Weiss tear
   c. Ulcer
   d. Varices

48. Regarding Upper GI bleed, true statement is:
   a. Most common cause is variceal bleeding
   b. It is bleeding upto ampulla of Vater *(Recent Question 2018)*
   c. Most commonly performed management is endoscopic banding
   d. Rockall scoring is used for risk stratification

MALLORY-WEISS TEAR

49. An old man presenting to the emergency following a bout of prolonged vomiting with excessive hematemesis following alcohol ingestion is likely to suffer from: *(MCI June 2018)*
   a. Mallory-Weiss syndrome
   b. Esophageal varices
   c. Gastric cancer
   d. Bleeding disorder

50. **Mallory-Weiss syndrome is partial thickness rupture occurs at:**
    (Recent Question 2017, Recent Question 2016, WBPG 2014, PGI Dec 97)
    a. Gastric cardia
    b. Esophagus mucosa
    c. Gastroesophageal junction
    d. Gastroduodenal junction

51. **Violent vomiting after forceful retching present with sudden severe hematemesis diagnosis is:** *(Recent Question 2018)*
    a. Haemangioma
    b. Carcinoma oesophagus
    c. Mallory-Weiss syndrome
    d. Esophageal varices

■ DIEULAFOY'S LESION

52. **Dieulafoy's lesion is:** *(Recent Question 2016, MHSSMCET 2006)*
    a. Prolapse gastropathy
    b. Gastric antral vascular ectasia
    c. Gastric hemorrhagic telengectasias
    d. Aberrant vessel in the mucosa that bleeds form a mucosal defect

■ GASTRIC ANTRAL VASCULAR ECTASIA

53. **'Watermelon stomach' is:** *(MHSSMCET 2008)*
    a. Prolapse gastropathy
    b. Gastric antral vascular ectasia
    c. Gastric hemorrhagic telengectasias
    d. Aberrant vessel in the mucosa that bleeds form a mucosal defect

54. **What is the most probable diagnosis on the basis of given endoscopy image?** *(Recent Question 2016)*
    a. Dieulafoy's lesion b. Gastric antral vascular ectasia
    c. Menetrier's disease   d. Mallory-Weiss syndrome

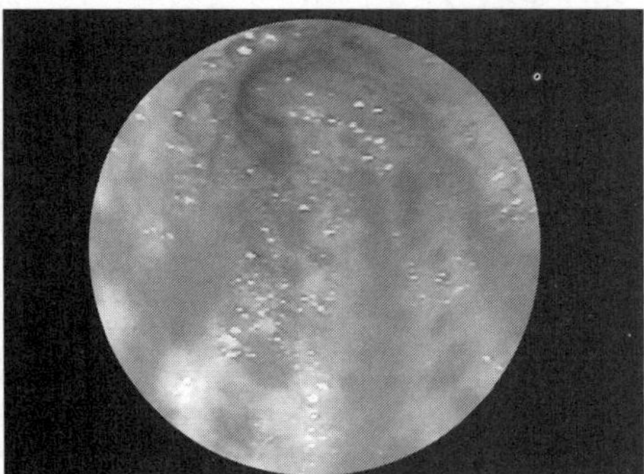

■ MENETRIER'S DISEASE

55. **A 50 years old male presented with the history of epigastric pain, anorexia, weight loss and pedal edema. On laboratory examination, total protein and albumin was low. Endoscopy was performed and the image is given below. What is the most probable diagnosis?**

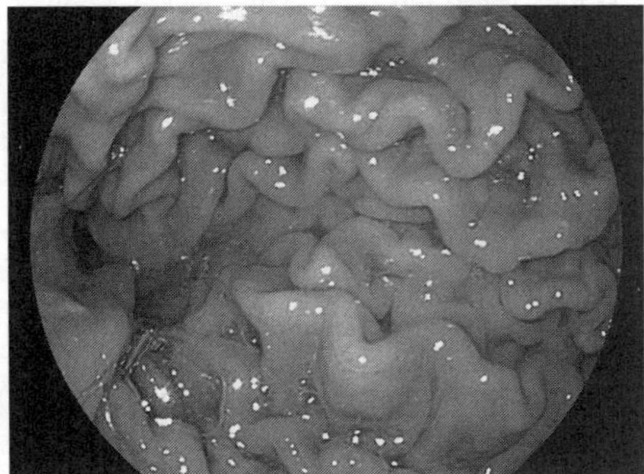

a. Gastric varices
b. Carcinoma stomach
c. Hamartomatous polyp
d. Menetrier's disease

56. **Menetrier's disease is characterized by all of the following except:** *(COMEDK 2006)*
    a. Giant folds in the pyloric antrum
    b. Foveolar hyperplasia
    c. Hypoalbuminaemia
    d. Hypochlorhydria

■ GASTRIC POLYPS

57. **Most common benign tumour of the stomach is:**
    a. Adenoma
    b. Lipoma
    c. Hamartoma
    d. Leiomyoma

58. **The commonest gastric polyp is:** *(COMEDK 2008)*
    a. Hyperplastic polyp
    b. Inflammatory polyp
    c. Adenomatous polyp
    d. Part of familial polyposis

■ CARCINOMA STOMACH PREDISPOSING FACTORS

59. **Due to popularity of refrigeration reducing the need to preserve food, which cancer's incidence has dramatically declined?** *(AIIMS May 2013)*
    a. Esophagus
    b. Stomach
    c. Colon
    d. Oropharyngeal malignancies

60. **E-cadherin is more often mutated in:** *(COMEDK 2010)*
    a. Diffuse type of gastric cancer
    b. Intestinal type of gastric cancer
    c. Malignant ulcer of stomach
    d. Erosive gastritis

61. **Which of the following anemia is a risk factor for the development of gastric carcinoma?**
    a. Pernicious anemia
    b. Megaloblastic anemia
    c. Aplastic anemia
    d. Hemolytic anemia

62. **All of the following predispose to gastric carcinoma except:** *(All India 1990)*
    a. Achlorhydria
    b. 'O' blood group
    c. Pernicious anaemia
    d. Postgastrectomy

63. **All are true about gastric carcinoma except:** *(DNB 2006)*
    a. More in low socioeconomic group
    b. Most common at fundus
    c. H. pylori infection increases risks
    d. Vitamin C protects

64. **AKT-1 amplification is seen in:** *(Recent Question 2016)*
    a. CA bladder
    b. CA colon
    c. Breast cancer
    d. Gastric cancer

■ CA STOMACH CLINICAL FEATURES AND TREATMENT

65. **All of the following are true about diffuse gastric cancer according to Lauren's classification except:**
    a. Familial *(Recent Question 2017)*
    b. More common in males
    c. Undifferentiated
    d. More common in the proximal part

66. **Hereditary diffuse gastric carcinoma is associated with:**
    a. Ductal carcinoma NOS subtype *(Recent Question 2017)*
    b. Lobular carcinoma
    c. Ductal carcinoma in-situ
    d. Metaplastic carcinoma

67. Type 1 gastric cancer according to Bormann's classification: *(Recent Question 2017)*
a. Protruding
b. Ulcerated
c. Flat
d. Excavated

68. GE junction tumor is: *(Recent Question 2017)*
a. Siewert type I
b. Siewert type II
c. Siewert type III
d. Siewert type IV

69. Sister Joseph's nodule may indicated cancer of all the following except: *(COMEDK 2004)*
a. Somach
b. Large bowel
c. Rectum
d. Ovary

70. A 20-years-old female, previously diagnosed with adenocarcinoma stomach and on examination following is seen. What is the most probable diagnosis? *(MCI Dec 2019)*

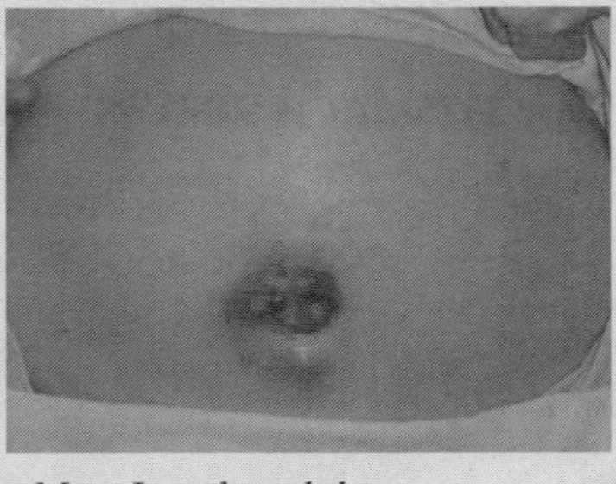

a. Sister Mary Joseph nodule
b. Ulcer
c. Infected umbilical hernia
d. Irish node

71. Most common site of carcinoma of stomach is: *(JIPMER 2010)*
a. Proximal stomach
b. Gastric antrum
c. Lesser curvature
d. Greater curvature

72. An ulcero-proliferative lesion in the antrum of the stomach 6 cm in diameter, invading the serosa, with 10 enlarged lymph nodes around and pylorus with no distant metastasis, the TNM staging is: *(COMEDK 2011)*
a. T2N1M0
b. T3N2M0
c. T4N1M0
d. T1N3M0

73. Troisier's sign is: *(MHPGMCET 2008, 2006, APPG 96)*
a. Metastatic left supraclavicular lymphadenopathy
b. Carpopedal spasm in hypocalcemia
c. Migratory thrombophlebitis
d. Any of the above

74. Irish node is most commonly seen in: *(WB PG 2015)*
a. Ca stomach
b. Ca lung
c. Ca larynx
d. CA endometrium

75. When carcinoma of stomach develops secondarily to pernicious anemia, it is usually situated in the:
a. Pre-pyloric region
b. Pylorus *(All India 2006)*
c. Body
d. Fundus

76. The best prognosis in carcinoma stomach is with:
(Bihar PG 2014, UPSC 2008, All India 95)
a. Superficial spreading type
b. Ulcerative type
c. Linnitis plastica type
d. Polypoidal type

77. All the following indicates early gastric cancer except:
(Recent Question 2015, DNB 2006, All India 2002, AIIMS Feb 97)
a. Involvement of mucosa
b. Involvement of mucosa and submucosa
c. Involvement of mucosa, submucosa and muscularis
d. Involvement of mucosa, submucosa and adjacent lymph nodes

78. Linnitis plastica is commonly seen in:
(Recent Question 2014, DNB 2005, 2001, 2000, All India 91)
a. Carcinoma stomach
b. Sarcoidosis
c. Lymphoma
d. Leiomyosarcoma

79. Peritoneal dissemination of gastric cancer is best detected by:
a. USG
b. Laparoscopy
c. CT
d. MRI *(COMEDK 2014)*

80. Locally invasive gastric carcinoma. Investigation of choice to know depth of cancer invasion: *(Recent Question 2013)*
a. CECT
b. MRI
c. Barium
d. EUS

81. Most common cause of Krukenberg's tumor is: *(DNB 2014)*
a. Ovary
b. Liver
c. Stomach
d. Kidney

■ GASTROINTESTINAL STROMAL TUMOR

82. Which of the following is false about GIST?
a. More common in female *(Recent Question 2017)*
b. >5 cm in size is high-risk
c. Mesodermal origin
d. Treatment of choice is segmental resection

83. For high-risk cases of GIST of size >10 cm, imatinib therapy is given for: *(Recent Question 2017)*
a. 1 year
b. 2 years
c. 3 years
d. 5 years

84. Treatment of choice for localized GIST: *(Recent Question 2017)*
a. Segmental resection
b. Total gastrectomy
c. Distal gastrectomy
d. Imatinib mesylate

85. Imatinib used in treatment of: *(Recent Question 2017, 2016)*
a. GIST
b. GI lymphoma
c. CA esophagus
d. CA colon

86. Most common site of GIST: *(Recent Question 2016)*
a. Esophagus
b. Stomach
c. Small intestine
d. Colon

87. Sunitinib is used in: *(KGMC 2011)*
a. GIST
b. Rectal cancer
c. Colonic carcinoma
d. Pancreatic carcinoma

88. A 50 years old male presents with obstructive symptoms. Biopsy of stomach reveals gastrointestinal stromal tumor (GIST). Most appropriate market for GIST is:
(Recent Question 2017, 2016, AIIMS May 2011)
a. CD-34
b. CD-117
c. CD-30
d. CD-10

89. Gold standard investigation for recurrent gastrointestinal stromal tumor is: *(AIIMS May 2011)*
a. MRI
b. MIBG
c. USG
d. PET-CT

90. True about GIST all except: *(Recent Question 2015, AIIMS Nov 2010)*
a. Most common in duodenum
b. Necrosis and ulceration present
c. PET is used to assess response to therapy
d. Cell circumscribed

91. Most common type of gastric sarcoma: *(MCI June 2018)*
a. Lipoma
b. Glomus tumour
c. Leiomyosarcoma
d. Leioblastoma

■ GASTRIC LYMPHOMA

92. The commonest site of lymphoma in the gastrointestinal system is: *(COMEDK 2007)*
a. Small bowel
b. Stomach
c. Large intestine
d. Oesophagus

93. False about gastric lymphoma is: *(AIIMS May 2008)*
a. Stomach is the most common site
b. Associated with H. pylori infection
c. Total gastrectomy with adjuvant chemotherapy is treatment of choice
d. 5 years survival rate after treatment is 60%

■ DUODENAL ATRESIA

94. Anomaly associated with duodenal atresia is: *(DNB 2010)*
a. Down's syndrome
b. Duodenal adenomas
c. Limb defects
d. Autoimmune disorders

95. Antenatal double bubble appearance on ultrasound is due to: *(Bihar PG 2014, PGI June 97)*
a. Diaphragmatic hernia
b. Duodenal atresia
c. Gastric volvulus
d. Intussuception

96. Double Bubble sign is seen with: *(Recent Question 2016, PGI Dec 2006, DNB 2007, 2003, AIIMS May 2009)*
a. Pyloric stenosis
b. Duodenal atresia
c. Ileal atresia
d. Esophageal atresia

97. A newborn baby was brought with the history multiple episodes of bilious projectile vomiting. X-ray abdomen was done. What is the diagnosis? *(Recent Question 2016)*
a. Duodenal atresia
b. Jejunal atresia
c. Ileal atresia
d. Hypertrophic pyloric stenosis

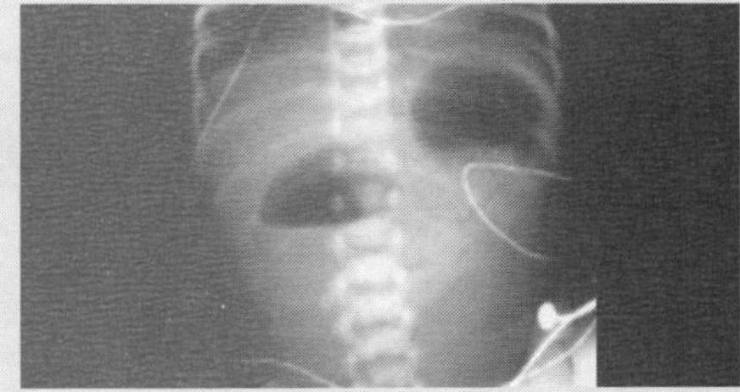

98. Which is the treatment of choice for duodenal atresia? *(DNB, 2011, 2002 MHSSMCET 2005)*
a. Duodenoduodenostomy
b. Duodenojejunostomy
c. Bishop-Koop Procedure
d. Gastroduodenostomy

99. Duodenal atresia is associated with: *(Recent Question 2017)*
a. Down's syndrome
b. Patau's syndrome
c. Turner's syndrome
d. Edward's syndrome

■ HYPERTROPHIC PYLORIC STENOSIS

100. Investigation of choice to diagnose hypertrophic pyloric stenosis in infants is: *(Recent Question 2015, 2014, COMEDK 2011)*
a. Contrast radiology
b. Gastroscopy
c. Ultrasound abdomen
d. CT abdomen

101. Hypertrophic pyloric stenosis presents as:
a. Mass in epigastriumv *(Recent Question 2014, GB Pant 2011)*
b. More common in girls
c. Congenital
d. Present at birth with bilious vomiting

102. Ramsted's operation is performed for:
a. Hirschsprung's disease
b. CHPS *(Bihar PG 2014, MHSSMCET 2005, Kerala 94)*
c. Duodenal atresia
d. Anorectal malformation

103. In a case of hypertrophic pyloric stenosis, the metabolic disturbance is: *(Recent Question 2017, Recent Question 2016, Bihar PG 2014, JIPMER 2013, All India 2002)*
a. Respiratory alkalosis
b. Metabolic acidosis
c. Metabolic alkalosis with paradoxical aciduria
d. Metabolic alkalosis with alkaline urine

104. Metabolic abnormalities associated with infantile pyloric stenosis in early phase include all except: *(DNB 2012)*
a. Hypokalemia
b. Aciduria
c. Hypochloremia
d. None of the above

105. Hypochloremia, hypokalemia and alkalosis are seen in:
a. Congenital hypertrophic pylori stenosis
b. Hirschsprung's disease *(DNB 2012, AIIMS June 2003)*
c. Esophageal atresia
d. Jejunal atresia

106. True about hypertrophic pyloric stenosis is all except:
a. Present at 4 weeks *(DNB 2007)*
b. First born male is commonly affected
c. Ramstedt operation is done
d. Visible peristalsis is always seen

107. String sign on barium meal is seen in: *(Recent Question 2015)*
a. Duodenal atresia
b. Intestinal obstruction
c. Duodenal ulcer
d. Congenital hypertrophic pyloric stenosis

108. The abdominal mass is palpable in …. region in hypertrophic pyloric stenosis.: *(Recent Question 2018)*
a. Umbilical
b. Right hypochondrium
c. Epigastrium
d. Right iliac fossa

■ GASTRIC OUTLET OBSTRUCTION

109. When peptic ulcer leads to gastric outlet obstruction, the most likely site of obstruction is? *(Orissa 2011)*
a. Antrum
b. Pylorus
c. Lesser curvature
d. First part of duodenum

110. The most common cause of gastric outlet obstruction in India is: *(All India 2006)*
a. Tuberculosis
b. Cancer of stomach
c. Duodenal lymphoma
d. Peptic ulcer disease

111. All of the following are seen in chronic pyloric obstruction except: *(MCI March 2010)*
a. Alkaline urine
b. Acidic urine
c. Hypochloremia
d. Hypokalemia

■ BEZOARS

112. Bezoar in the stomach present as: *(Punjab 2009)*
a. Melena
b. Perforation
c. GI obstruction
d. Diarrhea

113. A female in her twenties presents with complaints of pain abdomen, abdominal distention and vomiting. On examination, she was found to have alopecia and a crepitus in the epigastrium. What is your diagnosis? *(AIIMS Nov 2014)*
a. Trichobezoar
b. Carcinoma pyloric antrum
c. Intestinal tuberculosis
d. Rectus sheath hematoma

114. True about trichobezoars are all except: *(MAHE 2006)*
a. It is caused by Trichuris
b. It is a psychiatric manifestation
c. Ball of hairs in the stomach
d. Pulling the hair and sucking of hair is usually seen

■ STRESS GASTRITIS

115. Cushing ulcers are: *(Recent Question 2019)*
a. Stress ulcers in burns
b. Stress ulcers in head injury
c. Stress ulcers in hiatus hernia
d. Stress ulcers in analgesic drug abuse

116. Stress-induced ulcers are most commonly found in the: *(COMEDK 2010)*
a. Fundus of stomach
b. Antrum of stomach
c. Pyloric channel
d. First part of duodenum

117. Common sites of for Cushing ulcers include all of the following except: *(All India 99)*
a. Esophagus
b. Stomach
c. 1st part of duodenum
d. Distal duodenum

118. Most common site of Curling's ulcer:
(Recent Question 2014, AIIMS Nov 2008)
a. Ileum
b. Stomach
c. Duodenum
d. Esophagus

119. Erosive gastritis commonly occurs at: *(JIPMER 93)*
a. Body
b. Fundus
c. Lesser curvature
d. Antrum

120. Curling's ulcer is seen in:
a. Burn patients *(NEET 2013, DNB 2008, All India 88)*
b. Patients with head injuries
c. Zollinger Ellison syndrome
d. Analgesic drug abuse

■ GASTRIC VOLVULUS

121. Borchardt's triad of acute epigastric pain violent retching and inability to pass a nasogastric tube is seen in patients with:
a. Achalasia cardia
b. Acute gastric volvulus
c. Jejunogastric intussusceptions *(J & K 2005)*
d. Hiatus hernia

Explanations

■ H. PYLORI

1. Ans. d. Gastric leiomyoma *(Ref: Harrison 20/e p2215)*

Diseases Associated with H. pylori		
Antral Predominant Gastritis	**Corpus Predominant Atrophic Gastritis**	**Non-atrophic Pangastritis (Chronic Superficial gastritis)**
• Duodenal ulcer[Q]	• Gastric ulcer[Q] • Gastric adenocarcinoma[Q]	• MALT lymphoma[Q]

2. Ans. b. Metaplastic polyp

3. Ans. a. Low grade MALT lymphoma

4. Ans. a. MALTomas

■ PEPTIC ULCER ETIOLOGY AND CLINICAL FEATURES

5. Ans. d. Pernicious anemia *(Ref: Sabiston 20/e p1918; Schwartz 11/e p1121-1123, 10/e p1053-1073; Bailey 27/e p1116; Shackelford 8/e p673-676)*

Specific Chronic Disorders Associated with PUD	
With strong associations	**With possible associations**
• Systemic mastocytosis[Q] • Chronic pulmonary disease[Q] • Chronic renal failure[Q] • **Cirrhosis**[Q] • Nephrolithiasis[Q] • Alpha1-antitrypsin deficiency[Q]	• **Hyperparathyroidism**[Q] • Coronary artery disease • Polycythemia Vera • Chronic pancreatitis[Q]

6. Ans. c. H. pylori *(Ref: Bailey 27/e p1115)*

7. Ans. c. Plummer-Vinson syndrome

8. Ans. a. 1st part of duodenum

9. Ans. d. Lesser curvature near incisura angularis *(Ref: Sabiston 20/e p1207)*

GASTRIC ULCERS

- **MC type: Type I gastric ulcer**, is located near **angularis incisura** on the lesser curvature.
- **NSAID ulcers (Type V)** typically occur in the **antrum** but may be located anywhere in the stomach and may be multiple in origin.
- Type II and III: **High acid secretion**[Q]
- Type I and IV: **Normal** or **low acid secretion**[Q]
- **Association:**
  - **Type I:** Blood group **'A'**[Q]
  - **Type II, III,** and **IV:** Blood group **'O'**[Q]

10. **Ans. c. Duodenal ulcer; d. Gastric ulcer** *(Ref: Harrison 20/e p2227)*

> ### CLINICAL FEATURES OF PEPTIC ULCER
>
> - **Epigastric pain** described as a **burning** or **gnawing discomfort** can be present in both **DU** and **GU**[Q].
> - The discomfort is also described as an ill-defined, aching sensation or as hunger pain.
>
> > - The **typical pain pattern in DU** occurs **90 minutes** to **3 hours after** a meal and is **frequently relieved by antacids** or **food**[Q].
> > - **Pain** that **awakes** the **patient from sleep** (between **midnight** and **3 A.M.**) is the **most discriminating symptom**, with **two-thirds of DU patients** describing this complaint[Q].
>
> - The **pain pattern** in **GU patients** may be different from that in DU patients, where **discomfort** may actually be **precipitated by food**[Q].
> - **Nausea** and **weight loss** occur **more commonly in GU patients.**

11. **Ans. c. Type 3**

12. **Ans. c. Prepyloric region** *(Ref: Sabiston 20/e p1208; Schwartz 11/e p1123, 10/e p1057)*

13. **Ans. d. Lesser curve** *(Ref: Sabiston 20/e p1208; Schwartz 11/e p1123, 10/e p1057)*

■ PEPTIC ULCER COMPLICATIONS

14. **Ans. b. Gastroduodenal artery** *(Ref: Sabiston 20/e p1202-1203; Schwartz 11/e p1125, 10/e p1053-1073; Bailey 27/e p1127; Shackelford 8/e p694, 7/e p711-714)*

15. **Ans. c. Perforation**   16. **Ans. b. Duodenum**

17. **Ans. b. 75%** *(Ref: Schwartz 11/e p1134, 10/e p1061)*

  - **Upright chest x-ray** shows **free air** in about **80%** of patients of perforated peptic ulcer.

18. **Ans. a. Omental bursa**   19. **Ans. a. Gastroduodenal artery**

20. **Ans. c. Proton pump inhibitors**

■ PEPTIC ULCER DIAGNOSIS AND TREATMENT

21. **Ans. a. Before breakfast** *(Ref: Sabiston 20/e p1201; Schwartz 11/e p1125, 10/e p971,972,979; Bailey 27/e p1119)*
PPIs are taken before breakfast.

22. **Ans. a. Billroth-I operation** *(Ref: Sabiston 20/e p1208; Schwartz 11/e p1130, 10/e p1120; Bailey 27/e p1123; Shackelford 8/e p683)*

23. **Ans. b. Carman's meniscus sign**   24. **Ans. c. Vitamin B_{12} deficiency**

25. **Ans. a. Proximal two-thirds of stomach**   26. **Ans. d. Highly selective vagotomy**

27. **Ans. c. Truncal vagotomy and antrectomy**   28. **Ans. b. Truncal vagotomy and antrectomy**

29. **Ans. c. Vagotomy + repair of perforation** *(Ref: Sabiston 20/e p1202-1205; Schwartz 11/e p1133, 10/e p1068; Bailey 27/e p1123; Shackelford 8/e p691-692)*

Complications	Treatment
Perforated	Type I: • **Distal gastrectomy** in stable patients[Q] • Biopsy and patch closure in unstable patients[Q] **Type II and III: Patch closure in unstable patients (Truncal vagotomy** with **antrectomy in stable patients)**[Q]
Obstruction	**Truncal vagotomy** with **antrectomy**[Q] (Rule out malignancy)

30. **Ans. d. Graham's omentum patch repair**

■ GASTRECTOMY AND COMPLICATIONS

31. **Ans. c. Vitamin B_{12} deficiency**

32. **Ans. b. Presence of hypertonic content in small intestine** *(Ref: Sabiston 20/e p1212; Schwartz 10/e p1090-1092; Bailey 27/e p1123; Shackelford 8/e p719)*

33. **Ans. b. Starch is beneficial**   34. **Ans. b. Early dumping syndrome** *(Ref: Bailey 27/e p1123, 1124)*

35. **Ans. b. 4th day** *(Ref: Shackelford 7/e p930, 944)*

36. **Ans. a. Billroth-II**

37. **Ans. a. Clean contaminated wound** *(Ref: Sabiston 20/e p245; Schwartz 10/e p148)*

38. **Ans. a. Hernia surgery**

39. **Ans. c. Billroth** *(Ref: Sabiston 20/e p1208; Schwartz 11/e p1130, 10/e p1120; Bailey 27/e p1120; Shackelford 8/e p683)*

■ UPPER GI BLEED

40. **Ans. c. Adherent clot** *(Ref: Sabiston 20/e p1143; Shackelford 8/e p694)*

41. **Ans. a. Endoscopy**

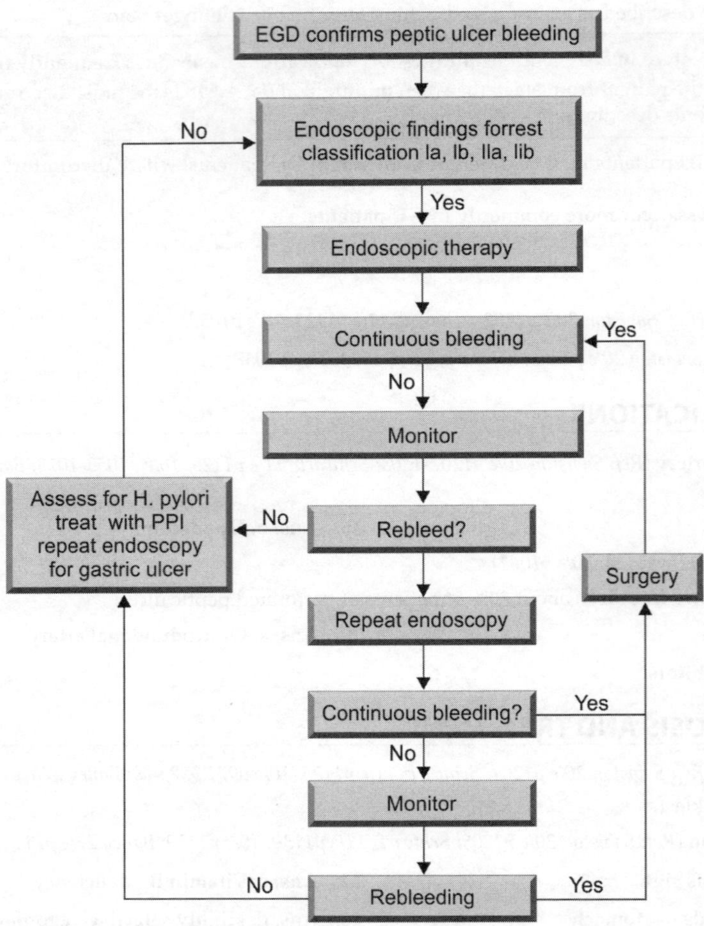

42. **Ans. b. Duodenal ulcer**

43. **Ans. a. Sclerotherapy** *(Ref: Sabiston 20/e p1149; Shackelford 8/e p1582, 7/e p1597; Harrison 20/e p2196)*

- Variceal Bleeding
- In addition to pharmacologic therapy **endoscopy** should be carried out **as soon as possible**
- If varices are found they are treated with either **endoscopic variceal ligation** or **sclerotherapy**[Q].
- **EVL** is the **treatment of choice** for **variceal bleeding**[Q].

44. **Ans. b. Radiolabelled erythrocyte scanning** *(Ref: Sabiston 20/e p1152)*

- **Radionuclide scanning** with **technetium-99m** (^{99m}Tc)-**labeled RBCs** is the **most sensitive** but **least accurate method** for **localization of GI bleeding**[Q].

45. **Ans. b. FII a**   46. **Ans. b. Peptic ulcer**

47. **Ans. a. Vascular ectasia**

48. **Ans. d. Rockall scoring is used for risk stratification** *(Ref: Sabiston 20/e p1142; Schwartz 11/e p1126, 10/e p1060)*

■ MALLORY-WEISS TEAR

49. **Ans. a. Mallory-Weiss syndrome**   50. **Ans. a. Gastric cardia**

51. **Ans. c. Mallory-Weiss syndrome**

■ DIEULAFOY'S LESION

52. **Ans. d. Aberrant vessel in the mucosa that bleeds form a mucosal defect**

■ GASTRIC ANTRAL VASCULAR ECTASIA

53. **Ans. b.** Gastric antral vascular ectasia

54. **Ans. b.** Gastric antral vascular ectasia *(Ref: Sabiston 20 /e p1146; Schwartz 11/e p115, 10/e p1088)*

■ MÉNÉTRIER'S DISEASE

55. **Ans. d.** Menetrier's disease   *(Ref: Sabiston 20/e p1231; Schwartz 11/e p1153, 10/e p1088; Bailey 27/e p1116)*

> • *History of epigastric pain, anorexia, weight loss and pedal edema and low total protein and albumin levels with massive gastric folds in the stomach giving rise to cobblestone or cerebriform appearance, which is characteristically seen in Menetrier's disease.*

56. **Ans. a** Giant folds in the pyloric antrum

■ GASTRIC POLYPS

57. **Ans. a. Adenoma** *(Ref: Sabiston 20/e p1215; Schwartz 11/e p1142, 10/e p1076-1077; Bailey 26/e p1045; Shackelford 8/e p764)*

> • Gastric Polyps
> • There are five types of gastric epithelial polyps inflammatory, hamartomatous, heterotopic, hyperplastic and adenoma. The first three types have negligible malignant potential.
>> • MC gastric polyp is the **hyperplastic**[Q] or **regenerative polyp**, which frequently occurs in the setting of gastritis.
>> • Polyps that are **symptomatic, > 2 cm** or **adenomatous** should be **removed**.
> • Among patients with **FAP, gastric polyps (33–60%)** are **more common** as compared to **gastric adenomas (15%)**.
> • **MC gastric polyp**[Q]: **Hyperplastic**
> • MC neplastic gastric polyp: Tubular

58. **Ans. a.** Hyperplastic polyp

■ CARCINOMA STOMACH PREDISPOSING FACTORS

59. **Ans. b.** Stomach

60. **Ans. a. Diffuse type of gastric cancer** *(Ref: Sabiston 20/e p1216; Schwartz 11/e p1140, 10/e p1216; Bailey 25/e p1068)*

61. **Ans. a.** Pernicious anemia

62. **Ans. b.** 'O' blood group

63. **Ans. b.** Most common at fundus

64. **Ans. d.** Gastric cancer

■ CA STOMACH CLINICAL FEATURES AND TREATMENT

65. **Ans. b. More common in males** *(Ref: Sabiston 20/e p1216; Schwartz 11/e p1144, 10/e p1079)*

66. **Ans. b. Lobular carcinoma** *(Ref: Devita 10/e p338)*

67. **Ans. a. Protruding** *(Ref: Sabiston 20/e p1216; Schwartz 11/e p1144, 10/e p1079; Bailey 27/e p1133)*

68. **Ans. b. Stiewert type II** *(Ref: Sabiston 20/e p1217)*

69. **Ans. c. Rectum** *(Ref: Sabiston 20/e p1216; Schwartz 11/e p1145, 10/e p1069; Bailey 27/e p1135)*

Sister Mary Joseph nodule	
Gastrointestinal malignancies	**Gynecological malignancies**
• **Gastric cancer (MC)**[Q] • **Colonic cancer**[Q] • **Pancreatic cancer** (mostly **body** and **tail**)[Q]	• **Ovarian cancer**[Q] • **Uterine cancer**[Q]

70. **Ans. a. Sister Mary Joseph nodule** *(Ref: Bailey 27/e p1044)*

71. **Ans. b.** Gastric antrum

72. **Ans.** None

> • T4a: Tumor invades serosa (visceral peritoneum)
> • N3a: Metastasis in 7-15 regional LNs
> • **Stage IIIC: T4aN3, T4bN2, T4bN3**

73. **Ans. a.** Metastatic left supraclavicular lymphadenopathy

74. **Ans. a.** Ca stomach

75. **Ans. d.** Fundus

76. **Ans. a.** Superficial spreading type

Most Common site of Gastric Malignancies	
CA stomach	Antrum[Q]
CA stomach in **pernicious anemia**	Fundus[Q]
Diifuse variety	Fundus[Q]
Gastric lymphoma	Antrum[Q]
Burkitt's lymphoma (by EBV)	**Cardia** or **body**[Q]

77. **Ans. c. Involvement of mucosa, submucosa and muscularis** *(Ref: Sabiston 20/e p1222; Schwartz 11/e p1144, 10/e p1216; Bailey 27/e p1132)*

EARLY GASTRIC CANCER

- Adenocarcinoma **limited to** the **mucosa** and **submucosa** of the stomach, **regardless of LN status**[Q].
- Approx. **10%** of patients will have **LN metastasis**[Q].
- Cancer of the lesser curve is more common than cancer of the greater curvature.

Treatment

- Treatment options: **Endoscopic mucosal resection**[Q], limited surgical resection or gastrectomy
- **Overall curative rate** with **adequate gastric resection** and **lymphadenectomy is 95%**[Q]
- **Best prognosis**[Q]

78. **Ans. a. Carcinoma stomach** *(Ref: Robbins 9/e p772; Sabiston 20/e p1227)*   79. **Ans. b. Laparoscopy**

80. **Ans. d. EUS** *(Ref: Schwartz 11/e p1145, 10/e p1080)*

- The best way to stage the tumor locally is via EUS, which gives fairly accurate (80%) information about the depth of tumor penetration into the gastric wall, and can usually show enlarged (> 5 mm) perigastric and celiac lymph nodes.

81. **Ans. c. Stomach**

■ GASTROINTESTINAL STROMAL TUMOR

82. **Ans. a. More common in female** *(Ref: Sabiston 20/e p1229, 1230)*

"Gastric GISTs can manifest at any age, although most typically they manifest in patients older than 50 years. They generally have an equal male-to-female ratio or a slight male predominance." (Sabiston 20/e p1229)

"High-risk GISTs: Defined as >10 cm tumor, mitotic count >10/50 HPF, tumor >5 cm and mitotic count ≥ per 50 HPF, or tumor rupture." (Sabiston 20/e p1230)

83. **Ans. c. 3 years** *(Ref: Sabiston 20/e p1230)*

"The Scandinavian Sarcoma Group (SSG) XVIII trial compared an extended 36-month course of adjuvant imatinib versus a 12-month course after resection for high-risk GISTs (defined as >10 cm tumor, mitotic count >10/50 HPF, tumor >5 cm and mitotic count > per 50 HPF, or tumor rupture). Patients in the extended treatment arm had higher recurrence-free survival (65.6% versus 47.9%) and overall survival (92.0% versus 81.7%) at 5 years after surgery. The results of this trial have established a 3-year course as the standard of care after surgical resection of high-risk GIST." (Sabiston 20/e p1230)

84. **Ans. a. Segmental resection** *(Ref: Sabiston 20/e p1230; Schwartz 11/e p1149, 10/e p1084; Bailey 27/e p1140)*

"GIST: Wedge resection with clear margins is adequate surgical treatment." (Schwartz 11/e p1149, 10/e p1084)

85. **Ans. a. GIST**   86. **Ans. b. Stomach**

87. **Ans. a. GIST**   88. **Ans. b. CD-117**

89. **Ans. d. PET-CT**   90. **Ans. a. Most common in duodenum**

91. **Ans. c. Leiomyosarcoma**

- Gastrointestinal stromal tumours (**GISTs**) are the **MC mesenchymal tumours** of the **GIT**.
- Formerly **GISTs** were commonly classified histologically as leiomyosarcomas; however, they are now known to **arise from** the **interstitial cells of Cajal.**
- **Majority** of GISTs overexpress **KIT** and have characteristic mutations within the gene, which are the targets of **drug treatment with tyrosine kinase inhibitors.**

> - **Leiomyosarcoma** is a **malignant tumour** of **smooth muscle differentiation** and falls into a **group of sarcomas** that show **complex karyotypic changes** with no consistent recurrent genetic abnormality.

- **Upper GI bleeding** is the **MC clinical manifestation** of **GISTs**[Q], manifesting as hematemesis or melena in **40-65%** of patients. Bleeding occurs because of an ulcer forming in the gastric mucosa overlying the tumor.
- **Bleeding** is **more commonly** seen **in GIST** as compared to **Leiomyosarcoma**[Q].

■ GASTRIC LYMPHOMA

92. Ans. b. Stomach

93. Ans. c. Total gastrectomy with adjuvant chemotherapy is treatment of choice

■ DUODENAL ATRESIA

94. Ans. a. Down's syndrome *(Ref: Sabiston 20/e p1870; Schwartz 11/e p1724-1725, 10/e p1612,1615-1616; Bailey 27/e p1293; Shackelford 8/e p774)*

95. Ans. b. Duodenal atresia

96. Ans. b. Duodenal atresia

97. Ans. a. Duodenal atresia

98. Ans. a. Duodenoduodenostomy

99. Ans. a. Down's syndrome *(Ref: Sabiston 20/e p1870; Schwartz 11/e p1724-1725, 10/e p1615; Bailey 27/e p133)*

■ HYPERTROPHIC PYLORIC STENOSIS

100. Ans. c. Ultrasound abdomen

101. Ans. a. Mass in epigastrium

102. Ans. b. CHPS

103. Ans. c. Metabolic alkalosis with paradoxical aciduria

104. Ans. b. Aciduria

105. Ans. a. Congenital hypertrophic pyloric stenosis

106. Ans. d. Visible peristalsis is always seen

107. Ans. d. Congenital hypertrophic pyloric stenosis

108. Ans. c. Epigastrium *(Ref: Sabiston 20/e p1869; Schwartz 11/e p1722, 10/e p1614; Bailey 27/e p128)*

> *"Palpation of the pyloric "olive" tumor in the epigastrium by an experienced examiner is pathognomonic for HPS. If the olive is confirmed, no additional diagnostic testing is necessary." (Sabiston 20/e p1869)*

■ GASTRIC OUTLET OBSTRUCTION

109. Ans. d. First part of duodenum

110. Ans. b. Cancer of stomach

111. Ans. a. Alkaline urine

■ BEZOARS

112. Ans. c. GI obstruction *(Ref: Sabiston 20/e p1233; Schwartz 11/e p1154, 10/e p1089; Bailey 27/e p1142; Shackelford 8/e p280)*

Symptoms of Trichobezoar: Pain from **gastric ulceration** and fullness from **gastric outlet obstruction** with occasional **gastric perforation** and **small bowel obstruction.**

113. Ans. a. Trichobezoar

114. Ans. a. It is caused by Trichuris

■ STRESS GASTRITIS

115. Ans. b. Stress ulcers in head injury *(Ref: Schwartz 11/e p1138, 10/e p1090; Sabiston 20/e p1211; Bailey 27/e p1142)*

116. Ans. a. Fundus of stomach

117. Ans. d. Distal duodenum

118. Ans. b. Stomach

119. Ans. b. Fundus

120. Ans. a. Burn patients

> - **Cushing ulcer:** Stress gastritis due to **intracranial injury/increased ICP[Q]**
> - **Curling ulcer: After burn injury (> 35%);** in the **body** and **fundus[Q]**; not in antrum and duodenum
> - **Cameron ulcers** or **riding ulcers:** Linear gastric erosions **in hiatal hernias[Q]**

■ GASTRIC VOLVULUS

121. Ans. b. Acute gastric volvulus

Peritoneum

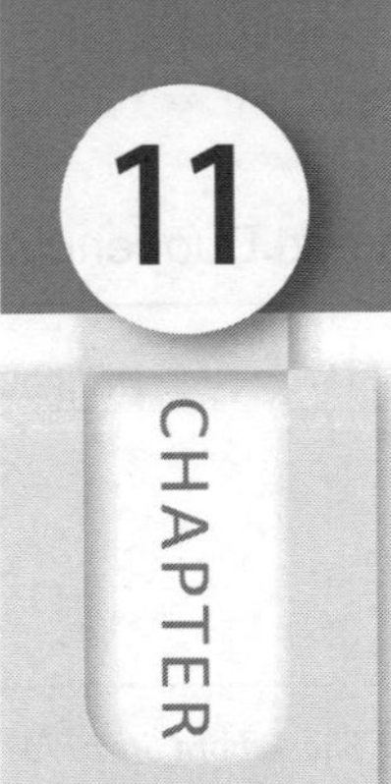

RETROPERITONEAL FIBROSIS

RETROPERITONEAL FIBROSIS

- Characterized by **proliferation of fibrous tissue** in the **retroperitoneum**[Q]
- Fibrosis is usually confined to **central & paravertebral spaces** between the **renal arteries & sacrum** and tends to **encase** the **aorta, IVC & ureters**[Q].
- Process usually **begins at the level** of aortic bifurcation & **spreads cephalad**[Q] up to renal artery generally.

Etiology

- Around **70% cases** are **primary** or **idiopathic (Ormond's disease)**[Q]

Causes of Secondary (30%)[Q] Retroperitoneal Fibrosis

- **Inflammatory conditions: CATH**[Q] **(Chronic pancreatitis, Actinomycosis, Tuberculosis, Histoplasmosis)**
- **Drugs: Methysergide (Most important)**
- **Malignancies:**
- **Autoimmune disorders: SLE, PAN & ankylosing spondylitis**
- **Radiation**

Clinical Features

- More common in **males of 40-60 years**[Q].
- **Early symptoms** are **vague & non-specific**[Q] (**abdominal** or **flank pain**, weight loss, malaise, & hypertension)
- **Obstructive uropathy** (dysuria, frequency, fever due to secondary infection of hydroneprotic kidney) is the **earliest and MC specific symptom**[Q].

> - **Ureters are MC involved, MC site is lower third of ureter.**
> - **Partial or complete obstruction** occurs in **75% patients**[Q].

Diagnosis: In absence of uremia, diagnosis is made by IVP.
- **IVP or RGP:**
  - Hydronephrosis with dilated tortuous upper ureter
  - **Medial pulling of ureters** or **pipestem ureters**[Q]
  - **Extrinsic ureteral compression**[Q]
- **CT scan is IOC** for retroperitoneal fibrosis[Q].
- **MRI is IOC** in cases of **compromised renal function**, because contrast cannot be given.

Treatment

- **Primary, idiopathic** retroperitoneal fibrosis: **Ureteral stenting** & **immunosuppression** (TAPS: Tamoxifen, Azathioprine, Penicillamine, Steroids)[Q]
- **Secondary retroperitoneal fibrosis: Midline transperitoneal ureterolysis** with **wrapping** the **ureter** with **omental flap** or **lateral retroperitoneal ureteral transposition**[Q].

SPONTANEOUS BACTERIAL PERITONITIS

SPONTANEOUS BACTERIAL PERITONITIS

- **SBP** is a common and severe complication of ascites characterized by **spontaneous infection of** the **ascitic fluid without an intra-abdominal source**[Q].

> - **MC organism in adults: E. coli**[Q] **>Klebsiella.**
> - **MC organism in children: Group A streptococci**[Q]

Contd...

Contd…

Mechanism

- **Bacterial translocation** with **gut flora traversing** the **intestine into mesenteric lymph nodes**, leading to **bacteremia** & **seeding of the ascitic fluid**[Q].
- **Predisposing Factors: Bowel preparation**, metabolic **alkalosis, dehydration** and **hypoproteinemia**[Q]

Clinical Features

- Patients with ascites may present with **fever, altered mental status, elevated WBC count**[Q], and **abdominal pain** or discomfort, or they may present without any of these features.
- **High degree of clinical suspicion** and **peritoneal taps** are important for making the **diagnosis.**

Diagnosis

- Presence of **>250**[Q] **polymorphonuclear cells** of ascitic fluid is consistent with SBP; with ascitic fluid **culture growing single organism**.
- If **more than two organisms** are identified, **secondary bacterial peritonitis** due to a **perforated viscus** should be considered[Q].

> - **Culture negative neutrocytic ascites** is diagnosed, when an ascitic fluid **PMN count of >250** is **unaccompanied by a positive ascitic fluid culture**[Q].
> - **Culture negative neutrocytic ascites** carries a **similar prognosis**[Q] to SBP and is **managed similarly.**

Treatment

- Treated with **cefotaxime** plus **albumin**[Q]

■ SECONDARY (ACUTE SUPPURATIVE) BACTERIAL PERITONITIS

SECONDARY (ACUTE SUPPURATIVE) BACTERIAL PERITONITIS

- When **bacteria contaminate** the peritoneum **as a result of spillage** from an intra-abdominal **viscus**[Q].
- Infection in secondary bacterial peritonitis is **polymicrobial**[Q]
- **E. coli** & **Bacteroides** are **MC organisms**[Q].
- The species of organism isolated vary with the source of the initial process and the normal flora present at the site.

■ PERITONITIS ASSOCIATED WITH CHRONIC AMBULATORY PERITONEAL DIALYSIS (CAPD)

PERITONITIS ASSOCIATED WITH CHRONIC AMBULATORY PERITONEAL DIALYSIS (CAPD)

- **Peritonitis is one of** the **MC complications** of CAPD[Q], occurring with an incidence of approximately **one episode every 1 to 3 years**[Q].
- **Refractory** or **recurrent peritonitis** is MC cause of **technical failure of CAPD**[Q].

> - **MC organism: Staphylococcus epidermidis**[Q] (30–50%).

Clinical Features

- Patients present with **abdominal pain, fever,** and **cloudy peritoneal dialysate** containing **>100 WBC/mm³**, with **>50%** of the cells being **neutrophils**[Q].

Treatment

- CAPD associated peritonitis is treated by the **intraperitoneal administration of antibiotics**, usually a **first-generation cephalosporin**[Q].
- **Recurrent** or **persistent peritonitis** requires **removal of** the **dialysis catheter** and resumption of **hemodialysis**[Q].

■ INTRA-ABDOMINAL ABSCESS

INTRA-ABDOMINAL ABSCESS

- **MC site** of **intra-peritoneal abscess: Pelvis**[Q]
- **Right subhepatic space** (lies between inferior surface of liver and hepatic flexure and transverse mesocolon) is the **most dependent portion** of the **abdominal cavity** in the **recumbent position**[Q].
- **Pelvic cavity** is the **most dependent area** of the **peritoneal cavity** in the **upright position**[Q].

Clinical Features

- **High spiking fevers, chills, abdominal pain, anorexia,** and **delay of return of bowel function**[Q] in the postoperative patient are typical presenting signs and symptoms of intraperitoneal abscess.

Diagnosis

- **CT scan: Investigation of choice** for diagnosis of intra-**abdominal abscess**[Q]

Treatment

- **Preferred treatment: CT guided percutaneous drainage**[Q]
- **Operative drainage:** If percutaneous drainage is not possible or contraindicated

PELVIC ABSCESS

- **Pelvis** is the **MC site of an intraperitoneal abscess**

Clinical Features

- Most characteristic symptoms are **diarrhea** & **passage of mucus** in the stools. [Q]
- **Rectal examination** reveals a **bulging** of the **anterior rectal wall**[Q], which, when the abscess is ripe, becomes softly cystic.

Diagnosis

- If any uncertainty exists, the **presence of pus** should be **confirmed by ultrasound** or **CT scanning with needle aspiration** if indicated[Q].

Treatment

> - In women, **vaginal drainage through** the **posterior fornix (Posterior colpotomy)** is often chosen[Q].
> - **In other cases**, when the abscess is definitely pointing into the rectum, **rectal drainage** is employed[Q].

- **Laparotomy** is **almost never necessary**[Q].
- **Rectal drainage** of a **pelvic abscess** is far **preferable to suprapubic drainage**, which risks exposing the general peritoneal cavity to infection[Q].
- **Drainage tubes** can also be **inserted percutaneously** or **via the vagina** or **rectum** under ultrasound or CT guidance[Q].

◼ DUODENAL STUMP BLOWOUT

DUODENAL STUMP BLOWOUT

- Duodenal stump blowout is **massive leakage** from **duodenal stump** following **Billroth-II gastrectomy**[Q].

Clinical Features

- Occurs on **4th to 7th** post-operative **day**[Q].
- Presents as **sudden intense thoracoabdominal pain, sudden elevation in pulse** and **temperature** or **generalized deterioration** of condition.

Treatment

- **Adequate drainage** must be instituted **immediately,** which is done by putting a **catheter** through an incision **below the right costal margin**[Q].
- TPN should be instituted and attention should be directed towards **fluid and electrolyte therapy**[Q].
- **Fistula closure** can be anticipated **within 2–3 weeks**[Q].

◼ MESENTERIC CYST

MESENTERIC CYST

- Mesenteric cyst is encountered **most frequently** in the **2nd decade of life**
- More common in **women**

Types of Mesenteric cysts	
• **Chylolymphatic (MC)**[Q] • Simple (**mesothelial**) • **Enterogenous**	• **Urogenital** remnant • **Dermoid** (teratomatous cyst)

Chylolymphatic Cyst	Enterogenous Cyst
• **MC type**, arises in **congenitally misplaced lymphatic tissue** that has **no efferent communication** with **lymphatic system**[Q] • Arises most frequently in **mesentery of ileum**[Q]. • **Thin wall** of cyst, **filled with clear lymph** or chyle. • Occasionally, the cyst attains a great size. • **Mostly unilocular** and **solitary**[Q] • Chylolymphatic cyst **blood supply is independent from** that of the **adjacent intestine**[Q] • **Enucleation** is possible without the need for resection of gut[Q].	• **Derived** either **from a diverticulum of** the **mesenteric border** of intestine or **from a duplication** of intestine[Q]. • **Thicker wall** than a chylolymphatic cyst and it is **lined by mucous membrane**, sometimes ciliated[Q]. • **Content** is **mucinous** and is either **colorless** or **yellowish brown** as a result of past hemorrhage. • **Muscle in** the **wall** of an **enteric duplication cyst** and **adjacent bowel** has a **common blood supply**[Q] • **Removal of the cyst** always entails **resection** of the **related portion of intestine**[Q].

Clinical Features

- A **painless abdominal swelling**[Q]
- **Recurrent attacks** of **abdominal pain**[Q] with or without vomiting (temporary impaction of a food bolus in a segment of bowel narrowed by the cyst or possibly from torsion of the mesentery)
- **Acute abdominal pain** may arises as a result of: **Torsion, rupture, hemorrhage, infection.**

Contd…

Gastrointestinal Surgery
Section 3

Contd…

> • **Tillaux triad:** Fluctuant swelling near the **umbilicus** + **moves freely** in a **plane perpendicular** to the **attachment of the mesentery** + **zone of resonance around the cyst**[Q].

Diagnosis

- **CT scan:** Investigation of choice for **diagnosis of mesenteric cyst**[Q]
- **USG:** Helpful in diagnosis

Treatment

- **Chylolymphatic cysts:** Enucleation is treatment of choice[Q]
- **Enterogenous cyst:** Resection & anastomosis is the treatment of choice[Q]
- **Aspiration alone** has a high rate of cyst recurrence[Q].

■ PSEUDOMYXOMA PERITONEI

PSEUDOMYXOMA PERITONEI

- Pseudomyxoma peritonei describes **mucinous ascites** arising from a **ruptured appendiceal** or **ovarian adenocarcinoma**[Q].
- **MC site** of **primary:** Appendix[Q]
- **Peritoneum** becomes **coated with a mucus-secreting tumor** that **fills the peritoneal cavity** with **tenacious semisolid mucus** and large, loculated cystic masses[Q].

Clinical Features

- Patients are **often asymptomatic**[Q] until late in the course of their disease.
- **On presentation, global deterioration in health** long before the diagnosis is made
- **Abdominal pain** & **distention** and **nonspecific complaints** are common.
- **Physical examination:** A new **hernia, ascites, distended abdomen** with **nonshifting dullness**[Q] and, occasionally, a palpable abdominal mass.

Diagnosis

- **CT (chest, abdomen & pelvis):** Information regarding the **diagnosis** and the **ability to resect the tumor completely** or **perform an adequate cytoreduction**[Q].
- **Preoperative colonoscopy:** Differentiate a **mucinous neoplasm** of the **appendix** from that **arising from the colon**[Q].
- Often, the **diagnosis** is **made at laparotomy** (peritoneal cavity containing **tenacious semisolid mucus** and **large, loculated cystic masses**)

Treatment

- **Cytoreduction** (Resection of as much of the tumor as possible) + **Intraperitoneal hyperthermic chemotherapy (IPHC)**[Q].

> • **Operative management:** Omentectomy, stripping of involved **peritoneum, resection of involved organs** and **appendectomy** with **right hemicolectomy**[Q]

■ ACUTE MESENTERIC LYMPHADENITIS

ACUTE MESENTERIC LYMPHADENITIS

- Syndrome of **acute right lower quadrant abdominal pain** associated with **mesenteric lymph node enlargement** and a **normal appendix**[Q].
- **Diagnosis is made upon exploration** of the abdomen of a **patient suspected of having acute appendicitis** at which time a **normal appendix** and **enlarged mesenteric lymph nodes**[Q] are discovered.
- Occurs **most commonly** in **children** and **young adults**[Q]
- **Etiology often remains unknown**
- Yersinia enterocolitica has been **associated with** this **syndrome in children**[Q].

Multiple Choice Questions

■ RETROPERITONEAL FIBROSIS

1. Ormond's disease is: *(MHPGMCET 2009, 2007)*
   a. Retractile testis
   b. Idiopathic retroperitoneal lymphadenopathy
   c. Idiopathic retroperitoneal fibrosis
   d. Idiopathic mediastinitis

2. Most common organ involved in retroperitoneal fibrosis is:
   (Recent Question 2014, AIIMS Nov 93)
   a. Aorta
   b. Ureter
   c. Inferior vena cava
   d. Sympathetic nerve plexus

■ PERITONITIS

3. Which of the following causes least irritation of the peritoneal cavity? *(All India 99)*
   a. Bile
   b. Blood
   c. Gastric enzyme
   d. Pancreatic enzyme

4. A 40-year-old male was brought to emergency with severe abdominal pain. On examination, pulse rate was 112/minute and systolic BP was 80 mm Hg. Chest X-ray is given below. What is the most appropriate management?
   (Recent Question 2019)
   a. Exploratory laparotomy
   b. Saline wash of stomach
   c. Intercostal tube drainage
   d. IV antibiotics

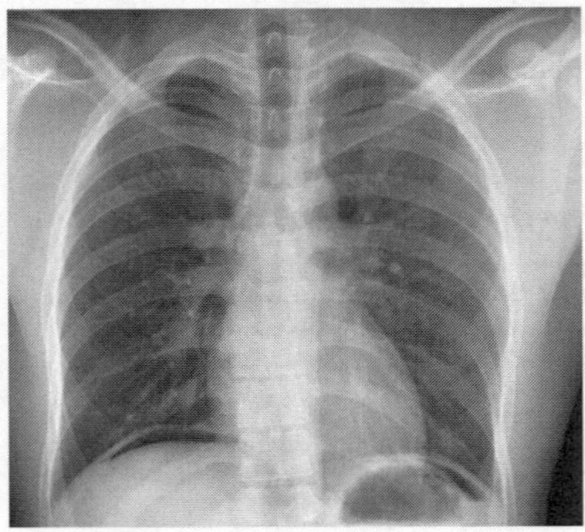

5. Most common cause of peritonitis in adult male is:
   (Recent Question 2014, All India 93)
   a. Duodenal ulcer perforation
   b. Abdominal tuberculosis
   c. Enteric perforation
   d. Perforated appendix

6. Apart from Escherichia coli, the other most common organism implicated in acute suppurative bacterial peritonitis is: *(Recent Question 2014, All India 2006)*
   a. Bacteroides
   b. Klebsiella
   c. Peptostreptococcus
   d. Pseudomonas

7. A 25-year-old female presents with pyrexia for ten days, develops acute pain in periumbilical region spreading all over the abdomen. What would be the most likely cause?
   (Recent Question 2014, UPSC 2007)
   a. Perforation peritonitis due to intestinal tuberculosis
   b. Generalized peritonitis due to appendicular perforation
   c. Typhoid enteric perforation and peritonitis
   d. Acute salpingo-oophoritis with peritonitis

8. Spontaneous peritonitis in cirrhosis patients; the polymorphonuclear cells are: *(NEET 2013, UPPG 2008)*
   a. More than 200 cells/cumm
   b. More than 300 cells/cumm
   c. More than 400 cells/cumm
   d. More than 500 cells/cumm

9. Which of the following is true regarding classical spontaneous bacterial peritonitis? *(NEET 2013, COMEDK 2010)*
   a. Ascitic fluid neutrophil count is 250/cumm
   b. Bowel perforation should be present
   c. Multiple organisms are isolated from ascetic fluid
   d. Board-like rigidity is present in abdomen

10. Sonu, a 15-year-old girl, a regular swimmer presents with sudden onset of pain in abdomen, abdominal distension and fever of 39°C and obliteration of the liver dullness. Most probable diagnosis is: *(Recent Question 2014, AIIMS June 2001, Nov 99)*
   a. Ruptured typhoid ulcer
   b. Primary bacterial peritonitis
   c. Ruptured ectopic pregnancy
   d. UTI with PID

11. All of the following regarding diagnosis of acute peritonitis are correct except: *(MCI March 2007)*
   a. Raised WBC count in peritoneal aspirate
   b. Moderately raised amylase levels are diagnostic of peritonitis
   c. CT scan may aid in diagnosis
   d. Upright films shows free air under the diaphragm

■ MESENTERIC CYST

12. Most common type of mesenteric cyst is: *(MHSSMCET 2005)*
   a. Enterogenous
   b. Chylolymphatic
   c. Urogenital
   d. Teratomatous

13. Mesenteric cyst whose removal entrails removals of part of gut: *(TN 95)*
   a. Chylolymphatic cyst
   b. Enterogenous cyst
   c. Dermoid
   d. All

14. All are mesenteric cyst except: *(DNB 2007)*
   a. Dermoid cyst
   b. Chylolymphatic cyst
   c. Gartner's cyst
   d. Enterogenous cyst

■ ASCITES

15. Serum-ascites albumin gradient >1.1 g/dL is seen in:
   (COMEDK 2005)
   a. Nephrosis
   b. Cirrhosis
   c. Pancreatic ascites
   d. Neoplasm

■ PSEUDOMYXOMA PERITONEI

16. In pseudomyxoma peritonei, mucinous cyst-adenocarcinoma of which following organ is involved: *(Orissa 2011)*
   a. Pancreas
   b. Ovary
   c. Kidney
   d. Abdominal testis

17. All are true about pseudomyxoma peritonei except:
   a. Associated with ovarian tumors *(DPG 2008)*
   b. Appendix is most common site of origin
   c. Yellow jelly collection of fluid
   d. Common in male

18. **False about pseudomyxoma peritonei is:** *(JIPMER May 2018)*
    a. Recurrence after surgery
    b. Refractory to drugs
    c. Hyperthermic intraperitoneal chemotherapy is treatment option
    d. Most commonly associated with appendiceal tumor

■ ABDOMINAL ABSCESS

19. **Commonest site of intraperitoneal abscess is:** *(Orissa 2011)*
    a. Lesser sac
    b. Greater sac
    c. Pelvis
    d. Paracolic gutter

20. **Most common site of intra-abdominal abscess:** *(MHPGMCET 2006)*
    a. Pelvic
    b. Subphrenic space
    c. Mesenteric
    d. Paracolic gutters

21. **Treatment of pouch of Douglas abscess is:** *(Recent Question 2016)*
    a. Laparotomy
    b. Posterior colpotomy
    c. Antibiotics
    d. Extraperitoneal drainage

22. **The most favored treatment for a pelvic abscess in cul-de-sac is:** *(DPG 96)*
    a. Laparotomy
    b. Colpotomy
    c. External I and D
    d. Antibiotics

23. **Most pathognomic in pelvic abscess is:** *(UPPG 2007)*
    a. Constipation
    b. Mucopurulent discharge
    c. Loose stool
    d. Bleeding

24. **A patient developed wound infection post laparotomy for pyoperitoneum, was treated conservatively. Now, granulation tissue is seen in the wound. Next step in management is:** *(Recent Question 2015)*
    a. Daily dressing
    b. Mesh repair
    c. Incision and drainage
    d. Re-suturing with interrupted stitches

■ PNEUMOPERITONEUM

25. **Best investigation for air in peritoneal cavity is:** *(CMC 98)*
    a. USG
    b. Laparotomy
    c. Laparoscopy
    d. X-ray abdomen-erect view

26. **The given finding of X-ray is rarely seen in which of the following?** *(Recent Question 2016)*
    a. Gastric perforation
    b. Duodenal perforation
    c. Ileal perforation
    d. Appendicular perforation

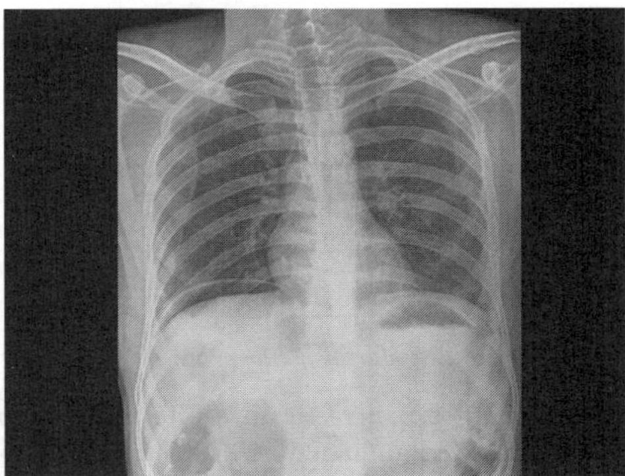

■ WOUND DEHISCENCE

27. **Burst abdomen most commonly occurs on the:** *(Recent Question 2014)*
    a. 2nd day
    b. 3rd day
    c. 7th day
    d. 9th day
    e. 5th day

28. **On 7th post operative day, abdominal wound shows pink serosanguinous discharge. It suggests:** *(DNB 2001)*
    a. Impending wound dehiscence
    b. Infection in the abdomen
    c. Stitch abscess
    d. Healing wound

■ MESENTERIC LYMPHADENITIS

29. **Acute mesenteric lymphadenitis is caused by:** *(All India 94)*
    a. E. coli
    b. α-hemolytic streptococci
    c. Hemophilus
    d. Yersinia

30. **The commonest cause of acute mesenteric adenitis is:** *(Recent Question 2016)*
    a. Tuberculosis
    b. Brucellosis
    c. Pneumococcal infection
    d. Idiopathic

Explanations

■ RETROPERITONEAL FIBROSIS

1. **Ans. c. Idiopathic retroperitoneal fibrosis** *(Ref: Sabiston 20/e p1087, Campbell 11/e p1143)*
2. **Ans. b. Ureter**

■ PERITONITIS

3. **Ans. b. Blood** *(Ref: Harrison 20/e p954)*

   - **Gastric juice, pancreatic juice, bile, urine** and **meconium irritate peritoneal cavity** and lead to **aseptic** or **chemical peritonitis**[Q].
   - **Chemical irritation** of the peritoneum **is greatest for acidic gastric juice** and **pancreatic enzymes**[Q].
   - **The chemical irritation caused by stomach acid & activated pancreatic enzymes is extreme and secondary bacterial infection may occur.**

4. **Ans. a. Exploratory laparotomy** *(Ref: Schwartz 11/e p1231, 10/e p1061; Sabiston 20/e p1134; Bailey 27/e p1051)*
5. **Ans. a. Duodenal ulcer perforation** *(Ref: Sabiston 20/e p1121)*

   MC cause of peritonitis in **adult male: Peptic** ulcer **perforation**

   #### PERITONITIS

   - The **most common cause is** a **perforation of** the **abdominal viscus-most commonly, a perforated ulcer**[Q], may occur as a result of perforation of any part of the bowel; other causes include a benign ulcer, a tumor, or trauma.
   - **MC cause** of **peritonitis** in **adult male: Peptic** ulcer **perforation**[Q]

6. **Ans. a. Bacteroides** *(Ref: Sabiston 20/e p1078; Bailey 27/e p1049)*
7. **Ans. c. Typhoid enteric perforation and peritonitis** *(Ref: Sabiston 20/e p1266-1267; Bailey 27/e p1248; Harrison 20/e p1176)*
8. **Ans. a. More than 200 cells/cumm**
9. **Ans. a. Ascitic fluid neutrophil count is 250/cumm**
10. **Ans. a. Ruptured typhoid ulcer**
11. **Ans. b. Moderately raised amylase levels are diagnostic of peritonitis**

■ MESENTERIC CYST

12. **Ans. b. Chylolymphatic** *(Ref: Sabiston 20/e p1082; Schwartz 11/e p1560, 10/e p1459-1460; Bailey 27/e p1063)*
13. **Ans. b. Enterogenous cyst**
14. **Ans. c. Gartner's cyst**

■ ASCITES

15. **Ans. b. Cirrhosis**

■ PSEUDOMYXOMA PERITONEI

16. **Ans. b. Ovary** *(Ref: Sabiston 20/e p1080; Schwartz 11/e p1340, 10/e p1258-1259; Bailey 27/e p1059)*
17. **Ans. d. Common in male**
18. **Ans. b. Refractory to drugs** *(Ref: Schwartz 11/e p1340, 10/e p1258-1259; Sabiston 20/e p1080; Bailey 27/e p1059)*

■ ABDOMINAL ABSCESS

19. **Ans. c. Pelvis** *(Ref: Maingot 11/e p179-184; Bailey 27/e p1055)*
20. **Ans. a. Pelvic**
21. **Ans. b. Posterior colpotomy**
22. **Ans. b. Colpotomy**
23. **Ans. b. Mucopurulent discharge**
24. **Ans. d. Re-suturing with interrupted stitches**

■ PNEUMOPERITONEUM

25. **Ans. d. X-ray abdomen-erect view** *(Ref: Bailey 27/e p1051)*

   - Bailey says "A **radiograph of** the **abdomen may confirm** the **presence of dilated gas-filled loops of bowel** (consistent with a paralytic ileus) or **show free gas**, although the **latter is best shown on an erect chest radiograph. If the patient is too ill for an 'erect' film** to demonstrate free air under the diaphragm, a **lateral decubitus film** is **just as useful, showing gas beneath the abdominal wall**."

26. **Ans. d. Appendicular perforation** *(Ref: Chapman 4/e p212)*
   Gas below right dome of diaphragm is rarely seen in appendicular perforation due to little amount of gas.

■ WOUND DEHISCENCE

27. **Ans. c. 7th day** *(Ref: CSDT 11/e p24; Bailey 27/e p299)*

28. **Ans. a. Impending wound dehiscence**

■ MESENTERIC LYMPHADENITIS

29. **Ans. d. Yersinia** *(Ref: Sabiston 20/e p1082-1083; Bailey 27/e p1062)*

30. **Ans. d. Idiopathic**

Intestinal Obstruction

■ SMALL BOWEL OBSTRUCTION

SMALL BOWEL OBSTRUCTION

- **Adhesions** secondary to previous surgery are the **MC cause of SBO**[Q].
- Causes: **Adhesions (60%) > Malignant tumors (20%) >Hernia (10%) > Crohn's disease (5%)**[Q]

> - **Metastatic** or **peritoneal carcinomatosis** are the **MC malignancies** leading to **SBO**[Q].

- Primary **colonic cancers** (particularly those arising from the **cecum & ascending colon**) **may present** as a **SBO**[Q].

Pathophysiology

- **Early in the course** of an obstruction, **intestinal motility** & **contractile activity increase** in an effort to **propel luminal contents**[Q] past the obstructing point.
- **Increase in peristalsis** early in the course of bowel obstruction is present **both above** and **below the point of obstruction**[Q] (diarrhea in partial or even complete small bowel obstruction **in the early period)**
- **Later in the course** of obstruction, the **intestine becomes fatigued & dilates**[Q], with contractions becoming less frequent & less intense.
- As the **bowel dilates, water** & **electrolytes accumulate** both **intraluminally** & in the **bowel wall**[Q] itself.

> - This **massive third-space fluid** loss accounts for the **dehydration & hypovolemia**[Q].
> - **Metabolic effects** of **fluid loss depend on** the **site** & **duration** of the obstruction.

- As the **intraluminal pressure increases** in the **bowel,** a **decrease in mucosal blood flow** can occur.

Clinical Features

- **Cardinal symptoms** of intestinal obstruction: **Colicky abdominal pain (1st symptom)**[Q], nausea, vomiting, **abdominal distention,** and a **failure to pass flatus & feces** (i.e., **obstipation)**[Q].
- **Typical crampy abdominal pain** occurs **in paroxysms at 4- to 5-minute intervals** & occurs **less frequently with distal obstruction**[Q].

> - **Nausea & vomiting** are **more common** with **proximal obstruction.**
> - **Cramping abdominal pain** is the **initial** and **most prominent symptom** in **distal obstruction**[Q]
> - **Abdominal distention** is **more common** in **distal obstruction**[Q]

- **Abdominal distention** occurs as the obstruction progresses, and the **proximal intestine becomes increasingly dilated**[Q].
- Patient may present with **tachycardia** & **hypotension**[Q], demonstrating the severe dehydration that is present.
- **Fever suggests** the possibility of **strangulation**[Q].
- **Abdominal distention** is dependent **on the level of obstruction**[Q].

> - **Early in the course** of bowel obstruction, **peristaltic waves** can be observed, particularly **in thin patients,** and auscultation of the abdomen may demonstrate **hyperactive bowel sounds** with **audible rushes** associated with **vigorous peristalsis**[Q] (i.e., borborygmi).
> - **Late** in the obstructive course, **minimal** or **no bowel sounds** are noted.

- **Localized tenderness, rebound,** & **guarding** suggest **peritonitis** and the likelihood of **strangulation**[Q].
- **Rectal examination:** To assess for **intraluminal masses** and to **examine the stool** for **occult blood**[Q] (an indication of malignancy, intussusception, or infarction)

Diagnosis

- **X-ray Abdomen: Confirm** the **clinical suspicion** and **define** more accurately the **site of obstruction (60% diagnostic accuracy)**[Q]

> - **Supine radiographs: Dilated loops** of **small intestine**[Q] without evidence of colonic distention, **diagnose site & level of obstruction**[Q]
> - **Erect radiographs: Multiple air-fluid levels**, which often layer in a **stepwise pattern**[Q] (up to **3-5 air fluid levels <2.5 cm** in length is **normal)**
> - **Supine films** are **better than erect** for **diagnosis of intestinal obstruction**[Q]

Contd...

Contd…

CT Scan
• **Highly sensitive** for **diagnosing complete** or **high-grade obstruction** of **the small bowel and for determining the location** and **cause of obstruction.** • Useful for **extrinsic cause** of bowel obstruction and **determining bowel strangulation**

- Enteroclysis is **investigation of choice** in low-grade, intermittent SBO[Q]
- **Ultrasound:** Useful in **pregnant patients**[Q]

■ TREATMENT OF ACUTE INTESTINAL OBSTRUCTION

Treatment of Acute Intestinal Obstruction

- **Fluid Resuscitation & Antibiotics**[Q]: Aggressive intravenous (IV) replacement with an isotonic saline solution such as lactated Ringer's.
- **Urine output** should be monitored by the placement of a Foley catheter.
- **Elderly patients** may require **central venous assessment**[Q]
- **Tube Decompression**[Q]: Nasogastric suction **reduces** the **risk of pulmonary aspiration** of vomitus and minimizing further **intestinal distention** from preoperatively swallowed air.

• Patients with a **partial intestinal obstruction** may be **treated conservatively** with **resuscitation** and **tube decompression** alone[Q]. • **Resolution of symptoms** and discharge **without** the need for **surgery** has been reported in **60–85%** of patients with a **partial obstruction**[Q].

- **Clinical deterioration** of the patient or **increasing small bowel distention** on abdominal radiographs **during tube decompression** warrants **prompt operative intervention**[Q].

Operative Management

- **Complete SBO** requires **operative intervention**[Q].
- **Adhesiolysis:** In cases of intestinal obstruction secondary to an **adhesive band**[Q]
- **Incarcerated hernias** can be managed by **manual reduction** of the herniated segment of bowel and **closure of the defect**[Q].

Consideration of laparoscopic management in patients with	
• **Mild abdominal distention**[Q] allowing adequate visualization • **Proximal** obstruction[Q]	• **Partial** obstruction[Q] • Anticipated **single-band** obstruction[Q]

Simple Obstruction	Strangulating Obstruction
• Simple obstructions that involve **mechanical blockage** of the flow of **luminal contents**[Q] • **Vascular supply** is **not compromised**[Q]	• Usually involves a **closed-loop obstruction**[Q] • **Vascular supply** to a segment of intestine is **compromised**[Q], can lead to intestinal infarction. • Associated with an **increased morbidity** and **mortality risk**[Q] • **Classic signs:** Tachycardia, fever, leukocytosis, and a constant, noncramping abdominal pain[Q]. • **CT scan:** Useful only in **detecting** the **late stages** of **irreversible ischemia** (e.g. **pneumatosis intestinalis, portal venous gas**)[Q].

Paralytic Ileus	Mechanical Obstruction
• **Pain** is **not a feature of paralytic ileus** and if present a steady, diffuse discomfort[Q]. • **Bowel sounds** are hypoactive or absent[Q] • **Presence of gas in colon & rectum**[Q] in paralytic ileus on abdominal X-ray	• Pain is **colicky**[Q] in mechanical obstruction • **Hyperactive bowel sounds**[Q] in mechanical obstruction • **Absence of gas** in **colon & rectum** in mechanical (**complete**)[Q] small bowel obstruction

■ POSTOPERATIVE ILEUS

Postoperative Ileus

- Following most abdominal operations or injuries, the motility of the GI tract is transiently impaired.
- **Proposed mechanisms** responsible for this dysmotility are **surgical stress-induced sympathetic reflexes, inflammatory response** mediator release, and **anesthetic/analgesic effects**[Q]; each of which can inhibit intestinal motility.

• **Return of normal motility: Small intestine**[Q] (within **24 hours**) >Gastric (48 hours)[Q] > Colonic (3-5 days)[Q] • **Post-operative ileus** is most pronounced in **colon**[Q]

- **Characteristic sequence** of return of normal motility: **Small intestinal motility** returning to normal **within the first 24 hours, gastric motility** within **48 hours** and **colonic motility** returning to normal **3 to 5 days**[Q].
- Because **small bowel motility** is **returned before colonic** and **gastric motility**, listening for **bowel sounds** is **not a reliable indicator** that **ileus has fully resolved**[Q].

Contd…

Contd…

Management of Postoperative Ileus
- The **essence of treatment** is **prevention**, with the **use of nasogastric suction** and **restriction of oral intake until bowel sounds** and the **passage of flatus return**[Q].
- **Following general principles** should be applied:
  - The **primary cause** must be **removed**[Q].
  - **Gastrointestinal distension** must be **relieved by decompression**[Q].
  - Close attention to **fluid** and **electrolyte balance**[Q] is essential.
  - There is no place for the routine use of peristaltic stimulants.
- **Rarely, in resistant cases, medical therapy** with an **adrenergic blocking agent** in association with **cholinergic stimulation**, e.g. **neostigmine (Catchpole regimen)**[Q], may be used, provided that an intraperitoneal cause has been excluded.

> - If **paralytic ileus** is **prolonged** and **threatens life**, a **laparotomy should be considered to exclude a hidden cause** and **facilitate bowel decompression**[Q]

■ INTUSSUSCEPTION

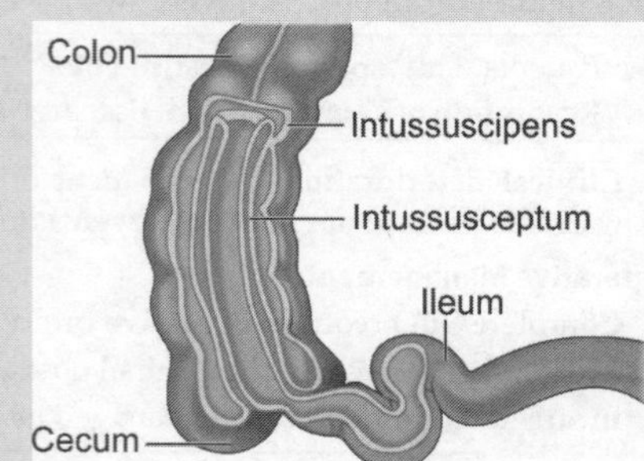

- **Telescoping** of one portion of the intestine into the other.
- **Middle layer** is **isolated between two sharp bends** and **first to become gangrenous**[Q].

> - **Apex is most prone to gangrene**
> - **Highest incidence** between 4 and **10 months**[Q] of age
> - Approx **80–90%** of cases occur **between 3 and 36 months**[Q]

- **Mostly idiopathic** in **infants** and **toddlers**[Q] (no clear etiology).
- **MC type: Ileocolic**[Q] > **Ileo-ileocolic > Ileo-ileal > Colocolic**[Q]

Etiology and Predisposing Factors
- **Upper respiratory tract infections** or **gastroenteritis**[Q] (adenovirus and rotavirus have been implicated) have been **thought to be contributory** to the development of "idiopathic" intussusception. **Hypertrophy** of **Peyer's patches**[Q] can be seen at surgery, but no single etiologic factor predominates.

> - Approximately **5–10%** of cases have a true **pathologic lead point**. The **older the toddler**, the **more likely** there will be a **lead point**[Q]
> - **MC lead point is Meckel's diverticulum**[Q] > **Polyp**[Q]

Clinical Features
- **Typical history: Sudden, short-duration, cyclic crampy abdominal pain**[Q].
- **During** these **episodes** the infant cries inconsolably with the **knees drawn up**[Q].
- **Between episodes** the infant is **asymptomatic**[Q].

> - **Vomiting** is almost **universal**[Q]
> - **Initially the passage of stools may be normal while later on blood mixed with mucus is evacuated-** red currant jelly stool

- An abdominal mass may be palpated- a **sausage shaped abdominal mass**[Q] (increase in size & firmness during the paroxysm of pain)
- There may be an **associated feeling of emptiness** in the **right iliac fossa (Sign of Dance)**[Q]
- **Occult or gross blood in 60–90%** of cases on rectal examination[Q]
- **Apex** may be **palpable** or even **protrude from anus** in extensive **ileocolic** or **colocolic intussusception**[Q]

Diagnosis
- **USG: Kidney-shaped mass** in the longitudinal view or a **target sign** in the transverse view

> - **Hydrostatic reduction** by **contrast agent** or **air enema (preferred) is the diagnostic** & **therapeutic procedure of choice**[Q]
> - **Successful reduction** is **confirmed** by **reflux of air**[Q] **(or barium)** into the small bowel

Treatment
- **Hydrostatic reduction** by **contrast agent** or **air enema** is the **diagnostic** & **therapeutic procedure of choice**[Q].
- The success rate with air or barium reduction should exceed 70%[Q].

> - **Failure of reduction** or the **presence of peritonitis** mandates **operative intervention**[Q], which can be performed laparoscopically or by a standard approach
> - **Definitive surgical procedure: Ileocolectomy with primary anastomosis**[Q]

Recurrence
- **Recurrence** after **successful hydrostatic reduction** is **5–10%**, recurrence rate after operative reduction is 1–4%.
- **Recurrence** is usually **managed by hydrostatic reduction**[Q].
- **Third recurrence**[Q] is an **indication for operative intervention** to look for a **lead point**.

Radiological Investigations in Intussusception

Plain X-ray Film	Barium Enema	Ultrasound
• Features of **small intestinal obstruction**[Q] • **Abdominal soft tissue density** in some cases which may show: • **Target sign**[Q]: Soft tissue mass with concentric area of lucency due to mesenteric fat. • **Meniscus sign**[Q]: Crescent of gas within colonic lumen that outlines the apex of intussusception	• **Claw sign**[Q]: Rounded apex of intussusception protrudes into the contrast column • **Coiled spring sign**[Q]: Edematous mucosal folds of returning limb of intussusception outlined by contrast material.	• **Target sign** or **Bull's eye sign** on **transverse scan**[Q] • **Pseudokidney sign** on **longitudinal scan**[Q]

■ ACUTE MESENTERIC ISCHEMIA

Acute Mesenteric Ischemia	

• **Emboli** (50%)[Q]:
   – **Arrhythmia, Valvular disease**[Q], Myocardial infarction
   – Cardiac aneurysm, Aortic atherosclerotic disease
	– Hypokinetic ventricular wall

Thrombosis (25%): Atherosclerotic disease	
• **Nonocclusive** (5–15%): – **Pancreatitis, Heart failure, Sepsis**[Q]	– Cardiac bypass, **Burns, Renal failure**[Q]
• **Venous occlusion:** – Hypercoagulable state	– Sepsis Compression, Pregnancy, Portal hypertension

ACUTE MESENTERIC ISCHEMIA

Clinical Features
- **Early diagnosis** is the **key to successful management** of AMI[Q].
- Most patients have **nonspecific symptoms** of **abdominal pain**[Q].
- **Abdominal pain out of proportion** to the findings on physical examination and persisting **beyond 2 to 3 hours** is the classic picture.
- Diarrhea, nausea, vomiting, and anorexia can also be part of the initial symptom complex.
- **Melena** or **hematochezia** in **15%**, and **occult fecal blood** is found in **half** of the patients.

Diagnosis

• IOC in AMI is **mesenteric arteriography**[Q]

- **CT scan: Wall hyperdensity**, absence of **wall enhancement**, wall thickening, bowel dilation, **pneumatosis**, **gas** in **mesenteric vein branches** and in **portal vein** branches.

Treatment
- Effective management: **Early diagnosis, aggressive resuscitation, early revascularization**, and ongoing supportive care.
- **Mucosal layer** is the **most sensitive to ischemia, bacterial translocation** should be anticipated and **intravenous antibiotics**[Q] used to treat the associated bacteremia.

• **Catheter-directed papaverine** to **reverse** the **severe mesenteric vasospasm**[Q] is initiated early after arteriography
 • **Anticoagulation** is given to **prevent propagation**[Q] of mesenteric thrombus

- In addition to aggressively correcting the low cardiac output, terminating vasoconstrictor use, and discontinuing digitalis preparations, **intra-arterial papaverine infusion** is the **treatment of choice**[Q].
- In the **absence of peritonitis**, supportive care with **anticoagulation** and **continued papaverine** infusion is recommended.
- **Evidence of peritonitis: Exploratory laparotomy**, with conservative resection of necrotic bowel.

Investigation of Choice	
Acute mesenteric ischemia[Q]	**Angiography**[Q]
Mesenteric venous thrombosis[Q]	**CECT**[Q]
Chronic mesenteric ischemia[Q]	**Aortography**[Q]

■ MESENTERIC VENOUS THROMBOSIS

MESENTERIC VENOUS THROMBOSIS

- MVT accounts for 5–15% of patients with mesenteric ischemia.
- **SMV** is **MC involved**, frequently with **extension of thrombus into portal vein**[Q].

• **IMV** is most often **spared**[Q]

Contd…

Contd…

Clinical Features
- Most commonly, patients complain of **midabdominal colicky pain**[Q]
- Nausea, vomiting, diarrhea, and anorexia frequently accompany their abdominal discomfort.
- Occult blood in the stool in half of the patients, gross bleeding such as hematemesis, hematochezia, or melena occurs in approximately 15%.
- Family history of venous thromboembolism[Q] in half of the patients
- **Bowel infarction** ultimately develops in **30–60%**[Q].

Diagnosis

> - **CECT** with IV contrast is the **diagnostic test of choice**[Q] for patients with suspected **acute MVT**

Treatment
- Rapid initiation of **systemic anticoagulation**[Q] is important.
- Exploratory laparotomy in localized or diffuse peritoneal irritation,
- Acute thrombus in large veins: Thrombectomy followed by recombinant tissue plasminogen activator solution.
- The patient is treated with heparin intraoperatively and anticoagulation is continued postoperatively[Q].

Prognosis
- **MVT** have a **high risk of recurrence (35–70%)**[Q], most frequently within 30 days, need for early & persistent anticoagulation.
- **Mortality rate** is high, **up to 50%.**

■ COLONIC PSEUDO-OBSTRUCTION

COLONIC PSEUDO-OBSTRUCTION
• **Pseudo-obstruction** of the colon describes the condition of **distention of the colon,** with **signs** and **symptoms** of **colonic obstruction,** in the **absence of** an actual **physical cause** of the obstruction[Q] • **Acute colonic pseudo-obstruction** is also known as **Ogilvie's syndrome**[Q] • Two types: Primary and secondary • **Secondary pseudo-obstruction is more common**[Q]

Pathophysiology
• **Mechanism** thought to play: **Sympathetic overactivity overriding the parasympathetic system**[Q] • Indirect support for this theory has been derived from the **success in treating** the **syndrome with neostigmine, a parasympathomimetic agent**[Q] • **Further support** comes from reports of **immediate resolution of** the **syndrome after administration of an epidural anesthetic** that provides sympathetic blockade

Primary Pseudo-obstruction
- It is a motility disorder:
  - A **familial visceral myopathy** (hollow visceral myopathy syndrome) or
  - A **diffuse motility disorder involving** the **autonomic innervation** of the intestinal wall.

Causes of secondary Pseudo-obstruction	
• **Neuroleptic medications**[Q]	• **Uremia**[Q]
• **Opiates**[Q]	• **Lupus, scleroderma, dermatomyositis**[Q]
• Severe metabolic illness	• **Parkinson's disease**[Q]
• **Myxedema** (Hypothyroidism[Q])	• Traumatic **retroperitoneal hematomas**[Q]
• **Hyperparathyroidism**[Q]	• **Diabetes mellitus**[Q]

Clinical Features
- **Acute form:** Most commonly affects patients with **chronic renal, respiratory, cerebral, or cardiovascular disease, involves only** the **colon**[Q].
- **Chronic form:** Affects other parts of the gastrointestinal tract, usually presents as bouts of **subacute** and **partial intestinal obstruction,** and tends to **recur periodically.**

> - **Acute colonic pseudo-obstruction** should be suspected when a **medically ill patient** suddenly **develops abdominal distention**[Q]
> - **The abdomen is** tympanitic, **usually** nontender, **and bowel sounds** are **usually present**

Diagnosis
- **Abdominal X-ray: Distended colon,** with the **right** and **transverse segments**[Q] tending to be **most dramatically affected** (radiologic appearance of large bowel obstruction). **Transition point** is frequently present, usually at or near the splenic flexure[Q].

> - **Most useful investigation: Water-soluble contrast enema**[Q]

Treatment
- **Initial treatment:** Nasogastric decompression, replacement of extracellular fluid deficits, and correction of electrolyte abnormalities[Q].
- **All medications** that **inhibit bowel motility,** such as opiates, **should be discontinued.**
- **Most patients improve with this regimen**[Q].

> - Treat this condition with **neostigmine**[Q]
> - **Mechanical obstruction should be excluded** (either by water-soluble contrast enema or colonoscopy) **before** the **administration of neostigmine**[Q]

■ LARGE BOWEL OBSTRUCTION

LARGE BOWEL OBSTRUCTION

- Classified as **dynamic (mechanical)** or **adynamic (pseudo-obstruction).**
- **Mechanical obstruction** is characterized by **blockage** of the **large bowel** (luminal, mural, or extramural), resulting in **increased intestinal contractility**[Q]
- **Pseudo-obstruction** is characterized by the **absence of intestinal contractility,** often associated with **decreased** or **absent motility** of the **small bowel** and **stomach**[Q]

> - MC cause of LBO: Colorectal cancer[Q] (CA Rectum > sigmoid)

Pathophysiology

- **Colon becomes distended as gas** (about **two thirds is swallowed air,** the remainder includes the products of bacterial fermentation), **stool**, and **liquid accumulate** proximal to the site of blockage.

> - In **obstructed hernia** or **volvulus**, the **blood supply** can become **compromised,** or **strangulated; initially**, the **venous return is blocked**[Q]
> - **Vascular compromise** of the **obstructed colon** can occur due to **excessive distention**[Q]

- **Closed-loop obstruction:** When **both** the **proximal** and **distal parts** of the bowel are **occluded**[Q] (strangulated hernia or volvulus)

Clinical Features

- **Cancers** of **rectum** or **left colon** are **more likely to obstruct**[Q] than those arising in the more capacious proximal colon.
- **Failure to pass stool** and **flatus** associated with **increasing abdominal distention** and **cramping abdominal pain**[Q].

Diagnosis

- **Abdominal X-ray: Distended colon**[Q]
- **CT scan:** Helpful in revealing an **inflammatory process** such as **diverticulitis.**
- **Water-soluble contrast enema:** For the **diagnosis of** suspected case of **volvulus** or **distal sigmoid cancer**[Q]

Treatment

- Virtually **all patients with complete acute large bowel obstruction** require **prompt surgical intervention**[Q] and should not undergo a trial of non-operative management.
- **Acute large bowel obstruction** in patients **with competent ileocecal valve** is a **true surgical emergency** because of **high chances of perforation (MC site: Cecum)**[Q].
- Once diagnosis has been made, **surgical exploration** should be undertaken **as soon as possible after appropriate resuscitation**[Q]

Treatment of Large Bowel Obstruction	
Site of Obstruction	**Procedure**
Right-sided colonic obstruction (cancer or volvulus)	• **Resection** with **ileo-transverse anastomosis**[Q]
Cancer of sigmoid colon	• **Hartmann's operation**[Q] (sigmoidectomy with descending colostomy & closure of the rectal stump), • **Sigmoidectomy** with **primary colorectal anastomosis**[Q] • **Abdominal colectomy** with **ileorectal anastomosis**[Q]
Cancer of **distal** or **mid rectum**	• **Loop colostomy** or **defunctioning colostomy**[Q] (to relieve obstruction) followed by **neoadjuvant chemoradiation**[Q], (with the plan to resect the primary lesion at a later time)

■ SIGMOID VOLVULUS

SIGMOID VOLVULUS

- Volvulus can occur in any segment of **large bowel attached to a long** & **floppy mesentery**[Q] or **fixed to the retroperitoneum by a narrow base of origin**[Q]

> - MC site of volvulus: Sigmoid colon
> - **More commonly anticlockwise** (can be both clockwise or anticlockwise)

- Equal frequency in both sexes[Q]

Associated Predisposing Factors

- **Age: 60–70 years**[Q].
- **Chronic constipation**[Q]
- **Institutionalized** or **neurologically impaired** or **psychiatric patients**[Q] (their medication may decrease intestinal motility, or they may fail to pass stool regularly, leading to fecal loaded large bowel predisposing to volvulus)
- **Diet high in fibre** and **vegetables**[Q] (as in **third world countries**)

Contd…

Contd…

Clinical Features
- Present as **acute** or **subacute intestinal obstruction**
- **Sudden onset** of **severe abdominal pain, vomiting, & obstipation.**
- **Abdomen is markedly distended** and **tympanitic,** with the **distention** often **more dramatic**[Q] than would be associated with other causes of obstruction.
- Severe abdominal pain, **rebound tenderness, & tachycardia** are **ominous signs**[Q].

Radiological (X-ray) Characteristics
- **Markedly dilated sigmoid colon** with the **appearance of a bent inner tube** or **coffee bean appearance**[Q].
- **Inferior convergence** of the dilated loop **points towards left side** of pelvis. Whorl sign on CT scan.

> - **Contrast enema demonstrates the point of obstruction with the pathognomic 'birds beak' or 'bird of prey' or 'ace of spades' sign**[Q]

Management of Sigmoid Volvulus
- **Initial management: Resuscitation**[Q] followed by **endoscopic decompression** and **detorsion**[Q].
- If detorsion/decompression cannot be achieved with either the rectal tube or colonoscope, **laparotomy with resections of the sigmoid colon**[Q] is done.
- Any evidence of **bowel gangrene** or **perforation contraindicates non-operative decompression** and an **immediate surgical exploration**[Q] is done.

■ CECAL VOLVULUS

CECAL VOLVULUS

- Cecal volvulus is **actually** a **cecocolic volvulus**[Q]
- Consists of an **axial rotation** of the **terminal ileum, cecum,** and **ascending colon**[Q] with concomitant twisting of the associated mesentery.
- Cause: Lack of fixation of the cecum to the retroperitoneum.[Q]

> - **Cecal volvulus** occurs in **clockwise direction**[Q]
> - **More common** in **women**[Q]
> - Affects a **younger age group** as compared to sigmoid volvulus, in **5th decade**[Q]

Predisposing Factors for Cecal volvulus	
- **Previous surgery**[Q]	- **Malrotation**[Q]
- **Pregnancy**[Q]	- **Obstructing lesions of the left colon**[Q]

Clinical Features
- Sudden onset of **abdominal pain & distention.**
- Presents with **features of small bowel obstruction.**
- **Asymmetric distention** of the abdomen, with a **tympanitic mass palpable** in either **the left upper quadrant** or **midabdomen**[Q].

Diagnosis
- **Abdominal X-ray:** Dilated cecum, displaced to the left side of the abdomen.
- **Distended cecum** assumes a **gas-filled comma shape** or **kidney bean shape**[Q], the **concavity** of which faces **inferiorly** and to the **right.**
- **Haustral markings** in the **distended loop** indicate that the dilated bowel is colon.
- **Torsion results in small bowel obstruction**[Q] (radiographic pattern of SBO)

> - Contrast enema is used to confirm the diagnosis and to exclude a carcinoma of the distal bowel as a precipitating cause of the volvulus[Q]

Treatment
- **Most cases require operation to correct** the **volvulus & prevent ischemia**[Q].
- **If ischemia** has already occurred, **immediate operation** is obviously required.

> - **Right colectomy** with **primary anastomosis** is the **procedure of choice**[Q]
> - In **frankly gangrenous bowel, resection** of the gangrenous bowel **with ileostomy** is a safar approach

- **Recurrence rates are high with ceropoxy,** and **right colectomy** remains the **procedure of choice for cecal volvulus.**

Multiple Choice Questions

■ ACUTE INTESTINAL OBSTRUCTION

1. **Best investigation for acute intestinal obstruction is:**
   (Recent Question 2014)
   - a. Barium studies
   - b. X-ray
   - c. USG
   - d. ERCP

2. **The most common cause of small intestinal obstruction is:**
   (Recent Question 2014)
   - a. Intussusception
   - b. Iatrogenic adhesions
   - c. Trauma
   - d. Carcinoma

3. **Commonest cause of acute intestinal obstruction is:**
   (Recent Question 2016)
   - a. Adhesions
   - b. Volvulus
   - c. Inguinal hernias
   - d. Internal hernias

4. **While doing emergency laparotomy for an intestinal obstruction, which organ would you first visualize to say whether it is small bowel or large bowed obstruction?**
   (AIIMS Nov 2018)
   - a. Ileum
   - b. Sigmoid colon
   - c. Cecum
   - d. Rectum

5. **A women of 35-years, comes to emergency department with symptoms of pain in abdomen and bilious vomiting but no distension of bowel. Abdominal X-ray showed no air fluid level. Diagnosis is:** *(Recent Question 2014; AIIMS June 2009)*
   - a. CA rectum
   - b. Duodenal obstruction
   - c. Adynamic ileus
   - d. Pseudo-obstruction

6. **The first to appear in a cause of acute intestinal obstruction is:**
   (Recent Questions 2016)
   - a. Constipation
   - b. Colicky pain
   - c. Vomiting
   - d. Distension

7. **For intestinal obstruction immediate operation should not be done in case of:** *(Kolkata 2000)*
   - a. Postop adhesion
   - b. Appendix perforation
   - c. Volvulus
   - d. Obstructed hernia

8. **Which of the following is most suggestive of neonatal small bowel obstruction?** *(All India 2003)*
   - a. Generalized abdominal distension
   - b. Failure to pass meconium in the first 24 hours
   - c. Bilious vomiting
   - d. Refusal of feeds

9. **What is the sure sign of intestinal obstruction?**
   (Recent Question 2013)
   - a. Vomiting and distension
   - b. Jelly like stool
   - c. Diarrhoea
   - d. Localized tenderness

10. **Ileal obstruction due to round worm obstruction treatment is:** *(Recent Question 2013)*
   - a. Resection with end to end anastomosis
   - b. Resection with side to side anastomosis
   - c. Enterotomy, removal of worms and primary closure
   - d. Diversion

11. **Investigation of choice for intermittent GI obstruction:**
   (Recent Question 2017)
   - a. X-ray
   - b. USG
   - c. Enteroclysis
   - d. Barium meal follow-through

12. **Step ladder pattern of gas shadow is seen in:**
   (Recent Question 2017)
   - a. Duodenal obstruction
   - b. Intestinal obstruction
   - c. Gastric outlet obstruction
   - d. Sigmoid volvulus

■ INTUSSUSCEPTION

13. **A neonate presents with colicky pain and vomiting with sausage-shaped lump in the abdomen, diagnosis is:**
   (UPPG 2009)
   - a. Enterocolitis
   - b. Perforation of the abdomen
   - c. Intussusception
   - d. Acute appendicitis

14. **Intussusception usually begins from:** *(DNB 2007)*
   - a. Jejunum
   - b. Terminal ileum
   - c. Colon
   - d. Rectum

15. **The most common type of intussusception:** *(MCI June 2018, DNB 2009, 2005, 2001, 2000, MHPGMCET 2009)*
   - a. Ileocolic
   - b. Colocolic
   - c. Ileoileal
   - d. Retrograde

16. **A child was operated for small intestine mass with intussusception and after the operation the tumor was diagnosed in histological section. Which is the most likely tumor associated?** *(AIIMS Nov 2012)*
   - a. Carcinoid
   - b. Villous adenoma
   - c. Lymphoma
   - d. Smooth muscle tumor

17. **What is intussuscipiens?** *(Recent Question 2014)*
   - a. The entire complex of intussusception
   - b. The entering layer
   - c. The outer layer
   - d. The process of reducing the intussusception

18. **Comment on the diagnosis of a film shown of a 65-year-old man with acute abdomen:** *(MCI Dec 2018)*

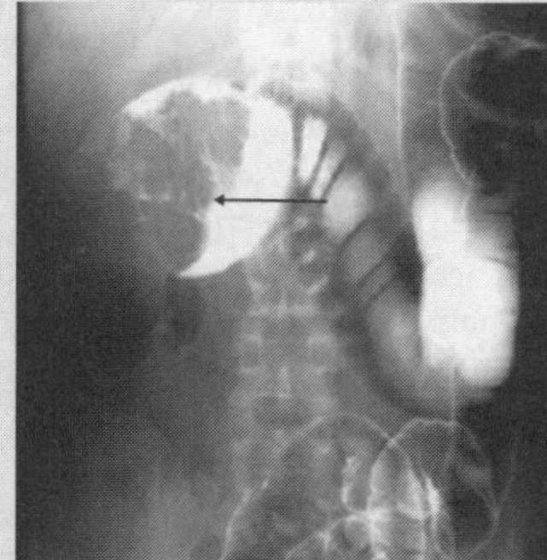

   - a. Ileocolic intussusception
   - b. Sigmoid volvulus
   - c. Toxic megacolon
   - d. Colocolic intussusception

19. **What is the name of sign in this barium enema done in the patient of intussusception?**
   - a. Meniscus sign
   - b. Claw sign
   - c. Coiled spring sign
   - d. Target sign

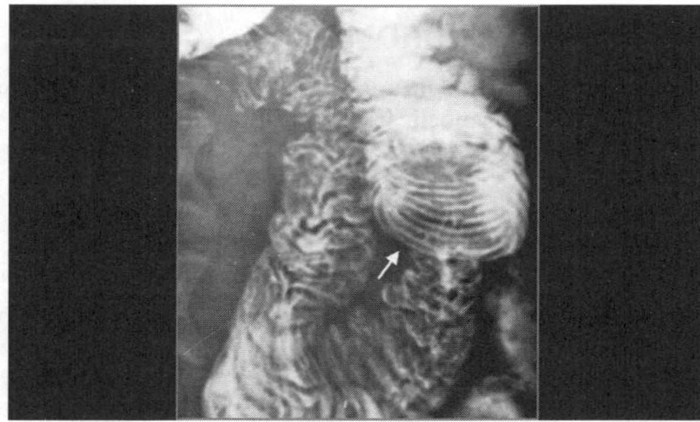

20. A 10-month-old infant presents with acute intestinal obstruction. Contrast enema X-ray shows the intussusceptions. Likely cause is: *(All India 2002)*
    a. Payers patch hypertrophy
    b. Meckel's diverticulum
    c. Mucosal polyp
    d. Duplication cyst

21. Recurrent obstruction, mass per rectum and diarrhea in child: *(Recent Question 2014)*
    a. Intussusception
    b. Rectal prolapsed
    c. Internal hernia
    d. Hemorrhoids

22. Commonest cause of intussusception is: *(WBPG 2015)*
    a. Submucous lipoma
    b. Meckel's diverticulum
    c. Hypertrophy of submucous Peyer's patches
    d. Polyp

23. Intussusception is frequently associated with: *(JIPMER 2014, 2012)*
    a. Submucosal lipoma
    b. Intramural lipoma
    c. Subserusal lipoma
    d. Subfascial lipoma

24. Which of the following is true about intussusception?
    a. Common in neonates *(DPG 2005)*
    b. Fever always present
    c. Not associated with tumors of intestine
    d. Usually relieved by barium enema

25. The least common type of intussusception is: *(Recent Question 2016)*
    a. Multiple
    b. Colocolic
    c. Ileoileal
    d. Ileoilecolic

26. Claw sign seen in: *(APPG 2008)*
    a. Intussusception
    b. Volvulus
    c. Both
    d. None

27. Which of the following is true about intussusception in children? *(Recent Question 2017)*
    a. Most common type is ileocecocolic
    b. Most common type is colocolic
    c. Entering tube is intussuscipiens
    d. Contrast enema is not useful in the management

28. A patient has acute abdominal pain with blood and mucus in stool with palpable mass per abdomen is due to: *(Recent Question 2014; AIIMS June 2000)*
    a. Meckel's diverticulum
    b. Volvulus
    c. Intussusception
    d. Hypertrophic pyloric stenosis

29. A 9-month-old child presents with excessive cry, right iliac fossa sausage shaped lump and blood in stools. What is the best treatment? *(MCI Nov 2017)*
    a. IV fluids-antibiotics-NG tube
    b. IV fluids-antibiotics-air enema
    c. IV fluids-antibiotics-barium enema
    d. IV fluids-antibiotics-warm saline enema

■ MECONIUM SYNDROME

30. A new born child has not passed meconium for 48 hours. What is the diagnostic procedure of choice? *(All India 2008)*
    a. USG
    b. Contrast enema
    c. CT
    d. MRI

31. Snow storm ascites is seen in: *(APPG 2005)*
    a. Meconium ileus
    b. Hirschsprung's disease
    c. Ileocaecal tuberculosis
    d. Pseudomyxoma peritonei

32. Meconium ileus is a presentation in which of the following disease? *(MCI June 2019)*
    a. Mucoviscidosis
    b. Hirschsprung's disease
    c. Ileal atresia
    d. Congenital aganglionosis

33. A new born girl not passed meconium for 48 hours, has abdominal distention and vomiting. Initial investigation of choice would be: *(AIIMS Nov 2007)*
    a. Manometry
    b. Genotyping for cystic fibrosis
    c. Lower GI contrast study
    d. Serum trypsin immunoblot

■ MESENTERIC ISCHEMIA

34. Occlusion to superior mesenteric artery affects jejunum and: *(UPPG 2010)*
    a. Pyloric antrum
    b. Fundus of stomach
    c. Duodenum distal to the opening of CBD
    d. Greater curvature
    e. Descending colon

35. Most common cause of acute mesenteric ischemia is: *(AIIMS May 2011, Nov 2008)*
    a. Arterial thrombosis
    b. Venous thrombosis
    c. Embolism
    d. Non occlusive disease

36. All are causes of dynamic intestinal obstruction except:
    a. Gallstones
    b. Bands
    c. Intussusception *(JIPMER 2010)*
    d. Mesenteric vascular occlusion

37. Ischemia of which of the vessel would cause least damage?
    a. Renal artery
    b. SMA *(AIIMS Nov 2011)*
    c. IMA
    d. Celiac trunk

38. String of lakes appearance on angiography is seen in:
    a. Chronic mesenteric ischaemia *(Recent Question 2016)*
    b. Non-occlusive mesenteric ischemia
    c. Mesenteric venous thrombosis
    d. Mesenteric arterial thrombosis

39. A 65-years old Ramdeen presents with abdominal pain and distension of abdomen. His stools were maroon colored and he gives a past history of cerebrovascular accident and myocardial infarction. What will be the probable diagnosis? *(AIIMS Nov 2000, Nov 97)*
    a. Ulcerative colitis
    b. Acute mesenteric ischemia
    c. Irritable bowel syndrome
    d. Crohn's disease

40. A man aged 60 years has history of IHD and atherosclerosis. He presents with abdominal pain and maroon stools. Most likely diagnosis: *(All India 2001)*
    a. Acute intestinal obstruction
    b. Acute mesenteric ischemia
    c. Peritonitis
    d. Appendicitis

■ PARALYTIC ILEUS

41. First to recover from post-operative ileus: *(Recent Question 2016, DNB 2014, 2008)*
    a. Small intestine
    b. Stomach
    c. Colon
    d. None

42. Routine management of paralytic ileus includes all of the following except: *(MCI March 2005)*
    a. Electrolyte correction
    b. Nasogastric aspiration
    c. Parasympathomimetics
    d. IV fluids

43. First to recover from paralytic ileus: *(Recent Question 2017)*
    a. Stomach
    b. Small intestine
    c. Rectum
    d. Colon

44. Most common electrolyte imbalance that causes paralytic ileus is: *(DNB 2014)*
    a. Hyponatremia
    b. Hypernatremia
    c. Hypokalemia
    d. Hyperkalemia

■ LARGE BOWEL OBSTRUCTION

45. Most common cause of colonic obstruction is:
(Recent Question 2016)
- a. Volvulus
- b. Hernia
- c. Adhesions
- d. Neoplasm

■ PSEUDO-OBSTRUCTION

46. Ogilvie's syndrome results from the denervation of the colon distal to the: *(COMEDK 2006)*
- a. Hepatic flexure
- b. Mid-transverse colon
- c. Splenic flexure
- d. Descending colon

47. True about Ogilvie's syndrome are all except:
(Recent Question 2016, 2015; AIIMS Nov 2007)
- a. It is caused by mechanical obstruction of the colon
- b. It involves entire/part of the large colon
- c. It occurs after previous surgery
- d. It occurs commonly after narcotic use

48. Colonic Pseudo-obstruction occurs in all, except:
(AIIMS June 94)
- a. Diabetes mellitus
- b. Dermatomyositis
- c. Scleroderma
- d. Hyperthyroidism

49. Ogilvie's syndrome: *(Recent Question 2017)*
- a. Acute colonic pseudo-obstruction
- b. Chronic colonic pseudo-obstruction
- c. Fecal obstruction
- d. Intussusception

50. Most common cause of Ogilvie's syndrome:
(Recent Question 2017)
- a. Head injury
- b. Electrolyte abnormalities
- c. Carcinoma
- d. Drugs

51. A 56-year-old woman has not passed stools for the last 14 days. X-ray shows no air fluid levels, Probable diagnosis is:
- a. Paralytic ileus   *(Recent Question 2014; All India 2001)*
- b. Aganglionosis of the colon
- c. Intestinal pseudo-obstruction
- d. Duodenal obstruction

52. Acute pseudo-obstruction of the colon known as:
(DNB 2012, UPPG 2007)
- a. Sjogren's syndrome
- b. Gardener's syndrome
- c. Ogilvie's syndrome
- d. Peutz-Jegher's syndrome

■ VOLVULUS

53. Most common site of volvulus: *(DNB 2012, GB PANT 2011)*
- a. Sigmoid colon
- b. Caecum
- c. Transverse colon
- d. Stomach

54. This characteristic appearance is seen in:
- a. Gastric volvulus
- b. Small intestinal volvulus
- c. Cecal volvulus
- d. Sigmoid volvulus

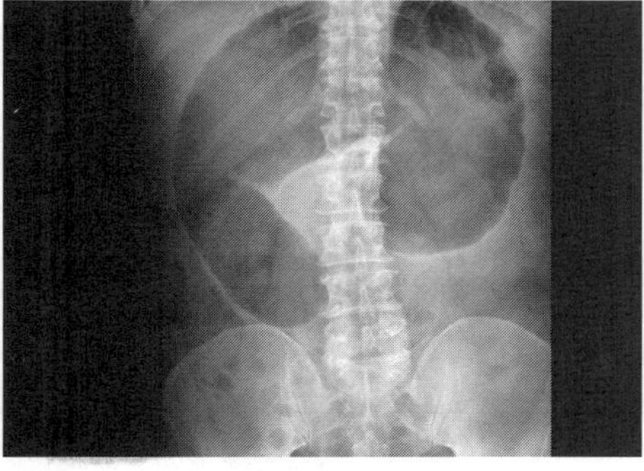

55. Which of the following statement about volvulus is false?
- a. More common in psychiatric patients   *(All India 2008)*
- b. Sigmoid volvulus is more common than caecal volvulus
- c. Lower GI scopy is contraindicated in sigmoid volvulus
- d. Volvulus of caecum is managed by conservative methods

56. This characteristic appearance is seen in: *(Recent Question 2017)*
- a. Gastric volvulus
- b. Small intestinal volvulus
- c. Cecal volvulus
- d. Sigmoid volvulus

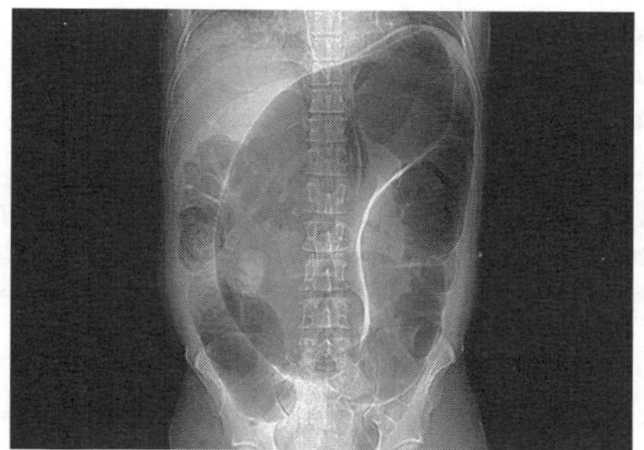

57. Sigmoid volvulus rotation occurs: *(UPPG 2007, 2005)*
- a. Clockwise
- b. Anticlockwise
- c. Both clockwise and anti clockwise
- d. Axial in direction

58. Which of the following statements abut sigmoid volvulus is incorrect? *(DPG 2009 March)*
- a. More common with laxative abuse
- b. Non-operative treatment has no role
- c. Recurrence rate around 40%
- d. Sigmoid resection is definitive treatment

59. All are predisposing factors for sigmoid volvulus except:
(DNB 2007)
- a. Hirschprung's diseases
- b. Chagas diseases
- c. Chronic constipation
- d. Tuberculosis

60. Least common volvulus site in neonate is: *(JIPMER 2013)*
- a. Ilioileal
- b. Large bowel volvulus
- c. Small bowel volvulus
- d. Gastric volvulus

61. Midgut volvulus symptoms appear at: *(Recent Question 2017)*
- a. 1st week
- b. 2nd week
- c. 3rd week
- d. 4th week

■ MALROTATION

62. Child presents with recurrent abdominal pain and bilious vomiting. Condition was diagnosed by barium follow through. Surgery was done, mesenteric widening, appendectomy, cutting the Ladd's band. What is the diagnosis?
(AIIMS Nov 2010)
- a. Recurrent cecal volvulus
- b. Malrotation
- c. Recurrent appendicitis
- d. Stricture TB

63. A 7-day-old infant presents with bilious vomiting and gross abdominal distention with absent bowel sounds. X-ray abdomen shows multiple gas filled loops. Diagnosis is:
- a. Hirschsprung's disease   *(MCI June 2019)*
- b. Congenital hypertrophic pyloric stenosis
- c. Duodenal atresia
- d. Malrotation of gut

64. The cecum is found to be placed below the stomach and in the midline. Which of the following abnormality must have taken place while rotation of the gut? *(AIIMS Nov 2010)*
- a. Non-rotation
- b. Malrotation
- c. Reversed rotation
- d. Mixed rotation

Explanations

■ ACUTE INTESTINAL OBSTRUCTION

1. Ans. b. X-ray	2. Ans. b. Iatrogenic adhesions

3. Ans. a. Adhesions

4. Ans. c. Cecum *(Ref: Bailey 27/e p1294)*

> *"After full resuscitation, the abdomen should be opened through a midline incision. Care should be taken to ensure that the loss of tamponade of the abdominal wall does not lead to increased caecal distension and rupture (this starts with splitting along the line of the taenia coli on the antimesenteric border).* **Distension of the caecum will confirm large bowel involvement. Identification of a collapsed distal segment of the large bowel and its sequential proximal assessment will readily lead to identification of the cause."** *–Bailey 27/e p1294*

5. Ans. b. Duodenal obstruction *(Ref: Sabiston 20/e p1249; Schwartz 11/e p1229, 10/e p1147; Bailey 27/e p1285-1286)*
   - Abdominal pain, bilious vomiting without abdominal distention is suggestive of proximal small intestinal obstruction, distal to ampulla of Vater (Duodenal obstruction).

> - Nausea and **vomiting** are **more common** with **proximal obstruction**[Q]
> - **Abdominal distention** is **more common in distal obstruction**[Q]

6. Ans. b. Colicky pain *(Ref: Bailey 27/e p1285)*	7. Ans. a. Postop adhesion
8. Ans. c. Bilious vomiting	9. Ans. a. Vomiting and distension

10. Ans. c. Enterotomy, removal of worms and primary closure *(Ref: Schwartz 11/e p1231, 10/e p1149; Farquharson's 8/e p470; Sabiston 20/e p1253)*

> - Resection of small bowel is done when the affected bowel segment is of questionable viability.
> - Diversion is the first step in case of colonic obstruction, followed by resection and anastomosis of affected segment and then closure of diversion colostomy at a later date.
> - Intestinal luminal obstruction such as due to Bezoars or fecolihs of worm intestations are dealt with by enterotomy and removal followed by primary closure.

11. Ans. c. Enteroclysis

12. Ans. b. Intestinal obstruction *(Ref: Sabiston 20/e p1242)*

> *"Characteristic findings of small bowel obstruction on supine radiographs are dilated loops of small intestine, without evidence of colonic distention. Upright radiographs demonstrate multiple air-fluid levels, which often layer in a stepwise fashion."*
> *–Sabiston 20/e p1242*

■ INTUSSUSCEPTION

13. Ans. c. Intussusception *(Ref: Sabiston 20/e p1879; Schwartz 11/e p1731, 10/e p1622; Bailey 27/e p1287; Shackelford 8/e p986)*

14. Ans. b. Terminal ileum	15. Ans. a. Ileocolic

16. Ans. c. Lymphoma *(Ref: Sabiston 20/e p1879; Schwartz 11/e p1731, 10/e p1622; Bailey 27/e p1284; Shackelford 8/e p986)*

17. Ans. c. The outer layer

18. Ans. d. Colocolic intussusception *(Ref: Bailey 27/e p1289)*

19. Ans. c. Coiled spring sign

20. Ans. a. Payers patch hypertrophy	21. Ans. a. Intussusception
22. Ans. c. Hypertrophy of submucous Peyer's patches	23. Ans. a. Submucosal lipoma

24. Ans. d. Usually relieved by barium enema

25. Ans. a. Multiple *(Ref: Bailey 27/e p1284)*

Types of Intussusception (in decreasing order)	
1. Ileocolic (77%)[Q]	**4. Colocolic (2%): MC in adults**
2. Ileo-ileo-colic (12%)	**5. Multiple (1%)**
3. Ilioileal (5%)	6. Retrograde (0.2%)

26. Ans. a. Intussusception

27. **Ans. a.** Most common type is ileocecocolic *(Ref: Sabiston 20/e p1879; Schwartz 11/e p1731, 10/e p1622; Bailey 27/e p1283)*

28. **Ans. c.** Intussusception

29. **Ans. b.** IV fluids-antibiotics-air enema *(Ref: Sabiston 20/e p1879; Schwartz 11/e p1731; Bailey 27/e p1287)*

■ MECONIUM SYNDROME

30. **Ans. b.** Contrast enema *(Ref: Sabiston 20/e p1876; Schwartz 11/e p1726, 10/e p1617-1619; Shackelford 8/e p979)*
    - **Failure to pass meconium in the first 2 days** of life (48 hours) is typically **suggestive of a lower GI tract obstruction** such as **Hirschprung's disease, meconium plug syndrome or anorectal malformation. A contrast enema** is the **most suitable primary investigation to make the diagnosis,** amongst the options provided.

31. **Ans. a.** Meconium ileus *(Ref: Sabiston 20/e p1875; Schwartz 11/e p1726, 10/e p1617-1619; Bailey 27/e p1294, 134; Shackelford 8/e p978)*

32. **Ans. a.** Mucoviscidosis *(Ref: Bailey 27/e p134, 1294)*

33. **Ans. c.** Lower GI contrast study

■ MESENTERIC ISCHEMIA

34. **Ans. c.** Duodenum distal to the opening of CBD *(Ref: Bailey 27/e p1253)*

SUPERIOR MESENTERIC ARTERY

- **SMA supplies** the **midgut,** from **distal part of duodenum** to **proximal 2/3rd of transverse colon**[Q].

35. **Ans. c.** Embolism *(Ref: Sabiston 20/e p1155; Schwartz 11/e p929, 10/e p859-866; Bailey 27/e p1253; Shackelford 8/e p1028)*

36. **Ans. d.** Mesenteric vascular occlusion

37. **Ans. c.** IMA *(Ref: Grays 40/e p1141)*
    - Grays Anatomy: **Occlusion of IMA does not always result in irreversible ischemia** of the **descending** and **sigmoid colon,** because the **marginal artery of colon** usually **receives an adequate supply** from the **left branch of the middle colic artery**[Q]

38. **Ans. b.** Non-occlusive mesenteric ischemia

39. **Ans. b.** Acute mesenteric ischemia *(Ref: Sabiston 20/e p1155; Schwartz 11/e p929, 10/e p859-866; Bailey 27/e p1253; Shackelford 8/e p1028)*

40. **Ans. b.** Acute mesenteric ischemia

■ PARALYTIC ILEUS

41. **Ans. a.** Small intestine

42. **Ans. c.** Parasympathomimetics *(Ref: Bailey 25/e p1202)*
    - **Rarely, in resistant cases, medical therapy with an adrenergic blocking agent in association with cholinergic stimulation, e.g. neostigmine (the Catchpole regimen**[Q]**), may be used, provided that an intraperitoneal cause has been excluded.**

43. **Ans. b.** Small intestine *(Ref: Sabiston 20/e p306; Bailey 27/e p1296)*   44. **Ans. c.** Hypokalemia

■ LARGE BOWEL OBSTRUCTION

45. **Ans. d.** Neoplasm

■ PSEUDO-OBSTRUCTION

46. **Ans. c.** Splenic flexure *(Ref: Sabiston 20/e p1336; Bailey 27/e p1297)*
    - **Ogilvie's syndrome: Distended colon,** with the **right** and **transverse segments** tending to **be most dramatically affected. Transition point** is frequently present, usually **at or near** the **splenic flexure.**

47. **Ans. a.** It is caused by mechanical obstruction of the colon

48. **Ans. d.** Hyperthyroidism

49. **Ans. a.** Acute colonic pseudo-obstruction *(Ref: Sabiston 20/e p1337; Schwartz 11/e p1308, 10/e p1221; Bailey 27/e p1297)*

    "Colonic pseudo-obstruction: This may occur in an acute or a chronic form. The former, also known as Ogilvie's syndrome, presents as acute large bowel obstruction."-Bailey 27/e p1297

50. **Ans. b.** Electrolyte abnormalities *(Ref: Sleisenger 10/e p1877; Sabiston 20/e p1337; Schwartz 11/e p1233, 10/e p1221; Bailey 27/e p1297)*

51. **Ans. c.** Intestinal pseudo-obstruction   52. **Ans. c.** Ogilvie's syndrome

▪ VOLVULUS

53. **Ans. a. Sigmoid colon**

54. **Ans. c. Cecal volvulus** *(Ref: Sabiston 20/e p1335; Schwartz 11/e p1307, 10/e p1220; Bailey 27/e p1289)*
   - **Cecal volvulus: Distended cecum** assumes a **gas-filled comma shape** or **kidney bean shape**[Q], **the concavity of** which faces **inferiorly and to the right.**

55. **Ans. c. Lower GI scopy is contraindicated in sigmoid volvulus d. Volvulus of cecum is managed by conservative methods**

56. **Ans. d. Sigmoid volvulus** *(Ref: Sabiston 20/e p1335; Schwartz 10/e p1219; Bailey 27/e p1284)*
   - **Sigmoid volvulus: Markedly dilated sigmoid colon** with the **appearance of a bent inner tube** or **coffee bean appearance**[Q].

57. **Ans. c. Both clockwise and anti-clockwise**

   - **Sigmoid volvulus** is **more commonly anticlockwise** (can be **both clockwise** or **anticlockwise**)[Q]
   - **Cecal volvulus** and **small intestine volvulus** are mostly **clockwise**[Q]

58. **Ans. b. Non-operative treatment has no role**

59. **Ans. d. Tuberculosis** *(Ref: Schwartz 11/e p1306, 10/e p1221)*
   - Hirschsprung's disease and Chagas disease can lead to megacolon, a risk factor for sigmoid volvulus.

60. **Ans. b. Large bowel volvulus**
   - Small bowel volvulus is most common form of volvulus in neonates. Colonic volvulus is very rare.

61. **Ans. a. 1st week** *(Ref: Bailey 25/e p85)*

   "Midgut volvulus can occur at any age, although it is seen most often in the first few weeks of life."

▪ MALROTATION

62. **Ans. b. Malrotation** *(Ref: Sabiston 20/e p1871; Schwartz 11/e p1725-1726, 10/e p1616-1617; Shackelford 8/e p970; Bailey 27/e p134-135)*

63. **Ans. d. Malrotation of gut** *(Ref: Bailey 27/e p134, 1284)*

64. **Ans. d. Mixed rotation** *(Ref: Sabiston 20/e p1871; Schwartz 11/e p1725-1726, 10/e p1616)*
   Mixed rotation of gut:
   - The intestine doesn't rotate as it re-enters the abdomen after physiological hernia.
   - **Caecum lies just inferior to the pylorus of the stomach.** It may result in volvulus (twisting) of intestine, which leads to obstruction further

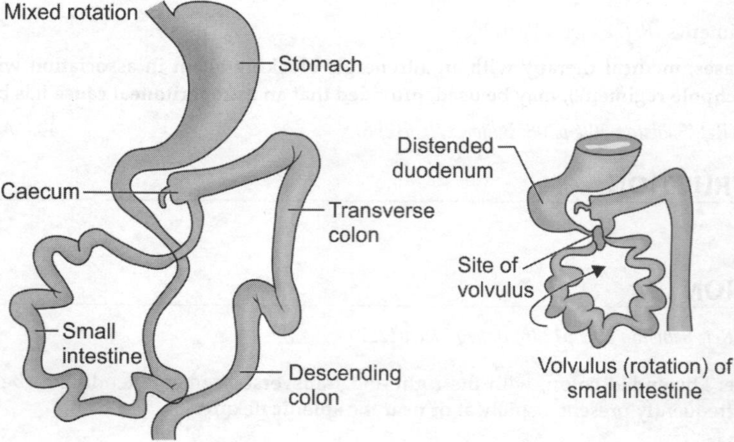

Small Intestine

■ MECKEL'S DIVERTICULUM

MECKEL'S DIVERTICULUM

- **Most commonly** encountered **congenital anomaly** of the **small intestine**[Q]
- Occur **2% of the population**[Q].

Rule of two in Meckel's diverticulum	
• **2% prevalence**[Q] • **2 inch** in **length**[Q]	• Half of these who are **symptomatic** are **<2 years**[Q] of age • **2 feet** proximal to **ileocecal valve**[Q]

- **True**[Q] **diverticulum** as it has **all the 3 layers** of the intestine[Q].
- Located on the **antimesenteric border** of the ileum 45 to 60 cm proximal to the **ileocecal valve**
- Results from **incomplete closure** of **omphalomesenteric** or **vitellointestinal duct**.
- An **equal incidence** among **men & women**[Q].

> • **MC heterotopic tissue: Gastric mucosa** (50%)[Q] >Pancreatic mucosa (5%) >colonic mucosa (rarely)

Clinical Features

- **Most** are **entirely benign** & **incidentally discovered** during autopsy, laparotomy, or barium studies

> • **MC clinical presentation** is **GI bleeding** (25-50%)[Q]
> • **Hemorrhage: MC symptomatic** presentation in **children ≤2 years**[Q]

- **Intestinal obstruction** (31%): Due to **volvulus, intussusception**, or, rarely, incarceration of the diverticulum in an inguinal hernia (**Littre's hernia**)[Q].

Complications of Meckel's Diverticulum

> • **MC complication** in **children & young adults: Bleeding**[Q]   • **MC complication** in **adults: Intestinal obstruction**[Q]

> • When the **appendix** is found to be **normal** during exploration for suspected appendicitis, the **distal ileum** should be **inspected for** the presence of an **inflamed Meckel's diverticulum**[Q].

Diagnosis

- **Most accurate diagnostic test** in **children**: Scintigraphy with sodium **99mTc-pertechnetate**[Q].
- In **adults** with normal nuclear medicine findings, **barium studies** should be performed.

Treatment

- **Symptomatic Meckel's diverticulum: Diverticulectomy** or **resection** of the **segment of ileum**[Q] bearing the diverticulum.
- **Segmental intestinal resection** is required **for bleeding** because the **bleeding site** usually is in the **ileum** adjacent to the diverticulum[Q].
- **Asymptomatic diverticula** found in **children** during laparotomy should be **resected**[Q].

> • **Incidentally found Meckel's diverticulum** should be **removed at any age up to 80 years** as long as no additional conditions (e.g., peritonitis) made removal hazardous[Q].

■ INTESTINAL ATRESIA

INTESTINAL ATRESIA

- **MC site** of intestinal atresia: Duodenum[Q]
- **MC cause** of neonatal intestinal obstruction: Duodenal atresia[Q]

Contd...

Contd...

Jejunoileal Atresia

- **Atresia & stenosis** are among the **MC causes** of **neonatal intestinal obstruction**[Q].
- Incidence of jejunoileal atresia is **1 in 300 to 1500**[Q] live births.
- **Gender ratio** is **equal.**
- **Jejunal atresia** is slightly **more common** than ileal atresia.
- In **80-90%** of cases the atresia is **isolated**. However, in up to **20%** of cases **atresias are multiple**.

> - **Cystic fibrosis** is an important comorbid condition with **reported incidence is 10-20%. White infants** with **jejunoileal atresia** have **more than 210 times the risk for cystic fibrosis**[Q].

Clinical Features

- Infants with atresia or stenosis usually have **bilious vomiting** on the **first day of life.**
- The **higher the obstruction**, the **earlier the vomiting**.
- **Abdominal distention** is more pronounced with **distal obstruction.**
- More than 60% of these **infants fail** to **pass meconium** in the **first day** of life, may have **grayish mucoid contents** in the rectal vault[Q].

Diagnosis

- Can be diagnosed by **prenatal ultrasonography**[Q].
- Associated with **maternal polyhydramnios**[Q]
- **Abdominal radiographs** show **gas- and fluid-filled bowel loops** with **absence of gas distally**[Q].

Treatment

- Management includes **intravenous fluid, decompression** of the stomach, withholding of enteral feeding, and **antibiotics.**
- **After resuscitation** the infant is taken to the operating room for **exploratory laparotomy.**
- The goals of the operation are to **restore intestinal continuity after resection** of the **atretic segment** while preserving intestinal length.

■ GASTROINTESTINAL TUBERCULOSIS

GASTROINTESTINAL TUBERCULOSIS

- **Mycobacterium tuberculosis**[Q] is responsible for **all the cases** of GI tuberculosis
- M. bovis has largely been eliminated by public health measures

Pathogenesis

Primary Intestinal Tuberculosis	Secondary Intestinal Tuberculosis
- Ingestion of **contaminated food**[Q] may cause primary tuberculosis (this route of infection has decreased in recent years)	- Arises from **swallowed sputum**[Q] containing tuberculous bacilli - Influenced by **virulence & quantity of bacilli** and host resistance of infection[Q]

- When the intestines become infected by **lymphatic spread** from the mesenteric nodes, **nodal disease** is considered as the **primary site &** intestinal involvement is secondary.
- **Earliest intestinal lesions** are found in **submucosa**[Q], while the overlying mucosa is normal.

Sites of Intestinal Involvement

- **MC site** is **terminal ileum & ileocecal junction**[Q]
- Other regions in decreasing frequency are: colon, jejunum, rectum, anal canal, duodenum, stomach & esophagus
- **Site of predilection** is dictated by the factors: abundance of **lymphoid tissue**, rate of **absorption** of intestinal contents, **prolonged stasis & digestive activity** of intestinal contents[Q]

Pathology

Ulcerative Tuberculosis (60%)	Hyperplastic Tuberculosis (10%)	Sclerotic or Fibrotic Tuberculosis (30%)
- **Tuberculous** intestinal **ulcers** are usually **deep & transversely placed**[Q] in the direction of lymphatics - **Multiple ulcers** may be seen, most often in **terminal ileum**[Q]	- A **fibroblastic reaction** occurs in submucosa and subserosa resulting in **marked thickening** of the **bowel wall**[Q] - Involvement of adjacent mesentery, lymph nodes and omentum, results in **formation** of a **mass lesion** - Hyperplastic lesions are due to **reduced bacterial virulence & increased host resistance**	- Associated with **strictures** of intestine, typically described as "**napkin-ring strictures**" which may be **single** or **multiple**

Contd...

Contd…

Clinical Features

- **Initial symptoms** are vague & **non-specific**[Q]
- As the diseases progress, individual may develop **fever** (in **two third**), **night sweats**, malaise, weakness, **anorexia & weight loss**[Q].
- **MC symptom** of GI tuberculosis is **abdominal pain**[Q].
- **Diarrhea** is another common symptom.
- Abdominal distention suggests presence of ascites or subacute intestinal obstruction

Primary Small Bowel Disease	Colonic Tuberculosis
• **Stools** are large in amount, **foul smelling** and resemble those seen in patients with **malabsorption**[Q].	• **Stools** may be **watery, small** in amount and mixed **with blood** when disease affects predominantly the **colon**[Q].

Complications

- **Intestinal obstruction & malabsorption** are MC **complications**[Q]
- **Bowel perforation & GI hemorrhage** are less common

Diagnosis

- **Laboratory tests:** MC abnormality is **raised ESR (90% cases)**[Q]

Ascitic Fluid Showing	
• **Lymphocytosis**[Q] (WBC **>500**/mm^3)	• **SAAG <1.1**[Q]
• **High protein**[Q] content (>2.5 gm/dL)	• **Adenosine deaminase** is **raised**, (sensitivity & specificity of 95%[Q])

RADIOLOGICAL IMAGING

Ultrasound

- **Club-sandwich appearance**[Q]

CT Scan

- **High density appearance** of ascitic fluid due to **elevated protein content**[Q]
- **Thickening** of bowel wall and ileocecal valve

BARIUM STUDIES IN GI TUBERCULOSIS
• **Earliest feature** is **spasm & hypermotility** with **edema of valve**[Q]
• **Thickening of valve lips** with **narrowing** of **terminal ileum** (Fleishner or **umbrella sign**[Q]) is **characteristic of TB.**
• In advance disease, characteristic deformity includes **symmetric, annular, napkin ring stenosis**[Q] and obstruction or shortening and pouch formation.
• **Cecum** become **shrunken & retracted** out of the iliac fossa due to **contraction of mesocolon (pulled up cecum**[Q])
• **Loss of ileocecal angle** with **dilated terminal ileum** imparting **goose neck deformity**[Q]
• **Narrowing of terminal ileum** due to irritability, along with shortened rigid cecum called as **"Sterlein sign"**[Q]
• **Persistent narrow stream** of **barium** in the bowel indicates stenosis known as **String sign**[Q]

Remember: **String sign** & **Sterlein sign** are also seen in **Crohn's disease** and are **not specific for TB**[Q].

Treatment

- Treatment of GI tuberculosis is **ATT.**
- **Majority of patients** (70%) with symptoms of **subacute intestinal obstruction** and evidence of intestinal **strictures** show **complete resolution** of the **radiological abnormality**[Q]

Indications of Surgery in GI Tuberculosis	
• Intestinal obstruction secondary to stricture (MC)[Q]	• Severe GI hemorrhage[Q]
• Free perforation[Q]	• Intra-abdominal abscess[Q]
	• Internal or external fistula[Q]

■ ENTERIC FEVER OR TYPHOID

ENTERIC FEVER OR TYPHOID

- Enteric fever is a potentially life-threatening systemic disease characterized by **fever** and **abdominal pain**[Q]
- It is caused by **Salmonella typhi** or **paratyphi**[Q]
- **Typhoid** is the **MC cause of ileal perforation** in **tropical countries (India)**[Q].

Pathology

- **Ulceration & necrosis** of ileocecal Peyer's patches[Q]
- **Ulcer** is **parallel to the long axis** of gut and is usually situated in the **lower ileum (longitudinal ulcers)**[Q]
- **Perforation** of a **typhoid ulcer** usually occurs during the **third week**[Q] and is occasionally the first sign of the disease.

Contd...

Clinical Features

- **Fever & abdominal pain** are **hallmark symptoms**[Q]
- Non-specific symptoms: Headache, cough, sweating, myalgia, arthralgia, fatigue
- **Paralytic ileus** is the **MC complication**[Q] of typhoid.
- **Intestinal hemorrhage (2nd MC)**[Q] may be the leading symptom.

Complications of Enteric Fever	
• **Paralytic ileus (MC)**[Q]	• Phlebitis
• Intestinal **hemorrhage (2nd MC)**[Q]	• Genitourinary inflammation
• **Perforation**[Q]	• Arthritis
• **Cholecystitis**[Q]	• Osteomyelitis

Characteristic Signs

- **Rose spots, splenomegaly, leucopenia** with **shift to left**[Q]
- **Lipopolysaccharide endotoxin** is responsible for **leucopenia** and **splenomegaly**[Q]
- **Relative bradycardia** despite of **high fever**[Q]

■ ENTEROCUTANEOUS FISTULA

ENTEROCUTANEOUS FISTULA

- Enterocutaneous fistulas are **most commonly iatrogenic**, usually the result of a **surgical misadventure**[Q]

Surgical Misadventure Leading to Enterocutaneous Fistula

- **Anastomotic leakage**[Q]
- **Injury of** the **bowel** or **blood supply**[Q]
- **Laceration** of the **bowel** by **wire mesh** or **retention suture**[Q]

Etiology of Enterocutaneous fistula	
• **Iatrogenic (MC)**[Q]	• Inflammatory bowel disease
• **Erosion** by **suction catheters adjacent abscesses,** or **trauma**[Q]	• Mesenteric vascular disease
• **Previous radiation therapy**[Q]	• Intra-abdominal sepsis
• **Intestinal obstruction**[Q]	• **Crohn's disease**[Q] leading to spontaneous fistula in 2% cases

Clinical Features

Typical Clinical Presentation
• **Typical clinical presentation** is that of a **febrile, postoperative patient** with an **erythematous wound**[Q].
• When a **few skin sutures** are **removed,** a **purulent** or **bloody discharge** is **noted; leakage of enteric contents** then occurs, sometimes immediately, but **often within 1 or 2 days**[Q].

- If the **diagnosis** is **in doubt**, **confirmation** can be obtained by **oral administration** of a **nonabsorbable marker**, such as **charcoal** or **Congo red**, or by **injection of water-soluble contrast medium** into the fistula[Q].

• In general, the **more proximal the fistula** in the intestine, the **more serious the problem**, with **greater fluid** and **electrolyte loss**[Q].
• The **drainage** has a **greater digestive capacity**, and the **distal segment** is **not available** for **absorption of nutrients**[Q].

Diagnosis

- **Fistulogram**[Q] to determine:
  - **Presence** and **extent of** any **abscess cavities**
  - **Extent** of **bowel wall disruption**
  - Whether a **distal obstruction** is present
  - **Length of the tract**
  - **Location** of the fistula
- **CT** is helpful in determining whether **underlying collections** of **fluid** or **pus** are present.

Treatment

- Successful management requires establishment of **controlled drainage**, usually using a **sump suction apparatus; management of sepsis; prevention of fluid** and **electrolyte depletion; protection of the skin;** and **provision of adequate nutrition**[Q].
- When **sepsis** has been **controlled** and **nutritional therapy** has been instituted, a course of **conservative management**[Q] should be followed.

• **Most of these fistulas heal spontaneously** within **4-6 weeks** of **conservative management**[Q]. If closure is not accomplished after this time, surgery is indicated.

- This **period of conservative management** not only allows those **fistulas to heal spontaneously** but also **allows for optimization of nutritional status** and **control of the wound** and **fistula sites**[Q].
- Also, a **reasonable delay permits** the **peritoneal reaction** and **inflammation to subside**, thus **making a second operation easier** and **safer**[Q].

Contd…

> • **Preferred operation:** Fistula tract excision and **segmental resection** of the **involved segment of intestine** and **reanastomosis**[Q].

- **Simple closure** of the fistula after removing the fistula tract **almost always results in** a **recurrence** of the fistula.
- If an **unexpected abscess** is encountered or if the **bowel wall is rigid** and **distended** over a **long distance**, thus making primary anastomosis unsafe, **exteriorization of both ends** of the **intestine** should be accomplished.

Complications

- **Sepsis, fluid** and **electrolyte depletion**, **necrosis** of the **skin** at the site of external drainage, and **malnutrition**[Q].
- **Mortality rates** for patients with enterocutaneous fistulas remain high **(15-20%)**

Factors Preventing Spontaneous Fistula Closure	
• **High output (>500 mL/day)**[Q]	• **Radiation enteritis**[Q]
• **Severe disruption** of intestinal continuity[Q] **(>50%** of bowel circumference)	• **Distal obstruction**[Q]
	• **Undrained abscess cavity**[Q]
• **Active inflammatory bowel disease**[Q] of bowel segment	• **Foreign body**[Q] in the fistula tract
• **Cancer**[Q]	• **Fistula tract <2.5 cm** long[Q]
	• **Epithelialization** of fistula tract[Q]

■ SUPERIOR MESENTERIC ARTERY SYNDROME

SUPERIOR MESENTERIC ARTERY SYNDROME

- Vascular compression of **third portion**[Q] of duodenum by **superior mesenteric artery** as it passes over this portion of duodenum.
- Also known as **Wilkie's syndrome, cast syndrome**, and **arteriomesenteric duodenal ileus** or **compression**[Q]

THREE MECHANICAL FACTORS MUST BE PRESENT
• An abnormally **narrow, aortomesenteric angle**[Q]
• An abnormally **highly fixed transverse duodenum**[Q]
• An **abnormal course** of the **mesenteric artery**[Q] continuing inferiorly, anterior to the unyielding vertebral column

- **Most commonly** seen in **young asthenic individuals**, with **women** being more commonly affected than men[Q].
- **Normal aortomesenteric angle: 38-65°**[Q]
- **Aortomesenteric angle in SMA syndrome: <22°**[Q]
- **SMA** normally **leaves aorta** at an **acute angle (50-60°)**
- Normally a **mass of fat** and **lymphatics** near **origin of SMA** is believed to **protect duodenum from compression.**

Predisposing Factors	
• Rapid weight loss[Q]	• Scoliosis[Q]
• Supine immobilization[Q]	• Placement of a body cast[Q]
• Rapid growth of height[Q]	

Clinical Features

- Nausea and vomiting, **abdominal distention, weight loss,** & **postprandial epigastric pain**[Q].
- **Weight loss** usually occurs **before** the **onset of symptoms** and contributes to the syndrome.

Diagnosis

- **Barium** upper gastrointestinal series or **hypotonic duodenography**[Q].
- CT has been useful in certain instances.

Treatment

- **Conservative measures** are tried initially and have been **increasingly successful** as **definitive treatment.**
- **Operative treatment of choice** is **duodenojejunostomy**[Q].
- **Strong's Procedure**[Q]: Mobilization of 4th part of duodenum & division of ligament of Treitz

■ SMALL-BOWEL NEOPLASM

SMALL-BOWEL NEOPLASM

- **MC tumor** of **small bowel: Stromal tumor**[Q] **>Adenoma**[Q]
- **MC tumor** of **small bowel in children: Lymphoma**[Q]
- **MC malignant tumor** of **small bowel: Adenocarcinoma**[Q] **> Carcinoid**
- **MC site** of small bowel **malignancy, carcinoids, lymphoma: Ileum**[Q]

■ CARCINOID TUMORS

CARCINOID TUMORS

- **Distribution (BIRACS)**[Q]: Bronchus> Ileum > Rectum > Appendix > Colon > Stomach
- **Combined incidence of carcinoid tumor in duodenum + jejunum + ileum (small intestine) > Bronchus**[Q]
- **MC site of carcinoid tumor: GI tract >Respiratory tract**[Q]
- Arise from **enterochromaffin cells**[Q] at the **base** of the **crypts of Lieberkuhn** in the GI tract.

Foregut carcinoids	**Mostly argyrophilic**[Q] (silver staining only with the addition of a reducing agent)
Midgut carcinoids	**Argentaffinic**[Q] (silver staining)
Hindgut carcinoids	**Mixed (60-70% argyrophilic & 8-16% argentaffinic)**[Q]

- **MC foregut location** for carcinoid tumors: **Stomach**[Q]
- **Small bowel carcinoids** are **multiple in 25% of cases**[Q].
- **Appendiceal carcinoids** are **typically solitary** lesion[Q].

> - **Highest percentage** of **non-localized disease (PCS): Pancreatic**[Q] (91%) >colonic (77%) >small intestinal carcinoid tumors (75%)
> - Highest percentage **localized disease (LOAR)**[Q]: Laryngeal carcinoid tumors (100%) >**Ovary, appendix >rectum**

Pathology

- GIT carcinoids produce a variety of peptide hormones, the **most common is serotonin**[Q].
- **Foregut carcinoids** produce **low levels of serotonin**[Q] (5-hydroxytryptamine) but may secrete 5-hydroxytryptophan or adrenocorticotrophic hormone.
- **Hindgut carcinoids rarely produce serotonin**[Q] but may produce other hormones such as somatostatin and peptide YY.
- **Gastric carcinoid** patients are **deficient** in the **enzyme dopa-decarboxylase**, the enzyme responsible for **conversion** of **5-hydroxytryptophan** to **serotonin** (5-hydroxy tryptamine).

Malignant potential in Carcinoids depends on (LSD Growth)			
• **L**ocation[Q]	• **S**ize[Q]	• **D**epth of invasion[Q]	• **G**rowth pattern[Q]

- In small bowel carcinoid (**SBC**), frequent **coexistence** of a **second primary malignant neoplasm** of a **different histological type**, this usually is a **synchronous adenocarcinoma**, most commonly in the **colon & breast**[Q].
- **Associated with MEN-I in 10% of cases**[Q].

Clinical Features

- **MC symptom** of **SBC: Intermittent intestinal obstruction**[Q]

> ### MALIGNANT CARCINOID SYNDROME
>
> - Occur in fewer than **10%** of patients with carcinoid tumors.
> - **Midgut carcinoids** are the **MC source**[Q] of carcinoid syndrome.
> - Attacks may be spontaneous or precipitated by **stress, alcohol, a large meal** or **sexual intercourse**.
> - Common symptoms and signs include **cutaneous flush (80%)**[Q]; **diarrhea** (76%); **hepatomegaly** (71%); **cardiac lesions** (70%); **asthma** (25%).
>
> > - **Bright-red patchy flushing** which is **typically seen with gastric carcinoids**[Q]

- **Diarrhea** is directly **related to serum serotonin level** (serotonin stimulates secretin release), **episodic** usually occurring **after meals, watery** and often **explosive**.
- **MC cardiac lesions: TR > PR > TS > PS**

Diagnosis

- Elevated urinary levels of **5-HIAA**[Q] (5-hydroxyindoleacetic acid) measured **over 24 hours** with high-performance liquid chromatography are **highly specific**[Q].

> - Plasma concentration of **chromogranin A is 100% specific**[Q]

> - **Initial imaging procedure** to localize & stage the carcinoid tumors: **SRS**[Q]
> - **Best investigation for localization: DOPA-PET**[Q]

Treatment

> ### SURGERY
>
> - Carcinoid tumors of the **jejunum & ileum: segmental resection** and **en-bloc lymphadenectomy**[Q].

Prognosis

- Carcinoid tumors have the **best prognosis** of **all small bowel tumors**, whether the disease is **localized** or **metastatic**[Q].

> - **Most useful prognostic marker** is an elevated level of **chromogranin A**[Q].
> - **Midgut carcinoid** has the **best prognosis**[Q].

■ SHORT BOWEL SYNDROME

SHORT BOWEL SYNDROME

- **Malabsorptive condition** that arises secondary to **removal of significant segments of the small intestine**[Q].
- Most common causes are **Mesenteric infarction**[Q], **Crohn's disease**[Q], **Trauma**[Q], **Volvulus**[Q].
- **Normal length of small intestine: 600 cm**[Q].
- **Length <200 cm leads to short bowel syndrome**[Q].

Changes Seen in Terminal Ileal Resection	
• **Malabsorption** of **bile salts** and **vitamin B_{12}** (which are normally absorbed in this region) • Vitamin B_{12} Malabsorption → **Megaloblastic anemia**[Q] • **Bile salts Malabsorption** → **Unabsorbed bile salts** escape into **colon** and **stimulate fluid secretion** from the colon → **watery diarrhea**[Q]. • Decreased bile salts in the bile → **Cholesterol gall stones**[Q]	• **Reduction in bile salt pool** → **steatorrhea**[Q] and **Malabsorption** of **fat soluble vitamins** (due to fat malabsorption) • **Unabsorbed fatty acids** bind with **calcium** → Increased concentration of **free oxalates** (oxalates bind with calcium normally and therefore escape without intestinal absorption) → Free oxalates are absorbed → **Oxalate kidney stones**[Q].

Removal of Ileocecal Valve

- **Bacterial overgrowth**[Q] from the **colon** → **diarrhea** & **malabsorption**[Q]
- **Decrease** in **intestinal transit time**[Q]

Adaptive Response

- **Resection of up to 70%** of **small bowel** usually can be **tolerated** if the terminal ileum & ileocecal valve are preserved.

> - **Proximal bowel resection** is tolerated much **better than distal resection**[Q]
> - Because the **ileum can adapt** and **increase its absorptive capacity more efficiently than the jejunum**[Q].

Treatment

- **Early phase: Control diarrhea, replacement of fluid and electrolytes**, and **TPN**[Q]
- **H_2-receptor antagonists** or **PPI** for **acid hypersecretion**[Q]
- **Cholestyramine**[Q] for **cathartic effects** of **unabsorbed bile salts** in the colon.

> - **Hypergastrinemia** and **gastric hypersecretion** occur after massive small bowel resection and **greatly contribute to diarrhea** after a **massive small bowel resection**[Q].

Intestinal Lengthening Operation

- **Bianchi Procedure**[Q]: Longitudinal intestinal lengthening and tailoring
- **STEP: Serial transverse enteroplasty procedure**[Q]

Multiple Choice Questions

■ MECKEL'S DIVERTICULUM

1. **All are true statement about Meckel's diverticulum except:**
    (Recent Question 2014; PGI Nov 2010)
    a. Occurs in 2% of population
    b. Perforation occurs
    c. Common on anti-mesenteric border
    d. Contains ectopic gastric tissue
    e. Diarrhea very common

2. **Meckel's diverticulum follows the rule of 2. Which of the following is false?** *(Recent Question 2018)*
    a. Occurs in approximately 2% of population
    b. Approximately 2 inches in length
    c. Generally present 2 feet proximal to ileocecal valve
    d. 2% are symptomatic

3. **Most common presenting complication of Meckel's diverticulum:** *(Orissa 2011)*
    a. Hemorrhage
    b. Intussusception
    c. Meckel's diverticulitis
    d. Intestinal obstruction

4. **What does the intraoperative photograph above depicts?**
    (APPG 2015)
    a. Transverse colon
    b. Fallopian tube
    c. Meckel's diverticulum
    d. Intussusception

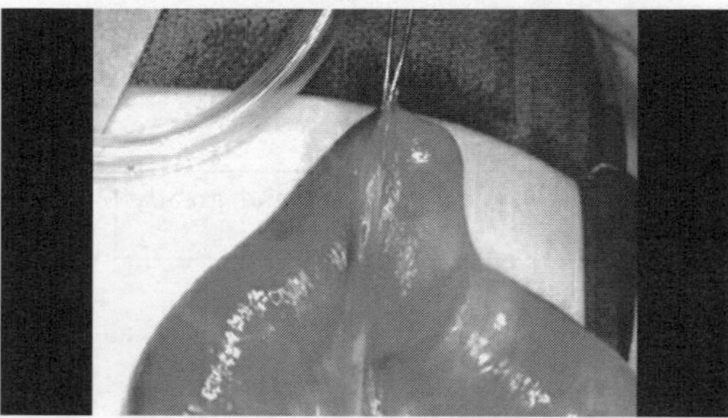

5. **Which one of the following statements is incorrect regarding Meckel's diverticulum?** *(Recent Question 2015)*
    a. Is found on the antimesenteric border of the small intestine
    b. Consists of mucosa without a muscle coat
    c. Heterotopic gastric mucosa can ulcerate and cause a brisk gastrointestinal bleed
    d. A fibrous band between the apex and umbilicus can cause intestinal obstruction

6. **Uncommon complication of Meckel's diverticulum:**
    (MCI Sept 2005)
    a. Intussusception
    b. Diverticulitis
    c. Malignancy
    d. Increased bleeding

7. **What is false about Meckel's diverticulitis?**
    a. Present in 3% of the population *(AIIMS Nov 2015)*
    b. Presents with periumbilical pain
    c. Remnant of proximal part of vitellointestinal duct
    d. Lies on the anti-mesenteric border

8. **Which of the following is true about Meckel's diverticula?**
    (Recent Question 2017)
    a. Most common congenital anomaly of the intestine
    b. Always contain heterotopic mucosa
    c. Pseudodiverticula
    d. Located on mesenteric border

■ GASTROINTESTINAL TUBERCULOSIS

9. **Which one is not true regarding hyperplastic ileocecal tuberculosis?** *(AIIMS June 97, All India 2001)*
    a. Mass in right iliac fossa
    b. Common site ileocecal region
    c. X-ray shows indrawing of caecum from ileum
    d. Conservative management is treatment of choice

10. **Not true about hyperplastic tuberculosis:** *(UPPG 2000)*
    a. Most common site is ileo-cecal region
    b. Presents as mass in right iliac fossa
    c. Surgery is the treatment of choice
    d. Barium studies are characteristic

11. **Kalu, 35-year-old male presented with the history of recurrent attacks of colicky abdominal pain. Barium meal follow through was done. What is the name of this radiological sign?** *(Recent Question 2016)*
    a. String sign of Kantor
    b. Goose neck appearance
    c. Fleischner sign
    d. Umbrella sign

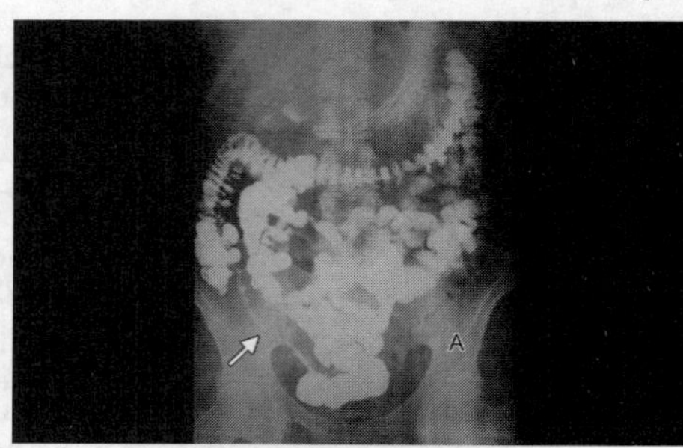

12. **Commonest site of tuberculosis of the intestines:**
    a. Stomach
    b. Ileum *(All India 89)*
    c. Jejunum
    d. Colon

13. **The most common cause of perforation of the distal ileum in India is:** *(UPSC 2005)*
    a. Tuberculosis
    b. Typhoid
    c. Amoebiasis
    d. Regional enteritis

14. **Pulled up cecum is seen in:** *(Recent Question 2014, 2013)*
    a. CA colon
    b. Carcinoid
    c. Ileocecal tuberculosis
    d. Crohn's disease

15. **Fleischner sign on barium study is seen in?** *(DNB 2014)*
    a. Ileocecal TB
    b. Crohn's disease
    c. Small bowel carcinoid
    d. Typhoid

■ SUPERIOR MESENTERIC ARTERY SYNDROME

16. **All are true regarding superior mesenteric artery syndrome, except:** *(All India 2000)*
    a. Caused by compression of distended duodenum
    b. Common in young females
    c. Does not occur in obese individuals
    d. Most common in 6th-7th decade

■ SHORT BOWEL SYNDROME

17. **Which one of the following gastrointestinal disorders predisposes to urolithiasis?** *(UPSC 2007)*
    a. Peutz-Jegher's syndrome
    b. Short bowel syndrome

c.   Familial polyposis coli
d.   Ulcerative colitis

18. **Which is not seen in massive resection of small bowel?**
     (AIIMS June 95, All India 98, PGI June 99, DPG 2008)
     a.   Hypogastrinemia   b.   Vitamin B12 deficiency
     c.   Malabsorption   d.   Oxalate stone

19. **Complications of short bowel syndrome:**   *(GB Pant 2011)*
     a.   Gall stones   b.   Oxalate renal stones
     c.   Cirrhosis   d.   All of the above

20. **Deficiency of which of the following vitamin is most commonly seen in short bowel syndrome with ileal resection?**
     (DNB 2012, All India 2012)
     a.   Vitamin B12   b.   Vitamin B1
     c.   Folic acid   d.   Vitamin K

21. **Distal ileum was removed in a 20 years old girl. Which of the following substance absorption will be affected?**
     (MCI Dec 2019)
     a.   Iron   b.   Bile salts
     c.   Folic acid   d.   Copper

22. **Mechanism of action of teduglutide in short bowel syndrome:**   *(Recent Question 2019)*
     a.   GLP-2 analogue   b.   HT1a inhibitor
     c.   GLP-1 analogue   d.   C-peptide analogs

■ ENTERIC FEVER

23. **Typhoid perforation occurs during:**
     (MHSSMCET 2005, MHPGMCET 2006, UPPG 2009, AIIMS 89)
     a.   1st week   b.   2nd week
     c.   3rd week   d.   4th week

24. **A 24-year-old male, who has been having fever for 15 days starts having acute pain and distension of abdomen. Abdominal examination reveals generalized tenderness with guarding. The most likely diagnosis is:**
     a.   Acute appendicitis   *(Recent Question 2015)*
     b.   Acute pancreatitis
     c.   Enteric perforation
     d.   Duodenal ulcer perforation

■ ENTERIC FISTULA

25. **All are associated with non-healing of fistula except:**
     (GB PANT 2011)
     a.   Contained abscess   b.   Distal obstruction
     c.   Non-epithelialization d.   Radiating enteritis

26. **Fistula leading to highest electrolyte in balance is:**
     a.   Gastric   b.   Duodenal   *(DNB 2009)*
     c.   Sigmoid   d.   Rectal

■ INTESTINAL ATRESIA AND DUPLICATION

27. **Commonest cause of intestinal obstruction in neonate is:**
     (MHPGMCET 2001)
     a.   Meconium ileus   b.   Intestinal atresia
     c.   Hirschsprung's disease d.   Volvulus

28. **Commonest site of intestinal atresia is in the:**   *(KGMC 2011)*
     a.   Duodenum   b.   Jejunum
     c.   Ileum   d.   Colon

29. **The treatment of choice in duodenal atresia:**   *(All India 89)*
     a.   Gastrojejunostomy
     b.   Duodenojejunostomy
     c.   Bishop koop procedure
     d.   Duodenoduodenostomy

30. **What is the type of given intestinal atresia?**

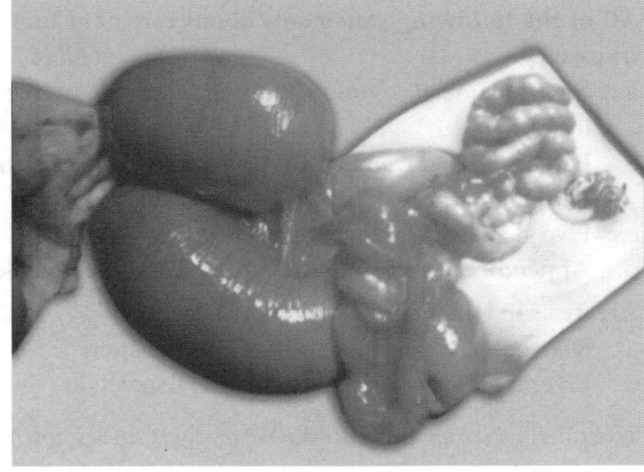

     a.   Type I   b.   Type II
     c.   Type III   d.   Type IV

31. **Duplication of the small intestine is associated with:**
     a.   Heterotopic mucosa   *(Recent Question 2017)*
     b.   Smooth muscle component
     c.   Spinal /vertebral defects
     d.   All are correct

32. **A newborn baby was brought with the history multiple episodes of bilious projectile vomiting. X-ray abdomen was done. What is the diagnosis?**   *(Recent Question 2017)*
     a.   Duodenal atresia
     b.   Jejunal atresia
     c.   Ileal atresia
     d.   Hypertrophic pyloric stenosis

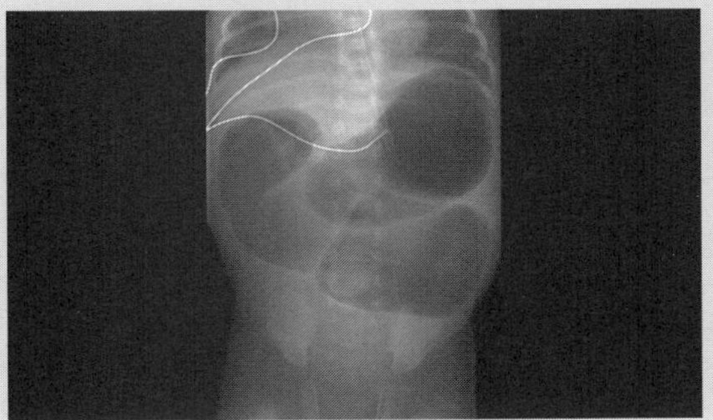

■ NEOPLASMS OF SMALL INTESTINE

33. **Most common tumor of small bowel in children:**
     (GB PANT 2011)
     a.   Lymphoma   b.   Carcinoma
     c.   Leiomyosarcoma   d.   Adenocarcinoma

34. **False statement regarding benign small bowel tumour is:**
     a.   Accidentally discovered during surgeries   *(JIPMER 2013)*
     b.   Most commonly asymptomatic
     c.   Cause hemorrhage
     d.   Causes malabsorption

35. **Most common malignancy of small bowel:**
     (Recent Question 2017)
     a.   Adenocarcinoma   b.   Carcinoid tumor
     c.   Leiomyosarcoma   d.   Lymphoma

36. **Aneurysmal dilatation of small bowel is seen in:**
     (Recent Question 2017)
     a.   Small bowel lymphoma
     b.   Gallstone ileus
     c.   Duodenal atresia
     d.   Sjogren syndrome

■ CARCINOID TUMORS

37. **All of the following statements about carcinoid tumors are true except:** *(All India 2012)*
    a. It is the most common malignant tumor of the small intestine
    b. Extensive involvement of small intestine is associated with higher probability of lung metastasis
    c. Five year survival for carcinoids tumors is > 60%
    d. Appendiceal carcinoids are more common in females

38. **All are seen in carcinoid syndrome except:** *(HPU 2005)*
    a. Diarrhea
    b. Constipation
    c. Liver metastasis
    d. 5-HT secretion

39. **The metabolite excreted in the urine carcinoid syndrome is:** *(MHCET 2016)*
    a. VMA
    b. 17-Ketosteroid
    c. Histamine
    d. 5-HIAA

40. **All of the following are associated with carcinoid syndrome except:** *(MCI Sept 2005)*
    a. Cyanosis
    b. Diarrhea
    c. Flushing
    d. Acute appendicitis

41. **Which of the following is true of small bowel carcinoids?**
    a. Most common site is duodenum *(AIIMS Nov 2006)*
    b. It does not cause endocardial fibroelastosis
    c. Increased risk of CA lung
    d. It is the most common malignancy of small intestine

42. **Increased level of 5 HIAA is seen in which disease?** *(Recent Question 2018)*
    a. Carcinoid tumor
    b. Phenylketonuria
    c. Pheochromocytoma
    d. Adenocarcinoma

43. **Most common site for carcinoid tumor is:** *(Recent Question 2013)*
    a. Esophagus
    b. Lung
    c. Appendix
    d. Ileum

Explanations

■ MECKEL'S DIVERTICULUM

1. **Ans. e. Diarrhea very common** *(Ref: Sabiston 20/e p1284; Schwartz 11/e p1247, 10/e p1163-1165; Bailey 27/e p1252; Shackelford 8/e p911)*

2. **Ans. d. 2% are symptomatic** *(Ref: Schwartz 11/e p1246, 10/e p1163; Sabiston 20/e p1284; Bailey 27/e p1252)*

3. **Ans. a. Hemorrhage**

4. **Ans. c. Meckel's diverticulum** *(Ref: Sabiston 20/e p1284; Schwartz 11/e p1247, 10/e p1164; Bailey 27/e p131)*

5. **Ans. b. Consists of mucosa without a muscle coat**

6. **Ans. c. Malignancy**

7. **Ans. a. Present in 3% of the population**

8. **Ans. a. Most common congenital anomaly of the intestine** *(Ref: Sabiston 20/e p1284; Schwartz 11/e p1247, 10/e p1164; Bailey 27/e p131)*

■ GASTROINTESTINAL TUBERCULOSIS

9. **Ans. d. Conservative management is treatment of choice** *(Ref: Sabiston 20/e p1079-1268; Bailey 27/e p1249)*

10. **Ans. c. Surgery is the treatment of choice**

11. **Ans. a. String sign of Kantor** *(Ref: Sabiston 20/e p1263; Bailey 27/e p1248)*

12. **Ans. b. Ileum**

13. **Ans. b. Typhoid** *(Ref: J Indian Med Assoc 199; 89:255-6)*

   - **Ileal perforation** is a common problem seen in **tropical countries**. The **commonest cause being typhoid fever**[Q].
   - In **western countries** the causes are **malignancy, trauma** and **mechanical etiology**, in the order of frequency[Q].

14. **Ans. c. Ileocecal tuberculosis**

15. **Ans. a. Ileocecal TB**

■ SUPERIOR MESENTERIC ARTERY SYNDROME

16. **Ans. d. Most common in 6th-7th decade** *(Ref: Sabiston 20/e p1292; Shackelford 8/e p782)*

■ SHORT BOWEL SYNDROME

17. **Ans. b. Short bowel syndrome** *(Ref: Sabiston 20/e p1291; Schwartz 11/e p1254, 10/e p1171-1173; Bailey 27/e p1256; Shackelford 8/e p921)*

18. **Ans. a. Hypogastrinemia**

19. **Ans. d. All of the above**

20. **Ans. a. Vitamin B12**

21. **Ans. b. Bile salts** *(Ref: Bailey 27/e p1256)*

22. **Ans. a. GLP-2 analogue** *(Ref: Sabiston 20/e p1292)*

   - "Randomized controlled trials have shown that *teduglutide, a GLP-2 analogue* that is *resistant to degradation by the proteolytic enzyme dipeptidyl peptidase 4 and therefore has a longer half-life than GLP-2*, is well tolerated and has led to the restoration of intestinal functional and structural integrity through significant intestinotrophic and proabsorptive effects. It is the *first targeted therapeutic agent to gain approval for use in adult short bowel syndrome with intestinal failure*."
   Sabiston 20/e p1292

■ ENTERIC FEVER

23. **Ans. c. 3rd week** *(Ref: Sabiston 20/e p1266; Bailey 27/e p1248; Harrison 20/e p1175)*

24. **Ans. c. Enteric perforation**

■ ENTERIC FISTULA

25. **Ans. c. Non-epithelialization** *(Ref: Sabiston 20/e p1287; Schwartz 11/e p1240, 10/e p1158; Bailey 27/e p1256; Shackelford 8/e p888)*

26. Ans. b. Duodenal *(Ref: Sabiston 20/e p1287)*

- In general, the **more proximal the fistula** in the intestine, the **more serious the problem**, with **greater fluid** and **electrolyte loss**[Q].
- The **drainage** has a **greater digestive capacity**, and the **distal segment** is **not available** for **absorption** of **nutrients**[Q].

■ INTESTINAL ATRESIA AND DUPLICATION

27. Ans. b. Intestinal atresia

28. Ans. a. Duodenum

29. Ans. d. Duodenoduodenostomy

30. Ans. c. Type III *(Ref: Sabiston 20/e p1871; Schwartz 11/e p1725, 10/e p1616; Bailey 27/e p133-134)*

- ***"Apple** peel" atresia or "Christmas tree" atresia is type IIIb of intestinal atresia.*

Classification of Intestinal Atresia	
Type **I**	**Membranous atresia** with **intact bowel** & **mesentery**
Type **II**	**Blind ends** separated by a **fibrous cord**
Type **IIIa**	**Blind ends** separated by a **V-shaped mesenteric defect**
Type **IIIb**	**"Apple peel" atresia**[Q] or **"Christmas tree"** [Q] **atresia**
Type **IV**	**Multiple atresias ("string of sausages")**[Q]

31. Ans. d. All are correct *(Ref: Schwartz 11/e p1724-1725, 10/e p1624; Bailey 27/e p136)*

32. Ans. b. Jejunal atresia

■ NEOPLASMS OF SMALL INTESTINE

33. Ans. a. Lymphoma *(Ref: Schwartz 11/e p1241, 10/e p1159; Bailey 27/e p1250; Shackelford 8/e p 965)*

34. Ans. d. Causes malabsorption

35. Ans. a. Adenocarcinoma *(Ref: Sabiston 20/e p1276; Schwartz 11/e p1241, 10/e p1159)*

"Adenocarcinomas constitute approximately 50% of the malignant tumors of the small bowel."-Sabiston 20/e p1276

36. Ans. a. Small bowel lymphoma *(Ref: Clinical Imaging of Small Intestine 2/e p415)*

"The typical presentation of a small bowel lymphoma is a thick walled infiltrating mass with aneurysmal dilatation without obstruction. Aneurysmal dilatation is based on destruction of small bowel wall and myenteric nerve plexus."

(Ref: Clinical Imaging of Small Intestine 2/e p415)

■ CARCINOID TUMORS

37. Ans. b. Extensive involvement of small intestine is associated with higher probability of lung metastasis *(Ref: Sabiston 20/e p1276; Schwartz 11/e p1242, 10/e p1162; Bailey 27/e p1250)*

Extensive involvement of **small intestine** by carcinoid tumor is associated with **higher probability** of **liver (not the lung) metastasis.**

- **MC malignant tumor** of small intestine: Adenocarcinoma[Q] > Carcinoid
- **Carcinoid tumors** have the **best prognosis of all small bowel tumors**, whether the disease is localized or metastatic.
- **Resection of a carcinoid tumor localized** to its **primary site** approaches a **100% survival rate**[Q].
- **Five-year survival rates** are about **65%** among patients **with regional disease** and 25% to 35% among those with distant metastasis.
- **Appendiceal carcinoids** are **more common in females**[Q].
- **Extensive involvement** of **small intestine** is associated with **higher probability** of **liver metastasis**[Q]

38. Ans. b. Constipation

39. Ans. d. 5-HIAA

40. Ans. d. Acute appendicitis

41. Ans. d. It is the most common malignancy of small intestine

42. Ans. a. Carcinoid tumor *(Ref: Sabiston 20/e p1273; Schwartz 11/e p1242, 10/e p1161; Bailey 27/e p1251)*

43. Ans. b. Lung

Large Intestine

■ HIRSCHSPRUNG'S DISEASE

HIRSCHSPRUNG'S DISEASE

- Occurs in **1** out of every **5000 live births**[Q]

> - **MC affected site: Rectosigmoid (75%)**[Q] > splenic flexure or transverse colon (17%) >**Entire colon** with **variable extension into** the **small bowel**[Q] (8%)

- **Increased Risk: Positive family history**[Q] & **Down syndrome**[Q]

Pathogenesis

- One type of **neurocristopathies**[Q]; Consequence of **defective migration of neural crest cell to colonic mucosa**[Q]
- **Absent ganglion cells** in the **myenteric (Auerbach's)** & **submucosal (Meissner's) plexus** with **hypertrophy of nerve trunks**[Q] in the plexus
- Associated with **muscular spasm** of **distal colon** & **internal anal sphincter** resulting in a **functional obstruction**[Q]
- **Abnormal bowel** is the **contracted distal segment**, whereas the **normal bowel** is **proximal, dilated portion**[Q].

Clinical Presentation		
Neonates	**First few weeks of life**	**Otherwise healthy children and adults**

• **Suspected in** all neonates presenting with:
  – **Delayed passage** of **meconium beyond** the **first 24 hours of life**[Q]
  – **Abdominal distension** following **feeds**[Q]
	• **Suspected in** any child presenting in first few weeks of life with:
	  – **Gross** abdominal **distension**[Q]
	  – **Chronic constipation**[Q]
	  – **Failure** to **thrive**[Q]
		• **Short segment Hirschsprung disease** should be suspected in **otherwise healthy children** and **adults**[Q] presenting with:
		  – **Severe constipation without fecal soiling**[Q]
		  – **Faecal soiling** is usually **not a feature** of this **condition.**

Digital Examination

- **Rectum** is **empty** on digital examination[Q];
- **Contracted rectal wall** can sometimes be appreciated by examining finger
- **Rapid expulsion of feces** often follows examination[Q]

Diagnosis		
Rectal biopsy	**Anorectal manometry**	**Radiology**

• **Gold standard for** the **diagnosis** of Hirschsprung's disease
• Confirms the diagnosis on demonstration of:
  – Aganglionosis[Q]
  – Hypertrophic nerve trunks[Q]
  – Increased acetylcholine esterase staining[Q]
	• Useful as a **screening test**[Q]
	• Rectoanal inhibitory **reflex** is **absent**[Q]
		• **Water soluble contrast enema** indi- cates the **length** and **site** of **involved intestine.**
		• Important positive findings include:
		  – **Coning down** of **transition zone**
		  – Irregularity in mucosa
		  – **Abnormal contraction** of intestine

- **Repeated tube decompression** and gentle **rectal washouts** with 30-50 mL of **normal saline** have a positive and significant clinical impact on these patients.

Treatment of Hirschsprung's Disease	
Short segment disease	**Long segment disease**
• **Extended myectomy**[Q] removing a **strip of rectal wall** up to the area where normal ganglion cells start may be sufficient	• **Temporary colostomy**[Q] for a few months to allow proximal intestine to return to its normal caliber followed by **definitive procedures**: – Swenson[Q] — Duhamel[Q] — Soave[Q]

Prognosis

- **MC postoperative problems: Constipation (MC)**[Q] >soiling >incontinence >enterocolitis.

■ COLONIC DIVERTICULA

COLONIC DIVERTICULA

- A **diverticulum** is an **abnormal sac or pouch protruding from the wall of a hollow organ**
- **True diverticulum** is composed of **all layers of the intestinal wall**[Q]
- **False diverticulum** (pseudodiverticulum) **lacks a portion** of the **normal bowel wall**[Q].

> - **Acquired diverticula** are the MC type[Q] and are mainly **false**[Q] diverticula
> - **MC site**[Q] of colonic diverticula: Sigmoid colon

Pathogenesis

- Diverticula are **herniation of mucosa through** the **muscularis propria**

> - **Protrusion** occurs **at the point** where the **nutrient artery penetrates** through **the muscularis propria**[Q], resulting in a break of the colonic wall, **mainly on mesenteric side**

- In some cases, the **arteriole** penetrating the wall can be **displaced over** the **dome** of **diverticulum** which results in **massive hemorrhage**[Q]

> - Another factor is **increased intraluminal pressure**[Q], **diets low in fiber** reduce the stool bulk which in turn leads to **increased peristaltic activity,** particularly in the **sigmoid colon.** This increases the intraluminal pressure.

- Diverticulosis is **more common in the western world**[Q], its **rare** in the **underdeveloped & developing countries**, where **diets include** more **fibre** and **roughage**[Q].

> - There is often a striking hypertrophy of the muscular layers of the colonic wall[Q] associated with diverticulosis.
> - This thickening of the colonic wall, most commonly affecting the sigmoid colon, may precede the appearance of diverticula[Q].

Diagnosis

- **Barium enema** is **investigation of choice** for **colonic diverticulosis**[Q].
- **Thickening** of the **circular muscle fibres** develops a **concertina** or **saw-tooth appearance** on **barium enema**[Q].
- **Investigation of choice** for **colonic diverticulosis: Barium enema**[Q]   • **Investigation of choice** for **diverticulitis: CT scan**[Q]

■ COLORECTAL POLYPS

Histological Classification of Colorectal Polyps	
Neoplastic Polyps	**Non-neoplastic polyps**

Adenomatous polyps or Adenomas:
• Tubular (MC)
• Tubulovillous
• Villous (most malignant)
	1. Hyperplastic polyps (MC)
	2. Hamartomatous polyps:
	  – Juvenile polyps
	  – PJS
	3. Inflammatory polyps

■ ADENOMATOUS POLYPS

ADENOMATOUS POLYPS

- **MC neoplastic polyp** is adenomatous, which harbors malignant potential[Q].
- Most colon cancers arise from adenomatous polyps (adenoma)[Q].
- Conditions associated with adenomatous polyps: Strong association with ureterosigmoidostomies[Q], acromegaly[Q] and streptococcus bovis bactermia[Q]

Probability of development of malignancy depends upon		
Gross Appearance of lesion	**Histology**	**Size**
• Pedunculated • **Sessile (Increased risk)**[Q]	• **Tubular (MC)**[Q] • Tubulovillous • **Villous (Highest risk)**[Q]	• <1 cm • 1-2 cm • **>2 cm (Increased risk)**[Q]

■ PEUTZ-JEGHER'S SYNDROME (AD)

PEUTZ-JEGHER'S SYNDROME (AD)

- **Hamartomatous polyps** (usually <100) throughout the GIT, **most common in jejunum**[Q]
- Associated with **hypermelanotic macule** in the **perioral region, buccal mucosa**[Q].
- **Mucocutaneous pigmentation** usually occurs during infancy and most commonly noted in **perioral** & **buccal region.**

> - **Pigmented macules** of PJS have **no malignant potential**[Q].

- Polyposis develops by age 20, occur most commonly in the jejunum (**jejunum**[Q] **>colon >stomach**).

Contd…

Gastrointestinal Surgery   Section 3

Contd…

Histology
- Smooth muscle extends into the superficial epithelial layer in a tree like manner known as **arborization**[Q].
- **Pseudoinvasion (epithelial cell trapping)**[Q]

Genetics
- It exhibits **autosomal dominant** inheritance[Q]
- Chromosome **19p13.3** encodes the serine threonine kinase **LKB1/STK11**[Q].

Extraintestinal Features
- **Increased risk** for **extraintestinal cancer** of the **pancreas, thyroid, breast** (may be bilateral), **lung, gallbladder, biliary tract (cholangiocarcinoma)**[Q].
- **Increased risk of gynecologic malignancies of the ovary (bilateral sex cord tumors** with annular features) & **uterus** (well-differentiated adenocarcinoma of the cervix, known as **adenoma malignum**)[Q]
- In men there is **increased risk** of **feminizing Sertoli cell tumors** of the testis[Q].

■ FAMILIAL ADENOMATOUS POLYPOSIS (AD)

FAMILIAL ADENOMATOUS POLYPOSIS (AD)

- FAP is an **autosomal dominant**[Q] inherited syndrome
- Results in the development of **>100 adenomatous polyps**[Q].
- Location of APC gene: **Long arm of chromosome 5q21.**
- Increased number of polyps predisposes patients to a greater risk of cancer[Q].
- Accounts for **<1%**[Q] of all cases of CRC
- **Earliest phenotypic change** present is known as **aberrant crypt formation**[Q]

> - **Average age of adenoma development** in FAP is **15 years**[Q], with approximately 15% manifesting polyps by 10 years, 75% by 20 years, and 90% by 30 years of age.
> - If left untreated, colorectal cancer develops in nearly **100%**[Q] of these patients **by age 40 years**[Q]

Extra-Intestinal Features		
• **Osteomas (mandible & skull)**[Q] • **Desmoid tumors**[Q]	• Thyroid papillary tumors • **Medulloblastomas**[Q] • Hypertrophic gastric fundic polyps[Q]	• **CHRPE**[Q] • Benign dental abnormalities • Epidermoid cyst

- Congenital hypertrophy of the retinal epithelium (CHRPEs) are asymptomatic and have no malignant potential; and are significantly larger, multiple, bilateral and with mixed pigment than sporadic CHRPE.

> - **After CRC, MC malignancy** diagnosed in patients with FAP is **periampullary adenocarcinoma of duodenum**[Q].
> - **After the CRC is eliminated by surgery, periampullary tumors**[Q] are **MC cause of death** among individuals with FAP.

- Others are tumors of the brain, hepatoblastoma, adrenal gland, thyroid, pancreas, biliary tree, stomach, & small intestine.

Diagnosis

> - **MC method used to screen for APC mutations** is the **APC gene testing** by protein truncation test[Q]

- A **positive screening test** should be **confirmed with a diagnostic modality**

Management
- **After the colorectal cancer is eliminated by surgery, periampullary tumors** are the **MC cause of death**[Q] among individuals with FAP.

> - **Prophylactic proctocolectomy** is recommended for patients with FAP, given the near 100% risk of early-onset CRC[Q].
> - **Treatment of choice: Total proctocolectomy with ileal pouch-anal anastomosis (IPAA)**[Q].

■ GARDNER'S SYNDROME (AD)

GARDNER'S SYNDROME (AD)

The combination of FAP with:
- Bony lesions (**osteomas**[Q], cortical thickening of long bones & ribs)
- Benign lymphoid polyposis of ileum[Q]
- **CHRPE**[Q]
- **Dental anomalies**[Q] (impacted tooth, supernumerary tooth, dental cyst)
- **Desmoid tumors & sebaceous cyst**[Q]

■ TURCOT'S SYNDROME (AR)

TURCOT'S SYNDROME (AR)

- **MC brain tumors** are **medulloblastoma** & particularly **glioblastoma**.
- Turcot's syndrome kindreds fall into two groups based on their types of brain tumor and particularly genetic alteration.
- **Medulloblastoma in FAP**[Q]
- **Glioblastoma multiforme in HNPCC**[Q]

■ HEREDITARY NONPOLYPOSIS COLORECTAL CANCER (AD)

HEREDITARY NONPOLYPOSIS COLORECTAL CANCER (AD)

- HNPCC is an **autosomal dominant**[Q] inherited syndrome
- **Defective mismatch repair genes** are located on chromosomes **2, 3 & 7**[Q].
- HNPCC is responsible for **3-5%**[Q] of **all cases of CRC**.
- **CRC** are mostly **poorly differentiated** & **mucinous** and have **signet ring histology** and **"Crohn's like" pattern** of tumor infiltrating lymphocytes[Q].
- Predominance of **right sided colon cancer** & **increased incidence of synchronous** & metachronous CRC.

  - **Lynch syndrome I: CRC only**[Q]
  - **Lynch syndrome II: CRC & associated malignancies**[Q]

Diagnosis

- **Gold standard for diagnosis** of HNPCC is the **detection of a germline mutation in MMR gene**[Q].
- Mismatch repair genes associated with HNPCC: (hMLH1, hMLH3, hPMS1, hPMS2) and (hMSH2, hMSH3, hMSH6)[Q].

  - **More than 90% of cases** are due to mutation in **hMLH1** or **hMSH2**[Q].

- **Revised Amsterdam criteria**: Used to **select at risk patients** for HNPCC[Q]
- **Bethesda guidelines**: To direct patient selection **for MSI testing**[Q]

Extraintestinal Features

- **Endometrial** (39-60%)[Q], **gastric** (13-19%)[Q], **ovarian** (6-12%)[Q], small intestine, pancreatic, thyroid, transitional cell epithelium of the urinary tract (renal pelvic, ureter, bladder); brain cancers.
- **MC extraintestinal feature: Endometrial cancer**[Q].
- **HNPCC associated tumor of the CNS: Glioblastoma**

  - Association with **benign** & **malignant tumors of sebaceous glands** & **keratocanthomas** is called **Muir-Torre syndrome**[Q]

■ SCREENING FOR COLORECTAL CANCER

SCREENING FOR COLORECTAL CANCER

- **American Cancer Society** suggests **fecal Hemoccult screening annually & flexible sigmoidoscopy every 5 years beginning at age 50 for asymptomatic individuals**[Q] having no colorectal cancer risk factors.

  - The American Cancer Society has also endorsed a **"total colon examination"** (i.e., **colonoscopy** or **double-contrast barium enema**) **every 10 years as an alternative**[Q] to Hemoccult testing with periodic flexible sigmoidoscopy.

- **Colonoscopy** has been shown to be **superior to double-contrast barium enema** and also to have a **higher sensitivity** for detecting villous or dysplastic adenomas or cancers[Q] than the strategy employing occult fecal blood testing & flexible sigmoidoscopy.

  - **Double-contrast barium enema** is done when **colonoscopy is contraindicated**[Q]

■ RISK FACTORS FOR COLORECTAL CANCER

Risk Factors for the Development of Colorectal Cancer	

1. Dietary Factors:
  – **High animal fat** diet[Q]
  – **Low fiber** diet[Q]
  – **Alcohol**[Q]
2. Hereditary syndromes:
  – **FAP**[Q]
  – **HNPCC**[Q]
	3. **Inflammatory bowel disease** (Both **UC** & **Crohn's disease**)[Q]
	4. **Streptococcus bovis** bacteremia[Q]
	5. **Ureterosigmoidostomy**[Q]
	6. **Smoking**[Q]
	7. **Acromegaly**[Q]
	8. **Pelvic irradiation**[Q]

■ CARCINOMA COLON

<u>CARCINOMA COLON</u>

- **Most common form of colon cancer** is sporadic[Q] in nature, without an associated strong family history.
- **MC site** of colon cancer: Sigmoid[Q]; **Least common site**: Hepatic flexure[Q]
- **MC site** of metastasis: Liver >Lung[Q]
- **Mucin production worsens** the prognosis since mucin aids tumor extension[Q]

> - **Incidence** of metastasis is related to depth of invasion[Q]
> - **Chemotherapy regimen**: FOLFOX-IV (5-FU, Leucovorin, Oxaliplatin)[Q]

Clinical Features

- **Symptoms** of colonic carcinoma are **non-specific** and generally **develop** when the **cancer** is **locally advanced**[Q].

Symptoms associated with colon cancer	
• **Abdominal pain (44%): MC**[Q]	• Hematochezia or melena (40%)
• Change in bowel habit (43%)	• Weakness or malaise (20%)

Right Colon	Left Colon
• **Fungating** or **cauliflower**[Q] type growth	• **Annular, constricting** or **stenosing** growth[Q]
• **Cancer** may become quiet **large without** any **obstructing symptoms** due to relative **liquid** stool **consistency**[Q]	• **Symptoms** of obstruction is **more common**[Q]
• **Lesions ulcerate** leading to **chronic insidious blood loss**[Q]	• Patients present with:
• Patients present with:	– **Decrease** in **stool caliber**[Q]
– **Melena, anemia, fatigue**[Q]	– **Alteration** of **bowel habbits (increasing constipation)**[Q]
– **Abdominal pain**[Q]	– **Palpable lump**[Q]
– **Mass** in **right iliac fossa**[Q]	• **Poor prognosis** (more **infiltrative**)[Q]
• **Good prognosis**[Q] as compared to left	

- **Lesions of transverse colon** are having **mixed symptoms** of bleeding and obstruction[Q].

Diagnosis

- **Barium enema**: "Apple core" or "napkin ring" lesion, caused by a **constricting carcinoma**[Q]

Colonoscopy
• **Gold standard for diagnosis** of **colon cancer**[Q].
• **Permits biopsy** of the tumor **to verify the diagnosis**[Q]
• Inspect entire colon to **exclude metachronous polyps** or **cancers**[Q]
• **Incidence** of a **synchronous cancer** is about 3%[Q]

- **Tumors causing complete obstruction**: Water-soluble contrast enema is useful in to **establish the anatomic level** of the **obstruction**[Q].
- IOC for staging of carcinoma colon: CECT[Q]

8th AJCC (2017) TNM Classification of Colorectal carcinoma	
Tis: Carcinoma in situ: intraepithelial or invasion of lamina propria	**N1**: Metastasis in **1-3** regional LNs **N1a**: Metastasis in **1** regional LN **N1b**: Metastasis in **2-3** regional LN
T1: Tumor invades **submucosa**[Q]	**N1c: Tumor deposits** in in the **subserosa, mesentery**, or **nonperitonealized pericolic** or **perirectal tissues without regional LN metastasis**[Q]
T2: Tumor invades **muscularis propria**[Q]	
T3: Tumor **invades subserosa or into non-peritonealized pericolic or perirectal tissues**[Q]	
T4a: Tumor **penetrates** the surface of **visceral peritoneum**[Q]	**N2a**: Metastasis in **4-6** regional LN[Q] **N2b**: Metastasis in **7 or more** regional LN[Q]
T4b: Tumor directly **invades** or is **adherent** to other **organs** or **structures**[Q]	**M1a**: Metastasis confined to **one organ or site** (e.g. Liver, lung, ovary, non-regional node) without peritoneal metastases[Q] **M1b**: Metastasis to **more than one organ**[Q] **M1c**: Metastasis to **peritoneum with or without other organ involvement**[Q]

Stage Grouping					
I	II	IIIA	IIIB	IIIC	IV
T1N0	IIA: T3N0	T1-T2, N1	T1-T2, N2b	T3-T4a, N2b	IVa: Tany Nany **M1a**
T2N0	IIB: T4aN0	T1, N2a	T2-T3, N2a	T4a, N2a	IVb: Tany Nany **M1b**
	IIC: T4bN0		T3-T4a, N1	T4b, N1-N2	IVC: Tany Nany **M1c**

Modified Duke's (Modified Astler-Collar) Classification	
Stage	**Description**
A	**Confined to the mucosa**
B1	**Partially penetrated** the **muscularis propria**[Q]
B2	**Fully penetrated**[Q] the muscularis propria
C1	**Lymph node invasion without penetration** of the entire bowel wall[Q]
C2	**Lymph node invasion with penetration**[Q] **of the entire bowel wall**
D	**Distant metastasis**[Q]

Treatment of Colon Cancer According to Stage	
Stage 0: (Tis, N0, M0)	• **Endoscopic polypectomy for** polyps containing **carcinoma in situ**
Stage I: (T1, N0, M0) **Malignant Polyp**	• Segmental colectomy[Q]
Stages I and II: (T1–3, N0, M0) **Localized Colon Carcinoma**	• Surgical resection[Q]
Stage III: (Tany, N1, M0) **Lymph Node Metastasis**	• **Surgical resection + Adjuvant chemotherapy**[Q] (routinely) • **Reference regimen: FOLFOX-IV**[Q] (5-FU, Leucovorin, Oxaliplatin)
Stage IV: (Tany, Nany, M1) **Distant Metastasis**	• **MC site of metastasis: Liver > Lung**[Q] • **Resection (metastasectomy)** for **isolated, resectable metastasis + adjuvant chemotherapy**[Q] • **Palliation** for unresectable disease

■ COLONIC ISCHEMIA

COLONIC ISCHEMIA

- **Intestinal ischemia** occurs **most commonly** in the **colon**[Q].
- **Most colonic ischemia** appears to **result from low flow** and/or **small vessel occlusion**[Q].

> • MC site of ischemic colitis: Splenic flexure[Q]

- **Ligation** of the **IMA during aortic surgery** predisposes **to colonic ischemia**[Q].

Risk factors for Colonic Ischemia	
• **Vascular disease**[Q]	• **Vasculitis**[Q]
• **Diabetes mellitus**[Q]	• **Hypotension**[Q]

Clinical Features

- Diagnosis of ischemic colitis is often based upon the **clinical history** and **physical examination**[Q].
- **Mild ischemia: Diarrhea** (usually bloody) **without abdominal pain**[Q].
- **Severe ischemia: Intense abdominal pain** (often out of proportion to the clinical examination), **tenderness, fever,** and **leukocytosis**[Q]
- **Peritonitis** and/or **systemic toxicity** are signs of **full-thickness necrosis** and **perforation.**

Diagnosis

- **Abdominal X-ray: Thumb printing**[Q] (due to **mucosal edema** and **submucosal hemorrhage**)[Q].
- **CT scan:** Nonspecific **colonic wall thickening** and **pericolic fat stranding**[Q].

> • **Sigmoidoscopy:** Characteristic **dark, hemorrhagic mucosa**[Q]
> • **Risk of precipitating perforation** is high, so **sigmoidoscopy** is **relatively contraindicated**[Q] in ischemic colitis.

Treatment

- **Majority** of patients with ischemic colitis **can be treated medically**[Q].
- **Bowel rest** and **broad-spectrum antibiotics** are the mainstay of therapy **(80% of patients recover**[Q] with this regimen)

Complications

- **Stricture** (10-15%): **MC site of stricture is sigmoid colon**[Q]
- **Chronic segmental ischemia** (15-20%).

■ PSEUDOMEMBRANOUS COLITIS

PSEUDOMEMBRANOUS COLITIS

- **PMC** is caused by C. **difficile,** a **gram-positive**[Q] bacillus.
- **C. difficile colitis** is the **leading cause of nosocomially acquired diarrhea**[Q].

Contd…

Contd…

Pathogenesis

- Colitis is thought to result from **overgrowth** of this **organism after depletion of** the **normal commensal flora** of the gut **with** the use of **antibiotics**[Q].

  - **Clindamycin**[Q] was the **first antimicrobial** agent associated with **C. difficile colitis**, almost **any antibiotic** may **cause this disease.**
  - Toxins produced: **Toxin A** (an **enterotoxin**) and **toxin B** (a **cytotoxin**)[Q].

- **Immunosuppression, medical comorbidities, prolonged hospitalization** or **nursing home residence**, and **bowel surgery increase** the **risk**[Q].

Clinical Features

- The **spectrum of disease** ranges from **watery diarrhea** to **fulminant, life-threatening** colitis

Diagnosis

- Diagnosis is made after **detection of one** or **both toxins by:**
  - **Stool cytotoxin assay**[Q]   – **ELISA**[Q]
- **Colonoscopy:** Characteristic **ulcers, plaques,** and **pseudomembranes**[Q]
- **CECT: Accordion sign**[Q] is seen

Treatment

- **Immediate cessation** of **offending antimicrobial agent**[Q].
- **Mild disease:**
  - **Oral metronidazole** (10-day course): **Drug of choice**[Q]
  - **Oral vancomycin: Second-line agent,** used in **metronidazole allergy** or in **recurrent disease**[Q]
- **Severe disease: Bowel rest, IV hydration,** and **IV metronidazole** or oral **vancomycin**[Q].

  - **Recurrent colitis** occurs in up to **20%** of patients and may be **treated by a longer course** of **oral metronidazole** or **vancomycin** (up to 1 month).
  - **Fulminant colitis,** characterized by septicemia and/or evidence of perforation, **requires emergent laparotomy**[Q].

■ LOWER GI BLEEDING

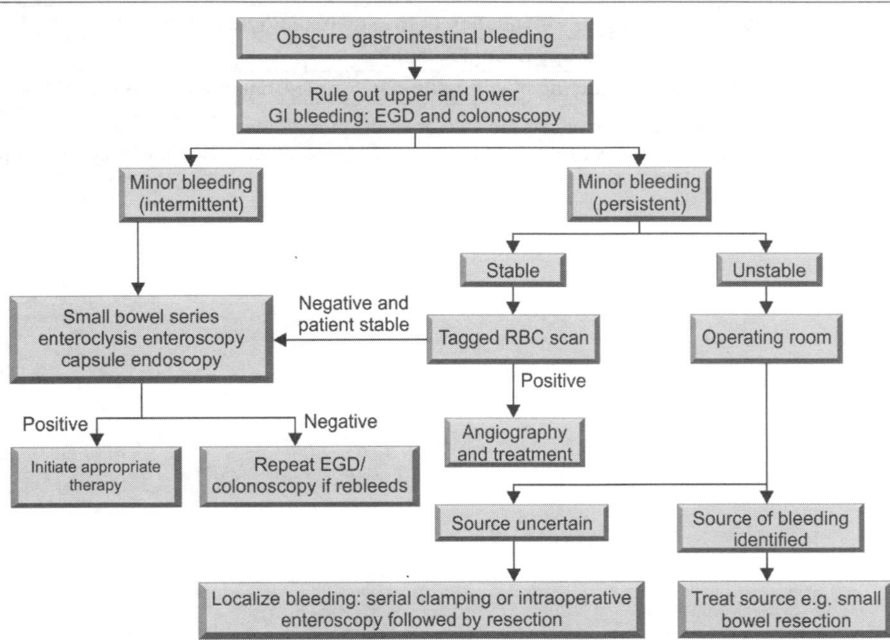

Lower Gastrointestinal Bleeding			
Colonic Bleeding (95%)	**%**	**Small Bowel Bleeding (5%)**	
Diverticular disease[Q]	30-40	**Angiodysplasias**	
Anorectal disease[Q]	5-15	Erosions or ulcers (potassium, NSAIDs)	
Ischemia	5-10	Crohn's disease	
Neoplasia	5-10	Radiation	
Infectious colitis	3-8	Meckel's diverticulum	

Contd…

Contd...

Postpolypectomy	3-7	Neoplasia	
Inflammatory bowel disease	3-4	Aortoenteric fistula	
Angiodysplasia	3		
Radiation colitis/proctitis	1-3		
Other	1-5		
Unknown	10-25		

LOWER GASTROINTESTINAL BLEED

- **Lower gastrointestinal bleed is defined as a bleeding from a site distal to the ligament of Treitz[Q].**
- MC site of lower GI bleed: colon (95%)[Q]
- MC cause of lower GI bleed in India: Hemorrhoids[Q] (Rarely massive bleeding)

• **MC cause of significant lower GI bleed: Diverticular disease (overall)[Q]**
• **MC cause of significant small bowel bleed: angiodysplasia[Q]**
• **MC cause of recurrent, obscure lower GI bleed: Vascular ectasia[Q]** (angiodysplasia)

■ VASCULAR ECTASIA (ANGIODYSPLASIA)

VASCULAR ECTASIA (ANGIODYSPLASIA)

- **MC vascular lesions** found in the **colon: Vascular ectasia[Q]**
- **MC cause** of **recurrent lower intestinal bleeding after 60 years** of age: **Vascular ectasia[Q]**
- Arise from **age-related degeneration of previously normal colonic blood vessels[Q]**.
- **Acquired condition[Q]**

• Almost **always occur in** the **cecum** or the **proximal ascending colon[Q]**
• **Usually multiple, are <5 mm[Q]** in diameter
• **Rarely identified** with **gross inspection** or **routine pathologic examination**
• **Diagnosed with colonoscopy** or **angiography**
• **Angiography: Slow emptying** of **vein[Q]** and dilation of **submucosal vessels[Q]**

- **Not associated with synchronous angiomatous lesions of the skin, mucous membranes, or other viscera[Q].**
- API: "Hemorrhoids and anal fissure are the most common cause of lower GI bleeding, however the bleeding is rarely **massive[Q]**."

Multiple Choice Questions

■ HIRSCHSPRUNG'S DISEASE

1. **Duhamel's operation is done for:** *(MHSSMCET 2005)*
   a. Hirschsprung's disease   b. Meconium ileus
   c. Annular pancreas   d. Imperforate anus

2. **Not true regarding Hirschsprung's disease is:**
   (Recent Question 2015; AIIMS Nov 97)
   a. Autosomal dominant
   b. Absent ganglionic cells in myenteric plexus
   c. Absent ganglionic cell in submucous plexus
   d. Rectal biopsy is diagnostic

3. **Aganglionic segment is encountered in which part of colon in case of Hirschsprung's disease?**
   a. Distal to dilated segment
   b. In whole colon   *(Recent Question 2014; AIIMS Nov 99)*
   c. Proximal to dilated segment
   d. In dilated segment

4. **Hirschsprung's disease involves which region of intestine?**
   (MCI March 2008)
   a. Colon   b. Rectum
   c. Rectosigmoid part   d. Terminal ileum

5. **Investigation of choice in Hirschsprung's disease is:** *(Recent Question 2017, AIIMS Nov 2005,DNB 2005, 2000, PGI Dec 98)*
   a. Rectal manometry   b. Rectal examination
   c. Rectal biopsy   d. Ba enema

6. **In Hirschsprung's disease, aganglionic segment is:**
   (DNB 2010)
   a. Normal or dilated   b. Normal or contracted
   c. Dilated or contracted   d. Always dilated

7. **Following procedures (except one) are done for correction of Hirschsprung's disease:** *(Recent Question 2016)*
   a. Duhamel's   b. Soave's
   c. Swenson's   d. Bayar's

8. **Most common presentation of Hirschsprung's disease:**
   (Recent Question 2017)
   a. Abdominal distention   b. Vomiting
   c. Failure to pass meconium   d. Failure to thrive

■ COLONIC DIVERTICULA

9. **Acquired diverticula are most commonly in seen in:**
   (Recent Question 2015; MHSSMCET 2007)
   a. Jejunum/ileum   b. Transverse colon
   c. Sigmoid colon   d. Ascending colon

10. **True regarding colovesical fistula is:** *(JIPMER 2013)*
    a. Commonly presents with pneumaturia
    b. Barium enema is diagnostic
    c. Common in Females
    d. May be a surgical complication

11. **Most common fistula in diverticulosis of colon"**
    (MHSSMCET 2010, 2006)
    a. Colocutaneous   b. Colovaginal
    c. Vesicovaginal   d. Colovesical

12. **Colonic diverticulosis is best diagnosed by:**
    (Recent Question 2015; AIIMS May 2007)
    a. Colonoscopy   b. Nuclear scan
    c. Barium enema   d. CT scan

13. **This characteristic appearance is seen on barium enema in:**
    (Recent Question 2018)
    a. Colonic polyps   b. Colonic diverticula
    c. Carcinoma colon   d. Ischemic colitis

14. **Massive colonic bleeding in a patient of diverticulosis is from:** *(All India 2000)*
    a. Inferior mesenteric artery
    b. Superior mesenteric artery
    c. Celiac artery
    d. Gastro-duodenal artery

15. **The most common site of bleeding diverticula is:** *(DPG 2008)*
    a. Sigmoid colon   b. Descending colon
    c. Rectum   d. Ascending colon

16. **Best investigation to diagnose colonic diverticulitis:**
    (Recent Question 2017)
    a. Barium enema   b. CECT
    c. Ultrasound   d. MRI

17. **Hinchey classification is used in cases of:** *(MHCET 2016)*
    a. Complicated diverticulitis   b. Complicated pancreatitis
    c. Complicated hepatitis   d. Complicated meningitis

■ COLORECTAL POLYPS

18. **Intestinal polyps that can potentially grow into cancer:**
    (DNB 2005, 2001, MHPGMCET 2007)
    a. Adenomatous polyp   b. Hyperplastic polyp
    c. Juvenile polyp   d. Hamartomatous polyp

19. **Diagnosis of colonic polyps is best done radiologically using:** *(COMEDK 2010)*
    a. Barium meal series
    b. Double-contrast barium enema
    c. Instant enema
    d. Water-soluble contrast enema

20. **Which polyp has maximum malignant potential?**
    (Recent Question 2015; AIIMS June 93)
    a. Sessile   b. Pedunculated
    c. Superficial spreading   d. Any of the above

21. **Incidence of malignancy is maximum in:** *(AIIMS Feb 97)*
    a. Villous adenoma   b. Juvenile polyps
    c. Hyperplastic polyps   d. Tubular adenoma

22. **All of the following are pre-malignant except:**
    (AIIMS Nov 2014)
    a. Crohn's disease   b. Ulcerative colitis
    c. Peutz-Jegher's syndrome   d. Barrett's esophagus

23. Polyp associated with highest risk of malignant transformation is: *(MHCET 2016)*
    a. Juvenile
    b. Villous adenoma
    c. Tubular adenoma
    d. Polyp of Peutz-Jegher's syndrome

24. Which of the following colonic polyps is not premalignant?
    a. Juvenile polyps   *(All India 2006, AIIMS Nov 2006)*
    b. Hamartomatous polyps associated with Peutz-Jegher's syndrome
    c. Villous adenoma
    d. Tubular adenomas

25. Metabolic abnormality seen in large colorectal villous adenoma: *(AIIMS May 2008)*
    a. Hypokalemic metabolic alkalosis
    b. Hypokalemic metabolic acidosis
    c. Chlorine sensitive metabolic acidosis
    d. Chlorine resistant metabolic alkalosis

26. Lalita, a female patient presents with pigmentation of the lips and oral mucosa and intestinal polyps. Her sister also gives the same history. Most probable diagnosis is:
    (DNB 2011, AIIMS June 2001, All India 2000)
    a. Carcinoid tumor
    b. Melanoma
    c. Villous adenoma
    d. Peutz-Jegher's syndrome

FAMILIAL ADENOMATOUS POLYPOSIS

27. "Gardner's syndrome" has all the following except:
    (COMEDK 2005)
    a. Colonic polyp
    b. Multiple epidermal cyst
    c. Bony exostosis
    d. Giant gastric folds

28. True about familial polyposis colon cancer syndrome except:
    a. Autosomal recessive   *(JIPMER 2011)*
    b. Associated with fibroma and osteomas
    c. Associated with brain tumors
    d. 100% incidence of colon carcinoma

29. Following genetic counseling in a family for Familial polyposis coli, next screening test is:
    (MCI June 2018, AIIMS Nov 2006)
    a. Flexible sigmoidoscopy
    b. Colonoscopy
    c. Occult blood in stools
    d. APC gene

30. Desmoid tumor is associated with: *(JIPMER 2014, 2013)*
    a. Colonic polyps
    b. Pancreatic cancer
    c. Ovarian cancer
    d. Gastric cancer

31. Which of the following is associated with FAP?
    (Recent Question 2017)
    a. Gardner's syndrome
    b. Peutz-Jegher's syndrome
    c. Juvenile polyps
    d. Hamartomatous polyp

HEREDITARY NON-POLYPOSIS COLON CANCER

32. Lynch syndrome is also known as: *(KGMC 2011)*
    a. FAP
    b. PJS
    c. HNPCC
    d. Cowden's syndrome

33. Multiple cutaneous sebaceous adenomas are seen in:
    (All India 2011)
    a. Gardner's syndrome
    b. Turcot's syndrome
    c. Muir-Torre syndrome
    d. Cowden syndrome

34. Patient with proximal CA colon with endometrial and ovarian carcinoma has:
    (Recent Question 2018, AIIMS GIS Dec 2006)
    a. Lynch syndrome
    b. Gardener's syndrome
    c. Cowden's disease
    d. Cronkhite-Canada syndrome

35. Most common mismatch repair gene mutation in HNPCC:
    a. MSH-2 and hMLH-1
    b. PMS-1   *(GB Pant 2011)*
    c. MSH-6
    d. PMS-2

COLORECTAL CANCER: RISK FACTORS

36. Based on epidemiological studies, which of the following has been found to be most protective against carcinoma colon?   *(DNB 2011, AIIMS May 2011, All India 2009)*
    a. High fiber diet
    b. Low fat diet
    c. Low selenium diet
    d. Low protein diet

37. All of the following genes may be involved in development of carcinoma of colon except: *(All India 2009)*
    a. APC
    b. Beta-Catenin
    c. K-ras
    d. Mismatch repair genes

38. Cholecystectomy may lead to increased risk of:
    (COMEDK 2004)
    a. Proximal colon cancer
    b. CA. pancreas
    c. Hepatic cancer
    d. Cholangiocarcinoma

CARCINOMA: CLINICAL FEATURES AND DIAGNOSIS

39. Most common site of colonic carcinoma:
    (GB Pant 2010, UPPG 2009; NEET 2013)
    a. Sigmoid
    b. Transverse
    c. Descending
    d. Ascending

40. Patient having diarrhea and colic on and of with mass in right iliac fossa. Most probable diagnosis is: *(DNB 2009)*
    a. Carcinoma rectum
    b. Carcinoma cecum
    c. Carcinoma sigmoid
    d. Carcinoma transverse colon

41. True regarding carcinoma colon is: *(AIIMS Nov 2000)*
    a. Lesion on left side of the colon presents with features of anemia
    b. Mucinous carcinoma has a good prognosis
    c. Duke's A stage should receive adjuvant chemotherapy
    d. Solitary liver metastasis is not a contraindication for surgery

42. On barium enema, this appearance is seen in:
    a. Ischemic colitis
    b. Carcinoma colon
    c. Colonic diverticula
    d. Colonic polyposis

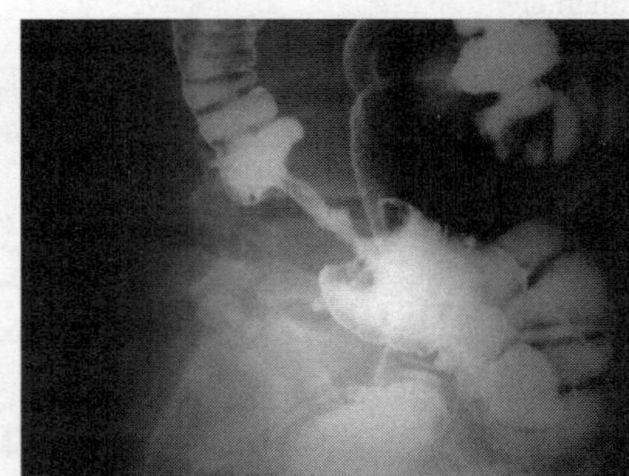

43. What is an acceptable screening technique for detecting recurrent colon cancer?   *(COMEDK 2004)*
    a. Screening sigmoidoscopy
    b. Screening the stool for occult blood
    c. Stool cytology
    d. Measurement of CEA levels

44. Most important prognostic factor for colorectal carcinoma is:
    a. Site of lesion   *(AIIMS May 2011)*
    b. Tumour size and characteristics
    c. Age of patient
    d. Lymph node status

45. The tendency of colonic carcinoma to metastasize is best assessed by: *(Recent Question 2014; AIIMS Nov 2003)*
    a. Size of tumor
    b. Carcinoembryonic antigen (CEA) levels
    c. Depth of penetration of bowel wall
    d. Proportion of bowel circumference involved

46. Metastatic liver disease is found in _______% of patients undergoing surgery for primary colorectal cancer:
(MCI Nov 2017)

a. 10% b. 15%
c. 33% d. 75%

■ CARCINOMA COLON TREATMENT

47. After undergoing surgery, for carcinoma of colon a patient developed single liver metastasis of 2 cm. What you do next?
(BIHAR PG 2014; All India 2002, All India 98)

a. Resection b. Chemoradiation
c. Acetic acid injection d. Radiofrequency ablation

48. Ramu is 60 years old male with CA descending colon presents with acute intestinal obstruction. In emergency department treatment of choice is:
(AIIMS Nov 99, Nov 98, Feb 97)

a. Defunctioning colostomy b. Hartman's procedure
c. Total colectomy d. Left hemicolectomy

■ COLONIC ISCHEMIA

49. Thumb printing appearance of colon on barium enema is seen in:
(COMEDK 2004)

a. Diverticulitis b. Ischemic colitis
c. Ulcerative colitis d. Carcinoma colon

50. This characteristic appearance is seen on barium enema in:

a. Colonic polyps b. Colonic diverticula
c. Ischemic colitis d. Carcinoma colon

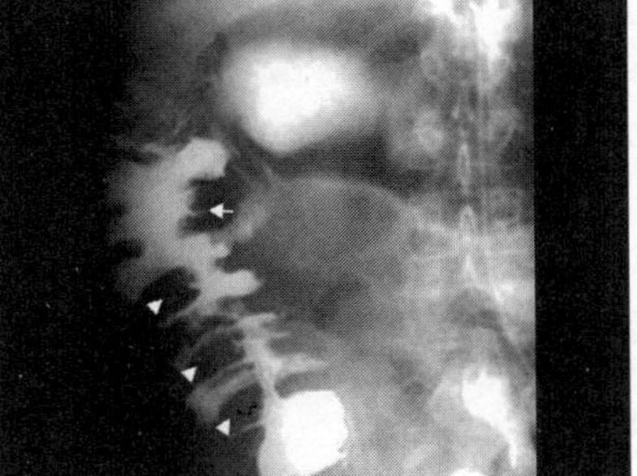

51. Commonest site for ischemic colitis is:
(AIIMS June 95, PGI Dec 97)

a. Hepatic flexure b. Splenic flexure
c. Descending colon d. Ascending colon

■ PSEUDOMEMBRANOUS COLITIS

52. Pseudomembranous colitis is associated with:
(COMEDK 2005)

a. Campylobacter b. Clostridium difficile
c. Clostridium retgari d. Salmonella typhi

53. Which among the following is the drug of choice for clostridium difficile-induced colitis? *(COMEDK 2009)*

a. Gentamicin b. Ciprofloxacin
c. Metronidazole d. Linezolid

54. A patient on antibiotics for treatment for peritonitis presents with mucus diarrhea. Most probable cause could be:

a. Ulcerative colitis *(MCI Sept 2009)*
b. Activation of latent tuberculosis
c. Antibiotic associated diarrhea
d. Gastritis

55. In a patient of pseudomembranous colitis, CECT was done. What is the name of sign seen on CECT? *(Recent Question 2017)*

a. Accordion sign b. Whorl sign
c. Central stellate scar d. Honeycombing

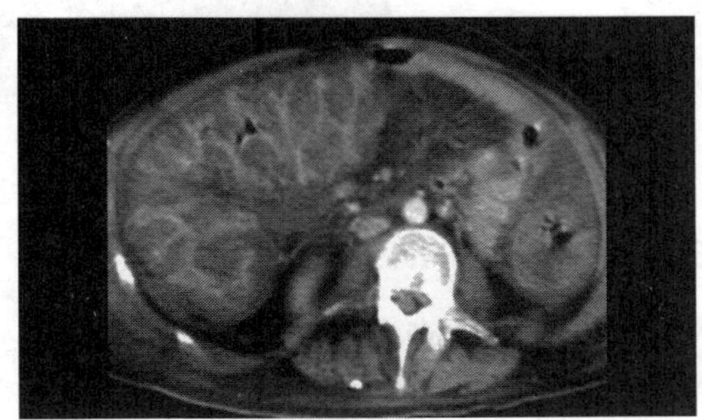

■ ENTERIC FISTULA

56. Most common cause of colonic fistula in India at age of 27 years: *(UPPG 2008)*

a. Crohn's disease b. Ulcerative colitis
c. Tuberculosis d. Carcinoma rectum

■ LOWER GI BLEED

57. Most common cause of heavy bleeding in 70 years old male:
(Recent Question 2014; KGMC 2011)

a. Colorectal carcinoma b. Colonic diverticulosis
c. Polyp d. Angiodysplasia

58. Which of the following is the least common possibility about angiodysplasia of colon? *(Recent Question 2015)*

a. Involvement of cecum
b. Involvement of rectum in 50% of cases
c. Affecting age group > 40 years
d. Cause of troublesome lower GI haemorrhage

59. Most common cause of lower GI bleed in India is:
(AIIMS Nov 94)

a. Benign tumour b. Non specific ulcer
c. Cancer rectosigmoid d. Hemorrhoids

60. The most useful investigation for profuse lower gastrointestinal bleeding is:
(UPSC 2005)

a. Proctosigmoidoscopy
b. Colonoscopy
c. Double contrast barium enema
d. Selective arteriography

61. Most common cause of lower gastro intestinal bleeding is:

a. Diverticulosis b. Colorectal carcinoma
c. Angiodysplasia d. Anal fissure *(UPPG 2007)*

62. The commonest cause of significant lower gastrointestinal bleed in a middle aged person with unknown reason is:
(DPG 2009 March)

a. Sigmoid diverticula b. Angiodysplasia
c. Ischemic colitis d. Ulcerative colitis

63. Most common site of angio dysplasia is: *(DNB 2007)*

a. Sigmoid colon b. Transverse colon
c. Ascending colon d. Descending colon

64. The commonest cause of significantly lower gastrointestinal bleed in a middle aged person without any known precipitating factor may be due to:

a. Ulcerative colitis *(MCI March 2008, Sept 2010)*
b. Ischemic colitis
c. Angiodysplasia
d. Diverticulum of sigmoid colon

65. Massive bleeding per rectum in a 70 years old patient is due to:
(DNB 2005, 2000, All India 2000)

a. Diverticulosis b. Carcinoma colon
c. Colitis d. Polyps

■ HIRSCHSPRUNG'S DISEASE

1. Ans. a. Hirschsprung's disease
2. Ans. a. Autosomal dominant
3. Ans. a. Distal to dilated segment
4. Ans. c. Rectosigmoid part
5. Ans. c. Rectal biopsy
6. Ans. b. Normal or contracted
7. Ans. d. Bayar's
8. Ans. a. Abdominal distention *(Sabiston 19/e p1848; Schwartz 10/e p1625)*

■ COLONIC DIVERTICULA

9. Ans. c. Sigmoid colon *(Ref: Sabiston 20/e p1330; Schwartz 11/e p1286, 10/e p1201; Bailey 27/e p1273; Shackelford 8/e p1827)*

10. Ans. a. Commonly presents with pneumaturia
11. Ans. d. Colovesical

12. Ans. c. Barium enema

- **Investigation of choice** for **colonic diverticulosis: Barium enema**[Q]
- **Investigation of choice** for **diverticulitis: CT scan**[Q]

13. Ans. b. Colonic diverticula *(Ref: Sabiston 20/e p1331; Schwartz 11/e p1286, 10/e p1201; Bailey 27/e p1274)*

14. Ans. b. Superior mesenteric artery *(Ref: Sabiston 20/e p1330; Schwartz 11/e p1286, 10/e p1201; Bailey 27/e p1273; Shackelford 8/e p1830)*
Although diverticular disease is much more common on the left side, right-sided disease is responsible for more than half episodes of bleeding (from SMA).

15. Ans. d. Ascending colon

16. Ans. b. CECT *(Ref: Sabiston 20/e p1331; Schwartz 11/e p1286, 10/e p1201; Bailey 27/e p1274)*

17. Ans. a. Complicated diverticulitis

■ COLORECTAL POLYPS

18. Ans. a. Adenomatous polyp *(Ref: Sabiston 20/e p1368; Schwartz 11/e p1290, 10/e p1205-1206; Bailey 27/e p1259; Shackelford 8/e p 1963)*

19. Ans. b. Double contrast barium enema *(Ref: Harrison 20/e p 574; Bailey 27/e p1260)*

- Best investigation for diagnosis of colorectal polyps: Colonoscopy >Double-contrast barium enema[Q]

20. Ans. a. Sessile
21. Ans. a. Villous adenoma

22. Ans. c. Peutz-Jegher's syndrome
23. Ans. b. Villous adenoma

24. Ans. a. Juvenile polyps

25. Ans. b. Hypokalemic metabolic acidosis *(Ref: Harrison 19/e p269)*

McKittrick-Wheelock Syndrome

- Villous adenoma causing profuse watery diarrhea and hypokalemia, hyponatremia, hypochloremia and metabolic acidosis[Q].
- Severe volume loss can lead to acute renal failure and cardiovascular collapse[Q].
- Treatment is resuscitation followed by resection[Q].

26. Ans. d. Peutz-Jegher's syndrome *(Ref: Sabiston 20/e p 1372; Schwartz 11/e p1242, 10/e p1202; Bailey 27/e p1250; Shackelford 8/e p 1972)*

■ FAMILIAL ADENOMATOUS POLYPOSIS

27. Ans. d. Giant gastric folds
28. Ans. a. Autosomal recessive

29. Ans. d. APC gene

- Most common method used to screen for APC mutations is the APC gene testing by protein truncation test[Q]

30. Ans. a. Colonic polyps

31. Ans. a. Gardner's syndrome *(Ref: Sabiston 20/e p1361; Schwartz 11/e p1292, 10/e p1207; Bailey 27/e p1259)*

■ HEREDITARY NON-POLYPOSIS COLON CANCER

32. Ans. c. HNPCC *(Ref: Sabiston 20/e p1370; Schwartz 11/e p1292-1293, 10/e p291-292,1183,1207; Bailey 27/e p1260; Shackelford 8/e p 1974)*

33. Ans. c. Muir-Torre syndrome   **34. Ans. a. Lynch syndrome**

35. Ans. a. MSH-2 and hMLH-1

■ COLORECTAL CANCER: RISK FACTORS

36. Ans. a. High fiber diet *(Ref: Maingot 11/e p626-627; Schwartz 11/e p1288, 10/e p1204)*

- **High fiber diet** has been found to have **protective effect** by **increasing** the **stool bulk, diluting** the **toxins,** and **reducing** the colonic transit time and thus **reducing exposure time to fecal carcinogens**[Q]

37. Ans. b. Beta-Catenin *(Ref: Sabiston 20/e p1360)*

Gene Mutations that Cause Colon Cancer	
Mutation type	**Genes Involved**
Germline	• **APC** and **MMR**[Q]
Somatic	• **Oncogenes: Myc, Ras, Src, erbB2**[Q] • **Tumor suppressor genes: p53, DCC, APC**[Q] • **MMR genes:** bMSH2, bMLH1, bPMS1, bPMS2, bMSH6, bMSH3[Q]
Genetic polymorphism	• APC[Q]

ADENOMATOUS POLYPOSIS COLI (APC) GENE

- APC gene is a tumor suppressor gene located on chromosome 5q21[Q].
- Its product is 2843 amino acids in length and forms a cytoplasmic complex with GSK-3β (a serine-threonine kinase), β-catenin, and axin[Q].

- **APC participates in cell cycle control by regulating the intracytoplasmic pool of β-catenin**[Q].
- **APC influences cell cycle proliferation by regulating Wnt expression**[Q].

- The **Wnt signaling proteins** are closely associated with the **APC-β-catenin pathway.**
- Under normal conditions, **reduced intracytoplasmic β-catenin levels inhibit Wnt expression.**
- When **APC** is **mutated** however, β-catenin levels rise, and **Wnt is activated.**

38. Ans. a. Proximal colon cancer *(Ref: Maingot 11/e p628)*

- **Bile acids can induce hyperproliferation of the intestinal mucosa**[Q] via a number of intracellular mechanisms.

    - **Cholecystectomy,** which alters the enterohepatic cycle of bile acids, has been associated with a **moderately increased risk** of **proximal colon cancers**[Q].
- It cannot be ruled out, however, that it is less the effect of the cholecystectomy than the impact of other, not yet identified factors in the lithogenic bile of such patients.
- A number of cofactors have been identified that **may enhance** or **neutralize the carcinogenic effects of bile acids,** e.g., the amount of **dietary fat, fiber, or calcium**[Q].
- **Calcium,** in fact, **binds bile acids** and thus may **reduce their negative impact**[Q].

■ CARCINOMA: CLINICAL FEATURES AND DIAGNOSIS

39. Ans. a. Sigmoid *(Ref: Bailey 27/e p1262)*

Site of Carcinoma	Frequency
• **Rectum (MC)**[Q]	• **38%**
• **Sigmoid colon (2nd MC)**[Q]	• **21%**
• **Cecum**	• **12%**
• Transverse colon	• 5.5%
• Ascending colon	• 5%
• Descending colon	• 4%
• Splenic flexure	• 3%
• **Hepatic flexure (LC)**[Q]	• **2%**

40. **Ans. b.** Carcinoma cecum
41. **Ans. d. Solitary liver metastasis is not a contraindication for surgery** *(Ref: Sabiston 20/e p 1377; Schwartz 11/e p1302, 10/e p1293-1294; Bailey 27/e p1264)*
42. **Ans. b. Carcinoma colon** *(Ref: Sabiston 20/e p1371; Bailey 27/e p1262)*

> • **Barium enema: "Apple core"** or **"napkin ring" lesion**, caused by a **constricting carcinoma**[Q]

43. **Ans. a.** Screening sigmoidoscopy
44. **Ans. d. Lymph node status** *(Ref: Schwartz 11/e p1295, 10/e p1203-1216)*
45. **Ans. c.** Depth of penetration of bowel wall   46. **Ans. c.** 33%

■ CARCINOMA COLON TREATMENT

47. **Ans. a.** Resection
48. **Ans. b.** Hartman's procedure

■ COLONIC ISCHEMIA

49. **Ans. b. Ischemic colitis** *(Ref: Sabiston 20/e p1356; Schwartz 11/e p1309, 10/e p1221; Bailey 27/e p1276; Shackelford 8/e p 1820)*
50. **Ans. c. Ischemic colitis** *(Ref: Sabiston 20/e p1356; Schwartz 11/e p1309, 10/e p1222; Bailey 27/e p1277)*
    • **Thumb printing**[Q] (due to **mucosal edema** and **submucosal hemorrhage)**[Q] **is characteristic feature of ischemic colitis.**
51. **Ans. b.** Splenic flexure

■ PSEUDOMEMBRANOUS COLITIS

52. **Ans. b. Clostridium difficile** *(Ref: Sabiston 20/e p1133; Schwartz 11/e p1309, 10/e p1222; Bailey 27/e p1273)*
53. **Ans. c.** Metronidazole
54. **Ans. c.** Antibiotic associated diarrhea
55. **Ans. a.** Accordion sign

■ ENTERIC FISTULA

56. **Ans. a.** Crohn's disease

■ LOWER GI BLEED

57. **Ans. b. Colonic diverticulosis** *(Ref: Sabiston 20/e p1151)*
58. **Ans. b.** Involvement of rectum in 50% of cases
59. **Ans. d. Hemorrhoids** *(Ref: API Medicine 6/e p509, 511)*

> • API: "Hemorrhoids and anal fissure are the most common cause of lower GI bleeding, however the bleeding is rarely **massive**[Q]**."**

60. **Ans. b.** Colonoscopy
61. **Ans. a.** Diverticulosis
62. **Ans. a.** Sigmoid diverticula
63. **Ans. c.** Ascending colon
64. **Ans. d.** Diverticulum of sigmoid colon
65. **Ans. a.** Diverticulosis

Ileostomy and Colostomy

■ STOMA

STOMA

- May be **colostomy** or **ileostomy**
- May be **temporary** or **permanent**
- **Temporary** or **defunctioning stomas** are usually fashioned as **loop stomas**
- An **ileostomy is spouted**; a **colostomy is flush**[Q]
- **Ileostomy effluent** is usually **liquid** whereas **colostomy effluent** is usually **solid**[Q]
- **Ileostomy patients** are more likely to develop **fluid & electrolyte problems**
- An **ileostomy** is usually sited in the **right iliac fossa**[Q]
- A **temporary colostomy** may be **transverse** and sited in the **right upper quadrant**[Q]
- **End-colostomy** is usually sited in the **left iliac fossa**[Q]
- All patients should be counseled by a stoma care nurse before operation

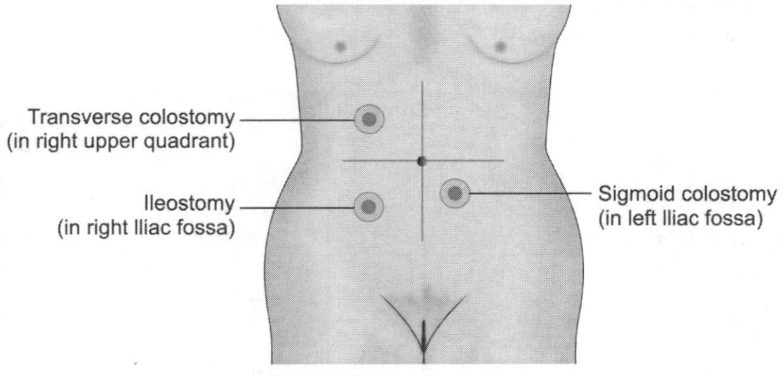

Sites of Stoma Formation

■ ILEOSTOMY

ILEOSTOMY

- **Opening** constructed **between** the **small intestine** and the **abdominal wall**, usually by **using distal ileum.**

  - **Indications of Permanent ileostomy:** For patients who require **removal of the entire colon** and **rectum** (**Crohn's disease** or **ulcerative colitis**[Q])
  - **Indications of loop ileostomy:** Cases where **multiple** and **complex anastomoses** must be **performed distally** (**Crohn's disease** or **CA rectum**[Q]).

- **Loop ileostomy use** is becoming **more frequent** (because of the complex sphincter-preserving operations being performed for **UC** and **FAP**)

Types of ileostomies	
• **End ileostomy (Brooke)**	• Continent ileostomy (Kock pouch)
• **Loop ileostomy**	• Urinary conduit
• **Loop-end ileostomy**	

Continent Ileostomy

- Continent ileostomy, or **Kock pouch,** has been used as an **alternative to** a **conventional ileostomy** for **selected patients** with **UC** or **FAP**[Q].

  - **Contraindicated in Crohn's disease**[Q] (risk of **recurrent disease**)
  - **Not recommended for well-functioning end ileostomy**[Q].

- It involves construction of an **internal pouch with** a **continent nipple valve.**

■ COLOSTOMY

COLOSTOMY

- **MC indication** for **fashioning a colostomy**: CA rectum[Q]
- Colostomies are also constructed as **treatment for obstructing lesions** of the **distal large intestine** and for **actual** or **potential perforations**[Q].

Type by Anatomic Location	
• **End-sigmoid colostomy (MC)**[Q] • **End-descending colostomy**[Q]	• Transverse colostomy • Cecostomy

> - However, **if the IMA is transected during an operation** for **CA rectum**, the **blood supply to the sigmoid colon is no longer dependable**, and it **should not be used** for stoma construction. Therefore, an **"end-descending" colostomy** is usually **preferable** to an end-sigmoid colostomy[Q].

- **Location** of the **colostomy** should **avoid any deep folds of fat**, **scars**, and **bony prominences** of the abdominal wall[Q].

Type by Function
• To **provide decompression of** the **large intestine**[Q]
• To **provide diversion of** the **feces**[Q]

■ STOMAL COMPLICATIONS

- **MC complication** of **both end & loop colostomy**: Parastomal hernia[Q]
- **Parastomal hernia** is **more common in end colostomy**[Q] as compared to loop colostomy.
- **Prolapse is more common in loop colostomy**
- **MC complication of ileostomy**: Skin irritation[Q]
- **MC early complication of ileostomy**: Ischemic necrosis[Q]

Stomal Complications				
	Early (RAPID-O)		**Late (SPF-GO)**	
Stoma	• Poor location • **Retraction*** • **Ischemic necrosis**[Q]	• Detachment • Abscess formation • Opening wrong end	• **Prolapse**[Q] • **Stenosis**[Q] • **Parastomal hernia**[Q]	• **Fistula formation**[Q] • Gas • Odor
Peristomal skin	• **Excoriation**[Q] • **Dermatitis***		• Parastomal varices • Dermatoses	• Cancer • Skin manifestations of IBD
Systemic	• **High output***		• **Bowel obstruction**[Q] • Nonclosure	

- *May also develop as a late complication

ILEOSTOMY AND COLOSTOMY

1. **Most common complication of end colostomy:** *(JIPMER 2011)*
   a. Parastomal hernia
   b. Prolapse
   c. Perforation
   d. Bleeding

2. **Known complication of stoma (e.g., Colostomy stoma):** *(MHPGMCET 2009)*
   a. Prolapse
   b. Stenosis
   c. Retraction
   d. All of the above

3. **Early postoperative complication of ileostomy:** *(AIIMS Nov 2006)*
   a. Obstruction
   b. Prolapse
   c. Diarrhea
   d. Necrosis

4. **Which of the following in a not a recognized complication of colostomy?** *(MHSSMCET 2011)*
   a. Prolapse
   b. Necrosis
   c. Stenosis
   d. Constipation

5. **Early postoperative complication of ileostomy:** *(JIPMER 2014, AIIMS May 2012)*
   a. Obstruction
   b. Prolapse
   c. Diarrhea
   d. Necrosis

6. **Parastomal hernia is most frequently seen with:** *(All India 2009)*
   a. End colostomy
   b. Loop colostomy
   c. End ileostomy
   d. Loop ileostomy

7. **Parastomal hernia is most frequently seen with:** *(Bihar PG 2016)*
   a. End colostomy
   b. Loop colostomy
   c. End ileostomy
   d. Loop ileostomy

8. **Prolapse is more frequently associated with:** *(Recent Question 2016)*
   a. End colostomy
   b. Loop colostomy
   c. End ileostomy
   d. Loop ileostomy

9. **Most common complication of ileostomy is:** *(Recent Question 2016)*
   a. Ischemic necrosis
   b. Skin irritation
   c. Prolapse
   d. Parastomal hernia

10. **Which of the following stoma is formed in Hartman's procedure?** *(Recent Question 2017)*
    a. End colostomy
    b. End ileostomy
    c. Loop ileostomy
    d. Cecostomy

11. **This complication is most commonly seen in which type of stoma?**

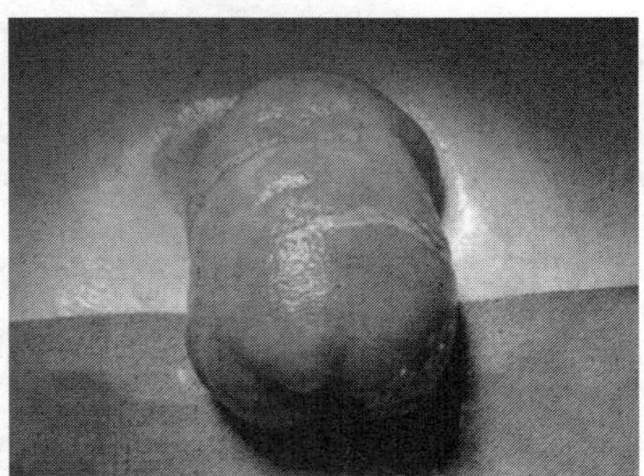

    a. End ileostomy
    b. Loop ileostomy
    c. End colostomy
    d. Loop colostomy

Explanations

ILEOSTOMY AND COLOSTOMY

1. **Ans. a. Parastomal hernia** *(Ref: Sabiston 20/e p1326-1330; Schwartz 11/e p1277, 10/e p1192-1193; Bailey 27/e p1278; Shackelford 8/e p2159; Maingot 11/e p141-148)*

2. **Ans. d. All of the above** *(Ref: Sabiston 20/e p1326-1330; Schwartz 11/e p1277, 10/e p1192-1193; Bailey 27/e p1278; Shackelford 8/e p2157; Maingot 11/e p153-154)*

3. **Ans. d. Necrosis** *(Ref: Sabiston 20/e p1328-1329; Schwartz 11/e p1277, 10/e p1193; Bailey 27/e p1255; Maingot 11/e p164-165)*
   - Schwartz says **"Stoma necrosis** may occur in the **early post-operative period** and usually is **caused by skeletonizing** the **distal small bowel** and/**creating an overly tight fascial defect"**.

4. **Ans. d. Constipation**

5. **Ans. d. Necrosis**

6. **Ans. a. End colostomy**

7. **Ans. a. End colostomy**

8. **Ans. b. Loop colostomy**

9. **Ans. b. Skin irritation**

10. **Ans. a. End colostomy**

11. **Ans. d. Loop colostomy** *(Ref: Sabiston 20/e p310-311; Schwartz 11/e p1277, 10/e p1193; Bailey 27/e p1277; Shackelford 8/e p2160; Maingot 11/e p141-148)*

Inflammatory Bowel Disease

■ CROHN'S DISEASE

CROHN'S DISEASE

- **Chronic, transmural inflammatory disease** of GIT for which the **cause is unknown**[Q].
- Can **involve any part of alimentary tract** from **mouth to anus** but most commonly affects **small intestine & colon**[Q].

  - Involvement of **both large** & **small intestine: 55%**[Q]
  - Involvement of **only small intestine: 30%**[Q]
  - Involvement of **only large intestine: 15%**[Q]

- Crohn's disease primarily **attacks young adults**[Q] in 2nd & 3rd **decades** of life.
- **More common** in smokers & **urban dwellers**[Q] & females taking OCPs
- **Strong familial association**[Q]

  - **Upper GI Crohn's disease** is most frequently found in **gastric antrum** & **duodenum**[Q].
  - In patients with **colonic disease, rectal sparing** is **characteristic**[Q].

Etiology: Unknown

- **Infectious agents** proposed as **potential causes: Mycobacterium paratuberculosis** & **measles virus**[Q].
- The identification of **CARD-15/NOD2 mutation**[Q] (on chromosome **16q,** also known as **IBD-1 locus**) provided the first definitive genetic link to the condition and is **relatively specific** for Crohn's disease.

IBD-1 (chromosome 16q)	Relatively specific for **Crohn's disease**[Q]
IBD-2 (chromosome 12q)	More common in **Ulcerative colitis**[Q]

Pathology

- **Diseased bowel** separated by areas of **grossly appearing normal bowel (skip areas)**[Q]
- **Extensive fat wrapping** caused by **circumferential growth** of **mesenteric fat**[Q] around the bowel wall (creeping fat).
- **Thickened, firm, rubbery,** & almost **incompressible bowel wall**[Q].
- **Involved segments** are **adherent to adjacent intestinal loops** or other viscera, with **internal fistulas**[Q].
- **Mesentery** of the involved segment is **thickened,** with **enlarged lymph nodes**[Q].

  - **Earliest gross pathologic lesion** is a **superficial aphthous ulcer**[Q] noted in the mucosa.

- **Linear ulcers** may coalesce to produce **transverse sinuses** with **islands of normal mucosa** in between **(cobblestone appearance**[Q])
- **Inflammatory reaction** is **characterized by extensive edema, hyperemia**[Q] **lymphangiectasia,** an intense infiltration of mononuclear cells, and **lymphoid hyperplasia**[Q].

  - **Characteristic histologic lesions** of Crohn's disease are **noncaseating granulomas** with **Langerhans' giant cells**[Q].
  - **Granulomas** are found in the **wall of bowel** or in **regional lymph nodes**[Q] in 60-70% of patients

Clinical Features

- **MC symptom** is **intermittent** & **colicky abdominal pain,** most commonly noted in **lower abdomen**[Q].
- **Diarrhea** is the next most frequent symptom and is present, at **least intermittently,** in about 85% of patients.
- In contrast to ulcerative colitis, patients with Crohn's disease **typically have fewer bowel movements,** & **stools rarely contain mucus, pus, or blood**[Q].

  - **Main intestinal complications** of Crohn's disease include **obstruction** & **perforation**[Q].
  - **Fistulas occur between** the **sites of perforation** & **adjacent organs,** usually **at the site of a previous laparotomy**[Q].

- **Long-standing Crohn's disease** predisposes to **cancer of small intestine** & **colon**[Q].
- **Perianal disease (fissure, fistula, stricture, or abscess**[Q]) is common

Contd...

Contd...

> • In **Crohn's disease, ileum** is **MC site** of **fistula (enterocutaneous & enterovesical)**, MC site of **perforation** and MC site of **carcinoma**[Q].

Diagnosis

- **IOC** for **diagnosis** of **Crohn's** disease: **CT Enteroclysis**[Q]
- **Serology:** Anti-Saccharomyces cerevisiae (**ASCA**[Q]) autoantibodies have **specificity of 92%** for **Crohn's disease.**

Radiological Findings of Crohn's Disease	
• **Aphthous ulceration: Earliest radiographic findings** in enteroclysis[Q] • **Deep ulcers**[Q] • **Cobble stone appearance**[Q] • **Fat halo sign**[Q] **on CT**: Low attenuation of submucosal fat around bowel • **Creeping fat sign**[Q]	• **Hose-pipe like appearance**[Q]: Long stricture extending up to ileocecal valve with thickened wall; corresponds to "**String sign of Kantor**"[Q] • **Raspberry thorn** or **rosethorn appearance**[Q]: Linear fissures throughout the bowel • **Comb sign**[Q]: Vascular jejunization of ileum

■ EXTRAINTESTINAL MANIFESTATIONS OF CROHN'S DISEASE

Extraintestinal Manifestations of Crohn's Disease	
• **Skin:** Erythema multiforme, **Erythema nodosum**, Pyoderma gangrenosum • **Eyes:** Iritis, Uveitis, Conjunctivitis • **Blood:** Anemia, **Thrombocytosis, Phlebothrombosis, Arterial thrombosis**	• **Joints: Peripheral arthritis**, Ankylosing spondylitis • **Liver:** Nonspecific triaditis, **Sclerosing cholangitis** • **Kidney: Nephrotic syndrome** • **Pancreas: Pancreatitis** • **General:** Amyloidosis

■ ULCERATIVE COLITIS

ULCERATIVE COLITIS

- UC occurs **more commonly** in developed countries[Q]
- More commonly affects patients **< 30 years; More common in females taking OCPs**
- **More common** in **whites, Jews,** and persons of **northern European ancestry**[Q]

Etiology

- Infectious agents, including **C. difficile & Campylobacter jejuni**[Q], have been implicated as playing a causative role in the pathogenesis, but such a role has not been confirmed.
- A **family history of IBD** is a **significant risk factor**[Q].

> - **Smoking** appears to confer a **protective effect**[Q]
> - Both **UC** and **Crohn's disease** are **more common in women** who **use OCPs**[Q]
> - Patients who have had an **appendectomy** appear to be at **decreased risk for developing UC**[Q].

Pathology

- Major **pathologic process involves mucosa & submucosa** of colon, with **sparing** of the **muscularis**[Q].
- **Typical gross appearance:** Hyperemic mucosa[Q]
- **Rectal involvement (proctitis)** is the **hallmark of disease**[Q], & diagnosis should be seriously questioned if the rectal mucosa is not affected.
- **Pseudopolyps,** or **inflammatory polyps** are seen in UC.
- **Diagnostic characteristic** of UC: **Continuous uninterrupted inflammation** of mucosa, **beginning in distal rectum & extending proximally**[Q] to a variable distance.

> - **Most characteristic lesion of UC: Crypt abscess**[Q] (collections of neutrophils fill & expand the lumina of individual crypts of Lieberkühn)
> - **Crypt abscesses** are **not specific for UC**[Q] and can be seen in Crohn's disease and infectious colitis.

- **Crypt branching** may be seen in **chronic UC** and is an **important characteristic**[Q].
- **Number of goblet cells** in the crypts **is diminished**, as is mucus production.

Clinical Features

- **Diarrhea** with **passage of mucus**[Q]
- **More urgency** than with Crohn's disease, because of **distal proctitis**[Q].
- **Rectal bleeding** is common in UC

Contd...

Contd...

> - **Rectal involvement** is present in almost **100%** of patients with UC, whereas **anal involvement is rare**.
> - **Crohn's disease** may have **normal rectal mucosa** (so-called **rectal sparing**[Q]), although **anal disease** (e.g. **fissures, fistulas, abscesses) is common**[Q].

Laboratory Investigations

- **Increased CRP, ESR & platelet count; Decreased hemoglobin**
- **Fecal lactoferrin**[Q]: **Highly sensitive & specific marker** for detecting **intestinal inflammation**[Q]
- **Fecal calprotectin**[Q] levels **correlate** well **with** histologic **inflammation, predict relapses & detect pouchitis**
- Both **fecal lactoferrin & calprotectin**[Q] are **integral part of management** & to **rule out active inflammation versus symptoms of irritable bowel or bacterial overgrowth**[Q]
- **p-ANCA** is having **92% specificity** for **UC**[Q].

Diagnosis

- In the **acute phase** of UC, **proctosigmoidoscopy** is sufficient because the rectum is invariably inflamed.
- **Colonoscopy**: If patient is **not having acute flare**, colonoscopy is used **to assess** the disease **extent & severity**[Q]
- **Earliest colonoscopic finding: Decreased vascularity** with **erythematous & edematous mucosa**[Q]
- **Disease severity** of UC can be graded by **Modified Truelove** and **Witts Classification**[Q]

Radiology

- **Earliest radiological change: Fine mucosal granularity**[Q]
- **Deep ulceration** appear as **"collar-button" ulcers**[Q] indicating that ulceration has penetrated the mucosa
- **Double contrast barium enema**: Primary radiologic tool **for confirming** the **diagnosis** & assessing the **extent** and **severity** of UC[Q].

End stage or Burned out UC is Characterized Radiographically by	
• **Shortening of colon**[Q] • **Loss of normal redundancy** in **sigmoid** region, at **splenic & hepatic flexures**[Q] • **Featureless mucosa**[Q] • Absence of discrete ulceration	• **Narrow caliber** of bowel[Q] • **Disappearance of haustral pattern**[Q]**/Ahaustral colon**[Q]**/Pipestem colon**[Q]**/Lead pipe sign**[Q]**/Garden hose appearance**[Q]**/Stove pipe appearance**[Q]

- Approximately **15–20%** of patients with **severe UC** have an associated **backwash ileitis**, characterized by a **fixed, patulous ileocecal valve** and a **dilated, granular terminal ileum** on **double contrast barium studies**[Q].

■ EXTRAINTESTINAL MANIFESTATIONS OF ULCERATIVE COLITIS

Extraintestinal Manifestations of Ulcerative Colitis	
• Arthritis • Ankylosing spondylitis • Erythema nodosum	• Pyoderma gangrenosum • Primary sclerosing cholangitis (PSC)

■ SURGICAL OPTIONS FOR ULCERATIVE COLITIS

Indications of Surgery in Ulcerative Colitis	
• **Intractability**[Q] • Dysplasia, **carcinoma**[Q]	• **Massive colonic bleeding**[Q] • **Toxic megacolon**[Q]

Surgical Options for Ulcerative Colitis	
• Total proctocolectomy with ileostomy • Restorative proctocolectomy with IPAA[Q] • Total proctocolectomy with a continent ileal reservoir (Kock pouch)[Q]	• Total abdominal colectomy with end-ileostomy

Indications of Surgical Options in Ulcerative Colitis
Total Proctocolectomy with End Ileostomy   • Total proctocolectomy has the advantage of removing all diseased mucosa, thereby preventing further inflammation and the potential for progression to dysplasia or carcinoma[Q].   • **Major disadvantage:** Need for a **permanent ileostomy**   • **Older patients**, those with **poor sphincter function**, and patients with **carcinomas in the distal rectum** may be candidates for this procedure[Q].

Contd...

Contd...

Total Proctocolectomy with Continent Ileostomy

- **Major problem with the Kock pouch** is the **high complication rate** necessitating **reoperation** in up to **50%** of patients[Q].
- **MC problem** is a **slipped valve**, which occurs when the intussuscepted limb everts and the continent nipple is lost.
- Procedure is **contraindicated in** patients with **Crohn's disease** because of **high incidence of its recurrence**, causing failure of pouch.

Total Proctocolectomy with Ileal Pouch-Anal Anastomosis (IPAA)

- Restorative proctocolectomy with IPAA has become the most common definitive operation for the surgical treatment of UC.

Complications of Total Proctocolectomy With IPAA	
• **Pouchitis** (7–33%)[Q]	• Anastomotic and pouch suture line **leaks**
• **Small bowel obstruction** (up to 27%)	• **Pouch-vaginal fistula**
• Pelvic sepsis	

■ DIFFERENCES BETWEEN CROHN'S DISEASE & ULCERATIVE COLITIS

Feature	Crohn's Disease	Ulcerative Colitis
A. Macroscopic features		
1. Distribution	Segmental with **skip areas**[Q]	**Continuous** without skip areas[Q]
2. Location	Commonly **terminal ileum** and/or **ascending colon**	Commonly **rectum,** sigmoid colon and extending upwards
3. Extent	Usually involves the **entire thickness** of the affected segment of bowel wall	Usually **superficial,** confined to mucosal layers
4. Ulcers	**Serpiginous ulcers**, that may develop into deep **Fissures**[Q]	**Superficial mucosal ulcers** without fissures
5. **Pseudopolyps**	Rarely seen	Commonly present[Q]
6. Fibrosis	Common	Rare
7. Shortening	Due to fibrosis	Due to contraction of muscularis
B. Microscopic features		
1. Depth of inflammation	Typically **transmural**[Q]	Mucosal[Q] and Submucosal
2. Type of inflammation	**Non-caseating granulomas**[Q] and infiltrate of mononuclear cells (lymphocytes, plasma cells and macrophage)	**Crypt abscess** and non-specific acute and chronic inflammatory cells (lymphocytes, plasma cells neutrophils, eosinophils, mast cells)
3. Mucosa	Patchy ulceration	Hemorrhagic mucosa with ulceration
4. Submucosa	Widened due to edema and lymphoid aggregates	Normal or reduced in width
5. Muscularis	Infiltrated by inflammatory cells	Usually spared, except in cases of **Toxic Megacolon**[Q]
6. Fibrosis	Present	Usually absent
C. Complications		
1. **Fistula formation**	**Internal** and **external fistulae** in 10% case	Extremely **rare**[Q]
2. Malignant changes	Less common but present	May occur in disease of more than 10 years duration (**more common**[Q])
3. **Fibrous strictures**	Common[Q]	Never[Q]
4. **Toxic megacolon**	–	Risk present[Q]
5. Named Features	**String Has CRF**	**GPL Stove Collar Button**
	• **S**tring sign of Kantor[Q]	• **G**arden hose appearance[Q]
	• **H**ose pipe appearance[Q]	• **P**ipestem colon[Q]
	• **C**reeping fat sign[Q]	• **L**ead pipe sign[Q]
	• **C**omb sign[Q]	• **Stove** pipe appearance[Q]
	• **R**aspberry thorn appearance[Q] or **R**osethorn appearance[Q]	• **Collar button** ulcer[Q]
	• **F**at halo sign on CT[Q]	

Remember

- **Earliest change** in Crohn's disease is Apthoid ulceration[Q].
- **Earliest Change** in Ulcerative colitis is Blurring of mucosal stripe and granular appearance[Q].
- **Surgery** is palliative in **Crohn's disease**[Q] whereas **curative in ulcerative colitis**[Q].
- Risk of **carcinoma colon: UC = CD**[Q]
- Risk of **small intestinal malignancies: CD > UC**[Q]
- Risk of **cholangiocarcinoma: UC > CD**[Q]

Multiple Choice Questions

■ INFLAMMATORY BOWEL DISEASE

1. **Crohn's disease can be seen in:** *(COMEDK 2007)*
   a. Jejunum only
   b. Colon only
   c. Terminal ileum and right side
   d. Mouth to anus

2. **Cobble stone appearance is seen in:**
   (Kerala PG 2015, COMEDK 2008, 2007)
   a. Ulcerative colitis
   b. Crohn's disease
   c. Appendicitis
   d. Carcinoma rectum

3. **String sign of Kantor seen in:** *(APPG 2008)*
   a. Crohn's disease
   b. Ulcerative colitis
   c. Both of the above
   d. None of the above

4. **True statement regarding anorectal Crohn's disease:**
   a. Ulceration, fistula is common
   b. Fistulas are painless and indurated
   c. Non-cutting setons are used in management
   d. All of the above

5. **Ulcerative colitis starts from:** *(GB Pant 2011)*
   a. Rectum
   b. Sigmoid colon
   c. Ascending colon
   d. Any part

6. **Skip lesions are seen in:**
   (Recent Question 2016, AIIMS May 2009)
   a. Ulcerative colitis
   b. Typhoid
   c. Crohn's disease
   d. Tuberculosis

7. **A patient gives chronic history of diarrhea and blood in stool presents with multiple fistulae in the perineum and multiple stricture in small intestine. The diagnosis is:**
   (AIIMS June 2000)
   a. In Crohn's disease
   b. Radiation enteritis
   c. Ulcerative colitis
   d. Ischemic bowel disease

8. **Histological difference between Ulcerative colitis and Crohn's disease is presence of:** *(Recent Question 2019)*
   a. Crypt abscess
   b. Diffuse distribution of pseudopolyps
   c. Mucosal edema
   d. Lymphoid aggregates in the mucosa

9. **In a 27 years old male, most common cause of a colovesical fistula would be:** *(All India 2001, 99)*
   a. Crohn's disease
   b. Ulcerative colitis
   c. TB
   d. Cancer colon

10. **The commonest site of involvement in the Crohn's disease is:** *(COMEDK 2005)*
    a. Jejunum
    b. Transverse colon
    c. Terminal ileum
    d. Rectum

11. **Crohn's disease is associated with:** *(COMEDK 2011)*
    a. NOD2/CARD-15 gene
    b. P53 suppressor gene
    c. Philadelphia chromosomes
    d. BRAC-1 gene

12. **Following statements regarding ulcerative colitis is true:**
    a. Smoking has a protecting effect *(COMEDK 2011)*
    b. Smoking does not have a protective effect
    c. There is no relation to smoking
    d. Smoking causes relapses

13. **Skip lesions are characteristic of:**
    (Recent Question 2016, JIPMER 2010)
    a. Typhoid
    b. Ischemic bowel disease
    c. Ulcerative colitis
    d. Crohn's disease

14. **Hose pipe appearance of intestine is a feature of:**
    (Recent Question 2013)
    a. Crohn's disease
    b. Malabsorption syndrome
    c. Ulcerative colitis
    d. Hirschsprung's disease

15. **Earliest gross pathologic lesion seen in Crohn's Disease:**
    (Recent Question 2018)
    a. Apthous ulcer
    b. Creeping fat
    c. Enlarged lymph nodes
    d. Strictures

16. **Which of the following is true about ulcerative colitis?**
    (Recent Question 2018)
    a. 20% end up in surgery in 1 year of diagnosis
    b. Extra intestinal problems are managed medically
    c. Steroid dependent cases need surgery
    d. Surgery is palliative in ulcerative colitis

17. **Which of the following statement is not true regarding Crohn's disease?** *(Recent Question 2018)*
    a. Rectum is not involved
    b. Continuous lesion visualized in endoscopy
    c. Noncaseating granulomas
    d. Cobblestone appearance

18. **True about Crohn's disease except:** *(MCI Dec 2019)*
    a. Recurrence is more common
    b. Rectum is involved
    c. Fissures are formed
    d. Transmural

19. **Which of the following is false about Crohn's disease?**
    a. No recurrence after surgery *(MCI Dec 2018)*
    b. Aphthous ulcer
    c. Skip lesions
    d. Fistula formation

■ IBD EXTRAINTESTINAL MANIFESTATIONS

20. **Pyoderma-gangrenosum is most commonly associated with:**
    (All India 99)
    a. Ulcerative colitis
    b. Crohn's disease
    c. Amoebic colitis
    d. Ischemic colitis

21. **The following are complications of ulcerative colitis except:**
    a. Peptic ulceration
    b. Arthritis *(All India 90)*
    c. Sclerosing cholangitis
    d. Toxic megacolon

22. **Type of renal stone formed in a patient with regional enteritis:** *(JIPMER 2011)*
    a. Calcium oxalate
    b. Cysteine
    c. Struvite
    d. Urate

23. **Most common stones in ulcerative colitis:** *(DPG 2007)*
    a. Oxalate
    b. Cysteine
    c. Uric acid
    d. Phosphate

■ IBD TREATMENT

24. **Treatment of choice in case of chronic ulcerative colitis is:**
    a. Colectomy with ileostomy *(AIIMS June 95)*
    b. Colectomy + manual proctectomy + ileoanal pouch anastomosis
    c. Proctocolectomy with ileoanal anastomosis
    d. Ileorectal anastomosis

25. **Sulfasalazine exerts its primary action in ulcerative colitis by inhibition of:** *(COMEDK 2004)*
    a. Folic acid synthesis
    b. Formation of prostaglandins (PG)
    c. Phospholipase C
    d. Formation of interleukins

26. **Procedure of choice in ulcerative colitis with acute perforation is:** *(Recent Question 2016)*
    a. Defunctioning ileostomy
    b. Closure of perforation
    c. Proximal diversion colostomy
    d. Total colectomy and ileostomy

27. **True statement regarding management of ileocaecal Crohn's disease is:** *(JIPMER, 2014, 2007)*
    a. Avoid antibiotics
    b. Avoid steroids in first week
    c. 5-ASA reduces small bowel obstruction
    d. Cholestyramine improves diarrhea, worsens steatorrhea

■ COLITIS ASSOCIATED CARCINOMA

28. **False about malignancy in ulcerative colitis:**
    a. Poorly differentiated with higher stage *(AIIMS GIS 2003)*
    b. Related to extent of disease
    c. Poor prognosis as compared to sporadic
    d. Evenly distributed

29. **Surgery is indicated in Ulcerative colitis in all except:**
    (MCI Dec 2018)
    a. Toxic megacolon
    b. Colonic polyp
    c. Colonic obstruction
    d. Refractory fistula

30. **All are true about colonic cancer in UC except:**
    a. In younger patients *(AIIMS GIS Dec 2010)*
    b. Depends upon duration of disease
    c. Depends on extent of UC in colon
    d. Risk of cancer irrespective of grade of dysplasia

■ IBD COMPLICATIONS

31. **Toxic megacolon is seen in:** *(COMEDK 2009)*
    a. Carcinoma colon
    b. Gastrocolic fistula
    c. Ulcerative colitis
    d. Amoebic colitis

32. **Treatment of choice in toxic megacolon:** *(MHSSMCET 2005)*
    a. Total colectomy
    b. Segmental resection
    c. Colostomy
    d. Clindamycin, Metronidazole, Steroids

33. **Toxic megacolon is seen in:** *(Orissa 2011)*
    a. Crohn's disease
    b. Ulcerative colitis
    c. Diverticulosis
    d. All of the above

34. **Most common cause of death in Crohn's disease is due to:**
    a. Sepsis *(AIIMS May 2009)*
    b. Thromboembolic complication
    c. Electrolyte disturbance
    d. Malignancy

35. **Most common postoperative complication of IPAA in ulcerative colitis is:** *(AIIMS Nov 2011)*
    a. Pouchitis
    b. Pelvic abscess
    c. Small bowel obstruction
    d. Perianal complications

Explanations

■ INFLAMMATORY BOWEL DISEASE

1. **Ans. d. Mouth to anus** (*Ref: Sabiston 20/e p1254; Schwartz 11/e p1285, 10/e p1153-1157; Bailey 27/e p1242-1243; Shackelford 8/e p865*)
2. **Ans. b. Crohn's disease**
3. **Ans. a. Crohn's disease**
4. **Ans. d. All of the above** (*Ref: Sabiston 20/e p1411; Schwartz 11/e p1283, 10/e p1153-1157; Bailey 27/e p1242-1243; Shackelford 8/e p865*)
5. **Ans. a. Rectum**
6. **Ans. c. Crohn's disease**
7. **Ans. a. In Crohn's disease**
8. **Ans. a. Crypt abscess** (*Ref: Sabiston 20/e p1340*)

> • *"The typical microscopic finding in ulcerative colitis is inflammation of the mucosa and submucosa. The most characteristic lesion is the crypt abscess, in which collections of neutrophils fill and expand the lumina of individual crypts of Lieberkühn."*
> — *Sabiston 20/e p1340*

9. **Ans. a. Crohn's disease** (*Ref: Sabiston 20/e p1350; Smith 17/e p581*)

COMMON CAUSES OF COLOVESICAL FISTULA

- **Diverticulitis (50–60%** More common in patients **> 40 years**[Q]
- **CA colon (20–25%** More common in patients **> 50 years**[Q]
- **Crohn's disease 10%** Seen in **2nd** to **3rd decade**[Q]

10. **Ans. c. Terminal ileum**
11. **Ans. a. NOD2/CARD-15 gene**
12. **Ans. a. Smoking has a protecting effect**
13. **Ans. d. Crohn's disease**
14. **Ans. a. Crohn's disease**
15. **Ans. a. Apthous ulcer** (*Ref: Sabiston 20/e p1350; Schwartz 11/e p1283, 10/e p1153; Bailey 27/e p1243*)

> • *"The earliest lesion characteristic of Crohn's disease is the aphthous ulcer."* Schwartz 11/e p1283, 10/e p1153

16. **Ans. b. Extra intestinal problems are managed medically** (*Ref: Sabiston 20/e p1341; Schwartz 11/e p1283, 10/e p1196; Bailey 27/e p1267*)
17. **Ans. b. Continuous lesion visualized in endoscopy**
18. **Ans. b. Rectum is involved** (*Ref: Bailey 27/e p1272*)
19. **Ans. a. No recurrence after surgery** (*Ref: Bailey 27/e p1246, 1247*)

■ IBD EXTRAINTESTINAL MANIFESTATIONS

20. **Ans. a. Ulcerative colitis**
21. **Ans. a. Peptic ulceration**
22. **Ans. a. Calcium oxalate**
23. **Ans. a. Oxalate** (*Ref: Harrison 20/e p2269*)

UROLOGIC MANIFESTATIONS OF IBD

- The **most frequent genitourinary complications** are calculi, ureteral obstruction, and **ileal bladder fistulas**[Q].
- **Calcium oxalate stones** develop **secondary to hyperoxaluria,** which results from **increased absorption of dietary oxalate**[Q].
- Normally, dietary calcium combines with luminal oxalate to form insoluble calcium oxalate, which is eliminated in the stool.
- In patients with **ileal dysfunction, nonabsorbed fatty acids bind calcium** and **leave oxalate unbound**[Q].
- The **unbound oxalate** is then **delivered to the colon,** where it is **readily absorbed,** especially **in the presence of inflammation**[Q].

■ IBD TREATMENT

24. **Ans. c. Proctocolectomy with ileonal anastomosis** (*Ref: Sabiston 20/e p1344; Schwartz 11/e p1283, 10/e p1187-1188; Bailey 27/e p1269; Shackelford 8/e p1919*)

Indications of Surgery in Ulcerative Colitis	
• **Intractability**[Q]	• **Massive colonic bleeding**[Q]
• Dysplasia, **carcinoma**[Q]	• **Toxic megacolon**[Q]

- Older patients or those with fecal incontinence should undergo a total proctocolectomy with an end ileostomy.
- Younger patients with no evidence of rectal dysplasia should undergo restorative proctocolectomy and IPAA with a double-stapled anastomosis and diverting loop ileostomy.
- Patients with confirmed rectal dysplasia should be treated with mucosectomy and a hand-sewn IPAA.
- Patients with significant debility who are poor operative candidates should undergo a total abdominal colectomy with a very low Hartmann closure and an end ileostomy.

25. **Ans. b. Formation of prostaglandins (PG)** *(Ref: Harrison 20/e p2270; Shackelford 8/e p1896)*

- **5-ASA** compounds exert its local anti-inflammatory effect by **inhibiting leukotriene production (PG synthesis)** by **inhibition of 5-lipooxygenase activity;** also inhibits the **production of IL-1 and TNF**[Q]

Commonly Used 5-ASA Formulations in IBD
• **Sulfasalazine**
• Oral **mesalamine** agents
• Azo compounds: **Balsalazide, Olsalazine**

26. **Ans. d. Total colectomy and ileostomy**

27. **Ans. c. 5-ASA reduces small bowel obstruction**

■ COLITIS ASSOCIATED CARCINOMA

28. **Ans. c. Poor prognosis as compared to sporadic**

29. **Ans. b. Colonic polyp** *(Ref: Bailey 27/e p1257, 1269)*

30. **Ans. d. Risk of cancer irrespective of grade of dysplasia**

■ IBD COMPLICATIONS

31. **Ans. c. Ulcerative colitis** *(Ref: Sabiston 20/e p1344; Schwartz 11/e p1282, 10/e p1195,1198,1199; Bailey 27/e p1267; Shackelford 8/e p1919)*

TOXIC MEGACOLON

- Toxic megacolon is a **serious life-threatening condition** that can occur in patients with **ulcerative colitis, Crohn's colitis,** and **infectious colitides** such as **pseudomembranous colitis**[Q]
- This **decompensation** results in a **necrotic thin-walled bowel** in which **pneumatosis**[Q] can often be seen radiographically.

Management
- **Medical treatment** is associated with a **high rate of recurrence** with subsequent **urgent operation**[Q] has been reported.
- **Aggressive preoperative stabilization** is required, using **volume resuscitation** with **crystalloid solutions** to prevent dehydration secondary to third-space fluid losses, stress-dose steroids for patients previously on steroid therapy, **and broad-spectrum antibiotics**[Q].

- **Total abdominal colectomy** with **ileostomy** and preservation of the rectum is **treatment of choice** for **toxic megacolon**[Q].
- It serves the **main purpose of removing the diseased colon** and **avoiding a difficult** and **morbid pelvic dissection**[Q].

32. **Ans. a. Total colectomy**

33. **Ans. b. Ulcerative colitis a. Crohn's disease**

34. **Ans. d. Malignancy** *(Ref: Sabiston 20/e p1265, 1352)*

- Long-term survival studies have suggested that patients with **Crohn's disease** have a **death rate** that is about **two to three times higher** than that in the general population.
- **Gastrointestinal cancer**[Q] remains the **leading cause of disease-related death** in patients with **Crohn's disease; other causes** of disease-related deaths include **sepsis, thromboembolic complications,** and **electrolyte disorders.**

35. **Ans. a. Pouchitis**

Vermiform Appendix

■ ACUTE APPENDICITIS

ACUTE APPENDICITIS

- Acute appendicitis is the MC general surgical emergency[Q]

Pathophysiology

- Obstruction of the lumen[Q] is believed to be the **major cause** of acute appendicitis[Q].
- Obstruction of the lumen may be **caused by inspissated stool** (fecalith[Q] or appendicolith[Q]), **lymphoid hyperplasia**[Q], **vegetable matter or seeds**[Q], **parasites**, or a **neoplasm**[Q].

Bacteriology

- MC bacteria isolated in **perforated appendicitis**: Bacteroides fragilis (80%) > E. coli (77%)[Q].

Clinical Features

- **Diagnosis** can be **made primarily** on the basis of the **history** & **physical examination** in **most cases**.
- **Typical presentation**: Periumbilical pain followed by anorexia & nausea.

> - The **pain** then **localizes to** the **right lower quadrant** as the inflammatory process progresses to involve the parietal peritoneum overlying the appendix.
> - This **classic pattern of migratory pain** is the **most reliable symptom of acute appendicitis**.
> - A **bout of vomiting** may occur. **Fever ensues, followed by** the development of **leukocytosis**.
> - **Occasional patients** have **urinary symptoms** or **microscopic hematuria**

- **Tenderness** is **directly over** the appendix, at **McBurney's point**.
- **Rectal** & **pelvic examinations** are **most likely** to be **negative** (Tenderness on examination in pelvic appendix)

Dunphy's sign[Q]	• **Pain on coughing**[Q]
Rovsing's sign[Q]	• **Pain in** the **right lower quadrant** during **palpation of** the **left lower quadrant**[Q]
Ten Horn sign	• Pain on gentle traction of right testis
Obturator sign[Q]	• **Pain on internal rotation of** the **hip**[Q] • Suggestive of **pelvic appendix**[Q]
Iliopsoas sign[Q]	• **Pain on extension** of the **right hip**[Q] • Suggestive of **retrocecal appendix**[Q]

Diagnosis

- IOC for diagnosis of acute appendicitis in children: USG[Q]
- Gold standard for diagnosis of acute appendicitis: CECT[Q]

Laboratory Studies

- **WBC count** is **elevated**, with **more than 75% neutrophils** in most patients[Q].
- **High WBC count (>20,000/mL)** suggests **complicated appendicitis** with **gangrene** or **perforation**[Q].
- **Microscopic hematuria** is **common in appendicitis** (**gross hematuria** may **indicate** the presence of a **kidney stone**)[Q]

Treatment

- Most patients are managed by prompt **appendectomy**[Q].

■ ALVARADO (MANTRELS) SCORES

Alvarado (MANTRELS) scores		
	Manifestations	**Score**
Symptoms	• Migratory RIF pain • Anorexia • Nausea and vomiting	1 1 1
Signs	• Tenderness (RIF) • Rebound tenderness • Elevated temperature	2 1 1
Laboratory	• Leuocytosis • Shift to left	2 1
	Total	10

Scores	Prediction
9–10	**Appendicitis** is **certain**
7–8	**High likelihood** of appendicitis
5–6	**Equivocal**
1–4	Appendicitis can be **ruled out**

- **CT scanning** is **appropriate for making diagnosis in** patients with **Alvarado scores** of 5 and 6 (in **equivocal cases**)[Q].

■ MANAGEMENT OF ACUTE APPENDICITIS

MANAGEMENT OF ACUTE APPENDICITIS

- Most patients are managed by **prompt surgical removal of** the **appendix**[Q].
- A **brief period of resuscitation**[Q] is usually sufficient to ensure the safe induction of general anesthesia.
- **Preoperative antibiotics**[Q] cover aerobic and anaerobic colonic flora.
- **Single** preoperative **dose of antibiotics** in **nonperforated appendicitis reduces postoperative wound infections** and **intra-abdominal abscess** formation[Q].
- **Perforated** or **gangrenous appendicitis:** Continue **postoperative IV antibiotics until** the **patient is** afebrile[Q].

> - **Appendectomies** are performed **laparoscopically,** particularly **in fertile women, obese patients,** and cases of **diagnostic uncertainty**[Q].
> - **Open appendectomy** is usually performed through a **transverse right lower quadrant incision (Davis-Rockey)** or an **oblique incision (McArthur-McBurney)**[Q].
> - For **uncomplicated cases,** a **transverse, muscle-splitting incision** lateral to the rectus abdominis muscle **over McBurney's point is preferred**[Q].

■ OCHSNER-SHERREN REGIME

MANAGEMENT OF APPENDICULAR MASS

- If an **appendix mass** is present and the **condition of the patient** is **satisfactory,** standard treatment is the **conservative Ochsner-Sherren regimen**[Q].
- This strategy is based on the premise that **inflammatory process** is **already localized** and that **inadvertent surgery is difficult**[Q] and **may be dangerous**. It may be impossible to find the appendix and, a **fecal fistula** may form.
- For these reasons, it is wise to observe a non-operative programme but to be prepared to operate should clinical deterioration occur.

> - **CECT abdomen** should be performed & **antibiotic therapy** (Metronidazole + 3rd generation cephalosporin or **single dose of ertapenem**) should be given[Q].
> - An **abscess**, if present, should be **drained radiologically**[Q].

- **Temperature & pulse rate** should be recorded **4-hourly** and a **fluid balance** record maintained.
- **Clinical deterioration** or **evidence of peritonitis** is an **indication for early laparotomy**[Q].

> - **Clinical improvement** is usually evident **within 24-48 hours**[Q].
> - **Failure of the mass to resolve** should raise **suspicion of a carcinoma** or **Crohn's disease**[Q].

- Using this regimen, approximately **90% of cases resolve without incident**.
- The **great majority of patients will not develop recurrence**, and it is **no longer considered advisable to remove** the **appendix** after an interval of 6–8 weeks[Q].

Criteria for stopping conservative treatment of an appendix mass		
• A **rising pulse rate**[Q]	• **Increasing** or **spreading abdominal pain**[Q]	• **Increasing size of** the **mass**[Q]

■ APPENDICULAR PERFORATION

APPENDICULAR PERFORATION

- **Immediate appendectomy** has long been the **recommended treatment** for acute appendicitis because of the presumed **risk of progression to rupture**[Q].
- The **overall rate of perforated appendicitis** is **25.8%**.
- **Children <5 years**[Q] of age and **patients > 65 years**[Q] of age have the **highest rates of perforation** (45 & 51%, respectively).

Risk Factors for Appendicular Perforation (Fecolith DIE in Pelvic Surgery)	
• **Fecalith**[Q]	• **Extremes of ages**[Q]
• Diabetes mellitus[Q]	• **Pelvic** appendix[Q]
• Immunosuppression[Q]	• Previous abdominal **surgery**[Q]

- It has been suggested that **delays in presentation** are **responsible for the majority of perforated appendices**[Q].
- **Appendiceal rupture** occurs **most frequently distal to** the **point of luminal obstruction along the antimesenteric border** of the appendix[Q].

> - **Rupture should be suspected** in the presence of **fever** with a **temperature of >39°C (102°F)** and a **WBC count of > 18,000 cells/mm³**.
> - **MC bacteria isolated** in perforated appendicitis: Bacteroides fragilis (80%) > E. coli (77%)[Q].

■ APPENDICEAL CARCINOID

APPENDICEAL CARCINOID

- **Appearance: Firm, yellow, bulbar mass** in the **appendix**[Q]
- **Majority of carcinoids** are **located in the tip**[Q] of the appendix.
- Carcinoid tumors **usually present with localized disease** (64%)[Q].

Clinical Features

- **Carcinoid syndrome** is **rarely associated**[Q] with appendiceal carcinoid unless widespread metastases are present.
- **Symptoms attributable directly to** the carcinoid are **rare**[Q]
- **Malignant potential is related to size**, with **tumors < 1 cm rarely resulting in extension outside of** the **appendix**[Q] or adjacent to the mass.

Treatment of Appendiceal Carcinoid	
Size	**Treatment option**
Up to 1 cm	• Appendectomy[Q]
> 1–2 cm	• **Appendectomy if located at tip or mid-appendix** • **Right hemicolectomy** if: – **Located at base**[Q] – **Invading mesoappendix**[Q] – **LN involvement**[Q]
> 2 cm	• **Right hemicolectomy**[Q]

■ APPENDECTOMY

CONVENTIONAL APPENDECTOMY

- When the preoperative diagnosis is considered reasonably certain, the incision that is widely used for appendectomy is the so called **gridiron incision** (gridiron: a **frame of cross-beams** to **support a ship** during repairs)[Q].

> - **Gridiron incision** (described first by McArthur[Q]) is **made at right angles** to a **line joining** the **anterior superior iliac spine** to the **umbilicus, its centre being along** the line at McBurney's point[Q].

- If **better access** is required, it is possible to **convert** the **gridiron to a Rutherford Morison incision**[Q] by **cutting** the **internal oblique** and **transversus muscles** in the line of the incision.

> - In recent years, a **transverse skin crease (Lanz**[Q]**)** incision has become **more popular**, as the **exposure is better** and **extension**, when needed, **is easier**.
> - **Lanz incision** is also known as: Modified McBurney incision/ Rocky Davis incision/ Bikini incision.
> - The **incision**, appropriate in length to the size and obesity of the patient, is made approximately **2 cm below** the **umbilicus centred on** the **mid-clavicular-midinguinal line**.
> - It is a **muscle splitting incision**[Q] along the **direction of fibers**.

Contd…

Contd…

- When the **diagnosis is in doubt**, particularly in the **presence of intestinal obstruction**, a **lower midline abdominal incision**[Q] is to be **preferred** over a right lower paramedian incision.
  - **Rutherford Morison's incision** is **useful if** the **appendix** is **para** or **retrocaecal & fixed**[Q].
  - It is **essentially an oblique muscle-cutting incision** with its **lower end over McBurney's point & extending obliquely upwards** and **laterally** as necessary. All layers are divided in the line of the incision[Q].

■ STEPS OF APPENDECTOMY

<table>
<tr><th>STEPS OF APPENDECTOMY</th></tr>
</table>

- **Cecum** is identified by the **presence of taeniae coli**, a turgid **appendix** may be **felt at the base** of the cecum[Q].
- **Base of** the **mesoappendix** is **clamped in artery forceps, divided** and **ligated**[Q].
- **Appendix** is **crushed near its junction with** the **cecum** in artery forceps, which is removed and reapplied just distal to the crushed portion[Q].
- An **absorbable ligature** is **tied around** the **crushed portion** close to the cecum[Q].
- **Appendix** is **amputated** between the artery forceps and the ligature.
- An **absorbable purse-string** or **'Z' suture** may then be **inserted into** the **cecum** about 1.25 cm from the base[Q].
- **Stump** of the appendix **is invaginated while** the **purse-string** or **'Z' suture is tied**, thus burying the appendix stump[Q].
- Many surgeons believe **invagination** of the appendiceal stump **is unnecessary**[Q].

Methods to be adopted in special circumstances	
Edematous and **inflamed cecal wall**	• **Purse string suture** is **not applied**[Q] • **Stump** is **not invaginated**[Q]
Inflamed base of appendix	• **Base** is **not crushed** for the fear of spread of infection by way of lymphatics and blood stream[Q]. • **Base** is **ligated close to the cecal wall**[Q], after which the appendix is amputated and the stump invaginated.
Gangrenous base of appendix	• **Neither crushing nor ligation**[Q] • Two **stitches** are **placed through** the **cecal wall close to the base** of the gangrenous appendix, which is **amputated flush with** the **cecal wall**[Q], after which these stitches are tied. **Further closure** is effected by means of a **second layer** of **interrupted seromuscular sutures**[Q].

■ COMPLICATIONS OF APPENDECTOMY

Complications of Appendectomy	

• **Wound infection: MC postoperative complication**[Q] (in **5-10%** of all patients).
 • **Intra-abdominal abscess**[Q]
 • **Ileus**[Q]
 • **Respiratory** complications (rare)[Q]
 • **Venous thrombosis** and **embolism**
 • **Portal pyaemia** (pylephlebitis)
 • **Adhesive intestinal obstruction:**
   – **MC late complication** of appendectomy[Q].
   – At operation, a **single band adhesion** is often **found to be responsible**[Q].
	• **Fecal fistula**[Q]
	   – **Leakage from** the **appendicular stump** occurs **rarely**, but may follow if the **encircling stitch** has been **put in too deeply** or if the **cecal wall was involved by edema** or **inflammation**[Q].
	   – Occasionally, a **fistula may result following appendicectomy** in **Crohn's disease**[Q].
	   – **Conservative management** with **low-residue enteral nutrition** will usually **result in closure**[Q].

■ ANATOMY OF APPENDIX

<table>
<tr><th>ANATOMY OF APPENDIX</th></tr>
</table>

- **Appendix, ileum,** and **ascending colon** are all **derived from** the **midgut**[Q].
- **Appendiceal artery (end artery)**, a **branch of** the **ileocolic artery**, supplies the appendix[Q].
- **Length: 2–20 cm** (average length is 9 cm in adults)[Q].
- **Base** of the appendix is **located at the convergence of the taeniae along** the **inferior aspect of** the **cecum**[Q]
- **MC location: Retrocecal**[Q]
- **Least common location: Post-ileal**[Q]

■ ACUTE APPENDICITIS

1. **Most dangerous position of appendix is:**
   (Recent Question 2015)
   - a. Retrocecal
   - b. Paracolic
   - c. Pelvic
   - d. Retroperitoneal

2. **In a case of retrocecal appendicitis which movement aggravates pain?** *(AIIMS Nov 2007)*
   - a. Flexion
   - b. Extension
   - c. Medial rotation
   - d. Lateral rotation

3. **Earliest symptoms in acute appendicitis is:** *(DNB 2003)*
   - a. Pain
   - b. Fever
   - c. Vomiting
   - d. Rise of pulse rate

4. **A patient with Crohn's disease was opened and an inflamed appendix found. The treatment of choice is:**
   - a. Appendectomy *(Recent Question 2016)*
   - b. Ileocolic resection and anastomosis
   - c. Close the abdomen and start medical treatment
   - d. None of the above

5. **When the rectum is inflated with air through a rectal tube, pain and tenderness occur in the right iliac fossa in case of appendicitis? This is known as:** *(Recent Question 2014)*
   - a. Aaron's sign
   - b. Battle's sign
   - c. Bastedo sign
   - d. MC Burney's sign

6. **The frequent mechanism in perforation of appendix is:**
   - a. Impacted faecolith *(DNB 89, 91)*
   - b. Tension gangrene due to the accumulating secretions
   - c. Necrosis of lymphoid patch
   - d. Retrocaecal infection

7. **Diffuse peritonitis following appendicitis is usually seen:**
   (Recent Question 2013, ICS 2000)
   - a. When appendicular perforation occurs early (within 24 hours)
   - b. When perforation occurs late (after 24 hours)
   - c. Particularly in non-obstructive appendicitis
   - d. When antibiotics are withheld

8. **False about appendicitis in children:** *(JIPMER 2011)*
   - a. Localized pain is the single most important symptom
   - b. Vomiting precedes abdominal pain
   - c. Perforation occurs in 80% of cases <5 years
   - d. 60% perforation occurs within 48 hours

9. **Which of the following clinical signs is not associated with acute appendicitis?** *(MHPGMCET 2009)*
   - a. Pointing sign
   - b. Rovsing's sign
   - c. Cullen's sign
   - d. Obturator sign

10. **"Ten horn" sign is a feature of:** *(MHSSMCET 2011)*
    - a. Rectus muscle hematoma
    - b. Acute pancreatitis
    - c. Choledocholithiasis
    - d. Acute appendicitis

11. **Alvarado scale is for:**
    (Recent Question 2017, DNB 2012, MHSSMCET 2011)
    - a. Diverticulitis
    - b. Mesenteric lymphadenitis
    - c. Acute appendicitis
    - d. Pelvic abscess

12. **From the surgery done below, name the scoring used to diagnose this condition:** *(Recent Question 2018)*

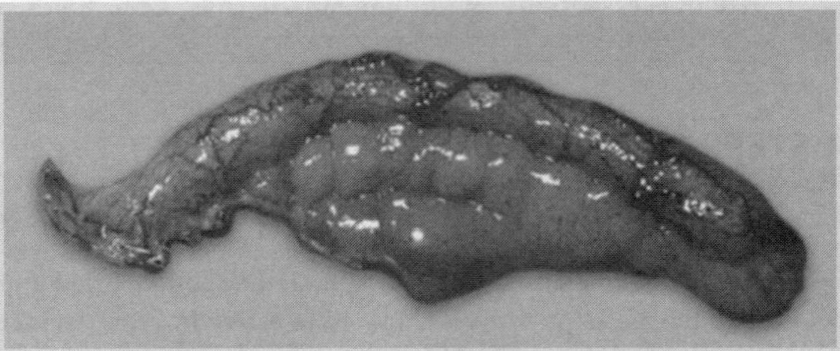

   - a. Alvarado
   - b. Ranson
   - c. Apache-II
   - d. BISAP

13. **Alvarado score consists of:** *(Recent Question 2013)*
    - a. Leucopenia
    - b. Anorexia
    - c. Diarrhea
    - d. Periumbilical pain

14. **Which of the following has score of 2 in ALVARADO score?**
    (MCI Dec 2019)
    - a. Temperature
    - b. Leukocytosis
    - c. Tenderness in left iliac fossa
    - d. Migratory pain

15. **Most common differential diagnosis for appendicitis:**
    (Recent Question 2013)
    - a. Gastroenteritis
    - b. Mesenteric lymphadenopathy
    - c. Intussusception
    - d. Meckel's diverticulitis

16. **Investigation of choice for acute appendicitis in children:**
    (AIIMS May 2015, Nov 2014, May 2013)
    - a. CT scan
    - b. Ultrasound
    - c. MRI
    - d. X-ray

■ APPENDICITIS IN PREGNANCY

17. **A pregnant female presents with pain in abdomen on examination, tenderness is found in right lumbar region. TLC is 12,000/cmm, and urine examination is normal, for diagnosis further test done is:** *(AIIMS June 99)*
    - a. Chest X-ray with abdominal shield
    - b. Ultrasound abdomen
    - c. Non contrast CT abdomen
    - d. Laparoscopy

18. **Which is the best test for diagnosis of acute appendicitis in a pregnant female?** *(MHSSMCET 2008)*
    - a. Alder's test
    - b. Aaron's test
    - c. Angell's test
    - d. Mc Burney's test

■ OCHSNER-SHERREN REGIME

19. **Ochsner-Sherren regimen is used for treatment of:**
    (DNB 2012, 2000, MHPGMET 2005)
    - a. Appendicular abscess
    - b. Appendicular mass
    - c. Acute appendicitis
    - d. Appendicular mucocele

20. A 26-year-old male presented with 4 day history of pain in the right sided lower abdomen with frequent vomiting. Patients general condition is fair and clinically a tender lump was felt in the right iliac fossa. Most appropriate management for this case would be: *(Recent Question 2014)*
    a. Exploratory laparotomy
    b. Immediate appendectomy
    c. Ochsner-Sherren regimen
    d. External drainage

21. A 25-year-old man presents with 3 days history of pain in the right lower abdomen and vomiting. Patient's general condition is satisfactory and clinical examination reveals a tender lump in right iliac fossa. The most appropriate management in this case would be: *(Recent Question 2015)*
    a. Immediate appendectomy
    b. Exploratory laparotomy
    c. Ochsner-Sherren regimen
    d. External drainage

22. A 30-year-old man presents with a four days history of the right iliac fossa pain. USG image is shown below. Which is the best management algorithm? *(MCI Dec 2018)*

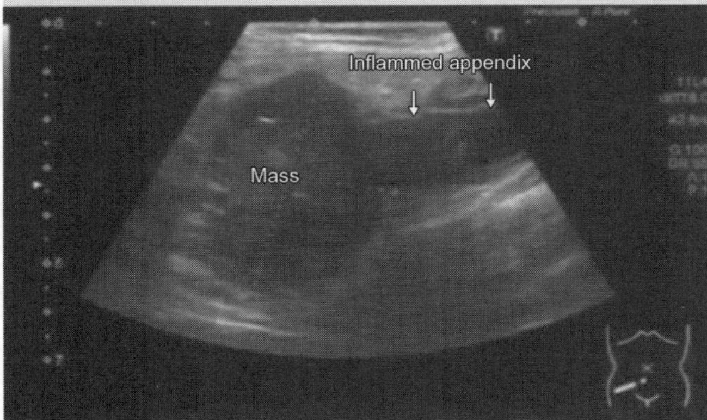

    a. Ochsner-Sherren regime
    b. Urgent appendectomy
    c. Extraperitoneal drainage and parenteral antibiotics
    d. Percutaneous drainage and parenteral antibiotics

■ NEOPLASM OF APPENDIX

23. Most common neoplasm of appendix is: *(Recent Question 2015, AIIMS Nov 93)*
    a. Lymphoma
    b. Adenocarcinoma
    c. Leiomyosarcoma
    d. Argentaffinoma

24. A 25-year-old patient presented with mass in right iliac fossa, which after laparotomy was found to be carcinoid of 2.5 cm in diameter. What will be next step in management? *(Recent Question 2013, AIIMS Nov 2000)*
    a. Segmental resection
    b. Appendectomy
    c. Right hemicolectomy
    d. Do yearly 5-HIAA assay

25. Treatment of an incidentally detected appendicular carcinoid measuring 2.5 cm is: *(MCI March 2009)*
    a. Right hemicolectomy
    b. Limits resection of the right colon
    c. Total colectomy
    d. Appendectomy

■ APPENDICULAR LYMPHOMA

26. Best treatment option for appendicular lymphoma:
    a. Right hemicolectomy *(Recent Question 2016)*
    b. Chemotherapy
    c. Right hemicolectomy + chemotherapy
    d. None

■ APPENDECTOMY

27. During appendectomy if it is noticed that base of appendix is inflamed then further line of treatment is: *(DPG 2011, PGI 96)*
    a. No appendectomy   b. No burying of stump
    c. Hemicolectomy   d. Cecal resection

28. The nerve commonly damaged during McBurney's incision is: *(Recent Question 2013, Bihar PG 2014, All India 2003)*
    a. Subcostal   b. Iliohypogastric
    c. 11th thoracic   d. 10th thoracic

29. A Gridiron incision becomes a Rutherford Morison's incision is extended by: *(Karnataka 94)*
    a. Splitting the muscles laterally
    b. Cutting the muscles laterally
    c. Cutting the muscles medially into the rectus sheath
    d. Incising vertically along the rectus muscle

30. Which of the following is a muscle splitting incision?
    a. Kocher's incision *(AIIMS Nov 2016)*
    b. Lanz incision
    c. Rutherford-Morrison incision
    d. Pfannenstiel incision

31. Incision at McBurney's point corresponds to: *(Recent Question 2017)*
    a. Tip of appendix
    b. Base of appendix
    c. Midpoint of appendix
    d. Base of cecum

■ APPENDIX ANATOMY AND PHYSIOLOGY

32. All are true about appendicular artery except: *(DPG 97)*
    a. Supplies only appendix
    b. Supplies terminal ileum also
    c. Is an end artery
    d. Branch of lower division of ileocolic artery

33. The commonest anatomical position of appendix is: *(Karnataka 2013, DNB 2012, MHPGMCET 2007, 2001)*
    a. Retrocaecal   b. Pelvic
    c. Paracecal   d. Preileal

ACUTE APPENDICITIS

1. Ans. c. Pelvic
2. Ans. b. Extension *(Ref: Sabiston 20th/e p1299; Schwartz 11/e p1336, 10/e p, 1259; Bailey 27/e p1304; Shackelford 8/e p1952)*
3. Ans. a. Pain
4. Ans. a. Appendectomy
5. Ans. c. Bastedo sign *(Ref: www.medilexicon.com)*

Bastedo Sign
• An **obsolete sign** in **chronic appendicitis**[Q]
• **Pain** and **tenderness** in **right iliac fossa** on **inflation** of the **colon with air**[Q]

6. Ans. b. Tension gangrene due to the accumulating secretions
7. Ans. a. When appendicular perforation occurs early (within 24 hours) *(Ref: Bailey 27/e p1303)*

- In **late stages, greater omentum** and **small bowel** becomes **adherent to inflamed appendix, walling off the spread** of **peritoneal contamination**[Q].

8. Ans. b. Vomiting precedes abdominal pain *(Ref: Sabiston 20/e p1297; Bailey 27/e p1303)*

- **Typical presentation: Periumbilical pain** followed by **anorexia** and **nausea**[Q].
- **Localized pain** is the **most important symptom**[Q]
- **Perforation** occurs in **80%** of cases < 5-years
- Approximately **60% perforation** occurs **within 48 hours**

9. Ans. c. Cullen's sign
10. Ans. d. Acute appendicitis
11. Ans. c. Acute appendicitis
12. Ans. a. Alvarado *(Ref: Schwartz 11/e p1333, 10/e p1245; Sabiston 20/e p1132; Bailey 27/e p1307)*
13. Ans. b. Anorexia
14. Ans. b. Leukocytosis *(Ref: Bailey 27/e p1307)*
15. Ans. b. Mesenteric lymphadenopathy
16. Ans. b. Ultrasound

APPENDICITIS IN PREGNANCY

17. Ans. b. Ultrasound abdomen
18. Ans. a. Alder's test *(Ref: www.ncbi.nlm.nlh.gov/.../PMC3398111)*

ALDER'S TEST
• **Localizing the area** of **maximal abdominal tenderness** and **maintaining constant pressure** on that point while the **patient** is **being turned to left**[Q].
• If the **pain is constant**, pain is of **extra-uterine origin**; if **pain disappears** it is more likely to be **uterine** or **tubal origin**[Q].
• This is a **very useful** and **important clinical test** which may be **employed in all cases** of an **acute abdomen in pregnancy**[Q].

OCHSNER-SHERREN REGIME

19. Ans. b. Appendicular mass
20. Ans. c. Ochsner-Sherren regimen
21. Ans. c. Ochsner-Sherren regimen
22. Ans. a. Ochsner-Sherren regime *(Ref: Bailey 27/e p1312)*

NEOPLASM OF APPENDIX

23. Ans. d. Argentaffinoma *(Ref: Sabiston 20/e p1308; Schwartz 11/e p1338, 10/e p1258; Bailey 27/e p1315; Shackelford 8/e p1956)*

- MC neoplasm of appendix: Carcinoid tumor

  - **MC malignant neoplasm of appendix (MAC):** Mucinous adenocarcinoma[Q] **(38%)** > Adenocarcinoma **(26%)** > **Carcinoid (17%)**.

24. **Ans. c. Right hemicolectomy** *(Ref: Sabiston 20/e p1308; Schwartz 11/e p1338, 10/e p1258; Bailey 27/e p1315; Shackelford 8/e p1956)*

25. **Ans. a. Right hemicolectomy**

■ APPENDICULAR LYMPHOMA

26. **Ans. c. Right hemicolectomy + chemotherapy**

■ APPENDECTOMY

27. **Ans. b. No burying of stump** *(Ref: Sabiston 20/e p1300; Schwartz 11/e p1336, 10/e p1251-1256; Bailey 27/e p1309; Shackelford 8/e p1955)*

28. **Ans. b. Iliohypogastric** *(Ref: Bailey 25/e p1213)*

- **Right inguinal hernia** is **more common** following a **gridiron incision** for appendectomy, and is **due to injury** to the **iliohypogastric nerve**[Q].
- **IH → IH** (IlioHypogastric nerve → Inguinal Hernia)

29. **Ans. b. Cutting the muscles laterally**

30. **Ans. b. Lanz incision**

31. **Ans. b. Base of appendix** *(Ref: Netter's Surgical Anatomy and Approaches E-Book By Conor P Delaney (2013)/p240)*

"An open incision is made at McBurney's point, located one-third the distance between the anterior superior iliac spine and the umbilicus. This area generally corresponds to the location of the base of the appendix."-Netter's Surgical Anatomy and Approaches E-Book By Conor P Delaney (2013)/p240

■ APPENDIX ANATOMY AND PHYSIOLOGY

32. **Ans. b. Supplies terminal ileum also** *(Ref: Sabiston 20/e p1296)*

33. **Ans. a. Retrocaecal**

Rectum and Anal Canal

■ HEMORRHOID

HEMORRHOID

- Recent theories regard hemorrhoids as **normal anatomical structures**[Q].
- These are **cushions of submucosal tissue** containing **venules, arterioles, smooth muscle fibres & elastic connective tissue (VASE)**.
- Three hemorrhoidal cushions are found in the **left lateral, right anterior & right posterior position (3, 7 & 11 O' Clock)**[Q]
- Hemorrhoids or **piles** are **symptomatic anal cushions.**

> - **More common** when **intra-abdominal pressure is raised, e.g. in obesity, constipation & pregnancy**[Q]
> - **Symptoms: bright-red, painless bleeding, mucus discharge & prolapse**
> - Hemorrhoids cannot be palpated, **best diagnosed by proctoscopy**[Q].

Internal Hemorrhoids	External Hemorrhoids
• Located **proximal to** the **dentate line**[Q] • **Painless,** can be **ligated**[Q] • **Banding** is **preferred**[Q]	• Located **distal to dentate line**[Q] • Also known as **5–days painful self curing lesion**[Q] • **Painful, not ligated**[Q] • **Excision is done**[Q] • Repeated thrombosis leads to **semi-ripe black currant appearance**

Classification of Internal Hemorrhoids	
1st degree	**Painless bleeding**[Q], no prolapse
2nd degree	**Prolapse** through the anus, on straining but **reduce spontaneously**[Q]
3rd degree	Prolapse through the anal canal and **require manual reduction**[Q]
4th degree	Permanently prolapsed and **cannot be manually reduced.**[Q]

Treatment

- Mere presence of hemorrhoids is not necessarily an indication of treatment.
- Treatment is **only indicated** if they are **symptomatic. Best treatment** is the **least invasive** one which is **possible to alleviate** the **symptoms**[Q].

Treatment of Hemorrhoids	
Medical therapy	• Bleeding from **1st & 2nd degree** hemorrhoids often improve with the addition of **dietary fibre, stool softeners** and other **diet regulation**[Q].
Rubber band ligation	• Done for **1st, 2nd & selected 3rd degree** hemorrhoids[Q]
Infrared photocoagulation	• Done for **1st & 2nd degree** hemorrhoids
Sclerotherapy	• Done for **1st, 2nd & selected 3rd degree** hemorrhoids[Q] • Most commonly used sclerosant is **5% phenol in almond** or **arachis oil.**
Operative hemorrhoidectomy[Q]	• **3rd & 4th degree** hemorrhoid[Q] • **2nd degree not cured by non-operative methods**[Q] • **Mixed** (combine internal/external hemorrhoids)[Q] • **Fibrosed hemorrhoids**

Operative Hemorrhoidectomy	
• **Milligan-Morgan open** hemorrhoidectomy[Q] • **Whitefield submucosal** hemorrhoidectomy[Q]	• **Ferguson closed** hemorrhoidectomy[Q] • **Longo's stapler** hemorrhoidectomy[Q]

■ RECTAL PROLAPSE

RECTAL PROLAPSE

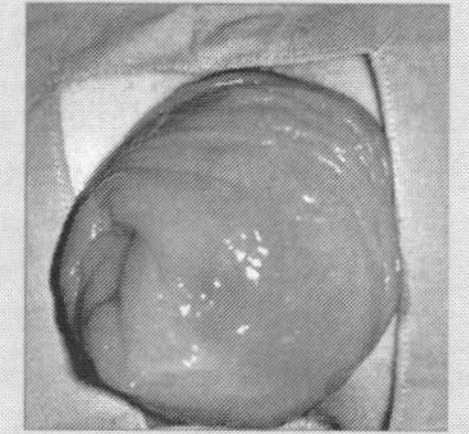

- **Mucous membrane** & **submucosa** of the rectum **protrude outside** the anus for approximately **1–4 cm**[Q].
- It may be **mucosal** or **full thickness** (whole wall of the rectum is included)
- Commences as a **rectal intussusception**[Q]
- In **children**, the prolapse is **usually mucosal** and should be **treated conservatively**
- In the **adult**, the prolapse is **often full thickness** and is frequently **associated with incontinence**[Q]
- **Surgery** is **necessary for full-thickness rectal prolapse**[Q]

Clinical Features

Children	• **Mucosal prolapse** often commences **after an attack of diarrhea**, or from **loss of weight** & **consequent loss of fat in** the **ischiorectal fossae**[Q]. • It may also be **associated with fibrocystic disease**, **neurological causes** & **maldevelopment of** the **pelvis**[Q].
Adults	• Often associated with **third-degree hemorrhoids**[Q]. • In the **female a torn perineum**, and in the **male straining from urethral obstruction**, predisposes to mucosal prolapse[Q]. • In **old age**, **both mucosal** & **full-thickness prolapse** are associated with **atony of** the **sphincter mechanism**[Q].

- **Prolapsed mucous membrane is pink** (prolapsed internal hemorrhoids are **plum colored, trifoliate** & **more pedunculated**)[Q]

Diagnosis

- Before operative intervention, a careful **history, physical examination,** & **colonoscopy** should be performed.
- **Manometry** should be done **in cases** associated **with incontinence**[Q].

Abdominal Procedures	Perineal Procedures

• Considered the **surgical procedures of choice** for **young** & **fit individuals**[Q]
• **Not suitable for elderly** & **infirm patients**[Q]
• Are most likely **to improve continence**[Q]
• Have **least recurrence rates**[Q]
• **Postoperative constipation** is the **MC side effect**[Q]
• Abdominal rectopexy
  – **Suture Rectopexy**
  – **Mesh Rectopexy**
    – Posterior (**Well's Ivalon's**)[Q]
    – Anterior (**Ripstein's**)[Q]
    – Lateral (**Orr-Loygue**)
    – Ventral
  – **Resection Rectopexy** (Frykman and Goldberg)
• **Anterior resection**[Q]
	• **Relatively minor procedures** that may be performed under local or regional anaesthesia
	• **Well tolerated by elderly**, **frail** & **unfit patients**[Q]
	• Less likely to improve continence
	• **Recurrence rates** varying from **5–35% higher than** following **abdominal rectopexy**[Q]
	• **Postoperative constipation** is **infrequent**[Q]
	
	Perineal Procedure
	• **Delorme's muscosectomy**[Q]
	• **Thiersh and encirclement**[Q]
	• **Altemeier rectosigmoidectomy**[Q]

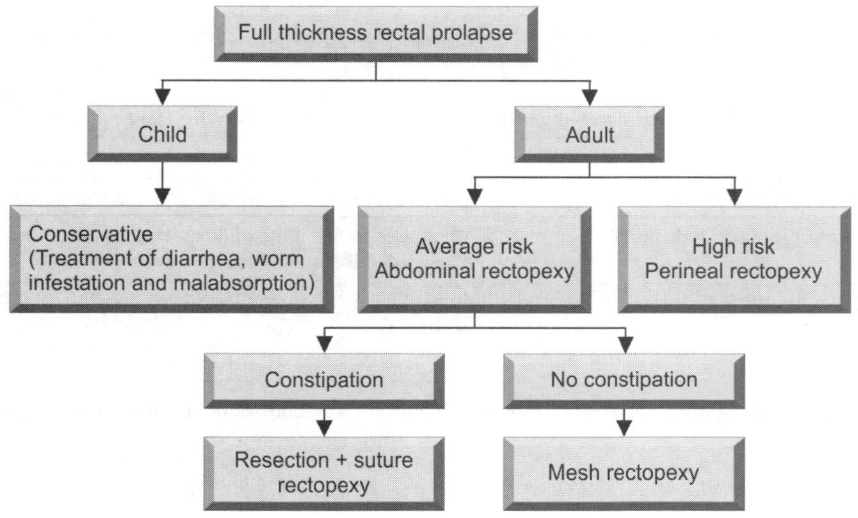

■ ANO-RECTAL ABSCESS

Ano-Rectal Abscess

- Acute sepsis in the region of the anus is common.
- **More common** in men[Q]
- **Subdivided into: Perianal (MC)[Q], Ischiorectal (2nd MC)[Q]**, submucous & pelvirectal
- **Underlying conditions: Fistula-in-ano (MC), Crohn's disease, diabetes, immunosuppression[Q]**

> **Cryptoglandular Theory of Intersphincteric Anal Gland Infection**
>
> • Upon **infection of a gland, pus**, which **travels along** the **path of least resistance**, may **spread caudally** to **present as** a **perianal abscess** or **ischiorectal abscess[Q]**

- **MC organism responsible: E. coli[Q] > Bacteroides[Q]**

Clinical Features

- Usually produces a **painful, throbbing swelling in** the **anal region** with **swinging pyrexia**
- Patients with infection in the larger **fatty-filled ischiorectal space**, in which **tissue tension is much lower,** usually **present later,** with **less well localized symptoms** but more constitutional upset & fever.

> • **Increased incidence of infection in ischiorectal fossa** is due to **poor blood supply[Q]**.

Treatment

- **Drainage of pus + Antibiotics[Q]**
- Always look for a **potential underlying problem[Q]**

> • For **perianal & ischiorectal sepsis** (with an **incidence of 60% & 30%** respectively), **drainage** is **through the perineal skin**, usually through a **cruciate incision** over the **most fluctuant point**, with excision of the skin edges to de-roof the abscess.

- **Modified Hanley's technique: Used for drainage of horseshoe ischiorectal abscess[Q]**

■ FISTULA-IN-ANO

Fistula-in-ano

- **Fistula-in-ano is a chronic abnormal communication, runs outwards** from the **anorectal lumen** to an **external opening** on the skin of the perineum or **buttock**
- Usually **results from anorectal abscess (cryptoglandular abscess[Q])**
- **Other causes**: Crohn's disease, tuberculosis, lymphogranuloma venereum, actinomycosis, rectal duplication, foreign body and malignancy
- **Types: High or Low** (according to whether **internal opening** is **below** or **above** the **anorectal ring[Q]**)

Clinical Presentation

- Non-specific anal fistulae are **more common in men** than women.
- Patients usually complain of **intermittent purulent discharge & pain[Q]** (which increases until temporary relief occurs when the pus discharges).
- There is a **previous episode of acute anorectal sepsis** that settled (**incompletely**) spontaneously or with antibiotics, or which was surgically drained.

> • **Passage of flatus or feces through** the **external opening** is suggestive of a **rectal** rather than an anal **internal opening[Q]**.

Parks Classification of Fistula-in-ano (ITS-E)	
Intersphincteric fistulae (45%): MC[Q]	Runs in intersphinteric space
Trans-sphincteric fistulae (30%)	Extends through both internal and external sphincters
Suprasphincteric fistulae (20%)	Originates in the Intersphincteric plane and tracks up and around the entire external sphincter
Extrasphincteric fistulae (5%)	Originates in the rectal wall and tracks lateral to both sphincters

Clinical Assessment

- A full **medical history & proctosigmoidoscopy** are **necessary** to gain information about **sphincter strength** and to **exclude associated conditions.**

Contd…

Contd…

Key Points to Determine	
• **Site** of the **internal opening**[Q] • **Site** of the **external opening**[Q] • **Course** of the **primary track**[Q]	• **Presence of secondary extensions**[Q] • Presence of **other conditions complicating** the **fistula**[Q]

- **Full examination under anesthesia** should be **repeated before surgical intervention**.
- **Dilute hydrogen peroxide**, instilled via the external opening, is a **very useful way** of demonstrating the **site of the internal opening**

> • **MRI** is the 'gold standard' for fistula imaging[Q]
> • Usually **reserved for difficult recurrent cases**[Q]

- **Fistulography** and **CT**: Useful techniques if an **extrasphincteric fistula** is suspected.

Treatment

- Treatment options: **Fistulotomy, fistulectomy, setons, advancement flaps** and **glues**, VAAFT
- **Laying open** is the **surest method of eradication**, but **sphincter division** may **result in incontinence**[Q]

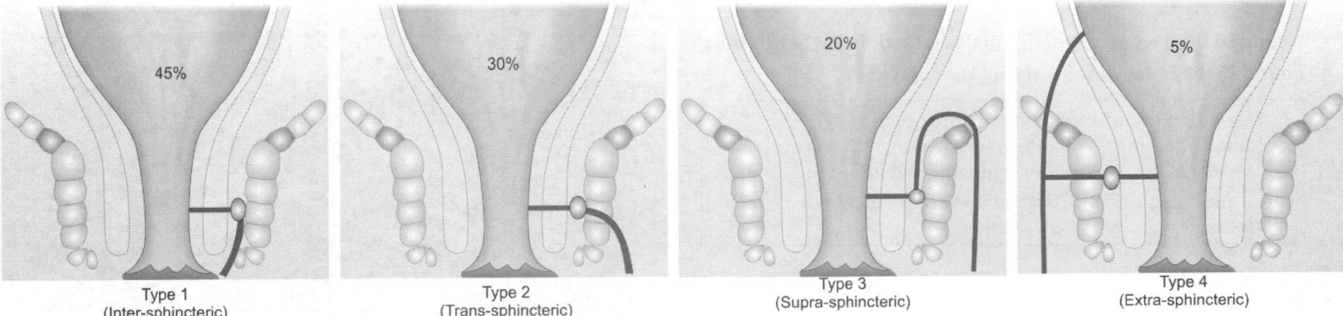

Goodsall's rule	

- Used to **indicate** the **likely position of** the **internal opening** according to the position of the external opening(s)

According to Goodsall's rule

- Fistulas with **external openings anterior** to horizontal imaginary line drawn across the mid-point of anus connect to the internal opening by **short straight track**[Q].
- Fistulas with **external openings posterior** to horizontal line run a **curvilinear course** and **open internally** into **posterior midline**[Q] (at 6 o'clock position[Q]).

- **Exceptions** of Goodsall's rule:
  - If an **anterior external opening** is **> 3 cm from** the **anal margin**. Such fistula track to the **posterior midline**.
  - When there is an **anterior** and also a **posterior opening** of the same fistula, **the rule of posterior opening** applies.

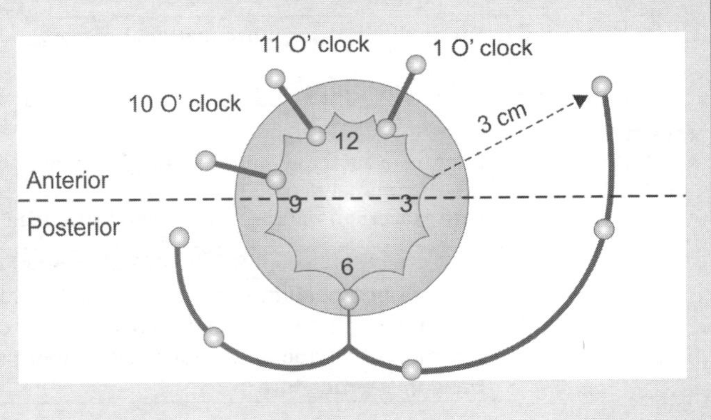

■ ANAL FISSURE (FISSURE-IN-ANO)

ANAL FISSURE (FISSURE-IN-ANO)

- An anal fissure is a **longitudinal split in** the **anoderm**, extending from **anal verge to dentate line**[Q].
- **MC site: Mid-line posteriorly**[Q] (6'O Clock Position)[Q]
- **MC symptom: Pain**[Q]

Etiology

- **Trauma caused by** the **strained evacuation** of a **hard stool** or from the **repeated** passage of **diarrhea**[Q].
- **Anterior anal fissure: More common in women**, arise **following vaginal delivery**.

Clinical Features

- **Acute fissure**: Characterized by **severe anal pain** associated **with defecation** with passage of fresh blood, normally noticed on the tissue after wiping.

> • **Chronic fissures:** Characterized by a **hypertrophied anal papilla** + Sentinel tag + Deep canoe shaped ulcer[Q]

- Mostly seen in **young adults, men & women** are **affected equally**[Q].

Contd…

Contd…

Treatment

- **Conservative initially**, consisting of **sitz bath** (in a basin containing **warm antiseptic lotion**), **stool-bulking agents** & **softeners**, **nitrates** and **calcium channel blockers to relax** the **anal sphincter** and **improve blood flow**[Q]
- **Surgery** if above fails, consisting of **lateral internal sphincterotomy** or **anal advancement flap**[Q]

Treatment of Anal Fissure
• **Chemical sphincterotomy: Nitroglycerine (0.2%**[Q]**)** or **diltiazem (2%**[Q]**)** for relaxation of anal sphincter
• **Lord's procedure: Dilatation** of **sphincter** under GA, not practiced due to **high rate of incontinence**[Q]
• **Notara's lateral sphincterotomy: Surgical procedure of choice** for anal fissure[Q]
• **Anal advancement flap:** An **inverted house-shaped flap** of **perianal skin** is carefully mobilized on its blood supply and **advanced without tension to cover** the **fissure**, and then sutured with interrupted absorbable sutures.

■ PILONIDAL SINUS

PILONIDAL SINUS

- **Acquired** disease, seen in **hairy males**[Q] **(Dark haired individuals)**
- **Found in** the **natal cleft overlying** the **coccyx**[Q]

> - Consisting of **noninfected, midline openings communicating with** a **fibrous track** lined by granulation tissue and containing hair lying loosely within the lumen.
> - **Common** among **military personnel**, also known as **'jeep disease'**[Q].

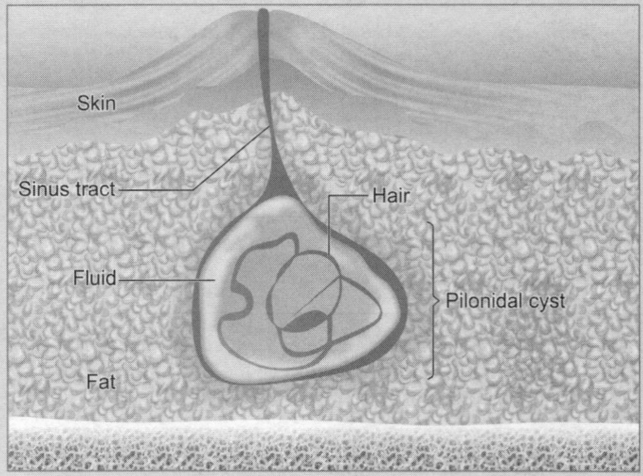

Clinical Features

- Patients complain of **intermittent pain, swelling** & **discharge** at the base of the spine
- **History of repeated abscesses** that have **burst spontaneously** or which have been incised, **usually away from** the **midline**[Q].

> - **Interdigital pilonidal sinus** is an **occupational disease of hairdressers**[Q]
> - Also seen in **axilla** & **umbilicus**[Q]

Treatment

- **Conservative treatment:** For minor symptoms, **simple cleaning out** of tracks & **removal of all hair**, with **regular shaving** of the area and **strict hygiene**, may be recommended[Q].
- **Treatment** of an **acute exacerbation (abscess):** Abscess drainage with **thorough curettage** of **granulation tissue** and **hair**[Q].

Surgical Treatment of Chronic Pilonidal Disease
• **Laying open of all tracks** with or without **marsupialisation**[Q]
• **Excision of all tracks** with or without primary closure[Q]
• **Excision of all tracks** & **closure by Limberg's flap**[Q], **Karydakis flap** or **rhomboid flap**[Q]
• **Bascom's procedure**[Q]:

■ CARCINOMA RECTUM

CARCINOMA RECTUM

- **MC site of colorectal cancer: Rectum**[Q]
- **MC type: Adenocarcinoma**[Q]
- **Multiple in 5% cases**[Q]
- Usually **present as an ulcer**, but polypoid and infiltrating types are also common.

> - **MC site of metastasis: Liver**[Q] (34%) >Lungs (22%) >Adrenals (11%)
> - With **improved response rates** to **modern chemotherapy** and advances in hepatic surgery, however, **more patients are now candidates for hepatectomy**[Q] than in the past.
> - **Dose of radiotherpay** given in CA rectum: **60 Gray**[Q]

Clinical Features

- **Age of presentation** in **CA rectum:** Above **55 years**
- **Bleeding** is the **earliest** and **MC symptom**[Q].
- **Sense of incomplete defecation**[Q]

Contd…

Gastrointestinal Surgery
Section 3

Contd…

Sense of Incomplete Defecation
• Sensation that there are more feces to be passed (**tenesmus**, a distressing **straining to empty** the **bowels without resultant evacuation**[Q]).
• This is a very important **early symptom** and is **almost invariably present in tumours of** the **lower half of the rectum**[Q].
• The patient may endeavor to **empty the rectum several times a day** (**spurious diarrhea**), often with the **passage of flatus** and **a little blood-stained mucus** ('bloody slime')[Q].

- **Alteration in bowel habit:** Patient has to **get up early in order to defecate**[Q], or one who **passes blood** & **mucus** in addition to feces ('**early-morning bloody diarrhea**'[Q]).
- Patient with an **annular carcinoma** at the **rectosigmoid junction** suffers with **increasing constipation**, and the one with a **growth in the ampulla** of the rectum who has **early-morning diarrhea**[Q].

• **Pain in the back,** or sciatica, occurs when the **cancer invades the sacral plexus**[Q].
• **Weight loss** is suggestive of **hepatic metastases**[Q].

Diagnosis

- **Sigmoidoscopy (rigid,** not flexible) and Biopsy: **Investigation of choice** for **diagnosis of CA rectum**[Q]
- **TRUS** (Transrectal ultrasound): **Best for ' T' staging**[Q]
- **Endorectal coil MRI: Best for** predicting **LN invasion and overall staging**[Q]
- **CECT:** Evaluation of **metastasis**

Treatment of Carcinoma Rectum	
Stage 0 (Tis, N0, M0)	• **Local excision**[Q]
Stage I: Localized Rectal Carcinoma (T1–2, N0, M0)	• **Polypectomy** with clear margins[Q] • **Radical resection** in good-risk patients with **unfavorable histologic characteristics** and located in the **distal third** of the rectum[Q]
Stage II: Localized Rectal Carcinoma (T3–4, N0, M0)	• **Preoperative chemoradiation + radical resection**[Q]
Stage III: Lymph Node Metastasis (Tany, **N1**, M0)	• **Preoperative chemoradiation + radical resection**[Q]
Stage IV: Distant Metastasis (Tany, Nany, **M1**)	• **Palliative procedures**[Q] • Resection to control pain, bleeding, or tenesmus

Treatment Options for Carcinoma Rectum	
Low Anterior Resection	• **Sphincter saving operation**[Q] • Performed for the **cancers of proximal third** to **two third of** the **rectum** (Located **> 5 cm above**[Q] the **anal verge**) • Descending colon is anastomosed with the distal rectum
Abdominoperineal Resection (APR or Miles Procedure)	• **Complete excision** of **rectum** and **anus**, by concomitant dissection through the abdomen and perineum with **creation of permanent colostomy**[Q]. • Performed for carcinoma of **lower rectum** (at or **below 5 cm** from **anal verge**)
Hartmann's Procedure	• When there is **too much destruction** or **sepsis** to allow a safe anastomosis[Q] • For **elderly** or **severely unstable patients**[Q] who would not stand a lengthy anterior resection or APR procedure

■ CARCINOMA ANAL CANAL

Carcinoma Anal Canal
• **MC type** of **CA anal canal: SCC >BCC >Melanoma**[Q]
• **Median age** at diagnosis: **60 years**[Q]

• **MC symptom: Bleeding PR**[Q]   • **MC site of metastasis: Lung**[Q]   • **MC site of LN metastasis: Inguinal LNs**[Q]

Risk Factors for Carcinoma Anal Canal	
• **HPV infection (16, 18, 31, 33)**[Q]	• **Sexual promiscuity**[Q]
• **HIV** or **immunosuppression**[Q]	• **Chronic inflammation**[Q]
• **Smoking**[Q]	• **Anal intra-epithelial neoplasia**[Q]
• **Anal receptive intercourse**[Q]	• History of **vulvar** or **cervical cancer**[Q]

Clinical Features

- **Most patients** present with **rectal bleeding** & **pain**[Q].
- Patients are **frequently misdiagnosed** as having a benign anorectal condition such as **hemorrhoids**[Q].

Contd…

Contd…

- **Additional symptoms: Incontinence, change in bowel habits, pelvic pain,** and **rectovaginal** or **rectovesical fistulas** are **ominous**[Q] suggest **advanced malignancy** with **infiltration into** the **sphincters** or **penetration into** the rectal wall[Q]

Diagnosis

- **Proctoscopy** with **biopsy: Investigation of choice** for diagnosis of **CA anal canal**[Q].
- **CT abdomen & pelvis: Mandatory** because **all of the draining lymph nodes** are **not palpable**[Q].
- **CT scan**: **Evaluate distant metastasis**

Treatment

- **Nigro regimen: Chemoradiation** is the **treatment of choice**[Q].
- More than **80%** are **cured by chemoradiation**. If any **residual tumor** is **left** behind after chemoradiation, **APR** is performed[Q].

- **Chemotherapy regimen: 5-FU + Mitomycin C/Cisplatin**[Q]
- First **chemotherapy** is given **followed by radiotherapy**[Q].

8th AJCC (2017) TNM Classification of Carcinoma of the Anal Canal & Anal Margin	
Tis: Carcinoma in situ (Bowen disease, high-grade squamous intraepithelial lesions (HSIL), anal intraepithelial neoplasia II-III (AIN II-III)	**N1a:** Metastases to **inguinal, mesorectal, and/or internal iliac LNs**[Q]
T1: Tumor **≤2 cm** in greatest dimension[Q]	**N1b:** Metastases to **external iliac LNs**[Q]
T2: **>2 cm** but **<5 cm** in greatest dimension[Q]	**N1c:** Metastases to **external iliac and in inguinal, mesorectal, and/or internal iliac LNs**[Q]
T3: **>5 cm** in greatest dimension[Q]	**M1:** Distant metastasis
T4: Invading adjacent structures: **vagina, urethra, or bladder**[Q] (involvement of the sphincter muscle alone, rectal wall, or perirectal subcutaneous tissue or skin is not classified as T4)	

Stage Grouping							
0	**I**	**IIA**	**IIB**	**IIIA**	**IIIB**	**IIIC**	**IV**
Tis N0M0	**T1** N0M0	**T2** N0M0	**T3** N0M0	**T1-2 N1** M0	**T4** N0M0	**T3-4** N1M0	Any T Any N **M1**

■ VILLOUS ADENOMA

1. **Villous polyp of rectum manifest:** *(Recent Question 2016)*
   a. Bleeding PR
   b. Mucus diarrhea with hypokalemia
   c. Prolapse rectum
   d. Obstruction

2. **In villous papillomas of the rectum which is lost:**
   a. Na⁺
   b. Mg²⁺ *(DNB 2007, 2003)*
   c. K⁺
   d. All

3. **The best surgical management for villous adenoma of the rectum is:** *(Recent Question 2016)*
   a. Local resection of lesion
   b. Repeated sigmoidoscopy
   c. Abdomino perineal resection
   d. Electrolyte infusion and chemotherapy

■ RECTAL POLYP

4. **Rectal polyps usually present with:** *(SGPGI 2005, UPPG 97)*
   a. Obstruction
   b. Perforation
   c. Bleeding
   d. Malignant change

5. **A toddler has few drops of blood coming out of rectum. Probable diagnosis is:** *(AIIMS May 2013, AIIMS May 2012)*
   a. Juvenile rectal polyp
   b. Adenomatous polyposis coli
   c. Rectal ulcer
   d. Piles

6. **Most common cause of fresh bleeding per rectum in a 5-years old child is:** *(WBPG 2012, AIIMS June 93)*
   a. Volvulus
   b. Trauma
   c. Worm infestation
   d. Rectal polyp

■ CARCINOMA RECTUM

7. **Dukes A stage of rectal carcinoma is managed by:**
   a. Surgical resection only *(DNB 2008)*
   b. Surgical resection + selective adjuvant chemotherapy
   c. Surgical resection + routine adjuvant chemotherapy
   d. Chemotherapy primarily

8. **Best treatment for a 4 cm moderate grade rectal cancer at the junction of lower and mid one thirds, with less than one third circumference of the rectum being involved?**
   a. Radiotherapy *(MHSSMCET 2008, 2006)*
   b. Anterior resection
   c. Transanal resection
   d. Abdomino-perineal resection

9. **Distal margins of clearance required for treatment of CA rectum is .... and lateral and proximal margins ....** *(MHSSMCET 2010)*
   a. 2 cm and 5 cm
   b. 3 cm and 5 cm
   c. 5 cm and 2 cm
   d. 5 cm and 3 cm

10. **A patient comes with rectal carcinoma situated 6 cm above dentate line with no nodal metastasis. Treatment of choice will be:** *(AIIMS Nov 97)*
    a. Anterior resection
    b. APR
    c. Radiotherapy
    d. Hartman's procedure

11. **For a rectal carcinoma at 5 cm from the anal verge, the best acceptable operation is:** *(All India 2004)*
    a. Anterior resection
    b. Abdominoperinereal resection
    c. Posterior resection
    d. APR done in lesion of upper zone

12. **Commonest presentation of CA rectum is:**
    a. Diarrhea *(JIMPER 2012, DPG 95)*
    b. Constipation
    c. Bleeding P/R
    d. Feeling of incomplete defecation

13. **In which case anterior resection is the method of treatment?** *(AIIMS Feb 97)*
    a. CA sigmoid colon
    b. CA rectum
    c. CA colon
    d. CA anal canal

14. **A punch biopsy shows carcinoma rectum with fixed mass and X-ray chest normal. Which of the following is least useful investigation?** *(UPPG 2008)*
    a. Rigid proctoscope
    b. Barium enema
    c. CT chest
    d. MRI-abdomen and pelvis

15. **Ideal management in an old and frail patient presenting with a mass situated 15 cm away from anal orifice:**
    a. Abdomino-perineal resection *(MCI March 2005)*
    b. Colonoscopic removal
    c. Hartman's operation
    d. Anterior resection

16. **Aim of surgery in carcinoma rectum is:** *(MCI March 2010)*
    a. Limited excision of the rectum
    b. Sacrificing gastrointestinal continuity
    c. Preserving the anal sphincter
    d. Preserving mesorectum

■ HEMORRHOIDS

17. **External hemorrhoids below the dentate line are:**
    a. Painful *(AIIMS May 2012, All India 2007, AIIMS Nov 2006)*
    b. Ligation is done as management
    c. Skin tag is not seen in these cases
    d. May turn malignant

18. **Injection sclerotherapy is ideal for the following:** *(All India 2004)*
    a. External hemorrhoids
    b. Internal hemorrhoids
    c. Posterior resection
    d. Local resection

19. **Commonest complication following haemorrhoidectomy is:** *(MHSSCET 2005, AIIMS 92)*
    a. Hemorrhage
    b. Infection
    c. Fecal impaction
    d. Urinary retention

20. **Five-day self subsiding pain is diagnostic of:** *(APPG 97)*
    a. Anal fissure
    b. Fistula-in-ano
    c. Thrombosed external hemorrhoids
    d. Thrombosed internal hemorrhoids

21. **The following are true of hemorrhoids except:**
    a. They are arteriolar dilatations *(JIPMER 2001)*
    b. They are common causes of painless bleeding
    c. They cannot be per rectally palpated
    d. They can be banded

22. **Most important disadvantage of cryosurgery for hemorrhoid is:** *(DPG 2005)*
    a. Pain
    b. Infection
    c. Profuse watery discharge
    d. Hemorrhage

23. **Which of the following is true about hemorrhoids?**
    a. More common with portal hypertension　　*(DNB 2008)*
    b. External hemorrhoids are proximal to dentate line
    c. Internal hemorrhoids bleed profusely and painless
    d. Internal hemorrhoids are covered by anoderm

24. **A patient with external hemorrhoids develops pain while passing stools. The nerve mediating this pain is:**
    (Recent Question 2015)
    a. Hypogastric nerve　　b. Sympathetic plexus
    c. Splanchnic visceral nerve　d. Pudendal nerve

■ SOLITARY RECTAL ULCER SYNDROME

25. **All are true regarding solitary rectal ulcer syndrome except:**
    a. Usually in anterior wall　　*(DNB 2002)*
    b. Associated with rectal prolapse
    c. Usually malignant
    d. Bowel training helps alot

26. **Most common site of SRUS:**　　*(GB Pant 2011)*
    a. Posterior, 7–10 cm from anal verge
    b. Anterior, 7–10 cm from anal verge
    c. Posterior, 2–3 cm from anal verge
    d. Anterior, 2–3 cm from anal verge

■ RECTAL PROLAPSE

27. **Treatment of rectal prolapse in childhood is:**
    a. Lahaut's operation　　*(AIIMS June 94)*
    b. Incision of prolapsed mucosa
    c. Thiersch wiring　　d. Ripstein operation

28. **Recurrent prolapse of the rectum in children is treated by:**
    (Recent Question 2015)
    a. Thiersch wiring　　b. Digital reposition
    c. Excision　　d. Ripstein's operation

29. **Delorme's procedure is used for:**
    (WBPG 2012, MHPGMCET 2007, SGPGI 2004)
    a. Rectal prolapse　　b. Solitary rectal ulcer
    c. Rectal bilharziasis　d. Proctalgia fugax

30. **In old age for rectal prolapse palliative surgery in a patient unfit for surgery is:**　　*(Recent Question 2013)*
    a. Delorme's procedure　b. Well's procedure
    c. Thiersch's operation　d. Low anterior resection

31. **Which of the following is a perineal procedure for rectal prolapse?**　　*(Recent Question 2017)*
    a. Delorme　　b. Ripstein
    c. Resection rectopexyd.Frykman Goldberg procedure

■ ANORECTAL ABSCESS

32. **Commonest type of anorectal abscess is:**　　*(DNB 2012)*
    a. Ischio rectal　　b. Submucous
    c. Pelvi-rectal　　d. Perianal

33. **Most common cause of anorectal abscess is:**
    a. Inflammation of anal gland　*(MAHE 2007, 2008)*
    b. Folliculitis
    c. Inflammation of rectal mucosa
    d. Rectum

■ FISTULA-IN-ANO

34. **An AIDS patient presents with fistula in ano. His CD$_4$ count is below 50. Treatment of choice is:** *(Punjab 2008, MAHE 2001)*
    a. Seton　　b. Fistulectomy
    c. Both　　d. Medical

35. **True statement regarding 'Fistula in ano' is :**
    a. Posterior fistulae have straight tracks　　*(All India 2001)*
    b. High fistulae can be operated with no fear of incontinence
    c. High and low divisions are made in relation to the pelvic floor
    d. Intersphincteric is the most common type

36. **The treatment of choice in fistula in ano:**　　*(JIPMER 93)*
    a. Anal dilatation　　b. Fissurotomy
    c. Fistulectomy　　d. Fistulotomy

37. **High or low fistula in ano is termed according to its internal opening present with reference to:**　　*(UPSC 2008)*
    a. Anal canal　　b. Dentate line
    c. Anorectal ring　　d. Sacral promontory

38. **Ideal investigation for fistula-in-ano is:**
    (Recent Question 2014, MCI March 2008)
    a. Endoanal ultrasound　b. MRI
    c. Fistulography　　d. CT scan

39. **Seton used in fistula in anosurgery is draining seton and:**
    (Recent Question 2014, 2013)
    a. Cutting seton　　b. Dissolving seton
    c. Dissecting seton　　d. Fibrosing seton

■ ANAL FISSURE

40. **All are treatment of acute fissure in ano except:**
    a. Conservative　　*(AIIMS Sept 96)*
    b. Dilatation under GA
    c. Lateral sphincterotomy
    d. External sphincterotomy

41. **Sitz Bath consists of which of the following?** *(Karnataka 96)*
    a. Patient bathed in normal saline
    b. Bathed in molten wax
    c. Sitz in a basin containing warm antiseptic lotion
    d. Sitz in a basin containing molten wax

42. **Rectal examination should not be done in:**　　*(JIPMER 90)*
    a. Anal fissure
    b. Fistula in ano
    c. Prolapsed piles with bleeding
    d. Anal stenosis

43. **Internal sphincterotomy is the treatment of choice for:**
    (Recent Question 2016)
    a. Piles　　b. Fistula
    c. Fissure-in-ano　　d. Carcinoma

44. **Anal fissure best diagnosed by:**
    a. Anoscopy　　*(Recent Question 2014, All India 2008)*
    b. History and superficial clinical examination
    c. PR examination
    d. USG

45. **Lateral internal sphincterotomy is useful for:**
    (Recebt Question 2014)
    a. Anal fistula　　b. Anal canal strictures
    c. Hemorrhoids　　d. Anal fissure

46. **A sentinel pile indicatess:**　　*(MHPGMCET 2008, 2007)*
    a. Internal hemorrhoids　b. Pilonidal sinus
    c. Fissure-in-ano　　d. Fistula-in-ano

47. **Most common site for anal fissure is:** *(Recent Question 2013)*
    a. 3 o'clock　　b. 6 o'clock
    c. 2 o'clock　　d. 10 o'clock

48. **Which of the following is not indicated in fissure-in-ano?**
    (Recent Question 2017)
    a. Botox injection
    b. Topical steroids
    c. Topical calcium channel blockers
    d. Topical nitroglycerine

PILONIDAL SINUS

49. The following statement about pilonidal sinus is true:
a. More common in females *(All India 2007)*
b. Mostly congenital
c. Prognosis after surgery is poor
d. Treatment of choice is surgical excision of sinus tract

50. Jeep's disease is also known as:
(Recent Question 2017 MCI March 2008)
a. Anal incontinence
b. Hemorrhoids
c. Pilonidal sinus
d. Anal fissure

51. All of the following are true regarding pilonidal sinus except: *(MCI Sept 2009)*
a. Seen predominantly in women
b. Occurs only in sacrococcygeal region
c. Tendency for recurrence
d. Obesity is a risk factor

CARCINOMA ANAL CANAL

52. Treatment of choice for squamous cell carcinoma of anal canal: *(Recent Question 2013, DNB 2012, JIPMER 2011,*
a. Abdominoperineal resection *MCI Dec 2018)*
b. Chemoradiation
c. Wide local excision
d. CO_2 laser

53. Most common surgical complication of condyloma acuminata? *(MHSSMCET 2008)*
a. Infection
b. Recurrence
c. Hemorrhage
d. Malignant change

54. Virus that has increased association with anal warts:
a. HPV
b. HIV *(MHPGMCET 2009)*
c. LMV
d. EBV

55. Quadrivalent vaccine available for HPV protects against:
(JIPMER 2010)
a. HPV 6, 11, 31, 32
b. HPV 11, 16, 30, 33
c. HPV 6, 11, 16 , 18
d. HPV 16, 18, 31, 35

56. Commonest type of carcinoma anal canal is:
(Recent Question 2014, AIIMS June 97)
a. Squamous cell carcinoma
b. Adenocarcinoma
c. Adenocanthoma
d. Papillary type

57. For CA Anal canal, treatment of choice is: *(DNB 2012,*
GB Pant 2011, AIIMS Feb 97, Nov 97, June 98, All India 2006)
a. Surgery
b. Surgery + Radiotherapy
c. Chemoradiation
d. Chemotherapy

58. In carcinoma of anus distal margin of clearance of anal canal of at least: *(Recent Question 2014, CMC 2001)*
a. 2 cm
b. 5 cm
c. 4 cm
d. 7 cm

PAGET'S DISEASE OF ANAL CANAL

59. Paget's disease of anal canal is: *(JIPMER GIS 2011)*
a. Squamous cell carcinoma in situ
b. Squamous cell adenoma
c. Intra-epithelial adenocarcinoma
d. Marginal anal cell carcinoma

60. Which of the following is true about extra-mammary Paget's disease? *(JIPMER 2011)*
a. MC site is vulva
b. MC site is penis
c. MC site is vagina
d. MC site is perianal region

ANORECTAL MALFORMATIONS

61. A newborn baby presents with absent anal orifice and meconuria. What is the most appropriate management:
a. Transverse colostomy *(MHCET 2016, All India 2008)*
b. Conservative
c. Posterior saggital anorectoplasty
d. Perineal V-Y plasty

62. Invertogram is taken after:
a. 2 hours after birth
b. 4 hours after birth
c. 6 hours after birth
d. 8 hours after birth

63. Anorectal anomalies are commonly associated with:
(JIPMER 2011)
a. Cardiac anomalies
b. Duodenal atresia
c. CNS malformations
d. Abdominal

Explanations

■ VILLOUS ADENOMA

1. **Ans. a. Bleeding PR, b. Mucus diarrhea with hypokalemia** *(Ref: Sabiston 20/e p1363; Schwartz 11/e p1291, 10/e p1205-1206; Bailey 27/e p1326; Harrison 20/e p264)*

   - Villous adenoma causes **profuse watery diarrhea** and **hypokalemia, hyponatremia, hypochloremia** and **metabolic acidosis**[Q].
   - **Best treatment: Submucosal resection** endoscopically or surgically (Provided cancerous change has been excluded)

2. **Ans. a. Na+, c. K+**

3. **Ans. a. Local resection of lesion**

■ RECTAL POLYP

4. **Ans. c. Bleeding**

5. **Ans. a. Juvenile rectal polyp**

6. **Ans. d. Rectal polyp**

RECTAL POLYPS

- Occur most commonly in **children < 5 years** of age[Q].
- Occur as a **single lesion** of the **rectum**[Q]
- Typical symptoms are **rectal bleeding, mucus discharge, diarrhea,** and abdominal pain[Q].

■ CARCINOMA RECTUM

7. **Ans. a. Surgical resection only**

8. **Ans. c. Transanal resection**

   Best treatment for this patient is **local resection,** as the **tumor** is **involving less than one third circumference of** the **rectum. Transanal resection** is the best among the provided options.

9. **Ans. a. 2 cm and 5 cm** *(Ref: Bailey 27/e p1332)*

   - Bailey says "Provided a **minimum distal margin of clearance** of **2 cm**[Q] can be secured, it is safe to restore gastrointestinal continuity (Williams). The **principles of the operation** involve **radical excision** of the **neoplasm, removal of the mesorectum** and **high proximal ligation** of the **inferior mesenteric lymphovascular pedicle**[Q]."
   - The **proximal** and **radial margin** should be **at least 5 cm**[Q].

10. **Ans. a. Anterior resection**

11. **Ans. b. Abdominoperineal resection**

12. **Ans. c. Bleeding P/R**

13. **Ans. b. CA rectum**

14. **Ans. b. Barium enema**

15. **Ans. c. Hartmann's operation**

16. **Ans. c. Preserving the anal sphincter**

■ HEMORRHOIDS

17. **Ans. a. Painful**

18. **Ans. b. Internal hemorrhoids**

19. **Ans. d. Urinary retention** *(Ref: Bailey 27/e p1360; Sabiston 20/e p1401, 19/e p1389-1391; Schwartz 11/e p1310, 10/e p1223-1224)*

Complications of Hemorrhoidectomy	
Early Complications	**Late Complications**
• **Pain (MC)**[Q] • **Acute retention** of urine (**2nd MC**)[Q] • Reactionary hemorrhage	• Secondary hemorrhage • Anal stricture • Anal fissure • Incontinence

20. **Ans. c. Thrombosed external hemorrhoids**

21. **Ans. a. They are arteriolar dilatations**

22. **Ans. a. Pain** *(Ref: Bailey 24/e p1259)*

    Most important disadvantage of cryosurgery for hemorrhoid is pain.

CRYOSURGERY

- The extreme cold (-196°C) of **liquid nitrogen** application causes **coagulation necrosis of the piles,** which subsequently separated and dropped off.
- **Cryosurgery for hemorrhoids cause:**
  - Pain[Q]
  - Mucous discharge[Q] (Not the watery discharge)

23. Ans. c. Internal hemorrhoids bleed profusely and painless 24. Ans. d. Pudendal nerve

■ SOLITARY RECTAL ULCER SYNDROME

25. Ans. c. Usually malignant 26. Ans. b Anterior, 7–10 cm from anal verge

■ RECTAL PROLAPSE

27. Ans. c. Thiersch wiring *(Ref: Bailey 27/e p1323)*

<table>
<tr><td colspan="2" align="center">Treatment of Rectal Prolapse in Childhood</td></tr>
<tr><td colspan="2">• Prolapse during childhood is best managed conservatively, the only exception is persistence of prolapse despite effective treatment of diarrhea, worm infestation and malabsorption[Q]. These cases are managed by surgery.</td></tr>
<tr><td align="center">Conservative Treatment</td><td align="center">Operative Treatment</td></tr>
<tr><td>• Effective control of diarrhea, worm infestation and correction of malnutrition[Q]
• Sclerotherapy:
• Usually reserved for prolapse of the redundant mucosa after an anoplasty or rectoplasty for an imperforate anus[Q]
• 5% phenol in olive oil is injected submucosally[Q]</td><td>• Thiersch operation[Q]:
  – Anal encirclement[Q]
• Ideally suited for prolapse in myelomeningocele and sacral agenesis[Q]
• Lockhart Mummery Rectopexy[Q]:
• Simplest and safest operation in childhood complete rectal prolapse[Q]
• Posterior rectal wall stiffening</td></tr>
</table>

28. Ans. a. Thiersch wiring 29. Ans. a. Rectal prolapse

30. Ans. c. Thiersch's operation 31. Ans. a. Delorme *(Ref: Sabiston 20/e p1397; Schwartz 11/e p1305, 10/e p1219; Bailey 27/e p1323)*

■ ANORECTAL ABSCESS

32. Ans. d. Perianal *(Ref: Sabiston 20/e p1406; Schwartz 11/e p1314, 10/e p1227; Bailey 27/e p1362; Schackelford 8/e p1871)*

33. Ans. a. Inflammation of anal gland

■ FISTULA-IN-ANO

34. Ans. a. Seton *(Ref: Sabiston 20/e p1408; Schwartz 11/e p1317, 10/e p1231; Bailey 27/e p1366; Schackelford 8/e p1881)*

<table>
<tr><td colspan="1" align="center">Setons</td></tr>
<tr><td>• A seton is a ligature of silk, nylon, silastic or linen[Q].
• Used for marking, draining, cutting or staging[Q].
• A high fistula may be converted into a low fistula by setons[Q]</td></tr>
</table>

Setons are Useful in the Management of
• Complex anorectal fistulas with risk of incontinence or poor healing[Q]
• Patients with Crohn's disease[Q]
• Immunocompromised (HIV) and incontinent patients[Q]
• Patients with chronic diarrheal states[Q]
• Anterior fistula in women[Q]

35. Ans. d. Intersphincteric is the most common type 36. Ans. d. Fistulotomy

37. Ans. c. Anorectal ring 38. Ans. b. MRI 39. Ans. a. Cutting seton

■ ANAL FISSURE

40. Ans. d. External sphincterotomy 41. Ans. c. Sitz in a basin containing warm antiseptic lotion

42. Ans. a. Anal fissure 43. Ans. c. Fissure-in-ano

44. Ans. b. History and superficial clinical examination 45. Ans. d. Anal fissure

46. Ans. c. Fissure-in-ano

<table>
<tr><td align="center">Atypical Fissures</td></tr>
<tr><td>• A fissure sited elsewhere around the anal circumference or with atypical features should raise the suspicion of a specific etiology[Q]
• Early examination under anesthesia, with biopsy and culture to exclude:
  – Crohn's disease, tuberculosis[Q]
  – STD (syphilis, Chlamydia, chancroid, lymphogranuloma venereum, HSV, CMV, Kaposi's sarcoma, B-cell lymphoma)
  – HIV-related ulcers[Q]
  – Squamous cell carcinoma[Q]</td></tr>
</table>

47. **Ans. b.** 6 o'clock
48. **Ans. b.** Topical steroids *(Ref: Sabiston 20/e p1405; Schwartz 11/e p1313, 10/e p1226; Bailey 27/e p1352)*

■ PILONIDAL SINUS

49. **Ans. d.** Treatment of choice is surgical excision of sinus tract
50. **Ans. c.** Pilonidal sinus
51. **Ans. a.** Seen predominantly in women

■ CARCINOMA ANAL CANAL

52. **Ans. b.** Chemoradiation *(Ref: Sabiston 20/e p1412-1413; Schwartz 11/e p1304, 10/e p1218; Bailey 27/e p1371; Schackelford 8/e p2095)*
53. **Ans. b.** Recurrence
54. **Ans. a.** HPV *(Ref: Sabiston 20/e p1412; Schwartz 11/e p1304, 10/e p485,1232,1233,1678,1680; Bailey 27/e p1368; Schackelford 8/e p2101)*

ANAL WARTS OR CONDYLOMATA ACCUMINATA

- HPV forms the **etiological basis of:** **Anal** and **perianal warts**, **AIN**, and **SCC** of the anus[Q].
- Subtypes **(16, 18, 31, 33)** are **associated with a greater risk of progression** to **dysplasia** and **malignancy**[Q].
- **Condylomata accuminata is the MC STD** encountered by colorectal surgeons[Q]
- Most frequently observed in **homosexual men**[Q].

Clinical Presentation

- **Many** are **asymptomatic** but **pruritus, discharge, bleeding** and **pain** are **usual presenting complaints**[Q].
- Rarely, **relentless growth results in giant condylomata (Buschke- Löwenstein tumour)**, which may obliterate the anal orifice[Q].
- **Diagnosis** is **confirmed by biopsy**[Q]

Treatment

- Application of **25% podophyllin**[Q]
- **Surgical excision**[Q]
- **Recurrence is common**[Q]

55. **Ans. c.** HPV 6, 11, 16, 18 *(Ref: Maingot 11/e p732)*

HPV VACCINES

- **Gardisil** is a **recombinant vaccine** against HPV **types 6, 11, 16, 18**[Q].
- It is **currently approved for** use in **females age 9–26 years** of age and requires a series of **three injections over a 6 month** period[Q].

> - Nearly **100% prevention rate** in **genital warts, vulvar, vaginal,** and **cervical precancerous lesions** caused by the **serotypes against** which the **vaccine is directed**[Q].

- **Vaccine** is **only effective in** patients **not previously exposed to the viruses included in** the vaccine, and it **confers no protection against viruses not covered** by the vaccine[Q]

56. **Ans. a.** Squamous cell carcinoma
57. **Ans. c.** Chemoradiation
58. **Ans. a.** 2 cm

■ PAGET'S DISEASE OF ANAL CANAL

59. **Ans. c.** Intra-epithelial adenocarcinoma *(Ref: Sabiston 20/e p1413-1414; Bailey 27/e p1372; Schackelford 8/e p 2101; Maingot 11/e p743-744)*
60. **Ans. a.** MC site is vulva

■ ANORECTAL MALFORMATIONS

61. **Ans. a.** Transverse colostomy *(Ref: Sabiston 20/e p1877-1879; Schwartz 11/e p1736, 10/e p1626-1628; Bailey 27/e p1345-1347)*

- The presence of **meconium in urine reflects** some form of **communication between** the **urinary tract** and **rectum**, and suggests a **high type of anorectal malformation**[Q].
- Such **patients require a diverting colostomy. The colostomy decompresses** the **bowel** and **provides protection during** the **healing of subsequent repair**[Q].
- **Posterior Saggital Anorectoplasty (PSARP)** is performed **after 4–8 weeks.**
- The presence of **meconium in urine** and a **flat bottom** are considered **indications of a protective colostomy**[Q].

62. **Ans. c.** 6 hours after birth
63. **Ans. a.** Cardiac anomalies

Hernia and Abdominal Wall

■ HERNIA

HERNIA

- **Hernia** is derived from the Latin word for **rupture**.
- A hernia is defined as an **abnormal protrusion** of an organ or tissue **through a defect**[Q] in its surrounding walls.

Nyhus Classification System	
Type I	• **Indirect hernia; internal ring normal**; typically **in infants, children, young adults**[Q]
Type II	• **Indirect hernia; internal ring enlarged**[Q] without impingement on the floor of the inguinal canal; does not extend to the scrotum
Type IIIA	• **Direct hernia**[Q] (size is not taken into account)
Type IIIB	• **Indirect hernia** enlarged enough to **encroach upon** the **posterior** inguinal **wall; indirect sliding** or **scrotal hernias** and **pantaloon hernias**[Q]
Type IIIC	• **Femoral hernia**[Q]
Type IV	• **Recurrent hernia**
A	• **Direct**[Q]
B	• **Indirect**
C	• **Femoral**
D	• **Combined**

Gilbert Classification System			
Type 1	**Small, indirect**	Type 5	**Diverticular**, direct
Type 2	**Medium**, indirect	Type 6	**Combined (pantaloon)**
Type 3	**Large**, indirect	Type 7	**Femoral**[Q]
Type 4	**Entire floor, direct**[Q]		

■ RISK FACTORS FOR HERNIA

Risk Factors for Hernia	
Weakness of Abdominal Muscles	**Increased Intra-abdominal Pressure**
• **Patent processus vaginalis**[Q] • Patent canal of nuck causing indirect inguinal hernia in females • **Connective tissue disorders**[Q] like Ehlers Danlos syndrome • Congenital conditions like **Extrophy of bladder, Prune Belly syndrome**[Q] • **Advancing age**[Q] • **Chronic debilitating disease**[Q] • **Defective collagen synthesis**[Q] • Previous **right lower quadrant incision**[Q] • **Cigarette smoking**[Q]	• **Chronic cough**[Q] (Bronchitis, tuberculosis) • **Chronic obstructive pulmonary disease**[Q] • **Obesity**[Q] • Chronic **constipation** with **straining** at stool • **Enlarged prostate** with **straining** at micturition • **Pregnancy**[Q] • **Cirrhosis** with **ascites**[Q] • **Heavy weight lifting**[Q] • Chronic ambulatory peritoneal dialysis • Intra-abdominal tumors • Chronically enlarged pelvic organs

- **MC type** of hernia **in males: Indirect inguinal hernia**[Q]
- **MC type** of hernia in females: **Indirect inguinal hernia**[Q]
- **Femoral hernia is more common in females**[Q].
- **Direct inguinal hernia is more common in the elderly**[Q]

■ INDIRECT INGUINAL HERNIA

Types of Indirect Inguinal Hernia

- **Bubonocele**: Hernia is **limited to inguinal canal**
- **Funicular: Processus vaginalis is closed just above** the **epididymis**, contents of sac can be felt separately from testis
- **Complete (Vaginal): Hernial sac is continuous with tunica vaginalis of testis. Testis** appear to **lie within** the **lower part of hernia**

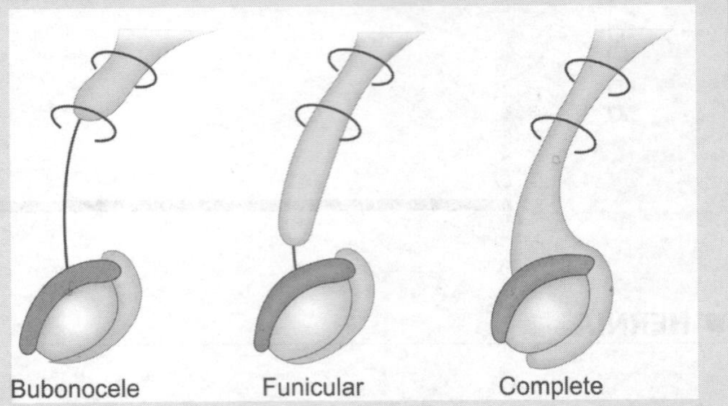

■ DIRECT INGUINAL HERNIA

DIRECT INGUINAL HERNIA

- In **adult males, 35% of inguinal hernias** are **direct**[Q]
- At presentation, **12%** of patients will have a **contralateral hernia**[Q]
- **Fourfold increased risk of** future **development of** a **contralateral hernia** if one is not present at the original presentation.
- **Always acquired**[Q]
- **Sac passes through** a **weakness** or **defect of transversalis fascia** in the **posterior wall** of the inguinal canal.
- Patient has **poor lower abdominal musculature**, presence of elongated bulgings (**Malgaigne's bulges**).

> - **Women** practically **never develop** a **direct inguinal hernia**[Q].

Predisposing Factors

- **Smoking**[Q]
- Occupations that involve **straining** and **heavy weight lifting**[Q]

> - **Damage** to the **iliohypogastric nerve (previous appendectomy)** is another cause, because of the resulting **weakness of** the **conjoined tendon**[Q].
> - IH → IH (IlioHypogastric nerve → Inguinal Hernia[Q])

Clinical Features

- Direct hernias **do not attain a large size** or **descend into the scrotum.**
- In contrast to an indirect inguinal hernia, a **direct inguinal hernia lies behind** the **spermatic cord.**
- Sac is often **smaller than hernial mass would indicate**, the **protruding mass** mainly consisting of **extraperitoneal fat**[Q].

> - As the **neck of the sac is wide, direct inguinal hernias do not often strangulate**[Q]

Management of Inguinal Hernia	

- **Objectives** of treatment:
  – **Treatment of hernia sac**
  – **Inguinal floor reconstruction**	

Treatment of Hernia Sac	**Inguinal Floor Reconstruction**

- Basic operation is **inguinal herniotomy**, which entails **dissecting out** & **opening** the **hernial sac, reducing any contents** and then **transfixing the neck** of the sac & **removing the remainder**[Q].
- **Direct sacs** are usually too broad for ligation and should not be opened but instead are simply **inverted into peritoneal cavity**[Q].
	- **Management of** the **hernia sac is sufficient for children** & **young adults**[Q]
	- **Reconstruction** (repair or strengthening) of the inguinal floor is **necessary in all adult hernias to prevent recurrence**[Q].
	- **Types of repair:**
	  – Primary **tissue repair**[Q]
	  – **Anterior tension-free mesh repair**[Q]
	  – **Preperitoneal repairs: Open** & **laparoscopic** approach[Q]

Section 3

Gastrointestinal Surgery

Inguinal Floor Reconstruction

Primary Tissue Repair	Anterior Tension-free Mesh Repair	Laparoscopic and Preperitoneal Repairs

• **Posterior wall** of inguinal wall is **strengthened by approximation of tissues with sutures**[Q].
• There is **no use of prosthetic material**[Q].
• **Advantages: Simplicity** of repair & **absence of** any **foreign body** in groin
• **Disadvantage: Higher recurrence rates** due to **tension** on the repair & **slower return to unrestricted physical activity**[Q].
 	
Types:
  – **Bassini repair**[Q]
  – Halsted repair
  – **McVay**[Q] (Cooper ligament) repair
  – **Shouldice repair**[Q]
  – Darn repair
	• Current practice in hernia management employ **synthetic mesh** to **bridge the defect**
	• **Recurrence** is **very low**
	• **Types:**
	  – **Lichtenstein repair**[Q]: Mesh is used to reconstruct the inguinal floor.
	  – **Patch & plug repair**[Q]: **Plug** of mesh is **inserted into** the hernia **defect** and sutured in place. Then another piece of **mesh** is **placed over** the **inguinal floor.**
		• Preperitoneal space is reached by either transabdominal laparoscopy (**TAPP**) or by totally extraperitoneal repair (**TEP**).
		• **Both techniques** are **similar in actual repair** but **differ in the manner** by which the **preperitoneal space is accessed.**
		• **TAPP (Transabdominal PrePeritoneal)** [Q]:
		  – Peritoneal space is reached by conventional laparoscopy and pre-peritoneum overlying the inguinal floor is dissected away as a flap.
		• **TEP (Totally ExtraPeritoneal)** [Q]:
		  – Preperitoneal space is accessed without entering the peritoneal cavity

Landmarks in Laparoscopic Repair

Triangle of Doom	Triangle of Pain	Corona Mortis

• Bounded **laterally** by **gonadal vessels**[Q]
• **Medially** by **vas deferens**[Q]
• **Apex** oriented superiorly at the **internal ring**[Q]
• Contain **external iliac vessels**[Q], deep circumflex iliac vein, femoral nerve & genital branch of genitofemoral nerve.
	• Also known as **Electrical hazard zone**[Q]
	• Bounded **medially** by **gonadal vessels**[Q]
	• **Superiorly** by **iliopubic tract**[Q]
	• **Laterally** by **peritoneum**[Q]
	• This triangle **contains** from lateral to medial:
	  – Lateral femoral cutaneous nerve[Q] (MC injured nerve in laparoscopic hernia repair)
	  – Anterior femoral cutaneous[Q]
	  – Femoral branch of the genitofemoral nerve[Q]
	  – Femoral nerve[Q]
		• Also known as **Crown of death**[Q]
		  – Vascular connections between the obturator and external iliac systems[Q]
		• **Aberrant obturator artery** arises from **inferior epigastric** artery, **arches over** the **Coopers ligament** and **joins** the **normal obturator artery**[Q] to complete a vascular ring
		• **Significant hemorrhage**[Q] may occur **if accidentally cut** and it is **difficult to achieve** subsequent **hemostasis**

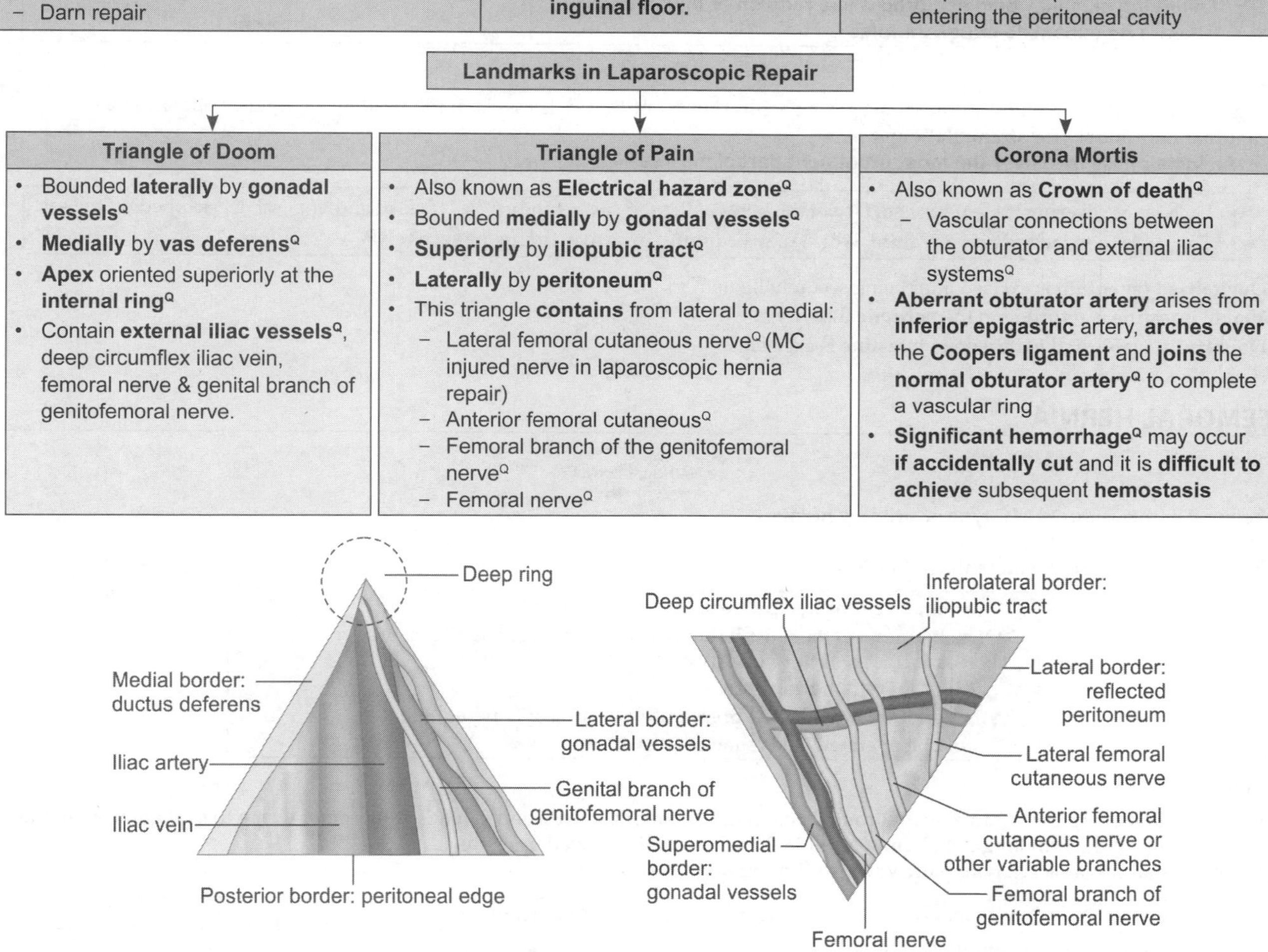

Complications of Groin Hernia Repairs

• **Recurrence** • Chronic groin pain • **Seroma** • Hematoma • **Ischemic orchitis** • **Testicular atrophy**	• Bladder injury • Wound infection • **Osteitis pubis** • Prosthetic complications (Contraction, Erosion, Infection)

- **MC injured nerve** in **laparoscopic** hernia repair: **Lateral cutaneous nerve of thigh**[Q] > **Genitofemoral nerve (GFN)**[Q]
- **MC injured nerve** in **open** hernia repair: **Ilio**inguinal nerve[Q] > **IlioH**ypogastric nerve[Q] > **G**enital branch of GFN[Q] (GHI in reverse sequence)

■ STRANGULATED INGUINAL HERNIA

STRANGULATED INGUINAL HERNIA

- **Indirect inguinal hernias strangulate more commonly**, the direct variety not so often because of wide neck of the sac.
- Strangulation occurs **more often in patients** who have **worn a truss for a long time** and in those with a partially reducible or an irreducible hernia.

> - **MC constricting agent: Neck of the sac**[Q] >External inguinal ring in children >Adhesions within the sac (rarely).
> - **MC contents: Small intestine**[Q] >Omentum

Diagnosis

- **Diagnosis of strangulation** is made **on clinical grounds.**

Clinical Features of Strangulated Inguinal Hernia
• In addition to patient having developed an **irreducible hernia** and an **intestinal obstruction**, patient develops **sudden pain**, at **first situated over hernia**, followed by **generalized abdominal pain.** • **Hernia** is **tense & extremely tender**[Q]. • **Overlying skin** may be **discolored** with a **reddish** or **bluish tinge**[Q]. • There is **no expansile cough impulse**[Q].

Treatment

- **Vigorous resuscitation** with IV fluids, **nasogastric aspiration & antibiotics** is **essential** followed by **emergency operation**[Q].
- **Inguinal herniotomy for strangulation:**
  - An **incision** is made **over the most prominent part** of the swelling.

> - **Each layer covering** the **anterior surface** of the body of the sac "**near fundus**"[Q] is **incised** and, if possible, stripped off the sac.
> - The sac is then incised and **any fluid**, which may be **highly infective, drained effectively**[Q].

- **Devitalised omentum** is **excised** after being securely ligated.
- **Viable intestine** is **returned to** the **peritoneal cavity**[Q].
- **Doubtfully viable** and **gangrenous intestine** is **excised**[Q].

■ FEMORAL HERNIA

FEMORAL HERNIA

- Femoral hernia is the **3rd MC type of primary hernia.**
- **More common** in **multipara**[Q]
- **More common** on **right side; Bilateral in 20%**[Q]

> - It **cannot be controlled by a truss**[Q]
> - Of all hernias it is the **most liable to become strangulated**[Q] because of:
>   - **Narrowness of the neck** of sac[Q]
>   - **Rigidity of femoral ring**[Q]
> - **Strangulation** is the **initial presentation** of **40% of femoral hernias**[Q]
> - Should be **operated on as soon as possible**[Q]

Anatomy

- **Femoral canal** occupies the **most medial compartment** of the **femoral sheath** and **extends from femoral ring** to **saphenous opening**[Q].
- **Femoral canal** is **1.25 cm long & 1.25 cm wide at its base**[Q], which is directed upwards.
- Femoral canal **contains fat, lymphatic vessels & lymph node of Cloquet**[Q].

Boundaries of Femoral Ring
• **Anteriorly** by the **inguinal ligament**[Q] • **Posteriorly** by Astley **Cooper's** (iliopectineal) **ligament, pubic bone & pectineus fascia**[Q] • **Medially** by **Gimbernat's** (lacunar) **ligament**[Q], which is also prolonged along the iliopectineal line, as Astley Cooper's ligament • **Laterally** by a **thin septum separating** it from the **femoral vein**[Q]

Clinical Features

- **Rare before puberty**
- Prevalence rises between **20-40 years**[Q] of age and this continues to old age.
- A small femoral hernia may be unnoticed by the patient or disregarded for years, perhaps **until the day it strangulates**[Q].
- **Mass** or **bulge below & lateral to pubic tubercle**[Q]

Contd…

Contd...

Treatment

- **Low inguinal** operation (**Lockwood**[Q])
- **Inguinal** operation (**Lotheissen**[Q])
- **High inguinal** operation (**McEvedy**[Q])
- Midline Abdominal Extraperitoneal Femoral Hernioplasty (**Henry Procedure**[Q]): This is now considered as the **procedure of choice**; does not damage the transversalis fascial floor; reducing the risk of a subsequent inguinal hernia.

Variants of Femoral Hernia	
Laugier's femoral hernia[Q]	• Hernia through a **gap in** the **lacunar** (Gimbernats) **ligament** • Diagnosis is based on **unusual medial position** of a **small femoral hernia sac** • **Always strangulated**
Narath's femoral hernia[Q]	• Occurs in patients with **congenital dislocation of hip** • Due to **lateral displacement of** the **psoas muscle** • Hernia lies hidden **behind** the **femoral vessels**
Cloquet's hernia[Q]	• **Sac lies under** the **pectineus** fascia

■ SPIGELIAN HERNIA

SPIGELIAN HERNIA

- Spigelian hernia **occurs through** the **spigelian fascia**[Q]
- **Spigelian fascia** is composed of **aponeurotic layer** between **rectus muscle** medially & **semilunar line** laterally[Q].

> - Nearly **all spigelian hernias** occur at or **below the arcuate line**[Q].
> - **Absence of posterior rectus fascia** may **contribute to** an **inherent weakness** in this area[Q].
> - These hernias are **often interparietal**, with the **hernia sac dissecting posterior to external oblique aponeurosis**[Q].
> - **Spigelian hernia** sac **always penetrates** the **spigelian aponeurosis** & **usually penetrates** the **internal oblique** musculature[Q].

Clinical Features

- **Most spigelian hernias** are **small** (1-2 cm in diameter)
- Patients often present with **localized pain** in the area **without a bulge** because the **hernia lies beneath** the intact **external oblique aponeurosis**[Q].

Diagnosis

- **Ultrasound** or **CT** of the abdomen can be **useful to establish** the **diagnosis**[Q].

Treatment

- A spigelian hernia is **repaired** because of the **risk for incarceration**[Q] associated with its **relatively narrow neck**.
- **Larger defects** are repaired using a **mesh prosthesis**[Q].

■ SLIDING HERNIA (HERNIA EN GLISSADE)

SLIDING HERNIA (HERNIA EN GLISSADE)

- Hernias in which **posterior wall of** the sac is **formed by a viscus**[Q]
- **Viscera is liable to be injured,** if the **hernia sac is resected during surgery**[Q]
- **More common** on **left side**[Q]

Most Common Content	
• **Left side**: **Sigmoid colon**[Q] & its mesentery (**MC**)	• **Right side**: **Cecum**[Q]

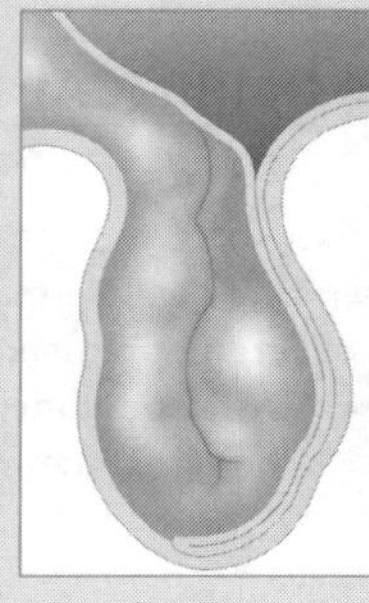

- **Other contents**: Appendix, urinary bladder, uterus, fallopian tube, ovary or ureter
- **Primary danger**: **Failure to recognize** the **visceral component** of hernia sac **before injury to** the bowel or bladder[Q].

Clinical Features

- **Occurs almost exclusively in men**[Q].
- **More common** on the **left side**[Q]; rarely bilateral
- Patient is **nearly always over 40 years of age**, the **incidence rising with age**[Q].

> - Occasionally, **large intestine is strangulated** in a sliding hernia; more often, **non-strangulated large intestine** is **present behind the sac containing strangulated small intestine**[Q].

Treatment

- **Operation** is indicated
- **Sliding hernia contents** are **reduced into the peritoneal cavity,** and **any excess hernia sac** is **ligated & divided**[Q].

> - Sliding hernia is a cause of considerable discomfort, **impossible to control with a truss**[Q].

■ LUMBAR HERNIA

LUMBAR HERNIA

- Lumbar hernias can be either **congenital (20%)** or **acquired (80%)**[Q]
- **Occur in** the **lumbar region** of the **posterior abdominal wall**[Q].
- **More common** on **left side**, in **men**[Q]

> - Hernias through the **superior lumbar triangle (Grynfeltt's triangle)** are **more common**[Q].
> - **Grynfeltt's triangle** is bounded by the **12th rib, paraspinal muscles & internal oblique muscle**[Q].

- **Less common** are hernias through the **inferior lumbar triangle (Petit's triangle)**[Q]
- **Petit's triangle** is bounded by **iliac crest, latissimus dorsi muscle, & external oblique muscle**[Q].
- **Weakness of lumbodorsal fascia** through either of these areas results in **progressive protrusion of extraperitoneal fat** and a **hernia sac**[Q].

Clinical Features

- **MC presentation: Unilateral bulge** in the flank[Q].
- **Lumbar hernias are not prone to incarceration**[Q].

Treatment

- **Dowd's operation** is done for **lumbar hernia**[Q].
- **Repair** is **best done by placement of prosthetic mesh**, which can be sutured to the margins of the hernia[Q].

■ OBTURATOR HERNIA

OBTURATOR HERNIA

- Also known as **skinny old lady hernia** or **French hernia**[Q].
- **Thin, elderly, & debilitated women** are at greatest risk
- More common in **female** secondary to the **larger & more oblique** design of the **obturator canal**[Q].

Predisposing Factors	
• Women with **wider pelvis & more triangular** **obturator canal**[Q] • **Malnutrition**[Q]	• Chronic constipation, COPD, ascites, kyphoscoliosis[Q] • Multiparity[Q] • Age **70-79 years**[Q]

Clinical Features

- Patients present **most commonly with intestinal obstruction**[Q] (jejunum or ileum within the hernial sac).

Howship-Romberg Sign[Q]	• **Pain radiating down** the **medial thigh to** the **knee** due to **compression of obturator nerve** (anterior division) by the hernial sac • **Pathognomonic for** an **incarcerated hernia** • Present in **25-50%** cases
Hannington Kiff sign[Q]	• **Absence of** the **obturator reflex** in the thigh **due to compression of obturator nerve.**

Treatment

- **Operation is indicated**
- **Posterior approach** (either open or laparoscopic) **is preferred**[Q].

■ UMBILICAL HERNIA

UMBILICAL HERNIA

- Umbilical hernias **in infants** are **congenital**[Q] and are quite common.
- **Strong predisposition** in individuals of **African descent**.
- **Close spontaneously in most cases** by the **age of 2 years**[Q].
- **Complications** are **unusual**[Q]
- Those that **persist after the age of 5 years** are frequently **repaired surgically**[Q]

Indications of Surgery in Umbilical Hernia	
• Persisting **beyond 5 years**[Q] • **Symptomatic**[Q] • **Strangulated**[Q]	• Defect **size >2 cm**[Q] • **Progressive enlarging**[Q] hernia after the age 1-2 years

Treatment

- **Small defects: Closed primarily**[Q]
- **Defects >3 cm: Closed using prosthetic mesh**[Q].

Mayo's Repair
• **Vest-over-pants repair** proposed by Mayo employs **imbrication of superior** and **inferior fascial edges**[Q].
• Because of **increased tension on** the **repair** and **recurrence rates** of 30%, it is **rarely performed today**[Q].

Abdominal Wall Defects	
Omphalocele	**Gastroschisis**
• **Intestine fails to return**, abdominal **contents protruding** directly **through** the **umbilical ring** with a **sac covering** the **bowel**[Q]	• **Fetal gut** is **extruded** through a defect in abdominal wall
• **Abdominal contents** are **covered with peritoneum** on the **inside** & **amnion** on the **outside**[Q]	• **Defect** is **always on** the **right side of umbilical ring** with an intact umbilical cord[Q]
• **Size of defect** is **variable**, ranging from a small opening through which a **small portion of intestine** is herniated to a **large one** in which **entire bowel & liver** are included[Q].	• **Covering sac is absent**[Q]
	• **Risk for associated anomalies is low**[Q].
	• **Association with intestinal atresia** in up to 15%.
• **Chromosomal abnormalities**[Q] are present in roughly **30%** of infants, including **trisomies 13, 18 & 21**[Q].	• Atresias may involve the **small and large intestine**[Q].
• **More than half** of infants have other **major** or **minor malforma-tions**, with **cardiac** being the **most common**[Q], followed by musculo-skeletal, gastrointestinal & genitourinary.	• Babies are more often **small for gestational age** and **born to mothers with** a history of **cigarette, alcohol**, and **recreational drug use** and intake of **aspirin, ibuprofen**, and **pseudoephedrine** during the first trimester[Q]
	• **Increased** risk in **mothers younger than 20 years**[Q].
• Close association with **Beckwith-Wiedemann syndrome**[Q] (omphalocele, hyperinsulinemia, and macroglossia).	• In patients with gastroschisis, the **intestine** is often **thickened, edematous, matted together**, and **foreshortened**[Q].
• **Poor prognosis**[Q] due to **associated abnormalities**.	• **Good prognosis**[Q]

■ EPIGASTRIC HERNIA (FATTY HERNIA OF THE LINEA ALBA, EPIGASTRIC LIPOMA)

EPIGASTRIC HERNIA (FATTY HERNIA OF THE LINEA ALBA, EPIGASTRIC LIPOMA)

- About 3% to 5% of the population has epigastric hernias.
- **More common in men**[Q].
- **Located between** the **xiphoid process** & **umbilicus**[Q]

> - **Multiple in** up to **20%** of patients, and **about 80%** are **just off**[Q] the **midline**.

- Usually **within 5 to 6 cm** of the **umbilicus**.
- **Defects** are **small** and often **produce pain out of proportion** to their size owing to **incarceration of preperitoneal fat**[Q].

Clinical Features
- **Majority** of these hernias are **asymptomatic**
- Sometimes such a hernia gives rise to **attacks of local pain**. This may be because the **fatty contents become nipped sufficiently** to produce **partial strangulation**[Q].

> - **Referred pain**: It is not uncommon to find that the patient, who may not have noticed the hernia, complains of **pain suggestive of a peptic ulcer**[Q].

Treatment
- Repair usually consists of **excision of** the **incarcerated preperitoneal tissue** & **simple closure of the fascial defect**[Q].

■ INCISIONAL HERNIA

INCISIONAL HERNIA

- **Postoperative ventral abdominal wall hernia** or incisional hernia is the result of a **failure of fascial tissues to heal** & **close** following laparotomy[Q].
- As the approximated **fascial tissue separates, bowel & omentum herniates** through the opening, **covered by a peritoneal sac**[Q].

> - **Highest incidence** is seen with **large, midline, vertical, lower abdominal incisions**[Q].
> - **Incidence** seems to be **lower in smaller incisions**

Risk Factors for Incisional Hernia		
Surgery Related	**Surgeon Related**	**Patient Related**
• **Emergency surgery**[Q] • **Wound infection**[Q] • **Midline vertical incisions**[Q]	• Wounds closed under **excessive tension**[Q] • **Poor technique**[Q] • Use of **absorbable sutures**[Q]	• **Advanced age, malnutrition**[Q] • **Ascites, Steroid use**[Q] • **Diabetes, obesity**[Q] • **Smoking, coughing**[Q] • **Vomiting & distension**[Q]

Clinical Features
- **Bulge** in the abdominal wall originating deep to the skin scar.
- **Symptoms aggravated** by **coughing** or **straining** as the hernia contents protrude through the abdominal wall defect.
- In **large ventral hernias**, the **skin** may present with **ischemic** or **pressure necrosis** leading to **frank ulceration**[Q].

Contd…

Contd...

Treatment
- **Operative repair:** Primary **suture repair** of the hernia, **open repair** with prosthetic mesh, and **laparoscopic incisional hernia repair**[Q].

  - Laparoscopic incisional hernia repair (**IPOM**- Intraperitoneal onlay mesh repair) has the **lowest rate of recurrence**[Q]

- Incisional hernias with a **diameter >4 cm** should be **repaired with mesh**[Q].

■ UMBILICAL ADENOMA OR RASPBERRY TUMOUR

Umbilical Adenoma or Raspberry Tumour

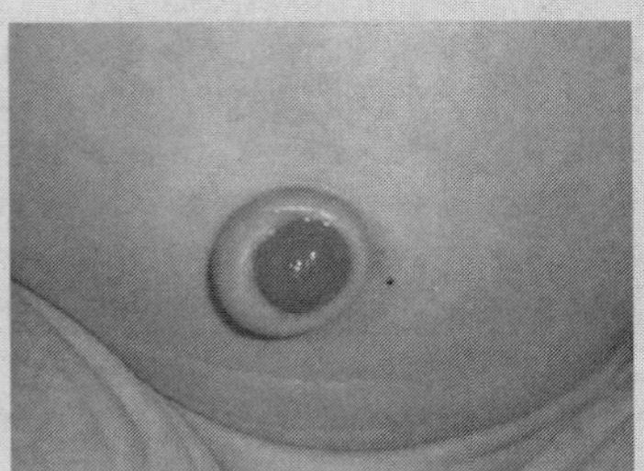

- **Commonly seen in infants** but only occasionally later in life[Q].
- Due to a **partially** (occasionally a completely) **unobliterated vitellointestinal duct**[Q].
- **Mucosa prolapsing through** the **umbilicus** gives rise to a **raspberry-like tumour**[Q]
- **Moist** and **tends to bleed**

Treatment
- **Pedunculated tumour:** A **ligature is tied around**[Q] it, in a few days, the polypus drops off.
- If tumour reappears after this procedure: **Umbilectomy**[Q]

■ DESMOID TUMOR

Desmoid Tumor

- **MC primary malignant neoplasm of the mesentery:** Desmoid tumor
- Arises from **musculoaponeurotic structures** of abdominal wall, especially **below** the **level of umbilicus**[Q].
- It is a **completely unencapsulated fibroma**[Q] and is **so hard** that it **creaks when** it is **cut**[Q].
- **Distribution: Extra-abdominal (60%), abdominal wall (25%), intra-abdominal (15%).**
- About **80% of cases** occur **in women**[Q], many of whom have borne children

  - Occurs **occasionally in scars**[Q] of old hernial or other abdominal **operation wounds**.
  - **Surgical trauma**[Q]: Important etiological factor
  - **Estrogens stimulate**[Q] desmoid growth
  - Occur in cases of **FAP**[Q] **(Gardener's syndrome)**

Pathology
- Tumour is composed of **fibrous tissue** containing **multinucleated plasmodial masses** resembling **foreign body giant cells**[Q].
- Usually of **very slow growth**, it **tends to infiltrate muscle** in the **immediate area**[Q].
- Eventually it **undergoes a myxomatous change** and it then **increases in size more rapidly**.
- **Metastasis does not occur**[Q], no sarcomatous change

Clinical Features
- **Desmoids classically arise in pregnancy** as an **abdominal mass independent of uterus**.
- **MC presentation: Abdominal mass**
- Affected patients may present with a **painful versus asymptomatic firm mass, bowel obstruction, or bowel ischemia**.

Diagnosis
- **MRI is investigation of choice** for **extremity & abdominal wall desmoids**[Q].
- **Biopsy** is required to **establish the diagnosis**.

Treatment
- **Wide local excision** (with **2 cm margin**) is **treatment of choice**[Q].
- **Surgery + Radiotherapy:** For **recurrent desmoid tumors**[Q]

■ CLASSIFICATION OF HERNIA

1. **Type IIIA in Nyhus classification of hernia:**
   (MCI Nov 2017, DNB 2011)
   a. Direct inguinal hernia   b. Indirect inguinal hernia
   c. Femoral hernia   d. Umbilical hernia

2. **Femoral hernia in Nyhus classification:** *(WBPG 2014)*
   a. IIIA   b. II
   c. IIIC   d. IV

■ RISK FACTORS FOR HERNIA

3. **The following are the risk factors for inguinal hernia:**
   a. Family history of inguinal hernia   *(PGI Dec 2007)*
   b. Weight lifter   c. COPD
   d. Female   e. Obesity

■ INGUINAL HERNIA

4. **Most common type of hernia in females is:**
   (AIIMS Feb 97, DPG 2005, JIPMER GIS 2011)
   a. Direct inguinal hernia   b. Indirect inguinal hernia
   c. Femoral hernia   d. Umbilical hernia

5. **For differentiating inguinal hernia and femoral hernia the landmark will be:** *(AIIMS Nov 98)*
   a. Public symphysis   b. Femoral artery
   c. Inferior epigastric level   d. Public tubercle

■ INDIRECT INGUINAL HERNIA

6. **All of the following statements are true about repair of groin hernias except:** *(AIIMS Nov 2004)*
   a. Lichtenstein tension free repair has a low recurrence rate
   b. TEP repair is an extraperitoneal approach to laparoscopic repair of groin hernia
   c. In Shouldice repair, non-absorbable mesh is used
   d. The surgery can be done under local anesthesia in selected cases

7. **The treatment of choice for inguinal hernia in infants is:**
   (MCI June 2018)
   a. Herniotomy   b. Herniorrhaphy
   c. Truss   d. Hernioplasty

8. **Which one of the following is not performed in Lichtenstein tension free hernioplasty?** *(Karnataka 2006)*
   a. High ligation of indirect hernia sac
   b. Mesh sutured to the conjoint tendon and inguinal ligament
   c. Conjoint tendon sutured to inguinal ligament
   d. Spermatic cord is placed in two tails of the internal ring

9. **True statement regarding direct inguinal hernia:**
   (UPPG 2008)
   a. Most common inguinal hernia in women is direct
   b. Direct hernia is medial to inferior epigastric artery
   c. Repair of the transversalis fascia and the internal ring
   d. Descends downwards and inwards towards the scrotum

10. **Content of epilocele is:** *(DNB 2011)*
    a. Omentum   b. Intestine
    c. Colon   d. Urinary bladder

11. **Triangle of Doom is bounded by all of the following except:**
    (AIIMS Nov 2008)
    a. Cooper's ligament   b. Vas deferens
    c. Gonadal vessels   d. Peritoneal reflection

12. **Which of the following is correct regarding the boundaries of triangle of Doom?** *(AIIMS May 2018)*
    a. Medially vas deferens, laterally gonadal vessels, inferiorly peritoneum
    b. Laterally vas deferens, medially gonadal vessels, inferiorly peritoneum
    c. Laterally medial umbilical ligament, medially gonadal vessels, inferiorly peritoneum
    d. Laterally gonadal vessels, medially lateral umbilical ligament, inferiorly peritoneum

13. **True regarding indirect inguinal hernia are all except:**
    a. Most common type of hernia   *(MCI March 2008)*
    b. Always unilateral
    c. Inguinal herniotomy is the basic operation
    d. Transillumination distinguishes it from hydrocele

14. **Most common type of hernia in the young age group:**
    (MCI Sept 2006)
    a. Femoral hernia   b. Direct inguinal hernia
    c. Indirect inguinal hernia   d. Umbilical hernia

15. **Least recurrence rate in incisional hernia repair is following:**
    (JIPMER 2010)
    a. On lay mesh repair   b. Intraperitoneal mesh repair
    c. Inlay mesh repair   d. Shouldice repair

16. **Inguinal herniotomy includes all of the following except:**
    a. Dissection and opening of the hernial sac   *(Orissa 2011)*
    b. Reduction of contents
    c. Transfixation of the neck and excision of redundant sac
    d. Repair of stretched inguinal ring and fascia transversalis

17. **Hesselbach's triangle is bounded by the following, except:**
    a. Rectus abdominis muscle   *(Orissa 2011)*
    b. Transversus abdominis muscle
    c. Inferior epigastric artery
    d. Inguinal ligament

18. **Ilioinguinal nerve is damaged while incising:**
    a. External oblique aponeurosis   *(MHSSMCET 2006)*
    b. Internal oblique muscle
    c. Transverse abdominis
    d. Linea alba

19. **Funicular hernia is type of:** *(DNB 2007)*
    a. Direct inguinal hernia   b. Indirect inguinal hernia
    c. Femoral Hernia   d. Umbilical hernia

20. **A 3-year-old child comes with hydrocele of the hernia sac. Management will include:** *(AIIMS May 2015)*
    a. Herniotomy   b. Herniorrhaphy
    c. Observation only   d. Operate after 5 years of age

21. **Triangle of doom is related to:** *(Recent Question 2014)*
    a. Laparoscopic Nissen's fundoplication
    b. Laparoscopic hernia surgery
    c. Endoscopic thyroidectomy
    d. Thoracoscopic thymectomy

22. **Inguinal hernia in a child is associated with:**
    Recent Question 2017
    a. Patent processus vaginalis   b. Ectopia vesicae
    c. Undescended testis   d. All are correct

23. **Triangle of doom is seen during which type of hernia surgery:** *(Recent Question 2017)*
    a. Laparoscopic
    b. Open
    c. Both
    d. None

■ COMPLICATIONS OF HERNIA

24. **During surgery of hernia, the sac of a strangulated inguinal hernia should be opened at the:**
    (AIIMS Nov 96, AIIMS June 2004)
    a. Neck
    b. Body
    c. Fundus
    d. Deep ring

25. **Treatment of strangulated hernia is:** *(Kerala 94)*
    a. Observation
    b. Immediate surgery
    c. Manual reduction
    d. Analgesics

26. **Which is the 1st sign of strangulation of inguinal hernia?**
    a. Tense
    b. Tenderness   *(UPPG 96)*
    c. Irreducible
    d. Redness

27. **During laparoscopic inguinal hernia repair a tacker was accidently placed below and lateral to the iliopubic tract. Postoperatively the patient complained of pain and soreness in the thigh. This is due to the involvement of:**
    (AIIMS Nov 2015, May 2015)
    a. Lateral cutaneous nerve of thigh
    b. Ilioinguinal nerve
    c. Genital branch of genitofemoral nerve
    d. Obturator nerve

28. **Most common nerve injured during hernia surgery:**
    (Recent Question 2017, 2014)
    a. Ilioinguinal nerve
    b. Iliohypogastric nerve
    c. Genitofemoral nerve
    d. None of the above

■ FEMORAL HERNIA

29. **Which structures live immediately lateral to femoral hernia?**
    (AIIMS Nov 2011)
    a. Lateral cutaneous nerve of thigh
    b. Femoral nerve
    c. Femoral artery
    d. Femoral vein

30. **Femoral hernia is characteristically ..... the public tubercle.**
    (MHPGMCET 2007, TN 89)
    a. Lateral and below
    b. Medial and above
    c. Lateral and above
    d. Medial and below

31. **In the treatment of femoral hernia, Lockwood's operation refers to:** *(Karnataka 2006)*
    a. Low inguinal operation
    b. High inguinal operation
    c. Inguinal operation
    d. Laparoscopic surgery

32. **Strangulation most commonly occurs in:**
    (DNB 2012, MCI Sept 2005)
    a. Femoral hernia
    b. Direct inguinal hernia
    c. Indirect inguinal hernia
    d. Lumbar hernia

33. **Medial boundary of femoral ring is formed by:**
    a. Inguinal ligament   *(JIPMER 2011)*
    b. Pectineal ligament
    c. Lacunar ligament
    d. Septum separating it from femoral vein

34. **A patient with femoral hernia can be managed by:**
    a. Bassini repair
    b. Hunters repair
    c. Shouldice repair
    d. McVay repair

35. **Hernia that lies under the fascia of pectineus muscle is:**
    (MHSSMCET 2006)
    a. Cloquet's hernia
    b. Laugier's hernia
    c. Narath's hernia
    d. Obturator hernia

36. **In Laugier's hernia opening is in the:** *(WBPG 2014)*
    a. Lacunar ligament
    b. Conjoint tendon
    c. External oblique
    d. Peritoneum

37. **Neck of sac of femoral hernia lies:** *(Recent Question 2013)*
    a. Below and lateral to pubic tubercle
    b. Above and lateral
    c. Above and medial
    d. Below and medial

■ SPIGELIAN HERNIA

38. **Spigelian hernia is seen in:** *(All India 99)*
    a. Lumbar triangle
    b. Subumbilical region
    c. Paraumbilical region
    d. Supraumbilical region

39. **Spigelian hernia is a type of hernia occurring at:**
    (Recent Question 2013 PGI June 95, PGI June 2000)
    a. Medial border of rectus abdominis
    b. Lateral border of rectus abdominis
    c. Lumbar region
    d. Femoral canal

40. **Spigelian hernia is:** *(MCI March 2005)*
    a. Passes through the obturator canal
    b. Hernia occurring through the linea alba
    c. Hernia through the triangle of Petit
    d. Hernia occurring at the level of arcuate line

41. **Spigelian hernia is a defect within the following muscle:**
    (COMEDK 2004)
    a. Rectus abdominis
    b. Internal oblique
    c. Transversalis abdominis
    d. External oblique

■ SLIDING HERNIA

42. **Most common content in 'Hernia en glissade' is:**
    (PGI June 96, All India 95)
    a. Omentum
    b. Urinary bladder
    c. Caecum
    d. Sigmoid colon

43. **Sliding constituent of a large direct hernia is:** *(All India 88)*
    a. Bladder
    b. Sigmoid colon
    c. Caecum
    d. Appendix

44. **Most useful investigation in sliding hernia in female:**
    a. Fluroscopy
    b. Barium-meal *(UPPG 2008)*
    b. Palpation method
    d. Ultrasound

45. **If caecum is involved as a part of the wall of hernia sac and is not its content, then it will be known as:**
    (Recent Question 2014, 2008)
    a. Richter's hernia
    b. Spigelian hernia
    c. Sliding hernia
    d. Interstitial hernia

■ LUMBAR HERNIA

46. **About lumbar hernia, false statements:**
    a. Superior triangle is Grynfeltt's triangle
    b. Inferior triangle is Petit's triangle
    c. Mostly acquired
    d. More common on right side

■ OBTURATOR HERNIA

47. **Howship-Romberg sign is seen in:**
    (JIPMER SS 2016, Recent Question 2016)
    a. Sliding hernia
    b. Obturator hernia
    c. Lumbar hernia
    d. Paraduodenal hernia

■ UMBILICAL HERNIA

48. **The covering over an omphalocele is:**
    a. Skin
    b. Amniotic membrane
    c. Chorionic membrane
    d. None of the above

49. Omphalocele is caused by: *(DNB 2010)*
    a. Duplication of intestinal loops
    b. Abnormal rotation of the intestinal loop
    c. Failure of gut to return to the body cavity from its physiological herniation
    d. Reversed rotation of the intestinal loop

50. Exomphalos major should be operated at: *(DNB 91)*
    a. Birth
    b. 3 months of age
    c. 1 year
    d. 3 years

51. Mayo's operation is done for: *(Recent Question 2016)*
    a. Spigelian hernia
    b. Femoral hernia
    c. Richter's hernia
    d. Umbilical hernia

52. What is the most probable diagnosis based on the given image?   *(Recent Question 2017)*

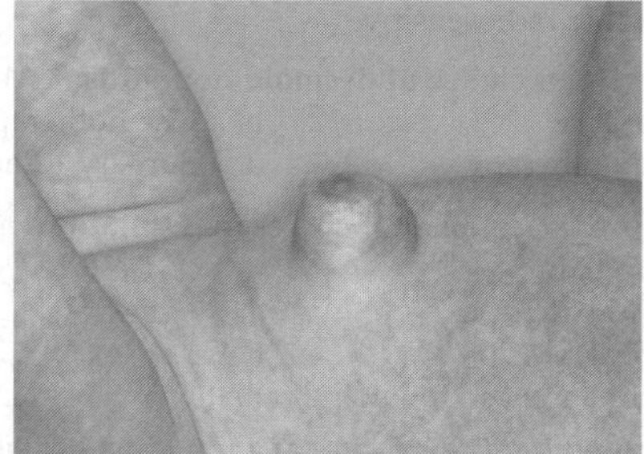

    a. Omphalocele
    b. Gastroschisis
    c. Umbilical hernia
    d. Ectopia vesicae

53. Umbilical hernia in a child - indication for surgery is/are:
    a. Failure to disappear by 3 years   *(MAHE 2007)*
    b. >2 cm size
    c. Symptomatic
    d. All of the above

54. A child of 6 months was presented with following presentation. What is the management protocol?   *(MCI Dec 2019)*

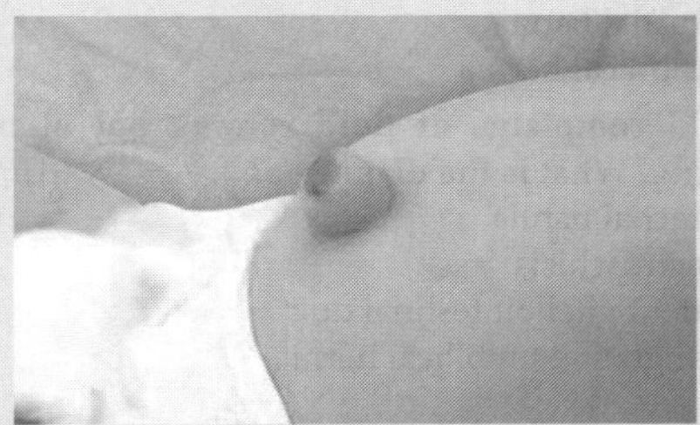

    a. Indication of surgery if not resolve by 2 years
    b. Surgery after 5 years
    c. Immediate surgery
    d. Hernioplasty

55. What is false regarding gastroschisis and omphalocele?   *(DNB 2012, AIIMS 2000)*
    a. Intestinal obstruction is common in gastroschisis
    b. Gastroschisis is associated with multiple anomalies
    c. Umbilical cord is attached in normal position in gastroschisis
    d. Liver is the content of omphalocele

56. Hernia that is least likely to strangulate is: *(AIIMS Nov 93)*
    a. Femoral hernia
    b. Direct inguinal hernia
    c. Indirect inguinal hernia
    d. Umbilical hernia

57. True regarding gastroschisis is: *(DNB 2003)*
    a. An omphalocele
    b. An anterior abdominal wall tumor
    c. A variant of gastric carcinoma
    d. Herniation of abdominal contents through body wall

58. What is the diagnosis based on the given image?
    a. Gastroschisis
    b. Omphalocele
    c. Umbilical hernia
    d. Ectopia vesicae

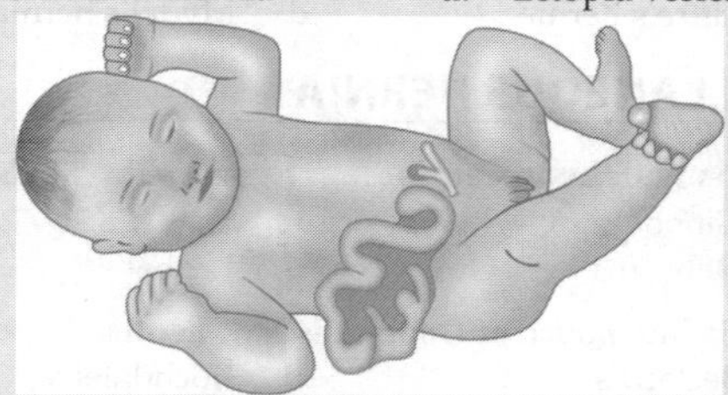

59. What is the diagnosis based on the given image?   *(Recent Question 2017)*
    a. Gastroschisis
    b. Omphalocele
    c. Umbilical hernia
    d. Epigastric hernia

60. In omphalocele abdominal wall defect is more than:
    a. 0.5 cm
    b. 2.5 cm   *(WBPG 2014)*
    c. 4 cm
    d. 6 cm

61. Omphalocele is caused by: *(Recent Question 2019)*
    a. Duplication of intestinal loops
    b. Abnormal rotation of intestinal loops
    c. Failure of gut to return to body cavity after its physiological herniation
    d. Reversed rotation of intestinal loops

■ EPIGASTRIC HERNIA

62. The hernia which often simulates a peptic ulcer is: *(WB PG 2015, MCI March 2007, Karnataka 94)*
    a. Umbilical hernia
    b. Fatty hernia of the linea alba
    c. Incisional hernia
    d. Inguinal hernia

63. True about epigastric hernia is: *(AIIMS May 2012)*
    a. Located below the umbilicus and always in the midline
    b. Located above the umbilicus and always in the midline
    c. Located above the umbilicus and on either side
    d. Can be seen anywhere on abdomen

■ RICHTER'S HERNIA

64. The sac contains only a portion of the circumference of the intestine: *(UPPG 2007, 2005)*
    a. Richter's hernia
    b. Littre's hernia
    c. Spigelian hernia
    d. Lumbar hernia

65. Strangulation without obstruction is seen in: *(DNB 2005)*
    a. Inguinal hernia
    b. Femoral hernia
    c. Richter's hernia
    d. Littres hernia

66. Richter hernia is most common in: *(Recent Question 2014)*
    a. Hiatus hernia
    b. Femoral hernia
    c. Lumbar hernia
    d. Direct inguinal hernia

■ LITTRE'S HERNIA

67. Which of the following is content of Littre's hernia?
    a. Urinary bladder   *(DNB 2012, MHPGMET 2005)*
    b. Meckel's diverticulum
    c. Circumference of intestinal wall
    d. Appendix

68. Hernia containing Meckel's diverticulum is:

(MHSSMCET 2005)

- a. Richter's hernia
- b. Pantaloon hernia
- c. Littre's hernia
- d. Mydel's hernia

■ MISCELLANEOUS HERNIA

69. Hernia with hydrocele is .... hernia. *(Recent Question 2016)*
- a. Gibbon's
- b. Fruber's
- c. Dobson's
- d. Leobel's

70. Hernia into pouch of Douglas is ...... hernia.
- a. Beclard's
- b. Bochdaleks
- c. Blandin's
- d. Berger's

71. The person whose work on the radical cure of hernia immortalised his name was: *(Karnataka 96)*
- a. William Halsted
- b. Eduardo Bassini
- c. Mc Vay
- d. Koontz

72. Truss cannot prevent progression of which type of inguinal hernia? *(UPPG 99)*
- a. Sliding
- b. Littre's
- c. Indirect
- d. Direct

■ INCISIONAL HERNIA

73. Which of the following does not predispose to abdominal wall dehiscence? *(JIPMER 92)*
- a. Faulty technique
- b. Malignancy
- c. Raised intra-abdominal pressure
- d. Old age

74. Ventral hernia is a/an: *(AMC 99)*
- a. Incisional hernia
- b. Umbilical hernia
- c. Femoral hernia
- d. Inguinal hernia

75. Incisional hernia, not true is: *(DPG 2006)*
- a. Faulty operative technique
- b. There is distension of abdomen
- c. Associated with infection of the wound
- d. Caused by use of local anesthesia

76. Hernia prone to re-occur apter primary repair: *(JIPMER 2013)*
- a. Femoral
- b. Epigastric
- c. Spigelian
- d. Incisional

■ UMBILICAL ADENOMA

77. Treatment of choice of umbilical adenoma in a new born is:
- a. Occlusion with a coin
- b. Strapping
- c. Surgery
- d. Masterly inactivity

78. "Raspberry tumour" is another name for:

(Recent Question 2013)

- a. Umbilical fistula
- b. Umbilical granuloma
- c. Umbilical adenoma
- d. Meckel's diverticulum

79. Raspberry tumour is: *(JIPMER 98)*
- a. Neoplastic
- b. Inflammatory
- c. Traumatic
- d. Congenital

■ DESMOID TUMOR

80. Regarding desmoid tumour which is not correct?
- a. Often seen below the umbilicus *(DNB 2002)*
- b. Unencapsulated
- c. More common in women
- d. Metastasis does not occur
- e. Highly radiosensitive

81. Treatment of choice of desmoid tumour is: *(AIIMS June 94)*
- a. Surgery
- b. Chemotherapy
- c. Radiotherapy
- d. Surgery + Radiotherapy

82. What is the treatment of choice in desmoid tumors?
- a. Irradiation *(DNB 2009, UPSC 2008)*
- b. Wide excision
- c. Local excision
- d. Local excision following radiation

83. Most common presentation of abdominal desmoid tumor is:

(AIIMS Nov 2017)

- a. Abdominal pain
- b. Abdominal mass
- c. Fever
- d. Rectal prolapse

■ PATENT URACHUS

84. A newborn presents with discharge of urine from the umbilicus for 3 days. Diagnosis is: *(UPPG 2008)*
- a. Meckel's diverticulum
- b. Mesenteric cysts
- c. Urachal fistula
- d. Umbilical hernia

85. A child complains of fluid coming out of umbilicus on straining. What is the diagnosis? *(AIIMS Nov 2014)*
- a. Urachal fistula
- b. Gastroschisis
- c. Patent vitellointestinal duct
- d. Congenital umbilical hernia

■ CLASSIFICATION OF HERNIA

1. **Ans. a. Direct inguinal hernia** *(Ref: Sabiston 20/e p1098; Schwartz 11/e p1602, 10/e p1634-1635)*
2. **Ans. c. IIIC**

■ RISK FACTORS FOR HERNIA

3. **Ans. a. Family history of inguinal hernia, b. Weight lifter, c. COPD, e. Obesity** *(Ref: Sabiston 20/e p1092; Schwartz 11/e p1604, 10/e p1500; Bailey 27/e p1023-1024)*

■ INGUINAL HERNIA

4. **Ans. b. Indirect inguinal hernia** *(Ref: Sabiston 20/e p1092; Schwartz 11/e p1606, 10/e p1634-1635; Bailey 27/e p1029; Schackelford 8/e p573)*

   - **MC type** of hernia **in males: Indirect inguinal hernia**[Q]
   - **MC type** of hernia **in females: Indirect inguinal hernia**[Q]
   - **Femoral hernia is more common in females**[Q].
   - **Direct inguinal hernia is more common in the elderly**[Q]

5. **Ans. d. Public tubercle** *(Ref: Sabiston 20/e p1092; Schwartz 11/e p1606, 10/e p1634-1635; Bailey 27/e p1029; Schackelford 7/e p561)*

Inguinal Hernia	Femoral Hernia
• **Neck of sac** lies **above** and **medial** to the **pubic tubercle**[Q]	• **Neck of sac** lies **below** and **lateral** to the **pubic tubercle**[Q]

■ INDIRECT INGUINAL HERNIA

6. **Ans. c. In Shouldice repair, non-absorbable mesh is used** *(Ref: Sabiston 20/e p1097-1102; Schwartz 11/e p1607, 10/e p1634-1635; Bailey 27/e p1032; Schackelford 8/e p603)*

   In **Shouldice repair**, inguinal floor is strengthened by approximation of tissues using non-absorbable sutures, **mesh is not used**.

7. **Ans. a. Herniotomy**

8. **Ans. c. Conjoint tendon sutured to inguinal ligament** *(Ref: Sabiston 20/e p1100; Schwartz 11/e p1612, 10/e p1508; Bailey 27/e p1032; Schackelford 8/e p602)*

   ### LICHTENSTEIN TENSION-FREE REPAIR

   - **Initial exposure** and **mobilization of cord structures** is identical to other open approaches.
   - Lichtenstein repair **does not include routine division** of the **transversalis fascia**[Q].
   - **Internal inguinal ring is not reconstructed** using canal structures.
   - **Floor** and **internal ring** are **reinforced through** the application of the **mesh.**[Q]
   - **Mesh is split to accommodate** the **spermatic cord**[Q].
   - **Rounded edge is attached** to the **anterior rectus sheath**[Q] just medial to the pubic tubercle
   - **Inferior margin** of the mesh is then **sutured to the shelving edge** of the **inguinal ligament**[Q]

9. **Ans. b. Direct hernia is medial to inferior epigastric artery** *(Ref: Sabiston 20/e p1092-1093; Schwartz 11/e p1607, 10/e p1503; Bailey 27/e p1029)*

	Indirect Hernia	Direct Hernia
Age	• **Any age**	• Common in **elderly**[Q]
Herniation	• **Protrusion** through **deep inguinal ring**; Herniation occurs latter[Q]	• **Herniation** through **posterior wall** of inguinal canal
Shape	• **Pyriform/oval** in shape[Q]	• **Globular/round** shape
Descent	• **Obliquely** and **downwards**	• **Directly forwards**
Descent to scrotum	• **Descent to** the **bottom of scrotum** and becomes **complete**[Q]	• **Rarely** descent to the bottom of the scrotum
Neck	• Narrow[Q]	• **Wide**[Q]
Sac	• **Lateral** to **inferior epigastric artery**	• **Medial** to **inferior epigastric artery**
Zieman's test	• **Cough impulse** on **index finger**[Q]	• **Cough impulse** on **middle finger**
Invagination test	• **Tip** of **finger**	• **Pulp** of **finger**

Ring occlusion test	• Does not bulge	• Bulge medial to occluding finger
Coverings (from inside out)	• Extraperitoneal tissue • **Internal spermatic fascia**[Q] • **Cremasteric fascia**[Q] • External spermatic fascia • Skin	• Extraperitoneal tissue • **Fascia transversalis** • **Conjoint tendon** • External spermatic fascia • Skin
	• Commonly **unilateral**	• Commonly **bilateral**[Q]
Obstruction/strangulation	• **Common**	• **Rare**
Sac	• Should be **opened during surgery**	• **Not necessary,** unless obstruction is present

10. **Ans. a. Omentum** *(Ref: Bailey 27/e p1031)*

11. **Ans. a. Cooper's ligament** *(Ref: Sabiston 20/e p1101-1102; Schwartz 11/e p1607, 10/e p1496)*

12. **Ans. a. Medially vas deferens, laterally gonadal vessels, inferiorly peritoneum** *(Ref: Schwartz 11/e p1605, 10/e p1496; Sabiston 20/e p1101-1102)*

13. **Ans. b. Always unilateral**

14. **Ans. c. Indirect inguinal hernia**

15. **Ans. b. Intraperitoneal mesh repair**

16. **Ans. d. Repair of stretched inguinal ring and fascia transversalis**

17. **Ans. b. Transversus abdominis muscle** *(Ref: Sabiston 20/e p1096; Bailey 27/e p1033; Schackelford 8/e p599)*

Hesselbach's Triangle		
Lateral Border	**Medial Border**	**Base**
• **Epigastric artery**[Q]	• **Lateral border** of **rectus abdominis**[Q] where it is attached to pubic crest	• **Inguinal ligament**

- **Indirect inguinal hernia** comes out of abdominal cavity **through deep inguinal ring**[Q], travel inguinal canal and becomes superficial through superficial inguinal ring.
- **Direct inguinal hernia** enters inguinal canal through **medial half** of **weak posterior wall (Hesselbach's triangle**[Q]) and becomes superficial through superficial inguinal ring.

18. **Ans. a. External oblique aponeurosis** *(Ref: Sabiston 20/e p1096; Schwartz 11/e p1605, 10/e p1495-1517, 1974; Bailey 27/e p1029)*

External oblique aponeurosis is in close relation to ilioinguinal nerve and hence during operation for inguinal hernia, prevention of injury to ilioinguinal nerve to avoid later development of incisional hernia is very important.

Nerves in Relation to Inguinal Hernia		
Ilioinguinal Nerve	**Iliohypogastric Nerve**	**Genitofemoral Nerve**

• **Pierces transversus abdominis** and **internal oblique** above the iliac crest and **inters inguinal canal**[Q].
• It **emerges from superficial** inguinal **ring to supply skin of**:
  – **Proximomedial skin** of **thigh**[Q]
  – **Skin** over **penile root**[Q]
  – **Upper part** of **scrotum**[Q]
	• **Pierces transversus abdominis**, travels **between transversus abdominis** and **internal oblique** until it **pierces** the aponeurosis of **both obliques**[Q] just above the external ring
	• It divides into two branches.
	  – **Lateral cutaneous** supplies **posterolateral gluteal skin**[Q]
	  – **Anterior cutaneous** supplies **suprapubic skin**[Q]
		• Divides into two branches
		  – **Genital branch** of genitofemoral nerve **enters** the **inguinal canal** at **deep ring** and **supplies**[Q] cremaster and scrotal skin
		  – **Femoral branch** of genitofemoral nerve **passes behind** the **inguinal ligament**, enters femoral sheath lateral to femoral artery, pierces the anterior layer of femoral sheath and fascia lata and **supplies** the **skin anterior** to **upper part of femoral triangle**[Q].

19. **Ans. b. Indirect inguinal hernia**

20. **Ans a. Herniotomy** *(Ref. Sabiston 20/e p1884; Schwartz 11/e p1607, 10/e p1634; Bailey 27/e p1503)*

21. **Ans. b. laparoscopic hernia surgery**

22. **Ans. d. All are correct** *(Ref: Campbell 11/e p3182)*

23. **Ans. a. Laparoscopic** *(Ref: Sabiston 20/e p1103; Schwartz 11/e p1613, 10/e p1499)*

■ COMPLICATIONS OF HERNIA

24. **Ans. c. Fundus**

25. **Ans. b. Immediate surgery**

26. **Ans. b. Tenderness**

27. **And. a. Lateral cutaneous nerve of thigh** *(Ref: Sabiston 20/e p1105; Schwartz 11/e p1619, 10/e p1514)*

28. **Ans. a. Ilioinguinal nerve**

■ FEMORAL HERNIA

29. **Ans. d. Femoral vein**

30. **Ans. a. Lateral and below**

31. **Ans. a. Low inguinal operation**

32. **Ans. a. Femoral hernia**

33. **Ans. c. Lacunar ligament**

34. **Ans. d. McVay repair** *(Ref: Schwartz 11/e p1610, 9/e p2514)*

McVay repair closes the femoral space, is effective for femoral hernia.

35. **Ans. a. Cloquet's hernia** *(Ref: Bailey 25/e p978-979)*

36. **Ans. a. Lacunar ligament**

37. **Ans. a. Below and lateral to pubic tubercle**

■ SPIGELIAN HERNIA

38. **Ans. b. Subumbilical region**

39. **Ans. b. Lateral border of rectus abdominis**

40. **Ans. d. Hernia occurring at the level of arcuate line**

41. **Ans. b. Internal oblique**

■ SLIDING HERNIA

42. **Ans. d. Sigmoid colon** *(Ref: Sabiston 20/e p1104; Bailey 27/e p1029)*

43. **Ans. b. Sigmoid colon**

44. **Ans. b. Barium-meal** *(Ref: CSDT 12/e p771)*

> An **upper GI barium series (Barium meal)** is the preferred examination in the **investigation of sliding hiatus hernia.** In this question, sliding hernia means sliding hiatus hernia.
>
> By the way, CSDT says "Finding a **segment of colon in** the **scrotum on barium enema** strongly suggests a **sliding hernia."**

45. **Ans. c. Sliding hernia**

■ LUMBAR HERNIA

46. **Ans. d. More common on right side** *(Ref: Sabiston 20/e p1115; Schwartz 11/e p1554, 10/e p1742; Bailey 27/e p1042; Schackelford 8/e p606)*

■ OBTURATOR HERNIA

47. **Ans. b. Obturator hernia**

■ UMBILICAL HERNIA

48. **Ans. b. Amniotic membrane** *(Ref: Sabiston 20/e p1883; Schwartz 11/e p1554, 10/e p1455,1631; Bailey 27/e p1037)*

49. **Ans. c. Failure of gut to return to the body cavity from the physiological herniation**

50. **Ans. a. Birth** *(Ref: Sabiston 20/e p1883; Schwartz 11/e p1554, 10/e p1453,1631,1632; Bailey 27/e p135)*

51. **Ans. d. Umbilical hernia** *(Ref: Sabiston 20/e p1107; Schwartz 11/e p1554, 10/e p1455,1631; Bailey 27/e p1037; Schackelford 8/e p579)*

52. **Ans. c. Umbilical hernia** *(Ref: Sabiston 20/e p1107; Schwartz 11/e p1554, 10/e p1631; Bailey 27/e p1037)*

53. **Ans. d. All of the above**

54. **Ans. b. Surgery after 5 years** *(Ref: Sabiston 20/e p1107; Schwartz 11/e p1554; Bailey 27/e p1037)*

55. **Ans. b. Gastroschisis is associated with multiple anomalies**

56. **Ans. b. Direct inguinal hernia**

57. **Ans. d. Herniation of abdominal contents through the body wall**

58. **Ans. a. Gastroschisis**

59. **Ans. b. Omphalocele**

60. **Ans. c. 4 cm**

> Omphalocele/exomphalos: Congenital herniation of abdominal contents at the umbilicus (i.e. into the umbilical cord). Occasionally divided into:
> - < 4 cm—Umbilical cord hernia
> - > 4 cm—Omphalocele

61. **Ans. c. Failure of gut to return to body cavity after its physiological herniation** *(Ref: Schwartz 11/e p1554, 10/e p1455; Sabiston 20/e p1883; Bailey 27/e p1037)*

■ EPIGASTRIC HERNIA

62. **Ans. b. Fatty hernia of the linea alba** *(Ref: Sabiston 20/e p1108; Schwartz 11/e p1554, 10/e p1455; Bailey 27/e p1039; Schackelford 8/e p573)*

63. **Ans. c. Located above the umbilicus and on either side**

> - **Epigastric hernias are multiple in** up to **20%** of patients, and **about 80%** are **just off the midline**[Q].

RICHTER'S HERNIA

64. Ans. a. Richter's hernia (*Ref: Bailey 27/e p1024*)

RICHTER'S HERNIA

- Richter's hernia is a hernia in which the **sac contains only a portion of** the circumference of the **intestine**[Q] (usually small intestine).
- It usually **complicates femoral** and, rarely, obturator hernias.

Strangulated Richter's Hernia

- **Operation** is frequently **delayed** because the **clinical features mimic gastroenteritis**[Q].
- The **local signs of strangulation** are often **not obvious**[Q]
- Patient may not vomit and, although colicky pain is present
- **Bowels** are often **opened normally** or there **may be diarrhea**[Q]
- **Absolute constipation** is **delayed** until paralytic ileus supervenes.
- For these reasons, **gangrene of the knuckle of bowel** and **perforation** have often **occurred before operation** is undertaken[Q].

65. Ans. c. Richter's hernia

66. Ans. b. Femoral hernia

LITTRE'S HERNIA

67. Ans. b. Meckel's diverticulum (*Ref: Bailey 27/e p1252*)

68. Ans. c. Littre's hernia

LITTRE'S HERNIA

- **Littre's hernia** is the **protrusion of a Meckel's diverticulum**[Q] through a potential abdominal opening.

MISCELLANEOUS HERNIA

69. Ans. a. Gibbon's

Gibbon's hernia	• Hernia with hydrocele[Q]
Berger's hernia	• **Hernia** into **pouch** of **Douglas**[Q]
Beclard's hernia	• **Femoral hernia** through **opening of saphenous vein**[Q]
Amyand's hernia	• Inguinal hernia **containing appendix**[Q]
Ogilve's hernia	• Hernia through the **defect in conjoint tendon** just lateral to where it inserts with the rectus sheath[Q]
Stammer's hernia	• **Internal hernia** occurring **through window in** the **transverse mesocolon after** retrocolic **gastrojejunostomy**[Q]
Peterson hernia	• Hernia **under Roux limb** after **Roux-en-Y gastric bypass**[Q]
Velpeau hernia	• Hernia **in front** of **femoral vessels**
Holthouse hernia	• Inguinal hernia with **extension of the loop of intestine along inguinal ligament**.

70. Ans. d. Berger's

71. Ans. b. Eduardo Bassini

72. Ans. a. Sliding

INCISIONAL HERNIA

73. Ans. d. Old age (*Ref: Sabiston 20/e p1109; Schwartz 11/e p1555, 10/e p1454-1455; Bailey 27/e p1039; Schackelford 8/e p574*)

Old age is a risk factor for incisional hernia, but not for wound dehiscence.

74. Ans. a. Incisional hernia

75. Ans. d. Caused by use of local anesthesia

76. Ans. d. Incisional

UMBILICAL ADENOMA

77. Ans. None (*Ref: Bailey 26/e p968*)

78. Ans. c. Umbilical adenoma

79. Ans. d. Congenital

DESMOID TUMOR

80. **Ans. e. Highly radiosensitive**

81. **Ans. a. Surgery**

82. **Ans. b. Wide excision** *(Ref: Devita 9/e p1573)*

- Devita says "In desmoid tumors, **postoperative radiation** is **not recommended** in patients **with negative margins. Residual tumor** from a primary lesion **does not invariably lead to treatment failure** and **adjuvant radiation may be omitted** as long as local progression would not cause significant morbidity."

83. **Ans. b. Abdominal mass** *(Ref: Sabiston 20/e p765, 1073, 1085; Schwartz 11/e p1557, 10/e p1454; Bailey 27/e p1045)*

- *"Patients with a desmoid tumor present with an asymptomatic mass or with symptoms related to mass effect from the tumor."* (Sabiston 20/e p1073)

PATENT URACHUS

84. **Ans. c. Urachal fistula** *(Ref: Bailey 27/e p1044)*

PATENT URACHUS

- A **patent urachus seldom reveals** itself **until maturity** or **even old age**[Q].
- This is because the **contractions of** the **bladder commence at the apex** of the organ and **pass towards the base**[Q].
- Because it opens into the apex of the bladder a **patent urachus is closed temporarily during micturition** and so the potential urinary stream from the bladder is cut off.
- Thus, the **fistula remains unobtrusive until a time when** the **organ is overfull**, usually due to **some form of obstruction**[Q].

Treatment
- **Remove the obstruction**[Q] in the lower urinary tract.
- If the **leak continues** or a **cyst develops** in connection with the urachus: **Umbilectomy** and **excision of the urachus**[Q]

85. **Ans. a. Urachal fistula**

Spleen

■ INDICATIONS OF SPLENECTOMY

- MC indication for splenectomy: Trauma[Q]
- MC indication for elective splenectomy: ITP[Q]

Indications for Splenectomy	
Splenectomy always indicated: • **Primary splenic tumor**[Q] • **Hereditary spherocytosis**[Q] **Splenectomy usually indicated:** • **Primary hypersplenism**[Q] • **Chronic ITP**[Q] • **Splenic vein thrombosis** causing **gastric varices**[Q] • **Splenic abscess**[Q]	**Splenectomy rarely indicated:** • Chronic leukemia • Splenic lymphoma • Macroglobulinemia • Thalassemia major • Sickle cell disease • Congestive splenomegaly and hypersplenism due to PHT • Felty's syndrome • Hairy cell leukemia • Chediak-Higashi syndrome • Sarcoidosis
Splenectomy sometimes indicated: • **Splenic injury**[Q] • **Autoimmune hemolytic disease**[Q] • Elliptocytosis with hemolysis • Nonspherocytic hemolytic anemia • **Hodgkin's disease (for staging**[Q]**)** • **Thrombotic thrombocytopenic purpura**[Q] • **Idiopathic myelofibrosis**[Q] • **Splenic artery aneurysm**[Q] • Wiskott-Aldrich syndrome • Gaucher's disease • Mastocytosis (aggressive disease)	**Splenectomy not indicated:** • Asymptomatic hypersplenism • Splenomegaly with infection • Splenomegaly associated with elevated IgM • Hereditary hemolytic anemia of moderate degree • Acute leukemia • Agranulocytosis

■ SPLENECTOMY

SPLENECTOMY

- **Most serious sequela** is **overwhelming postsplenectomy infection (OPSI)**, with meningitis, pneumonia, or bacteremia.
- **OPSI is typically caused by polysaccharide-encapsulated organisms**, such as **Streptococcus pneumoniae, Neisseria meningitidis, & Hemophilus influenzae**[Q].

  - When elective splenectomy is planned, **vaccination against encapsulated bacteria** should be given at least **2 weeks before surgery**[Q].
  - If spleen is removed in **emergency, vaccination** should be given **as soon as possible**[Q] following surgery.

- **Vaccines** should be given for **Streptococcus pneumoniae, Hemophilus influenzae type b & Meningococcus**[Q].
- In addition to above given 3 vaccines, **annual influenza immunization**[Q] is also advised as influenza has been implicated as a risk factor for secondary bacterial infections.
- **Booster injection** of **pneumococcal vaccine** should be given **every 5-6 years**[Q].

■ COMPLICATIONS OF SPLENECTOMY

<table>
<tr><td colspan="2" align="center">Complications of Splenectomy</td></tr>
<tr>
<td>Pulmonary Complications:
• Left lower lobe atelectasis: MC complication[Q]
• Pleural effusion
• Pneumonia</td>
<td>Thromboembolic Complications:
• DVT
• Portal vein thrombosis</td>
</tr>
<tr>
<td>Hemorrhagic Complications:
• Subphrenic hematoma</td>
<td></td>
</tr>
<tr>
<td>Infectious Complications:
• Subphrenic abscess
• Wound infection</td>
<td></td>
</tr>
<tr>
<td>Pancreatic Complications:
• Pancreatitis
• Pseudocyst
• Pancreatic fistula</td>
<td></td>
</tr>
</table>

■ OVERWHELMING POSTSPLENECTOMY INFECTION

OVERWHELMING POSTSPLENECTOMY INFECTION (OPSI)

- OPSI is **MC fatal late complication** of **splenectomy**.

  - **Mortality associated with OPSI: 40-50%**[Q]
  - **Infection may occur at any time after splenectomy**[Q], **Life long risk remains**[Q]
  - **Most infections occurr more than 2 years after splenectomy** usually after 5 years of splenectomy.
  - **Risk is greatest in thalassemia major & sickle cell anemia**[Q]

Clinical Features

- OPSI **typically begins with** a **prodromal phase** characterized by **fever, rigors** & chills and other **nonspecific symptoms**, including sore throat, malaise, myalgias, diarrhea, & vomiting.

  - **Progression of the illness is rapid, with the development of hypotension, DIC, respiratory distress, coma, & death within hours of presentation**[Q].
  - **Despite antibiotics and intensive care, the mortality rate is between 50-70% for florid OPSI**[Q].

- **Most frequently involved organism in OPSI is S. pneumoniae**[Q] (50-90% of cases)
- Other organisms involved in OPSI: **H. influenzae, N. meningitidis, Streptococcus** and **Salmonella spp**[Q].

  - **Risk for OPSI is greater in splenectomy for malignancy** or **hematologic conditions** than for those who underwent splenectomy for trauma[Q].
  - **Risk is greater for young children**[Q] (**<4 years** of age).

■ SPLENIC TUMORS

- **MC neoplasm of spleen: Lymphoma**[Q] (Non-Hodgkin's lymphoma)
- **MC primary tumor of spleen: Hemangioma**[Q]
- **MC primary malignant tumor of spleen: Angiosarcoma**[Q] (Hemangiosarcoma)

■ SPLENIC CYST

- **MC true splenic cyst: Parasitic** or **hydatid cyst:** Echinococcus[Q] (**10%**)
- **MC non-parasitic splenic cyst: Pseudocyst** (secondary to **trauma**)[Q] (**70–80%**)
- **MC congenital nonparasitic splenic cyst:** Epidermoid cysts[Q]

■ IDIOPATHIC THROMBOCYTOPENIC PURPURA

1. **An evidence that splenectomy might benefit a patient with idiopathic thrombocytopenic purpura includes which of the following?** *(UPSC 2007)*
   a. A significant enlargement of the spleen
   b. A high reticulocyte count
   c. Patients age less than five years
   d. An increase in platelet count on corticosteroid therapy

2. **A patient with ITP is being planned for splenectomy. What is the best time for platelet infusion in this patient:**
   a. 2 hours before surgery *(All India 2010, 2008)*
   b. At the time of skin incision
   c. After ligating the splenic artery
   d. Immediately after removal of spleen

3. **Which of the following is the best treatment for ITP?** *(Recent Question 2019)*
   a. Prednisolone
   b. Azathioprine
   c. Splenectomy
   d. Platelet transfusion

■ HYPERSPLENISM

4. **All are seen in hypersplenism except:** *(AIIMS GIS Dec 2011)*
   a. Anemia
   b. Thrombocytopenia
   c. Splenomegaly
   d. Hypocellular bone marrow

5. **Which of the following doesn't fit into definition of hypersplenism?** *(JIPMER GIS 2011)*
   a. Bone marrow hypoplasia
   b. Splenomegaly
   c. Pancytopenia
   d. Antiplatelet antibodies

■ SPLENECTOMY

6. **In contemporary world, most common indication for splenectomy is:** *(DNB 2005, 2000 JIPMER GIS 2011)*
   a. Trauma
   b. Hemolytic anemia
   c. ITP
   d. Infections

7. **Splenectomy can be curative in all of the following except:**
   a. Thalassemia *(DNB 2007, 2005, 2003, MHSSMCET 2005)*
   b. Sickle cell disease
   c. Hereditary spherocytosis
   d. ITP

8. **Splenectomy is done to tide over the acute crises of uncontrollable:** *(MHPGMCET 2006)*
   a. ITP
   b. TTP
   c. HUS
   d. All of the above

9. **Auto splenectomy is seen in one of the following hemolytic anemias:** *(MHCET 2016, COMEDK 2006)*
   a. Hereditary spherocytosis
   b. Sickle cell anemia
   c. Thalassemia
   d. Immunohemolytic anemia

10. **Vaccine for post splenectomy infection is given against all except:** *(MCI Sept 2009, Punjab 2007)*
    a. Streptococcus pneumonia
    b. Haemophilus influenza
    c. Neisseria meningitides
    d. E. coli

11. **Most common infection after splenectomy is:** *(Recent Question 2016, PGI May 2005, June 97, AIIMS Nov 93)*
    a. Anaerobic
    b. Staphylococcal
    c. Streptococcal
    d. Pneumococcal

12. **In which case pneumococcal vaccine is most effective?**
    a. When given preoperatively *(AIIMS Nov 97)*
    b. When given post operatively
    c. Against all strains of bacteria
    d. Against gram negative bacteria

13. **Which is the commonest postsplenectomy infection?** *(DNB 2003, 2002, 2001, All India 2000, AIIMS Nov 99; Recent Question 2013)*
    a. Streptococcus pyogenes
    b. Staphylococcus aureus
    c. Streptococcus pneumoniae
    d. Pseudomonas aeruginosa

14. **Splenectomy can lead to:** *(DNB 2012, MCI Sept 2005)*
    a. Leucopenia
    b. Thrombocytosis
    c. Thrombocytopenia
    d. Thrombocytopenia and leucopenia

■ SPLENIC TRAUMA

15. **The innovative method for treatment of moderate splenic injury:** *(Recent Question 2014, MHSSMCET 2006)*
    a. Conservative management
    b. Mesh repair
    c. Splenorraphy
    d. Splenectomy

16. **The most common immediate complication of splenectomy:** *(MCI Dec 2018)*
    a. Hemorrhage
    b. Fistula
    c. Bleeding gastric mucosa
    d. Pancreatitis

17. **Kehr sign is seen in:** *(Recent Question 2014, MHSSMCET 2009, AIIMS June 94)*
    a. Splenic injury
    b. Liver injury
    c. Renal injury
    d. Mesenteric hematoma

18. **All of the following are true regarding splenic-rupture except:** *(MCI Sept 2009)*
    a. Elevation of the left dome of diaphragm
    b. Obliterated psoas shadow
    c. Obliterated colonic gas shadow
    d. Obliterated splenic outline

■ SPLENIC TUMORS

19. **Most common tumor of spleen is:** *(All India 2000)*
    a. Lymphoma
    b. Sarcoma
    c. Hemangioma
    d. Metastasis

20. **Most common malignancy affecting spleen is:** *(UPSC 2008, PGI June 97)*
    a. Angiosarcoma
    b. Hamartoma
    c. Secondaries
    d. Lymphoma

21. **Most common cause of isolated splenic metastasis is:** *(All India 2012)*
    a. Carcinoma pancreas
    b. Carcinoma stomach
    c. Carcinoma ovary
    d. Carcinoma cervix

22. **True regarding hemangioma of the spleen:** *(MCI March 2005)*
    a. Least common benign tumour of the spleen
    b. May transforms into a haemangiosarcoma
    c. Malignant transformation may be managed conservatively
    d. None of the above

■ SPLENIC CYST

23. Most common cysts of the spleen are: *(All India 2010)*
   a. Hydatid cyst
   b. Dermatoid cyst
   c. Pseudocyst
   d. Lymphangioma

■ ACCESSORY SPLEEN

24. Commonest site of accessory spleen is:
   (Recent Questions 2017, DNB 2012, AIIMS Nov 93)

   a. Lienorenal ligament
   b. Hilum of spleen
   c. Gastro splenic ligament
   d. Around tail of pancreas

25. True about splenunculi:
   (JIPMER May 2018)

   a. It is encapsulated
   b. Most common site is tail of pancreas
   c. Often single
   d. Have more red pulp than spleen

Explanations

■ IDIOPATHIC THROMBOCYTOPENIC PURPURA

1. **Ans. d.** An increase in platelet count on corticosteroid therapy

2. **Ans. c.** After ligating the splenic artery

3. **Ans. c.** Splenectomy *(Ref: Sabiston 20/e p1560; Bailey 27/e p1182)*

■ HYPERSPLENISM

4. **Ans. d.** Hypocellular bone marrow *(Ref: Sabiston 20/e p1562; Schwartz 11/e p1528, 10/e p1427; Bailey 27/e p1184)*

HYPERSPLENISM

- Characterized by **splenic enlargement,** any combination of **anemia, leucopenia** or **thrombocytopenia, compensatory bone marrow hyperplasia & improvement after splenectomy**[Q].
- Careful clinical judgment is required to balance the long- and short-term risks of splenectomy against continued conservative management.

5. **Ans. a.** Bone marrow hypoplasia

■ SPLENECTOMY

6. **Ans. a.** Trauma *(Ref: Sabiston 20/e p1564; Schwartz 11/e p1538, 10/e p206-207; Bailey 27/e p1185)*

Overall, the **most common indication for splenectomy** is **trauma to** the **spleen,** whether external trauma (blunt or penetrating) or iatrogenic injury (e.g. during operative procedures for other reasons).

7. **Ans. b.** Sickle cell disease

Splenectomy is not curative in sickle cell disease.

8. **Ans. a.** ITP

9. **Ans. b.** Sickle cell anemia

Autosplenectomy	Sickle cell anemia[Q]
Autonephrectomy	Renal TB[Q]

10. **Ans. d.** E. coli *(Ref: Sabiston 20/e p1564; Schwartz 11/e p1538, 10/e p1429-1445; Bailey 27/e p1186; Shackelford 8/e p1649)*

11. **Ans. d.** Pneumococcal

12. **Ans. a.** When given preoperatively *(Ref. Sabiston 20/e p1567)*

- When elective splenectomy is planned, **vaccination against encapsulated bacteria** should be given **at least 2 weeks before surgery**.
- If spleen is removed in **emergency, vaccination** should be given **as soon as possible** following surgery.

13. **Ans. c. Streptococcus pneumoniae**

14. **Ans. b. Thrombocytosis**

■ SPLENIC TRAUMA

15. **Ans. a. Conservative management** *(Ref: Sabiston 20/e p435-437; Schwartz 11/e p227, 10/e p206; Shackelford 8/e p1624)*

    The innovative method for treatment of moderate splenic injury is conservative management.

    SPLENORRHAPHY

    - **Splenorrhaphy** represents a variety of **"spleen-sparing" techniques** aimed at **controlling the hemorrhage from a splenic injury**[Q] while sparing the patient the long-term immunologic consequences of splenectomy.

        - **Splenorrhaphy** is most appropriately considered in cases of **less severe splenic injury** (e.g., grades **I** and **II**, and occasionally grade **III**) [Q].
        - Splenorrhaphy **should not be attempted to** repair **extensive** or **complex shatter** or **crush-type injuries** of the spleen, **nor** is it well-**advised** to undertake splenorrhaphy **in** the face of **multiple concomitant traumatic injuries** or **associated hypotension**[Q].

    - The placement of a **simple monofilament suture** through the **splenic parenchyma** (often in a mattress technique and incorporating a **piece of Gelfoam** or an **omental patch** placed at the site of bleeding) will often **bring** about **satisfactory hemostasis**[Q].
    - **Wrapping** the **entire spleen** with **either absorbable** or **nonabsorbable mesh**[Q] has been described as a means of **effecting external tamponade** and **controlling bleeding** and has not been associated with significantly increased risk of infectious complications.

16. **Ans. a. Hemorrhage** *(Ref: Bailey 27/e p1186)*

17. **Ans. a. Splenic injury** *(Ref: Sabiston 20/e p436; Shackelford 8/e p1593)*

Kehr's sign[Q]	• **Pain** may **be referred to tip** of **left shoulder** in **splenic rupture (Kehr's sign)**[Q] • Due to **irritation of undersurface of diaphragm** with **blood** and pain is referred to the shoulder through the affected fibers of phrenic nerve (**C4 & C5**[Q]) • **Kehr's sign** can be **elicited by bimanual compression** of the **left upper quadrant**[Q] after the patient has been in Trendelenberg's position for about 10 minutes prior to maneuver.
Ballance's sign[Q]	• A fixed area of **percussible dullness** in the **left upper quadrant** due to **coagulation of blood from** the **injured spleen**[Q].

18. **Ans. c. Obliterated colonic gas shadow** *(Ref: emedicine.medscape.com/article/373694-overview)*

Signs of Splenic Injury in X-ray Abdomen	
• **Obliteration** of **spleen outline**[Q]	• **Obliteration** of **psoas shadow**[Q]
• **Intendation** of **gastric air bubble** on the **left side**[Q]	• **Elevation** of **left hemidiaphragm**[Q]
• Some of the **left lower ribs** may be **fractured**[Q]	• Increased **free fluid** in **between air filled intestinal coils**[Q]

■ SPLENIC TUMORS

19. **Ans. a. Lymphoma** *(Ref: Maingot 11/e p1085; Bailey 26/e p1094)*

20. **Ans. d. Lymphoma**

21. **Ans. c. Carcinoma ovary** *(Ref: Oncological Imaging by Paul Silvermann 2012/chapter 31/The spleen)*

    In case of **"isolated"** splenic metastasis, **ovarian** and **colorectal carcinomas** are the most common causes.

    - Causes of **isolated splenic metastasis: Carcinoma Ovary**[Q] (27%) >**Colorectal carcinoma** (26%) >**Uterine cancer** (17%)
    - **MC primary** for **metastasis to spleen: Malignant melanoma**[Q] (30-50%) > **CA Breast** (21%) > **CA Lung** (18%).

22. **Ans. d. None of the above** *(Ref: Shackelford 8/e p1643)*

■ SPLENIC CYST

23. **Ans. c. Pseudocyst** *(Ref: Sabiston 20/e p1563-1564; Schwartz 11/e p1530, 10/e p1436; Bailey 27/e p1178; Shackelford 8/e p1643)*

■ ACCESSORY SPLEEN

24. **Ans. b. Hilum of spleen**

25. **Ans. a. It is encapsulated** *(Ref: Schwartz 11/e p1533, 10/e p1425; Sabiston 20/e p1561; Bailey 27/e p1178)*

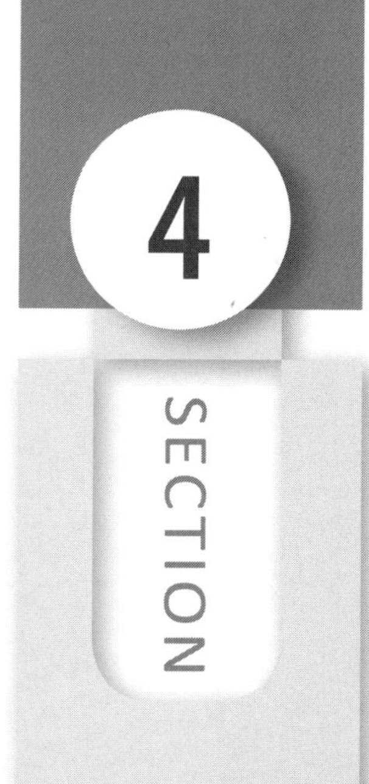

Urology

- Kidney and Ureter
- Urinary Bladder
- Prostate and Seminal Vesicles
- Urethra and Penis
- Testis and Scrotum

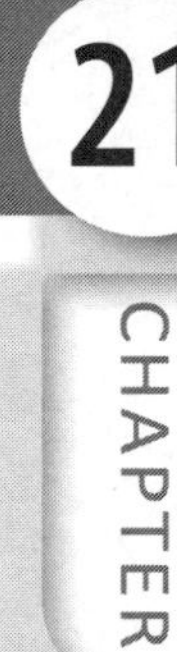

Kidney and Ureter

■ RENAL CALCULI

RENAL CALCULI

- Peak incidence 20–40 years, more common in **males**[Q]
- **Infectious stones** are more common in **females**[Q]
- For formation of stones, a period of **abnormal crystalluria** is required. Urine must be supersaturated with salt of the stone forming crystal (**Supersaturation & crystallization**)[Q]

Clinical Features
- **MC symptom** is **pain**[Q].
- **Severity of pain** is **not related** to **size of stone**[Q]

  - Stone in **upper ureter** or **renal pelvis** → pain referred to **testis**[Q] in males, labia majora in females[Q]
  - Stone in **mid ureter** → referred along **iliohypogastric**[Q] nerve to **iliac fossa**, mimicking appendicitis
  - Stone in **lower ureter** → referred along **ilioinguinal**[Q] nerve to **thigh, scrotum and perineum**[Q].

- Stone approaching **bladder** → bladder symptoms (frequency, urgency & dysuria)
- Stone in the **intramural ureter** → **strangury**[Q].
- **Drug of choice** for **ureteric colic** is **diclofenac (voveran)**.

■ TYPES OF RENAL CALCULI

TYPES OF RENAL CALCULI

- **Calcium oxalate**
  - **MC** type of **kidney stone (85%)**[Q]
  - Risk factors are **hypercalciuria, hypercalcemia, hyperoxaluria**
  - Have **hard, small** and **jagged surface**
  - On section-wavy concentric laminae
- **Uric acid stones**
  - About **5–10 %** of all kidney stones, **MC radiolucent urinary calculi**[Q], formed in **acidic urine**
  - Patients with uric acid stones may have **gout, myeloproliferative disorders** or Lesch-Nyhan syndrome (hyperuricemia)

Uric Acid Stones Management
• Cornerstone of treatment: **Low purine diet, hydration** and **alkalization of urine**[Q]
• **Allopurinol**[Q] (Inhibits conversion of hypoxanthine & xanthine to uric acid)
• **Acetazolamide**[Q] (may be added if urine pH is <6.5)

- **Struvite stones (Infection stones)**
  - Composed of **calcium, ammonium, magnesium phosphate (Triple phosphate stones)**[Q]
  - Tend to grow in **alkaline urine**[Q], especially with **Proteus infection** and **fill whole** of the **PCS**, forming **staghorn calculi**[Q]
  - Formed in **high urinary concentration** of **ammonia**
  - More common in **women**[Q] (increased susceptibility for UTI)

Struvite Stones Management
• **PCNL + ESWL (best treatment option)**[Q]
• **Acetohydroxamic acid (irreversible inhibitor of urease)**[Q] decreases likelihood of precipitation

Contd…

Contd...

- **Cystine**
  - **Extremely hard stone,** formed in **acidic urine;** Radio-opaque due to double sulphur bonds[Q]
  - Relatively **resistant** to fragmentation by **ESWL**
  - Occur in cystinuria with typical **"ground glass" appearance** with a **round smooth outline**[Q]
  - Typical **benzene** or **hexagonal cystine crystals**[Q] in urine.

Cystine Stones Management
• **Stone removal**
• To lower cystine concentration in urine (**Low methionine diet** and **alkalization**)[Q]
• **Cystine complexing agents**: **D-Penicillamine**[Q] and **Alpha-mercaptopropionylglycine (MPG)**[Q]
• **Alpha-MPG is better tolerated than d-penicillamine**

- **Xanthine**
  - Seen in **xanthinuria, radioluscent**[Q]
  - Stones are **smooth, brick red colored, round** and show **lamination on cross section**[Q]
  - **Management: High fluid intake** (most effective therapy) and **Allopurinol**[Q]
- **Indinavir**
  - **A protease inhibitor** used in **AIDS patients,** resulting in **radioluscent calculi**[Q] in 6% patients.
- **Silicate:** Associated with **long term use of antacids** containing **silica**[Q]
- **Triamterene: Antihypertensive** medication, leading to **radioluscent**[Q] stones

■ RENAL CALCULI: INVESTIGATIONS

RENAL CALCULI

Laboratory Investigations

- **Urine:** pH, microscopic examination (RBCs, pus cells and crystalluria) and culture for splitting organisms

• **Acidic urine: CCU** (**C**alcium oxalate, **C**ystine, **U**ric acid)[Q]
• **Alkaline urine:** Calcium **Phosphate, Struvite**[Q]

Crystalluria: To Determine the Stone Composition	
Crystal	**Appearance**
Calcium oxalate monohydrate	**Dumbbell** or hourglass[Q]
Calcium oxalate dehydrate	**Enveloped or bipyramidal**[Q]
Calcium phosphate (apatite)	**Amorphous**[Q], Flat shaped plates or wedge-shaped prisms
Brushite	**Needle shaped**[Q]
Struvite	**Coffin lid**[Q]
Uric acid	Multifaceted, irregular plates or rosettes[Q]
Cystine	**Hexagonal** or benzene ring[Q]

Radiographic Investigations

- **X-ray KUB:**
  - **Ninety percent** are **radiopaque**[Q]
  - **Radiolucent stones (TIXU): Triamterene, indinavir, xanthine & uric acid**[Q]
- **USG:** A screening tool for hydronephrosis or stone within collecting system.
- **IVP:**
  - Early films (At 1 and 5 min for promptness of contrast excretion and Any obstruction along urinary tract)
  - Delayed films (Identifies cause of delayed contrast excretion)

• **Non-contrast spiral CT**[Q] is the **most sensitive investigation** for **renal/ureteric calculus**[Q].

- **Retrograde pyelogram (RGP):**
  - Better delineation of anatomy. Especially useful **if distal ureter not visualized**[Q] well.
  - **Excludes unsuspected** additional **ureteric calculi** and allows **assessment of coexistent ureteric disease** such as **stricture**[Q], which may complicate the operative and post operative course.

Radionuclide Evaluation

- **DMSA** (Dimercaptosuccinic acid): Renal **morphology**[Q] (scar)
- **DTPA** (Diethylene Triamine Pentacetic Acid): To assess **perfusion** (Effective renal plasma flow) & **function**[Q] (Total and differential GFR), less effective than MAG-3 for decreased renal function

Contd…

- **MAG-3 (Mercapto-acetyl glycine): Best** for **renal perfusion**[Q] (Assess renal plasma flow).

> - **Metabolic workup** should be done **in young** patients, with **recurrent** calculi, **multiple** calculi and in **nephrocalcinosis**[Q], **struvite stones, uric acid stones and cystine stones.**

■ MANAGEMENT OF RENAL AND URETERIC CALCULI

MANAGEMENT OF RENAL AND URETERIC CALCULI

Indications of Conservative Treatment (for 4-6 weeks)

(Feature of stone likely to pass spontaneously)

- **Single** stone ≤ **5 mm**[Q]
- Ureter is **undilated**[Q]
- Stone in **lower third** of **ureter**[Q]
- Evidence of **downward movement**[Q]

Surgical Intervention

- **ESWL** (Extracorporeal shock wave lithotripsy)
- **URS** (Ureteroscopy)
- OSS (Open stone surgery)
- **PCNL** (percutaneous nephrolithotomy)
- Laparoscopic stone surgery
- The **majority (80-85%)** of **simple renal calculi** are treated satisfactorily with **ESWL**[Q].
- **Rests** are managed by PCNL/URS
- OSS is the least common treatment modality now days.

■ INDICATIONS OF OPEN STONE SURGERY

INDICATIONS OF OPEN STONE SURGERY

- **Anatomic abnormality** requiring open operative intervention (e.g. PUJO)[Q]
- **Nonfunctioning kidney** with stone (nephrectomy)[Q]

■ TREATMENT DECISIONS BY STONE BURDEN

TREATMENT DECISIONS BY STONE BURDEN

- **Stone ≤ 2 cm: ESWL**[Q]
- Unless factors of stone composition, location, or renal anatomy shift the balance towards more invasive modalities (PCNL/URS).
- **Stone > 2 cm: PCNL**[Q]
- **Stag horn calculi: (PCNL + ESWL)** is TOC[Q]
- Initial approach is **PCNL, followed by ESWL,** as an adjunct to minimize the number of repeat PCNL accesses.

■ EXTRACORPOREAL SHOCK WAVE LITHOTRIPSY (ESWL)

EXTRACORPOREAL SHOCK WAVE LITHOTRIPSY (ESWL)

- **High energy shock waves**[Q] are produced outside the patient's body, which are focused on stones with help of fluoroscopy or ultrasound.
- The **change in density** between the **soft renal tissue** and **hard stone** causes **release of energy** at the stone surface which causes "**compression induced tensile cracking of stones**"[Q]
- Incoming shock wave result in fragmentation of stones from **erosion & shattering**[Q]
- The stone fragments into small pieces and may pass down the ureter.
- **Strongest** or **Gold standard lithotripter** for ESWL is **Dornier unmodified HM-3.**[Q]

> - **Difficult (hard) stones for ESWL:**
>   Brushite, Hydroxyapatite, Cystine,
>   Calcium oxalate monohydrate (BHC-2)[Q]

Contd…

Contd…

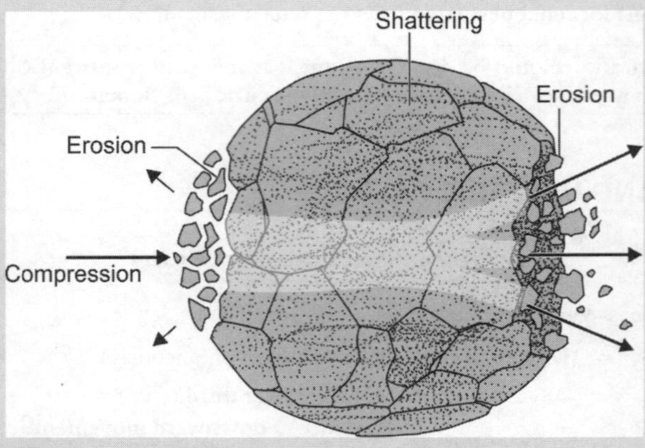

Factors Responsible for Decreasing the Chances of Stone Free Status

- **Stone burden: Multiple stones, > 2 cm** and **staghorn calculi**[Q]
- (ESWL is best suited for stone < 2 cm in renal pelvis or calyces with no distal obstruction)
- **Reduced clearance: Lower calyceal location**, marked **hydronephrosis or scarring**, **calyceal diverticulum** or **horseshoe kidney**[Q].
- **Stone composition:**
  - **Difficult:** Brushite, Hydroxyapatite, Cystine, Calcium oxalate monohydrate **(BHC-2)**[Q]
  - **Breakable:** Uric acid, struvite, Calcium oxalate dihydrate.

Contraindications of ESWL		
Absolute	**Relative**	
• **Pregnancy**[Q] • **Bleeding disorder**[Q]	• **UTI**[Q] • Unrelieved **distal obstruction**[Q] • Cardiac **pacemaker**[Q] • **Uncontrolled hypertension**[Q] • Severe **orthopaedic deformity**	• Weight **> 300 pounds** • Severe **renal failure**[Q] • **Aneurysm**

■ PERCUTANEOUS NEPHROLITHOTOMY (PCNL)

PERCUTANEOUS NEPHROLITHOTOMY (PCNL)

- Removal of kidney stone via a **'track'** developed **between** the **surface of skin** & **collecting system** of kidney.
- **Posterior approach**[Q] is most commonly used, **through the posterior calyx** rather than into the renal pelvis, as it **avoids damage** to **posterior branches of renal artery**[Q], which are closely associated with renal pelvis.

Indications of PCNL

- **Obstructive uropathy**[Q] (contraindication for ESWL)
- **Large volume stone (>2 cm), stag horn calculi**[Q]
- Other modalities failure (**Ureteroscopic failure or ESWL failure**)[Q]
- **Lower pole calyceal stone**[Q]
- Difficult (hard) stones for ESWL: **Brushite, Hydroxyapatite, Cystine, Calcium oxalate monohydrate (BHC-2)**[Q]

Complications

- **Bleeding, (MC complication)**
- **Urinary extravasation**
- **Sepsis**
- **Injury** to other viscera like **pleura (MC)**[Q]**, colon, spleen**
- **Retained fragments**

■ URETEROSCOPY

URETEROSCOPY

- Ureteroscopic stone extraction is **highly efficacious** for **lower ureteric calculi**[Q].
- The use of small-caliber ureteroscopes and the advent of balloon dilatation or ureteral access sheaths have increased **stone-free rates (66–100%)** dramatically.

Contd…

Contd…

Indications

- **Lower ureteric calculi**[Q]
- Upper ureteric calculi of **ESWL failure**[Q]
- Suspicion of **urothelial tumor**[Q] (filling defect, Brush cytology)
- **Ureteric dilatations** or DJ stents[Q]
- Retrieval of **foreign body**[Q]

Complications

- Iatrogenic injuries or **ureteric perforations**[Q]

■ URETERIC CALCULI

URETERIC CALCULI

Proximal and Mid-ureteral Stones

- Stone ≤ 1 cm: ESWL[Q] is primary approach. **Ureteroscopy** is preferred in **failed ESWL, distal obstruction** or **impacted stones.**
- Stone > 1 cm: Ureteroscopy[Q] is primary approach. PCNL for large proximal stones or impacted calculi.

Distal ureteral stones

- Stone ≤ 1 cm: ESWL and Ureteroscopy equally successful. **Ureteroscopy**[Q] is the primary approach
- Stone > 1 cm: Ureteroscopy[Q]

    Remember: For **all ureteric stones, ureteroscopy** is the **primary approach except ≤ 1 cm proximal** and **mid-ureteral stones**[Q].

■ PYONEPHROSIS

PYONEPHROSIS

- Bacterial infection of a **hydronephrotic, obstructed kidney**, which leads to **suppurative destruction** of the renal parenchyma and potential loss of renal function.
- Kidney is a **bag of pus**[Q].
- **MC cause: Renal stones**[Q]. Others are infected hydronephrosis, acute pyelonephritis.

Clinical Features

- Mostly **unilateral**[Q], characterized by triad of **anemia, fever** and **swelling in loin**[Q].

Diagnosis

- **USG** diagnose pyonephrosis.

Management

- Immediate institution of **antibiotic therapy** and **drainage**[Q] of the infected collecting system.
- Antibiotics should be started before manipulation of the urinary tract.
- In the **ill patient**, drainage of the collecting system with a **percutaneous nephrostomy**[Q] tube
- **Nephrectomy** in **destroyed** or **non-functioning kidney**

■ PERINEPHRIC ABSCESS

PERINEPHRIC ABSCESS

- Sources of perinephric abscesses are mainly **extension** of **cortical abscesses** or **hematogenous**[Q].
- Generally caused by **E. coli** or **Proteus**[Q] species.

Clinical Features

- **High grade swinging fever**[Q], abdominal tenderness and flank mass

Diagnosis

- **Urine cultures** (positive only if communication with collecting system is present, so most are usually negative) identify causative organisms in **one-third**[Q] and **blood cultures** in **half**[Q] of cases
- Accurately detected on **USG** or **CT scans.**

Management

- Appropriate **antibiotic therapy**[Q]. If the patient **does not respond within 48 hours** of treatment, **percutaneous drainage**[Q] under CT or ultrasound guidance is indicated.
- If the abscess still does not resolve, then **open surgical drainage** or **nephrectomy**[Q] may be necessary.

■ GENITOURINARY TUBERCULOSIS

GENITOURINARY TUBERCULOSIS

- Tubercle bacilli (**M. tuberculosis**) may invade one or more organs of genitourinary tract and cause **chronic granulomatous infection**[Q].
- More common in **males**[Q] (young adults of age **20-40** years)

Etiology

- M. tuberculosis reaches the genitourinary organs by **hematogenous route** from **lungs**[Q].
- The **primary site** is often **not symptomatic** or **apparent**[Q].

> - Tubercle bacilli lodge in **periglomerular capillaries** and form **cortical granulomas**[Q] after hematogenous spread from a distant focus.
> - These contain **dormant bacilli** that may remain stable, but have the potential to multiply, years later producing the disease.
> - **Spontaneous healing** is the **usual response**[Q].

- Development of **disease** depends on the **interaction between pathogen** & **immune response of host**[Q].
- In whole of genitourinary tract, **Kidney & prostate** is the **primary site of infection**[Q] (hematogenous). Rest organs are involved by ascent or descent.
- Generally **testis** is **not involved**[Q].

Pathogenesis

- **Granulomas** at **renal pyramid** → Enlarge (**tubercular abscess**) → Burst into **PC system** & **pus discharge** in urine (sterile pyuria[Q].
- **Vesical irritability** is an **early clinical manifestation**[Q].

Complications

> **Stenosis** of calyceal neck or pelvic ureteric junction → **Hydronephrosis & pyonephrosis** → **Perinephric abscess** → Kidney replaced by caseous material (**putty kidney**) → **Calcification (Cement Kidney)** → **Autonephrectomy** (a calcified non-functioning kidney, representing end-stage disease)[Q].

- **Autonephrectomy** is the final result of marked parenchymal fibrosis & obstructive uropathy.
- **Scarring** with **stricture formation**[Q] is one of the most typical lesions of tuberculosis and most commonly affects **juxtavesical portion** of ureter.
- **Inflammation** of **bladder mucosa** in early stages → **tubercle formation** (seen endoscopically as **white** or **yellow raised nodules**[Q] surrounded by halo of hyperemia) → Mural fibrosis (**Thimble bladder**)[Q]
- **Large calcifications** in the **prostate** & **beaded appearance** of **vas deferens**[Q]

Clinical Features

> - **Earliest symptom** is **urinary frequency**[Q]

- **Active tuberculosis** elsewhere in the **body** is found in **less than half** of patients with **genitourinary tuberculosis**[Q].
- In tuberculosis of epididymis, an abscess may drain spontaneously through the scrotal wall. A **chronic draining sinus** should be regarded as **tubercular** until proved otherwise.

Diagnosis

- Diagnosis rest on **demonstration** of **tubercle bacilli** in the **urine** by **culture** or **PCR**[Q].

> **Urine: Pyuria** with **acid urine**, **sterile** on ordinary culture (**Persistent pyuria without organisms** on culture means **tuberculosis** until proved otherwise), culture for tubercle bacilli from the **first morning urine sample** is positive in high percentage of patients.

- **Plain X-ray**: May show **calcified lesions** or **punctate calcifications**[Q] in renal parenchyma
- **IVP: IOC for diagnosis of early renal TB**[Q]

> **IVP in Tuberculosis**
> - **Earliest sign** is **"moth-eaten" calyx**[Q] (Obliteration of clear cut outline of renal papilla) due to erosion.
> - **Obliteration** of one or more **calyces** (calectasis, hydronephrosis)
> - SOL in pelvis (**TB abscess**) seen as **splaying of calyces**[Q]
> - **Ureteric strictures**[Q] (single or multiple)
> - **Shrunken bladder** with irregular wall (**Thimble bladder**)[Q]
> - Absence of function of kidney due to complete ureteral occlusion and renal destruction (**autonephrectomy**)[Q]

- **RGP**: Extensive calcification or thickness of the ureter (**Pipe-stem ureter**)[Q], are usually associated with **pyonephrosis**.

> **Cystoscopy in Tuberculosis**
> - **Earliest sign** is **pallor**[Q] around ureteric orifice.
> - Other features are **tubercular ulcer** and **golf hole ureteric orifice**[Q].

- **CECT is IOC for genitourinary tuberculosis**[Q].
- **MRI:** Diffuse, radiating streaky areas of low signal intensity in the prostate (watermelon skin sign)

Treatment

- **ATT** and **Surgery (for complications)**[Q]

Contd…

Contd…

<table>
<tr><td colspan="2" align="center">Surgery in Genitourinary Tuberculosis</td></tr>
<tr><td colspan="2" align="center">Optimal time of surgery is 3-6 weeks[Q] after ATT is started.</td></tr>
<tr><td colspan="2">Procedures
• Ureteral dilatations offer >50% chances of cure in ureteric strictures[Q]
• Pyeloplasty for PUJ obstruction
• Boari operation or bowel interposition for ureteral strictures[Q]
• Augmentation or substitution cystoplasty for bladder contracture[Q]
• Nephroureterectomy for nonfunctioning kidney (as the ureters are usually refluxing)
• Partial nephrectomy for polar lesions not responding to ATT</td></tr>
</table>

■ HYDRONEPHROSIS

<table>
<tr><td align="center">HYDRONEPHROSIS</td></tr>
</table>

• Hydronephrosis is an **aseptic dilatation** of the kidney caused by **obstruction to the outflow of urine.**

Unilateral Hydronephrosis		
Extramural Obstruction	**Intramural Obstruction**	**Intraluminal Obstruction**
• **Tumour** from **adjacent structures[Q]**, e.g. carcinoma of the **cervix, prostate**, rectum, colon or cecum • **Idiopathic retroperitoneal fibrosis[Q]** • **Retrocaval ureter[Q]**	• **Congenital stenosis** (PUJ obstruction)[Q] • **Ureterocele** and congenital small ureteric orifice • **Inflammatory stricture[Q]** • **Neoplasm** of the **ureter** or **bladder** cancer **involving** the **ureteric orifice[Q]**	• **Calculus** in the **pelvis** or **ureter[Q]** • **Sloughed papilla** in **papillary necrosis[Q]** (especially in **diabetics[Q], analgesic abusers[Q]** and those with **sickle cell disease[Q]**) may obstruct the ureter

Bilateral Hydronephrosis	
Congenital	**Acquired**
• **Posterior urethral valves[Q]** • **Urethral atresia[Q]**	• **BPH** or **CA prostate[Q]** • Postoperative **bladder neck scarring[Q]** • **Urethral stricture[Q]** • **Phimosis[Q]**

Pathology

• There is **calyceal dilatation & renal parenchyma** is **destroyed by pressure atrophy[Q]**.
• A **kidney** destroyed by longstanding hydronephrosis is a **thin-walled, lobulated, fluid-filled sac.**
• **Urethral obstruction** tends to lead to **detrusor hypertrophy**, which can lead to **obstruction of the ureters** in their **intramural course[Q]**.

Clinical Features

Unilateral Hydronephrosis

• Unilateral hydronephrosis is more common in women and on the right.
• **Presenting features** include the following:
  – **Mild pain** or **dull aching** in the **loin**, often with a sensation of dragging heaviness made worse by excessive fluid intake. The **kidney may be palpable[Q]**.
  – **Attacks of acute renal colic** may occur with no palpable swelling.
  – **Intermittent hydronephrosis (Dietl's crisis)[Q]**. A **swelling in the loin** is associated with **acute renal pain**. Some hours later the **pain is relieved** and the **swelling disappears** when a **large volume of urine is passed[Q]**.

Bilateral Hydronephrosis
• From lower urinary obstruction symptoms of **bladder outflow obstruction[Q]** predominate. • The kidneys are unlikely to be palpable[Q] because renal failure intervenes before the kidneys become sufficiently large.

Diagnosis

• **Ultrasound[Q]** is the least invasive means of detecting hydronephrosis and is regularly used to diagnose **PUJ obstruction** in utero.
• **Excretion urography** is only helpful if there is **significant function** in the **obstructed kidney**.
• **Isotope renography (DTPA scan)[Q]** is the **best test** to establish that dilatation of the **renal collecting system** is **caused by obstruction.**
• Very occasionally, a **Whitaker test** is indicated.

Treatment

• The **indications for operation** are **bouts of renal pain, increasing hydronephrosis, evidence of parenchymal damage** and **infection[Q]**.
• **Conservation of renal tissue[Q]** is the aim; nephrectomy should be considered only when the renal parenchyma has been largely destroyed.
• **Mild cases** should be **followed by serial USG** and **operated upon if dilation is increasing[Q]**.

■ PERCUTANEOUS NEPHROSTOMY

PERCUTANEOUS NEPHROSTOMY

- **Percutaneous nephrostomy** is **occasionally essential**, if not life saving, in the treatment of **acute** or **chronic upper urinary tract obstruction**[Q].
- It is the **first step** in **obtaining antegrade access to the kidney**[Q] for various procedures.

Indications of Percutaneous Nephrostomy	
• **Acute** or **chronic upper urinary tract obstruction**[Q] in which access to the kidney is impossible from the lower urinary tract • **Creatinine level** is **rising above the reference range**[Q] and the urine cannot be drained through the ureter. • **Renal pelvis disorders** (UPJ obstruction, horseshoe kidneys, ureter duplex, ureter fissures, double renal collecting systems)[Q] • **Hydronephrosis in renal transplant allografts**[Q] • **Treatment of staghorn calculi** and **large** or **lower-pole kidney stones**[Q]	• **Contraindications to ESWL**[Q] • **Stones** or **tumors associated with distal obstruction** or a **foreign body**[Q] that cannot be removed through the ureter • When **rapid dilation of the nephrostomy tract** is **required**[Q] • To diagnose ureteral obstruction, filling defects , and anomalies via antegrade radiography • Tumors, such as sarcomas, ovarian tumors, and other retroperitoneal tumors

■ ANGIOMYOLIPOMA

ANGIOMYOLIPOMA

- **AML** is a **benign** clonal neoplasm consisting of varying amounts of **mature adipose tissue, smooth muscle & thick-walled vessels**[Q]

  - Approximately **20–30%** are found in patients with **tuberous sclerosis (TS)**[Q]
  - **AML in TS** is more likely to be **bilateral & multicentric**, presents with **accelerated growth rates & symptomatic presentation**[Q]

- Who do not have TS **(70-80%)**, pronounced **female predominance**, present **later** during **5th** or **6th decade**[Q]
- **Massive retroperitoneal hemorrhage** from AML **(Wunderlich's syndrome)**[Q] is seen in **10%** of patients. It's the most significant and feared complication.
- **Pregnancy** appears to **increase the risk of hemorrhage**[Q] from AML

Diagnosis

- **CT scan: Presence of fat**[Q] within a renal lesion virtually **excludes the diagnosis of RCC** and is considered **diagnostic of AML.**
- **Lack of calcification**[Q]

- **USG:** Well circumscribed, **highly echogenic lesion**, often associated with **shadowing.**
- **Angiography: Aneurysmal dilation**[Q] is found in **50% of AMLs**
- Positive immunoreactivity for **HMB-45**[Q], is **characteristic** for **AML** (used to differentiate AML from sarcoma)

Treatment

- **Asymptomatic AML** upto **4 cm: Follow up** with imaging at 6-12 months.
- **Symptomatic** or **> 4 cm:** Intervention is required.
  - **Nephron sparing approach** for small symptomatic AML by selective **embolization**[Q] (most preferred) or **partial nephrectomy**
  - **Total nephrectomy** for larger lesions or **life threatening hemorrhage**[Q]

■ CLASSIFICATION OF RCC

CLASSIFICATION OF RCC

- Clear cell carcinoma:
  - **MC type** of RCC, **mainly sporadic**[Q].

    - Both sporadic & familial cases are associated with **loss of sequence** on **chromosome 3** either by **translocation (3:6, 3:8, 3:11)** or **deletion**[Q].
    - This region harbors the **VHL gene**[Q]

  - Arise from **proximal convoluted tubule (PCT)** particularly of **cortex**[Q].
  - Occurs as **solitary unilateral lesion**[Q], often a pseudocapsule is formed around tumor by compression of surrounding tissue.
  - Tumor cells are **clear** and contain **glycogen & lipids**[Q].
  - Most are **well differentiated**[Q].

Contd...

Contd…

- **Papillary carcinoma:**
  - Characterized by **papillary growth pattern**[Q].

  > - MC cytogenetic abnormalities are **trisomies 7, 16, & 17**[Q].
  > - Loss of 18 in sporadic form, trisomy 7 in familial form.
  > - This is due to **mutated MET gene** on chromosome **7**[Q].

  - **Arise from proximal convoluted tubule (PCT)**[Q], can be **multifocal & bilateral**[Q]
  - Typically **hemorrhagic & cystic.**
  - Papillary carcinoma is the **MC type** of RCC in patients with **dialysis associated cystic disease**[Q].
  - Composed of **cuboidal & low columnar cells**[Q].
  - **Psammoma bodies** may be present.
- **Chromophobe renal carcinoma:**
  - Represent 5% of RCC, composed of cells with **prominent cell membrane & eosinophilic cytoplasm** with a **halo around nucleus.**
  - Relative **transparent cytoplasm** with a **fine reticular pattern** described as 'Plant cell' appearance.
  - Associated with **best prognosis**

  > - These tumors exhibit **multiple chromosome loss & extreme hypodiploidy**[Q].
  > - Loss of multiple chromosomes **1**[Q], **2**[Q], 6, 10, 13, 17, 21 & **Y**[Q].

  - Arises from **intercalated cells** of collecting duct[Q].
  - Composed of **pale eosinophilic cells** often with a **perinuclear halo**[Q].
- **Collecting duct (bellini duct) carcinoma:**
  - **Rarest type** of RCC[Q], composed of malignant cells enmeshed within a prominent fibrotic stroma typically in medullary location.
  - Arise from **collecting duct cells** in the **medulla**[Q].   - **Hobnail pattern** on histology[Q]
  - Has got **very aggressive course**[Q].   - Associated with **desmoplastic reaction**[Q]
- Remember: **Medullary cell carcinoma** is seen **almost exclusively** in association with **sickle cell trait.**

> **RENAL CELL CARCINOMA**
>
> - **MC type** of RCC: **Clear cell carcinoma**[Q]
> - **MC type** seen with **dialysis associated cystic disease: Papillary carcinoma**[Q]
> - **Exclusively** associated with **sickle cell trait: Medullary cell carcinoma**[Q]
> - **Best prognosis: Chromophobe carcinoma**[Q]

■ RENAL CELL CARCINOMA

> **RENAL CELL CARCINOMA (GRAVITZ TUMOR, HYPERNEPHROMA, INTERNIST'S TUMOR, RADIOLOGIST'S TUMOR)**[Q]

- **MC malignant tumor** of adult kidney and **most lethal**[Q] of all malignancies
- More common in **males**, in 6th & 7th decade
- Majority are **sporadic**
- Hereditary variants are **VHL syndrome, Hereditary clear cell carcinoma** and **Hereditary papillary carcinoma**[Q]
- Tumor usually involve **upper pole**[Q]

Risk Factors

- **Most significant risk factors** are **smoking & tobacco chewing**[Q]
- Other risk factors are obesity, hypertension, exposure to **Asbestos**, petroleum products and **cadmium**, chronic renal failure (specially due to **analgesic nephropathy**)[Q]

Spread

- Characteristic feature of RCC is tendency to **invade renal vein.** Further extension produces a **continuous cord of tumor** in **IVC** and even in **right side of heart**[Q].
- **MC route is hematogenous**[Q]

  > - MC sites of distant metastasis are **lungs (cannon ball deposits & pulsating secondaries)**[Q] > bone> liver> brain.

- **Lymphatic spread** occurs when tumor extends beyond renal capsule.

Notable Features of RCC

- Encapsulated in spite of being malignant (**pseudocapsule**)   - **Response** to biological response modifiers (IL-2 & IFN-alpha)[Q]
- **Spontaneous regression**[Q]   - **Prolonged** period of **stable disease**[Q]
- **Refractoriness** to cytotoxic agents[Q]

Contd…

Contd…

Clinical Features

- Classical triad of **gross hematuria, abdominal mass & pain** is seen in 10% cases[Q] **(Too late triad)**
- MC and **consistent presentation** is hematuria[Q].
- Other symptoms are fever, weight loss, malaise, **acute & non-reducing varicocele, lower limb edema** due to IVC obstruction.

RCC: Paraneoplastic Syndromes (20%)

• **Raised ESR: MC** paraneoplastic manifestation[Q]
• **Hypercalcemia:**
  – Due to production of **PTH-rp**[Q]
  – **Only paraneoplastic syndrome** in which **medical therapies** are proven **useful.**
• **Hypertension**[Q] (**Renin** production from tumor)
• **Polycythemia**[Q] (**Erythropoietin** production from tumor)
• **Stauffer's syndrome:**
  – **Non-metastatic hepatic dysfunction**[Q] due to raised **IL-6**[Q] leading to **increased ALP, PT** and **bilirubin**
  – Hepatic function **normalizes after nephrectomy**[Q]
• Others are: **Cushing syndrome**, hypoglycemia, anemia, gynecomastia, amenorrhea

Diagnosis

• **Diagnostic IOC: CT** (95% accurate)[Q] • **MRI** is **most accurate** non-invasive investigation for detecting **tumor thrombus** in **renal vein** or **IVC.** **Distinguishes tumor thrombus** from **bland thrombus**[Q] • **Inferior venocavogram**[Q] is **most sensitive & specific** but **invasive** means to detect involvement of **IVC.**

- **Renal arteriography** is done before **renal sparing surgery** (partial nephrectomy), but 3-D helical CT is also sufficient.
- Specific **plain X-ray** finding is **central calcification**[Q].

FNAC is not Routinely done in RCC, Indications are	
• Suspected **secondaries**[Q] • Suspected **lymphoma**[Q]	• Clinical suspicion of **renal abscess**[Q] • To prove pathological diagnosis in **disseminated** or **unresectable disease**[Q]

Treatment

Localized RCC
• **TOC** is **open radical nephrectomy**[Q] • Chemotherapy & radiotherapy is not effective

- Patient with **Stauffer's syndrome** are also candidate for **radical nephrectomy**[Q].
- **Radical nephrectomy** or **debulking** is done **for cytoreduction** in both **locally advanced** and **metastatic RCC**[Q].

Indications of Nephron Sparing Surgery
• **Bilateral RCC** or **VHL syndrome**[Q] • RCC involving a **solitary functioning kidney**[Q] • Unilateral carcinoma and a functioning opposite kidney affected by a condition that might threaten its future function (e.g. RAS) • Low stage or **≤ 4 cm RCC**[Q] **at any location**

Locally Advanced and Metastatic RCC
• **Sunitinib** is the **first line treatment** for **metastatic RCC** (response rate: **31%**)[Q] • Combined **IL-2 & IFN-alpha** is the **2nd line** treatment for **metastatic RCC** (response rate: **15%**)[Q] • Chemotherapy with **vinblastine**[Q], as it is single most effective agent

Prognostic Factors

- **Pathologic stage**[Q] is single **most important** prognostic factor
- **Lymph node involvement** is a **poor** prognostic factor

Staging and Grading

- **TNM** (preferred) and **Robson's**[Q] staging are used for RCC.
- **Fuhrman**[Q] histological system is used for **grading.**
- **Leibovich prognostic score** (0–11) **for RCC:** Based on **tumor stage, grade, size**, involvement of **LN & tumor necrosis** histologically[Q].

Contd…

8th AJCC (2017) TNM Staging for Renal Cell Carcinoma	
T: Primary tumor	**N: Regional lymph nodes**
T1a: Tumor **≤4 cm** and confined to the kidney[Q] **T1b**: Tumor **>4 cm** and **≤7.0 cm** and confined to the kidney[Q]	N0: No regional lymph nodes metastasis N1: Metastasis in regional lymph node
T2a: Tumor **>7 cm** but **≤10 cm** and confined to the kidney[Q] **T2b**: Tumor **>10 cm** and confined to the kidney[Q]	
T3a: Tumor grossly extends into **renal veins** or its **segmental (muscle containing) branches, or tumor invades perirenal and/or renal sinus fat** but **not beyond Gerota's fascia**[Q]	M: Distant metastases
T3b: Tumor grossly extents into **vena cava below diaphragm**[Q]	M0: No distant metastasis M1: Distant metastasis present
T3c: Tumor extends into the **vena cava above** the **diaphragm** or **invades** the **wall of vena cava**[Q]	
T4: Tumor invades **beyond Gerota's fascia**[Q] (including contiguous extension into ipsilateral adrenal gland)	

Stage I	Stage II	Stage III	Stage IV
T1N0M0	T2N0M0	**T1-3 N1** M0 **T3 N0** M0	**T4** anyN M0 AnyT anyN **M1**

Pediatric Tumors	
• **MC malignant** tumor of infancy • **MC extracranial solid** tumor in children • **MC abdominal** malignancy in children	• **Neuroblastoma**[Q]
• **MC primary malignant renal** tumor of **childhood**	• **Wilms' tumor**[Q]
• **MC renal tumor** of **infancy**	• **Congenital mesoblastic nephroma**[Q]
• **MC soft tissue** tumor in **infants & children**	• **Rhabdomyosarcoma**[Q]
• **MC solid tumor** of **childhood**	• **Brain tumor**[Q]
• **MC cancer** of **childhood**	• **Leukemia**[Q] (30%) **>Brain tumors**[Q] (22%)

■ WILMS' TUMOR

WILMS' TUMOR

- Wilms' tumor: **MC primary renal tumor** of **childhood (2-5 years)**[Q].
- Wilms' tumor: **2nd MC malignant abdominal tumor** in **children (MC is neuroblastoma).**
- Arise from kidney, composed of **three elements- Blastema, Epithelium & Stroma**[Q]. (BESt)
- **MC presenting feature** is **asymptomatic abdominal mass or swelling**[Q].
- Mostly **unilateral.**

> • Characterized by **triad of abdominal mass, fever & microscopic hematuria**[Q].

- Fever typically resolve after tumor resection

Associated Malformations

- **WAGR Syndrome**[Q]: It consists of **aniridia, genital anomalies & mental retardation.** The risk of **Wilms' tumor is increased** by **33%** in this syndrome[Q]. Associated with **WT-1 gene deletion** located on chromose[Q] **11p 13**
- **Denys-Drash Syndrome**[Q]: It consists of **gonadal dysgenesis** (Male pseudohermaphroditism), **nephropathy** leading to **renal failure. Majority** of patients with this syndrome **have renal failure.**
- **Beckwith-Wiedmann Syndrome**[Q]: It consists of **enlargement of body organs, hemi-hypertrophy, renal medullary cysts** and **abnormal large cells** in **adrenal cortex,** macroglossia, omphalocele, hepatoblastoma. Associated with **WT-2 gene deletion** located on chromosome **11p 15.5.**

Diagnosis

- **USG (first investigation)**[Q] or CT abdomen for staging.
- **MRI** is **superior** to other imaging modalities in **delineating nephroblastomatosis elements.**
- **Calcification** tends to be more **crescent shaped, discrete & peripheral**[Q] in comparison of finely stippled calcification of neuroblastoma.

Contd…

Treatment

- **Surgical excision (transperitoneal radical nephrectomy)** is treatment of choice.
- **Routine exploration** of **contralateral kidney** is **not necessary** if imaging is satisfactory and doesn't suggest bilateral process.

> - In unfavorable histology, **Radiation therapy** should be **started within 10 days[Q]** after nephrectomy, Chemotherapy should be **started 5 days after surgery[Q]**.

- **Chemotherapy:** *VCD* (Vincristine + Cyclophosphamide + Doxorubicin or dactinomycin)
- **Whole lung irradiation** is recommended for **pulmonary metastasis.**

Preoperative Treatment should be Considered	
• **Solitary kidney[Q]**	• Tumor **thrombus** in **IVC above** the level of **hepatic veins[Q]**
• **Bilateral[Q]** renal tumors	
• Tumor in **horse shoe kidney[Q]**	• **Respiratory distress** due to **metastatic[Q]** disease

Prognosis

- **Histology[Q]** of Wilms' tumor & **tumor stage** is identified as most important **determinant of prognosis[Q]** (Histology > Stage).
- The **postchemotherapy based staging system** is the **'SIOP' staging** system developed by the **International society of oncology.**
- Two Staging Systems are currently being used for the staging of Wilm's Tumor.

Prechemotherapy Staging System	Postchemotherapy Staging System
• Developed by the **National Wilms' Tumor staging Group (NWTSG** - Staging system)	• Developed by the **International Society of Pediatric Oncology (SIOP** - Staging system)
• This staging system is widely used in **North America** and **Canada**	• This staging system is widely used in Europe
• 'NWTSG' approach involves **employment of 'primary surgery'.**	• 'SIOP' approach involves employment of **preoperative chemotherapy without histological confirmation** of Wilms' tumor.
• **Chemotherapy** with or without **Radiation therapy** is given **after surgery**	• **Primary chemotherapy** for **all patients** regardless of extent
• **Staging** is done **at time of surgery (Prechemotherapy)**	• **Staging** is done **at time of surgery (Postchemotherapy)**

■ RENAL INJURIES

RENAL INJURIES

- **Kidney** is the **most commonly injured** part of **urinary tract[Q]**
- **Hematuria** is the **best indicator[Q]** of traumatic urinary system injury.
- **More than 80%** of patients sustaining **penetrating renal injuries** have **other intra-abdominal injuries[Q]**.
- Blunt renal injuries are generally divided into minor and major injuries.
- **Minor injuries** account for approximately **85%[Q]** of cases.
- MC cause of blunt renal injury is **motor vehicle accident[Q]**.

> **Penetrating wounds** causing **small parenchymal injuries** are generally treated by **débridement, primary repair,** and **drainage[Q]**.

- **Injuries involving the hilum** are **seldom repaired primarily[Q]**, and in most circumstances total nephrectomy is necessary.

Imaging Studies

Contrast enhanced CT is the IOC for Renal Injuries[Q]
Indications
• Gross hematuria[Q]
• Microscopic hematuria with hypotension[Q] anytime during initial resuscitation

- **IVP** should be done to see the **function of the opposite kidney[Q]**
- **Arteriography** is used to **define arterial injuries** suspected on CT or to **localize arterial bleeding** that can be controlled by **embolization[Q]**.

Grade	Type	Description
I	Contusion	Microscopic **(>3 RBCs/HPF)[Q]** or gross hematuria, urological studies normal
	Hematoma	**Subcapsular,** nonexpanding without parenchymal laceration.
II	Hematoma	Nonexpanding **perirenal** hematoma, confined to renal retroperitoneum
	Laceration	**<1 cm** parenchymal depth of renal cortex **without urine extravasation[Q]**.
	Laceration	**>1 cm** parenchymal depth of renal cortex **without collection system rupture or urinary extravasation[Q]**
IV	Laceration	Parenchymal laceration **extending through collecting system[Q]**
	Vascular	**Main renal artery** or **vein injury** with contained hemorrhage
V	Laceration	Completely **"Shattered kidney"[Q]**
	Vascular	**Avulsion of renal hilum,** devascularising the kidney.

Note: **Advance one grade for bilateral injuries upto grade III.**

Section 4

Urology

MANAGEMENT

Nonoperative

- **Most (>95%)** of **renal injuries** can be **managed non-operatively**[Q].
- Significant renal injuries (Grade II–V) are found only in **5%** of renal trauma.
- A **hemodynamically stable patient** with an **injury well staged by a CT scan** can usually be **managed without renal exploration**[Q]. Hospital admission, bed rest, vital monitoring and repeated CT scan is required.

Renal Exploration in Injuries	
Renal exploration should be done by transabdominal approach in order to have a control on the renal vessels first[Q].	
Absolute Indications	**Relative Indications**
• Persistent renal bleeding[Q] • Expanding or pulsatile perirenal hematoma[Q]	• Urinary extravasation • Non viable tissue (>20% necrosis) • Segmental arterial injury

Indications of Nephrectomy
• Hemodynamically **unstable patient**, with **low body temperature** and **poor coagulation**, with a **normal contralateral kidney**[Q]. • **Extensive renal injuries**[Q] when the patient's life would be threatened by an attempt at renal repair. • Already **poorly functioning hydronephrotic kidney**[Q] with continuous bleeding

■ COMPLICATIONS AFTER RENAL TRAUMA

COMPLICATIONS AFTER RENAL TRAUMA

- **Complication rate** after renal trauma is **3–10%**[Q]
- **Urinoma** is the **MC complication**[Q] after renal trauma
- **Delayed bleeding** usually occurs **within 1–2 weeks**[Q] after injury

Early Complications	Late Complications
• Urinoma, delayed bleeding • Urinary fistula, abscess • Hypertension	• Hydronephrosis, pyonephrosis • Stone formation, AV fistula • Delayed hypertension

■ ADULT POLYCYSTIC KIDNEY DISEASE (AD)

ADULT POLYCYSTIC KIDNEY DISEASE (AD)

- Inheritance is **autosomal dominant**[Q] with 100% gene penetrance, 50% offsprings are affected.
- **Chromosome** affected: **16 & 4**[Q]; **Protein abnormality: Polycystin**[Q]
- Usually **bilateral**[Q]
- An important cause of **renal failure**, accounting for **10-15%** of patients **who receive hemodialysis**.

Pathology

- Kidneys are **grossly enlarged**[Q] with multiple cysts
- Cyst are distributed **uniformly**[Q] throughout cortex & medulla
- Cysts contain straw colored fluid that may become hemorrhagic
- **Renal arteriolar thickening** is a prominent finding in **adults**

Presentation

- Usually occurs in 3rd or 4th decade
- MC clinical feature is **hypertension (75% adults & 25% children)**[Q] due to activation of rennin angiotensin system[Q].
- **Pain** due to infection (pyelonephritis)/obstruction/sudden hemorrhage.
- **Hematuria**[Q], **nocturia** (due to impaired concentrating ability), **nephrolithiasis** (15–20%)[Q]
- Progressive decline in renal function leading CRF
- **MC cause of death: Cardiovascular disorders**[Q]

ADPKD Extra-renal manifestations	
• Cysts: **Liver (MC)**[Q], **spleen, pancreas** and **ovaries**	• **Colonic diverticulosis**[Q]
• **Berry aneurysms** (10–40%)[Q]	• **Mitral valve prolapse**[Q]
• Cyst in seminal vesicles (40%), Arachnoid membrane (8%)	

Contd…

Contd…

Diagnosis

- **USG:** Enlarged kidney with uniformly increased medullary echogenecity

IVP in ADPKD	
• Stretching of the calyces by the cysts (**spider leg** or **bell like deformity**)[Q]	• **Bubble appearance**[Q] (calyceal distortion) • **Swiss cheese appearance**[Q]

- **CT scan** is **IOC**[Q] in ADPKD

Management

- Treatment is mainly aimed to control UTI, hypertension, calculi & general measures for uremia (low protein diet)
- Pain relief by percutaneous aspiration with instillation of sclerosing agent or **Rovsing's operation (deroofing of the cyst)**[Q]
- **Dialysis** or **renal transplantation** (only definitive treatment) for renal failure[Q].

■ PELVIURETERIC JUNCTION (PUJ) OBSTRUCTION

Pᴇʟᴠɪᴜʀᴇᴛᴇʀɪᴄ Jᴜɴᴄᴛɪᴏɴ (PUJ) Oʙsᴛʀᴜᴄᴛɪᴏɴ

- A blockage of the ureter at the junction with the renal pelvis resulting in restriction of urine flow
- **MC cause** of **fetal hydronephrosis**[Q]
- More common in **boys**[Q], mainly **left sided**, **bilateral** in **10–15%** cases

Causes of PUJ Obstruction	
Congenital	**Acquired**
• **Aperistaltic segment**[Q] due to disorganization of smooth muscle or collagen deposition • Crossing **aberrant renal vessel**[Q]	• **Calculus**[Q] • **Instrumentation**[Q] • **Infection**[Q]

Associated Abnormalities

- **PUJ Obstruction** of **opposite kidney (MC)**[Q] in 40%
- **VUR**[Q]
- **VATER defects**[Q] (Vertebral anomalies, anorectal malformations, TE fistula, Radial and renal dysplasia)

Clinical Presentation

- Most infants are **asymptomatic**[Q]
- Most infants are discovered by **palpable abdominal mass** or **prenatal USG**[Q].

Diagnosis

- **USG:** Diagnoses **hydronephrosis**, but does not diagnose whether it is obstructive.
- **IVP:** It was the primary radiological study to define PUJO but now **replaced by DTPA scan**[Q].

DTPA Scan
• **Investigation of choice for PUJO** to establish that hydronephrosis is due to obstruction.

Treatment

- **Conservative** in children with **good renal function without any complication**
- Pyeloplasty or nephrectomy
- Treatment of choice: Anderson hynes (dismembered) pyeloplasty

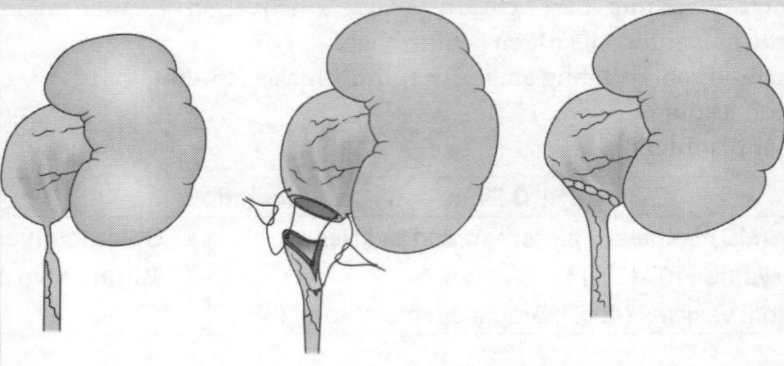

Anderson-Hynes dismembered pyeloplasty

■ RETROCAVAL URETER

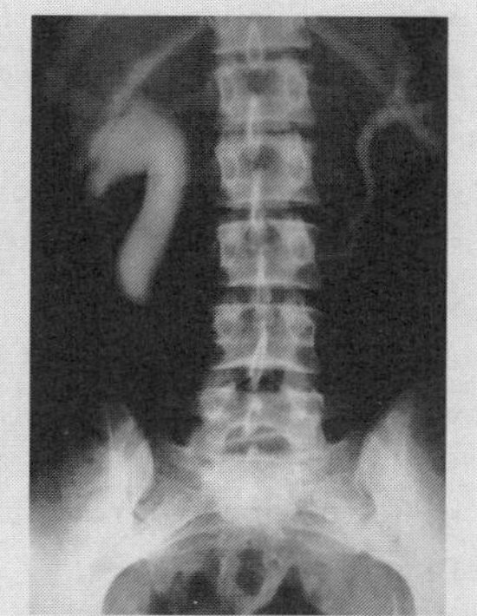

RETROCAVAL URETER (CIRCUMCAVAL URETER)

- An **embryologically normal ureter** becomes **entrapped behind IVC**[Q]
- Because of **abnormal persistence of right posterior subcardinal**[Q] (as opposed to the supracardinal) **vein**. This forces the right ureter to encircle the vena cava from behind (**Altered development of IVC**)[Q]
- **Right ureter** typically **deviates medially behind** the **IVC**[Q], winding about and crossing in front of it from medial to lateral direction, to resume a normal course to the bladder.
- More common in **males**[Q]

Clinical Features

- Signs & Symptoms of **ureteric obstruction**[Q]

Diagnosis

- **MRI is IOC** to delineate anatomy clearly and **non-invasively**[Q]
- IVP: "Reverse J", "Fish Hook" or **"Shepherd crook"**[Q] deformity.
- Retrograde ureterography

Surgical Management

- Ureteral division with **relocation ureteroureterostomy** in cases of obstruction.

■ HORSESHOE KIDNEY

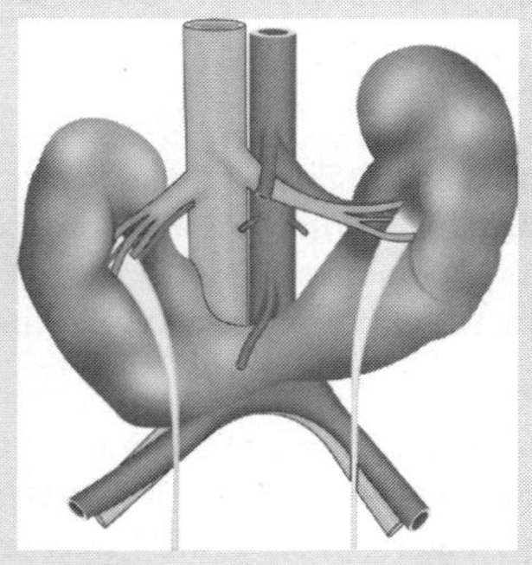

HORSESHOE KIDNEY

- **MC renal fusion abnormality**[Q] with incidence of **1:400**[Q], more common in **males**[Q]
- Fusion at the **lower poles**[Q] by a parenchymatous or fibrous isthmus

Etiopathogenesis

- Fusion occurs before kidneys have rotated at their long axes
- The axes of these masses are **vertical**[Q] whereas axes of normal kidneys are oblique to spine, because they lie along the edges of the psoas muscle
- **Pelvis and ureters** are usually **anteriorly placed**[Q] or anteromedial, crossing anteriorly to isthmus
- **Calyces** point **posteriorly**[Q]. **Lowermost calyx** extends **caudally** or even **medially**[Q]
- **Migration** is **incomplete**. Inferior mesenteric artery (IMA) **prevents full ascent**[Q]
- **Isthmus** usually located adjacent to **L3-L4** vertebra, just below the origin of IMA from aorta
- **Ureteral compression** can occurs due to **anteriorly displaced ureter**[Q] or from obstruction by **aberrant vessels** leading to hydronephrosis and infection.

Associated Abnormalities (Present in one-third[Q] cases)	
• **CVS (VSD)** and **CNS** involvement • **Anorectal malformations**[Q] • **Unicornuate or bicornuate uterus**[Q]	• Renal: **VUR** and **PUJ** obstruction in **one third**[Q] cases • **Hypospadias, undescended testis**[Q]

Clinical Features

- Most are **asymptomatic**[Q], mostly it is an autopsy finding
- **MC symptom: vague abdominal pain**[Q]
- **Rovsing syndrome: abdominal pain, nausea** and **vomiting**[Q] on hyperextension of spine

Diagnosis is usually made on IVP showing
• **Low lying kidneys**[Q], closed to vertebral column • **Vertical axes**[Q] through kidneys point towards the LS spine • Characteristic orientation of the calyces, directed posterior to each renal pelvis, with the **lowermost calyx** pointing **caudally** or **even medially (Hand joining sign)**[Q] • High insertion of the ureter appears to drape over a midline mass (**Flower vase-like curves of ureters**)[Q]

• **Angiography** is done before surgery as **blood supply is unpredictable**[Q] but not needed usually as helical CT is useful.

Treatment

- **Pyeloplasty** is done only in symptomatic cases, **isthmus is not divided**[Q].

■ URETEROCELE

URETEROCELE

- Cystic dilation of terminal ureter
- More common in **females**[Q]

Types

- **Intravesical (20%)**: Most often with **single ureter**[Q]
- **Ectopic (80%)**: Nearly always involve the **upper pole** of **duplicated ureters**[Q].

Clinical Features

- **MC presentation** is **UTI** or **urosepsis**[Q]
- Palpable abdominal mass (due to **hydronephrosis**)
- **Prolapse** through female urethra as a cyst
- **Calculi** due to urinary stasis, mostly in distal ureter

Diagnosis

- **USG**: Hydroureteronephrosis, cyst in bladder
- **IVP**: Typical **Adder head** or **Cobra head** or **Spring onion appearance**[Q] is diagnostic of ureterocele
- **MCU**: A **smooth filling defect**[Q] in the trigonal area
- **Cystoscopy**: **Enlarging & collapsing cysts**[Q] as urine flows

Treatment

- Significant upper pole function: **Endoscopic incision** or **cyst excision & reimplantation**[Q]
- Poor upper pole function: Upper pole nephrectomy and partial ureterectomy.

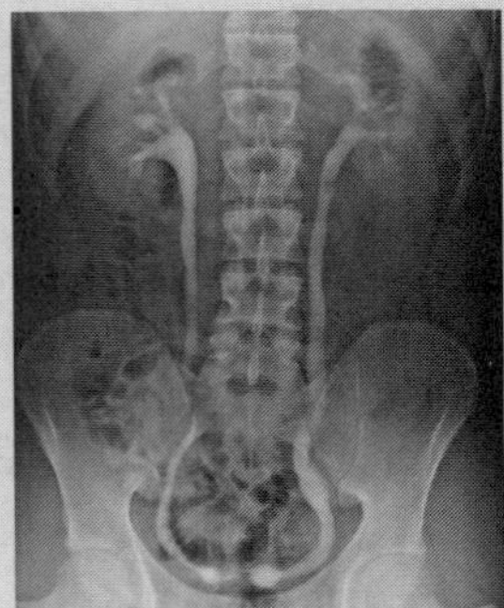

■ DUPLICATION OF URETER (AD)

DUPLICATION OF URETER (AD)

- **MC congenital anomaly** of **upper urinary tract**[Q]
- Mode of inheritance is **autosomal dominant**[Q]
- More common in **females** and often **bilateral**[Q]
- **"Yo-Yo" effect**[Q] in **fused ureter** (incomplete duplication) is seen.

Types

- **Incomplete duplication**: Both ureters join together and a single ureteric opening
- **Complete duplication**: Both ureters open separately
  - **Weigert-Meyer's rule**[Q]: In cases of complete duplication, the upper pole ureter and the lower pole ureter rotate on their long axes so that the **upper pole ureteric orifice** is **medial & caudal** to the **lower pole orifice**[Q].
  - **Upper pole ureter** becomes **ectopic & obstructed**[Q], whereas the **lower pole ureter** end laterally and have a **short intravesical tunnel** leading to **VUR**[Q].

Clinical Features

- Many patients are **asymptomatic**[Q]
- A common presentation is **persistent** or **recurrent infections**[Q].

> - In **females**, the **upper pole ureter** may be **ectopic**, with an **opening distal** to the **external sphincter**[Q] or even **outside the urinary tract**.
> - Such patients have **classic symptoms**: **incontinence** characterized by **constant dribbling** with a **normal pattern of voiding**[Q].

- In **males**, because the mesonephric duct becomes the vas and seminal vesicles, the **ectopic ureter** is **always proximal** to the **external sphincter**[Q], and associated **incontinence does not occur**[Q].

Diagnosis

- **IVP**: Shows **duplication** in most of cases
- **MCU** discloses **VUR** (in lower pole ureter) and demonstrate presence of **ureterocele** (in upper pole ureter).

Treatment

- Treatment of reflux alone is not influenced by duplication in most of the cases.
- Lower grade reflux is treated medically and higher grade surgically
- **Surgery** is reserved for **upper pole obstruction** or **ectopy**[Q]. If renal function in one segment is very poor, **heminephrectomy** is the most appropriate treatment.

> - **MC congenital anomaly** of **upper urinary tract**: Duplication of **ureter**[Q]
> - **MC congenital anomaly** of **genitourinary tract**: **VUR**[Q]

■ VESICOURETERIC REFLUX (VUR)

Vesicoureteric Reflux (VUR)

- VUR is the **most common inheritable disease**[Q] of the genitourinary tract.
- **Autosomal dominant** mode of transmission.
- **Majority** of cases (75%) are **asymptomatic**[Q].
- Major cause of VUR is **attenuation of trigone**[Q] and its contiguous **intravesical ureteric musculature**[Q].

Types

Primary	Secondary
• The length of **submucosal ureter** may be **short** • **Deficiency** of the **longitudinal muscle**[Q] of the intravesical ureter resulting in an inadequate valvular mechanism	• Caused by **elevated pressures** in the bladder • **MC anatomical cause: Posterior urethral valves (50%** have **VUR)**[Q] • Other causes: **Neurogenic bladder** or bladder dysfunction

Investigations

- **MCU is IOC for VUR**[Q]
- **DMSA scan: IOC** for **pyelonephritis** and **cortical renal scarring**[Q]
- Urine culture

MCU Grading of VUR (International classification)	
Grade I	Reflux into **non dilated ureter**[Q]
Grade II	Reflux into **pelvis & calyces**[Q] without dilation
Grade III	**Mild to moderate dilation** of the **ureter, renal pelvis & calyces**[Q] with minimal blunting of the fornices
Grade IV	**Dilation** of the **pelvis & calyces** with **blunting**[Q].
Grade V	**Gross dilation** of the **ureter, pelvis & calyces**; loss of papillary impression and **ureteral tortuosity**[Q].

Natural History

- With **bladder growth** and **maturation, most low-grade** reflux **resolves spontaneously**[Q].
- **Severe grades** of reflux are **less likely to resolve**[Q].
- **Mean age** of reflux resolution is **6-7 years**[Q].

> • Resolution rates: Grades I & II: 80–84%, Grade III: 50%, Grade IV: 20-30%, Grade V: 0-5%[Q]

- Younger children, especially the **neonates**, are **more likely to have spontaneous resolution**[Q]
- Reflux of **infected urine** cause **pyelonephritis**. Repeated such episodes lead to **renal scarring** and **nephropathy** resulting in **hypertension** and **azotemia**[Q].
- If urine is kept sterile, significant nephropathy rarely occurs.

Management

- **Medical management: Keep** the **urine sterile**[Q] and wait for spontaneous resolution

Medical Management Recommended as the Initial Management for
• All prepubertal children with **grade I-III reflux**[Q] as most of the cases usually resolve.
• **Unilateral grade IV reflux**, especially in **young children**[Q].

Drugs used in VUR
• **Age up to 6 weeks**: **Amoxicillin** or **Ampicillin**[Q].
• **Age after 6 weeks**: The biliary system is mature enough to handle **TMP-SMX (DOC** for **prophylaxis)**[Q]. Usually **nighttime doses** are given. Other option is **nitrofurantoin**.

- **Periodic cultures** every **3 months**[Q] for evaluation of breakthrough infections.
- **DMSA scan** if recurrent bouts of **pyelonephritis**[Q] are suspected. Yearly radiographic studies for resolution.
- **Surgical management: Ureterovesicoplasty** or **ureteric reimplantation**[Q] and **STING**[Q] (Subureteric transurethral injection of teflon paste) are the treatment options.

Methods of Ureteric Implantation
• **Lich-Gregoir technique**[Q] by direct implantation of ureter
• **Leadbetter-Politano technique**[Q] involves creation of a submucosal anti-reflux tunnel.

Indications of Surgical Management in VUR
• **Breakthrough UTIs**[Q] despite prophylactic antibiotics
• Severe grades of reflux- **grade V** or **bilateral grade IV**[Q]
• **New renal scars** or **deterioration of renal function**[Q] as on serial USG of DMSA scan.
• Reflux that **persist in girls** at full linear growth (**at puberty)**[Q]
• Reflux **associated with** congenital abnormalities (**Bladder diverticula)**[Q].
• **All secondary reflux**, which **persist**[Q] after correction of the primary cause e.g. fulguration of posterior urethral valves or management of uninhibited detrusor.

Multiple Choice Questions

■ RENAL AND URETERIC CALCULI

1. Renal calculi associated with proteus infection:
   (All India 2011, 2009)
   a. Uric acid
   b. Triple phosphate
   c. Calcium oxalate
   d. Xanthine

2. Nephrolithiasis occurs with the toxicity of: *(COMEDK 2005)*
   a. Ritonavir
   b. Saquinavir
   c. Indinavir
   d. Nelfinavir

3. Not true about 'Struvite Stones' is: *(AIIMS Nov 2001)*
   a. Better known as staghorn calculus
   b. These are triple phosphate stones
   c. Common in infected urine
   d. Usually seen in acidic urine

4. Randall's plaques causes: *(Recent Question 2014)*
   a. Bile stones
   b. Urinary stones
   c. Premalignant lesions
   d. Bacterial infections

5. Staghorn calculus is made of:
   (Recent Question 2017, DNB 2012, UPSC 97)
   a. Oxalate
   b. Phosphate
   c. Uric acid
   d. Cystine

6. Renal stones which are laminated and irregular in outline
   are: *(Recent Question 2013)*
   a. Uric acid
   b. Calcium oxalate
   c. Struvite
   d. Cystine

7. Most common renal stone: *(Recent Question 2017)*
   a. Calcium oxalate stone
   b. Uric acid stone
   c. Staghorn calculi
   d. Cystine stone

8. Chronic laxative abuse can result in the formation of which
   type of stone?   *(Recent Question 2018)*
   a. Xanthine
   b. Cysteine
   c. Ammonium urate
   d. Struvite

9. Potent producer of urease is: *(Recent Question 2017)*
   a. E. coli
   b. Proteus
   c. Klebsiella
   d. Pseudomonas

■ RENAL AND URETERIC CALCULI:
CLINICAL FEATURES

10. Locate the renal stone with pain radiating to medial side of
    thigh and perineum due to slipping of stone in males:
    a. At pelvic brim   *(AIIMS June 2010, All India 96)*
    b. Intramural opening of ureter
    c. Junction of ureter and renal pelvis
    d. At crossing of gonadal vessels and ureter

11. Triad of renal colic, swelling in loin which disappears after
    passing urine is called: *(All India 96)*
    a. Kocher's triad
    b. Saint's triad
    c. Dietl's crisis
    d. Charcot's triad

12. Ureteric colic due to stone is caused by:
    (UPPG 2010, All India 2008)
    a. Stretching of renal capsule due to back pressure
    b. Increased peristalsis of ureter to overcome the obstruction
    c. Irritation of intramural ureter
    d. Extravasation of urine

13. Ureteric colic characterized by all except: *(UPPG 2007)*
    a. Acute onset
    b. Stillness of the patient
    c. Responds to antispasmodics
    d. Radiates to the groin

14. Treatment of choice of ureteric colic is: *(GB Pant 2010)*
    a. Nitrites
    b. Pethidine
    c. Adrenaline
    d. Diclofenac

■ RENAL AND URETERIC CALCULI:
DIAGNOSIS AND TREATMENT

15. All are radioopaque except one: *(AIIMS June 2000)*
    a. Oxalate
    b. Uric acid
    c. Cystine
    d. Mixed

16. Which of the following stones is hard to break by ESWL?
    a. Calcium oxalate monohydrate   *(All India 2010)*
    b. Calcium oxalate dehydrate
    c. Uric acid
    d. Struvite

17. Ramesh, 30-year-old male presented with repeated attacks of
    renal colics. X-ray KUB was done. Findings are suggestive of:
    a. Calcium oxalate stone
    b. Uric acid stone
    c. Struvite stone
    d. Cystine stone

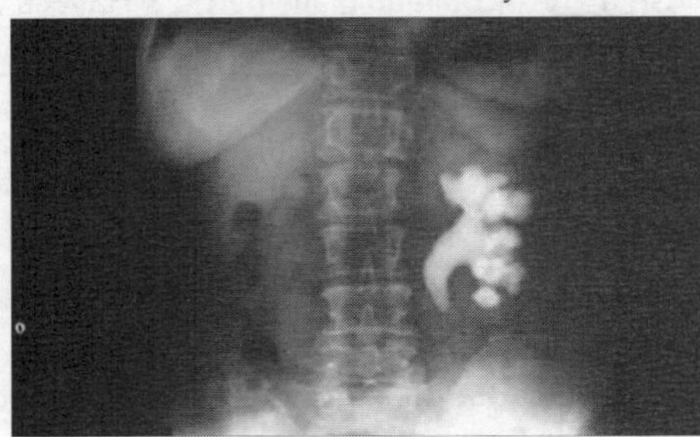

18. What complication should one expect when PCNL is done
    through 11th intercostals space?   *(All India 2010)*
    a. Hydrothorax
    b. Hematuria
    c. Damage
    d. Remnants fragments

19. Which of the following is not a contraindication for extra
    corporeal shockwave lithotripsy (ESWL) for renal calculi?
    a. Uncorrected bleeding diathesis   *(AIIMS June 2003)*
    b. Pregnancy
    c. Ureteric stricture
    d. Stone in a calyceal diverticulum

20. Treatment used for lower ureteric stone is: *(AIIMS June 98)*
    a. Endoscopic removal
    b. Diuretics
    c. Drug dissolution
    d. Laser

21. Correct order of stones on the basis of images of crystals:
    a. Calcium oxalate, struvite, uric acid, cystine
    b. Calcium oxalate, uric acid, struvite, cystine
    c. Uric acid, calcium oxalate, struvite, cystine
    d. Struvite, uric acid, calcium oxalate cystine

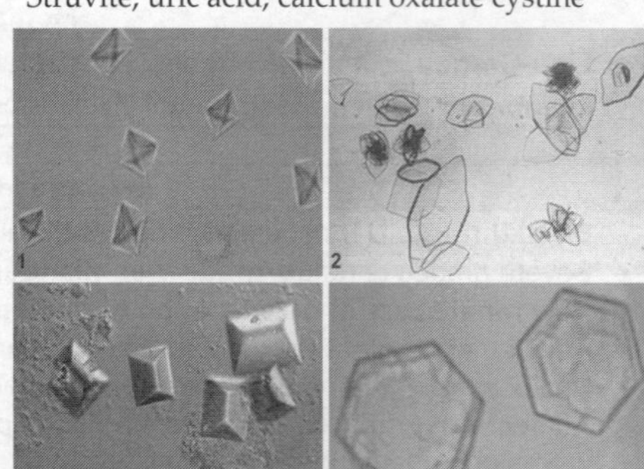

22. **Steinstrasse is:** *(Recent Questions 2017, HPU 2001)*
    a. Staining of stones   b. Stones
    c. Failure of ESWL
    d. Ureteric obstruction due to fragments in ureter

23. **Identify the crystals depicted in urine microscopy.**
    (APPG 2015)
    a. Oxalate crystals   b. Cystine crystals
    c. Struvite crystals   d. Uric acid crystals

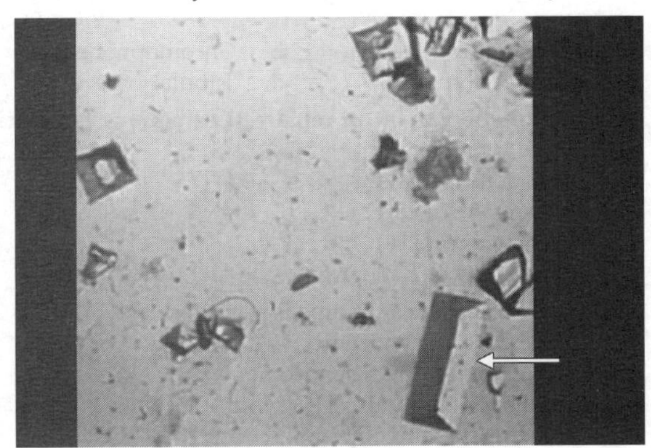

24. **All are indicated in a patient with cystinuria with multiple renal stones except:** *(AIIMS Nov 2012)*
    a. Cysteamine   b. Increase fluid intake
    c. Alkalinization of urine   d. Penicillamine

25. **Identify this crystal found in urine analysis.**
    a. Calcium carbonate stone   *(AIIMS Nov 2015)*
    b. Ammonium phosphate stone
    c. Uric acid   d. Calcium oxalate stone

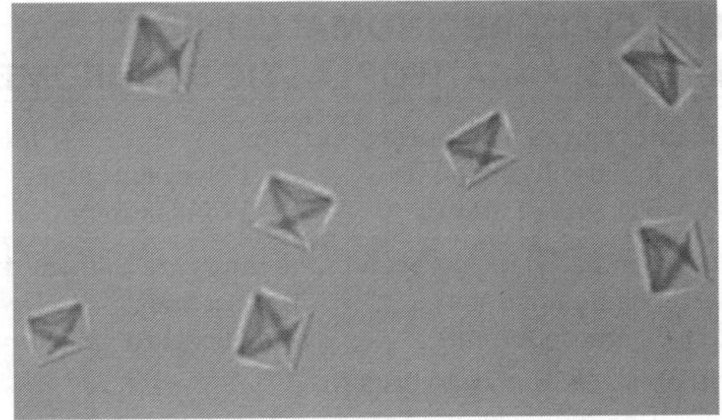

26. **Which one of the following is radiolucent stone?**
    (Recent Question 2017, 2015, GB Pant 2010, MCI Sept 2007)
    a. Calcium oxalate   b. Cystine
    c. Uric acid   d. Phosphate

27. **Treatment of choice for 0.5 mm renal calyx stone is:**
    a. ESWL   b. PCNL   *(DNB 2007)*
    c. Ureteroscopy   d. Cystoscopy

28. **All are risk factors for nephrolithiasis except:** *(DNB 2007)*
    a. Renal tubular acidosis   b. High protein intake
    c. High calcium intake   d. Hypercalciuria

29. **Commonest cause of ureteric obstruction:**
    a. Stone   b. Clot   *(MHSSMCET 2006)*
    c. Cast   d. Carcinoma

30. **LASER used in treatment of ureteric calculi:**
    (MHSSMCET 2008, 2006, All India 2003)
    a. Holmium   b. Nd-Yag
    c. Argon   d. CO_2

31. **A patient is passing stones recurrently in urine for past few years. All are to be restricted in diet except:** *(AIIMS Nov 2010)*
    a. Protein restriction   b. Calcium restriction
    c. Salt restricted   d. Phosphate restriction

32. **Management of 4 cm size renal staghorn calculus:**
    (AIIMS Nov 2017)
    a. ESWL   b. PCNL
    c. Intra renal repair surgery   d. Open pyelolithotomy

33. **A 62-year-old female has kidney stone and treated with PCNL. After 2 days, she again comes to OPD with chills and fever. What is the complication?** *(MCI Dec 2019)*
    a. Bacterial sepsis   b. Acute pancreatitis
    c. Splenic injury   d. Ureteric stricture

34. **Which of the following is the best for the management of a 3 cm stone in renal pelvis without evidence of hydronephrosis?** *(MCI Dec 2018)*
    a. ESWL   b. PCNL
    c. Anterograde pyeloplasty
    d. Retrograde pyeloplasty

■ RENAL INFECTIONS

35. **Most common cause of emphysematous pyelonephritis:**
    (GB Pant 2011, COMEDK 2008)
    a. E. coli   b. Proteus
    c. Klebsiella   d. Pseudomonas

36. **Xanthogranulomatous pyelonephritis is often associated with infection by:** *(DNB 2010, COMEDK 2009)*
    a. Proteus   b. E. coli
    c. H. influenza   d. Klebsiella

37. **Most common predisposing factor for chronic pyelonephritis is:** *(DNB 2004, 2000)*
    a. Diabetes mellitus   b. Renal stone
    c. Posterior urethral valve   d. Vesicoureteric reflux

■ GENITOURINARY TUBERCULOSIS

38. **Most common route of infection in kidney tuberculosis:**
    (Recent Question 2015, All India 93)
    a. Ascending spread   b. Hematogenous
    c. Lymphatic spread   d. Direct invasion

39. **The most sensitive imaging modality to detect early renal tuberculosis is :** *(Recent Questions 2017)*
    a. Intravenous urography
    b. Computed tomography
    c. Ultrasound
    d. Magnetic resonance imaging

40. **Renal tuberculosis originates in the:** *(Recent Questions 2017)*
    a. Renal papilla
    b. Renal medulla
    c. Afferent tubules
    d. Efferent arteriole of glomerulus

41. **"Golf-hole" ureter is seen in:** *(WBPG 2015, 2014; Karnataka 94)*
    a. Ureteric calculus   b. Ureteral polyp
    c. Tuberculosis of ureter   d. Retroperitoneal fibrosis

42. **Earliest and often the only presentation of TB kidney is:**
    (DNB 2005, 2001)
    a. Increased frequency   b. Pain
    c. Hematuria   d. Renal calculi

43. **Genitourinary TB in a male patient presents with:**
    a. Painful and tender epididymis   *(JIPMER 2011)*
    b. Bacteriuria without pyuria
    c. Renal cysts (unilateral)
    d. Microscopic hematuria

44. **Sterile pyuria is characteristically seen in:** *(All India 2011)*
    a. Renal tuberculosis   b. Chronic Hydronephrosis
    c. Wilm's Tumor   d. Neuroblastoma

■ HYDRONEPHROSIS

45. Unilateral hydronephrosis is due to: *(AMC 99)*
- a. Bladder neck contracture
- b. Stricture urethra
- c. Carcinoma of prostate
- d. Ureterocele

46. A 60-year-old male with poor stream of urine, post void residual urine is 400 mL, bilateral hydronephrosis and prostate weighing 70 g. His urea is 120 and creatinine 3.5. Ideal "next immediate" step: *(AIIMS Nov 2010)*
- a. Catheterize with Foley catheter
- b. Bilateral PC nephrostomies
- c. CT to rule out carcinoma
- d. MRI pelvis

47. Hydronephrosis due to obstruction of ureter is best diagnosed by: *(MHPGMCET 2008)*
- a. IVU
- b. Radioisotope scan
- c. Retrograde pyelography
- d. Whitaker test

■ DIAGNOSTIC AND LABORATORY INVESTIGATIONS

48. After a single episode of painless gross hematuria in a boy. Doctor performed an excretory urogram showing a filling defect towards the lower renal infundibulum 1.5 cm in size. What will be the next investigation to be done? *(Karnataka 2003, AIIMS Nov 2000)*
- a. Cystoscopy
- b. Urine cytology
- c. USG
- d. Retrograde pyelography

49. The investigation of choice for renal scarring defect in kidney: *(Recent Question 2016, All India 2012)*
- a. DMSA scan
- b. DTPA scan
- c. Dexa scan
- d. MCU

50. The substance present in the gallbladder stones or the kidney stones can be best identified by the following techniques:
- a. Fluorescence spectroscopy *(All India 2003)*
- b. Electron microscopy
- c. Nuclear magnetic resonance
- d. X-ray diffraction

51. Reflux nephropathy is diagnosed mainly by:
- a. X-ray KUB
- b. Micturating cystourethrogram *(MCI Sept 2005)*
- c. CT scan
- d. MRI

52. A patient presents with hematuria of several days and dysmorphic RBC casts in urine. The site of origin is:
- a. Kidney
- b. Ureter *(AIIMS Nov 2001)*
- c. Bladder
- d. Urethra

53. Percutaneous nephrostomy is indicated in: *(DNB 2001)*
- a. Polycystic kidney disease
- b. Solitary adenocarcinoma
- c. Simple hydronephrosis
- d. Pyonephrosis

54. Most useful investigation in a child, who recovered from the bout of pyelonephritis: *(Recent Question 2017)*
- a. DTPA scan
- b. DMSA scan
- c. MCU
- d. IVP

■ BENIGN RENAL TUMORS

55. Regarding angiomyolipoma of kidney, what is incorrect?
- a. Pain in the loin *(AIIMS Nov 94)*
- b. Presents with hypertension
- c. Bleeding is self limited
- d. Nephrectomy is the treatment of choice

56. Central stellate scar on CT scans are seen in: *(COMEDK 2008)*
- a. Renal hemangioma
- b. Renal oncocytoma
- c. Wilm's tumour
- d. Papillomas

■ RENAL CELL CARCINOMA: TYPES

57. Renal cell carcinoma histopathologicaly showing 'perinuclear halo' and "Plant like" structure in malignant cells is seen in:
- a. Clear cell tumor *(PGI Dec 2000)*
- b. Papillary carcinoma
- c. Collecting duct carcinoma
- d. Chromophobe cell carcinoma

58. The most common histological variant of renal cell carcinoma is: *(Bihar PG 2016)*
- a. Clear cell type
- b. Chromophobe type
- c. Papillary type
- d. Tubular type

59. Chromophobe variant to renal cell carcinoma is associated with: *(All India 2010)*
- a. VHL gene mutations
- b. Trisomy of 7 and 17 (+7, +17)
- c. 3 p deletions (3 p-)
- d. Monosomy of 1 and Y (-1, -Y)

60. Bilateral renal cell carcinoma is seen in: *(COMEDK 2008)*
- a. Eagle-Barett's syndrome
- b. Beckwith-Weidman syndrome
- c. von-Hippel Lindau (VHL) syndrome
- d. Bilateral angiomyolipoma

61. Most common site of origin of RCC: *(MHSSMCET 2008)*
- a. PCT
- b. DCT
- c. Collecting ducts
- d. Loop of Henle

62. Sickle cell anemia is associated with which type of renal cell carcinoma? *(JIPMER Nov 2017)*
- a. Medullary
- b. Papillary
- c. Chromophobe
- d. Colloid

■ RENAL CELL CARCINOMA: CLINICAL FEATURES, PARANEOPLASTIC SYNDROMES

63. Painless gross hematuria occurs in: *(All India 94)*
- a. Renal cell carcinoma
- b. Polycystic kidney
- c. Stricture of urethra
- d. Wilm's tumor

64. Cannon ball deposits seen in the lungs are characteristic of:
- a. Seminoma testis
- b. Carcinoid *(DNB 2003)*
- c. Hypernephroma
- d. Pheochromocytoma

65. Bilateral RCC may be seen in: *(DNB 2002)*
- a. Tuberous sclerosis
- b. von-Willebrand's disease
- c. von-Hippel Lindau disease
- d. von-Recklinghausen disease

66. All are true about renal cell carcinoma except: *(DPG 2006)*
- a. Invasion of renal vein means inoperability
- b. Presents with abdominal pain, hematuria
- c. Arises from tubular epithelium
- d. More common in males

67. Not correct regarding renal cell carcinoma: *(Recent Questions 2017)*
- a. May be associated with varicocele
- b. May invade renal vein
- c. More common in female
- d. Arises from proximal convoluted tubule

68. A 55-year-old male with 35 pack years presented with painless mass in left scrotal sac and microscopic hematuria. On laboratory investigation, Alpha-fetoprotein and lactate dehydrogenase was negative. What is the diagnosis? *(AIIMS May 2013)*
- a. Epididymitis
- b. Seminoma
- c. Renal cell carcinoma
- d. Carcinoma lung

69. **Most common presentation of renal adenocarcinoma:**
(COMEDK 2005)
   a. Hematuria
   b. Local pain
   c. Mass
   d. Fever

■ RENAL CELL CARCINOMA: DIAGNOSIS AND TREATMENT

70. **A patient presented with renal cell carcinoma invading IVC and renal vein. False statement is:**
(AIIMS Nov 2001, June 2001)
   a. Pre operative biopsy is not necessary
   b. IVC involvement indicates inoperability
   c. Pre-op radiotherapy is not essential
   d. Chest X-ray should be done to rule out pulmonary metastasis

71. **Most important prognostic indicator for renal cell carcinoma:**
(AIIMS May 2009)
   a. Nuclear grade
   b. Histological type
   c. Size
   d. Pathological staging

72. **A 60 years old male, who is a chronic smoker, presented with 'too late' triad. Chest X-ray film image is given below. What is the most probable diagnosis?** *(Recent Question 2016)*
   a. Carcinoma bladder
   b. Carcinoma renal pelvis
   c. Choriocarcinoma
   d. Renal cell carcinoma

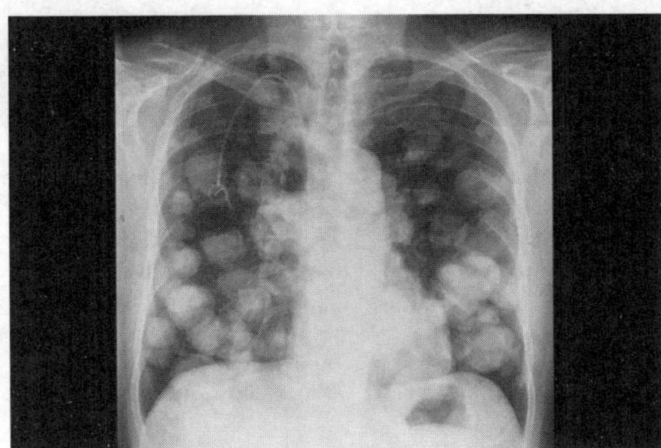

73. **The treatment of choice in renal cell carcinoma with the tumor If less than 4 cm in size is:** *(AIIMS Nov 2004)*
   a. Partial nephrectomy
   b. Radical nephrectomy
   c. Radical nephrectomy + post operative radiotherapy
   d. Radical nephrectomy + chemotherapy

74. **False regarding hypernephroma is:**
(Recent Question 2014, AIIMS Nov 93)
   a. Radiosensitive
   b. Arise from cortex usually from pre existing adenoma
   c. May present with rapidly developing varicocele
   d. Usually adenocarcinoma

75. **The commonest systemic abnormality associated with renal cell carcinoma is:** *(COMEDK 2009)*
   a. Hypertension
   b. Polycythemia
   c. Elevated ESR
   d. Pyrexia

76. **In radical nephrectomy, following structures are removed except:** *(Recent Question 2017)*
   a. Gerota's fascia
   b. Ipsilateral adrenal gland
   c. Surrounding hilar nodes
   d. Para-aortic nodes

77. **Best investigation for diagnosis and extension of IVC thrombus in renal cell carcinoma:** *(Recent Question 2016)*
   a. MRI
   b. CT
   c. Venacavagraphy
   d. USG

78. **Stage T3 renal cell carcinoma:** *(Recent Question 2017)*
   a. Tumor invades beyond Gerota's fascia
   b. Contiguous extension into the ipsilateral adrenal gland
   c. Tumor grossly extends into the inferior vena cava
   d. Confined to the kidney

■ WILMS' TUMOR

79. **Commonest presentation of Wilm's tumour is:**
(Recent Questions 2017)
   a. Hematuria
   b. Abdominal lump
   c. Hydronephrosis
   d. Pain in abdomen

80. **The most important determinant of prognosis in Wilm's tumor is:** *(All India 2006)*
   a. Stage of disease
   b. Loss of heterozygosity of chromosome 1p
   c. Histology
   d. Age less than 1 year at presentation

81. **The ideal timing of radiotherapy for Wilm's tumor after surgery is:** *(All India 2006)*
   a. Within 10 days
   b. Within 2 weeks
   c. Within 2 months
   d. Anytime after surgery

82. **Neuroblastoma differs from Wilm's tumor radiologically by all except:** *(AIIMS June 2001)*
   a. Calcification
   b. Aorta and IVC are not eroded but pushed aside
   c. Same location
   d. Intraspinal extension of tumor

83. **Earliest symptom of Wilm's tumour:** *(Recent Questions 2017)*
   a. Hematuria
   b. Pyrexia
   c. Abdominal mass
   d. Metastases

84. **The triad of Wilm's tumour is:**
   a. Hematuria
   b. Mass abdomen
   c. Pain
   d. Fever
   e. Weight loss

85. **Commonest site of metastasis of Wilm's tumour is:**
   a. Bones
   b. Lungs *(AIIMS 94)*
   c. Liver
   d. Brain

86. **Which of the following is the treatment of choice for stage I Wilm's tumor?** *(All India 2012)*
   a. Laparoscopic nephrectomy
   b. Open nephroureterectomy
   c. Chemotherapy
   d. Observation

87. **Wilm's tumor chromosome is:** *(JIPMER 2012)*
   a. 13 q
   b. 13 p 14
   c. 11 p 13
   d. 17

■ TUMORS OF RENAL PELVIS

88. **Commonest type of cancer of the renal pelvis and upper ureter is:** *(Recent Questions 2017)*
   a. Transitional cell carcinoma
   b. Adenocarcinoma
   c. Squamous cell carcinoma
   d. Nephroblastoma

89. **'Stipple sign' in transitional cell carcinoma of the renal collecting system is best demonstrated by:** *(COMEDK 2009)*
   a. Intravenous urography
   b. Retrograde pyeloureterography
   c. Radionuclide scan
   d. Ultrasound scan

90. **Nephroureterectomy is indicated in:** *(DNB 2011)*
   a. Renal cell carcinoma
   b. Chronic pyelonephritis
   c. Polycystic kidney disease
   d. Transitional carcinoma of the pelvis extending till ureter

91. Gold standard treatment of TCC involving renal pelvis:
a. Radical nephroureterectomy   *(Recent Question 2016)*
b. Pelviureterectomy
c. Radical nephrectomy
d. Conservative Nephrectomy

■ RENAL TRAUMA

92. Which of the following is true about renal trauma?
a. Urgent IVP is indicated   *(All India 95)*
b. Exploration of the kidney to be done in all cases
c. Lumbar approach to kidney is preferred
d. Renal artery aneurysm is common

93. All except one are correct regarding renal trauma:
a. Observation is best   *(AIIMS June 95)*
b. IVP is indicated
c. Exploration indicated in all cases
d. Hematuria is a cardinal sign

94. During renal rupture the nephrectomy is not attempted until: *(UPPG 2010)*
a. Fluid replacement
b. Antibiotics covers
c. Contralateral renal function is ascertained
d. Renal angiogram

95. Absolute indication for surgical exploration after renal trauma?   *(MHSSMCET 2008)*
a. Hematuria   b. Pulsatile hematoma
c. Cortical renal contusion   d. Delayed arterial injury

■ URETERIC INJURY

96. Inadvertent surgical injury of the ureter leads to:
a. Complete renal atrophy   b. Hematuria
c. Renal failure   d. Hydronephrosis
e. Hypertension

97. Commonest cause of ureteric injury during surgical operation is: *(UPPG 2007, 2006)*
a. Abdominoperineal resection
b. Hysterectomy
c. Prostatectomy   d. Colectomy

■ POLYCYSTIC KIDNEY DISEASE

98. All of the following are features of adult polycystic kidney disease except: *(COMEDK 2005)*
a. Autosomal recessive trait   b. Present as renal mass
c. Haematuria   d. Renal failure

99. Polycystic kidney disease is associated with all of the following except: *(COMEDK 2010)*
a. Cerebral aneurysms   b. Mitral valve prolapsed
c. Renal cell carcinoma   d. Hepatic cysts

100. Image of kidney in a patient having polycystin 2 mutation is given below. What is the inheritance mode in this disease?
(Recent Question 2016)
a. Autosomal dominant   b. Autosomal recessive
c. X-linked dominant   d. X-linked recessive

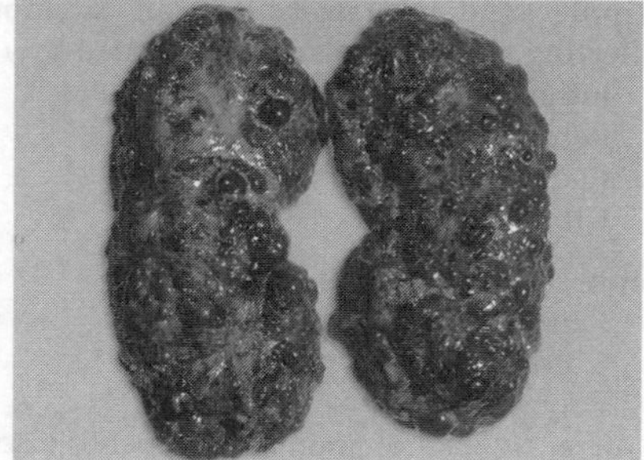

101. In adult polycystic kidney, all are true except:
a. Hypertension is rare   *(AIIMS June 2001)*
b. Hematuria is a common symptom
c. Cysts are seen in liver spleen and pancreas
d. Autosomal dominant transmission is seen

102. Polycystic kidney may be associated with cyst in all the sites except: *(Bihar PG 2014, All India 91)*
a. Lung   b. Liver
c. Pancreas   d. Brain

103. IVP was done in the patient of ADPKD. What is the name of this sign?   *(Recent Question 2016)*
a. Spider leg appearance   b. Swiss cheese appearance
c. Bubble appearance
d. Bristles of brush appearance

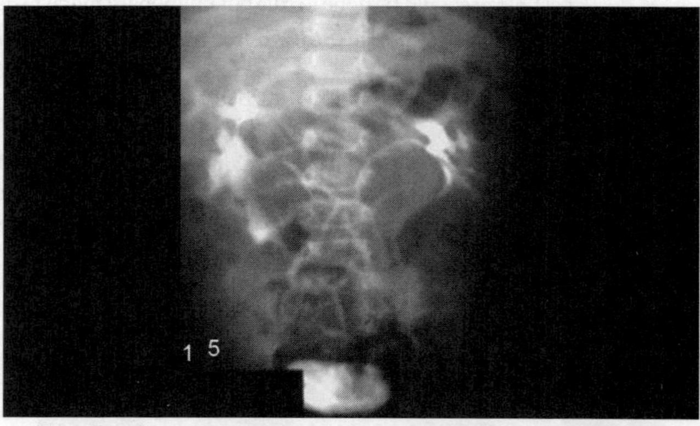

104. The typical appearance of "spider leg" on excretory urography is seen in: *(Recent Question 2016, UPSC 2008)*
a. Hydronephrosis   b. Polycystic kidney
c. Medullary sponge kidney d. Renal cell carcinoma

105. All the following are features of polycystic disease of kidneys except: *(MCI June 2018)*
a. Hematuria   b. Hypertension
c. Renal failure   d. Erythrocytosis

■ PUJ OBSTRUCTION

106. Not true about congenital PUJ obstruction is:
a. Can be associated with renal agenesis   *(AIIMS Nov 2001)*
b. Can be diagnosed antenatally
c. Bilateral in 10–15% of cases
d. Aberrant vessel is the most common cause

107. Anderson-Hynes operation is performed for:
a. Achalasia cardia   *(MCI June 2018)*
b. Pyloric stenosis   c. Pseudopancreatic cyst
d. Pelviureteric junction obstruction

108. Investigation of choice for documentation of obstructive nature of pelvicalyceal system dilatation:
(Recent Questions 2017)
a. IVP   b. DTPA scan
c. Whittaker test   d. Ultrasound

109. Distention of abdomen with passage of large amount of urine is known as: *(MHPGMCET 2001)*
a. Dietl's crisis   b. Anderson-Hynes crises
c. Meteriorism   d. Strangury

■ CONGENITAL ANOMALIES OF KIDNEY

110. A symptom of medullary sponge kidney disease is:
a. Nocturia   b. Anemia   *(All India 95)*
c. Azotemia   d. UTI

111. **Which of the following is the most common renal vascular anomaly?**   *(All India 2010)*
    a. Supernumerary renal arteries
    b. Supernumerary renal veins
    c. Double renal arteries
    d. Double renal veins

112. **Persistent fetal lobulation of adult kidney is due to:**
    a. Congenital renal defect   *(AIIMS Nov 2007)*
    b. Obstructive uropathy
    c. Intrauterine infections and scar
    d. Is a normal variant

■ ABERRANT RENAL ARTERY

113. **Aberrant renal artery, all true except:**
    a. More common in women
    b. Usually towards left
    c. May cause hydronephrosis
    d. Usually divided to gain access to renal pelvis

114. **All are true of aberrant renal artery except:**   *(PGI 93)*
    a. Bilateral   b. Leads to hydronephrosis
    c. Common in females   d. More common on left side

■ RETROCAVAL URETER

115. **'Reverse J' deformity on IVP is seen in:**
    a. Congenital megaureter   b. Ureterocele
    c. Retrocaval ureter   d. VUR

116. **Retrocaval ureter occurs due to persistence of:**
    (Recent Question 2016)
    a. Azygous vein   b. Hemiazygous
    c. Anterior cardinal vein   d. Posterior cardinal vein

■ HORSESHOE KIDNEY

117. **Isthmus of horses is located at what level?**
    (Recent Questions 2017)
    a. L1-L2 vertebra   b. L3-L4 vertebra
    c. L4-L5 vertebra   d. L2-L3 vertebra

118. **"Hand joining sign" and 'Flower vase' pattern of uteters is characteristic of:**   *(Recent Questions 2017)*
    a. Sigmoid kidney   b. Horseshoe kidney
    c. Crossed ectopia   d. L-shaped kidney

119. **Horseshoe kidney ascent is prevented by:**
    a. Superior mesenteric artery   *(Recent Question 2017)*
    b. Superior mesenteric vein
    c. Inferior mesenteric artery
    d. Inferior mesenteric vein

■ RENAL CYST

120. **Spider leg appearance in IVP is suggestive of:**
    a. Renal cyst   b. Renal carcinoma
    c. Renal Tb   d. Hydronephrosis
    e. Chronic renal failure

121. **Which of the following is the most common renal cystic disease in infants is?**
    a. Polycystic kidney   b. Simple renal cyst
    c. Unilateral renal dysplasia   d. Calyceal cyst

■ URETEROCELE

122. **Cobra head appearance on excretory urography is suggestive of:**   *(MCI March 2010)*
    a. Horseshoe kidney   b. Duplication of renal pelvis
    c. Simple cyst of kidney   d. Ureterocele

123. **Treatment of choice for ureterocele?**   *(MHSSMCET 2009)*
    a. DJ stent   b. Laparoscopic repair
    c. LASER ablation   d. Endoscopic diathermy

124. **A 3-year-old girl presents with recurrent UTI. On USG shows hydronephrosis with filling defect and negative shadow of bladder with no ectopic orifice:**   *(UPPG 2004)*
    a. Vesicoureteric reflux   b. Hydronephrosis
    c. Ureterocele   d. Sacrococcygeal teratoma

125. **This characteristic appearance is seen on IVP in:**
    (Recent Question 2019, 2017)
    a. Tuberculosis   b. VUR
    c. Ureterocele   d. Ureteric stone

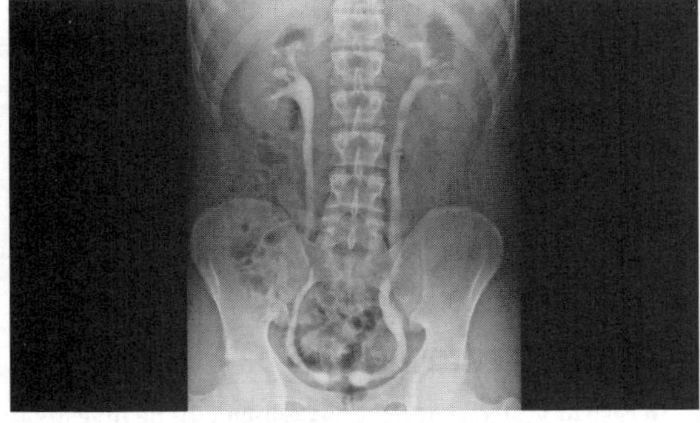

■ URETERIC ABNORMALITIES

126. **Ectopic ureter opening is not located in:**
    (MAHE 2005, AIIMS Nov 98)
    a. Bulbar urethra   b. Prostatic urethra
    c. Seminal vesicle   d. Bladder neck

127. **Most common congenital anomaly of the upper renal tract is:**   *(Recent Questions 2017)*
    a. Duplication of renal pelvis
    b. Duplication of ureter
    c. Ectopic ureteric orifice
    d. Congenital megaureter

128. **On the basis of given IVP image, what is the most probable diagnosis?**   *(Recent Question 2016)*
    a. Bilateral duplication of ureter
    b. Right bifid and left complete duplication of ureter
    c. Right bifid and left incomplete duplication of ureter
    d. Left bifid and right complete duplication of ureter

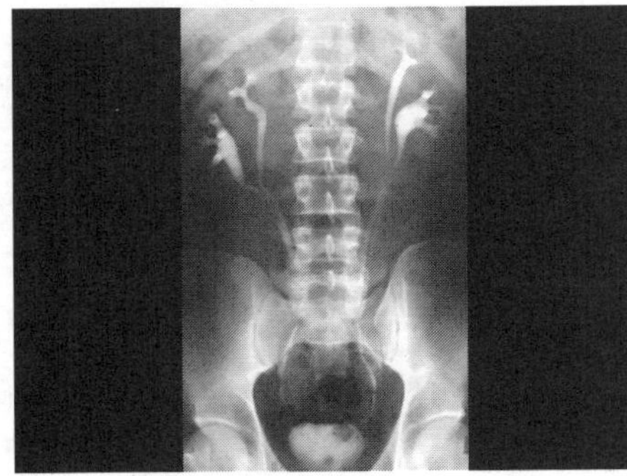

129. **True statement about duplex draining system of urinary tract are all except:**   *(Recent Question 2015, Punjab 2007)*
    a. It is most common anomaly of the upper urinary tract
    b. Upper moiety drains lower in the bladder
    c. Lower pole moiety is more prone to obstruction and upper pole more prone to reflux
    d. Yo-Yo Reflux may occur if ureters get fused

130. Yo-Yo reflux is seen in: *(Recent Question 2017)*
    a. Duplication of ureter
    b. Polycystic kidney disease
    c. Medullary sponge kidney
    d. Ureterocele

131. According to Weigert-Meyer's rule of duplication of ureter, the lower pole ureter in urinary bladder is:
                                          (JIPMER Nov 2017)
    a. Lateral and cephalad to the upper pole ureter
    b. Lateral and caudal to the upper pole ureter
    c. Medial and cephalad to the upper pole ureter
    d. Medial and caudal to the upper pole ureter

132. In the female, the most common site of termination of the ectopic ureter is the: *(Recent Question 2016)*
    a. Vestibule   b. Fallopian tube
    c. Ovary   d. Uterus

133. Classic symptom of ectopic ureter in females:
    a. Painful defecation   *(Recent Question 2016)*
    b. Urinary frequency
    c. Ureteral incontinence with otherwise normal voiding
    d. Labial swelling

■ VESICOURETERIC REFLUX

134. In case of vesicoureteric reflux which will be investigation of choice: *(AIIMS Nov 98)*
    a. Micturating cystourethrogram
    b. IVP
    c. Cystography
    d. Radionuclide study

135. In a patient suspected to be suffering from vesicoureteric reflex, which one of the following radiological investigations may confirm the diagnosis?   *(UPSC 2007)*
    a. Intravenous urography
    b. Micturating cystourethrography
    c. Pelvic ultrasound
    d. Antegrade pyelography

136. Treatment of choice for grade IV vesicoureteric reflux with recurrent UTI: *(AIIMS June 2000)*

    a. Cotrimoxazole
    b. Bilateral reimplantation of ureter
    c. Injection of collagen in the ureter
    d. Endoscopic resection of ureter

■ RENAL ARTERY ANEURYSM

137. The risk of rupture in renal artery aneurysms is:
    a. Less than 1%   b. 5%
    c. 20%   d. 75%
    e. None of the above

■ HEPATORENAL SYNDROME

138. Which of the following statements are incorrect with regard to hepatorenal syndrome in a patient with cirrhosis?
    a. Creatinine clearance 40 ml/min   *(All India 2003)*
    b. Urinary sodium < 10 mEq/L
    c. Urine osmolality lower than plasma osmolality
    d. No sustained improvement in renal function after volume expansion

■ DIALYSIS

139. The following are the complications of hemodialysis except:
    a. Hypotension   b. Peritonitis
    c. Hypertension   d. Bleeding tendency

■ RENAL TRANSPLANT

140. First autologous renal transplantation was done:
    a. Hardy   b. Kavosis   *(All India 2010)*
    c. Higgins   d. Studor

141. After renal transplant, the commonest malignancy is:
                                          (AIIMS June 97)
    a. Lymphoma   b. Renal cell carcinoma
    c. Skin cancer   d. Adrenal cancer

142. Not true about right kidney is: *(DNB 2003, AIIMS June 2001)*
    a. Right kidney is preferred over the left for transplantation
    b. It is lower than the left kidney
    c. Right renal vein is shorter than the left
    d. Right kidney is related to the duodenum

Explanations

■ RENAL AND URETERIC CALCULI

1. **Ans. b. Triple phosphate** *(Ref: Smith 18/e p255; Campbell 11/e p1182-1196; Bailey 27/e p1406)*
2. **Ans. c. Indinavir**
3. **Ans. d. Usually seen in acidic urine**
4. **Ans. b. Urinary stones** *(Ref: Campbell 11/e p1175)*

RANDALL'S PLAQUES

- **Randall's plaques** are **soft tissue calcifications**[Q] found in the **deep renal medulla** skirting the surface of the epithelium of the papilla, where they **act as nucleating elements** for **renal calculi** or **stones**[Q].

5. **Ans. b. Phosphate**
6. **Ans. b. Calcium oxalate**
7. **Ans. a. Calcium oxalate stone** *(Ref: Campbell 11/e p1209; Smith 18/e p252; Bailey 27/e p1406)*
8. **Ans. c. Ammonium urate** *(Ref: Campbell 11/e p1195, 1196)*

"Conditions associated with ammonium acid urate crystallization include laxative abuse, recurrent urinary tract infection, recurrent uric acid stone formation, and inflammatory bowel disease."-Campbell 11/e p1195

"The underlying pathophysiologic mechanism of ammonium acid urate stone formation due to laxative abuse has been postulated to be the result of dehydration due to gastro-intestinal fluid loss causing intracellular acidosis and enhanced ammonia excretion. Because urinary sodium is low in the setting of laxative use, urate complexes with abundant ammonia, thereby leading to urinary supersaturation of ammonium acid urate."- Campbell 11/e p1196

9. **Ans. b. Proteus** *(Ref: Campbell 11/e p1194; Smith 18/e p255; Bailey 27/e p1406)*

■ RENAL AND URETERIC CALCULI: CLINICAL FEATURES

10. **Ans. a. At pelvic brim** *(Ref: Smith 18/e p257; Campbell 1/e p1-2; Bailey 27/e p1407)*
11. **Ans. c. Dietl's crisis** *(Ref: Bailey 27/e p1411)*

DIETL'S CRISIS

- **Intermittent hydronephrosis (Dietl's crisis):** A **swelling** in the **loin** is associated with **acute renal pain**. Some hours later the **pain is relieved** and the **swelling disappears** when a **large volume of urine is passed**[Q].

12. **Ans. b. Increased peristalsis of ureter to overcome the obstruction** *(Ref: Smiths 18/e p257)*
    - The **severity** and **colicky nature** of **ureteric colic pain** are **caused by** the **hyperperistalsis** and **spasm** of **smooth muscles** of the **ureter** as it **attempts to rid** itself of a **foreign body** or **to overcome obstruction**.

PAIN FROM ACUTE OBSTRUCTION OF URETER (STONE OR BLOOD CLOT)

- **Ureteral pain** is typically **stimulated by acute obstruction** (passage of a **stone** or a **blood clot**)[Q].
- **Back pain** from **renal capsular distention**[Q] combined with **severe colicky pain** (due to **renal pelvic** and **ureteral muscle spasm**[Q] that radiates from the costovertebral angle down toward the lower anterior abdominal quadrant, along the course of the ureter.
- The **severity** and **colicky nature** of this pain are caused by the **hyperperistalsis**[Q] and **spasm**[Q] of this **smooth muscle organ** as it attempts to **rid itself of a foreign body** or to **overcome obstruction**.

13. **Ans. b. Stillness of the patient**
14. **Ans. d. Diclofenac**

■ RENAL AND URETERIC CALCULI: DIAGNOSIS AND TREATMENT

15. **Ans. b. Uric acid**
16. **Ans. a. Calcium oxalate monohydrate** *(Ref: Smith 18/e p268; Campbell 11/e p1268; Bailey 27/e p1408)*

    - *"Calculi composed of cystine, callium oxalate monohydrate are known to be resistant to fragmentation (ESWL)"*

17. **Ans. c. Struvite stone** *(Ref: Smith 18/e p255; Campbell 11/e p1182-1196; Bailey 25/e p1295-1300)*
18. **Ans. a. Hydrothorax** *(Ref: Smith 18/e p272; Campbell 11/e p1282; Bailey 27/e p1409)*

    - **PCNL** done through the **11th intercostals space** traverses the **lower aspect of pleura** and can **result in significant hydrothorax** from **large amount of irrigative fluid**.

19. **Ans. d. Stone in a calyceal diverticulum** *(Ref: Smith 17/e p264-268; Campbell 11/e p1278, 10/e p1380-1381)*

20. **Ans. a. Endoscopic removal** *(Ref: Campbell 11/e p1283; Bailey 27/e p1408)*

21. **Ans. b. Calcium oxalate, uric acid, struvite, cystine** *(Ref: Smith 18/e p 255; Campbell 11/e p1182-1196; Bailey 27/e p1406)*

22. **Ans. d. Ureteric obstruction due to fragments in ureter**   23. **Ans. c. Struvite crystals**

24. **Ans. a. Cysteamine** *(Ref: Harrison 19/e p1871; Smith 18/e p256; Campbell 11/e p1229)*

- **Patient with cystinuria with multiple renal stones** should be **treated with increase urine volume** (high fluid intake), **alkalinization of urine, Penicillamine** and **tiopronin. (α-Mercaptopropionyl glycine).**

25. **Ans. d. Calcium oxalate stone**   *(Ref: Smith 18/e p255; Campbell 11/e p1182-1196, 10/e p1296-1302; Bailey 25/e p1295-1300)*

In the given image, which shows enveloped or bipyramidal crystals are seen in calcium oxalate (dihydrate) stones.

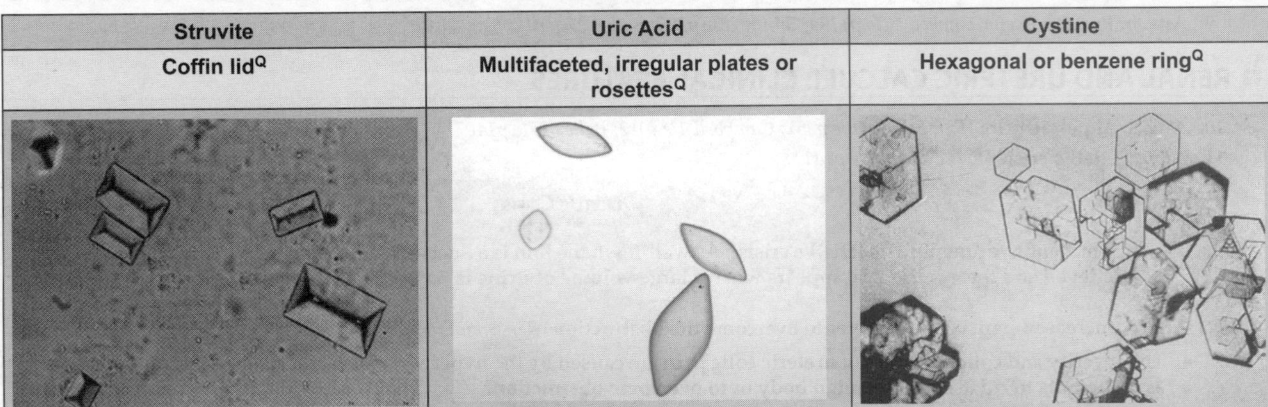

Calcium Oxalate	Calcium Oxalate Monohydrate	Brushite
Enveloped or bipyramidal[Q]	Dumbbell or hourglass[Q]	Needle shaped[Q]

Struvite	Uric Acid	Cystine
Coffin lid[Q]	Multifaceted, irregular plates or rosettes[Q]	Hexagonal or benzene ring[Q]

26. **Ans. c. Uric acid**   27. **Ans. a. ESWL**   28. **Ans. c. High calcium intake**

29. **Ans. a. Stone**

- **MC cause** of **ureteric obstruction: Stone**[Q]
- **MC cause** of **ureteric colic in hematuria: Clot**[Q]

30. **Ans. a. Holmium**   31. **Ans. b. Calcium restriction** *(Ref: Smith 18/e p253)*

32. **Ans. b. PCNL** *(Ref: Campbell 11/e p1240; Smith 18/e p272; Bailey 27/e p1409)*

33. **Ans. a. Bacterial sepsis** *(Ref: Campbell 11/e p1240; Smith 18/e p272; Bailey 27/e p1409)*

34. **Ans. b. PCNL** *(Ref: Bailey 27/e p1408)*

■ RENAL INFECTIONS

35. **Ans. a. E. coli** *(Ref: Smith 18/e p206; Campbell 11/e p279-280)*

36. **Ans. a. Proteus**

37. **Ans. d. Vesicoureteric reflux** *(Ref: Bailey 27/e p1404)*

- **Chronic pyelonephritis** is so often **associated with vesicoureteric reflux** that some feel that it is **better named "Reflux nephropathy".** It is important cause of renal damage and death from end-stage renal failure.

■ GENITOURINARY TUBERCULOSIS

38. Ans. b. Hematogenous *(Ref: Smith 18/e p223-225; Campbell 11/e p422; Bailey 27/e p1405)*

39. Ans. a. intravenous urography *(Campbell 11/e p425)*

- IVU is the gold standard for imaging early renal TB.

> **Intravenous urography:** The majority of cases will show positive findings on excretary urography, **the most common findings being hydrocalycosis, hydronephrosis or Hydroureter due to stricture formation. Early signs include the moth-eaten appearance of calyceal erosion and papillary irregularity.** These signs are best seen on early excretary **films because they are often masked by increasing density of the contrast on later films of the IVU.** Cavitory lesions communicating with the collecting system are characteristic of TB.

40. Ans. a. Renal papilla *(Ref: Smith 18/e p223; Campbell 11/e p422; Bailey 27/e p1405)*

PATHOGENESIS OF GENITO-URINARY TUBERCULOSIS

- **Granulomas** at **renal pyramid** → Enlarge (**tubercular abscess**) → **Burst** into **PC system** and **pus discharge** in urine (sterile pyuria[Q]).
- **Vesical irritability** is an **early clinical manifestation**[Q].

41. Ans. c. Tuberculosis of ureter

CYSTOSCOPY IN TUBERCULOSIS

- **Earliest sign** is **pallor**[Q] around ureteric orifice.
- Other features are **tubercular ulcer** and **golf hole ureteric orifice**[Q].

42. Ans. a. Increased frequency   **43. Ans. d. Microscopic hematuria**   **44. Ans. a. Renal tuberculosis**

■ HYDRONEPHROSIS

45. Ans. d. Ureterocele

46. Ans. a. Catheterize with Foley catheter *(Ref: Bailey 27/e p1412, 1349; CSDT 13/e p922)*

- **Catheterization** is **mandatory for acute urinary retention**[Q]. Spontaneous voiding may return, but a **catheter** should be **left indwelling for 3 days** while detrusor tone returns.

47. Ans. b. Radioisotope scan

■ DIAGNOSTIC AND LABORATORY INVESTIGATIONS

48. Ans. c. USG

- Causes of **filling defect** on **IVP: Stone, mass, cyst**[Q].
- After excretory urogram, **next best investigation** will be **USG** for **lesion characterization**[Q].

49. Ans. a. DMSA scan *(Ref: Bailey 27/e p1392)*

- **Renal scarring** or **structure of kidney** is best demonstrated by a **DMSA scan**.

Investigation of Choice	
ADPKD (Retroperitoneal Fibrosis)	CT scan[Q]
Medullary Sponge Kidney	IVP[Q]
VUR	MCU[Q]
Retrocaval ureter	MRI[Q]
PUJ Obstruction	DTPA scan[Q]
Renal structure or **surface**	DMSA scan[Q]

50. Ans. d. X-ray diffraction *(Ref: www.imaging.robarts.ca/.../2005pmb50)*

X-RAY DIFFRACTION

- The **X-ray diffraction** is dedicated to **materials identification** and characterize through single crystal and power X-ray diffraction analysis.
- Monoenergetic **X-ray diffraction (XRD) analysis** is an **established standard** for the assessment of **urinary stone composition**[Q].
- For the **precise determination** of true **stone composition**, x-ray diffraction analysis has often been the **method of first choice**[Q].

51. **Ans. b. Micturating cystourethrogram**

52. **Ans. a. Kidney** *(Ref: Smith 18/e p528; Campbell 11/e p23)*

Clinical Significance of Different Casts	
1. **Hyaline casts**	• **A normal constituent[Q] of urine** and has no attached significance[Q] • **Tom Horsfall protein[Q]** is protein secreted by **epithelial cells** of **loop of henle**. This protein may be excreted as Hyaline cast[Q]
2. **RBC cast**	• Are suggestive of **glomerular injury[Q]** or **acute glomerulonephritis**
3. **WBC casts**	• Are suggestive of **interstitial injury** and may be seen in **interstitial nephritis[Q]** • **WBC cast** with **bacteria** indicate **pyelonephritis[Q]**
4. **Brood granular casts**	• Are seen in **CRF[Q]** and suggests interstitial fibrosis and dilatation of tubules.
5. **Pigmented muddy brown granular casts**	• Are suggestive of ischemic or nephrotoxic injury[Q] **(Tubular Necrosis)**

53. **Ans. d. Pyonephrosis**

54. **Ans. b. DMSA scan** *(Ref: Campbell 11/e p285, 2940; Smith 18/e p206; Bailey 27/e p1404)*

■ BENIGN RENAL TUMORS

55. **Ans. c. Bleeding is self limited, d. Nephrectomy is the treatment of choice** *(Ref: Smith 18/e p331; Campbell 11/e p1309; Bailey 27/e p1416)*

56. **Ans. b. Renal oncocytoma** *(Ref: Smith 18/e p330; Campbell 11/e p1305)*

Central Stellate Scar is seen in	
• **FNH[Q]**	• **Serous cystadenoma[Q]** (pancreas)
• **Fibrolamellar HCC[Q]**	• Renal **oncocytoma[Q]**

■ RENAL CELL CARCINOMA: TYPES

57. **Ans. d. Chromophobe cell carcinoma** *(Ref: Smith 18/e p333; Campbell 11/e p1329; Bailey 27/e p1417)*

58. **Ans. a. Clear cell type**

59. **Ans. d. Monosomy of 1 and Y (-1, -Y)** *(Ref: Smith 18/e p333; Campbell 11/e p1329; Bailey 27/e p1417)*

- These tumors exhibit **multiple chromosome loss** and **extreme hypodiploidy[Q]**.
- Loss of multiple chromosomes **1[Q], 2[Q],** 6, 10, 13, 17, 21 and **Y[Q]**.

60. **Ans. c. von-Hippel Lindau (VHL) syndrome**

61. **Ans. a. PCT** *(Ref: Smith 18/e p333; Campbell 11/e p1329; Bailey 27/e p1417)*

62. **Ans. a. Medullary** *(Ref: Campbell 11/e p1333)*

- *"Renal medullary carcinoma is a subtype of RCC that occurs almost exclusively in patients with the sickle cell trait. It is typically diagnosed in young African-Americans, often in the third decade of life, and many cases are both locally advanced and metastatic at the time of diagnosis."-Campbell 11/e p1333*

■ RENAL CELL CARCINOMA: CLINICAL FEATURES, PARANEOPLASTIC SYNDROMES

63. **Ans. a. Renal cell carcinoma**

64. **Ans. a. Seminoma testis, c. Hypernephroma** *(Ref: Smith 18/e p333)*

- **Cannon-Ball pulmonary metastases** are **characteristic feature of RCC and testicular carcinoma.** As a rule, RCC produces spherical or round cannon-ball metastases.

65. **Ans. c. von-Hippel Lindau disease**

66. **Ans. a. Invasion of renal vein means inoperability**

67. **Ans. c. More common in female**

68. **Ans. c. Renal cell carcinoma**

69. **Ans. a. Hematuria**

■ RENAL CELL CARCINOMA: DIAGNOSIS AND TREATMENT

70. **Ans. b. IVC involvement indicates inoperability** *(Ref: Smith 18/e p340; Campbell 11/e p1355; Bailey 27/e p1419)*

- **45–70% of patients with RCC and IVC thrombus can be cured with an aggressive surgical approach including radical nephrectomy and IVC thrombectomy.**

71. **Ans. d.** Pathological staging
72. **Ans. d.** Renal cell carcinoma *(Ref: Campbell 11/e p1340; Harrison 19/e p578)*

Renal Cell Carcinoma
• **Cannon-Ball pulmonary metastases** are **characteristic feature of RCC**[Q].   • As a rule, **RCC produces spherical or round cannon-ball metastases**[Q].

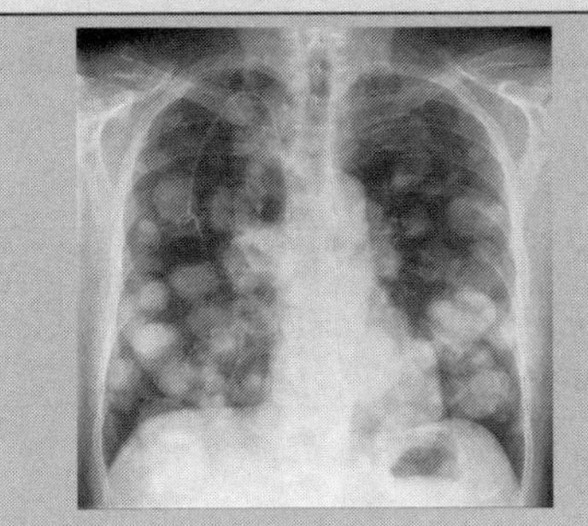 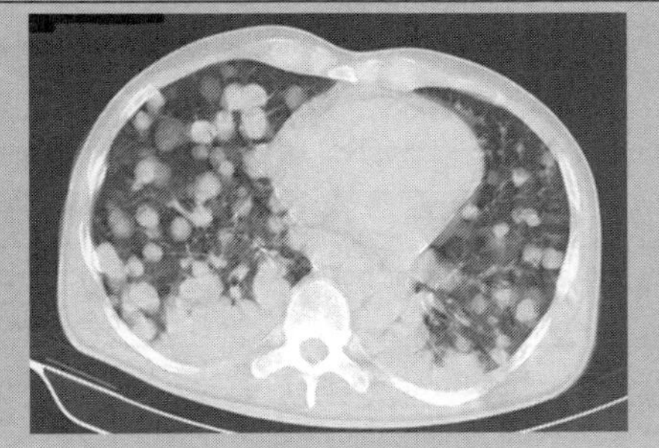 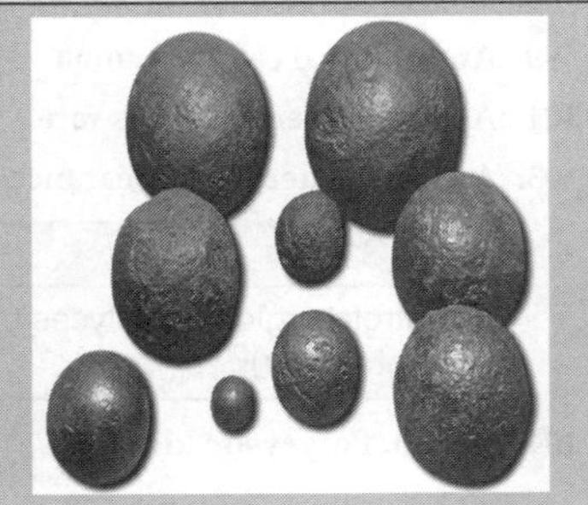

73. **Ans. a.** Partial nephrectomy
74. **Ans. a.** Radiosensitive
75. **Ans. c.** Elevated ESR
76. **Ans. d.** Para-aortic nodes *(Ref: Campbell 11/e p1345)*
77. **Ans. c.** Venacavagraphy
78. **Ans. c.** Tumor grossly extends into the inferior vena cava *(Ref: Campbell 11/e p1337; Smith 18/e p334)*

■ WILMS' TUMOR

79. **Ans. b.** Abdominal lump *(Ref: Smith 18/e p342; Campbell 11/e p3572; Bailey 27/e p1421)*
80. **Ans. c.** Histology
81. **Ans. a.** Within 10 days
82. **Ans. c.** Same location
83. **Ans. c.** Abdominal mass
84. **Ans. a.** Hematuria, b. Mass abdomen, d. Fever
85. **Ans. b.** Lungs
86. **Ans. b.** Open nephrourecterectomy *(Ref: Campbell 11/e p3574)*

- The **treatment of choice** for **satge I Wilm's tumor** is **transperitoneal radical nephrectomy (radical nephroureterectomy)**[Q] followed by **chemotherapy with or without radiotherapy** depending upon tumor histology.

87. **Ans. c.** 11 p13

■ TUMORS OF RENAL PELVIS

88. **Ans. a.** Transitional cell carcinoma *(Ref: Smith 18/e p322; Campbell 11/e p1370)*

- **Urothelial (transitional cell) carcinoma make up > 90% of upper urinary tract tumors**

89. **Ans. b.** Retrograde pyeloureterography *(Ref: Smith 18/e p324; Campbell 11/e p1371)*

- **Goblet sign** and **Stipple sign** describe the **appearance of ureteral dilation below** the **site** of an **intraluminal ureteral filling defect**, **best seen at** retrograde pyelography **(RGP)**[Q].
- The **Stipple sign** refers to the **pointillistic end-on appearance**[Q] on IVP or RGP of **contrast material tracking into the interstices** of a papillary lesion.
- Because maturity of TCC have a papillary configuration, **presence of this sign** should **raise** the **suspicion of TCC**, while the **Stipple sign** is **best seen in large papillary bladder tumors**[Q], it can occur anywhere in urothelial tumor, which expresses papillary architecture.

90. **Ans. d.** Transitional carcinoma of pelvis extending till ureter
91. **Ans. a.** Radical nephroureterectomy

■ RENAL TRAUMA

92. **Ans. a.** Urgent IVP is indicated *(Ref: Smith 18/e p286; Campbell 11/e p1151; Bailey 27/e p1413)*
93. **Ans. c.** Exploration indicated in all cases
94. **Ans. c.** Contralateral renal function is ascertained
95. **Ans. b.** Pulsatile hematoma

■ URETERIC INJURY

96. Ans. a. Complete renal atrophy, d. Hydronephrosis *(Ref: Smith 18/e p288; Bailey 27/e p1414)*   **97.** Ans. b. Hysterectomy

■ POLYCYSTIC KIDNEY DISEASE

98. Ans. a. Autosomal recessive trait *(Ref: Smith 18/e p537; Campbell 11/e p3017; Bailey 27/e p1402)*

99. Ans. c. Renal cell carcinoma   **100.** Ans. a. Autosomal dominant *(Ref: Campbell 11/e p3017; Smith 18/e p537)*

101. Ans. a. Hypertension is rare   **102.** Ans. a. Lung

103. Ans. a. Spider leg appearance *(Ref: Smith 18/e p537; Campbell 11/e p3017; Bailey 27/e p1402)*

IVP in ADPKD	
• Stretching of the calyces by the cysts (**spider leg** or **bell like deformity**)[Q]	• **Bubble appearance**[Q] (calyceal distortion) • **Swiss cheese appearance**[Q]

104. Ans. b. Polycystic kidney   **105.** Ans. d. Erythrocytosis *(Ref: Campbell 11/e p3017; Smith 18/e p537; Bailey 27/e p1402)*

■ PUJ OBSTRUCTION

106. Ans. d. Aberrant vessel is the most common cause *(Ref: Smith 18/;e p575; Campbell 11/e p1105; Bailey 26/e p1290-1292)*

107. Ans. d. Pelviureteric junction obstruction *(Ref: Campbell 11/e p1105; Smith 18/e p575)*

108. Ans. b. DTPA scan   **109.** Ans. a. Dietl's crisis

■ CONGENITAL ANOMALIES OF KIDNEY

110. Ans. d. UTI *(Ref: Smith 18e p522; Campbell 11/e p3037)*

- MSK is usually a benign process, and it may remain asymptomatic and undetected for life. Clinical presentation usually occurs after age 20 years with most common presentation being renal colic (50-60%), followed by urinary tract infection (20-30%) and gross hematuria (10-18%)

111. Ans. a. Supernumerary renal arteries *(Ref: Campbell's 10/e p26; Smith 18/e p522)*

- Vascular anomalies involving the kidney are very common being present in 25% to 40% of kidneys.
- **Supernumerary renal arteries** with two or more renal arteries supplying each kidney are the **most common renal vascular anomaly**.

ABNORMALITIES OF RENAL VASCULATURE

- **MC renal vascular anomaly** is the **presence of supernumerary renal arteries**[Q].
- **Variations** of the **main renal artery** and **vein** are common, present in **25% to 40%** of kidneys.
- **MC variation** is **occurrence of supernumerary renal arteries** (two or more arteries to a **single kidney**[Q])
- **MC sub-group** of **supernumerary renal arteries** is a **duplicated renal artery** (**double renal artery**)[Q] involving a second dimunitive renal artery supplying each kidney
- Supernumerary renal veins are also common, but occur about half as commonly as supernumerary renal arteries.

112. Ans. d. Is a normal variant *(Ref: www.ajronline.org/content/188/5/1380.full)*

PERSISTENT FETAL LOBULATION

- **Persistent fetal lobulation** is a **normal variant** seen occasionally **in adult kidneys**.
- It occurs when there is **incomplete fusion** of the **developing renal lobules**[Q].
- Embryologically, the kidneys originate as distinct lobules that fuse as they develop and grow.
- It is often seen on **ultrasound, CT or MRI** as **smooth indentations of the renal outline in between renal pyramids**[Q].
- They should be **distinguished from renal cortical scarring**, which **generally overlie the pyramids**[Q].

■ ABERRANT RENAL ARTERY

113. Ans. d. Usually divided to gain access to renal pelvis *(Ref: Smith 18/e p522)*

ABERRANT RENAL ARTERY

- Arteries that originate from vessels other than aorta or the main renal artery
- **Unilateral**[Q], more common on **left side**[Q], involving **lower pole**[Q] of kidney
- May cause **hydronephrosis** due to **extrinsic compression**[Q]
- These are **end arteries**[Q], therefore any injury or division may lead to lower pole infarction.

- The **renal arteries** are **end-arteries, division** leads to **infarction** of parenchyma[Q].
- **Renal veins** have **extensive collaterals** and an aberrant vein **can be divided** with impunity[Q].

114. **Ans. a.** Bilateral

■ RETROCAVAL URETER

115. **Ans. c.** Retrocaval ureter *(Ref: Smith 18/e p575; Campbell 11/e p1125; Bailey 27/e p1402)*

116. **Ans. d.** Posterior cardinal vein

■ HORSESHOE KIDNEY

117. **Ans. b.** L3-L4 vertebra

118. **Ans. b.** Horseshoe kidney

119. **Ans. c.** Inferior mesenteric artery *(Ref: Campbell 11/e p2293; Smith 18/e p520; Bailey 27/e p1399)*

■ RENAL CYST

120. **Ans. a.** Renal cyst *(Ref: Smith 18/e p515; Campbell 11/e p1300; Bailey 27/e p1402)*

121. **Ans. a.** Polycystic kidney *(Ref: Smith 18/e p514; Campbell 11/e p3017)*

- **Incidence of polycystic kidney: 1 in 400[Q] (0.25%)**
- **Simple renal cyst** is MC cystic disease in **human kidney** (incidence is **0.22% from birth to 18 years**)[Q]

■ URETEROCELE

122. **Ans. d.** Ureterocele *(Ref: Smith 18/e p571; Campbell 11/e p3076; Bailey 27/e p1401)*

123. **Ans. d.** Endoscopic diathermy   124. **Ans. c.** Ureterocele

125. **Ans. c.** Ureterocele *(Ref: Smith 18/e p571; Campbell 11/e p3076; Bailey 26/e p1286)*

- **IVP:** Typical **Adder head** or **Cobra head** or **Spring onion appearance**[Q] is diagnostic of ureterocele

■ URETERIC ABNORMALITIES

126. **Ans. a.** Bulbar urethra *(Ref: Smith 18/e p570; Campbell 11/e p3098; Bailey 27/e p1400)*

127. **Ans. b.** Duplication of ureter

- **MC congenital anomaly** of **upper urinary tract:** Duplication of **ureter**[Q]
- **MC congenital anomaly** of **genitourinary tract:** VUR[Q]

128. **Ans. b.** Right bifid and left complete duplication of ureter *(Ref: Campbell 11/e p3075; Smith 18/e p578)*

Right Incomplete (bifid) with Left Complete Duplication of Ureter

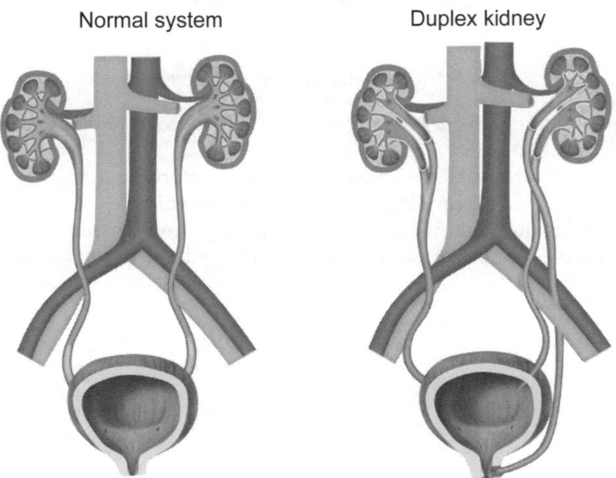

129. **Ans. c.** Lower pole moiety is more prone to obstruction and upper pole more prone to reflux

130. **Ans. a.** Duplication of ureter *(Ref: Smith 18/e p570; Campbell 11/e p3098; Bailey 27/e p1400)*

131. **Ans. a.** Lateral and cephalad to the upper pole ureter *(Ref: Campbell 11/e p3098; Smith 18/e p570; Bailey 27/e p1400)*

132. **Ans. a.** Vestibule

133. **Ans. c.** Ureteral incontinence with otherwise normal voiding

■ VESICOURETERIC REFLUX

134. **Ans. a. Micturating cystourethrogram** *(Ref: Smith 18/e p191; Campbell 11/e p3141)*

135. **Ans. b. Micturating cystourethrography**

136. **Ans. a. Cotrimoxazole**

■ RENAL ARTERY ANEURYSM

137. **Ans. b. 5%** *(Ref: Smith 18/e p523; Campbell 11/e p2999)*

■ HEPATORENAL SYNDROME

138. **Ans. c. Urine osmolality lower than plasma osmolality**
- **Hepatorenal syndrome** is associated with **urine osmolality greater than plasma osmolality[Q]**.

■ DIALYSIS

139. **Ans. b. Peritonitis, c. Hypertension** *(Ref: Harrison 19/e p1824)*

COMPLICATIONS DURING HEMODIALYSIS

- **Hypotension** is the **MC acute complication** of **hemodialysis**, particularly among patients with diabetes mellitus.
- **Muscle cramps** during dialysis are also a common complication of the procedure.
- **Anaphylactoid reactions** to the dialyzer, particularly on its first use, have been reported most frequently with the **bioincompatible cellulosic-containing membranes**.
- **Cardiovascular disease** constitutes the **major cause of death in patients with ESRD. Cardiovascular mortality** and **event rates are higher in dialysis patien**ts than in patients post-transplantation, although rates are extraordinarily high in both populations.

■ RENAL TRANSPLANT

140. **Ans. a. Hardy** *(Ref: Campbell 11/e p1087)*

First autologous renal transplantation was performed by 'Hardy' in 1963[Q]
'In 1963, Hardy performed the first renal autotransplantation to resolve on extensive ureteral lesion'.

141. **Ans. c. Skin cancer** *(Ref: Bailey 27/e p1542)*

142. **Ans. a. Right kidney is preferred over the left for transplantation** *(Ref: Bailey 27/e p1549)*

If the left kidney has a single renal artery (10% of kidneys have two or more renal arteries) it is usually chosen for transplantation because it has a longer renal vein, which simplifies the transplant operation[Q].

RENAL TRANSPLANTATION

- **Before the donation** it is essential to **perform imaging** (usually **MR angiography** or **CT angiography**) to **delineate the anatomy** of the **arterial supply to the kidneys[Q]**.
- If the **left kidney** has a **single renal artery** (10% of kidneys have two or more renal arteries) it is **usually chosen for transplantation** because it has a **longer renal vein**, which **simplifies the transplant operation[Q]**.
- The presence of **multiple arteries does not necessarily preclude donation** although implantation of living donor kidneys with multiple arteries may **increase the chances of vascular complications** developing **after implantation[Q]**.

Urinary Bladder

■ EXSTROPHY OF BLADDER (ECTOPIA VESICAE)

EXSTROPHY OF BLADDER (ECTOPIA VESICAE)

- Extrophy of bladder is **complete ventral defect** of Urogenital sinus and the **overlying skeletal system**[Q].
- **Defect in the infraumbilical part** of **anterior abdominal wall,** associated with **incomplete development** of **anterior wall of the bladder**[Q].

Embryology

- **Basic defect** is **abnormal overdevelopment** of the **cloacal membrane** and **its rupture.**
- **Timing of this rupture** of this **defective cloacal membrane determines the variant** of the extrophy-epispadias complex that results.

Clinical Features

- **Posterior wall of the bladder protrudes through the defect** with mucosal edges fused with skin and **urine spurts** onto the abdominal wall from the **ureteral orifices**[Q].
- **Rectus muscles** which are inserted on the pubic rami are also **widely separated**[Q].
- An **umbilical hernia**[Q] though usually small is present along with extrophic bladder.

  - In males, **complete epispadias** with a **wide & shallow scrotum. Undescended testis & inguinal hernias**[Q] are common.
  - **Females** also have **epispadias** with **bifid clitoris** and **wide separation** of the **labia**[Q].

- **Anus** is **dislocated anteriorly** in both sexes and there may be **rectal prolapse**[Q].

Complications

- Consequences of untreated bladder exstrophy are **total urinary incontinence**[Q] and an increased incidence of bladder cancer, usually **adenocarcinoma.**

Treatment

- **Enterocystoplasty**[Q] is the method of choice to augment bladder capacity and aid in reservoir function.
- **Urinary diversion with cystectomy**[Q] is treatment of choice for small, fibrotic or inelastic bladder.
- **Complete reconstruction** is achieved by:
  - Bladder closure with **sacral osteotomy** and **lengthening of penis**[Q] (Posterior iliac osteotomy[Q] is done in ectopia vesicae)
  - Antiureteral reflux procedure with **bladder neck reconstruction**[Q]
  - **Repair** of **epispadiac penis**[Q]

■ BLADDER STONE

Vesical Calculus	
Primary Bladder Calculi	**Secondary Bladder Calculi**
• Develop in **absence of** any **known functional, anatomic** or **infectious factors**[Q]	• Develop in concert with **bladder outlet obstruction**[Q], infection, impaired bladder emptying or a **foreign body.**

MIGRANT BLADDER CALCULI

- Found in **upper urinary tract, passed into bladder** and **retained**
- Most stones migrate out of ureter into bladder are **< 1 cm** and easily **passed into urethra**
- Calculi that are **retained,** are associated with **small bladder outlet** or **bladder outlet obstruction**
- Retained upper tract stones may grow to large size in bladder

■ PRIMARY BLADDER CALCULI (ENDEMIC BLADDER CALCULI)

PRIMARY BLADDER CALCULI (ENDEMIC BLADDER CALCULI)

- Mainly seen in **underdeveloped countries**[Q] (North Africa, Thailand, Myanmar, Indonesia), in **pediatric age** group.

> - **Most common in children <10 years, with a peak incidence at 2 to 4 years of age**.

- **More common in boys** than in girls.
- Common in **Rajasthan, Andhra Pradesh**[Q] and some north-eastern states of **India**.

> - Related to **chronic dehydration** and **low protein, low phosphate, exclusive milk & high carbohydrate diet**[Q].
> - Low phosphate diet increases urinary ammonium excretion leading to **ammonium urate stones**[Q].

Diagnosis
- USG bladder: Identifies the stone with its **characteristic shadowing** and **stone moves** with **changing body position.**

Treatment
- **Small stones:** Removed or crushed transurethrally **(Cystolitholapexy)** [Q]
- **Larger stones:** Disintegrated by **transurethral electrohydraulic lithotripsy** or **Cystolithotomy**[Q]

> - Primary bladder calculi **rarely recur after treatment**[Q].

■ SECONDARY BLADDER CALCULI

SECONDARY BLADDER CALCULI

- **Most** bladder stones are secondary, more common in **older males**[Q] (>50 years), usually because of **bladder outlet obstruction**[Q].
- **MC type:** Uric acid (sterile urine) > **Struvite stones**[Q] (Infected urine)
- Bladder stones are **usually solitary**[Q], multiple in 25% patients.

Etiology
- Bladder outlet obstruction (MC cause)[Q]
- **Neurogenic bladder**[Q]
- Foreign body (**Foley's catheter**, forgotten DJ stents)[Q]
- Bladder **diverticula**[Q]

Clinical Features
- Typical symptoms are **intermittent, painful voiding** and **terminal hematuria** with **severe pain** at the end of micturition[Q].
- **Pain** may be referred to the **tip of the penis** or to the **labia majora**[Q].

Diagnosis
- A large percentage of bladder stones are **radiolucent (uric acid)**[Q].
- **USG bladder:** Identifies the stone with its **characteristic shadowing** and **stone moves** with **changing body position**[Q].

Treatment
- **Small stones:** Removed or crushed transurethrally **(Cystolitholapexy)**[Q]
- **Larger stones:** Disintegrated by **transurethral electrohydraulic lithotripsy** or **Cystolithotomy**[Q]

Stones of Genitourinary Tract	
MC renal stone: **Calcium oxalate**[Q]	**MC primary bladder** stone: **Ammonium urate**[Q]
MC bladder stone: **Uric acid**[Q] **>Struvite**	**MC prostate** stone: **Calcium phosphate**[Q]

■ SCHISTOSOMIASIS (BILHARZIASIS)

SCHISTOSOMIASIS (BILHARZIASIS)

- Schistosomiasis is an infection with **Schistosoma haematobium**[Q].
- More common in **Males**[Q]

Lifecycle
- **Man**[Q] is the **only definitive host** & **intermediate host** is **snail**[Q].
- Life cycle begins with the passage of **eggs** into **freshwater** regions through **urine**[Q].
- When the **eggs** are hatched, **miracidia** are produced. These **penetrate** the **snail** and eventually form into **cercariae.**

> - **Eggs → Miracidium**[Q] (penetrate the snail) → **Cercaria**[Q] (penetrate skin of man) → Migrate to **vesical venous plexus**[Q] for reproduction → **Eggs in urine**[Q]

Contd…

Contd…

- Fluke embryos (**cercariae**) **penetrate** the **skin** of man from infected water and migrate to the **vesical venous plexus**, where **sexual reproduction** takes place[Q].
- **Eggs** are laid in the **submucosal veins** & **penetrate** the **bladder wall** to enter **urine**[Q].

Pathology

- Schistosoma **eggs** are **highly antigenic** and induce **intense granulomatous reaction** in bladder resulting in **bladder fibrosis** with **ureteric** or **urethral strictures**[Q].
- **Calcification** of **dead eggs** within bladder can produce a **calcified bladder** or **bladder stones**[Q].

Complications

- **Bladder calcification: Schistosomiasis** is the **MC cause**[Q] of bladder calcification worldwide.
- Urolithiasis, ascending urinary tract infection, urethral & ureteric stricture with subsequent hydronephrosis, & renal failure.
- **Squamous cell carcinoma**[Q] (Most serious complication)

Symptoms

- **MC symptom** of urinary schistosomiasis is **urinary frequency**[Q].

> - **Swimmer's itch** is the **first clinical sign** due to local inflammatory response from **cercarial penetration (<24 hours)**[Q]
> - **Katayama fever** (Acute schistosomiasis)[Q]: Generalized allergic reaction associated with onset of egg laying, which includes fever, urticaria, lymphadenopathy, hepatosplenomegaly & eosinophilia (**3 weeks to 4 months**)

- Acute inflammation phase when eggs are deposited, penetrate tissues and excreted (**hematurea, frequency & terminal dysurea**)
- Fever, rigor, toxemia & uremia are manifestations of renal involvement
- Signs:
  - In early uncomplicated cases, there are essentially no clinical findings.
  - In **advanced cases**, rectal examination may reveal a **fibrosed prostate, enlarged seminal vesicle** or **thickened bladder base**[Q].

Diagnosis

- Demonstration of schistosomal **eggs** in **early morning urine sample**[Q]
- **Sandy patches** (eggs in trigone) on **cystoscopy**[Q]
- IVU, RGU or cystography may show **mucosal irregularity**, inflammatory pseudo polyps, ureterits cystica, **ureteral dilation & stricture, reduced bladder capacity**[Q]

> - **Calcification** in the **wall of the bladder** or distal ureters on **plain radiographs (Fetal head appearance)**[Q]
> - **Calcifications** of the **distal ureters** have a characteristic pattern of **linear or parallel calcifications**[Q] on plain radiographs

Treatment

- **Praziquantel**[Q] **(DOC), metrifonate**[Q] or **oxaminiquine**[Q] are the drugs used in schistosomiasis.
- Surgery to treat the bladder contraction or for resection of the bladder cancer.

■ BLADDER RUPTURE

BLADDER RUPTURE

- Bladder injuries occur most often from **external force** to **full bladder** and often associated with **pelvic fractures**[Q].
- **Pelvic fracture** accompanies bladder rupture in **90%**[Q] cases.
- Classic triad suggestive of bladder rupture: **Suprapubic pain and tenderness + Difficulty in ability to pass urine + Hematuria**[Q]

Extraperitoneal (80%)

- **MC cause** is **pelvic fracture**[Q].
- Diagnosed by **cystogram** or **CT cystography**[Q]

> - **Flame sign** or **pear sign**[Q] (pattern of contrast extravasation) or **tear drop bladder**[Q] is seen
> - Treated by **simple catheter drainage**[Q] (Typically **10 days** of catheter drainage will provide adequate healing time)

- **Surgical repair** is indicated in cases of **repeated blockade** of catheter due to bleeding, **projecting bone fragment** or **tear extending** to the **bladder neck**[Q].

Intraperitoneal (20%)

- **Blow, kick or fall** on **fully distended bladder**[Q] leads to intraperitoneal rupture
- Usually seen in **males, MC site of rent** is **dome**[Q] of bladder.

> - Apart from classic triad suggestive of bladder rupture (Suprapubic pain and tenderness + Difficulty in ability to pass urine + Hematuria) patients develop **peritonism** and **abdominal distention**[Q].

Contd…

Contd…

- Diagnosis is made by **retrograde cystography** or **CT cystography**.
- **X-ray** abdomen shows **ground glass appearance**[Q] (due to fluid in abdomen).
- **Laparotomy** with **peritoneal lavage and bladder repair** with **SPC**[Q] should be done.
- **Cystography (gold standard)**[Q] reveals **distorted bladder** with **extravasation** of **contrast** in **perivesical space** and **streaks of contrast** into **fascial planes** giving rise to typical **"sun-burst" appearance**[Q].
- **USG** shows **bladder in bladder appearance**[Q] due to **perivesical collection** and rent may be detected.

■ RISK FACTORS FOR CARCINOMA URINARY BLADDER

Transitional Cell Carcinoma	Squamous Cell Carcinoma
• **Cigarette smoking**[Q]: **main etiological factor**, account for about 50% bladder cancer • Occupational exposure to chemicals: **Naphthylamine, benzidine, acrolein, aniline dyes, hydrocarbons**[Q] • **Schistosoma hematobium**[Q]: Risk factor **for both TCC** and **SCC, more for SCC** • Drugs: **Phenacetin and Chlornaphazine**[Q] • **Cyclophosphamide**[Q] • **Pelvic irradiation**[Q] • Occupations associated with increased risk: **Chemical, dye, rubber, petroleum, leather and printing industry workers**[Q]	• **Schistosoma hematobium**[Q]: Risk factor for both TCC and SCC, more for SCC • **Chronic irritation: Urinary calculi, long term indwelling catheters, chronic urinary tract infections**[Q] • **Bladder diverticula**[Q]

Types of Carcinoma Urinary Bladder		
Transitional Cell Carcinoma	Squamous Cell Carcinoma (Bilharzial carcinoma)[Q]	Adenocarcinoma Urinary Bladder
• More than **90%** of bladder cancer are **TCC**[Q] • Most commonly appear as **papillary** or **exophytic lesions**[Q]	• Account for **5–10%**, arise from **lateral bladder wall** and **dome**[Q] • Often **nodular** and **invasive**[Q] at the time of diagnosis • Do not respond to TURBT, partial cystectomy or chemotherapy • Treatment is **Radical cystectomy**[Q] • Stage to stage and grade to grade prognosis is same as TCC	• Account for **< 2%** bladder cancer • **Urachal remnants** and **ectopia vesicae** are **risk factors**[Q] • Three types: **primary vesical, urachal** and **metastatic**[Q] • Adenocarcinoma also occur in **intestinal urinary conduits, augmentations, pouches and ureterosigmoidostomies**[Q] • **Primary adenocarcinoma** arise along the **floor** whereas adenocarcinoma arising from **urachus** occur at the **dome** • **Treatment: Radical cystectomy** with **pelvic lymphadenectomy**[Q] • Poor response to chemotherapy and radiotherapy

- **MC benign mesenchymal** tumor of urinary bladder: **Leiomyoma**[Q]
- MC **malignant** mesenchymal tumor of urinary bladder: **Leiomyosarcoma**[Q]
- MC malignant mesenchymal tumor of urinary bladder in **children: Embryonal rhabdomyosarcoma**[Q]

■ CARCINOMA URINARY BLADDER

CARCINOMA URINARY BLADDER

- More common in **whites, higher socio-economic status** and in **males**[Q], in **6th & 7th** decade
- **75%** are **localized** to bladder and **25%** have **spread to regional nodes** or **distant sites** at the time of presentation
- Most tumors develop at **trigone & adjacent posterolateral wall**[Q] with ureteral involvement
- Tumors tend to be **multifocal**[Q] in bladder

Pathology

- MC type grossly is papillary & histologically, TCC.[Q]

Clinical Features

- **MC symptom: Painless hematurea**[Q] (85% cases)
- Hematuria is **gross** or microscopic, **intermittent**[Q] rather than constant
- **Vesical irritability**[Q]: Frequency, urgency and dysurea
- Bone pain & abdominal pain in advanced disease
- **MC** site of **lymphatic metastases: Pelvic lymph nodes (obturator is MC)**[Q]
- MC site of **hematogenous spread: Liver**[Q] > lung

Cystoscopy

- Diagnosis and initial staging is made by **cystoscopy and transurethral resection (TUR)**[Q]
- **Urinary Cytology**
- Cytologic examination of exfoliated cells are useful in **detecting cancer in symptomatic patients** and **assessing response to treatment**[Q]
- Most useful for **early diagnosis of recurrence in TCC**[Q]
- CT and MRI: used for staging[Q]

Contd…

Contd…

Management

- **Cystoscopy** and **TUR** or **biopsy; further management** is based on **stage, grade, size, multiplicity** and **recurrence pattern**[Q]
- **Systemic chemotherapy: MVAC** (Methotrexate + Vinblastine + Adriamycin + Cisplatin)
- **Drugs used for Intravesical chemotherapy:** BCG, mitomycin-c, epirubicin, thiotepa

8th AJCC (2017) TNM Staging for CA Bladder	
T: Primary tumor	**N: Regional lymph nodes**
Ta: Non-invasive papillary carcinoma[Q] **Tis:** Carcinoma in situ **"Flat tumor"**[Q]	**N1: Single** regional **LN** in true **pelvis** (hypogastric, obturator, external iliac or presacral LN)[Q]
T1: Tumor invades **subepithelial connective tissue**[Q]	**N2: Multiple** regional **LN** in true **pelvis** (hypogastric, obturator, external iliac or presacral LN)[Q]
T2a: Superficial muscularis propria **invasion (inner half)**[Q] **T2b: Deep** muscularis propria **invasion (outer half)**[Q]	**N3:** LN metastasis to **common iliac LNs**[Q]
T3a: Microscopic extension into perivesical fat[Q] **T3b: Macroscopic extension** into perivesical fat[Q]	**M: Distant metastases**
T4a: Cancer invading **pelvic viscera** (e.g., prostatic stroma, vaginal wall, rectum, uterus)[Q] **T4b:** Extension to **pelvic sidewalls, abdominal walls**, or **bony pelvis**[Q]	**M0:** No distant metastasis **M1:** Distant metastasis present

Treatment of CA Bladder	
Tis	**Intravesical BCG**[Q]
Ta (single, low to moderate grade, not recurrent)	**Complete TUR**[Q]
Ta (large, multiple, high grade or recurrent) and **T1**	**Complete TUR** followed by **intravesical chemo or immunotherapy**[Q]
T2-T4	• **Radical cystectomy**[Q] • **Neoadjuvant chemotherapy** followed by **radical cystectomy**[Q] • Radical cystectomy followed by adjuvant chemotherapy • Neoadjuvant chemotherapy followed by concomitant chemotherapy and irradiation
Any T, N+,M+	**Systemic chemotherapy** followed by selective **surgery** or **irradiation**

<h1 style="text-align:center">Multiple Choice Questions</h1>

■ ECTOPIA VESICAE

1. **Ectopic vesicae includes all except:** *(COMEDK 2005)*
   a. Hypospadias
   b. Extrophy of bladder
   c. Defective abdominal wall
   d. Bifid clitoris

2. **What is the diagnosis based on the given image?** *(JIPMER Nov 2017)*
   a. Gastroschisis
   b. Omphalocele
   c. Umbilical hernia
   d. Ectopia vesicae

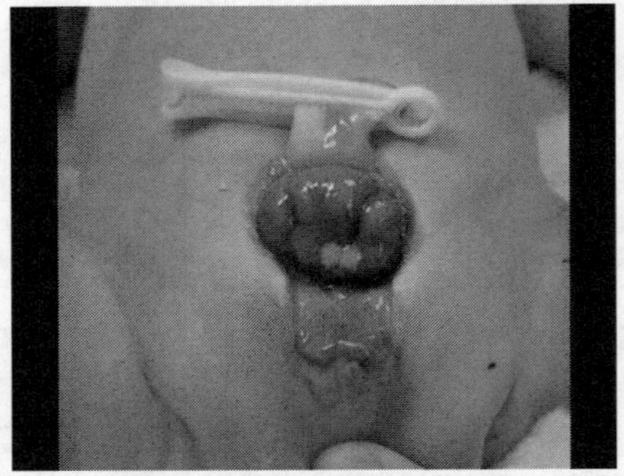

3. **All of the following are features of exstrophy of the bladder except:** *(All India 97)*
   a. Epispadias
   b. Cloacal membrane is present
   c. Posterior bladder wall protrudes through the defects
   d. Umbilical and inguinal hernia

4. **Which is not seen in complete ectopic vesicae:** *(Recent Quetsion 2016)*
   a. Umbilical hernia
   b. Visible uretero vesical efflux
   c. Hypospadias
   d. Waddling gate

■ URINARY BLADDER STONES

5. **Secondary vesical calculus refers to stones formed due to:** *(Karnataka 2006)*
   a. Hypercalciuria
   b. Injury
   c. Infection
   d. Migrating from above

6. **A 60-year-old man presented with intermittent painful voiding of urine. What is the diagnosis based on clinical picture and the given image?** *(Recent Question 2018)*
   a. Bladder stone
   b. Ureteric stone
   c. Prostate calcification
   d. Schistosomiasis

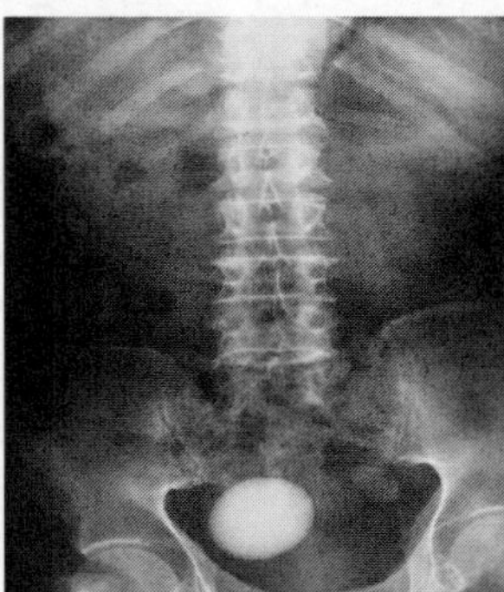

7. **The commonest bladder stone is:** *(Recent Question 2016)*
   a. Triple phosphate
   b. Xanthine
   c. Uric acid
   d. Cysteine

■ URINARY BLADDER: TUBERCULOSIS

8. **Thimble bladder is seen in:** *(MCI Dec 2018, Recent Question 2015, All India 91)*
   a. Acute tuberculosis
   b. Chronic tuberculosis
   c. Neurogenic bladder
   d. Schistosomiasis

9. **Treatment of 'Thimble bladder' is:** *(Recent Question 2015)*
   a. Anti-tubercular treatment
   b. Corticosteroids
   c. Ileocystoplasty
   d. Anti-tubercular drugs + steroids

■ SCHISTOSOMIASIS

10. **One of the following disease will show urinary bladder calcification radiologicaly which resemble fetal head in pelvis:** *(AIIMS June 2000)*
    a. Tuberculosis
    b. Schistosomiasis
    c. Chronic cystitis
    d. Malignancy

11. **Metrifonate is effective against:** *(COMEDK 2008)*
    a. Amebiasis
    b. Leishmaniasis
    c. Schistosomiasis
    d. Giardiasis

■ CARCINOMA URINARY BLADDER: RISK FACTORS

12. **Carcinoma common in dye industry workers:** *(MHPGMCET 2001)*
    a. Skin
    b. Scrotum
    c. Urinary bladder
    d. Maxilla

13. **Most common site of prostatic cancer:** *(MCI Dec 2019)*
    a. Posterior lobe
    b. Lateral lobe
    c. Medial lobe
    d. Anterior lobe

14. **Transitional cell carcinoma can be seen in:** *(MHSSMCET 2006)*
    a. Analgesic nephropathy
    b. Urate nephropathy
    c. Pulmonary infections
    d. Myocardial infarction

15. **All are precancerous for carcinoma bladder except:** *(Recent Question 2015, All India 91)*
    a. Tuberculosis bladder
    b. Aniline dyes
    c. Schistosomiasis
    d. Chronic ulcer

16. **Associated with urinary bladder carcinoma are all of the following except:** *(MCI Sept 2009)*
    a. Smoking
    b. HPV infection
    c. Schistosomiasis
    d. Cyclophosphamide

17. **Which of the following drug causes carcinoma bladder?** *(Recent Question 2017)*
    a. Cyclophosphamide
    b. Cisplatin
    c. Taxane
    d. Tamoxifen

■ CARCINOMA URINARY BLADDER: TYPES

18. **SCC of bladder is best treated by:** *(GB Pant 2011)*
    a. Chemotherapy
    b. Radical cystectomy
    c. Radiotherapy
    d. TUR

19. **Most common tumor of urinary bladder is:**
    a. Squamous cell carcinoma   *(DNB 2008, PGI June 97)*
    b. Adenocarcinoma
    c. Transitional carcinoma
    d. Stratified squamous carcinoma

20. **Bladder tumors mostly arises from:**   *(All India 91)*
    a. Mucosa   b. Submucosa
    c. Muscularis mucosa   d. Serosa

■ CARCINOMA URINARY BLADDER: CLINICAL FEATURES AND DIAGNOSIS

21. **A 67-year-old chronic heavy smoker presents with 2 weeks history of frank hematuria. Ultrasound pelvis shows a filling defect. Most probable diagnosis:**   *(JIPMER May 2018)*
    a. Bladder diverticula
    b. Adenocarcinoma of bladder
    c. Squamous cell carcinoma of bladder
    d. Transitional cell carcinoma of bladder

22. **An elderly male presents with one episode of gross heematuria. All of the following investigations are recommended for this patient except:**   *(All India 2007)*
    a. Cystoscopy
    b. Urine microscopy for malignant cells
    c. Urine tumor markers
    d. Intravenous pyelogram

23. **Urinary cytology is a useful screening test for the diagnosis of:**   *(Recent Question 2016)*
    a. Renal cell carcinoma   b. Wilms' tumour
    c. Urothelial carcinoma   d. Carcinoma prostate

24. **Which of the following is a tumor marker for bladder cancer?**   *(Recent Question 2017)*
    a. AFP   b. CEA
    c. Bladder surface protein   d. NMP-22

25. **A 60-year-old smoker male patient presents with painless gross hematuria for 1 day. IVU shows 1.2 cm filling defect at the lower pole of infundibulum. Which is the next best investigation to be done?**   *(MCI Nov 2017)*
    a. Cystoscopy   b. Urine cytology
    c. USG abdomen   d. DMSA scan

■ CARCINOMA URINARY BLADDER: TREATMENT

26. **Treatment of choice for low grade superficial bladder carcinoma:**   *(JIPMER 2011)*
    a. Local excision   b. Radical cystectomy
    c. Intravesical BCG   d. Chemotherapy

27. **BCG is used in the treatment of:**   *(MHPGMCET 2006)*
    a. Carcinoma cervix
    b. Carcinoma colon
    c. Carcinoma of urinary bladder
    d. All

28. **Which of the following is the most effective intravesical therapy for superficial bladder cancer?**   *(AIIMS Nov 2005)*
    a. Mitomycin   b. Adriamycin
    c. Thiotepa   d. BCG

29. **A 65-year-old male smoker presents with gross total painless hematuria. The most likely diagnosis is:**   *(All India 2003)*
    a. Carcinoma of urinary bladder
    b. Benign prostatic hyperplasia
    c. Carcinoma prostate
    d. Cystolithiasis

30. **Laser used in carcinoma bladder:**   *(Recent Question 2017)*
    a. Carbon dioxide laser
    b. Nd-YAG laser
    c. Ho-YAG laser
    d. Argon laser

31. **Chemotherapy used for metastatic bladder cancer:**
    a. AC (Adriamycin and Cisplatin)   *(Recent Question 2016)*
    b. Interferon
    c. MVAC (Methotrexate, Vinblastine, Adriamycin and Cisplatin)
    d. Cisplatin alone

■ URINARY BLADDER INJURY

32. **True about extraperitoneal urinary bladder rupture is all except:**
    a. Associated with fracture   *(MHPGMCET 2002)*
    b. More common than intraperitoneal bladder rupture pelvis in about 70% cases
    c. Commonly associated with anterior urethral rupture
    d. Can be managed conservatively without surgical intervention

33. **In extraperitoneal rupture of bladder, urine extravasates in:**
    a. Groin   *(AIIMS Nov 94, All India 93)*
    b. Intraperitoneal region
    c. Extraperitoneal region
    d. Perivesical space

34. **Intraperitoneal bladder rupture management:**
    a. Requires laparotomy   *(Recent Question 2017)*
    b. Antegrade cystogram is needed
    c. Simple catheter drainage is the treatment
    d. Conservative management

Explanations

■ ECTOPIA VESICAE

1. Ans. a. Hypospadias
2. Ans. d. Ectopia vesicae
3. Ans. b. Cloacal membrane is present
4. Ans. c. Hypospadias

■ URINARY BLADDER STONES

5. Ans. c. Infection *(Ref: Smith 18/e p275; Campbell 11/e p1292; Bailey 27/e p1434)*
6. Ans. a. Bladder stone *(Ref: Bailey 27/e p1435; Smith 18/e p276; Campbell 11/e p1291-1292)*
7. Ans. c. Uric acid

■ URINARY BLADDER: TUBERCULOSIS

8. Ans. b. Chronic tuberculosis
9. Ans. c. Ileocystoplasty

■ SCHISTOSOMIASIS

10. Ans. b. Schistosomiasis
11. Ans. c. Schistosomiasis

■ CARCINOMA URINARY BLADDER: RISK FACTORS

12. Ans. c. Urinary bladder *(Ref: Smith 18/e p312; Campbell 11/e p2187-2188; Bailey 27/e p1446)*
13. Ans. a. Posterior lobe *(Ref: Bailey 27/e p1469)*
14. Ans. a. Analgesic nephropathy
15. Ans. a. Tuberculosis bladder; d. Chronic ulcer
16. Ans. b. HPV infection
17. Ans. a. Cyclophosphamide *(Ref: Campbell 11/e p2188; Smith 18/e p310; Bailey 27/e p1446)*

■ CARCINOMA URINARY BLADDER: TYPES

18. Ans. b. Radical cystectomy *(Ref: Smith 18/e p313; Campbell 11/e p2225; Bailey 27/e p1451)*
19. Ans. c. Transitional carcinoma
20. Ans. a. Mucosa

■ CARCINOMA URINARY BLADDER: CLINICAL FEATURES AND DIAGNOSIS

21. Ans. d. Transitional cell carcinoma of bladder
22. Ans. c. Urine tumor markers
23. Ans. c. Urothelial carcinoma
24. Ans. d. NMP-22
25. Ans. a. Cystoscopy

■ CARCINOMA URINARY BLADDER: TREATMENT

26. Ans. a. Local excision *(Ref: Smith 18/e p316; Campbell 11/e p2207; Bailey 27/e p1450-1451)*
27. Ans. c. Carcinoma of urinary bladder
28. Ans. d. BCG *(Ref: Smith 18/e p318, 17/e p316; Campbell 11/e p2212-2216; Bailey 27/e p1450, 26/e p1334)*

Drugs used in Intravesical Chemotherapy			
• Mitomycin C[Q]	• Epirubicin[Q]	• Thiotepa[Q]	• BCG (most effective)[Q]

29. Ans. a. Carcinoma of urinary bladder
30. Ans. b. Nd-YAG laser *(Ref: Campbell 11/e p2210)*

> *"Laser coagulation allows minimally invasive ablation of tumors up to 2.5 cm in size. The neodymium : yttrium-aluminum-garnet (Nd : YAG) laser has the best properties for use in bladder cancer."* -Campbell 11/e p2210

31. Ans. c. MVAC (Methotrexate, Vinblastine, Adriamycin and Cisplatin)

■ URINARY BLADDER INJURY

32. Ans. c. Commonly associated with anterior urethral rupture *(Ref: Smith 18/e p290; Campbell 11/e p2368; Bailey 27/e p1425)*

Bladder Rupture	
Extraperitoneal (80%)	**Intraperitoneal (20%)**
• **MC cause** is **pelvic fracture**[Q]. • Classic triad: **Suprapubic pain and tenderness + Difficulty** in ability **to pass urine + Hematuria**[Q] • Diagnosed by **cystogram** or **CT cystography**[Q] • **Flame sign** or **pear sign**[Q] (pattern of contrast extravasation) is seen • Treated by **simple catheter drainage** (Typically **10 days** of catheter drainage will provide adequate healing time)[Q] • **Surgical repair** is indicated in cases of **repeated blockade** of catheter due to bleeding, **projecting bone fragment** or **tear extending** to the **bladder neck**[Q].	• **Cause: Blow, kick** or **fall** on **fully distended bladder**[Q] • Usually seen in **males, MC site of rent** is **dome** of bladder[Q]. • Apart from classic triad suggestive of bladder rupture (Suprapubic pain and tenderness + Difficulty in ability to pass urine + Hematuria) patients develop **peritonism** and **abdominal distention**[Q]. • Diagnosis is made by **retrograde cystography** or **CT cystography**[Q]. • **X-ray** abdomen shows **ground glass appearance**[Q] (due to fluid in abdomen) • **Laparotomy** with **peritoneal lavage and bladder repair** with **SPC** should be done[Q].

33. Ans. d. Perivesical space

34. Ans. a. Requires laparotomy *(Ref: Campbell 11/e p2387; Smith 18/e p291; Bailey 27/e p1425)*

Prostate and Seminal Vesicles

■ BENIGN PROSTATIC HYPERPLASIA (BPH)

BENIGN PROSTATIC HYPERPLASIA (BPH)

Incidence and Epidemiology

- **BPH** originates in the **transition zone**[Q], **incidence** is **age related**[Q]
- The prevalence of BPH is **20%** in **41–50** years, **50%** in **51–60** years, **> 90%** older than **80** years.

Etiology

- Seems to be **multifactorial** and **endocrine controlled**[Q].
- Prostate is composed of **stromal & epithelial elements**[Q], and each, either alone or in combination, can give rise to **hyperplastic nodules**[Q] and symptoms associated with BPH.

Pathology

- **BPH** develops in the **transition zone**. It is truly a **hyperplastic process**[Q].
- Nodular growth pattern is composed of varying amounts of **stroma & epithelium**.
- **Stroma** is composed of **collagen & smooth muscle**[Q].

> - **Alpha-blocker** therapy result in **excellent responses**[Q] in patients with BPH having significant component of **smooth muscle**, while those with BPH predominantly composed of **epithelium** might respond better to **5-alpha-reductase inhibitors**[Q].
> - **Effects starts early** with **alpha-blockers** whereas **effect starts after 1 month** and may **take 6 months for maximum effect** with **5-alpha-reductase inhibitors**[Q].

- Patients with significant components of **collagen** in the stroma **may not respond** to **either form** of medical therapy.
- As **BPH nodules** in the transition zone enlarge, **compress** the outer zones of the prostate, resulting in the formation of a **surgical capsule** separating the transition zone from the peripheral zone, and serves as a **cleavage plane** for **open enucleation**[Q] of the prostate.

Pathophysiology

- **Prostatic size on DRE correlates poorly with symptoms** because the **median lobe** is **not** readily **palpable**[Q].

> - **Prostatic stroma**, composed of **smooth muscle & collagen**, is rich in **adrenergic nerve supply**. The level of autonomic stimulation thus sets a tone to the prostatic urethra. Use of **alpha-blocker therapy decreases this tone**, resulting in a decrease in outlet resistance[Q].
> - **Irritative voiding complaints** of BPH result from the **secondary response** of **bladder** to the **increased outlet resistance**[Q].

- Bladder outlet obstruction leads to **detrusor muscle hypertrophy, hyperplasia & collagen deposition**[Q] (collagen deposition is most likely responsible for a decrease in bladder compliance).

Symptoms

- **Obstructive symptoms** include **hesitancy, decreased force** & caliber of stream, sensation of incomplete bladder emptying, **double voiding** (urinating a second time within 2 hours of the previous void), **straining to urinate & post-void dribbling**[Q].
- **Irritative symptoms** include **frequency, urgency & nocturia (FUN)** [Q]
- **IPSS (International Prostatic Symptom Score)**: score can range from 0–35. **Mild: 0–7, moderate: 8–19, severe: 20–35.**

Signs

- **Size & consistency** of the prostate is noted.
- BPH usually results in a **smooth, firm, elastic enlargement** of the prostate.
- **Induration** is suggestive of **cancer** and the need for further evaluation (**PSA, TRUS and biopsy**)[Q].

Imaging

- **IVP or ultrasound** is recommended only in the **presence of concomitant urinary tract disease** or **complications** from BPH (hematuria, urinary tract infection, renal insufficiency, history of stone disease).
- **Uroflowmetry: (Q_{max} >15 ml/sec is normal,** 10–15 ml/sec is equivocal and **< 10 ml/sec** is suggestive of **obstruction**)[Q]
- **Cystometrograms** and **urodynamic profiles** are reserved to differentiate outflow obstruction from neurogenic bladder (**voiding pressure > 80 cm H_2O signifies outlet obstruction**)[Q]

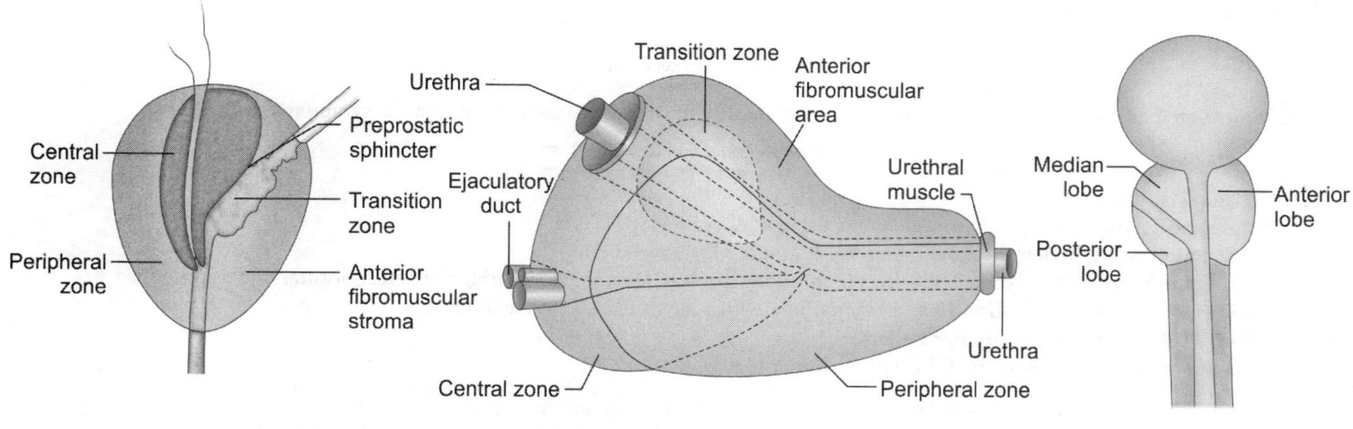

Anatomy of the prostate gland

MEDICAL THERAPY IN BPH

MEDICAL THERAPY IN BPH

- **Alpha-blockers:** (Prazosin, terazosin, doxazosin, tamsulosin, alfuzosin, **silodosin**[Q])
  - **Relaxes smooth muscle** & **decreases urethral resistance**[Q].
  - **Side effects**: orthostatic hypotension, dizziness, tiredness, retrograde ejaculation, rhinitis & headache[Q].
- **5-Alpha-reductase inhibitors:** (Finasteride, dutasteride, triptorelin pamoate)
  - **Blocks** the conversion of **testosterone** to **dihydrotestosterone**, affecting the **epithelial component**[Q] of the prostate, resulting in a **reduction in the size of gland**[Q] and improvement in symptoms.

  > - **Six months of therapy** are **required** to see the **maximum effects** on prostate size (**20% reduction**)[Q] and symptomatic improvement. However, **symptomatic improvement** is seen **only in** men with **enlarged prostates (> 40 cm³)**[Q].

  - **Side effects**: decreased libido, decreased ejaculate volume and impotence[Q].
- **Combination therapy**
  - The **reduction in risk** associated with **combination therapy** (66% risk reduction) is **greater than** that associated with **doxazosin or finasteride alone**[Q].
  - Patients most likely to benefit from combination therapy: whom **baseline risk of progression** is **very high**, generally patients with **larger glands** and **higher PSA values**[Q].

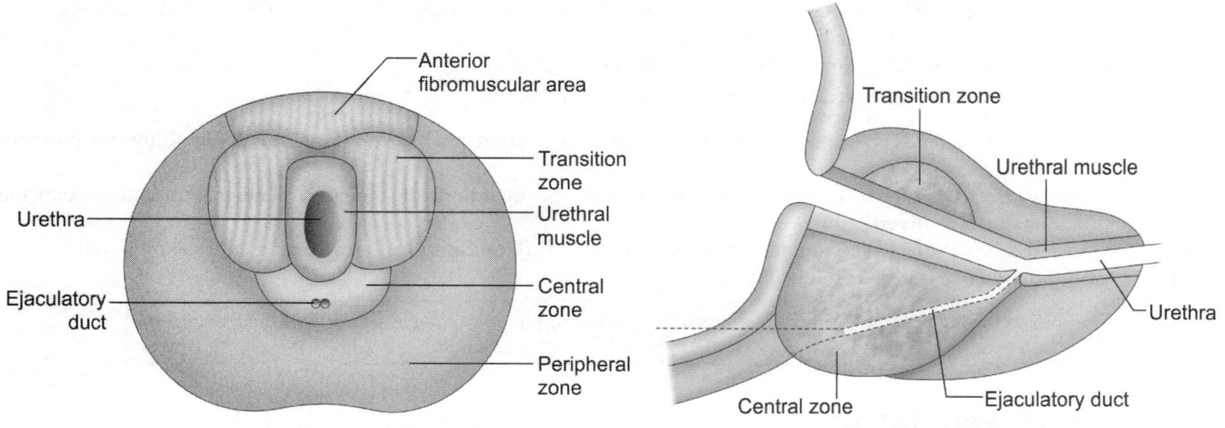

Absolute Indications for Surgery in BPH

1. **Refractory urinary retention**[Q] (failing at least one attempt at catheter removal)
2. **Recurrent UTI**[Q]
3. **Recurrent gross hematuria**[Q]
4. Bladder **stones**[Q]
5. **Renal insufficiency**[Q]
6. Minimal improvement on medical treatment[Q]

■ TREATMENT OF BPH

TREATMENT OF BPH

- **MC indication** for surgery is **symptoms interfering** with **quality of life**[Q] (bothersome symptoms & symptoms of BOO).

CONVENTIONAL SURGICAL THERAPY

- **TURP (Gold standard)**[Q]:
  - Cystoscopic removal of strips of prostatic tissue using diathermy loop.
  - **Two techniques: NESBIT technique** (preferred) & Mauer Mayer technique
  - **Best irrigant fluid is 1.5% glycine**[Q] (**Electrolyte solutions** like NaCl are **not compatible** with **electrocautery**, so **not used**).
  - **Glycine** is composed of **glycolic acid** and **ammonium,** which can **cause CNS (visual) toxicity.**[Q]
  - TURIS: TUR in saline using bipolar cautery[Q]
  - **Chips of prostate are removed by Ellik's evacuator.**

  > - **Verumontanum** is the single most important anatomical **landmark** in TURP[Q].
  > - **Verumontanum** lies immediately **proximal to external sphincter** and serve as the **distal landmark for prostate resection** to prevent injury to the external sphincter.
  > - **Verumontanum: Distal landmark** for **prostate resection**[Q].
  > - **Verumontanum:** Landmark for **proximal limit** of **external sphincter**[Q].

  - **Resection** proceeds at **1 gm/minute** for **an hour**.
  - **Risks of TURP:** Retrograde ejaculation (75%)[Q], impotence (5–10%)[Q] & incontinence (< 1%)[Q].
  - **Complications:** Bleeding, **urethral stricture** or **bladder neck contracture**[Q], perforation of the prostate capsule with extravasation, and if severe, TUR syndrome.

  > **TUR syndrome (Dilutional hyponatremia or water intoxication)**
  > - **TUR syndrome (Dilutional hyponatremia** or **water intoxication)**[Q] resulting from a hypervolemic, hyponatremic state due to **absorption of** the **hypotonic irrigating solution**.
  > - **Clinical Features:** Nausea, vomiting, confusion, hypertension, bradycardia, & **visual disturbances**[Q].
  > - The risk increases with **resection times > 90 minutes** or **gland size > 75 gm**.
  > - **Treatment** includes **diuresis** (furosemide) and in **severe cases, hypertonic saline** (3%) administration.

  > **Late Complications of TURP**
  > - **Bladder neck stenosis** (4%) **> Urethral stricture** (3.6%)
  > - **Bladder neck stenosis** is seen more often with **small (< 30 gm) fibrotic prostates**.

- **Transurethral incision of the prostate (TUIP):**
  - For posterior commissure hyperplasia (elevated bladder neck), involves two incisions using the Collins knife at the 5- and 7-o'clock positions.
  - The **incisions** are started **just distal** to the **ureteral orifices** and are **extended** outward **to the verumontanum**.

  > - **TUIP** lowers the **incidence** of **bladder neck contracture** when **compared to TURP**, so **TUIP** should be strongly **considered** in patients with **smaller gland** in place of TURP.
  > - **TUIP** is used for **smaller (20 gm) prostate, young patients**.
  > - **Decreased incidence** of **retrograde ejaculation** as compared to TURP.

- **Open simple prostatectomy: Glands > 75 gm**, concomitant bladder **diverticulum** or a bladder **stone** or if **dorsal lithotomy** positioning is **not possible**.
  - **Suprapubic prostatectomy:** Performed **transvesically (Frayer's)**[Q] and **operation of choice** in dealing with concomitant bladder pathology **(Bladder stones** or **diverticulum)**[Q].
  - **Retropubic prostatectomy (Millin's)**[Q]: Transverse incision is made in surgical capsule of prostate and enucleation is done.
  - **Perineal prostatectomy (Youngs)**[Q]: Abandoned now

  > - **Carcinoma prostate** originates in **peripheral zone** of prostate, so prostatectomy for **BPH confers no protection** for subsequent cancer[Q].

■ ACUTE BACTERIAL PROSTATITIS

ACUTE BACTERIAL PROSTATITIS

- Acute inflammation of prostate associated with UTI
- Caused by **ascending urethral infection** or **reflux** of **infected urine**[Q] into prostatic ducts
- MC organism: **E. coli**[Q]

Contd…

Contd…

- Patients present with sudden onset **high grade fever** with **chills** and **rigors**, severe **irritative symptoms** and **enlarged, tender** and **boggy prostate**[Q]
- **Catheterization** and **prostatic massage** is **contraindicated**[Q]
- MC used antibiotics are: **TMP-SMX** and **Ciprofloxacin** (Both are having better **concentration in prostatic tissue**)[Q]
- Around **4-6 weeks**[Q] of antibiotic therapy is used to avert chronic bacterial prostatitis.

■ CHRONIC BACTERIAL PROSTATITIS

CHRONIC BACTERIAL PROSTATITIS

- Due to **persistent bacterial infection**[Q] of prostate
- Insidious in onset, characterized by **relapsing or recurrent UTI**[Q] caused by persistence of pathogen in prostatic fluid despite of antibiotic therapy
- **Diagnosis** is made by **microscopic examination** and **culture** of prostatic expressate and culture of urine obtained before and after prostatic massage[Q]
- **Treated** by **chronic antibiotic suppression (3–4 months).**[Q]

■ PROSTATIC ABSCESS

PROSTATIC ABSCESS

- Most cases result from **complications** of **acute bacterial prostatitis**[Q]
- **Fluctuation** is a **very late sign**[Q]
- **Predisposing factors:** Diabetes, **renal insufficiency, immunosuppression, urethral instrumentation, chronic indwelling catheter**[Q]
- **Diagnosis: TRUS** or **pelvic CT scan** is crucial for diagnosis and treatment
- Treated by **transurethral drainage** and **antibiotics**[Q]

■ PROSTATIC CALCULI

PROSTATIC CALCULI

- Thought to represent **calcified corpora amylacea**[Q], which is composed of **calcium phosphate**[Q]
- Usually **phosphate**, seen on **TRUS** in **nearly all elderly males**[Q]
- Lie at the **periphery** of **transition zone** (posterior and posterolateral zones of prostate)
- Usually **asymptomatic** due to peripheral location, tend to **occur in clusters**[Q]
- **Calculi do not predispose** to **infections**[Q]
- But if **infections** occurs **in the presence of calculi**, it is almost **impossible to eradicate**[Q] the as the calculi may get infected and serve as a source of bacterial persistence and recurrent UTI.

■ PROSTATE CANCER

PROSTATE CANCER

- **MC cancer** of **males, MC** cause of **bone secondaries**[Q]
- **African-American men** have highest incidence, **less common in Asians**[Q]
- **Best screening protocol** for CA prostate: **PSA + DRE**[Q]

Risk Factors

- **Advancing age & increased fat intake**[Q] increase the risk
- **Lycopene, Vitamin A & E** and **selenium** decrease the risk[Q]
- **MC genetic alteration** in CA prostate is **hypermethylation of glutathione transferase (GSTP-1)**[Q] gene promoter located on **chromosome 11**[Q].

Pathology

- **MC type** is **adenocarcinoma**[Q] >TCC
- **Site:** Peripheral zone- **75%**[Q], Transition zone- **15%**, Central zone- **10%**

Contd…

Contd…

Spread
- Spread occurs by direct local invasion and through hematogenous and lymphatics
- **Local invasion** most commonly involves **seminal vesicles & base of bladder**[Q]

> - **Hematogenous spread** occurs mostly to **bone** (axial skeleton is MC site with **lumbar spine**[Q] being most frequently implicated) forming **osteoblastic secondaries**[Q]
> - **Visceral metastasis** most commonly involve **lungs**[Q] > liver > adrenal glands
> - **Lymphatic metastasis** are most often identified in **obturator nodes**[Q]

- **CNS involvement** is usually a result of **direct extension** from **skull metastasis**[Q]

Clinical Features
- Most patients with **early-stage** CA prostate are **asymptomatic**, being **peripheral**[Q].
- Presence of **symptoms** suggest **locally advanced** or **metastatic disease**
- **DRE: Hard, irregular, nodular** prostate with **median sulcus obliteration**[Q]

Laboratory Findings
- **Azotemia** (bilateral ureteral obstruction), **anemia** in metastatic disease, **raised ALP** in bony metastasis
- **PSA velocity >0.75 ng/ml/yr** indicates carcinoma[Q]

Prostate Biopsy
- **TRUS guided biopsy** is done in patients with **abnormal DRE** or **elevated PSA** or **both**[Q].
- **Differentiation of tumor** is graded by **Gleason score**[Q]. A sum of 7 or more suggests an aggressive cancer.

Imaging
- **TRUS** is used for **staging**, most lesions are **hypoechoic**[Q].

Endorectal MRI in CA Prostate
• **Most optimal imaging** to appreciate the **prostate anatomy**[Q]

Axial imaging in CA Prostate
• **CT scan** is mainly used to detect **LN metastasis**
• Intravenous administration of **superparamagnetic nanoparticles**, which gain access to lymph nodes by means of interstitial-lymphatic fluid transport, at the time of high resolution MRI, appears to **improve visualization** of **small nodal metastasis**[Q]

Bone Scan
- Patients with **PSA ≥ 15 ng/ml** or greater, **locally advanced disease (T3b, T4)** are at **higher risk** for **bone metastasis**, and should be considered for bone scan[Q].

■ GLEASON SCORE AND GRADING SYSTEM

GLEASON SCORE AND GRADING SYSTEM

- **Gleason score** is the **MC used histological grading system** for **prostate cancer**[Q].
- The **two most predominant histological patterns** of the prostate cancer are assigned a **Gleason grade** ranging from **1–5**[Q].

> - **Primary grade** is assigned to the **pattern of cancer** that is **most commonly observed** in the histological slides of the specimen[Q].
> - **Secondary grade** is assigned to the **second most commonly observed pattern** in the specimen.
> - **Gleason score** is the **sum of the two grades**. Thus it is also known as **Gleason sum**[Q].

- If the entire specimen has only one pattern present, then both the primary and secondary grades are reported as the same grade.

> - The **Gleason grade** ranges from **1 to 5**, with 5 having the **worst prognosis**[Q].
> - The **Gleason score** ranges from **2 to 10**[Q].

- The **Gleason score** is used to help **evaluate the prognosis** of men with prostate cancer. Together with other parameters, the Gleason score is incorporated into a strategy of prostate cancer staging which predicts prognosis and help guide therapy.

> - A point of importance is that the **primary Gleason grade** is **most important**[Q] with respect to placing patients in prognostic groups.
> - For example in patients with a **Gleason score 7**, a Gleason 4+3 is a **more aggressive cancer** than a **Gleason 3+4**.

■ TUMOR MARKERS OF CA PROSTATE (APART FROM PSA)

TUMOR MARKERS OF CA PROSTATE (APART FROM PSA)

- **Prostatic acid phosphatase:**
  - PAP activity is **1000 fold greater** in the **prostate**[Q] than any other tissue

Contd…

Contd…

- – PAP is **not prostate specific**[Q] and detectable levels are noted after prostatectomy
- – **Increased in renal, liver** and **bony malignancies**[Q]
- **Alkaline phosphatase:**
  - – **Raised** in **liver involvement** or **bony metastasis**[Q]
- **Alpha-methyl co-A racemase**[Q]
- **Hepsin**[Q]
- **DD3**[Q]

■ PROSTATE SPECIFIC ANTIGEN (PSA)

PROSTATE SPECIFIC ANTIGEN (PSA)

- It is a **glycoprotein**, serine protease.[Q]
- **Free: 10–40%;**[Q] **Complexed** to antiprotease: **60–90%**[Q]
- **Formed in prostate**[Q], secreted in seminal fluid
- Causes **liquefaction of seminal coagulum**[Q]

> - **Normal value: ≤ 4 ng/ml**[Q] (in > 50 years); Value > **20 ng/ml** is **diagnostic of CA prostate**[Q]
> - PSA is the single test with **highest positive predictive value for CA prostate**[Q].
> - PSA is **prostate specific, not** the **cancer specific**[Q]
> - **Level of PSA** is directly related to **tumor burden**[Q]

- **Best use of PSA** is **monitoring** after **radical prostatectomy**[Q]

PSA related Investigations		
PSA Density	**PSA Velocity**	**Free PSA**
• **PSA/Prostate volume** • If **≥ 0.15, biopsy**[Q] recommended	• **Rate of change** of **PSA** per year[Q] • **≥ 0.75 ng/ml/year** indicates **carcinoma**[Q] • Assessment at every 18 months	• **Free PSA** (in %) appears to be **most useful** in **distinguishing** between those with and without **CA prostate** when total **PSA levels** fall in the range of **4–10 ng/ml**[Q]

8ᵗʰ AJCC (2017) TNM Staging for CA Prostate	
T: Primary tumor	**N: Regional lymph nodes**
Tis: Carcinoma in situ (**PIN**)	**N0:** No regional LN metastasis
T1a: ≤5% of tissue in resection for benign disease has cancer, normal DRE[Q] **T1b: >5%** of tissue in resection for benign disease has cancer, normal DRE[Q] **T1c:** Tumor identified by **needle biopsy** (e.g., because of elevated PSA)[Q]	**N1:** Metastasis in a regional LNs[Q] (**obturator, internal iliac, external iliac, presacral LNs**)
T2a: Tumor involves **one half of one lobe** but not both lobes[Q] **T2b:** Tumor involves **more than one half of one lobe** or less **T2c:** Tumor involves **both lobes**[Q]	**M: Distant metastases**
	M1a: Distant metastasis in **non-regional** lymph nodes[Q]
T3a: Extracapsular extension on one or both sides including bladder neck involvement[Q] **T3b: Seminal vesicle** involvement[Q]	**M1b:** Distant metastasis to **bone**[Q] **M1c:** Distant metastasis to **other sites**[Q]
T4: Tumor is fixed or invades adjacent structures other than seminal vesicles: **external sphincter, rectum, levator muscles and/or pelvic wall**[Q]	

Treatment of CA Prostate	
T1a	• **Incidentally found tumors** at TURP, by definition **low volume (≤5%),** usually **well-differentiated** associated with **very slow growth rate**[Q]. • Managed by **watchful waiting** (Regular follow up with **DRE & PSA**)[Q]
T1b, T1c and T2	• Management depends on patient's age, life expectancy, performance status and patient's preference. • In **younger, fitter men (<70 years): Radical prostatectomy**[Q] or **radiotherapy**[Q], if surgery is contraindicated • **Elderly (>70 years)** with **life expectancy <10 years: Watchful waiting**[Q] (**Progress rate** is **very slow,** 10% at 10 years)
Advanced disease (T3, T4 or any metastasis)	• Palliative treatment, androgen ablation or palliative radiotherapy • **Androgen ablation** (Hormone therapy) is **first line of treatment: Orchiectomy + Flutamide** or **LHRH + Flutamide**[Q] • **Palliative radiotherapy**[Q]

New Drugs in metastatic, castration resistant CA Prostate
• **Cabazitaxel** and **Sipuleucel-T**[Q]

■ BENIGN PROSTATIC HYPERPLASIA

1. **In BPH most common lobe involved is:**
   (Recent Question 2016, WBPG 2015, AIIMS June 2000)
   - a. Lateral
   - b. Posterior
   - c. Median
   - d. Anterior

2. **Most common site of BPH:** *(Recent Question 2017)*
   - a. Peripheral zone
   - b. Middle zone
   - c. Transition zone
   - d. Central zone

3. **Which is the earliest symptom of benign hypertrophy of prostate?** *(Karnataka 94, 96)*
   - a. Frequency
   - b. Hematuria
   - c. Incontinence
   - d. Strangury

4. **The following statements regarding finasteride are true except:** *(All India 2005)*
   - a. It is used in the medical treatment of benign prostatic hypertrophy
   - b. Impotence is well documented after its use
   - c. It blocks the conversion of dihydrotestosterone to testosterone
   - d. It is a 5-α reductase inhibitor

5. **Indication for surgery in benign prostatic hypertrophy are all except:** *(Recent Question 2016)*
   - a. Prostatism
   - b. Chronic retention
   - c. Hemorrhage
   - d. Enlarged prostate

■ TURP AND COMPLICATIONS

6. **The most common complication of transurethral resection of prostate (TURP):** *(COMEDK 2007, 2008, 2009)*
   - a. Erectile dysfunction
   - b. Retrograde ejaculation
   - c. Urinary incontinence
   - d. Impotence

7. **Delirium, mental confusion and nausea in patients who had undergone transurethral resection of prostate suggests:** *(MCI Nov 2017, Sept 2009)*
   - a. Hypernatremia
   - b. Sepsis
   - c. Hepatic coma
   - d. Water retention

8. **During TURP, surgeon takes care to dissect above the verumontanum to prevent injury to:** *(All India 2011)*
   - a. External urethral sphincter
   - b. Urethral crest
   - c. Prostatic utricle
   - d. Trigone of bladder

9. **TURP was done in an old patient of BHP, after which he developed altered sensorium cause is?** *(MCI June 2018, AIIMS June 2001, AIIMS June 99)*
   - a. Hypernatremia
   - b. Hypokalemia
   - c. Hyponatremia
   - d. Hypomagnesemia

10. **Which of the following substances is not used as an irrigant during transurethral resection of the prostate?** *(AIIMS Nov 2003)*
    - a. Normal saline
    - b. 1.5% glycine
    - c. 5% dextrose
    - d. Distilled water

11. **Which one of the following is used as an irrigation solution during transurethral resection of the prostate?** *(COMEDK 2014)*
    - a. 1.5% glycine
    - b. Physiological Saline
    - c. Ringer's lactate
    - d. 5% dextrose

■ CARCINOMA PROSTATE

12. **Most common site of development of carcinoma of prostate is:** *(Recent Question 2015, DNB 2012, Orissa 2011, MHPGMCET 2002, 2001)*
    - a. Peripheral zone
    - b. Central zone
    - c. Transitional zone
    - d. Fibromuscular stroma

13. **On MRI, origin of carcinoma prostrate is seen in:** *(Recent Question 2017)*
    - a. Peripheral zone
    - b. Central zone
    - c. Transition zone
    - d. Periurethral zone

14. **Transrectal ultrasonogram in evaluation of carcinoma prostate is most useful for:** *(All India 2008)*
    - a. Taking guided biopsy
    - b. Identifying seminal vesicle invasion
    - c. Nodal sampling
    - d. Measuring the extent of invasion

15. **Secondary deposits form prostatic carcinoma is commonest in:** *(Recent Question 2015)*
    - a. Bone
    - b. Kidney
    - c. Liver
    - d. Brain

16. **In carcinoma prostate with metastasis which is raised?** *(Recent Question 2016)*
    - a. ESR
    - b. Alkaline phosphatase
    - c. Acid phosphatase
    - d. Bilirubin

17. **Serum acid phosphatase is raised in:** *(MCI June 2018)*
    - a. Osteosarcoma
    - b. Prostatic carcinoma
    - c. Paget's disease
    - d. Hyperparathyroidism

18. **Normal level of PSA in males is:** *(DNB 2011)*
    - a. < 4 ng/ml
    - b. 4–10 ng/ml
    - c. > 10 ng/ml
    - d. PSA is not produced by normal males

19. **Gleason scoring is done for:** *(Recent Question 2017, DNB 2009)*
    - a. Prostatic cancer
    - b. Lung cancer
    - c. Bladder cancer
    - d. Hodgkins lymphoma

20. **Gleason score: all are true except:** *(AIIMS May 2011, Nov 2008)*
    - a. Used for grading prostate cancer
    - b. Scores range from 1–10
    - c. Higher the score, poorer the prognosis
    - d. Helps in planning management

21. **Osteoblastic metastasis commonly arise from:** *(JIPMER 2014, 2013, AIIMS May 2013)*
    - a. Breasts
    - b. Prostate
    - c. Lung
    - d. RCC

22. **Best screening marker of prostate cancer is:** *(UPPG 2009)*
    - a. AFP
    - b. Prostate specific antigen
    - c. CA 19-20
    - d. CA 125 to 26

23. **Treatment for metastatic CA Prostate:** *(JIPMER 2011)*
    - a. GnRH analogue
    - b. Estrogen therapy
    - c. Radiotherapy with chemotherapy
    - d. Radiotherapy

■ CARCINOMA PROSTATE TREATMENT

24. Treatment of metastatic prostate carcinoma is: *(JIPMER 2011)*
    a. Radiotherapy
    b. Estrogen only
    c. GnRH analogs
    d. Radiotherapy with chemotherapy

25. Which of the following drugs is useful for treatment of advanced prostate cancer? *(AIIMS Nov, May 2014)*
    a. Goserelin
    b. Ganirelix
    c. Cetrorelix
    d. Abarelix

26. Sipuleucel-T is a vaccine for: *(Recent Question 2017)*
    a. RCC
    b. Testicular tumor
    c. Carcinoma prostate
    d. Carcinoma bladder

27. Ketoconazole action in prostate carcinoma is: *(Recent Question 2017)*
    a. Pituitary inhibition
    b. Adrenal ablation
    c. Inhibits DHT formation
    d. Androgen antagonist

■ PROSTATITIS

28. Complication which commonly accompanies acute prostatitis: *(Recent Question 2016)*
    a. Epididymitis
    b. Orchitis
    c. Seminal vesiculitis
    d. Sterility

29. A 60-year-old male presented with fever, chills and dysuria. Patient was hospitalized in emergency for 5 days. PSA level was 7.4. Next best step in this patient: *(AIIMS Nov 2013)*
    a. Repeat PSA
    b. TURP
    c. TRUS guided biopsy
    d. Antibiotics and admit

30. Most common organism responsible for acute bacterial prostatitis: *(Recent Question 2018)*
    a. E. coli
    b. Peptostreptococci
    c. Enterococci
    d. Streptococci agalactiae

Explanations

■ BENIGN PROSTATIC HYPERPLASIA

1. Ans. c. Median
2. Ans. c. Transition zone *(Ref: Campbell 11/e p2433; Smith 18/e p350; Bailey 27/e p1458)*
3. Ans. a. Frequency
4. Ans. c. It blocks the conversion of dihydrotestosterone to testosterone
5. Ans. d. Enlarged prostate

■ TURP AND COMPLICATIONS

6. Ans. b. Retrograde ejaculation *(Ref: Smith 18/e p354; Campbell 11/e p2515; Bailey 27/e p1466)*
7. Ans. d. Water retention
8. Ans. a. External urethral sphincter
9. Ans. c. Hyponatremia
10. Ans. a. Normal saline *(Ref: Campbell 11/e p2510)*
    The use of an ionic solution (i.e., normal saline) leads to dissipation of the cutting current and poor cutting efficacy
11. Ans. a. 1.5% glycine *(Ref: Campbell 11/e p2510)*

■ CARCINOMA PROSTATE

12. Ans. a. Peripheral zone *(Ref: Smith 18/e p357; Campbell 11/e p2594; Bailey 27/e p1469)*
13. Ans. a. Peripheral zone *(Ref: Campbell 11/e p2396; Smith 18/e p357; Bailey 27/e p1469)*
14. Ans. a. Taking guided biopsy
15. Ans. a. Bone
16. Ans. c. Acid phosphatase
17. Ans. b. Prostatic carcinoma
18. Ans. a. < 4 ng/mL
19. Ans. a. Prostate cancer
20. Ans. b. Scores range from 1 to 10 *(Ref: Smith 18/e p362; Bailey 27/e p1472; Campbell 11/e p2595)*
    Gleason score ranges from 2 to 10.
21. Ans. b. Prostate *(Ref: Harrison 19/e p580; Devita 9/e p2512-2513; CSDT 12/e p1202)*
    Osteoblastic metastasis commonly arises from carcinoma prostate.

    - **MC site of primary** for **bone metastasis: CA Breast**[Q]
    - **MC cause of osteoblastic secondaries** in males: **CA Prostate**[Q]
    - **MC cause of osteoblastic secondaries** in females: **CA Breast**[Q]
    - **MC tumor metastasize to bone** in females: **CA Breast**[Q]

22. Ans. b. Prostate specific antigen
23. Ans. a. GnRH analogue *(Ref: Smith 18/e p372)*

    - **In metastatic CA prostate, Androgen ablation** (Hormone therapy) is **first line of treatment: Orchiectomy + Flutamide** or **LHRH + Flutamide**[Q].
    - **Leuprolide** and **goserelin** are **GnRH analogues,** which are **used primarily** for the treatment of **hormone-responsive prostate cancer**[Q].

■ CARCINOMA PROSTATE TREATMENT

24. Ans. c. GnRH analogs
25. Ans. a. Goserelin *(Ref: Katzung12/e p972; Goodman and Gilman 12/e p1763-1764; Smith 18/e p372; Campbell 11/e p291)*
    Goserelin is useful for the treatment of advanced prostate cancer.

    *"The **treatment of choice** for patients with **advanced prostate cancer** is **elimination of testosterone production** by the testes through either **surgical** or **chemical castration**. Bilateral orchiectomy or estrogen therapy in the form of diethylstibestrol was previously used as first-line therapy. Presently, the use of **GnRH agonists-including leuprolide** and **goserelin**, alone or in combination with anti-androgen (e.g. **flutamide, bicalutamide or nilutamide**) is the preferred approach."- Katzung12/e p972*

26. Ans. c. Carcinoma prostate *(Ref: Campbell 11/e p2813; Smith 18/e p373)*

> *"In prostate cancer, several immunologic strategies have been under clinical development. **The most important of these include the sipuleucel-T (Provenge) autologous prostatic acid phosphatase (PAP)-loaded dendritic cell vaccine, the GVAX allogeneic recombinant whole cell vaccine, and CTLA-4 inhibitory approaches.**"- Campbell 11/e p2813*

27. Ans. b. Adrenal ablation *(Ref: Campbell 11/e p2787; Smith 18/e p372; Bailey 27/e p1474)*

■ PROSTATITIS

28. Ans. c. Seminal vesiculitis *(Ref: Smith 18/e p218; Campbell 11/e p310, 313; Bailey 27/e p1474)*

29. Ans. d. Antibiotics and admit *(Ref: Smith 18/e p218; Campbell 11/e p310, 313; Bailey 27/e p1475)*

> - *A 60-year-old male presented with fever, chills and dysuria. Patient was hospitalized in emergency for 5 days. PSA level was 7.4. This patient is most probably suffering from acute bacterial prostatitis and treated by antibiotics.*

30. Ans. a. E. coli *(Ref: Campbell 11/e p305; Smith 18/e p218; Bailey 27/e p1474)*

> *"**The most common cause of bacterial prostatitis is the** Enterobacteriaceae **family of gram- negative bacteria, which originate in the gastrointestinal flora. The most common organisms are strains of** Escherichia coli**, which are identified in 65% to 80% of infections.**"- Campbell 11/e p305*

Urethra and Penis

■ HYPOSPADIAS

HYPOSPADIAS

- Hypospadias results when **fusion of urethral folds is incomplete**, and urethral **meatus opens** on the **underside of penis** or **perineum (ventral surface of penis)**[Q].

> - Occurs in **1:250 male births** and **multifactorial**[Q] in inheritance.
> - **Hypospadias** is MC congenital malformation of urethra[Q].

- Estrogens & progestins given during pregnancy increase the risk.
- **Anterior forms** are **more** common[Q] then posterior because fusion of urethral folds is from posterior to anterior.
- **70% cases** are **distal penile** or **coronal**[Q].
- **Circumcision is not done** in patients with hypospadias, as the prepuce can later be **used in surgical repair**[Q].

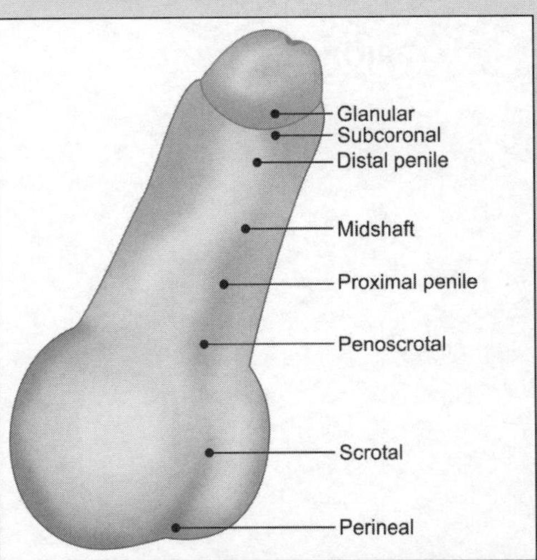

Types of Hypospadias		
• Glanular	• Penile	• Scrotal
• Coronal	• Penoscrotal	• Perineal
• Subcoronal		

- **Surgical pathology** in addition to ventrally placed ectopic meatus, hypospadias has:
- **Chordee** ventral curvature of penis due to contracture of fibrous cord which has replaced the distal urethra and corpus spongiosum. **Severity of chordee** is proportional to **degree of hypospadias**[Q].
- **Hooded prepuce** deficient on ventral aspect and excess **on dorsal aspect**[Q].
- **Stenosis of ectopic meatus**[Q]
- **Flattening of glans**[Q]
- Multiple urethral orifices
- Microphallus

Associated Abnormalities
- **Undescended testis**[Q] (10%) with or without sexual ambiguity
- **Inguinal hernia**[Q] (10%)
- Urinary tract abnormality (upper and lower)

Associated Problems
- **Abnormal stream, painful erection** (chordee) & **infertility** (in proximal or posterior types)[Q]

Management
- Treatment is not required in anterior variety. (repair is done for cosmetic reasons only)
- **Optimal time** of repair is **6–12 months**[Q].
- **Meatal advancement** or **local skin flap advancement**[Q] is the surgical procedure done along with removal of chordee.

Named Procedures in Hypospadias
• **Dennis-Brown** technique (Two stage) [Q]
• **MAGPI**[Q] (Meatal advancement and glanuloplasty integrated) for coronal or subcoronal
• **Mathiew procedure**[Q] (Perimeatal based flap, one stage) for distal penile
• **Asopa** or **Duckett**[Q] technique using vascularized preputial island (one stage)
• **Thiersch-Duplay** or **Bracka**[Q] technique for proximal penile

Complications of Surgery
- MC complications is **urethral fistula**[Q] (10%)
- **Meatal stenosis**[Q] due to devascularisation of distal neourethra
- **Urethral stricture and stenosis** due to poor vascularity of flap, **persistent chordee**[Q]

> - Incidence of **hypospadias: 1 in 250**[Q]
> - Incidence of **horse-shoe kidney: 1 in 400 (0.25%)**[Q]
> - Incidence of **renal agenesis: 1 in 1000**[Q]

■ EPISPADIAS

EPISPADIAS

- Urethra opens on the **dorsum (upper aspect)** of the penis in males, in females there is a **fissure in the wall**[Q] of the urethra which opens above the clitoris

Associated Anomalies

- **Extrophy of bladder**[Q] (ectopia vesicae) with pubic diastasis and waddling gait
- **Dorsal Chordee**[Q]
- **VUR** in 40% cases[Q]

Clinical Features

- **Females: Bifid clitoris** & **separation of the labia. Most** are **incontinent**[Q] because of maldevelopment of the urinary sphincters.
- **Males:** Patients with **glandular epispadias seldom have urinary incontinence.** However, incontinence in **penopubic** is **95%** and **penile epispadias** is **75%**[Q].
- Epispadias is a mild form of bladder exstrophy, and in severe cases, exstrophy and epispadias coexist.

Management

- **Surgery** is required to **correct the incontinence, remove the chordee** to straighten the penis, and **extend the urethra** out onto the glans penis[Q].
- **Bladder augmentation** combined with the **artificial sphincter** may be required in patients in whom incontinence cannot be corrected.

■ POSTERIOR URETHRAL VALVE

POSTERIOR URETHRAL VALVE

- **Symmetrical folds of urothelium** extending **distally from prostatic urethra to external urinary sphincter**[Q].

  - **Exclusively** an anomaly of **male urethra**[Q].
  - Four types, **Type 1 is MC** (lies just **distal to the verumontanum** or **at the verumontanum**)[Q]

- Acts as a **flap valve**[Q] (one way valve)- allows catheter, but balloons out during micturition and obstructs stream.

Clinical Features

- **Newborns** may present with **palpable abdominal masses (distended bladder, hydronephrotic kidneys & ascites)**[Q]
- Infants with **urinary infection** & **sepsis**[Q].
- **Sometimes,** the **valves** are **incomplete**[Q] and the patient remains **without symptoms** until adolescence or adulthood.
- Approximately **30%** of patients experience **end stage renal disease**.[Q]
- **Vesicoureteral reflux** occurs in **50% of patients**[Q].

Associated with

- Oligohydramnios[Q]
- Renal parenchymal dysplasia (**most important factor** in overall **prognosis**)[Q]
- Abnormal bladder function (25%)[Q]
- **Pulmonary hypoplasia (MC cause of death)**[Q]

Investigations

- **Investigation of choice: MCU**[Q] (shows proximal urethral dilatation with distal stricture)

- **Cystoscopy:** Shows dilation of urethra above valve.
- **Prenatal diagnosis by ultrasound,** showing **bilateral hydroureteronephrosis with enlarged thickened bladder** as early as **28 weeks**[Q] of gestation (**Keyhole** sign on **prenatal** USG).

Management

- First a small polyethylene **feeding tube** is **inserted** in the bladder and left for several days. Then further management is done according to serum creatinine level.
  - **Normal serum creatinine** - transurethral ablation (**endoscopic fulgration**)[Q] of the valves
  - **Increased serum creatinine** and the worsening of condition – **vesicostomy (Blockson's technique is best)** to bypass the obstruction and **when normal creatinine levels** are achieved, transurethral ablation (**endoscopic fulgration**)[Q] is done.

Prognosis

- **Bladder dysfunction** and **renal hypoplasia** is associated with **poor prognosis** and is major cause of progressive renal failure[Q].
- **Pulmonary hypoplasia** is **MC cause** of **death**[Q].

■ PHIMOSIS

PHIMOSIS

- Phimosis is a condition in which the **contracted foreskin cannot be retracted over the glans**[Q].
- **Chronic infection** from **poor local hygiene** is its **most common cause**[Q].
- Most cases occur in **uncircumcised males**, although excessive skin left after circumcision can become stenotic and cause phimosis.

Types
- Congenital
- **Acquired:** Usually presents late in life and associated with **inflammation, balanitis xerotica obliterans, trauma** or **cancer**[Q].

Clinical Features
- **Difficulty in micturition**[Q] is the main symptom.
- **Ballooning of prepuce during micturition**[Q] is suggestive of phimosis.
- Edema, erythema, and tenderness of the prepuce and the presence of purulent discharge usually cause the patient to seek medical attention.
- Inability to retract the foreskin is a less common complaint.

Complications
- Balanoposthitis, **H**ydronephrosis or hydroureter
- **Prepucial calculi, carcinoma under foreskin**[Q]

Treatment
- **Local steroid** cream for **4–6** weeks[Q].

> - **Circumcision** should be done if **no response to steroids, recurrent balanitis** or **balanoposthitis, age > 16–18 years**[Q].

- If phimosis is associated with considerable **infection**, it should be treated with **broad-spectrum antimicrobial drugs**. The **dorsal slit of foreskin**[Q], if improved drainage is necessary.
- **Circumcision** for phimosis should be **avoided in children requiring general anesthesia; except** in cases with **recurrent infections**[Q].
- The procedure should be **postponed until** the child reaches an age when **local anesthesia** can be used.

■ PARAPHIMOSIS

PARAPHIMOSIS

- **Acquired** condition in which the **foreskin**, once retracted over the glans, **cannot be replaced** in its normal position.
- It is uncommon for the urethra to be compressed, so the **micturition** is normally **not affected**[Q].

Pathology
- **Chronic inflammation** under the redundant foreskin leads to **contracture** of **preputial opening** (phimosis) and formation of a **tight ring of skin** when the foreskin is retracted behind the glans.
- The **skin ring** causes **venous congestion** leading to **edema** and **enlargement** of the **glans**[Q].
- As the condition progresses, **arterial occlusion & necrosis of the glans**[Q] may occur.

Treatment
- **Ice bags, gentle manual compression**[Q] and injection of a solution of **hyaluronidase** in normal saline may help to reduce swelling.
- **Circumcision:** If conservative method fails

■ PRIAPISM

PRIAPISM

- **Painful, persistent erection**[Q] not normally associated with sexual excitement or desire, which does not subside after sexual excitement or desire.
- Most patients present with an **erection of at least 24 hours**[Q] duration.
- **Priapism is an emergency**, if therapy is delayed for 36–48 hours, then marked tissue damage (due to ischemia) is likely to occur with **cavernosal fibrosis** and **impotence**[Q].

Types
- **High flow (non-ischemic) priapism**[Q]: Occurs secondary to **penile or perineal trauma**, arterial sinusoidal shunt within corpus cavernosum.
- **Low flow (ischemic) priapism**[Q]: **Painful priapism**, can lead to **compartment syndrome**, **more common** than high flow Priapism, caused by **Sickle cell anemia, leukemia**, spinal cord lesions, fat emboli, **malignant penile inflammation**[Q], autonomic neuropathy, drugs (Trazadone)[Q]
- Majority due to **vasoactive intracorporeal injections**[Q]

Contd…

Contd…

Clinical Presentation: Two peak ages
- **Children 5–10 years old**: Most common due to **sickle cell disease**[Q], attacks are usually nocturnal and the patient awakens with painful erection.
- **Adults 20–50 years**: **Mostly iatrogenic**[Q], priapism involves only corpora cavernosa. The spongiosum and glans are flaccid.

Diagnosis
- Diagnosis is **mainly clinical**[Q], only investigation useful to supplement clinical examination is **doppler**.

Treatment
- If present early, **within 4–6 hours: Ketamine**[Q] (dissociative anesthesia) causes 50% detumescence.

> - **Aspiration** and **saline irrigation** till the aspirate is bright red, followed by injection of diluted **phenylephrine**[Q].
> - **Active treatment** in **high flow priapism** as it represents a **compartment syndrome**[Q].

- **Selective internal pudendal arteriography** and **selective embolization of** the **artery** feeding the shunt for **high flow non-ischemic priapism**[Q]
- **Operative intervention:**
- **Winter's procedure** (percutaneous **cavernoglandular** shunt)[Q]
  - Corpora spongiosa shunt
  - Corpora saphenous shunt

■ PEYRONIE'S DISEASE

PEYRONIE'S DISEASE

- Peyronie's disease (**plastic induration of penis/ penile fibromatosis**[Q]) usually seen **over 40 years** of age.

> - It is due to **fibrous plaques** in one or both corpus cavernosum of varying sizes **involving tunica albuginea**[Q] which may later calcify or ossify.

- Cause remains obscure, the dense fibrous plaque is microscopically consistent with **findings of severe vasculitis.**
- Palmar fibromatosis (**Dupuytren's contracture**), plantar fibromatosis and penile fibromatosis (**Peyronie's disease**) are components of the same pathological process called **superficial fibromatosis**[Q].
- **Galezia's Triad: (DPR) Dupuytren's contracture + Peyronie's disease + Retroperitoneal fibrosis**[Q]

Clinical Features
- **Painful erection, curvature of penis** and **poor erection distal to involved area**[Q].
- No pain when the penis is in nonerect state.
- **Palpable induration** or **mass** appears usually on the **dorsolateral aspect**[Q] of the penis.

Treatment
- **Spontaneous remission** occurs in about **50% cases**[Q], so observation & emotional support advised initially.
- If the penile deformity is distressing, **Nesbitt's operation**[Q] can be performed to straighten the penis.
- **Nesbitt operation**: Straightening of penis by **placing non-absorbable sutures** in **corpus cavernosum opposite** to the **plaque**.

■ URETHRAL INJURY

URETHRAL INJURY

- Urethral injuries occur most often in **men**, usually associated with **pelvic fractures** or **straddle type falls.**
- Urethra is separated in two anatomic divisions:
  - **Posterior urethra: Prostatic urethra + Membranous urethra**[Q]   –   **Anterior urethra: Bulbous urethra + Penile urethra**[Q]

■ INJURIES TO POSTERIOR URETHRA

INJURIES TO POSTERIOR URETHRA

Etiology
- The part of urethra **most likely injured in pelvic fracture** is **membranous urethra**[Q].
- Membranous urethra is **sheared** at the bulbomembranous or **prostatomembranous junction**[Q].
- **Bulbomembranous junction** is **more prone than prostato membranous junction** during pelvic fracture (posterior urethra is densely adhered to pubis via urogenital diaphragm & puboprostatic ligaments)

Clinical Features
- **Retention of urine + Blood at urethral meatus + Pelvic hematoma** and **High lying prostate**[Q]
- Presence of blood at external urethral meatus indicates that **immediate urethrography**[Q] is **necessary to establish the diagnosis.**

Section 4

Urology

Contd…

Contd…

- Associated with **deep extravasation** of **urine** in pelvis & retroperitoneal tissues[Q].
- **Pie in sky appearance**[Q] on **IVP** in **membranous urethral injury**.
- **Superior displacement** of **prostate does not occur** if the **puboprostatic ligaments** remain **intact**.

Instrumental Examination

- The only instrumentation involved should be for **urethrography**[Q].

> - **Catheterization or urethroscopy** should **not** be **done in every case** (as its associated with an **increased risk** of **hematoma, infection**, and **conversion of partial urethral tear** into **complete transection** of **urethra**)[Q].
> - In suspected **partial injury, gentle single attempt** to **catheterize** the patient **acts as** a **stent** over which **urethra heals**[Q].

Complications

- **Bladder rupture** may be associated with posterior urethral injuries in **20% of cases**[Q].
- **Stricture, impotence,** and **incontinence**[Q] are complications of prostatomembranous disruption.

> - **Stricture** following **primary repair** and **anastomosis** occurs in about **50%** of cases, with **delayed repair** incidence of stricture can be reduced to about **5%**[Q].

- The incidence of **impotence after primary repair** is **30–80%** , can be **reduced to 30–35%** by **delayed urethral reconstruction**[Q].

Diagnosis

- When blood is noticed at meatus, **immediate RGU** should be done to rule out urethral injury.

TREATMENT

Immediate Management

- **No urethral instrumentation** or **manipulation** and **suprapubic cystostomy**

> - In suspected **partial injury, gentle single attempt** to **catheterize** the patient **acts as** a **stent** over which **urethra heals**.

- **Incomplete laceration** of the posterior urethra **heals spontaneously**, and the **suprapubic cystostomy** can be **removed within 2–3 weeks**[Q].
- **SPC** remains the **gold standard** for **initial management, endoscopic alignment** can be done **over guidewire** if patient presents **within 7–10 days**[Q].

Delayed Urethral Reconstruction

- **Reconstruction** of the urethra after prostatic disruption can be undertaken **within 3 months**[Q].

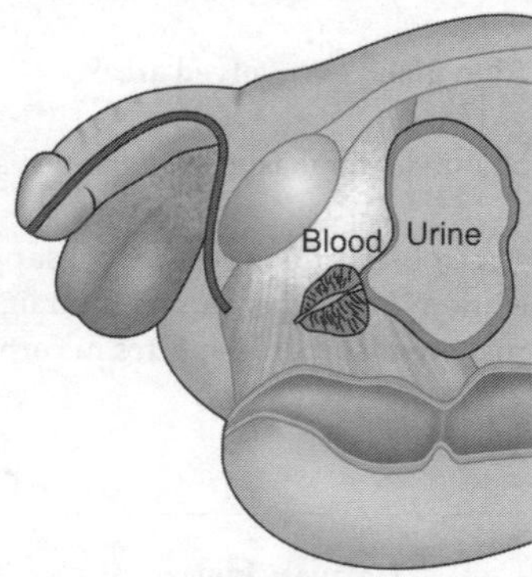

Injury to the posterior (membranous) urethra

■ INJURIES TO ANTERIOR URETHRA

INJURIES TO ANTERIOR URETHRA

Etiology

- **Direct blow to the perineum**[Q] is the mechanism of injury.
- **Self-instrumentation** or **iatrogenic instrumentation** may cause **partial disruption**[Q].
  MC site is bulbar urethra
- **Straddle injury**[Q] may cause laceration or contusion of the urethra.

Clinical Features

- **Retention of urine + Blood at urethral meatus + Perineal hematoma** and **Normal prostate** on P/R[Q]

> - **Superficial extravasation** of **urine**, urine collects in **scrotum, anterior perineum**, beneath **superficial fascia** of **penis** and spreads **under fascia scarpa**[Q].

- **Massive urinary extravasation** and **infection** in the perineum and scrotum in delayed presentation

Contd…

Contd…

Complications

- **Heavy bleeding** from **corpus spongiosum** injury and urethral **meatus**[Q].
- **Sepsis** and **infection**[Q] due to **urinary extravasation** (**Aggressive debridement** and **drainage** for infection)
- **Stricture** at the **site of injury**[Q]

Treatment

- **Urethral contusion:**
  - After urethrography, if the voiding occurs normally, without pain or bleeding, no additional treatment.
- **Urethral lacerations:**
  - **Suprapubic cystostomy**[Q] for complete urinary diversion while the urethral laceration heals.
- **Urethral laceration with extensive urinary extravasation:**
  - Suprapubic cystostomy for urinary diversion and antibiotic therapy for Infection and abscess formation

■ STRICTURE URETHRA

STRICTURE URETHRA

- Area of narrowing in the caliber of urethra due to formation of scar in the tissues surrounding the urethra
- **Male urethra** is **more prone** to **trauma** & **stricture**[Q] formation.
- **Large catheters** and **instruments** are more likely than small ones to cause **ischemia, internal trauma** leading to **stricture**[Q].

Etiology

- **Traumatic (MC)**[Q], straddle injuries for anterior and pelvic fracture for posterior urethra
- **Inflammatory** or **infectious** (Infection from **long-term catheter use**[Q] is a major cause, gonococcal urethritis is seldom a cause of strictures today)
- **Ischemia**
- **Malignant**
- Congenital (**Fossa navicularis** and **membranous urethra** is **MC site**[Q] of congenital urethral stricture)

Clinical Features

Obstructive voiding symptoms

- **Decreased force** of urinary stream, improving with pressure **(MC)**[Q]
- **Spraying** or **double stream**[Q]
- **Incomplete emptying** of the bladder, **terminal dribbling** and urinary **intermittency**[Q]
- Urinary retention, dilation of proximal urethra and prostatic ducts, urinary tract infections

Diagnosis

- **Location, length, depth** and **density** of stricture should be evaluated for appropriate treatment.
- **Retrograde urethrogram** or **MCU**[Q] to demonstrate location and extent of stricture

RGU

- **MCU and RGU, both are required for adequate assessment**
- **MCU for posterior urethra, RGU for anterior urethra**
- **High frequency ultrasound** for **short bulbar strictures** (more accurate in measuring stricture length than RGU and is helpful in determining whether to excise or graft)
- **MRI** for defining the **distorted pelvic anatomy** associated with **posterior urethral strictures**[Q] resulting from trauma.

Management

- **Periodic urethral dilations** to stretch the scar without producing additional scarring.
- **Internal urethrotomy:** Incising the stricture transurethrally using endoscopic equipment to release scar tissue. The incision is made under direct vision at **12 O'clock** position with urethrotome, with curative success rate of **20–35%** (**Good** success in **short strictures without spongiofibrosis**[Q])

Open Reconstruction

- **Excision & re-anastomosis** for strictures ≤ 2 cm[Q]: Complete excision of the fibrotic segment with a widely spatulated **tension-free re-anastomosis**, most dependable technique
- **Excision & tissue transfer** for strictures > 2 cm[Q]: Full-thickness skin graft tissue is harvested from the desired non-hair bearing location, **penile skin, bladder epithelium**, or **buccal mucosa** (**MC** and **best results**)[Q].

■ CARCINOMA PENIS

CARCINOMA PENIS

- Most commonly occur in **6th decade**[Q] of life, but "**40% patients** are **less than 40 years**"
- Most commonly associated etiologic factor is **poor hygiene**[Q]
- **Phimosis**[Q] is commonly associated (**50%**)

> - **Neonatal circumcision** confers **immunity**[Q] against **CA penis, HIV** or **STDs**, but **not if done later.**

- Most important **carcinogens** are **smegma** and **HPV infection (16, 18, 31, 33)**[Q].

Premalignant Lesions

- **Buschke-Lowenstein tumour**[Q] (Verrucous carcinoma): Tumour destroy adjacent tissue by compression, no metastasis usually. (Locally Malignant)
- **Balanitis Xerotica Obliterans**[Q]: Whitish patch on glans, meatus and urethra, meatal stenosis.
- **Leukoplakia**[Q] (more common in **diabetics**)
- Cutaneous horn
- Long standing genital warts

Carcinoma in Situ

- **Bowen's disease**[Q]: Intraepithelial skin neoplasm (solitary thickened, grey white plaque with ulceration and scabbing) with HPV association in 80% cases. Converts into infiltrating **SCC in 10%. No high incidence of visceral malignancy.** When it involves **glans** and **prepuce**, it is called **Erythroplasia of Queyrat**[Q]
- **Erythroplasia of Queyrat**[Q]: **Red velvety plaques** over **glans** or **prepuce**, treated by **5% 5-FU cream** or ND YAG laser.

Clinical Features

- **Squamous cell carcinoma (80%)**[Q] is the **MC type, most commonly originates from glans**[Q]>prepuce>sulcus>shaft (GPS).
- Others are **transitional cell carcinoma (15%)**, basal cell carcinoma, malignant melanoma, sarcoma.
- **MC symptom** is **lesion itself** associated with foul smelling discharge.
- **Phimosis** is associated in **50%.**
- There is **little or no pain.**
- Lesions are typically confined to penis at the time of presentation.

> - **More than 50% patients** of CA Penis presents with **enlarged inguinal lymph nodes**[Q].
> - 50% of patients presenting with **enlarged lymph inguinal lymph nodes are reactive** (non-metastatic), used to **subside after 4-6 weeks of antibiotics**[Q].
> - Priapism is the MC and earliest symptom of metastatic CA penis[Q].
> - MC cause of death is bleeding caused by **erosion of femoral artery** by **metastatic inguinal lymph nodes**[Q].
> - **2nd MC** cause of death is **sepsis.**

- **Hypercalcemia**[Q] is seen **in absence** of **osseous metastasis** in **20%** of patients, appears to **correlate with volume of disease**[Q].

Patterns of Spread

- **Buck's fascia**[Q] and **tunica albuginea** represents a **barrier to corporal invasion** and **hematogenous spread**.
- Primary dissemination is to **inguinal, femoral** and **iliac** LNs.

> - **Prepuce** and **shaft skin** drain into the **superficial inguinal LNs**[Q] (Superficial to tensor fascia lata).
> - **Glans** and **corporal bodies** drain to **both superficial** and **deep inguinal LNs**[Q] (deep to tensor fascia lata).
> - **Anterior urethra** to **inguinal LN** and **posterior urethra** to **internal iliac LNs.**
> - **Penile drainage** is **bilateral** because of **multiple croos-connections**[Q].

- Penetration of buck's fascia and tunica albiginea leads to invasion of vascular corpora and vascular dissemination (rare).
- **Distant metastases** in **< 10% cases,** may involve **lung,** liver bone or brain.

Diagnosis

- **Good incisional biopsy**[Q] from the periphery of the lesion from its junction with the normal tissue for grade and depth of invasion is **mandatory for diagnosis.**

> - **Sentinel lymph node biopsy (CABANA procedure)** is done for inguinal LN status.

Radiological Investigations

- Assessment of depth by **USG** or **MRI**[Q] (CT is not effective)

> - **MRI** is **IOC for staging in CA penis.**

Contd...

Contd…

Treatment

- Without any treatment of invasive carcinoma, **death within 2 years**.
- **Small non-invasive lesion involving prepuce: 5-FU cream, Nd-YAG laser, radiotherapy + close follow-up** is mandatory/ Wide excision or circumcision

  - Lesions involving **glans or distal shaft**: Partial penectomy with **2 cm margin**[Q]
  - Lesions involving **proximal shaft** or 2 cm margins are not achieved: **Total penectomy** with **perineal urethrostomy**[Q].
  - **Bilateral Ilioinguinal LN dissection**[Q] for metastatic lymph nodes.

- Chemotherapy used are **Bleomycin**, 5-FU, **Cisplatin**, methotrexate.
- **Radiotherapy** for selected **superficial small lesions**.

Prognosis

- Survival correlates with **presence** or **absence of nodal disease**[Q].

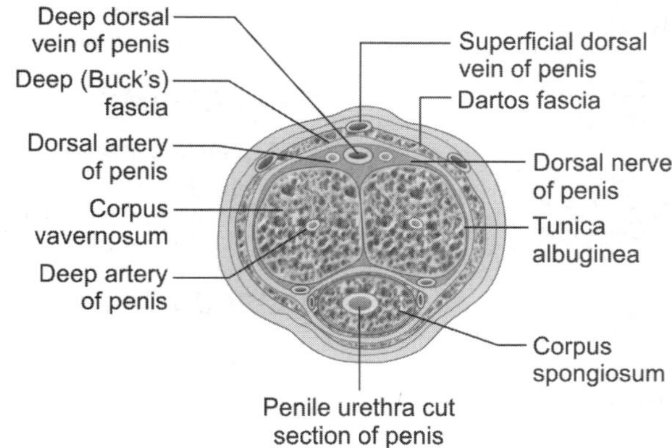

8th AJCC (2017) TNM Staging for CA Penis	
T: Primary tumor	**N: Regional lymph nodes**
Tis: Carcinoma in-situ[Q] **Ta: Noninvasive verrucous carcinoma**[Q]	**N1**: Palpable mobile **unilateral inguinal LN**[Q]
T1a: Invades subepithelial connective tissue without lymphovascular invasion and is not poorly differentiated[Q]	**N2**: Palpable mobile **multiple** or **bilateral inguinal LNs**[Q]
T1b: Invades subepithelial connective tissue **with lymphovascular invasion** or **poorly differentiated**[Q]	**N3: Fixed inguinal nodal masses or pelvic lymphadenopathy unilateral or bilateral**[Q]
T2: Invades **corpus spongiosum** with or without invasion of urethra[Q]	
T3: Invades **corpus cavernosum** with or without invasion of urethra[Q]	**M: Distant metastases**
T4: Invades **other adjacent structures**[Q]	M0: No distant metastasis M1: Distant metastasis present

Stage 0	Stage I	Stage IIA	Stage IIB	Stage IIIA	Stage IIIB	Stage IV
Tis N0M0 **Ta** N0M0	**T1a** N0M0	**T1b** N0M0 **T2** N0M0	**T3** N0M0	**T1-3 N1** M0	**T1-3 N2** M0	**T4** anyN M0 Any T **N3** M0 Any T any N **M1**

Multiple Choice Questions

■ HYPOSPADIAS

1. **True about hypospadias:** *(JIPMER 2011)*
   a. Associated with chordee
   b. 50% associated with undescended testis
   c. Due to failure of fusion of posterior wall of urethra
   d. Circumcision done immediately

2. **Circumcision is contraindicated in:**
   (NEET 2013; WBPG 2012; GB Pant 2010)
   a. Paraphimosis   b. Meatal stenosis
   c. Hypospadias   d. Phimosis

3. **Most common congenital anomaly of urethra:**
   (MHSSMCET 2008)
   a. Hypospadias   b. Epispadias
   c. Meatal stenosis   d. PU valve

4. **Commonest hypospadias is:**
   (DNB 2011, 2001, AIIMS Dec 95)
   a. Penile   b. Glandular
   c. Scrotal   d. A or C

5. **Features of hypospadias are all except:**
   a. Chordee   *(WBPG 2014, All India 98)*
   b. Hooded prepuce
   c. No-treatment required with glandular variety
   d. Cryptorchidism

6. **Penis is curved in downward direction in all types of hypospadias except:** *(Recent Question 2016)*
   a. Glandular   b. Coronal
   c. Penile   d. Perineal

7. **Best age for hypospadias repair:** *(Recent Question 2017)*
   a. Before 1 year   b. 2 years
   c. 4 years   d. 5 years

8. **Name of surgery in hypospadias:** *(Recent Question 2017)*
   a. Dennis-Brown   b. Ombridann's
   c. Ladd and Gross   d. Keetley-Torek

■ EPISPADIAS

9. **Epispadias is associated with:** *(All India 2008)*
   a. Bifid pubic symphysis   b. Chordee
   c. Anal atresia   d. Intestinal obstruction

■ POSTERIOR URETHRAL VALVE

10. **A three years old boy presents with poor urinary stream. Most likely cause is:** *(AIIMS June 2003)*
    a. Stricture urethra   b. Neurogenic bladder
    c. Urethral calculus   d. Posterior urethral valve

11. **A male child with recurrent UTI with dribbling of urine most likely cause is:** *(Punjab 2011)*
    a. VUR   b. Posterior urethral valves
    c. Stricture urethra   d. Neurogenic bladder

12. **For posterior urethral valve—investigation of choice is:**
    (BIHAR PG 2014; AIIMS June 97, PGI Dec 2002, Dec 2003, June 2003)
    a. Cystoscopy   b. MCU
    c. Cystourethroscopy   d. Retrograde urethroscopy

13. **Posterior urethral valve is usually seen:**
    a. Above verumontanum   *(MHSSMCET 2005, 2006, 2008)*
    b. Below verumontanum
    c. At the level of bladder neck
    d. At the level of verumontanum

■ PHIMOSIS

14. **The recommended treatment for preputial adhesions producing ballooning of prepuce during micturition in a 2 years old boy is:** *(AIIMS June 2003)*
    a. Wait and watch policy   b. Circumcision
    c. Dorsal slit
    d. Preputial adhesions release and dilatation

■ PARAPHIMOSIS

15. **Not true about paraphimosis is:** *(AIIMS June 98)*
    a. Iatrogenic   b. Seen in diabetes mellitus
    c. Gangrene of glans
    d. Circumcision is the treatment

■ CIRCUMCISION

16. **Circumcision is done in a child in which of the following conditions:** *(TN 91)*
    a. Phimosis   b. Recurrent balanitis
    c. Paraphimosis   d. All of the above

17. **Indications of circumcision are all except:** *(MHPGMCET 2002)*
    a. Chronic balanoposthitis   b. Jew religion
    c. Carcinoma penis   d. Paraphimosis

18. **All are true regarding circumcision except:**
    (JIPMER Nov 2017)
    a. Hemorrhage due to bleeding from frenular artery
    b. Increases sexual drive
    c. Avoid correction of congenital anomaly
    d. Reduces sexually transmitted infections

■ PRIAPISM

19. **Persistent priapism is rarely seen as a consequence of:**
    (COMEDK 2010)
    a. Sickle cell disease   b. Leukemia
    c. Spinal cord disease   d. Prolonged sexual activity

20. **Priapism in a polytrauma patient signify:**
    (Recent Question 2017)
    a. Penile injury   b. Spinal cord injury
    c. Significant head injury   d. Pelvic injury

21. **Cut off duration for diagnosis of priapism is:**
    (MCI Dec 2018)
    a. 1 hour   b. 2 hours
    c. 3 hours   d. 4 hours

■ PEYRONIE'S DISEASE

22. **Peyronie's disease is:** *(MHPGMCET 2007)*
    a. Browning of penis
    b. Ectopic opening of urethra
    c. Curved deformity of penis due to fibrous plaque
    d. Absent glans penis

23. **Nesbitt's operation is done for:**   *(MHPGMCET 2009, 2005)*
   a. Ectopic testis   b. Hypospadias
   c. Peyronie's disease   d. Any of the above

24. **Dupuytren's contracture is seen in:** *(Recent Question 2014; 2013)*
   a. Peyronie's disease   b. Hypospadias
   c. Epispadias   d. Exstrophy

■ URINARY TRACT INFECTION

25. **What will be next investigation to be done in case of a 2 years old female child with 1st episode of UTI?**   *(AIIMS June 98)*
   a. Abdominal ultrasound   b. DMSA scan
   c. 6 monthly urine culture   d. Nothing actively needed

26. **A child with recurrent urinary tract infection is most likely to show:**   *(All India 2005)*
   a. Posterior urethral valves   b. Vesicoureteric reflux
   c. Neurogenic bladder   d. Renal and ureteric calculi

27. **Which fruit juice helps in preventing UTI?**
                           (AIIMS Nov 2011, Nov 2006)
   a. Grape   b. Raspberry
   c. Cranberry   d. Orange

28. **Commonest organism giving rise to urinary tract infection:**
                               (Recent Question, 2017)
   a. E. coli   b. Proteus
   c. Staphylococcus   d. Streptococcus

■ URINARY RETENTION

29. **Acute urinary retention in a male child may be due to:**
                              (Recent Question 2016)
   a. Prostatic radiotherapy   b. Urethral stricture
   c. Hysteria   d. Meatal ulcer with scabbing

30. **Most frequent causes of acute retention of urine include all except:**   *(DPG 2009 March)*
   a. Meatal ulcer with scabbing in children
   b. Haemorrhoidectomy
   c. Herniorrhaphy   d. Fecal impaction

■ URETHRAL INJURY

31. **Not true about urethral injuries is:**   *(AIIMS Nov 2001)*
   a. Catheterize the patient immediately
   b. Can be associated with fracture pelvis
   c. Bladder injury is associated with post urethral injuries
   d. Blood at the external urethral meatus is an imp feature

32. **Membranous urethral rupture causes collection of blood in:**
   a. Ischiorectal fossa   *(Recent Question, 2014; AIIMS Nov 93)*
   b. Deep perineal pouch
   c. Superficial inguinal region
   d. Pelvic diaphragm

33. **All are true about bulbar urethral rupture, except:**
   a. Perineal hematoma   *(DNB 2011, AIIMS June 93)*
   b. Floating prostate on per rectal examination
   c. Collection of urine in perineum
   d. Bleeding per urethra

34. **Urine extravasation occurs in the following in case of penile urethral rupture, except:**   *(JIPMER 2003)*
   a. Ischiorectal fossa
   b. Scrotum
   c. Abdomiadias
   d. Below superficial fascia of penis

35. **A young man gets into a fight after taking beer and is kicked by the lower abdomen. There was pelvic fracture. Blood at meatus. Most likely cause is:**   *(MCI Nov 2017)*
   a. Rupture of membranous urethra
   b. Bulbar urethral injury
   c. Kidney laceration   d. Ureteric injury

36. **All the features of membranous urethral injury except:**
   a. Blood of meatus   b. Retention of urine
   c. Pelvic fracture   d. None *(MAHE 2007, 2008)*

37. **With the knowledge of anatomy of the pelvis and perineum, which of the following is true regarding collection of urine in urethral rupture above deep perineal pouch?**
                               (AIIMS Nov 2012)
   a. Medial aspect of thigh   b. Scrotum
   c. True pelvis only   d. Anterior abdominal wall

38. **Following urethral rupture, immediate procedure to be done is:**   *(MCI Sept 2008, March 2009)*
   a. Urinary catheterization b. Suprapubic cystostomy
   c. Referral to a urologist   d. Observation

■ URETHRAL STRICTURE

39. **The commonest cause of an obliterative stricture of the membranous urethra is:**   *(All India 2003)*
   a. Fall-astride injury
   b. Road-traffic accident with fracture pelvis and rupture urethra
   c. Prolonged catheterization
   d. Gonococcal infection

40. **What is the location of stricture in the given RGU?**

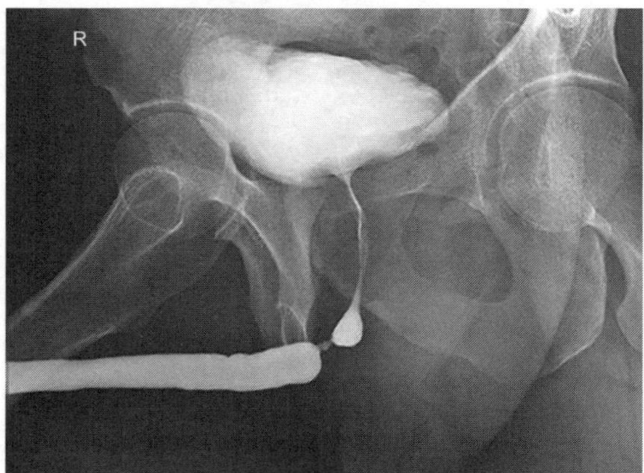

   a. Membranous urethra   b. Bulbar urethra
   c. Penile urethra   d. Prostatic urethra

41. **Commonest cause of urethral stricture in a young person is:**
   a. Trauma   b. Gonococcal *(Karnataka 96)*
   c. Syphilis   d. Tuberculosis

42. **Post gonococcal stricture urethra is most commonly situated in the:**   *(Recent Questions 2015)*
   a. Bulbar urethra
   b. Penoscrotal junction
   c. Distal part of spongy urethra
   d. Just distal to external meatus

43. **Most common cause of urethral stricture is:**
                           (Recent Questions 2013)
   a. Trauma   b. Infection
   c. Congenital   d. Post endoscopy

44. **A 40 years old patient of pelvic injury presents with stricture of bulbar urethra of 1.5 cm length. Best management:**
   a. Urethral dilatation   *(Recent Question 2017)*
   b. Excision with end-to-end urethroplasty
   c. Partial graft urethroplasty
   d. Urethrotomy

■ CARCINOMA PENIS

45. True about verrucous carcinoma is all except: *(Punjab 2009)*
   a. Locally aggressive form of condyloma acuminate
   b. Also known as Buschke-Lowenstein Tumor
   c. They frequently metastasize
   d. Wide excision is the treatment of choice

46. Buschke-lowenstein tumor is: *(MHCET 2016)*
   a. Malignant transformation in plantar wart
   b. Malignant transformation in anogenital wart
   c. Malignant transformation in common wart
   d. Malignant transformation in seborrheic wart

47. In CA penis, soft tissue planes are best delineated by:
   a. MRI   b. CT scan *(GB PANT 2011)*
   c. X-ray   d. USG

48. The most common cause of death in carcinoma penis:
(MHPGMCET 2008, AIIMS Nov 94)
   a. Uremia   b. Urinary sepsis
   c. Lung metastases   d. Erosion of femoral vessels

49. Cabana procedure is done in: *(GB PANT 2010)*
   a. CA testis   b. RPLND
   c. Sentinel LN biopsy in penile carcinoma
   d. None

50. Sentinel lymph node of carcinoma penis: *(MHSSMCET 2006)*
   a. Cabana   b. Virchow
   c. Delphian   d. Darwins

51. Erythroplasia of Queyrat occurs in: *(MCI Sept 2008)*
   a. Scrotum   b. Testes
   c. Penis   d. Bladder

52. Features of carcinoma penis are all except:
(Recent Question 2017)
   a. Circumcision soon after birth provides total immunity
   b. Metastatic to inguinal nodes
   c. Surgery is treatment of choice
   d. Transitional cell carcinoma

53. Treatment of choice of small preputial penile carcinoma is:
(Recent Question 2016)
   a. Total penectomy   b. Partial penectomy
   c. Emasculation   d. Wide excision

54. Sentinel lymph node biopsy was first done in:
(Recent Question 2017, DNB 2012)
   a. Carcinoma breast   b. Carcinoma colon
   c. Carcinoma penis   d. Melanoma

55. All are true about carcinoma penis except:
(Recent Question 2013)
   a. Most common type is verrucous
   b. Spreads by blood borne metastasis
   c. Leads to erosion of artery
   d. Slowly progressive

■ URETHRAL CARCINOMA

56. Most common site of urethral carcinoma in men is:
(Recent Question 2016, All India 2010)
   a. Bulbomembranous urethra
   b. Penile urethra
   c. Prostatic urethra
   d. Fossa navicularis

Explanations

■ HYPOSPADIAS

1. Ans. a. **Associated with chordee** *(Ref: Smith's 18/e p637; Campbell 11/e p3399-3401; Bailey 27/e p1478)*
2. Ans. c. **Hypospadias**   3. Ans. a. **Hypospadias**   4. Ans. b. **Glandular**
5. Ans. d. **Cryptorchidism**   6. Ans. a. **Glandular**
7. Ans. a. **Before 1 year** *(Ref: Campbell 11/e p3401; Smith 18/e p639; Bailey 27/e p1478)*
8. Ans. a. **Dennis-Brown** *(Ref: Campbell 11/e p3410)*

■ EPISPADIAS

9. Ans. b. **Chordee** *(Ref: Smith 18/e p639; Campbell 11/e p3221; Bailey 27/e p1478)*

■ POSTERIOR URETHRAL VALVE

10. Ans. d. **Posterior urethral valve**   11. Ans. b. **Posterior urethral valves**
12. Ans. b. **MCU**   13. Ans. b. **Below verumontanum**

■ PHIMOSIS

14. Ans. a. **Wait and watch policy** *(Ref: Smith 18/e p640; Campbell 11/e p3370; Bailey 27/e p1486)*

■ PARAPHIMOSIS

15. Ans. b. **Seen in diabetes mellitus** *(Ref: Smith 18/e p641; Campbell 11/e p3364-3370; Bailey 27/e p1489)*

■ CIRCUMCISION

16. Ans. d. **All of the above** *(Ref: Smith 18/e p641; Bailey 27/e p1487)*
    Circumcision is indicated in patients with infection, phimosis or paraphimosis.
17. Ans. c. **Carcinoma penis** *(Ref: Smith 18/e p641)*

Indications of Circumcision	
• **Phimosis**[Q]	• **Religion (Jews** and **Muslims)**[Q]
• **Paraphimosis**[Q]	• **Balanitis** or **balanoposthitis**[Q]
• **Recurrent UTI**[Q]	• **BXO** (balanitis xerotica obliterans)

18. Ans. b. **Increases sexual drive** *(Ref: Smith18/e p641; Bailey 27/e p1487)*

■ PRIAPISM

19. Ans. c. **Spinal cord disease** *(Ref: Bailey 27/e p1491; Campbell 11/e p671)*
    Priapism is **rarely seen** as a consequence of **spinal cord disease**.

PERSISTENT PRIAPISM

- The **penis** remains **erect** and becomes **painful.**
- This is a **pathological erection** and the **glans penis** and **corpus spongiosum** are **not involved**[Q].
- The condition is **usually seen as a complication of** a **blood disorder** such as **sickle cell disease** or **leukaemia**[Q].
- However, it can sometimes follow **therapeutic injection of papaverine** or even an **abnormally prolonged bout** of otherwise **normal sexual activity**[Q].
- A **tiny proportion** is caused by **malignant disease** in the **corpora cavernosa** or the **pelvis.**
- **Priapism** is **rarely seen** as a consequence of **spinal cord disease**[Q].

20. Ans. b. **Spinal cord injury**
21. Ans. d. **4 hours** *(Ref: Bailey 27/e p1491)*

> *"Priapism means a persistent erection lasting longer than 4 hours and it is a surgical emergency."*- Bailey 27/e p1491

■ PEYRONIE'S DISEASE

22. Ans. c. **Curved deformity of penis due to fibrous plaque**
23. Ans. c. **Peyronie's disease**   24. Ans. a. **Peyronie's disease**

■ URINARY TRACT INFECTION

25. Ans. a. Abdominal ultrasound *(Ref: Smith 18/e p198; Campbell 11/e p253)*

This patient must be having anatomic genitourinary abnormalitis (VUR), and the next best investigation is USG.

Epidemiology of UTI by Age Group and Sex			
Age (years)	Incidence (%)		Risk Factors
	Female	Male	
< 1	0.7	2.7	Foreskin, **anatomic GU abnormalities**
1–5	4.5	0.5	**Anatomic** genitourinary **(GU) abnormalities**
6–15	4.5	0.5	Functional GU abnormalities
16–35	20	0.5	Sexual intercourse, diaphragm use
36–65	35	20	Surgery, prostate obstruction, catheterization
> 65	40	35	Incontinence, catheterization, prostate obstruction

ULTRASOUND

- **Ultrasound study** is an important renal imaging technique because it is **noninvasive, easy to perform,** and **rapid** and **offers no radiation** or **contrast agent risk** to the patient[Q].

26. Ans. b. Vesicoureteric reflux

27. Ans. c. Cranberry *(Ref: Smith 18/e p204)*

- **Alternatives to antibiotic therapy** in the **treatment of recurrent cystitis/UTI** include **intravaginal estriol, lactobacillus vaginal** suppositories, and **cranberry juice taken orally**[Q].
- **Cranberry juice** is traditionally **used for prophylaxis** and **treatment of UTI**[Q].

28. Ans. a. E. coli *(Ref: Smith 18/e p199)*

URINARY TRACT INFECTION

- **Most UTIs** are caused **by a single bacterial species**[Q].
- At least **80%** of the **uncomplicated cystitis** and **pyelonephritis** are due to **E. coli**[Q], with most of pathogenic strains belonging to the **O serogroups**.
- Other less common uropathogens include Klebsiella, Proteus, and Enterobacter spp. and enterococci.
- In **hospital acquired UTIs,** a wider variety of causative organisms is found, including **Pseudomonas** and **Staphylococcus** spp[Q].

> - **UTIs** caused by **S. aureus** often result from **hematogenous dissemination**[Q].
> - **Group B beta-hemolytic streptococci** can cause **UTIs** in **pregnant women**[Q].
> - **In children, Klebsiella** and **Enterobacter spp.** are **common causes of UTI**[Q].

- **Anaerobic bacteria, lactobacilli, corynebacteria, streptococci** (not including enterococci) and **S. epidermidis** are found in **normal periurethral flora.** They do not commonly cause UTIs in healthy individuals and are considered common **urinary contaminants**[Q].

■ URINARY RETENTION

29. Ans. d. Meatal ulcer with scabbing *(Ref: Bailey 27/e p1426)*

Acute urinary retention in a male child may be due to local inflammatory causes like meatal ulcer with scabbing.

Etiology of Urinary Retention in Children	
Neurological processes (**17%**)	Locally invading neoplasms (6%)
Severe voiding dysfunction (15%)	Benign obstructing lesions (6%)
UTI (13%)	Idiopathic (6%)
Constipation (13%)	Combined UTI and constipation (2%)
Adverse drug effect (13%)	Incarcerated inguinal hernia (2%)
Local inflammatory causes (7%)	

30. Ans. c. Herniorrhaphy

■ URETHRAL INJURY

31. Ans. a. Catheterize the patient immediately

32. Ans. b. Deep perineal pouch

33. Ans. b. Floating prostate on per rectal examination *(Ref: Smith 18/e p294; Campbell 11/e p2391; Bailey 27/e p1481)*

34. Ans. a. Ischiorectal fossa *(Ref: Smith 18/e p292; Campbell 11/e p2391; Bailey 27/e p1479-1481)*

	Bulbar Urethral Injury	Membranous Urethral Injury
Incidence	• **More common**[Q]	• Less common
Mechanism of injury	• **Direct blow** to the perineum (**Straddle injury**)[Q]	• **Blunt pelvic trauma** with **fracture pelvis**[Q]
Signs and symptoms	• Retention of urine[Q] • Blood at urethral meatus[Q] • **Perineal** hematoma[Q] • Normal prostate[Q]	• Retention of urine[Q] • Blood at urethral meatus[Q] • **Pelvic** hematoma[Q] • **High lying prostate**[Q]
Urine extravasation	• **Superficial extravasation**[Q]	• **Deep extravasation**[Q]

35. Ans. a. Rupture of membranous urethra

36. Ans. d. None

37. Ans. c. True pelvis only

38. Ans. b. Suprapubic cystostomy

■ URETHRAL STRICTURE

39. Ans. b. Road-traffic accident with fracture pelvis and rupture urethra

40. Ans. b. Bulbar urethra (*Ref: Sabiston 20/e p2093; Schwartz 10/e p1665; Bailey 27/e p1483*)

Retrograde Urethrogram

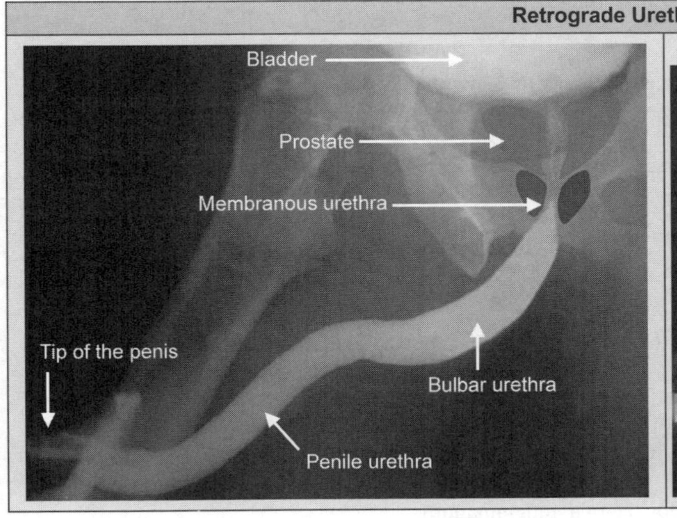

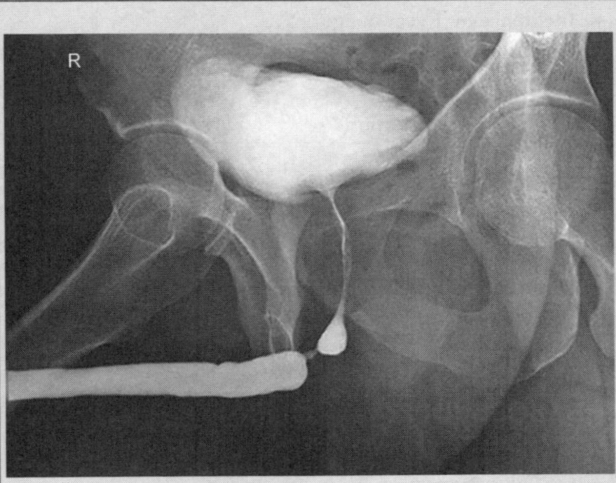

41. Ans. a. Trauma   42. Ans. a. Bulbar Urethra   43. Ans. a. Trauma

44. Ans. b. Excision with end-to-end urethroplasty (*Ref: Campbell 11/e p921*)

"Excision with primary anastomosis has proved to be the gold standard form of repair for anterior urethral strictures. In years past, excision with primary anastomosis was thought to be a relatively limited procedure and applicable only for strictures less than 1.5 to 2.0 cm. However, with better understanding of the anatomy, longer and longer strictures have been successfully addressed with excision and primary anastomosis." –Campbell 11/e p921

■ CARCINOMA PENIS

45. Ans. c. They frequently metastasize (*Ref: Smith 18/e p389; Campbell 11/e p849; Bailey 27/e p1492*)

46. Ans. b. Malignant transformation in anogenital wart (*Ref: Campbell 11/e p848*)

47. Ans. a. MRI (*Ref: Campbell 11/e p851*)   48. Ans. d. Erosion of femoral vessels (*Ref: Campbell 11/e p849*)

49. Ans. c. Sentinel LN biopsy in penile carcinoma (*Ref: Campbell 11/e p850*)

50. Ans. a. Cabana (*Ref: Campbell 11/e p850*)   51. Ans. c. Penis (*Ref: Campbell 11/e p848*)

52. Ans. d. Transitional cell carcinoma   53. Ans. d. Wide excision

54. Ans. c. Carcinoma penis (*Ref: Mastery of Surgery 5/e p1531*)

• "The historic contribution by **Cabana** in 1977 (Cancer 1977; 39:456) **established the importance, lymphatic histology with sentinel lymph node mapping** of patients with **penile carcinoma.** This approach identified the **sentinel lymph node** as the **first site of residual nodal metastasis** and is **predictive of the nodal status of the remaining node basin."**

55. Ans. a. Most common type is verrucous

■ URETHRAL CARCINOMA

56. Ans. a. Bulbomembranous urethra (*Ref: Smith 18/e p322; Campbell 11/e p882*)

Testis and Scrotum

■ UNDESCENDED TESTIS

UNDESCENDED TESTIS

- UDT affects 3% of **full-term**[Q] newborns.
- **Incidence** by **1 year** of age is **1%.**
- Approximately **70% to 77%** of UDT will **spontaneously descend**, usually by **3 months**[Q] of age.

> - **Birth weight**[Q] may be the **principal determinant** of UDT **at birth** and at **1 year** of life, **independent** of the **length of gestation.**

- In UDT, **80%** are **palpable** and **20%** are **nonpalpable**[Q].
- **MC location** for an ectopic UDT is within the **superficial pouch**[Q].

Pathology

- **Germ cell histology** of **both the testes** is **abnormal.**
- **Hypoplasia of the Leydig cells**, observed from the **1st month**[Q] of life, is the **earliest postnatal histologic abnormality**[Q] in UDT.

Associated Anomalies

- **Epididymal anomalies** and **patent processus vaginalis** up to **90%**[Q] cases of UDT.
- **Renal Anomalies** in **10% cases** (Renal hypoplasia, agenesis, horse shoe kidney, PUJ obstruction)
- **Hypospadias**
  Hazards: (SATHI- Sterility, Atrophy, Trauma, Tumor, Torsion, Hernia, Inflammation)

Neoplasia
• Relative risk of testicular tumor is increased **17 times**.
• MC tumor that develops is **seminoma**[Q].
• **Higher the testis, greater the risk**[Q] (Abdominal testis has higher risk than inguinal)
• **Orchiopexy does not decrease the risk, it helps in early detection only**[Q].

- **Hernia: Patent processus vaginalis**[Q] is seen in **90%** cases of UDT.
- **Torsion:** Increased susceptibility

Diagnosis

- **Inguinal exploration** is IOC for UDT[Q].

Diagnostic Laparoscopy
• **IOC** for **'non-palpable'** UDT[Q].
• **MC application** of laparoscopy in children is for UDT.
• **Vas** and **testicular artery** is traced in pelvis.
• **Blind ended vas doesn't conclude** the **absence of testis**[Q], whereas **blind ended testicular artery** is a **definitive investigation** for an **absence of testis**[Q].

Management: Orchiopexy, Ideal time: **6-12 months**[Q] of age. (**Best time** is **6 months**[Q])

Types of Orchiopexy	
1. **Fowler-Stephens** orchiopexy[Q]	4. **Ombridann's** orchiopexy[Q]
2. **Microvascular testicular autotransplantation (Best results)**[Q]	5. **Placing testis in Dartos pouch**[Q]
3. **Ladd and Gross** orchiopexy[Q]	6. **Keetley-Torek** orchiopexy[Q]

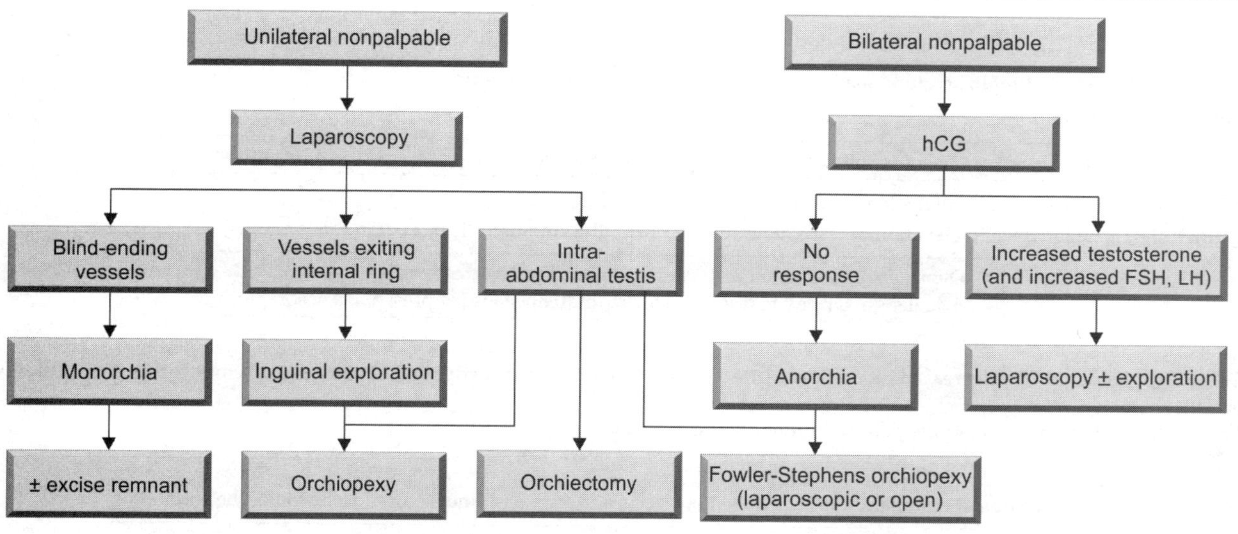

■ ECTOPIC TESTIS

ECTOPIC TESTIS

- An ectopic testicle **descends normally through the inguinal canal** but then **moves into an abnormal position** in the **groin area**[Q].
- An **ectopic testis** is usually[Q]. **Fully developed**[Q]. The **main hazard** is **liability to injury**[Q].

Locations of Ectopic Testis
• **Superficial inguinal pouch (MC location)**[Q]
• **Femoral canal**[Q] (the inner portion of the thigh near the groin)
• **Perineum**[Q] (below the scrotum)
• **Suprapubic region**[Q] (above the penis)
• **Contralateral scrotum (Least common)**[Q]

Embryology
- Ectopic testis are likely related to **abnormalities of** the **gubernaculum**[Q], which is a fibrous, cord-like membrane that runs through the inguinal canal from the abdomen to the scrotum.
- The **gubernaculum helps to guide the descent** of the **testicles**[Q] and has branches that attach to these other locations.
- **Most ectopic testicles** can be felt **(are palpable)**[Q].

Treatment
- **Surgical treatment** to place an ectopic testicle in its normal position any time **after about age 6 months** but **no later than 2 years of age**[Q].

■ TESTICULAR TORSION

TESTICULAR TORSION

- Twisting of testis on the spermatic cord, resulting in strangulation of the blood supply and infarction of testis.
- Types of testicular torsion: Intravaginal and Extravaginal.

INTRAVAGINAL TESTICULAR TORSION

- **Torsion** occurs **within the space of tunica vaginalis**, which is **highly invested**[Q], resulting in lack of normal fixation of testis & epididymis to the fascial & muscular coverings (scrotal parietal wall)
- **MC age group** affected is **10-25 years**, with peak in **prepubertal age**[Q]
- **Cremaster fibers** have a **spiral attachment over the cord**, it favors rotation **when cremaster reflex is strong**[Q].

Predisposing Factors
- **Inversion of the testis** (testis lies transversely or upside down) is **MC predisposing factor**[Q]
- **High investment of tunica vaginalis** causes the **testis to hang within the tunica like a clapper in a bell**[Q]
- **Separation of the epididymis from the body of testis**[Q] permit torsion of testis without involving cord

Clinical Features
- **Sudden agonizing scrotal pain** with **nausea or vomiting**[Q]
- **Dysuria** or other **bladder symptoms** are usually **absent**[Q]

Contd…

Contd...

Urology

Section 4

- Affected **testis high-riding in scrotum**, may have **abnormal transverse orientation**[Q]
- **Cord** is usually **thickened**[Q]

> - **Absent cremasteric reflux**[Q] is **highly suggestive** of torsion testis (**present in epididymitis**)

- After several hours massive scrotal edema may obliterate all the findings
- **Prehn's sign** is **negative**[Q] (On elevation of testis, pain relieved in epididymo-orchitis but not in torsion testis)

> - **Deming sign: Affected testis** at **higher level** because of twisting of cord[Q]
> - **Angel sign: Opposite testis lies horizontally** because of present of mesorchium[Q]

Imaging
- **Color Doppler** detects the **decreased blood flow** to the testis in torsion and is **investigation of choice**[Q] to exclude torsion from epididymo-orchitis.
- **Tc99 pertechnate scan** demonstrate **poor radionuclide tracer uptake**[Q]

Treatment
- Testicular torsion is **urological emergency** as ischemic injury occurs as soon as **4 hours**[Q] after occlusion of the cord.

> - **Immediate surgical exploration**[Q] is indicated if testicular torsion is suspected because if treated within first 4 hours, the chances of testicular salvage are high.

- Even if manual detorsion is done, it may not totally correct the rotation and prompt exploration is still indicated.
- Viable as well as testis of marginal viability are preserved, and **orchiopexy** is done either by **placing into dartos pouch without suture fixation or suture fixation of tunica albuginea with the parietal wall**[Q].

> - **Exploration of contralateral hemiscrotum** must be carried. In almost all cases, a **bell clapper deformity is found.**
> - **Contralateral testis** must be **fixed** to **prevent subsequent torsion**[Q].

- **Risk of autoimmunization** against own sperms is **low in children <10 years**, because there is no blood testis barrier and spermatogenesis is dormant.
- Current recommendation is **preserve a compromised testis in children <10 years**, proceed with orchidectomy in older children.

EXTRAVAGINAL TESTICULAR TORSION

- There is **no anatomical defect**[Q]
- Occurs in **perinatal period**, as there is **no testicular fixation**[Q] (adherence of tunica vaginalis to the dartos layer) by that time, and as a result the spermatic cord and tunica vaginalis **rotate as one unit**[Q]

Prenatal torsion	Postnatal torsion
• A **hard non-tender testis** at birth, **fixed to the overlying skin**[Q]	• **Swelling and tenderness of scrotum**, usually **no fixation**[Q] of the skin
• **Salvage rate is nil**[Q]	• **Prompt surgical exploration** is indicated
• **Contralateral scrotal exploration** is **not recommended**[Q] as it is not associated with a testicular fixation defect	• **Exploration of contralateral testis** should be done as **20% cases** are associated with **bell clapper deformity**[Q]

- **Blue dot sign**: seen in **torsion** of **appendage of testis**[Q].

■ VARICOCELE

VARICOCELE

- Dilated & tortuous veins of pampiniform plexus (veins draining testis & epididymis)[Q] lying **posterior & above the testis**
- Most common **surgically correctable cause** of male **subfertility**[Q]
- Surgical **correction** can **reverse atrophy** in **adolescents**[Q]

Etiology
- **Absent or incompetent valves** in the internal spermatic or **left testicular vein (MC)**[Q] and it joins left renal vein at right angles.
- Increased venous pressure in left renal vein (**Nutcracker phenomenon**[Q]- caused by compression of left renal vein between aorta and superior mesenteric artery)
- Collateral venous anastomosis
- Compression by sigmoid colon

Contd...

Contd…

Clinical Features

- MC seen in **young adults**[Q], **tall thin men**[Q] are frequently affected
- **Painless**, compressible mass lying **posterior and above the testis**
- **Bag of worms** like feel on palpation in standing position[Q]
- Marked **left side predominance**[Q] (90%)
- Varicocele **do not regress spontaneously**[Q], associated with testicular atrophy
- **Suspicious varicoceles:** May be **secondary to RCC**, as growth from renal cell carcinoma **blocks the renal vein by venous permeation**. In RCC, varicocele **does not decompress in supine position**[Q].
  - **Right sided** varicoceles[Q]
  - **Rapidly evolving** varicoceles[Q]
  - Varicoceles in **elderly**[Q]
  - Varicocele that **does not decompress** in supine position[Q]

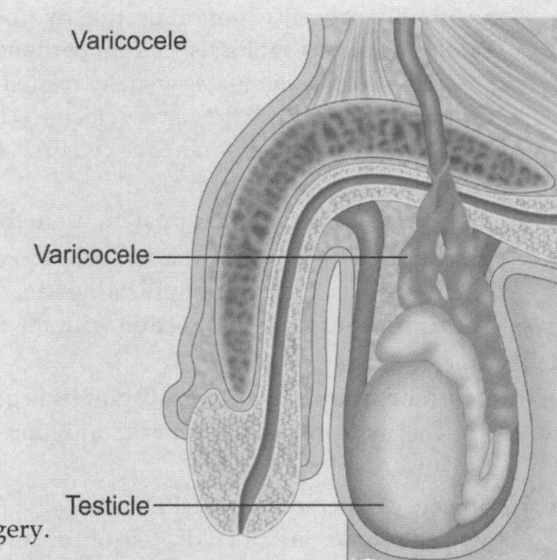

Effect on Spermatogenesis

- Varicocele **increases the temperature of scrotum**[Q] and this decreases spermatogenesis
- Abnormal semen analysis (**decreased sperm motility & number**), normalizes after surgery.

Diagnosis

- Diagnosis is made by **clinical examination** and **confirmed by color Doppler analysis** (**reflux/reverse flow** is characteristic of varicoceles)[Q].
- **Venography: Most accurate** method of varicocele diagnosis, done for varicocele in the **postsurgical patients**[Q].

Indications for surgery	
1. Infertility[Q]	4. Significant discomfort
2. Poor testicular growth in adolescents[Q]	5. Recruitment to police or armed forces
3. Defective sperm count or motility[Q]	

Treatment

- **Ligation** of **testicular vein above** the **inguinal ligament**[Q] where the pampiniform plexus has coalesced into one or two vessels. (**Venous drainage** after ligation is by **cremasteric veins**[Q])

> - **Best surgical option is microscopic subinguinal ligation**[Q].

- Other procedures are open inguinal/subinguinal, laparoscopic or retroperitoneal (**Palomo's operation**) ligation or embolization.

■ SPERMATOCELE

SPERMATOCELE

- **Unilocular retention cyst derived from** some portion of the **sperm-conducting mechanism** of the **epididymis**[Q].

Clinical Features

- **Typically lies in the epididymal head, above** and **behind** the **upper pole** of the **testis.**
- **Usually small** and **unobtrusive**[Q].
- Usually **softer** and **laxer than other cystic lesions** in the scrotum but, like them, it **transilluminates**[Q]
- The **fluid contains spermatozoa**[Q] and resembles **barley water appearance**[Q].

Treatment

- Small spermatoceles can be ignored.
- **Larger ones** should be **aspirated** or **excised** through a scrotal incision.

■ HYDROCELE

HYDROCELE

An accumulation of fluid in layers of tunica vaginalis

Types:

- **Vaginal hydrocele (MC)**[Q]
  - Abnormal accumulation of serous fluid within the tunica vaginalis.
- **Infantile hydrocele:**
  - Does not necessarily appear in infants.
  - Tunica & processus vaginalis are distended to the inguinal ring **without any connection** with **peritoneal cavity**[Q].

Contd…

Contd…

- **Congenital hydrocele** (Communicating hydrocele):
  - **Patent processus vaginalis**[Q] allows peritoneal fluid to freely communicate.
  - Size of hydrocele fluctuates, usually related to activity
  - Congenital hernia has the same defect. UDT are commonly associated.
  - **Wait for 2 years** for **spontaneous closure**[Q]. Otherwise the treatment is **herniotomy**[Q].
- **Funicular hydrocele:**
  - Processus vaginalis remains **patent up to** the **top** of the **testis**[Q], where it is shut off from the tunica vaginalis.
- **Hydrocele En bisac or Bilocular hydrocele:**
  - Hydrocele has **2 intercommunicating sacs**, one **above** and one **below** the **neck**[Q] of scrotum.
  - The upper sac has **no connection with** the **processus vaginalis**[Q] and it is in fact the herniated tunica vaginalis.
- **Hydrocele of the cord:**
  - **Central portion** of **processus vaginalis** is **patent**[Q], but its upper & lower parts are obliterated.
  - Presents as **painless groin mass** contiguous with cord structures, moves downward and becomes less mobile if testis is pulled gently downwards.
- **Hydrocele of the canal of Nuck:**
  - Female counterpart of Hydrocele of the cord. It is seen in relation to the round ligament.
- **Hydrocele of hernial sac: Neck of hernial sac** becomes **closed by adhesions** or **plugged by omentum** with **retention of fluid secreted by peritoneum of hernial sac**[Q]

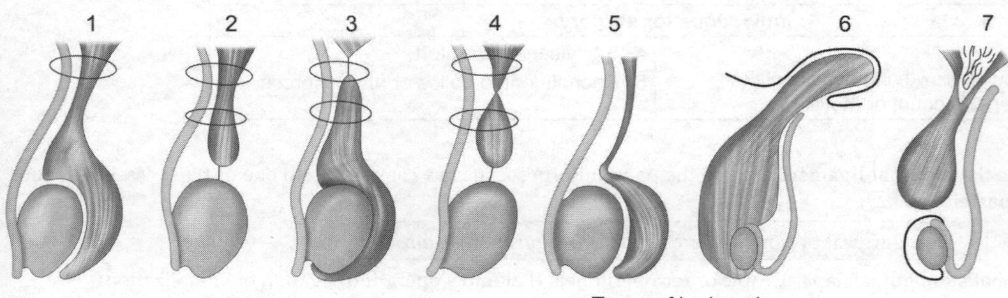

Types of hydrocele

Secondary Hydrocele
• **Causes** are acute or chronic **epididymo-orchitis (MC)**[Q], testicular tumors, torsion of testis
• Usually **lax** and of **small size** with **palpable underlying testis**[Q]
• Subsides with resolution of epididymo-orchitis

Treatment of Vaginal Hydrocele
1. **Small** hydrocele: **Lord's** procedure (**Plication** of sac)[Q]
2. **Medium** hydrocele: **Jaboulay's** procedure (**Eversion** of sac)[Q]
3. **Large** hydrocele: **Excision** of sac[Q]

■ ACUTE EPIDIDYMO-ORCHITIS

Acute Epididymo-orchitis

- **Inflammation** of **epididymis & testis**, from an **ascending infection**[Q] from the lower urinary tract.
- Initially epididymis is involved, after that there is involvement of testis.
- Most cases of epididymitis in **men younger than 35 years** are due to **sexually transmitted organisms** [C. trachomatis (MC)[Q] and **N. gonorrhoe**]
- In **children** and **older men** are due to **urinary pathogens** such as **E. coli**[Q].
- In **homosexual men**, **E. coli**[Q] and other coliform bacteria are common causative organisms.

Clinical Features

- Patient presents with **fever, swollen, red & tender scrotum**[Q].
- The epididymis and testis are swollen (**Thickened cord** with **reactive hydrocoele**)[Q]
- Symptoms of **urethritis, cystitis or prostatitis**[Q]
- Urine analysis typically demonstrates **WBCs and bacteria** in the **urine or urethral discharge**[Q]

Contd…

Contd…

Diagnosis

- Scrotal USG showing enlarged epididymis with increased blood flow with reactive hydrocoele.
- **Prepubertal children** diagnosed with epididymitis **require radiologic investigation** for **urinary tract anomalies** such as reflux or ureteral Ectopia[Q].

Treatment

- Antibiotics, rest , scrotal elevation and NSAIDs[Q].

> - **MC organism** causing epididymo-orchitis in **<35** and **sexually active males: Chlamydia**[Q]
> - **MC organism** causing epididymo-orchitis in **children, elderly, homosexuals: E. coli**[Q]

■ FOURNIER'S GANGRENE (IDIOPATHIC SCROTAL GANGRENE)

FOURNIER'S GANGRENE (IDIOPATHIC SCROTAL GANGRENE)

- A form of **necrotizing fasciitis**, with **abrupt onset** of a **rapidly fulminating genital gangrene** of idiopathic origin and **gangrene up to deep fascia**[Q].

Predisposing Factors	
• **Diabetes mellitus (MC)**	• Anal infections
• Local trauma	• **Immunosuppression**[Q]
• Paraphimosis	

- **Multiple organisms (aerobes + anaerobes)**[Q] results in fulminating inflammation of the subcutaneous tissues which results in **obliterative arteritis** of arterioles of the scrotal skin. (**Polymicrobial**)[Q]

Clinical Features

- History of **recent perineal trauma**, **instrumentation**, urethral **stricture** or a **rectal source** of infection is frequently present[Q].
- Infection commonly starts as cellulitis. Involved area swollen, erythematosus and tender as the infection begins to involve the deep fascia.

> - Areas of **purplish** and **blackish discoloration, dishwater** like **discharge, fetid odour** and **skin necrosis**.
> - **Pain** is predominant with **fever** and **marked systemic toxicity**[Q]. Crepitus is present[Q].

- **Skin, superficial fascia, deep fascia** is **destroyed**, while **corpora cavernosa, urethra, testis, cord structures** are **preserved**[Q].

Management

- **Prompt diagnosis** and **aggressive treatment**[Q] is the initial treatment to limit the spread.

> - **IV hydration, antibiotics, surgical debridement** of the necrotic fat and fascia[Q]
> - **Mortality** without treatment: **7-75%**[Q] (Average-20%)

- **Surgical debridement** is cornerstone, **serial debridement**[Q] is usually required.

■ CLASSIFICATION OF TESTICULAR TUMORS

CLASSIFICATION OF TESTICULAR TUMORS

- **Germ cell tumors:**
  - Seminomas
  - **Non-seminomas:**
    - Embryonal cell carcinoma
    - Teratoma
    - Yolk sac tumour
    - Choriocarcinoma
- **Sex cord/gonadal stromal tumors:**
  - Leydig cell tumour
  - Granulosa cell tumor
  - Sertoli cell tumor
  - Thecoma/fibroma
- **Tumors containing both germ cell and sex cord/gonadal stromal elements:**
  - Gonadoblastoma
- **Lymphoid and Hematopoetic tumour:**
  - Lymphoma, Leukemia, Plasmacytoma
- **Miscellaneous:**
  - Carcinoid, Adenoma, Carcinoma

■ PREDISPOSING FACTORS FOR TESTICULAR GCTs

PREDISPOSING FACTORS FOR TESTICULAR GCTs

- **Cryptorchidism**
  - Of the predisposing factors, **cryptorchidism** has the **strongest association** with the **testicular carcinoma**[Q].
  - **Higher the testis, greater the risk**[Q]. Abdominal cryptorchid testis is at higher risk than inguinal cryptorchid testis.

  > - **Increased risk** is seen in **both the testis (cryptorchid** and **normally descended testis)**[Q]
  > - **MC tumour seen: Seminoma** > Embryonal cell carcinoma

  - **Orchidopexy does not decrease the risk of malignancy**[Q], however it facilitates examination and tumour detection.
- **Testicular feminization syndrome**
- **GCT** of **one testis** for other testis
- **Testicular carcinoma** in **sibling**
- **Klinefelter's syndrome** (increases risk of both **testicular** and **mediastinal GCT**) and **male CA breast**[Q].
- **Administration of DES (estrogen)** in utero

■ TESTICULAR TUMORS: MOST COMMON TYPE

TESTICULAR TUMORS

- MC **histological type** of testicular tumour: **Mixed**[Q] (if option is there, otherwise seminoma)

  > - **MC tumour** of testis: **Seminoma**[Q]
  > - **MC bilateral primary testicular tumour: Seminoma**[Q]
  > - **Most radiosensitive** testicular tumor: **Seminoma**[Q]

- MC testicular tumor in **infant & children up to 3 years: Yolk sac tumour**[Q]
- MC testicular tumor in **prepubertal children: Teratoma**[Q]

  > - **MC testicular tumor in patients >60 years: Lymphoma**[Q]
  > - **MC bilateral testicular tumour: Lymphoma**[Q]
  > - **MC secondary testicular tumour: Lymphoma**[Q]

- MC **histologic type** of testicular lymphoma: **Diffuse large B-cell lymphoma (DLBL)**
- Testicular tumour with **best prognosis: Yolk sac tumour**[Q]
- Testicular tumour with **worst prognosis: Hurricane tumour** (Type of **choriocarcinoma**)[Q]

■ TESTICULAR TUMORS

TESTICULAR TUMORS

- **MC tumour** of testis: **Seminoma**[Q]
- **MC histological type** of testicular tumour: **Mixed**[Q] (if option is there, otherwise seminoma)
- **Genomic change** found in all **germ cell tumors** is an **isochromosome** of **short arm** of chromosome **12**[Q].

Clinical Features

- **MC presentation** is a **nodule or painless swelling of one gonad**[Q].
- 10% patients present with acute pain or manifestation due to secondaries like neck or abdominal masses, GI disturbances, respiratory or CNS symptoms, bone pain or lumbar backache due to nerve roots involvement by bulky retroperitoneal disease.
- **Secondary hydrocele** is also seen in **5-10%**[Q] cases.

  > - **5% GCT** may present with **gynecomastia**[Q] as a systemic endocrine manifestation.
  > - **Gynecomastia is more commonly** seen with **sex cord** or **gonadal stromal tumors (Leydig cell tumor, Sertoli cell tumor, Granulosa/Theca cell tumor)**[Q].

- **Majority (2/3rd) of seminoma** are **confined to testis**[Q] at the time of presentation, whereas majority of **non-seminomatous GCT** have **widespread metastasis** at presentation.
- Any patient with a **solid firm intratesticular mass** must be considered to have **testicular tumour** unless proved otherwise.

Investigations

- **USG:** Any hypoechoic area within tunica albuginea is markedly suspicious.

  > - **FNAC is Contraindicated (Scrotal seedlings** may result in **inguinal LN metastasis)**[Q]

Contd…

Contd…

- **Histopathological Diagnosis: Radical orchiectomy** by inguinal canal approach, the **cord is ligated** at **deep inguinal ring (high inguinal orchiectomy)**[Q].
- **Trans-scrotal Orchidectomy** is **contraindicated** as it permits the development of alternate **lymphatic channel pathway** to **inguinal** and **pelvic lymph nodes.**

<table>
<tr><td>Chevassu maneuver[Q]</td></tr>
<tr><td>• First a soft clamp is applied to the cord, suspicious area is biopsied and sent for frozen section. If malignant, formally ligate the cord and send the orchiectomy sample for final histopathology.</td></tr>
</table>

- **CECT abdomen** for evaluation of **retroperitoneum** and **lymph nodes**[Q].

Spread of Disease

- **Germ cell tumors** of the testis typically **spread** in a **stepwise lymphatic fashion (MC mode)**[Q].

> - **Primary landing site for right testis** is **interaortocaval area**[Q] at the level of right renal hilum, and **for the left testis is para-aortic area**[Q] at the level of left renal hilum.
> - In the absence of disease on the left side, no crossover metastases to the right side have ever been identified. However, **right-to-left crossover metastases**[Q] are common.

- **Retroperitoneum** is the **most commonly involved site**[Q] in metastatic disease.
- Most **blood borne metastasis** occurs following LN involvement, **Lung** is **MC organ**[Q] involved.
- **Choriocarcinoma** is the exception and characterized by **early hematogenous spread**, especially to the **lung**[Q].

Chemotherapy

- Chemotherapy for **extragonadal GCT:** Combination of **Bleomycin + Etoposide**[Q]**+ Cisplatin (BEP)**[Q]

8th AJCC (2017) TNM Staging for Testicular Tumors	
T: Primary tumor	**N: Regional lymph nodes**
pTis: Intratubular germ cell neoplasia (carcinoma in situ)	**N1**: LN mass ≤2 cm or multiple LN masses, none >2 cm
pT1: Limited to the **testis & epididymis** and no vascular/lymphatic invasion; Tumor may **invade tunica albuginea** but not tunica vaginalis[Q]	**N2**: LN mass, **>2 cm** but **<5 cm** or multiple LN masses, any one mass >2 cm but not <5 cm[Q]
pT2: Limited to the testis & epididymis **with vascular/lymphatic invasion** or extending through **tunica albuginea** with **involvement of tunica vaginalis**[Q]	**N3**: LN mass >5 cm[Q]
pT3: Invades the **spermatic cord** with or without vascular/lymphatic invasion[Q]	**M: Distant metastases**
pT4: Invades the **scrotum** with or without vascular/lymphatic invasion[Q]	**M1: Non-regional nodal** or **pulmonary metastases**[Q] **M2: Non-pulmonary visceral masses**[Q]

Serum Tumor Markers (S)			
	LDH	**hCG (mIU/mL)**	**AFP (ng/mL)**
S0	≤N	≤N	≤N
S1	**<1.5 × N**	**<5,000**	**<1,000**
S2	**1.5–10 × N**	**5,000–50,000**	**1,000–10,000**
S3	**>10 × N**	**>50,000**	**>10,000**

Staging and Treatment			
Stage	**Extent of disease**	**Seminoma**	**Nonseminoma**
IA	**Testis only**, without vascular or lymphatic invasion (**T₁**)	Radiation therapy[Q]	RPLND or observation[Q]
IB	Testis with **vascular or lymphatic invasion (T₂)**, or extension through **tunica albuginea (T₂)**, or involvement of **spermatic cord (T₃)**, or **scrotum (T₄)**	Radiation therapy[Q]	RPLND[Q]
IIA	Nodes ≤ 2 cm (**N₁**), S0/S1	Radiation therapy	RPLND or chemotherapy followed by RPLND[Q]
IIB	Nodes >2-5 cm (**N₂**), S0/S1	Radiation therapy[Q]	**RPLND** ± adjuvant chemotherapy or chemotherapy followed by RPLND[Q]
IIC	Nodes > 5 cm (**N₃**), S0/S1	**Chemotherapy**[Q]	**Chemotherapy** followed by RPLND[Q]
III	Distant metastasis	**Chemotherapy**[Q]	**Chemotherapy** followed by surgery (biopsy or resection)[Q]
Is	Only serum tumor markers are raised (**S₁** to **S₃**)[Q]	**Chemotherapy**[Q]	**Chemotherapy**[Q]

Tumour Markers	
Oncofetal substances	**Cellular Enzymes**

1. **α-FP:** (Increases in **YET**)[Q]
  – Produced by **trophoblastic cells**
  – **Increases** in **Yolk sac tumour, embryonal carcinoma and terato carcinoma. (YET)**
  – **Does not increase** in **pure choriocarcinoma** and **pure seminoma**[Q]
  – Metabolic **half life: 5-7 days**[Q]
	1. **LDH:**
	  – Not a specific tumour marker
	  – Most useful as a marker for **"bulk' disease**
	  – Raised serum LDH has poor prognosis

2. **β-hCG:** (Increases in **CES**MINOMA)
  – Produced by **syncytiotrophoblastic cells**[Q]
  – **Increases in all choriocarcinomas, 50% embryonal carcinoma and 5-10% of pure seminoma** (as they contain syncytiotrophoblast like giant cells).
  – Serum **half life: 24-36 hours**[Q]
	2. **PLAP** (Placental alkaline phosphatase):
	  – Most useful as a marker for **"bulk' disease**
	  – Elevated in **seminoma**[Q]
	3. **GGT** (Gamma glutamyl transpeptidase):
	  – Marker of **seminoma testis**[Q]
	  – Marker for **"bulk" disease**

■ CARCINOMA SCROTUM (CHIMNEY SWEEP'S CANCER)

Carcinoma Scrotum (Chimney Sweep's Cancer)

- Squamous cell carcinoma of scrotum[Q], most commonly resulted from exposure to environmental carcinogens including **chimney soot, tars, paraffin** and petroleum products[Q].
- **Superficial inguinal lymph nodes** are the **first lymph nodes involved.**[Q]

Risk Factors

- Most cases results from **poor hygiene** and **chronic inflammation**[Q].

Diagnosis

- **Diagnosis** is established by **biopsy of scrotal skin**[Q].

Treatment

- **Wide excision** with **2 cm margins**[Q] should be performed for malignant tumors.
- **Prognosis** correlates with **presence or absence of nodal involvement**[Q].

> - MC common **benign lesion** of scrotum: **Sebaceous cyst**[Q]
> - MC common **malignant tumor** of scrotum: **Squamous cell carcinoma**[Q]

Multiple Choice Questions

■ UNDESCENDED TESTIS

1. **Best time for surgery of undescended testis is:**
   (Recent Question 2014, 2015; All India 2010)
   a. Just after birth
   b. 6 months of age
   c. 12 months of age
   d. 24 months of age

2. **Most common tumors in undescended testis:**
   (DNB 2005, Punjab 2009)
   a. Seminoma
   b. Teratoma
   c. Embryonal carcinoma
   d. None

3. **Best investigation for undescended testis in 1-year-old child is:** *(Recent Question 2017)*
   a. USG abdomen
   b. CT
   c. MRI
   d. Laparoscopy

4. **True about incompletely descended testis are all of the following except:** *(MCI March 2008)*
   a. Early repositioning can preserve function
   b. It may lead to sterility, if bilateral
   c. Poorly developed secondary sexual characters
   d. May be associated with indirect inguinal. hernia

5. **In cryptorchidism, hallmark histological changes appear in testis at:** *(Recent Question 2016)*
   a. 4 months
   b. 6 months
   c. 8 months
   d. 1 year

6. **Fowler-Stephen surgery is done in:** *(Recent Question 2017)*
   a. Epispadias
   b. Hypospadias
   c. Exstrophy of bladder
   d. Cryptorchidism

■ ECTOPIC TESTIS

7. **Most common site of ectopic testis:** *(GB PANT 2010)*
   a. Superficial inguinal pouch
   b. Root of penis
   c. Femoral triangle
   d. Perineum

8. **Ectopic testis is found in all location except:**
   (Recent Questions 2016)
   a. Lumbar
   b. Perineal
   c. Intra abdominal
   d. Inguinal

■ TESTICULAR TORSION

9. **True about torsion of testis is all except:** *(AIIMS Nov 2001)*
   a. Presents with sudden pain in testis
   b. Commonly associated with pyuria
   c. Doppler U/S shows decreased blood flow to the testis
   d. Simultaneous orchiopexy of the other side should also be done

10. **Bell-clapper testis predisposes to:** *(MCI Dec 2018)*
    a. Torsion testis
    b. Varicocele
    c. Cancer of testis
    d. Hydrocele

11. **All are true regarding torsion of the testis, except:** *(Orissa 2011)*
    a. Common in adolescents and young adults
    b. Inversion of testis is the most common predisposing cause
    c. Elevation of testis reduces the pain
    d. If diagnosis is doubtful, prompt exploration is the rule

12. **In testicular torsion, surgery within how much time can save viability of testis?** *(Recent Question 2013)*
    a. 6 hours
    b. 12 hours
    c. 24 hours
    d. 1 weeks

13. **Identify the abnormal condition given below:**
    (MCI Dec 2019)

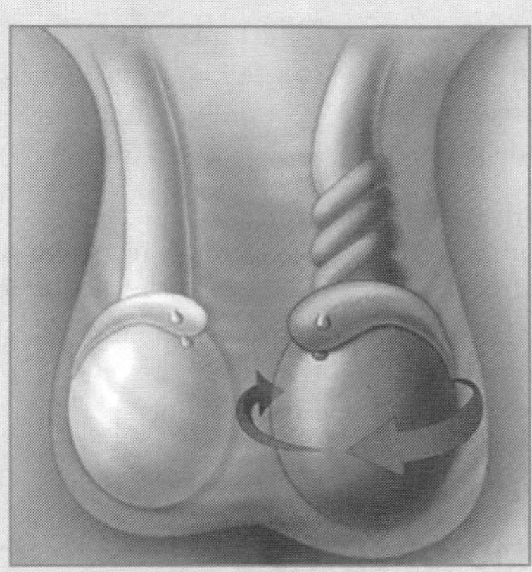

    a. Testicular torsion
    b. Hydrocele
    c. Varicocele
    d. Testicular atrophy

■ VARICOCELE

14. **Not true about varicocele is:** *(AIIMS Nov 2001)*
    a. Common on the right side
    b. Can present as a later sign of renal cell carcinoma
    c. Has bag of worm like feeling
    d. Can lead to infertility

15. **A 58-years old male presenting with acute onset of varicocele on left side most probable cause:** *(CMC 98)*
    a. CA testes
    b. Epididymitis
    c. Inguinal lymph nodes
    d. CA kidney

16. **True about varicocele is:** *(DNB 2007)*
    a. More common on right side
    b. Can cause oligospermia
    c. No effect on valsalva
    d. Lies anterior to testis

17. **Bag of worm like sensation is felt in:** *(Recent Question 2015)*
    a. Varicocele
    b. Hydrocele
    c. Torsion of testis
    d. Congenital hernia

18. **A 40-year-old man is suffering from heaviness in scrotum. A bag of worms feel is observed on scrotal examination and the swelling is seen to reduce in supine position. What is the best treatment?** *(MCI June 2019)*
    a. Suction drainage
    b. Varicocelectomy
    c. Jaboulay's procedure
    d. Herniotomy

■ SPERMATOCELE

19. **Chinese lantern on transillumination seen in:**
    (Recent Question 2014)
    a. Spermatocele
    b. Epididymal cyst
    c. Hydrocele of cord
    d. Secondary Hydrocele

20. **Spermatoceles are most commonly found at:**
    (Recent Question 2017)
    a. Head of epididymis
    b. Testes
    c. Prostate
    d. Seminal vesicle

■ HYDROCELE

21. **Hydrocele is labeled 'vaginal' when it is:** *(AIIMS 96)*
    a. Limited to scrotum
    b. Upto inguinal canal
    c. Communicating into coelomic cavity
    d. Upto deep inguinal ring

22. **Congenital hydrocele is best treated by:**
    (DNB 2009, 2008, 2005, 2001, Punjab 2011, AIIMS June 2001)
    a. Eversion of sac
    b. Excision of sac
    c. Lords procedure
    d. Herniotomy

23. **Lords plication is done for:** *(All India 2010)*
    a. Inguinal hernia
    b. Testicular cancer
    c. Hydrocele
    d. Testicular varices

24. **Classical treatment of hydrocoele:** *(DPG 2008)*
    a. Aspiration
    b. Aspiration and sclerosant agent
    c. Surgery
    d. Tapping

■ EPIDIDYMO-ORCHITIS

25. **Most common cause of acute epididymitis in males:**
    (COMEDK 2010, GB PANT 2011)
    a. E. coli
    b. Proteus
    c. Chlamydia trachomatis
    d. N. gonorrhoea

26. **Positive Prehn's sign is:** *(DNB 2010)*
    a. Elevation of testis increases pain of epididymitis
    b. Elevation of testis reduces pain of epididymitis
    c. Depression of testis increases pain of epididymitis
    d. Depression of testis reduces pain of epididymitis

27. **Acute orchitis all are seen except:** *(Recent Question 2013)*
    a. Increased local temperature
    b. Decreased blood flow
    c. Etythematous scrotum
    d. Raised TLC

28. **Prehn sign is seen in:** *(Recent Question 2015; 2013)*
    a. Acute orchitis
    b. Chronic orchitis
    c. Testicular torsion
    d. None

■ FOURNIER'S GANGRENE

29. **All are features of Fournier's gangrene except:** *(MAHE 2008)*
    a. Testicles are involved
    b. Obliterative arteritis seen
    c. Hemolytic streptococci
    d. Necrotising fasciitis
    e. E. coli, staphylococci, Cl. welchii can be isolated

30. **Fournier's gangrene is seen in:** *(MCI Sept 2008)*
    a. Scrotum
    b. Shaft of penis
    c. Base of penis
    d. Glans penis

■ TESTICULAR CARCINOMA PREDISPOSING FACTORS

31. **Testicular cancer is common in:** *(All India 91)*
    a. Ectopic testis
    b. Undescended abdominal testis
    c. Atrophic testis
    d. Anteverted testis

■ TESTICULAR CARCINOMA

32. **Most radiosensitive testicular tumour is:** *(MCI March 2008)*
    a. Seminoma
    b. Teratoma
    c. Interstitial tumours
    d. Lymphoma

33. **Most common testicular tumour in 4th decade:**
    (MCI Sept 2008)
    a. Teratoma
    b. Dermoid
    c. Seminoma
    d. All of the above

34. **Most common testicular tumor in prepubertal adults is:**
    (AIIMS May 2008)
    a. Yolk sac tumor
    b. Embryonal cell Ca
    c. Seminoma
    d. Teratoma

35. **Germ cell tumor not seen in males:** *(MCI Dec 2018)*
    a. Choriocarcinoma
    b. Seminoma
    c. Sertoli cell tumor
    d. Teratoma

36. **Testicular teratoma in adults is:** *(DNB 2011)*
    a. Benign
    b. Malignant
    c. Locally aggressive
    d. Border line

37. **Most common testicular tumor in prepubertal adults is:**
    (AIIMS May 2008)
    a. Yolk sac tumor
    b. Embryonal cell Ca
    c. Seminoma
    d. Teratoma

38. **Most malignant testicular tumour is:** *(DNB 2004)*
    a. Seminoma
    b. Teratoma
    c. Choriocarcinoma
    d. Embryonal carcinoma

39. **A 20-year-old male presents with scrotal mass. The first investigation to be done is:**
    (Recent Question 2014; JIPMER 2011)
    a. Clinical evaluation (Palpation and transillumination)
    b. USG
    c. Biopsy
    d. AFP

40. **Most radiosensitive testicular tumor is:**
    (UPSC 2005, MHPGMCET 2002)
    a. Seminoma
    b. Teratoma
    c. Lymphoma
    d. Sertoli cell tumor

41. **Most common testicular tumor in children:**
    (Recent Question 2017)
    a. Yolk sac tumor
    b. Leydig cell tumor
    c. Seminoma
    d. Choriocarcinoma

42. **A 12-year-old boy presents with serotal mass. The next best things to do in this patent is:** *(JIPMER 2011)*
    a. Clinical evaluation
    b. USG
    c. Biopsy
    d. Immenate surgery

■ TESTICULAR CARCINOMA STAGING

43. **High inguinal orchidectomy specimen showed tumor testis with involvement of epididymis without vascular invasion; stage is:** *(MAHE 2007)*
    a. T1
    b. T2
    c. T3
    d. T4

44. **High inguinal orchiectomy specimen showed teratoma testis with involvement of epididymis; stage is:**
    (DNB 2011, MAHE 2008)
    a. T1
    b. T2
    c. T3
    d. T4b

■ TESTICULAR CARCINOMA TREATMENT

45. **Stage I seminoma testis, treatment of choice is:**
    a. High inguinal orchidectomy *(AIIMS Nov 2001)*
    b. High inguinal orchidectomy and radiotherapy

c. Radiotherapy and chemotherapy
d. Trans-scrotal orchidectomy

46. Treatment of extragonadal germ cell tumour is: *(All India 99)*
    a. Chemotherapy
    b. Radiotherapy
    c. Surgery
    d. Immunotherapy

47. Stage-II testicular teratoma is treated by:
    a. Orchidectomy + RPLND   *(DNB 2008, 2005, AMU 05)*
    b. Orchidectomy + Chemotherapy
    c. Orchidectomy
    d. Radiotherapy

48. Treatment of stage I teratoma is: *(MCI Sept 2008)*
    a. Chemotherapy
    b. Radiotherapy
    c. Chemotherapy plus Radiotherapy
    d. Observation /RPLND

■ SEX CORD/GONADAL STROMAL TUMORS

49. Not true of sertoli cell tumour: *(Punjab 2009)*
    a. Poor response to radiotherapy
    b. Prominent lymphocytes in section
    c. Common in adults
    d. Can be malignant in 10–20% of cases

■ CARCINOMA SCROTUM

50. The lymph nodes first involved in cancer of the skin of the scrotum are: *(Karnataka 96)*
    a. Superficial inguinal
    b. External iliac
    c. Para aortic
    d. Gland of Cloquet

Explanations

■ UNDESCENDED TESTIS

1. **Ans. b. 6 months of age** *(Ref: Smith 18/e p380; Campbell 11/e p3443; Bailey 27/e p1498)*

   If spontaneous testicular descent does not occur, surgical treatment after 6 months of (corrected gestational) age is indicated.

2. **Ans. a. Seminoma** *(Campbell 11/e p3451)*

3. **Ans. d. Laparoscopy** *(Ref: Campbell 11/e p3441; Bailey 27/e p125)*

   - *"Laparoscopy is the procedure of choice to confirm or exclude the presence of a viable or remnant abdominal testis, unless a prominent scrotal nubbin is palpable with other clinical signs of monorchism." –Campbell 11/e p3441*

4. **Ans. c. Poorly developed secondary sexual characters**   5. **Ans. d. 1 year**

6. **Ans. d. Cryptorchidism** *(Ref: Campbell 11/e p3447)*

■ ECTOPIC TESTIS

7. **Ans. a. Superficial inguinal pouch** *(Ref: Smith 18/e p25; Bailey 27/e p1498)*

8. **Ans. a. Lumbar, c. Intra abdominal**

■ TESTICULAR TORSION

9. **Ans. b. Commonly associated with pyuria** *(Ref: Smith 18/e p707; Campbell 11/e p3391; Bailey 27/e p1500)*

10. **Ans. a. Torsion testis** *(Ref: Bailey 27/e p1500)*   11. **Ans. c. Elevation of testis reduces the pain**

12. **Ans. a. 6 hours** *(Ref: Campbell 11/e p3391)*   13. **Ans. a. Testicular torsion** *(Ref: Bailey 27/e p1498)*

■ VARICOCELE

14. **Ans. a. Common on the right side** *(Ref: Smith 18/e p707; Campbell 11/e p3393; Bailey 27/e p1501)*

15. **Ans. d. CA kidney**   16. **Ans. b. Can cause oligospermia**

17. **Ans. a. Varicocele** *(Ref: Campbell 11/e p3393)*   18. **Ans. b. Varicocelectomy** *(Ref: Bailey 27/e p1502)*

■ SPERMATOCELE

19. **Ans. b. Epididymal cyst**

20. **Ans. a. Head of epididymis**

■ HYDROCELE

21. Ans. a. Limited to scrotum *(Ref: Campbell 11/e p3384; Bailey 27/e p1503)*

22. Ans. d. Herniotomy

23. Ans. c. Hydrocele

24. Ans. c. Surgery *(Ref: Campbell 11/e p3386)*

■ EPIDIDYMO-ORCHITIS

25. Ans. c. Chlamydia trachomatis *(Ref: Smith 18/ep241; Campbell 10/e p3117-3118; Bailey 27/e p1505)*

26. Ans. b. Elevation of testes reduces pain of epididymitis

27. Ans. b. Decreased blood flow

28. Ans. a. Acute orchitis

■ FOURNIER'S GANGRENE

29. Ans. a. Testicles are involved

30. Ans. a. Scrotum

■ TESTICULAR CARCINOMA PREDISPOSING FACTORS

31. Ans. b. Undescended abdominal testis

■ TESTICULAR CARCINOMA

32. Ans. a. Seminoma *(Ref: Smith 18/e p381; Campbell 11/e p784; Bailey 27/e p1506; CSDT 11/e p1071)*

33. Ans. c. Seminoma

34. Ans. d. Teratoma *(Ref: Smith 18/e p381; Campbell 11/e p788)*

> - MC testicular tumour in **prepubertal adults**: Teratoma[Q]
> - MC testicular tumor of **infants** and **children**: Yolk sac tumor[Q]

35. Ans. c. Sertoli cell tumor *(Ref: Bailey 27/e p1506; Robbin's 9/e p975)*

"Germ cell tumours (90–95%): These include seminoma, embryonal cell carcinoma, yolk sac tumour, teratoma, and choriocarcinoma." - Bailey 27/e p1506

36. Ans. b. Malignant

37. Ans. d. Teratoma

38. Ans. c. Choriocarcinoma

39. Ans. b. USG

40. Ans. a. Seminoma

41. Ans. a. Yolk sac tumor *(Ref: Campbell 11/e p3594)*

42. Ans. a. Clinical evaluation

■ TESTICULAR CARCINOMA STAGING

43. Ans. a. T1 *(Ref: Campbell 11/e p791)*

44. Ans. a. T1

■ TESTICULAR CARCINOMA TREATMENT

45. Ans. b. High inguinal orchidectomy and radiotherapy

46. Ans. a. Chemotherapy

47. Ans. a. Orchidectomy + RPLND *(Ref: Smith 18/e p385; Campbell 11/e p796; Bailey 27/e p1508)*

48. Ans. d. Observation /RPLND

■ SEX CORD/GONADAL STROMAL TUMORS

49. Ans. b. Prominent lymphocytes in section *(Ref: Smith 18/e p387; Campbell 11/e p811)*

■ CARCINOMA SCROTUM

50. Ans. a. Superficial inguinal *(Ref: Smith 18/e p391)*

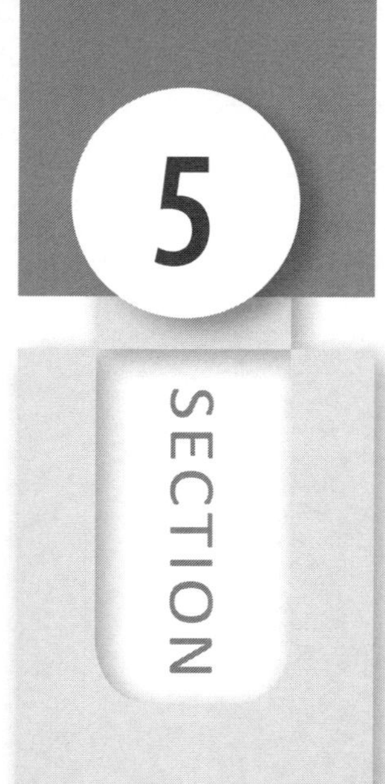

Cardiothoracic Vascular Surgery

- Arterial Disorders
- Venous Disorders
- Lymphatic System
- Thorax and Lung

Arterial Disorders

■ ARTERIAL OCCLUSION

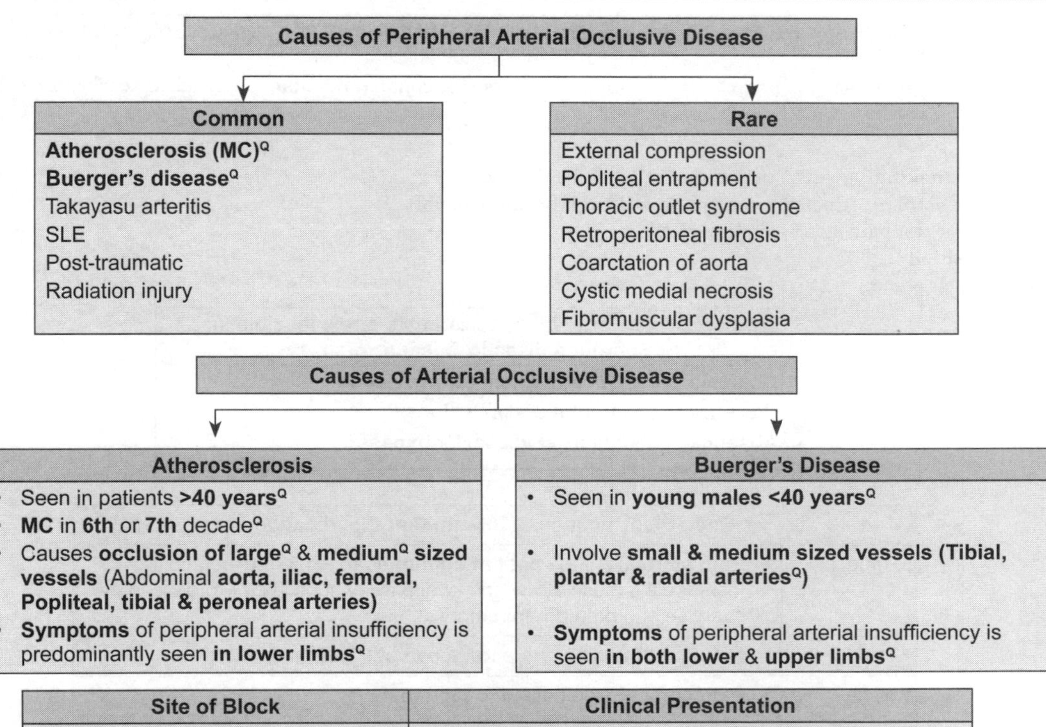

The table for "Causes of Arterial Occlusive Disease":

Atherosclerosis	Buerger's Disease
• Seen in patients **>40 years**^Q • **MC in 6th or 7th decade**^Q • Causes **occlusion of large**^Q **& medium**^Q **sized vessels** (Abdominal **aorta, iliac, femoral, Popliteal, tibial & peroneal arteries**) • **Symptoms** of peripheral arterial insufficiency is predominantly seen **in lower limbs**^Q	• Seen in **young males <40 years**^Q • Involve **small & medium sized vessels (Tibial, plantar & radial arteries**^Q**)** • **Symptoms** of peripheral arterial insufficiency is seen **in both lower & upper limbs**^Q

Site of Block	Clinical Presentation
Aorto-iliac disease	• **Buttock, thigh & calf** claudication^Q • Leriche syndrome^Q
Common femoral disease	• **Thigh & calf** claudication^Q
Superficial femoral disease	• Calf claudication^Q
Popliteal artery disease	• Calf claudication^Q
Crural artery disease	• Calf claudication^Q

■ BUERGER'S DISEASE (THROMBOANGIITIS OBLITERANS)

BUERGER'S DISEASE (THROMBOANGIITIS OBLITERANS)

- Segmental inflammatory disease^Q, affecting small & medium sized^Q arteries in upper & lower^Q extremities
- **Inflammatory process** involves **neighboring veins & nerves**^Q
- **Definite relationship with smoking**^Q

Histopathology

- Sharply segmental acute & chronic vasculitis of small & medium vessels with thrombosis of lumen which may undergo organization & recanalization^Q
- Thrombus contains microabscesses

- **Inflammatory process** extends to involve **neighboring veins & nerves**^Q
- With time, **all three structures (artery, vein & nerve)** become **incased in fibrous tissue**^Q

Contd...

Contd…

Clinical Features (RIM)
- Characterized **by triad of Intermittent claudication, Raynaud's phenomenon & Migratory superficial vein thrombophlebitis**[Q]

> - Typically seen in **young (<40 years), male smokers**[Q]

- **Not seen** in **females & non-smokers**[Q]
- Patient initially presents with **foot, leg, arm or hand claudication** progressing to **rest pain and ulcerations** on the toes, feet or fingers

> - **TAO** principally **affects distal (small + medium) vessels**[Q], so **claudication** is usually confined to **calves & feet or forearm & hands**

Diagnosis
- **Angiography of all four limbs**[Q] (multiple limbs may be involved)
- Even if symptoms are not yet present in a limb, angiographic findings may be demonstrated.

> - **Characteristic angiographic findings: Disease confinement to the distal circulation**, usually **infrapopliteal** and **distal to the brachial artery**[Q].
> - **Occlusions** are segmental and **show "skip" lesions with extensive collateralization**, the so-called **"corkscrew collaterals**[Q]**."**

Treatment
- **Abstinence from smoking**[Q] arrests, but does not reverse, the disease.
- **Vasodilators (Xanthinol nicotinate**[Q]**/complamina & Pentoxifylline**[Q]**/trental)**
- **Sympathectomy** for **rest pain** and **ulcerations**[Q]
- **Omental transposition**[Q]
- **Amputations**[Q] in gangrene

Surgical bypass or revascularization is rarely feasible in Buerger's disease, because of:
1.   **Occlusion of small & medium sized vessels**[Q]
2.   Presence of **segmental & skip lesions**[Q]
3.   **Absence** of **distal target vessel** for **bypass**[Q]

Boyd Classification of Intermittent Claudication	
Grade **1**	• **Pain starts** but if the **patient continues to walk**, the metabolites increase the muscle flow and sweep away substance P produced by exercise and **pain disappears**[Q].
Grade **2**	• **Pain continues** but the **patient can still walk** with effort[Q]
Grade **3**	• **Pain compels** the patient **to take rest**[Q]
Grade **4**	• **Rest pain**[Q]

■ LUMBAR SYMPATHECTOMY

Lumbar Sympathectomy

- **Open sympathectomy** is done preferably **through extraperitoneal approach**[Q].
- **Sympathetic chain** lies on the **sides of body of vertebra**, sometimes inside **psoas muscle sheath.**

> - In **unilateral surgeries**, sympathetic ganglia **L1, L2, L3** and sometimes **L4** are removed[Q].
> - In **bilateral surgeries, L1** of one side is **preserved to avoid retrograde ejaculation**[Q].

- **Lumbar chain** can be **mistaken** with **lymphatic chain, genitofemoral nerve, psoas sheath, psoas minor** leading to technical failure[Q].

Indications of Sympathectomy (BARA CHEF)	
• **Buerger's disease**[Q]	• **Erythrocyanosis**[Q]
• **Atherosclerosis** producing ischemia of limbs[Q]	• **Frost bite**[Q]
• **Raynaud's disease**[Q]	• **Hyperhydrosis**[Q]
• **Acrocyanosis**[Q]	• Peripheral vascular insufficiency
	• **Causalgia**[Q]

■ ANKLE BRACHIAL INDEX (ABI)

ANKLE BRACHIAL INDEX (ABI)

- **ABI** = Systolic **BP** at the **ankle** / Systolic **BP** in the **arms**
- Compared to the arm, **lower blood pressure in** the leg is an **indication of blocked arteries (peripheral vascular disease).**
- ABI is calculated by dividing the systolic blood pressure at the ankle by the systolic blood pressures in the arm.

ABI	Interpretation
>1.2	Noncompressible, severely calcified vessel (in DM & ESRD)[Q]
1.0-1.2	**Normal vessels**[Q]
0.5-0.9	Intermittent claudication[Q] (mild to moderate ischemia)
0.1-0.4	**Critical limb ischemia**[Q] (Ischemic ulceration, gangrene)

Fontaine Classification of Limb Ischemia	
Stage **I**	Asymptomatic[Q]
Stage **IIa**	**Mild** claudication[Q]
Stage **IIb**	**Moderate to severe** claudication[Q]
Stage **III**	Ischemic **rest pain**[Q]
Stage **IV**	**Ulceration** or **gangrene**[Q]

■ ARTERIAL ULCER

ARTERIAL ULCER

- **Arterial insufficiency ulcers ischemic ulcers** are mostly located on the **lateral surface of** the **ankle** or the **distal digits**[Q].
- **Most common** on **distal ends** of limbs[Q].

Etiology

- Caused by **lack of blood flow** to the capillary beds of lower extremities.
- Most often **endothelial dysfunction** is causative factor in **diabetic microangiopathy & macroangiopathy**[Q]

Characteristic Features

- **Punched-out appearance**[Q]
- **Intensely painful**[Q]
- **Pulses** are **not palpable**[Q]
- Associated **skin changes (thin shiny skin, absence of hair, brittle nails**[Q])

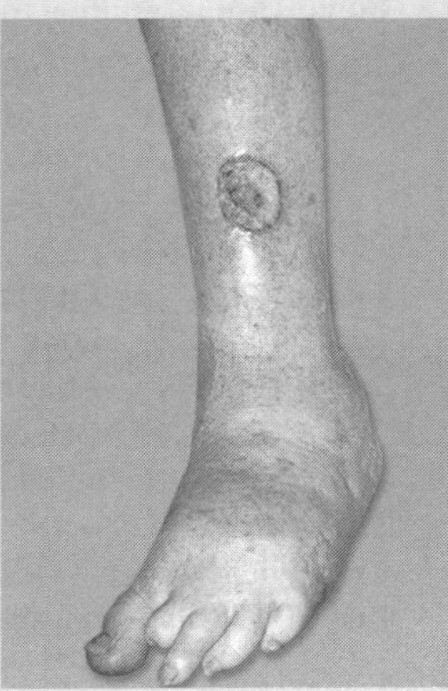

Diagnosis

- The lesion can be easily identified clinically.
- **Arterial doppler** & **pulse volume recordings** for baseline assessment of blood flow.
- **Radiographs** may be necessary **to rule outosteomyelitis.**

Treatment

- **Vascular surgery** to revascularize the area.
- In **infection: Antibiotics + Debridement**[Q]

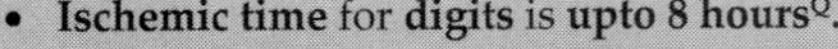

- **Ischemic time** for **digits** is **upto 8 hours**[Q].
- **Ischemic time** for **extremities** is **4-6 hours**[Q].
- **Organ containing bag** should be **placed in** a solution of **saline with ice**[Q].

■ ARTERIOVENOUS FISTULA (AVF)

ARTERIOVENOUS FISTULA (AVF)

- **AVF (**communication between an **artery** & vein) may be **congenital or acquired** (penetrating trauma **or** surgically created **for hemodialysis**)

Contd…

Contd…

- MC type of AVF: Congenital[Q]
- MC cause of acquired AVF: Penetrating trauma[Q]

- **Structural effects on veins:** Veins are **arterialized** (become **dilated, tortuous & thick walled**[Q])

Physiological Effects of AVF

- **Increased pulse pressure**[Q] (Increased systolic & decreased diastolic)
- **Increased venous return** leading to **increased HR & increased CO**[Q]
- **Left ventricular enlargement**[Q] and later **cardiac failure**[Q] may occur

- A **congenital fistula** in the young patient may cause **overgrowth of** the **limb**[Q]
- In the leg **indolent ulcers** may result from **relative ischemia below** the **short circuit**[Q]

Clinical Signs

- A **pulsatile swelling**[Q]
- **Thrill** on palpation[Q]
- **Continuous bruit** on auscultation[Q]

- **Nicoladoni's or Branham's sign:** Pressure on artery **proximal to fistula** causes the swelling to diminish in size, a **thrill** or **bruit to cease**, the **pulse rate** to **fall** & the **pulse pressure** returns to **normal**[Q].

Diagnosis

- **Duplex scan** and/or **angiography** confirm the diagnosis[Q].

Treatment

- Treatment is by **embolization**[Q].
- **Excisional surgery** (rarely) **for severe deformity** or **recurrent hemorrhage**[Q].

■ THORACIC OUTLET COMPRESSION SYNDROME (TOS)

THORACIC OUTLET COMPRESSION SYNDROME (TOS)

- **TOS** refers to **compression of subclavian vessels** & nerves of **brachial plexus** in the region of **thoracic inlet**[Q].
- Divided into: **Vascular forms** (Arterial and /or Venous) & **Neurogenic forms**
- **Compression** resulting from TOS **is dynamic & best evaluated clinically by mechanical provocative maneuvers**[Q]

- **Symptoms most commonly** develop **secondary to neural compromise**[Q]
- **Middle-aged women**[Q] are most commonly affected

Neurovascular structures of the upper extremity may be compressed by	
• **Cervical rib**[Q]	• Trauma (neck hematoma, **bone dislocation**[Q])
• **Long transverse process of C7**[Q]	• **Fibrous bands**[Q] (congenital and acquired)
• **Abnormal first rib**[Q]	• **Neoplasms**[Q]
• Osteoarthritis	• **Scalenes muscle**[Q]

Clinical Features

- Symptoms vary depending on the anatomic structure that is compressed[Q].
- In > 90% of cases, neurogenic manifestations are reported[Q].

- **Ulnar nerve (C8-T1) involvement is most common**[Q].
- It is **associated with:**
  - **Motor weakness & atrophy of the hypothenar & interosseous muscles**[Q]
  - **Pain & paresthesia along the medial aspect of the arm, hand, 5th finger & medial aspect of 4th finger**[Q].

- Symptoms of **subclavian artery compression:** Fatigue, weakness, coldness, ischemic pain, & paresthesia. **Thrombosis with distal embolization** rarely can occur, producing vasomotor symptoms **(Raynaud's phenomenon)** in the hand or **ischemic changes**[Q].
- **Venous compression: Edema, venous distention, collateral formation, & cyanosis** of the affected limb[Q]

Diagnosis

- **Compression** resulting from TOS **is dynamic** and **best evaluated clinically by mechanical provocative maneuvers**[Q]
- **Specific investigations** (CT scan, MRI, Angiography, X-ray) **are used to exclude other conditions** and to **establish the associated diagnosis**[Q].

Contd…

Contd…

Treatment
- Approx. **50-90%** of patients can be **successfully treated** by **improvements** in **postural sitting, standing & sleeping positions, behavior modification** at work and **muscle stretching & strengthening exercises**[Q].

Indications for Surgical Intervention
• **Failure of conservative management**[Q]
• **Progression of** sensory or motor **symptoms**[Q]
• Presence of **excessively prolonged ulnar or median nerve conduction velocities**[Q]
• **Narrowing** or **occlusion** of the **subclavian artery**[Q]
• **Thrombosis** of the **axillary** or **subclavian vein**[Q]

- **Operation for TOS: Complete removal** of the **first rib**, with **division of scalenus** anticus & medius[Q].
- **Large aneurysms** or thrombosis of the **subclavian artery: Graft reconstruction**[Q]
- **Subclavian vein thrombosis: Thrombolytic & anticoagulant therapy** and simultaneous **surgical decompression**[Q].

Provocative Clinical Tests to establishing the diagnosis of Thoracic Outlet Syndrome (TOS)		
Provocative Test	**Instruction**	**Inference**
Adson's Test[Q] **(Scalene Test)**	Patient is instructed to: • Take a **deep breath and hold it** • **Extend** the **neck fully** • **Turn faZce towards** the **side**	• Maneuver **tightens** the **anterior & middle scalene muscles,** thus decreasing the interscalene space & magnifying any preexisting compression. • **Obliteration** or diminution **of radial pulse** suggests the diagnosis
Costoclavicular Test[Q] **(Military Position or Halsted Test)**	Patient is instructed to: • Draw shoulders downwards and backwards	• Maneuver narrows the costoclavicular space by approximating the clavicle to the first rib thus tending to compress the neurovascular bundle • Obliteration of radial pulse or reproduction of symptoms indicates compression
Hyperabduction Test[Q] **(Wright Test)**	Patient is instructed to: • **Hyperabduct** (Raise) the **arm to 180°**	• Maneuver causes the neurovascular structures to be pulled around the pectoralis minor tendon, coracoid process and head of humerus • Obliteration or diminution of radial pulse suggests the diagnosis
Roos Test[Q] **(Arm Claudication Test)**	Patient is instructed to: • Draw shoulders backwards • Rise **arms to horizontal position** with **elbows flexed to 90°** • Exercise the hands	• **Numbness** or **pain in** the **hands with exercise** suggests the diagnosis

■ ANEURYSM

ANEURYSM

- **Aneurysm:** Permanent & irreversible localized dilatation of blood vessel with at least **50% increase** in diameter
- **Ectasia:** dilatation <50% of normal diameter
- **AAA** (abdominal aortic aneurysm) is diagnosed if diameter **>3 cm** in males or **>2.6 cm** in **females**

• **MC vessel involved in aneurysm: Circle of Willis**[Q]
• **MC location of extra-cranial aneurysm: Aorta >Iliac >Popliteal >Femoral (AIPF)**[Q]
• **MC site of extra-cranial arterial aneurysm** is **infrarenal aorta**[Q]
• **MC site of peripheral aneurysm: Popliteal aneurysm**[Q]
• **Degenerative aneurysms (caused by atherosclerosis)** are **MC AAA (90%)**[Q]

- **Width of aneurysm** is **most important** predicting **factor** of **rupture**[Q].
- **Juan Parodi**[Q] introduced endovascular aortic aneurysm repair **(EVAR).**

Classification
- **True** (all three layers of vessel are involved), **false** (do not have all three layers of vessel)
- **Infected (mycotic) aneurysm** are false aneurysm
- **Dissecting aneurysm** (dissection with aneurysmal dilatation of false lumen)
- **Fusiform (symmetrical enlargement** involving whole circumference of artery)
- **Saccular** (affect **only part** of the arterial circumference) have **higher risk of rupture**[Q]

■ MYCOTIC ANEURYSM

MYCOTIC ANEURYSM

- **Mycotic aneurysms** are **focal dilatation of arteries** occurring at **points in the arterial wall weakened by infection**

Contd…

Contd...

Mycotic aneurysms may originate
1. As a result of **embolization from bacterial endocarditis**[Q]
2. As an **extension of** an **adjacent suppurative process**[Q] **(extravascular source)**, ex. Osteomyelitis, sinus infection, meningitis etc.
3. By **circulating organisms** directly **infecting arterial wall**[Q]

- MC location: Femoral artery >Aorta[Q]
- MC organisms: Staphylococcus >Salmonella[Q]

Minimum Size for Surgery (**AIPF**: All India Police Force)
Abdominal **A**ortic Aneurysm (**5.5 cm**) = **I**liac aneurysm (**3.5 cm**) + **P**opliteal/**F**emoral aneurysm (**2.0 cm**)

Indications of Surgery in Aneurysms on the basis of Size (diameter)	
• Descending thoracic aorta	• ≥6.5 cm[Q]
• Ascending thoracic aorta	• ≥5.5 cm[Q]
• Abdominal aorta	• ≥5.5 cm[Q]
• Iliac artery	• ≥3.5 cm[Q]
• Femoral & Popliteal artery	• ≥2.0 cm[Q]

■ SUBCLAVIAN ARTERY STENOSIS

Subclavian Artery Stenosis

- MC cause of subclavian artery stenosis: Atherosclerotic disease
- Left[Q] subclavian artery stenosis is significantly more common than right

> - **MC site** of stenosis: **First part**[Q] of subclavian artery
> - Stenosis **typically occurs just distal to origin of subclavian artery & lies proximal to origin of vertebral artery**[Q].

- **Stenosis of first part** of subclavian artery may give rise to **subclavian steal syndrome**[Q]
- **Subclavian steal syndrome** is characterized by **reversed flow in vertebral artery** to compensate for a proximal stenosis in the ipsilateral subclavian artery there by **stealing blood from** the **'brain'** to feed the **'arm'**[Q].

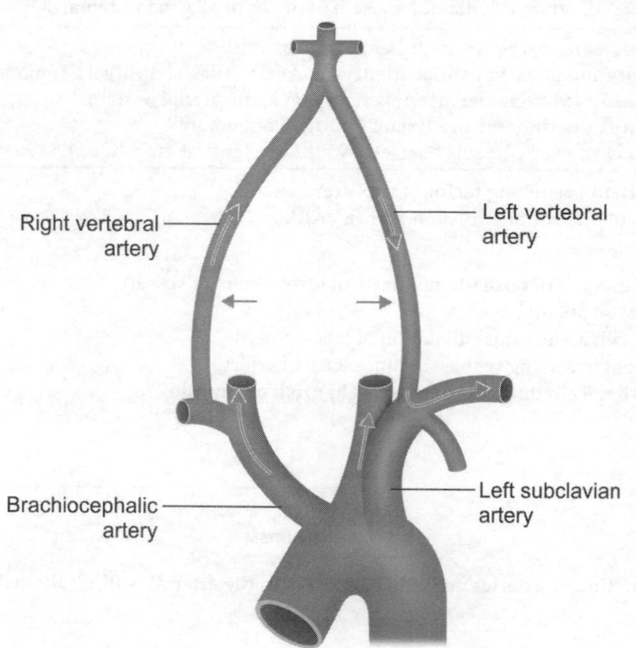

■ SUBCLAVIAN STEAL SYNDROME

SUBCLAVIAN STEAL SYNDROME

- **Occlusion of** either the **innominate (brachiocephalic)** or the **subclavian artery before the origin of vertebral artery reverses the direction of blood flow** in the **ipsilateral vertebral artery**[Q].

  - This **reversal of flow** often is **asymptomatic** but **may cause ischemia** in the **posterior circulation**[Q].
  - **Neurological features** are weakness, vertigo, visual complaints, & syncope[Q].
  - Classically **symptoms occur** when **arm exercise increase** the **steal of blood flow from** the **brainstem**[Q].

- The **exercise reduces peripheral resistance** in the affected arm, **lowering blood pressure distal to occlusion.** This in turn results in **increased retrograde flow from** the **vertebral artery**[Q].
- If the contralateral vertebral artery cannot keep up with the demand, the **arm** may **steal blood from the basilar artery,** lowering the pressure in the **posterior cerebral circulation**[Q].
- The result may be transient vertebrobasilar ischemia[Q].

■ VASCULAR GRAFT

Vascular Graft	
Bioprosthetic	**Synthetic**

• **Autograft**[Q]
• **Homograft (allograft)**
• **Heterograft (Xenograft)**
• **Tissue engineered**
	• **Textile:**
	  – **Dacron**[Q]
	• **Non-textile:**
	  – **ePTFE**[Q]
	  – **Polyurethane**[Q]

Best natural vascular graft: Reversed saphenous vein[Q]
Best **synthetic** vascular graft: **Dacron**[Q]
Best vascular graft for **suprainguinal bypass: Dacron**[Q]
Best vascular graft for **infrainguinal bypass: Saphenous vein**[Q]
Best vascular graft for **aorta: Dacron**[Q]
Most preferred graft for CABG: LIMA (left internal mammary artery) > Saphenous vein[Q]
MC used graft for CABG: Saphenous vein[Q]

Multiple Choice Questions

■ ARTERIAL OCCLUSION

1. The most common cause of peripheral limb ischemia in India is: *(AIIMS Nov 2005)*
   a. Trauma
   b. Atherosclerosis
   c. Buerger's disease
   d. Takayasu disease

2. Which among the following is not a feature of peripheral arterial occlusion? *(Recent Question 2016)*
   a. Shock
   b. Pallor
   c. Pain
   d. Pulselessness

3. Not a feature of acute arterial occlusion: *(DNB 2010, AIIMS Nov 98)*
   a. Cyanosis
   b. Pallor
   c. Paralysis
   d. Paraesthesia

4. Fogarty's catheter is used for: *(Recent Question 2015; UPSC 2007)*
   a. Drainage of urinary bladder
   b. Parenteral hyperalimentation
   c. Removal of embolus form blood vessels
   d. Ureteric catheterization

5. Intermittent claudication is defined as: *(All India 2009)*
   a. Pain in muscle at rest only
   b. Pain in muscle on first step
   c. Pain in muscle on exercise only
   d. Pain in muscle on last step

6. In a subclavian artery block at outer border of 1st rib, all of the following arteries help in maintaining the circulation to upper limb except: *(AIIMS May 2011)*
   a. Subscapular artery
   b. Superior thoracic artery
   c. Thyrocervical trunk
   d. Suprascapular artery

7. Intermittent claudication at the level of the hip indicates:
   a. Popliteal artery occlusion *(Recent Question 2016)*
   b. Bilateral iliac artery occlusion
   c. Common femoral occlusion
   d. Superficial femoral artery occlusion

8. Intermittent claudication is defined as pain__________?
   a. At rest *(MCI Nov 2017)*
   b. On first step of walking
   c. Relieved on standing still
   d. Increase on limb dependency

9. Which of the following is true about Leriche syndrome?
   a. Caused by aortoiliac occlusion *(Recent Question 2017)*
   b. Erection or impotence problems
   c. Gluteal claudication is seen
   d. All of the above

10. Fontaine and Rutherford classification of peripheral arterial disease is based on: *(Recent Question 2017)*
    a. Clinical
    b. Arterial stenosis on imaging
    c. Both clinical and arterial stenosis on imaging
    d. All of the above

11. A 45-years-old policeman comes from duty with complain of pain in right buttock and right leg. On examination, pulse in right popliteal fossa was absent, whereas on the left side it was normal. The block is at which level?
    a. Femoral
    b. Iliac *(MCI Dec 2019)*
    c. Aortoiliac
    d. Popliteal

■ BUERGER'S DISEASE

12. Buerger's disease usually affects all of the following except: *(Recent Question 2014; MCI Sept 2009, 2010)*
    a. Small sized arteries
    b. Medium sized arteries
    c. Large arteries
    d. Deep veins

13. Superficial thrombophlebitis is seen in: *(MCI March 2005)*
    a. AV fistula
    b. Raynaud's disease
    c. Buerger's disease
    d. Aneurysm

14. Which of the following is true about Buerger's disease?
    a. Atherosclerotic *(AIIMS Nov 2012)*
    b. Neural involvement present
    c. Ulnar artery and peroneal arteries involved
    d. Only arteriole is involved

15. What is the diagnosis based on the given image? *(Recent Question 2016)*
    a. Dry gangrene
    b. Raynaud's disease
    c. Wet gangrene
    d. Gas gangrene

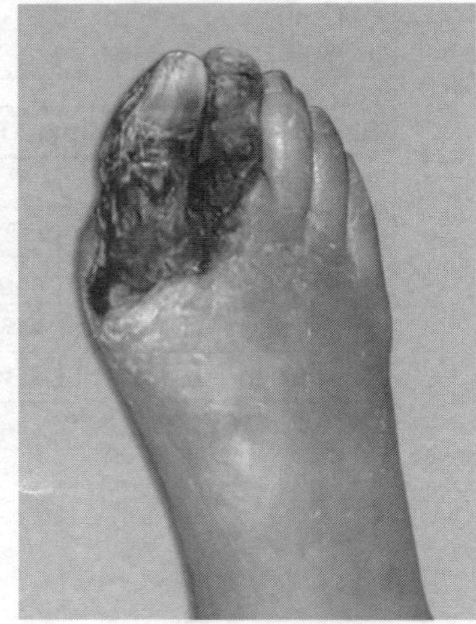

16. Identify the lesion shown below: *(MCI Dec 2018)*
    a. Wet gangrene
    b. Dry gangrene
    c. Frost-bite
    d. Ainhum

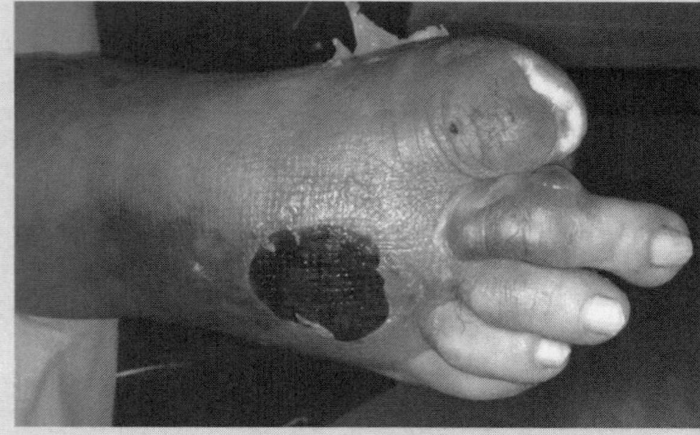

17. Buerger's disease affects all except: *(Recent Question 2015; DNB 2009)*
    a. Lymphatics
    b. Small vessels
    c. Nerves
    d. Veins

■ LUMBAR SYMPATHECTOMY

18. Lumbar sympathectomy is of value in the management of:
   a. Intermittent claudication   *(All India 2009, 2005)*
   b. Distal ischemia affecting the skin of the toes
   c. Arteriovenous fistula
   d. Back pain

19. Sympathectomy is indicated in all following conditions except: *(All India 2009, 2003, Punjab 2007)*
   a. Ischemic ulcers   b. Intermittent claudication
   c. Anhidrosis   d. Acrocyanosis

20. Which of the following is spared in lumbar sympathectomy?   *(Recent Question 2015, JIPMER Nov 2017)*
   a. L1   b. L2
   c. L3   d. L4

■ CRITICAL LIMB ISCHEMIA

21. An adult patient with leg pain and gangrene of toe. His ankle to brachial arterial pressure ratio would be less than:
   a. 1   b. 0.3   *(DNB 2011)*
   c. 0.5   d. 0.8

22. Normal value of ankle brachial index is: *(Recent Question 2014, 2013)*
   a. 0.8   b. 1
   c. 1.2   d. 1.4

23. ABPI in imminent necrosis: *(Recent Question 2015)*
   a. < 0.3   b. < 0.6
   c. < 0.9   d. > 1.2

24. False elevation of ABPI is seen in: *(Recent Question 2018)*
   a. DVT
   b. Acute limb ischemia
   c. Chronic venous insufficiency
   d. Calcified vessel walls

■ ARTERIAL ULCER

25. Foot ulcers secondary to arterial insufficiency are successfully treated by all of the following techniques except:
   a. Debridement of devitalized tissue   *(COMEDK 2004)*
   b. Elevation of the affected extremity
   c. Antibiotic administration
   d. Bed rest

■ AMPUTATION

26. Re-implantation time for lower limb is: *(Kerala 97)*
   a. 6 hours   b. 4 hours
   c. 8 hours   d. 10 hours

27. For reimplantation surgery, the detached digit or limb is best preserved in cold: *(Recent Question 2014; UPSC 2000)*
   a. Glycerol   b. Distilled water
   c. Hypertonic saline   d. Isotonic saline

28. Amputated finger is transported in: *(Recent Question 2017)*
   a. Plastic bag with wet ice
   b. Plastic bag with dry ice
   c. Plastic bag with cold saline
   d. Plastic bag with cold water

■ ARTERIOVENOUS FISTULA

29. Nicoladoni sign is also known as: *(AIIMS Nov 2008)*
   a. Murray sign   b. Frei sign
   c. Darrier sign   d. Branham sign

30. The most common cause of acquired arteriovenous fistula is: *(All India 2006)*
   a. Bacterial infection   b. Fungal infection
   c. Blunt trauma   d. Penetrating trauma

31. Commonest cause of A-V fistulae is: *(Recent Question 2013, DNB 2000)*
   a. Congenital   b. Traumatic
   c. Surgical creation   d. Tumor erosion

■ THORACIC OUTLET SYNDROME

32. Thoracic outlet syndrome is primarily diagnosed by:
   a. Clinical evaluation   b. CT scan   *(All India 2009)*
   c. MRI   d. Angiography

33. Adson's test is positive in: *(MHSSMCET 2005)*
   a. Cervical spondylosis   b. Fracture ribs
   c. Cervical rib   d. All of the above

34. Which is not true about thoracic outlet syndrome?   *(Recent Question 2016, AIIMS Nov 98)*
   a. Radial nerve is commonly affected
   b. Neurological features are most common
   c. Resection of 1st rib relieves symptom
   d. Positive Adson's test

35. Commonest symptom associated with thoracic outlet syndrome is: *(Recent Question 2016)*
   a. Intermittent claudication   b. Pain on radial distribution
   c. Pain in ulnar distribution   d. Gangrene

36. Adson's test is used for determining vascular insufficiency. It is useful in: *(Recent Question 2013)*
   a. Peripheral vascular disease
   b. Varicose veins
   c. Cervical rib
   d. AV fistula

37. All of the following are predisposing factors for thoracic outlet syndrome except: *(Recent Question 2017)*
   a. Scalene muscle
   b. Long transverse process of C7
   c. Spondylosis
   d. Cervical rib

■ RAYNAUD'S DISEASE

38. Raynaud's syndrome occurs in all of the following except:
   a. SLE   *(DNB 2009, MCI Sept 2007)*
   b. Rheumatoid arthritis
   c. Osteoarthritis   d. Cryoglobulinemia

39. Sequence of colour changes observed in Raynaud's disease: *(MCI Sept 2009)*
   a. Red, blue, white   b. White, blue, red
   c. Blue, red, white   d. White, red, blue

40. If a patient with Raynaud's disease immersed his hand in cold water, the hand will: *(All India 2003)*
   a. Become red   b. Remain unchanged
   c. Turn white   d. Become blue

■ DIABETIC FOOT

41. Diabetic gangrene is due to: *(Kerala 94)*
   a. Ischemia   b. Increased blood glucose
   c. Altered defense by host and neuropathy
   d. All of the above

42. Etiopathogenesis of diabetic foot include the following except: *(UPSC 2007)*
   a. Myelopathy   b. Osteoarthropathy
   c. Microangiopathy   d. Infection

■ AORTIC DISSECTION

43. The most common site of acute aortic dissection is:
    a. Right lateral wall of ascending aorta
    b. Arch of aorta   *(DNB 2013, COMEDK 2010)*
    c. Suprarenal abdominal aorta
    d. Infrarenal abdominal aorta

■ AORTIC ANEURYSM

44. Most common cause of abdominal aortic aneurysm is:
    a. Atherosclerosis   b. Trauma   *(All India 2010)*
    c. Syphilis   d. Vasculitis

45. The most common site of rupture of abdominal aortic
    aneurysm is: *(All India 2009)*
    a. Laterally into the left retroperitoneum
    b. Laterally into the right retroperitoneum
    c. Posteriorly into the posterior retroperitoneum
    d. Anteriorly into the peritoneum (Intraperitoneal)

46. Abdominal aortic aneurysm is operated when the size is
    more than: *(Recent Question 2018)*
    a. 35 mm   b. 45 mm
    c. 55 mm   d. 65 mm

47. Mycotic aneurysm is aneurysm infected because of:
    a. Fungal infection   *(All India 2006)*
    b. Blood borne infection (Intravascular)
    c. Infection introduced from outside (Extravascular)
    d. Both intravascular and extra-vascular infection

48. The procedure of choice for the evaluation of aortic aneurysm is:
    a. Ultrasonography   *(Recent Question 2013, All India 2006)*
    b. Computed tomography
    c. Magnetic resonance imaging
    d. Arteriography

49. Which of the following is true about coeliac plexus block?
    a. Located retroperitoneally at the level of L3
    b. Usually done unilaterally   *(AIIMS May 2013)*
    c. Useful for the painful conditions of lower abdomen
    d. Most common side effect is diarrhea and hypotension

50. In the abdomen, aneurysms of the commonly occur ...... next
    only to the aorta: *(Recent Question 2016)*
    a. Internal iliac artery   b. External iliac artery
    c. Splenic artery   d. Inferior mesenteric artery

■ FEMORAL ARTERY ANEURYSM

51. Treatment of femoral artery aneurysm: *(PGI June 2007)*
    a. Ultrasound guided compression of the neck of aneurysm
    b. Thrombin injection
    c. Bypass graft repair
    d. Ligation of involved vessel

■ POPLITEAL ARTERY ANEURYSM

52. Most common site of peripheral aneurysm: *(MCI June 2018,
    Nov 2017; Recent Question 2015; AIIMS Nov 2008)*
    a. Femoral artery   b. Radial artery
    c. Popliteal artery   d. Brachial artery

■ PSEUDOANEURYSM

53. Pseudoaneurysms are most commonly due to:
                (Recent Question 2015; JIPMER 93)
    a. Atherosclerosis   b. Trauma
    c. Congenital deficiency   d. Infections

■ SUBCLAVIAN STEAL SYNDROME

54. Commonest part of subclavian artery to be affected by
    stenosis is: *(All India 2009)*
    a. First part   b. Second part
    c. Third part   d. Equally affected

55. Which of the following statement is true regarding subcla-
    vian steal syndrome?   *(AIIMS Nov 2005)*
    a. Reversal of blood flow in the ipsilateral vertebral artery
    b. Reversal of blood flow in the contralateral carotid artery
    c. Reversal of blood flow in the contralateral vertebral artery
    d. Bilateral reversal of the flow in the vertebral arteries

■ VASCULAR GRAFT

56. Best graft for femoropopliteal bypass:
                (JIPMER May 2018; MHSSMCET 2007)
    a. Autologous vein   b. Dacron
    c. Teflon   d. PTF

57. Best material for below inguinal arterial graft is:
    a. Saphenous vein graft (upside-down)
    b. PTFE   *(WBPG 2015; All India 2009)*
    c. Dacron
    d. Teflon

58. Neointimal hyperplasia causes vascular graft failure as a
    result of hypertrophy of: *(All India 2006)*
    a. Endothelial cells   b. Collagen fibers
    c. Smooth muscle cells   d. Elastic fibers

59. Dacron vascular graft is:
                (Recent Question 2013, All India 2006)
    a. Nontextile synthetic   b. Textile synthetic
    c. Nontextile biologic   d. Textile biologic

60. Preferred material for femoro-popliteal bypass:
                (Recent Question 2018, 2017, 2014)
    a. Dacron   b. PTFE
    c. Saphenous vein   d. Gortex

61. Best graft for aortic dissection: *(JIPMER May 2018)*
    a. Dacron   b. Autologous vein
    c. Autologous artery   d. PTFE

62. Most preferred vascular graft for CABG:
                (Recent Question 2017)
    a. LIMA   b. RIMA
    c. Long saphenous vein   d. PTFE

■ VASCULAR TRAUMA

63. Management of subclavian artery injury due to inadvertent
    central catheter insertion include all of the following except:
                (Recent Question 2018)
    a. Closure device   b. Mechanical compression
    c. Covering stent   d. Track embolization

■ ANGIOGRAPHY AND COMPLICATIONS

64. Seldinger needle is used for: *(MCI March 2010)*
    a. Suturing muscles   b. Arteriography
    c. Pulmonary biopsy   d. Lymphangiography

■ TAKAYASU ARTERITIS

65. In Takayasu arteritis most common artery involved is:
                (Recent Question 2017, JIPMER 2014)
    a. Common carotid artery   b. Subclavian artery
    c. Renal artery   d. Inferior mesenteric artery

■ MISCELLANEOUS

66. Allen's test is useful in evaluating:
(APPG 2015, DNB 2011, All India 2006)
- a. Thoracic outlet compression
- b. Presence of cervical rib
- c. Integrity of palmar arch
- d. Digital blood flow

67. The artery commonly involved in cirsoid aneurysm is:
(Recent Question 2016)
- a. Occipital
- b. Superficial temporal
- c. Internal carotid
- d. External carotid

68. The Hunterian ligature operation is performed for:
(Recent Question 2014; DNB 2003, AIIMS Nov 2008, All India 2003)
- a. Aneurysm
- b. Varicose veins
- c. AV fistulas
- d. Acute arterial ischemia

69. Mycotic aneurysm occurs due to: *(MHSSMCET 2007)*
- a. Fungus
- b. Syphilis
- c. Salmonella
- d. Medial necrosis of arteries

70. Butcher's thigh is: *(DNB 2010)*
- a. Vastus lateral rupture
- b. Subcutaneous lipodermatosclerosis
- c. Bursa in adductor canal
- d. Accidental injury to major vessels in thigh or groin

71. What is the best way to control external hemorrhage?
- a. Direct pressure
- b. Elevation *(DNB 2012)*
- c. Proximal torniquet
- d. Artery forceps

72. Which of the following is the best management for radiation induced occlusive disease of carotid artery? *(MCI Nov 2017)*
- a. Low dose aspirin
- b. Carotid angioplasty and stenting
- c. Carotid endarterectomy
- d. Carotid bypass procedure

Explanations

■ ARTERIAL OCCLUSION

1. **Ans. b. Atherosclerosis** *(Ref: ASI Surgery/1333)*

   - ASI says **"Most common cause** of **peripheral limb ischemia in adults in India is atherosclerosis**[Q].

2. **Ans. a. Shock**

3. **Ans. a. Cyanosis**

4. **Ans. c. Removal of embolus form blood vessels** *(Ref: Sabiston 20/e p1778; Schwartz 11/e p956, 10/e p877; Bailey 27/e p955)*

FOGARTY BALLOON CATHETER

   - **Fogarty balloon catheter** is used for **removal of embolus** form blood vessels[Q]
   - **Embolectomy:**
     - Artery (usually the **femoral**), **bulging with clot**, is exposed and held in slings.
     - Through a longitudinal or transverse incision the **clot** begins to extrude and is **removed, together with** the **embolus, with** the help of a **Fogarty balloon catheter**[Q].
     - Catheter, with its balloon tip, is introduced both proximally and distally until it is deemed to have passed the limit of the clot.
     - **Balloon is inflated and catheter withdrawn slowly,** together with any obstructing material.
     - **Procedure** is **repeated until bleeding occurs.**

5. **Ans. c. Pain in muscle on exercise only** *(Ref: Sabiston 20/e p1765; Schwartz 11/e p954, 10/e p828,882; Bailey 27/e p943,947)*

   - **Intermittent Claudication**: Crampy pain in muscles induced by exercise (walking) and **relieved by rest.**

INTERMITTENT CLAUDICATION

   - **Crampy pain in muscles that is:**
     - **Brought on by walking**[Q] (exercise)
     - **Relieved by standing still/rest**[Q] (unlike pseudoclaudication)
     - **Not present on** taking the **first step**[Q] (unlike osteoarthritis)

6. **Ans. b. Superior thoracic artery** *(Ref: BDC 4/e pvol I/56, 82)*

   A rich anastomosis exists around the scapula between branches of subclavian artery (first part) and the axillary artery (third part). This anastomosis provides a collateral circulation through which blood can flow to the limb when the distal part of subclavian artery or the proximal part of axillary artery is blocked.

Anastomosis around Scapula
• Formed by branches of: – **First part** of **subclavian artery**[Q] (**Suprascapular**[Q] and deep branches of **transverse cervical** artery[Q]) – **Third part** of **axillary artery**[Q] (**Subscapular** and its **circumflex scapular** branch[Q])

7. **Ans. b. Bilateral iliac artery occlusion** *(Ref: Sabiston 20/e p1756-1758; Schwartz 11/e p941, 10/e p874; Bailey 27/e p943-944)*

8. **Ans. c. Relieved on standing still** *(Ref: Bailey 27/e p943, 947)*

9. **Ans. d. All of the above** *(Ref: Sabiston 20/e p1738; Schwartz 11/e p941, 10/e p874; Bailey 27/e p943)*

10. **Ans. a. Clinical** *(Ref: Sabiston 20/e p1757; Schwartz 11/e p952, 10/e p883)*

11. **Ans. c. Aortoiliac** *(Ref: Bailey 27/e p943)*

■ BUERGER'S DISEASE

12. **Ans. c. Large arteries**

13. **Ans. c. Buerger's disease**

14. **Ans. b. Neural involvement present** *(Ref: Robbins 9/e p512; Sabiston 20/e p1780; Schwartz 11/e p974, 10/e p906,1822; Bailey 27/e p567; Harrison 20/e p1925)*

15. **Ans. a. Dry gangrene** *(Ref: Sabiston 20/e p1780)*

16. **Ans. a. Wet gangrene** *(Ref: Bailey 27/e p952)*

   "Wet gangrene occurs when superadded infection and putrefaction are present. Crepitus may be palpated as a result of infection by gas-forming organisms, commonly in diabetic foot problems, and should be considered a surgical emergency with urgent tissue debridement or amputation required." - Bailey 27/e p952

17. **Ans. a. Lymphatics**

■ LUMBAR SYMPATHECTOMY

18. **Ans. b. Distal ischemia affecting the skin of the toes** *(Ref: Sabiston 20/e p1780; Schwartz 11/e p974, 10/e p906; Bailey 27/e p968)*
    - **Lumbar sympathectomy is indicated** in the management of distal ischemia affecting skin of the toes.
    - Arteriovenous fistula, back pain and intermittent claudication are not included amongst the indications for lumbar sympathectomy.

    - MC indication of sympathectomy is ischemic disorders mainly of the limbs[Q].
    - MC ischemic condition for which sympathectomy is carried out is peripheral vascular occlusive disease of the young male smokers[Q].
    - Lumbar sympathectomy is not of value in the management of intermittent claudication[Q]

19. **Ans. b. Intermittent claudication c. Anhidrosis** *(Ref: Sabiston 20/e p1780; Schwartz 11/e p974, 10/e p906; Bailey 27/e p968)*
    - **Sympathectomy is used for the treatment of hyperhydrosis. It would worsen anhydrosis rather than treating it.**

20. **Ans. a. L1** *(Ref: Sabiston 20/e p1780; Bailey 25/e p924)*

■ CRITICAL LIMB ISCHEMIA

21. **Ans. b. 0.3**   22 **Ans. b. 1**

23. **Ans. a. < 0.3**   24. **Ans. d. Calcified vessel walls** *(Ref: Sabiston 20/e p1758; Schwartz 11/e p958, 10/e p830; Bailey 27/e p945)*

■ ARTERIAL ULCER

25. **Ans. b. Elevation of the affected extremity**

■ AMPUTATION

26. **Ans. a. 6 hours** *(Ref: Essential Emergency Trauma by Kaushal Shah, Daniel Egan, Joshua Quaas– 2010/679)*

    - Ischemic time for digits is upto 8 hours[Q].
    - Ischemic time for extremities is 4-6 hours[Q].
    - Organ containing bag should be placed in a solution of saline with ice[Q].

27. **Ans. d. Isotonic saline**

    - A phantom limb is the sensation that an **amputated or missing limb** (even an organ appendix) is **still attached to the body** and is moving appropriately with other body parts based upon **"Law of Projection"**.
    - It states that no matter where a sensory pathwayis stimulated alongsts coure, the sensation produced is referred back to site of receptor.

28. **Ans. a. Plastic bag with wet ice** *(Ref: Sabiston 20/e p1996; Schwartz 11/e p1938, 10/e p1800)*

    "If it is anticipated that the amputated part will be considered for replantation, it is critical to transport the patient and the part in an appropriate manner. The amputated part is placed in a clean, dry, plastic bag, which is sealed and placed on top of ice in a Styrofoam container. This keeps the part sufficiently cool at 4° C to 10° C without freezing. The amputated part is wrapped in a lightly moistened saline gauze to prevent tissue drying."- Sabiston 20/e p1996

    "In preparation for replantation, the amputated part and proximal stump should be appropriately treated. The amputated part should be wrapped in moistened gauze and placed in a sealed plastic bag. This bag should then be placed in an ice water bath. Do not use dry ice, and do not allow the part to contact ice directly; frostbite can occur in the amputated part, which will decrease its chance of survival after replantation. Bleeding should be controlled in the proximal stump by as minimal a means necessary, and the stump should be dressed with a non-adherent gauze and bulky dressing."-Schwartz 11/e p1938, 10/e p1800

■ ARTERIOVENOUS FISTULA

29. **Ans. d. Branham sign**   30. **Ans. d. Penetrating trauma**   31. **Ans. a. Congenital**

■ THORACIC OUTLET SYNDROME

32. **Ans. a. Clinical evaluation** *(Ref: Sabiston 20/e p1604; Bailey 26/e p872)*
    - **Thoracic outlet syndrome is diagnosed primarily by clinical evaluation and the diagnosis is based on reproducibility of symptoms (resulting from compression of neurovascular bundle at the thoracic outlet) during mechanical provocative maneuvers (Adson's test or costoclavicular test or Hyperabduction test or Roos Arm Claudication test)**
    - **Specific investigations (CT scan, MRI, Angiography, X-ray) are used to exclude other conditions and to establish the associated diagnosis.**

33. **Ans. c. Cervical rib**   34. **Ans. a. Radial nerve is commonly affected**

35. **Ans. c. Pain in ulnar distribution**   36. **Ans. c. Cervical rib**

37. **Ans. c. Spondylosis** *(Ref: Sabiston 20/e p1603; Schwartz 11/e p899, 995, 10/e p829; Bailey 27/e p991)*

■ RAYNAUD'S DISEASE

38. Ans. c. Osteoarthritis   39. Ans. b. White, blue, red   40. Ans. c. Turn white

■ DIABETIC FOOT

41. Ans. d. All of the above   42. Ans. a. Myelopathy

■ AORTIC DISSECTION

43. Ans. a. Right lateral wall of ascending aorta *(Ref: Harrison 20/e p1919; Sabiston 20/e p1746; Schwartz 11/e p882-884, 10/e p806-816; Bailey 27/e p909-911)*

■ AORTIC ANEURYSM

44. Ans. a. Atherosclerosis *(Ref: Harrison 20/e p1919, 19/e p1637; Sabiston 20/e p1722; Schwartz 11/e p919, 10/e p850-859; Bailey 27/e p961)*
    - **"90% all abdominal aortic aneurysms are related to atherosclerotic disease and most of these aneurysms are below the level of renal arteries."**

45. Ans. a. Laterally into the left retroperitoneum

46. Ans. c. 55 mm *(Ref: Sabiston 20/e p1725; Schwartz 11/e p925, 10/e p852; Bailey 27/e p961)*

    "Surgical treatment is generally recommended for aneurysms more than 5.5 cm in maximal diameter, those demonstrating more than 5 mm of growth in 6 months or more than 1 cm in a year, and aneurysms with a saccular rather than the typical fusiform anatomy."-Sabiston 20/e p1725

47. Ans. d. Both intravascular and extra-vascular infection *(Ref: Harrison 20/e p1922; Sabiston 20/e p1908)*
    - **A mycotic aneurysm is an infected aneurysm resulting from either an extravascular or an intravascular source of infection.**

48. Ans. b. Computed tomography   49. Ans. d. Most common side effect is diarrhea and hypotension

50. Ans. c. Splenic artery *(Ref: Sabiston 20/e p1788; Schwartz 11/e p1531, 10/e p1425; Bailey 27/e p961)*
    - **MC site of intra-abdominal aneurysm: Aorta >Splenic artery**[Q]
    - **MC site of splanchnic artery aneurysm: Splenic artery**[Q]

■ FEMORAL ARTERY ANEURYSM

51. Ans. a. Ultrasound guided compression of the neck of aneurysm, b. Thrombin injection, c. Bypass graft repair *(Ref: Sabiston 20/e p1782; Bailey 27/e p966)*

■ POPLITEAL ARTERY ANEURYSM

52. Ans. c. Popliteal artery *(Ref: Sabiston 20/e p1782; Bailey 27/e p966)*

■ PSEUDOANEURYSM

53. Ans. b. Trauma
    - **MC cause of pseudoaneurysm: Trauma (Penetrating** trauma or iatrogenic by **catheterization)**[Q]

■ SUBCLAVIAN STEAL SYNDROME

54. Ans. a. First part *(Ref: Grainger Diagnostic Radiology 4/e p 773; Bailey 27/e p952)*
    MC site of subclavian artery stenosis is the first part of the subclavian artery.

55. Ans. a. Reversal of blood flow in the ipsilateral vertebral artery *(Ref: Bailey 27/e p952)*

■ VASCULAR GRAFT

56. Ans. a. Autologous vein
57. Ans. a. Saphenous vein graft (upside-down) *(Ref: Bailey 27/e p890, 949; Washington Manual of surgery 5/e p322)*
58. Ans. c. Smooth muscle cells *(Ref: Vascular.surgery.duke.edu/files/.../Vascular_Grafts_2-27-09.pdf; Schwartz 9/e p762-764)*

VASCULAR GRAFT FAILURE

- Smooth muscle cells in the middle layer (media) of the vessel wall become activated, divide, proliferate and migrate into the inner layer (intima)[Q].
- The resulting abnormal neointimal cells express pro-inflammatory molecules, including cytokines, chemokines, and adhesion molecules that further trigger a cascade of events that lead to occlusive neointimal hyperplasia and eventually graft failure[Q].

59. Ans. b. Textile synthetic *(Ref: Sabiston 20/e p234; Schwartz 11/e p924, 10/e p4; Bailey 27/e p949, 950, 951)*

60. Ans. c. Saphenous vein **61.** Ans. a. Dacron **62.** Ans. a. LIMA

■ VASCULAR TRAUMA

63. Ans. b. Mechanical compression

> **Adequate manual compression of the subclavian artery** to obtain hemostasis is often **not possible** because of **the interposing subcutaneous tissue** and **bony structure**, as well as **lack of structural support** around subclavian artery.

■ ANGIOGRAPHY AND COMPLICATIONS

64. Ans. b. Arteriography *(Ref: Sabiston 20/e p1762; Schwartz 11/e p965-966, 10/e p832-833, 918; Bailey 26/e p190)*

- **Seldinger needle** is **used for angiography** (arteriography).

ARTERIOGRAPHY

> - **Aortic and lower extremity arteriograms are generally performed by needle puncture of the femoral[Q] or brachial arteries[Q]** followed by guidewire placement and catheter insertion using the Seldinger technique.

■ TAKAYASU ARTERITIS

65. Ans. b. Subclavian artery

■ MISCELLANEOUS

66. Ans. c. Integrity of palmar arch

67. Ans. b. Superficial temporal

CIRSOID ANEURYSM

> - A cirsoid aneurysm is the **dilation of a group of blood vessels** due to **congenital malformations** with AV **(arteriovenous) shunting[Q]**.
> - **Cirsoid means** resembling a **varix**.
> - **Most commonly occurs over** the **head** usually the **superficial temporal artery.**
> - **Superficial temporal artery** is the **most commonly involved artery[Q]**.

68. Ans. a. Aneurysm Endovascular Hunterian Ligation

HUNTERIAN LIGATION

> - **Hunterian ligation** refers to one of the **oldest successful interventions** for **arterial aneurysms: Ligation of** the **femoral artery to treat a popliteal aneurysm[Q]** by **John Hunter** in 1785.

69. Ans. c. Salmonella

70. Ans. d. Accidental injury to major vessels in thigh or groin *(Ref: Bailey 18/e p69, 147)*

BUTCHER'S THIGH

> - Butchers thigh is **penetrating wound of femoral triangle** due to **knife slipping while boning meat**.
> - Penetrating wound involving main veins in the thigh or groin are **potentially fatal**, as exsanguination may follow the first aid dressing which has apparently controlled the bleeding.

71. Ans. a. Direct pressure *(Ref: Advanced Assessment and Treatment of Trauma by Americans (2010)/71)*

EXTERNAL BLEEDING

> - Control of external hemorrhage during the early phase (circulation) of resuscitation is imperative.
> - **External bleeding is best controlled by direct digital pressure.**
> - **Direct pressure assists in** the process of **coagulation** by slowing the flow of blood out of the vessels and **giving clot time to form.**
> - In most cases of external bleeding, if pressure is applied quickly to the area of hemorrhage **(direct pressure)** or to the blood vessel supplying the bleed **(indirect pressure)**, the volume of blood escaping will be greatly reduced.
> - To be effective, direct pressure must be at least equal to the pressure of the blood attempting to escape.
> - Arterial bleeding is often difficult to control and may require up to 5 minutes of firm direct pressure to be successful.

72. Ans. b. Carotid angioplasty and stenting

Section 5

Cardiothoracic Vascular Surgery

Venous Disorders

■ RISK FACTORS FOR HYPERCOAGULABLE STATES/THROMBOSIS

Risk Factors for Hypercoagulable States/Thrombosis	
Inherited	**Acquired**

• Defective inhibition of coagulation factors:
  – **Factor V Leiden**[Q] (resistant to inhibition by activated protein C)
  – **Antithrombin III deficiency**[Q]
  – **Protein C or S deficiency**[Q]
  – **Prothrombin gene mutation**[Q] (G20210A)
	• Diseases or syndromes:
	  – Lupus anticoagulant/anticardiolipin syndrome[Q]
	  – **Malignancy**[Q], **recent MI**[Q], **infection**[Q]
	  – **Myeloproliferative disorder**
	  – **Thrombotic thrombocytopenic purpura**[Q]
	  – **Estrogen**[Q] treatment
	  – Hyperlipidemia, **Diabetes mellitus**[Q]

• Impaired clot lysis:
  – Dysfibrinogenemia
  – **Plasminogen deficiency**[Q]
  – **t-PA deficiency**[Q]
  – **PAI-I excess**[Q]
	– Hyperviscocity, **polycythemia**[Q]
	  – **Nephrotic syndrome**[Q]
	  – **Paroxysmal nocturnal hemoglobinuria**[Q]
	  – **Inflammatory bowel disease**[Q]
	  – **Behcet's syndrome**[Q]

• Uncertain mechanism:
  – **Homocystinuria**[Q]
  – **High homocysteine** levels due to **MTHFR mutation**[Q]
	• Physiological states:
	  – **Pregnancy** (especially post-partum[Q])
	  – **Obesity**[Q], **Immobilization**[Q], **Old age**[Q]
	  – **Postoperative state**[Q]

- MC genetic cause for thrombophilia: Factor V Leiden
- MC congenital cause of venous thrombosis: Factor V Leiden
- MC genetic hereditary blood coagulation disorder: Factor V Leiden

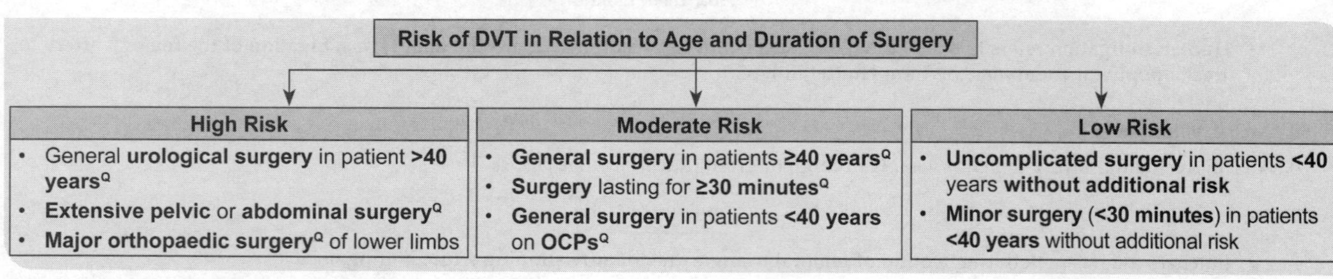

Risk of DVT in Relation to Age and Duration of Surgery

High Risk	Moderate Risk	Low Risk
• General **urological surgery** in patient >40 years[Q] • **Extensive pelvic** or **abdominal surgery**[Q] • **Major orthopaedic surgery**[Q] of lower limbs	• **General surgery** in patients ≥40 years[Q] • **Surgery** lasting for ≥30 minutes[Q] • **General surgery** in patients <40 years on **OCPs**[Q]	• **Uncomplicated surgery** in patients <40 years **without additional risk** • **Minor surgery** (<30 minutes) in patients <40 years without additional risk

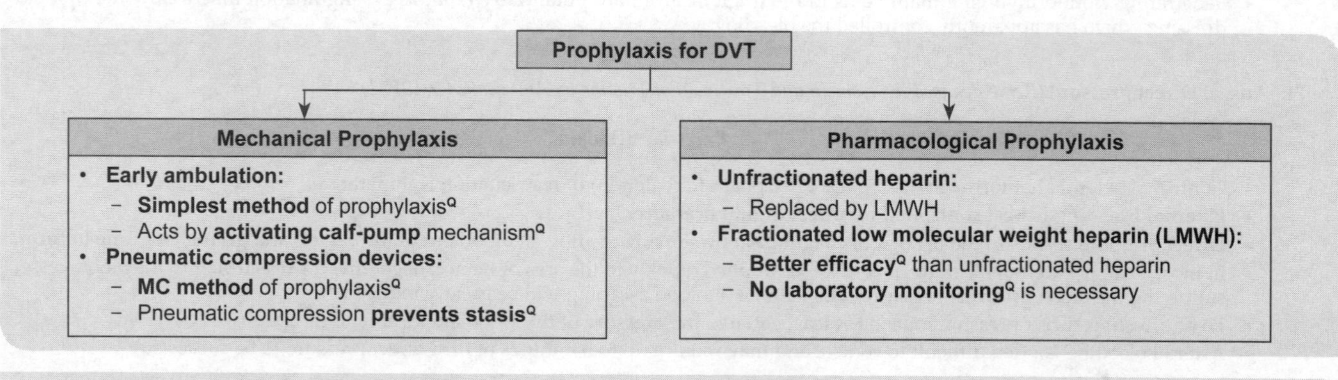

Prophylaxis for DVT

Mechanical Prophylaxis	Pharmacological Prophylaxis

• **Early ambulation:**
  – **Simplest method** of prophylaxis[Q]
  – Acts by **activating calf-pump** mechanism[Q]
• **Pneumatic compression devices:**
  – **MC method** of prophylaxis[Q]
  – Pneumatic compression **prevents stasis**[Q]
	• **Unfractionated heparin:**
	  – Replaced by LMWH
	• **Fractionated low molecular weight heparin (LMWH):**
	  – **Better efficacy**[Q] than unfractionated heparin
	  – **No laboratory monitoring**[Q] is necessary

- Unfractionated heparin & warfarin are **rarely used** in the **prophylaxis of DVT**[Q].

■ DEEP VENOUS THROMBOSIS

DEEP VENOUS THROMBOSIS

- **DVT of** the **leg** is complicated by the **immediate risk of pulmonary embolus & sudden death**[Q].
- Patients are at **risk of** developing a **post-thrombotic limb & venous ulceration**[Q].

Virchow's Triad

- Three factors described by Virchow are important in the development of venous thrombosis. These are:
  - **Endothelial injury**[Q] (**vascular injury**)   -   **Stasis** or turbulence of blood flow[Q]
  - **Hypercoagulability** of blood[Q] (**thrombophilia**)

- **Most important predisposing factor: Hospital admission**[Q] for the treatment of a medical or surgical condition.

Pathology

- **MC site of DVT: Calf or soleal vein**[Q]
- **MC site of DVT leading to pulmonary embolism: Femoropopliteal vein**[Q]
- A **thrombus develops in** the **soleal veins** of the calf, this is likely to **extend up** to the next large venous branch and is **more likely to break off** and **embolize**[Q] to the lung as a pulmonary embolism.
- **Acute right heart obstruction** may lead to **sudden collapse & death**[Q].

  - **Lung infarction is rare**[Q] as the **lung** has a **dual blood supply** (**bronchial & pulmonary arteries**).

Clinical Features

- **MC presentation** of DVT: **Pain & swelling**, especially in the **calf** of one lower limb[Q].
- **Bilateral DVT** is common, occurring in up to **30%**[Q].
- **Many patients** have **no symptoms of thrombosis** and **may first present with** signs of a **pulmonary embolism**, e.g. pleuritic chest pain, hemoptysis & shortness of breath[Q].
- **Physical signs: Mild pitting edema** of the ankle, **dilated surface veins**, a **stiff calf** and **tenderness** over the course of the deep veins.
- **Earliest sign of DVT: Calf tenderness**[Q]

  - **Low-grade fever** may be present, especially in a patient who is having **repeated pulmonary emboli**[Q].

- **Homan's sign: Resistance** (not pain) of the **calf muscles to forcible dorsiflexion** is not discriminatory and should be abandoned.

Homan's sign	• **Resistance** (not pain) **of** the **calf muscles to forcible dorsiflexion**[Q]
Phlegmasia alba dolens	• **Painful white leg**[Q] • Obstruction of major **deep venous channel**[Q]
Phlegmasia cerulea dolens	• **Painful blue leg**[Q] • Obstruction of **both collaterals & deep venous channel**[Q]
Moses sign (Bancroft's sign)	• **Calf tenderness** on **direct pressure on** the **calf**[Q]
Pratt's sign	• **Calf tenderness** on **squeezing** the **calf** from the sides[Q]

Diagnosis

- **D-dimer measurement: If normal, no indication for further investigation**[Q] but, if raised, a duplex ultrasound examination of the deep veins should be performed.
- **Duplex ultrasound: Investigation of choice** for diagnosis of **DVT** (**Filling defects** in flow and **lack of compressibility** indicate the presence of a thrombosis[Q]).
- **Ascending venography:** Shows **thrombus as a filling defect**, is now **rarely required**[Q].

Treatments

- **Confirmed DVT on duplex imaging:** Start **subcutaneous LMWH** and **rapid anticoagulation with warfarin** unless there is a specific contraindication[Q].

  - **Duration of heparin** should be **at least 5 days**[Q].
  - **Warfarin** is usually started at a dose of **10 mg** on **day one**, **10 mg** on **day two** and **5 mg** on **day three**[Q].
  - **PT on day 3** guides the **maintenance dose** of warfarin.

- **Thrombolysis:** In iliac vein thrombosis, especially if **seen early** and limb is **extremely swollen**[Q].
- A **minimum treatment time of anticoagulation** advocated in **DVT** is **3 months**[Q].
- **Palma operation: Surgical treatment of DVT**[Q]

■ VARICOSE VEINS

VARICOSE VEINS

- **Varicose veins** are **dilated, tortuous elongated superficial veins**[Q] ≥3 mm in diameter measured in upright position with demonstrable reflux.
- **Most develop in** the tributaries of the **greater** and **lesser saphenous veins**, which are **usually dilated** but rarely varicose themselves.

> - **Usual distribution** of varicose veins is **below** the **knee in branches of greater saphenous system**[Q].

- **Varicosities in** the **thigh: Long saphenous** incompetence[Q]
- **Varicosities on** the **back of** the leg: **Short saphenous** incompetence[Q]

Primary Varicose Veins	Secondary Varicose Veins
• **More common**[Q] • Due to **congenital predisposition** with **occupational reinforcement**[Q] • **Decreased number or defective valves**[Q]	• Less common • Arises from **destruction** or **dysfunction of valves** caused by: – **Trauma**[Q] – **DVT**[Q] – **AV fistula**[Q] – Non-traumatic proximal venous obstruction (pregnancy, pelvic tumor)

Risk Factors for Varicose Veins	
• **Female sex**[Q] • **Pregnancy** (especially **multiparity**[Q]) • **Pelvic tumors**[Q] • **Family history**[Q]	• **AV fistula**[Q] • **DVT**[Q] • **Prolonged standing**[Q] • **Obesity**[Q]

Pathophysiology

- **Defective connective tissue** & **smooth muscle** in the **vein wall** leading to a **secondary incompetence** of the valves[Q]

Clinical Features

- **MC symptom: Dull aching pain in** the **veins** at the **end of** the **day, after prolonged standing**[Q]
- Other symptoms: **Ankle swelling**, itching, bleeding, **superficial thrombophlebitis, eczema, lipodermatosclerosis** and **ulceration**[Q].

Diagnosis

- **Duplex ultrasound: Investigation of choice** for diagnosis of **varicose veins**[Q]
- **Varicography:** Useful investigation in **recurrent varicose veins** or **complex anatomy**[Q]
- **Venography:** Not used as a standard investigation in varicose veins, **useful if** the **duplex scan indicates, but cannot confirm**, the **presence** of post-thrombotic change[Q].

Treatment

- **Gold standard treatment for varicose vein: Endothermal ablation**[Q]
- Patients **without symptoms** or **signs of lipodermatosclerosis** or **ulceration: Reassurance**[Q]
- **Elastic compression stockings:** For **varicose veins with post-thrombotic damage**[Q]

> - **Bisgard's Regime: Limb elevation + Compression stockings + Massage** for varicose ulcers[Q]

Indications for Varicose Vein Intervention	
• **Cosmesis**[Q] • Symptoms **refractory to conservative therapy**[Q] • **Bleeding** from a varix	• Superficial **thrombophlebitis**[Q] • **Lipodermatosclerosis**[Q] • Venous stasis **ulcer**[Q]

- A previous **DVT** usually **contraindicates varicose vein surgery**[Q]

> - **DVT** is a **contraindication for** the **treatment of varicose veins**[Q].
> - **Varicose vein surgery** should **never be attempted** in a case **where DVT exists along** with **varicose veins**, because in these cases, **superficial veins** are the **only valved venous pathway** and excising them will only aggravate the condition[Q].

Endothermal Ablation of Varicose Veins
• **Endothermal ablation (replaced surgical ligation & stripping) is now considered as the gold standard treatment for varicose vein**[Q]. • Cost effective & can be performed under local anesthesia. • Methods used: Endovenous laser ablation & RFA[Q]

Contd…

Contd…

Treatment of Varicose Veins	
Injection sclerotherapy	• **Sodium tetradecyl sulphate** is **most commonly used**[Q] • **Destroys lipid membranes** of endothelial cells causing them to shed, leading to **thrombosis, fibrosis** and **sclerosis**[Q]. • **Not effective** at **eradicating varicosities** in the presence of **major saphenous incompetence**[Q] • Useful for dealing with **minor varicosities (<3 mm**[Q]) and **recurrences** in the **calf** and **lower leg** • **Tesari method: Most widely used method for foam sclerotherapy**[Q]
Surgical Treatment	• **Ligate** the **saphenofemoral** and/or **saphenopopliteal junctions** and **remove major part of** the **incompetent trunk**[Q]
Radiofrequency ablation	• **Destroy** the **endothelial lining**[Q]
Endovenous laser ablation	• Causes endothelial damage[Q]

Complications of varicose vein surgery

- **Recurrence (MC): Incidence of recurrence** after surgery is upto **10%**[Q].
- **Hematoma** or **Ecchymosis: MC cause of discomfort**[Q] after varicose vein surgery
- Sensory nerve injury

  - **Greater saphenous vein** should only be **stripped** to **just below the knee to avoid damage** to the accompanying **saphenous nerve**[Q]
  - **Sural nerve** must be **carefully dissected off** the **lesser saphenous vein** at the **ankle**[Q].

'CEAP' Classification of Chronic Lower Extremity Venous Disease	
C	**Clinical signs** (grade$_{0-6}$), supplemented by **"A"** for **asymptomatic** and **"S"** for **symptomatic** presentation
E	**Etiologic classification** (**c**ongenital, **p**rimary, **s**econdary)
A	**Anatomic distribution** (**s**uperficial, **d**eep, or **p**erforator, alone or in combination)
P	**Pathophysiologic dysfunction** (**r**eflux or **o**bstruction, alone or in combination)

Tests for Varicose Veins	
Morrissey's test	• Cough impulse test[Q]
Perthe's test	• Affected lower extremity is wrapped with elastic bandage and patient is instructed to move around and exercise. • **Increase in size** of the varices indicates **incompetence of deep venous system**[Q] • **Severe crampy pain** is suggestive of **deep venous obstruction**[Q]
Modified Perthes test	• Tourniquet is applied around the upper part of the thigh and patient is asked to walk quickly with tourniquet in the place • **Severe crampy pain** is suggestive of **deep venous obstruction**[Q]
Schwartz test	• In long standing varicose veins if the **lower part of varicosity is tapped**, an **impulse is felt at** the **saphenous opening**[Q]
Fegans test	• Palpation to find the **fascial defects** to **locate incompetent perforators**[Q]

■ BRODIE-TRENDELENBURG TEST

BRODIE-TRENDELENBURG TEST

- **Brodie-Trendelenburg test** is **positive** in:
  - Incompetent saphenofemoral junction (SFJ)[Q]
  - **Incompetent perforators** or **communicating veins**[Q]

Procedure

- Test is performed in two ways.
- In both the methods the patient is first placed in the recumbent position and his legs are raised to empty the veins.
- The SFJ is now compressed with the thumb of the clinician and the patient is asked to stand up quickly.

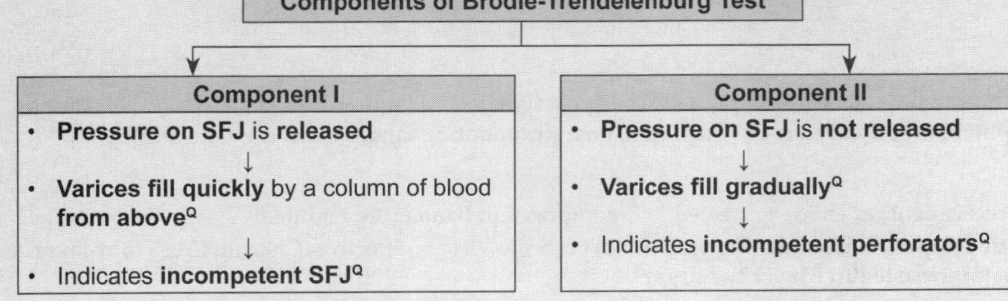

■ TRENDELENBURG OPERATION

Trendelenburg Operation

- Consists of **saphenofemoral junction flush ligation** & **greater saphenous vein (GSV) stripping**[Q]
  - **All four tributaries (superficial inferior epigastric, superficial circumflex iliac, deep & superficial external pudendal veins) is divided**[Q]
- **Ligate** the **GSV** deep to all tributaries **flush with** the **common femoral vein**[Q]
- **Greater saphenous vein** should only be **stripped** to **just below the knee to avoid damage** to the accompanying **saphenous nerve**[Q]

■ VENOUS ULCERS

Venous Ulcers

- **Venous disease** is responsible for **60-70% of all ulcers** in the **lower leg.**

Causes of Leg Ulcers	
• **Venous disease**: Superficial incompetence; deep venous damage (post-thrombotic)	• Traumatic ulcers
• **Arterial ischemic ulcers**	• **Neuropathic ulcers** (diabetes)
• Rheumatoid ulcers	• Neoplastic ulcers (**SCC** and **BCC**)

Etiology

- **Fibrin cuff theory**: High venous pressure → Pericapillary infiltrate → Fibrin → Fibrosis → Cuffs → Diffusion block → Tissue damage[Q]
- **White cell trapping**: White cell 'trapping' → Reactive oxygen species → Free radicals → Tissue damage[Q].

  - At present, **ambulatory venous hypertension** is the **only accepted cause of ulceration**[Q].

Clinical Features

- **Venous ulcer: Sloping edge, base** contains **granulation tissue**[Q] covered by slough and exudate.
- **Any elevation** of the **ulcer edge** should indicate the **need for a biopsy to exclude a carcinoma** (SCC or BCC).

  - Venous ulcer of the leg **characteristically develops in** the skin of the **gaiter region**[Q], the **area between** muscles of the calf & ankle
  - **Majority of ulcers** develop on the **medial side** of the **calf**[Q]
  - **Ulcers associated with lesser saphenous incompetence** often develop on the **lateral side** of the leg[Q].

- Almost **all venous ulcers have** surrounding **lipodermatosclerosis (thickening, pigmentation, inflammation & induration** of calf skin[Q])
- **Pigmentation** comes **from hemosiderin & melanin**

  - Presence of an **ankle flare suggests venous hypertension**[Q].
  - **Inverted Champagne bottle leg** is seen in **varicose veins**[Q].

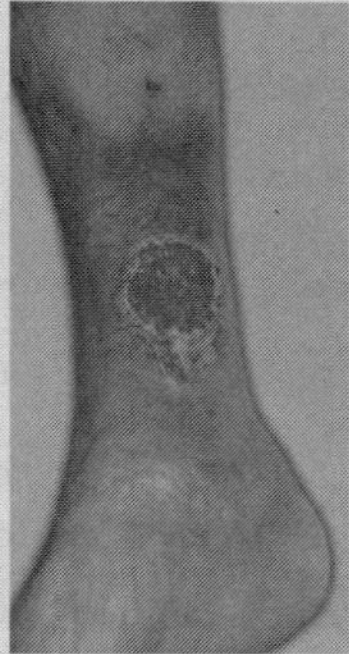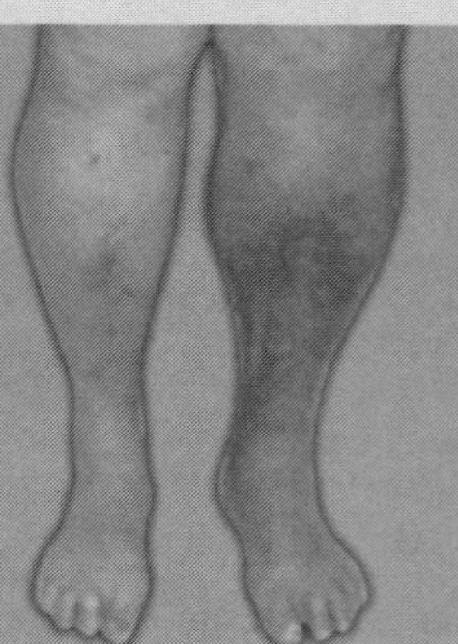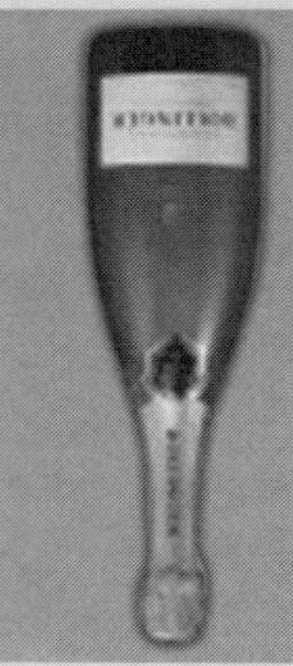

Diagnosis

- **Duplex ultrasound**: Assess the state of deep & superficial veins (IOC)[Q]
- **Bipedal ascending phlebography: Detect obstruction** & **post-thrombotic changes missed by** the **duplex scan**[Q]

Management

- **Probable venous ulcer:** Patients are initially treated by a **compression bandaging regimen**[Q]
- A **multilayered elastic compression bandaging system** has been shown to be effective (**Charing Cross four-layer bandage**), as has a **rigid multilayered system (Steripaste three layer bandage)**[Q].

■ ARTERIO-VENOUS MALFORMATION

Klippel-Trenaunay Syndrome

Characterized by	
• Congenital **AV fistula**[Q]	• **Hypertrophy** of involved **extremity**[Q]
• **Cutaneous hemangioma**[Q]	• **Absence of deep venous system**[Q]
• **Varicose veins**[Q]	

Management

- **Most patients** with Klippel-Trenaunay syndrome should **be treated conservatively with elastic compression** hosiery[Q]
- **Pathological superficial veins should not be removed**[Q] without evidence of an intact deep system.

Kasabach-Merritt Syndrome

- **Characterized by:**
  - Thrombocytopenia[Q]
  - Consumptive coagulopathy[Q]
  - Microangiopathic hemolytic anemia[Q]
  - Enlarging vascular lesion (Hemangioma or AV malformation[Q])

Pathology

- Vascular lesion (**Hemangioma** or **AV malformation**) **triggers** an **intravascular coagulation** with **platelet trapping** and consequent **thrombocytopenia,** and an **activation** and **consumption of coagulation factors**[Q].

Management

- Treatment options: **Embolization, external compression bandages**[Q]
- Drugs: Corticosteroids, vincristine

Malignancies Associated with Migratory Thrombophlebitis	
• **CA pancreas (MC)**[Q]	• **Prostate cancer**[Q]
• **CA lung**[Q]	• **Ovarian** cancer[Q]
• **GI malignancies**[Q]	• **Lymphoma**[Q]

Multiple Choice Questions

■ HYPERCOAGULABLE STATES AND DVT RISK FACTORS

1. All the following disorders are inherited except:
a. Protein S deficiency *(Recent Question 2017, JIPMER 2010)*
b. Antiphospholipid antibody syndrome
c. Protein C deficiency
d. Factor V Leiden mutation

2. Congenital cause of hypercoagulable states are all except:
(AIIMS Nov 2010)
a. Protein C deficiency　　b. Protein S deficiency
c. MTHFR mutation　　d. Lupus anticoagulant

3. All of the following are acquired causes of hypercoagulability, except: *(All India 2009)*
a. Infection
b. Inflammatory bowel disease
c. Myeloproliferative disorders
d. Prolonged surgery

■ DEEP VENOUS THROMBOSIS

4. Which of the following is associated with Virchow's triad?
a. Hypercoagulability *(MCI Sept 2005)*
b. Disseminated malignancy
c. DVT
d. All of the above

5. DVT, investigation of choice is:
(DNB 2005, 2001, PGI Dec 97, June 97)
a. Doppler　　b. Plethysmography
c. Venography　　d. X-ray

6. The patient falls in hish risk group for DVT and pulmonary embolism after: *(MHCET 2016)*
a. Major burns
b. Major surgery age < 40 years
c. Major medial illness/cancer
d. Major orthopedic surgery/fracture pelvis

7. Earliest sign of deep vein thrombosis is:
(DNB 2005, 2001, 2000, AIIMS 87)
a. Calf tenderness　　b. Rise in temperature
c. Swelling of calf muscle　　d. Homan's sign

8. A patient undergoes surgery in pelvic region. Which vein is most likely to result in thrombosis?
(JIPMER Nov 2017)
a. Iliac vein　　b. Femoral vein
c. Calf vein　　d. IVC

9. Patient had retrograde pelvic thrombophlebitis and it progressed to bilateral ileofemoral occlusion and now the presentation is: *(Recent Question 2018)*
a. Blue leg　　b. White leg
c. Red leg　　d. Purple leg

10. The initial therapy of documented deep venous thrombosis in a post-operative case is:
a. Subcutaneous heparin therapy
b. Intravenous heparin therapy
c. Thrombolytic therapy with urokinase
d. Aspirin therapy *(Recent Question 2013, Karnataka 2003)*

11. The device, whose image is given below, used for:
(AIIMS Nov 2018)

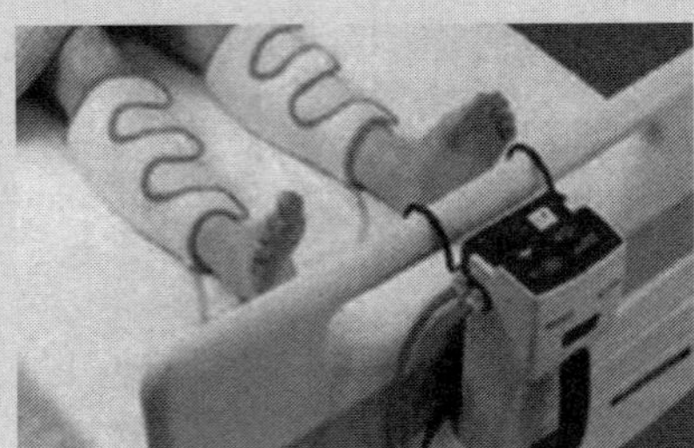

a. Pneumatic compression stocking to prevention of DVT
b. Varicose vein
c. Hypothermia
d. Cellulites

12. All of the following statements are correct about deep venous thrombosis except: *(Recent Question 2019)*
a. Clinical assessment is highly reliable
b. Mostly bilateral
c. Most common clinically presents as pain and tenderness in calf
d. Some cases may directly present as pulmonary thromboembolism

■ VARICOSE VEINS

13. 'SEPS' is a procedure used for: *(All India 2009)*
a. Veins　　b. Arteries
c. Lymphatics　　d. AV fistula

14. The most common complication of varicose vein stripping is:
a. Infection　　b. Hemorrhage *(DPG 2011)*
c. Ecchymosis　　d. Thromboembolism

15. Drug used for sclerotherapy of varicose veins are the following except: *(MCI Sept 2007)*
a. Ethanolamine oleate　　b. Polidocanol
c. Ethanol　　d. Sodium tetradecyl sulfate

16. Most commonly varicose veins are seen with:
a. Long saphenous vein *(AIIMS June 99)*
b. Short saphenous vein
c. Both
d. Popliteal and femoral vein

17. Surgery in varicose veins is not attempted in presence of:
a. Deep vein thrombosis *(AIIMS Nov 93, June 2000)*
b. Multiple incompetent perforators
c. Varicose veins with leg ulcer
d. All of the above

18. Perforators are not present at: *(AIIMS Nov 2007)*
a. Ankle　　b. Medial calf
c. Distal to calf　　d. Below inguinal ligament

19. The following is the commonest site for venous ulcer:
a. Instep of foot *(Recent Question 2014)*
b. Lower 1/3rd leg and ankle
c. Lower 2/3rd of leg
d. Middle 1/3rd of leg

20. Lipodermatosclerosis is most commonly seen at: *(DNB 2012)*
a. Anterior aspect of leg　　b. Medial aspect of leg
c. Anterior aspect of thigh　　d. Posterior aspect of thigh

21. **Gold standard diagnostic test in varicose veins is:**
    a. Photoplethysmography   *(JIPMER 2003)*
    b. Duplex imaging
    c. Ultrasonography
    d. Radio-labeled fibrinogen study

22. **Bisgard treatment is for:**   *(APPG 96)*
    a. Arterial ulcer   b. Venous ulcer
    c. TAO   d. Raynaud's phenomenon

23. **Treatment of choice for a patient presenting with venous ulcer and incompetent perforators:**   *(DNB 2005)*
    a. Stripping of saphenous vein
    b. Subfascial ligation of perforators
    c. Saphenofemoral ligation
    d. Conservative

24. **Patient presents with varicose vein with sapheno-femoral incompetence and normal perforator. Management options include all of the following except:**   *(AIIMS Nov 2012)*
    a. Endovascular stripping
    b. Sclerotherapy
    c. Sapheno-femoral flush ligation
    d. Saphenofemoral flush ligation with striping

25. **Contraindication for surgery in varicose veins:**
    a. DVT   *(Recent Question 2015)*
    b. Multiple incompetent perforators
    c. Ulcer at ankle
    d. None

26. **A patient of varicose veins came to hospital; intern was on duty. Which test he shall perform to rule out the DVT?**
    a. Brodie Trendelenberg test   *(MCI Dec 2019)*
    b. Perthes test
    c. Thomas test
    d. Ober's test

27. **Which complication is seen after varicose vein stripping procedure?**   *(MCI June 2019)*
    a. Neuralgia   b. Deep vein thrombosis
    c. Acrocyanosis   d. Telangiectasia

28. **Most common complication of below-knee stripping of varicose veins is:**   *(MCI Dec 2018)*
    a. Hemorrhage   b. Thromboembolism
    c. Neuralgia   d. Infection

■ AV MALFORMATIONS

29. **A patient presented with pulsating varicose veins of the lower limb. Most probable diagnosis is:**   *(AIIMS Nov 2001)*
    a. Klippel-Trenaunay syndrome
    b. Tricuspid regurgitation
    c. DVT
    d. Right ventricular failure

30. **Klippel-Trenaunay syndrome associated with all except:**   *(JIPMER Nov 2017)*
    a. Portwine stain   b. Varicose veins
    c. Limb lengthening   d. Fused vertebra

■ THROMBOPHLEBITIS

31. **Migratory thrombophlebitis is seen most commonly with:**   *(PGI June 2002)*
    a. Pancreatic carcinoma   b. Testicular carcinoma
    c. Gastric carcinoma   d. Breast carcinoma
    e. Liver carcinoma

32. **The most common cause of superficial thrombophlebitis is:**
    a. Intravenous catheters/infusion   *(All India 2009)*
    b. DVT
    c. Varicose veins   d. Trauma

■ HYPERCOAGULABLE STATES AND DVT RISK FACTORS

1. **Ans. b. Antiphospholipid antibody syndrome** (*Ref: Harrison 20/e p1910; Sabiston 20/e p1842; Schwartz 11/e p984, 10/e p761; Bailey 27/e p987*)
2. **Ans. d. Lupus anticoagulant**   3. **Ans. None**

■ DEEP VENOUS THROMBOSIS

4. **Ans. a. Hypercoagulability** (*Ref: Harrison 20/e p1910; Sabiston 20/e p1841; Schwartz 11/e p984, 10/e p918-927; Bailey 27/e p986-987*)
5. **Ans. a. Doppler**   6. **Ans. c. Major medial illness/cancer**   7. **Ans. a. Calf tenderness**
8. **Ans. c. Calf vein**   9. **Ans. a. Blue leg**
10. **Ans. b. Intravenous heparin therapy** (*Ref: Harrison 20/e p1913; Sabiston 20/e p1844; Schwartz 11/e p987, 10/e p199, 921-923; Bailey 27/e p990*)

Antithrombotic Therapy in DVT

- **Any venous thrombosis** involving the **femoropopliteal system** is **treated with full anticoagulation**[Q].
- Traditionally, the **treatment of DVT centers around heparin treatment** to maintain the PTT at 60 to 80 seconds, followed by **warfarin therapy** to obtain an **INR of 2.5 to 3.0**[Q].
- This **initial therapy** usually is **continued for at least 5 days**[Q], while oral vitamin K antagonists are being simultaneously administered.

Unfractionated Heparin
- **UFH therapy** is **most commonly administered** with an **initial IV bolus of 80 units/kg** or **5000 units**[Q].
- **Initial bolus** is **followed by a continuous IV drip**, initially at **18 units/kg per hour**[Q] or **1300 units per hour**[Q].
- The **half-life of IV UFH** ranges from **45-90 minutes** and is **dose dependent**[Q].
- **Level of antithrombotic therapy** should be **monitored every 6 hours using aPTT**, with the **goal range of 1.5 to 2.5 times control values**[Q].

11. **Ans. a. Pneumatic compression stocking to prevention of DVT** (*Ref: Schwartz 11/e p992, 10/e p925; Sabiston 20/e p1843; Bailey 27/e p989*)
12. **Ans. b. Mostly bilateral** (*Ref: Schwartz 11/e p986, 10/e p919; Sabiston 20/e p1842; Bailey 27/e p986-988*)

■ VARICOSE VEINS

13. **Ans. a. Veins** (*Ref: Sabiston 20/e p1841; Schwartz 11/e p996, 10/e p929-930; Bailey 27/e p982*)

Subfascial Endoscopic Perforator Vein Surgery (SEPS)

- **SEPS** is a **new endoscopic technique for** the management of **chronic venous insufficiency** due to **incompetent perforator veins**[Q].
- SEPS involves **insertion of** a **rigid endoscope** through the skin and superficial fascia to a **plane above** the **muscle**, such that perforator veins are visible as they exit the muscles.
- These **perforator veins** are **dissected** free from surrounding tissue and **closed** with the help of metal clips.

14. **Ans. c. Ecchymosis** (*Ref: Sabiston 20/e p1836; Schwartz 11/e p996, 10/e p929-930; Bailey 27/e p974-982*)
15. **Ans. c. Ethanol** (*Ref: Sabiston 20/e p1835; Schwartz 11/e p996, 10/e p929; Bailey 27/e p979*)

Sclerosing Agents

- These are **irritants** causing **inflammation, coagulation** and ultimately **fibrosis**, when injected into **hemorrhoids** or **varicose veins**[Q].
- Used only for **local injection**

Sclerosing Agents

• **Phenol**[Q] **(5%)** in **almond** oil or **peanut oil**[Q]	• **Sodium tetradecyl sulphate**[Q] **(3%)** with benzyl alcohol (2%)
• **Ethanolamine oleate**[Q] **(5%)** in 25% glycerin and 2% benzyl alcohol	
• **Polidocanol**[Q] **(3%)**	• **Hypertonic saline**[Q]

16. **Ans. a. Long saphenous vein** (*Ref: Sabiston 20/e p1831; Schwartz 11/e p996, 10/e p929; Bailey 27/e p975*)

- The **usual distribution** of varicose veins is **below** the **knee in branches of greater saphenous system**[Q].

17. **Ans. a. Deep vein thrombosis** *(Ref: Sabiston 20/e p1836; Schwartz 11/e p996, 10/e p929; Bailey 27/e p976)*

- **DVT** is a **contraindication for** the **treatment of varicose veins**[Q].
- **Varicose vein surgery** should **never be attempted** in a case **where DVT exists along** with **varicose veins**, because in these cases, **superficial veins** are the **only valved venous pathway** and excising them will only aggravate the condition[Q].

18. **Ans. d. Below inguinal ligament** *(Ref: Sabiston 20/e p1828; Schwartz 11/e p996, 10/e p915; Bailey 26/e p902)*

PERFORATORS LOCATION (IN CBD HUNTERS)

- **Below** the **medial malleolus** (**Infra**malleolar perforators/ **May or Kuster**)
- In the **medial calf** (**C**ockett's perforators[Q])
- Just **below** the knee (**B**oyd's perforators[Q])
- Just **above** the knee (**D**odd's perforators[Q])
- At the level of **adductor canal** (**H**unterian perforators[Q])

19. **Ans. b. Lower 1/3rd leg and ankle**

20. **Ans. b. Medial aspect of leg** *(Ref: Sabiston 20/e p1832; Bailey 27/e p973, 984, 986)*

LIPODERMATOSCLEROSIS

- Lipodermatosclerosis is the name given to the **skin changes seen in chronic venous insufficiency.**
- Components of lipodermatosclerosis:
  - **Pigmented skin**
  - **Inflamed subcutaneous tissue**
  - **Elevated venous pressure** facilitates the extravasation of the RBCs and fluid leading to inflammation
- The pigmentation is due to **fixation of hemosiderin** in the tissue
- It is most commonly seen **on gaiter area (above medial malleolus)**

21. **Ans. b. Duplex imaging**

22. **Ans. b. Venous ulcer**

23. **Ans. b. Subfascial ligation of perforators**

24. **Ans. b. Sclerotherapy** *(Ref: Sabiston 20/e p1835; Schwartz 11/e p996, 10/e p929-930; Bailey 27/e p979-780)*

Injection sclerotherapy is useful for dealing with **minor varicosities (<3 mm**[Q]**)** and **recurrences** in the **calf** and **lower leg.** Though it's a treatment option for varicose vein, but for a **patient of varicose vein with sapheno-femoral incompetence and normal perforator**, this will be least preferred amongst the given options.

Treatment of Varicose Veins
- **Saphenofemoral flush ligation** with **ligation of tributaries** and **stripping of major part of the incompetent trunk**[Q]

25. **Ans. a. DVT**

26. **Ans. b. Perthes test**

27. **Ans. a. Neuralgia** *(Ref: Bailey 27/e p982)*

"Complications (minor and major) are reported in up to 20% of patients who undergo traditional varicose vein surgery. Wound infections, the most common complication, are reduced by prophylactic antibiotics. Nerve injury is the most common serious complication. The incidence of saphenous nerve neuralgia is up to 7% following GSV stripping to the knee (the incidence is higher with stripping to the ankle). The incidence of sural nerve neuropraxia and common peroneal nerve injury may be as high as 20% and 4%, respectively, following SSV surgery. The incidence of venous thromboembolic complications is approximately 0.5% following varicose vein surgery; however, patient risk factors must be individually assessed and appropriate prophylaxis administered according to guidelines." - Bailey 27/e p982

28. **Ans. c. Neuralgia** *(Ref: Bailey 27/e p982)*

■ AV MALFORMATIONS

29. **Ans. a. Klippel-Trenaunay syndrome** *(Ref: Schwartz 11/e p2000, 10/e p1850; Bailey 27/e p972, 991, 1000)*

30. **Ans. d. Fused vertebra**

■ THROMBOPHLEBITIS

31. **Ans. a. Pancreatic carcinoma; c. Gastric carcinoma** *(Ref: Sabiston 20/e p1845; Schwartz 11/e p994, 10/e p927; Bailey 27/e p990)*

32. **Ans. a. Intravenous catheters/infusion**

Lymphatic System

■ LYMPHEDEMA

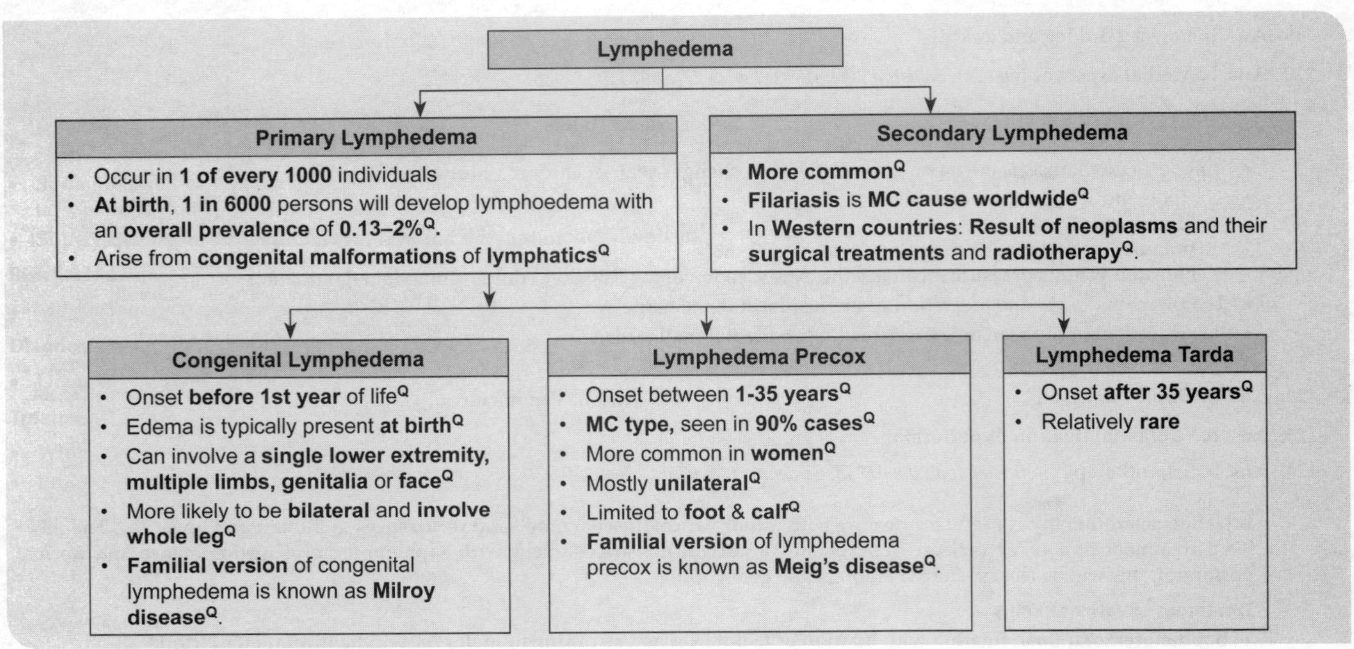

■ COMPLICATIONS OF LYMPHEDEMA

COMPLICATIONS OF LYMPHEDEMA

- **Limb swelling:** Cause discomfort and aching[Q]
- **Infections:** Recurrent bacterial and fungal infections, recurrent cellulitis or lymphangitis leading to **skin thickening**[Q]
- **Risk of malignancy:** Lymphangiosarcoma (Stewart-Treves' syndrome[Q])

Malignancies Associated with Lymphedema	
• **Lymphangiosarcoma**[Q]	• Malignant melanoma
• **(Stewart–Treves' syndrome)**	• Malignant fibrous histiocytoma
• **Kaposi's sarcoma** (HIV)	• Basal cell carcinoma
• Squamous cell carcinoma	• Lymphoma
• Liposarcoma	

Signs in Chronic Lymphedema	
Buffalo hump[Q]	• **Contour of** the **ankle is lost** through infilling of the submalleolar depressions, a 'buffalo hump' forms **on the dorsum of the foot**
Square toes[Q]	• **Toes appear 'square'** because of **confinement of footwear**
Stemmer's sign[Q]	• **Skin on** the **dorsum of the toes cannot be pinched** because of **subcutaneous fibrosis**

■ LYMPHEDEMA: INVESTIGATIONS

Direct-contrast lymphangiography provides the **finest details** of the lymphatic anatomy. However, it is an invasive study that **involves exposure** and **cannulation of lymphatics** at the **dorsum of the forefoot**, followed by **slow injection of contrast medium** (ethiodized oil). The procedure is tedious, the **cannulation often necessitates aid of magnification optics** (frequently an operating microscope is needed), and the dissection requires some form of anesthetic. **After cannulation of a superficial lymph vessel, contrast material is slowly injected** into the **lymphatic system.**

Lymphangiography

Direct Lymphangiography	Indirect Lymphangiography
• Involves the **injection of contrast medium** (**Isosulfan blue**[Q]) into a **peripheral lymphatic vessel** and radiographic visualization of the vessels and nodes[Q]. • **Gold standard for** showing **structural abnormalities of larger lymphatics and nodes**[Q] • **Technically difficult**, **unpleasant** for the patient • May cause **lymphatic injury** • **Reserved for preoperative evaluation** of megalymphatics being considered for **bypass** or **fistula ligation**[Q].	• Indirect lymphangiography involves the **intradermal injection** of **water-soluble, non-ionic contrast** into **a web space**, from where it is taken up by lymphatics and then **followed radiographically**[Q]. • It will **show distal lymphatics** but **not normally proximal lymphatics and nodes**[Q].

■ TREATMENT OF LYMPHEDEMA

TREATMENT OF LYMPHOEDEMA

- **Most** (95%) of patients can be **managed non-operatively**[Q]
- **Mainstay of treatment** is **nonsurgical measures:**
  - Use of **external compressive garments** and **devices**[Q]
  - **Limb elevation**[Q]
  - **Antibiotics** for episodes of cellulitis[Q]
  - Specialized complex **physical therapy**[Q]

> • **Efficacy** of surgical options is **generally poor**, and these are **reserved for** cases in which **aggressive nonsurgical measures** have **failed**[Q].

- **Surgical treatment** may be considered in cases of **severe functional impairment, recurrent lymphangitis** or **severe pain** despite medical therapy[Q].

Surgical Treatment of Lymphedema

Reconstructive Operations	Excisional Operations

• Indicated in patients with **proximal** (either primary or secondary) **obstruction** of the extremity, **lymphatic obstruction, dilated lymphatics distal to obstruction**[Q].
• **Bypass procedures:**
  – Omental pedicle
  – **Skin bridge (Gillies**[Q]**)**
  – Anastomosing **lymph nodes** to **veins** (**Neibulowitz**[Q])
  – **Ileal mucosal patch (Kinmonth**[Q]**)**
  – Direct lymphovenous anastomosis with the aid of operating microscope
	• Only viable option for patients **without residual lymphatics** of **adequate size** for reconstructive procedures
	• **Sistrunk**[Q]**:**
	  – A **wedge of skin** and **subcutaneous tissue** is **excised** and wound **closed primarily**[Q]
	  – **Most commonly carried out to reduce girth** of the thigh[Q].
	• **Kondoleon's or Homan's**[Q]**:**
	  – **Staged subcutaneous excision**[Q] underneath flaps
	• **Thompson**[Q]**:**
	  – **Denuded skin flap** is **sutured to deep fascia** and buried beneath the second skin flap ('**buried dermal flap'**[Q])
	• **Charles Procedure**[Q]**:**
	  – In **severe lymphedema** with **unhealthy** and **infected skin**[Q]
	  – Involves **complete** and **circumferential excision** of **skin, subcutaneous tissue** and **deep fascia** of the involved leg and dorsum of the foot[Q].

Multiple Choice Questions

■ LYMPHEDEMA

1. **Most common type of primary lymphedema is:** *(DNB 2010)*
   a. Lymphedema congenita   b. Lymphedema precox
   c. Lymphedema tarda   d. None

2. **In India, what is the most common cause of unilateral lymphedema of lower limb?** *(UPSC 2007)*
   a. Lymphedema tarda
   b. Carcinoma of penis with metastatic nodes
   c. Filariasis
   d. Tubercular lymphadenopathy

3. **Chronic lymphedema of limb is predisposed to all of the following except:** *(All India 2004)*
   a. Thickening of the skin
   b. Recurrent soft tissue infections
   c. Marjolin's ulcer   d. Sarcoma

4. **Commonest cause of unilateral pedal edema in India is:** *(All India 90)*
   a. Filariasis   b. Post traumatic
   c. Post irradiation   d. Milroy's disease

5. **All are true about congenital lymphedema except:**
   a. It is bilateral   *(Recent Question 2014; All India 91)*
   b. Involve lower limb
   c. Almost always manifests before puberty
   d. Acute lymphangitis may occur

6. **Milroy's disease is:** *(JIPMER 92)*
   a. Edema due to filariasis
   b. Post cellulitic lymphedema
   c. Congenital lymphedema
   d. Lymphedema following surgery

7. **Most common bacterial infection in lymphedema is:** *(DNB 2010)*
   a. Staphylococcus   b. Streptococcus
   c. E. coli   d. Pseudomonas

8. **Stemmer's sign is seen in:** *(Recent Question 2017)*
   a. Lymphedema   b. Venous disease
   c. Factitious lymphedema d. Arterial disease

9. **Diagnosis of lymphedema is usually done by:**
   a. History and clinical examination   *(Recent Question 2017)*
   b. Lymphangiogram
   c. MRI   d. CT scan

10. **Most common cause of lymphedema:**
    a. Filariasis   *(Recent Question 2017)*
    b. Lymph node dissection in malignancies
    c. Bacterial infection d. Congenital

■ MISCELLANEOUS

11. **True about lymphangioma is:**
    a. Common in puberty
    b. Respond in low doses to radiotherapy
    c. Lymphangioma progress slowly and may invade local tissue
    d. Predisposes to cancer

12. **Lymphangiosarcoma occurs in:** *(DNB 2010)*
    a. Lymphangiomas   b. Lymphomas
    c. Lymphedema   d. Serous cavity tumour

Explanations

■ LYMPHEDEMA

1. **Ans. b. Lymphedema precox**
2. **Ans. c. Filariasis**
3. **Ans. c. Marjolin's ulcer** *(Ref: Sabiston 20/e p1850; Schwartz 11/e p1001, 10/e p934-936, 1879-1880; Bailey 27/e p998-999)*
4. **Ans. a. Filariasis**
5. **Ans. None**
6. **Ans. c. Congenital lymphedema**
7. **Ans. b. Streptococcus**

> The **most common complication** of both **primary** and **secondary lymphedema is erysipelas** (**Acute Streptococcus bacterial infection** of the deep epidermis with lymphatic spread). Cellulites may occur concurrently in lymphedema because of **pooling of protein rich lymph fluid** makes it easier for the patient to develop an infection.

8. **Ans. a. Lymphedema** *(Ref: Bailey 27/e p998)*

> *"The contour of the ankle is lost through infilling of the submalleolar depressions, a 'buffalo hump' forms on the dorsum of the foot, the toes appear 'square' because of confinement of footwear and the skin on the dorsum of the toes cannot be pinched because of subcutaneous fibrosis (Stemmer's sign)."-Bailey 27/e p998*

9. **Ans. a. History and clinical examination** *(Ref: Bailey 27/e p1006)*

> *"It is usually possible to diagnose and manage lymphoedema purely on the basis of history and examination, especially when the swelling is mild and there are no apparent complicating features. In patients with severe, atypical and multifactorial swelling, investigations may help confirm the diagnosis, inform management and provide prognostic information."-Bailey 27/e p1006*

10. **Ans. a. Filariasis** *(Ref: Bailey 27/e p1003)*

■ MISCELLANEOUS

11. **Ans. c. Lymphangioma progress slowly and may invade local tissue**
12. **Ans. c. Lymphedema**

Thorax and Lung

■ MEDIASTINUM

MEDIASTINUM

Mediastinum is situated **between** the **lungs in** the **center of** the **thorax.**

Mediastinum is divided into 3 compartments		
Anterior or **Anterosuperior**	**Middle** or **Visceral compartment**	**Posterior** or **Paravertebral sulci**
Lies **in front of anterior pericardium** and **trachea**[Q]	Lies **within pericardial cavity**[Q] including trachea	Lies **posterior to posterior pericardium** and **trachea**[Q].

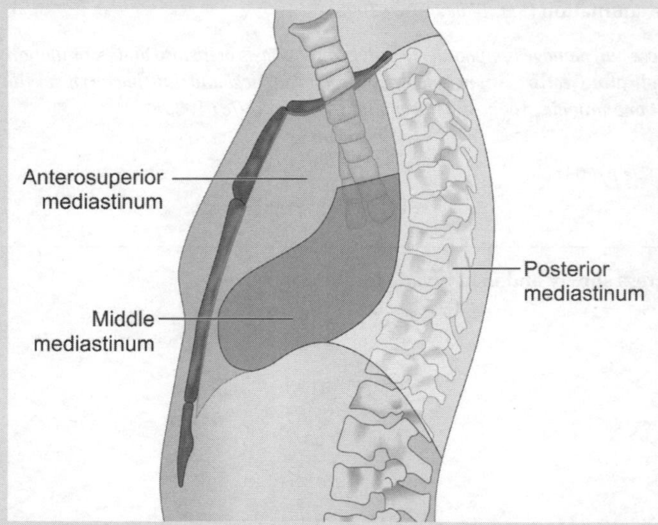

Locations of the Common Mediastinal Masses		
Anterior Mediastinum	**Middle Mediastinum**	**Posterior Mediastinum**

• **Thymoma**[Q] (**MC** in anterior mediastinum)
• **Lymphoma**[Q]
• **Germ cell tumors**[Q]
• **Thyroid** and **parathyroid masses**[Q]
• **Bronchogenic cyst**[Q]
• **Aneurysm**[Q]
	• **Cysts** (**MC** in middle mediastinum):
	  – **Pericardial (MC)**[Q]
	  – **Bronchogenic**[Q]
	  – Enterogenous
	  – **Neuroenteric**[Q]
	• Vascular masses (**aneurysm**[Q])
	• LN enlargement and **lymphoma**[Q]
	• Mesenchymal tumors
	• Pheochromocytoma
		• **Neurogenic tumors (MC overall**[Q])
		• **Meningoceles**[Q]
		• Mesenchymal tumors
		• Pheochromocytoma
		• **Lymphoma**[Q]
		• **Bochdalek hernia**[Q]
		• **Bronchogenic cyst**[Q]
		• **Enterogenous cyst**[Q]

Mediastinal Tumors in Adults		
Tumor Type	**Percentage of Total**	**Location**
Neurogenic tumors[Q]	21	**Posterior**
Cysts[Q]	20	All
Thymomas[Q]	19	**Anterior**

Contd…

Contd...

Tumor Type	Percentage of Total	Location
Lymphomas[Q]	13	**Anterior/middle**
Germ cell tumors	11	**Anterior**
Mesenchymal tumors	7	**All**
Endocrine tumors	6	Anterior/middle

Mediastinal Tumors in Children		
Tumor Type	**Percentage** of Total	**Location**
Neurogenic tumors	**40**[Q]	**Posterior**[Q]
Lymphomas	**18**[Q]	Anterior/middle
Cysts	18	**All**
Germ cell tumors	11	**Anterior**
Mesenchymal tumors	9	**All**
Thymomas	Rare	Anterior

MEDIASTINAL MASSES (MM)

- MC anterior MM: Thymoma[Q]
- MC middle MM: Cyst[Q] (Pericardial cyst is MC[Q])
- MC posterior MM: Neurogenic tumors[Q]
- MC MM (overall): Neurogenic tumors[Q]
- MM seen in **all three compartments** of mediastinum: Lymphoma, bronchogenic **cyst & m**esenchymal **tumors**[Q] (LYMB)
- IOC for diagnosis of MM (except neurogenic tumors): CT[Q]
- IOC for diagnosis of neurogenic tumors: MRI[Q]

■ THYMOMA

THYMOMA

- MC neoplasm of thymus; MC site: Anterior mediastinum[Q]
- Most frequently seen in **40-60 years** of age
- Most thymomas are **completely surrounded by a fibrous capsule**[Q]
- On the basis of cell types, divided into:
  - **Lymphocytic (25%)**
  - **Epithelial (25%)**
  - **Lymphoepithelial (50%)**[Q]

Clinical Features
- **Mostly asymptomatic**[Q], detected incidentally on chest X-ray
- May cause **dysphagia, dyspnea, SVC syndrome** and **paraneoplastic syndromes**[Q]

Paraneoplastic Syndromes		
Autoimmune	**Hematological**	**Neuromuscular**
• **SLE**[Q] • **Rheumatoid arthritis** • Polymyositis • Sarcoidosis	• **Cytopenias**[Q] • **Red cell aplasia**[Q] • **Hypogammaglobulinemia**[Q] • **Erythrocytosis**[Q]	• **Myasthenia gravis**[Q] **(MC)** • Neuromuscular disorders • Myotonic dystrophy • Myositis

Diagnosis
- **CT: Investigation of choice** for diagnosis of **thymoma**[Q].
- **Definitive diagnosis** is made on **histological study**[Q].

> - **Cytokeratin**[Q] is the **marker** that **best distinguishes thymomas** from lymphomas.
> - **CT scan: Most lymphomas** are associated with **marked lymphadenopathy** and **thymomas** most frequently appear as a **solitary encapsulated mass**[Q].

Staging
- **Masaoka staging**[Q] system is used.

Treatment
- **Treatment of choice: Total thymectomy** performed through **median sternotomy**[Q]
- **Large thymoma (>5 cm) with evidence of invasion: Thymectomy + Chemotherapy**[Q]
- **Myasthenia gravis** is treated with **thymectomy** and **anticholinesterase drugs**[Q].

■ PNEUMOTHORAX

PNEUMOTHORAX

- Pneumothorax is presence of **air within pleural space**
- **Spontaneous pneumothorax** is also known as **closed pneumothorax**, occurs when **visceral pleura ruptures without an external traumatic or iatrogenic cause**
- **Types**: Primary spontaneous pneumothorax & secondary spontaneous pneumothorax

■ PRIMARY SPONTANEOUS PNEUMOTHORAX

PRIMARY SPONTANEOUS PNEUMOTHORAX (PSP)

- **PSP** is spontaneous pneumothorax occurring **without underlying lung disease**
- **MC cause: Rupture of apical subpleural bleb**[Q]

Risk Factors for PSP	
• **Male sex**[Q]	• Family history
• **Smoking**[Q]	• **Marfan syndrome**[Q] (Tall thin body habitus[Q])

Clinical Features
- **Sudden in onset**, patient presents with **mild dyspnea**[Q]

Diagnosis
- **Best X-ray film** for diagnosis: **Chest X-ray PA view**[Q] (expiratory film)
- **Best investigation for diagnosis: NCCT**[Q]

Treatment
- **Initial treatment: Simple needle aspiration**[Q]   • **TOC: ICD insertion**[Q]

Thoracoscopic Management of PSP
• Thoracoscopic management includes **bleb resection** with **pleurodesis by talc** or **pleural abrasion**[Q]
• **100% successful in preventing recurrences**

Indications of Thoracoscopic Management of PSP	
• **Recurrences**[Q]	• **Complete lung collapse in first episode**[Q]

■ TENSION PNEUMOTHORAX

TENSION PNEUMOTHORAX

- A tension pneumothorax develops when a **'one-way valve' air leak** occurs either **from** the **lung** or **through** the **chest wall**[Q].
- **Air is forced into thoracic cavity** without any means of escape, **completely collapsing the affected lung**[Q].

> • **Mediastinum is displaced to the opposite side, decreasing venous return** and **compressing the opposite lung**[Q].

Common Causes of Tension Pneumothorax	
• **Penetrating chest trauma**[Q]	• **Iatrogenic lung punctures** (e.g. due to subclavian central venepuncture)
• **Blunt chest trauma**[Q] (with **parenchymal injury** and **air leak** that did not spontaneously close)	• Mechanical **positive pressure ventilation**[Q]

Clinical Features
- **Clinical presentation is dramatic.**
- The patient is panicky with **tachypnoea, dyspnoea** and **distended neck veins** (similar to pericardial tamponade)[Q].
- **Clinical examination** can reveal **tracheal deviation** (a **late finding** – not necessary to clinically confirm diagnosis), **hyperresonance** and **absent breath sounds over the affected hemithorax**[Q].

Diagnosis
- Tension pneumothorax is a **clinical diagnosis** and **treatment should not be delayed**[Q] by waiting for radiologicalconfirmation.

Treatment
- Treatment consists of **immediate decompression** by **rapid insertion** of a **large-bore needle** into the **2nd intercostal space** in the **mid-clavicular line**[Q] of the affected hemithorax.
- This is **immediately followed** by **insertion of a chest tube** through the **5th intercostal space** in the **anterior axillary line**[Q].

> • If the **tension in the pleural space is not relieved**, the **patient** is likely to **die from inadequate cardiac output** or **marked hypoxemia**[Q].

- **ATLS updates (2018)** says "Recent evidences support insertion of wide bore needle in 5th intercostal space slightly anterior to mid axillary line in adults"[Q]

■ HEMOTHORAX

HEMOTHORAX

- **Causes:** Trauma (MC), tumor, tuberculosis[Q]
- **Massive hemothorax** is usually the **result of major pulmonary vascular injuries** or **major arterial wounds** while minor injuries can cause small hemothorax.
- **MC cause of massive hemothorax in blunt injury:** Torn intercostal vessels because of rib fracture[Q]

Diagnosis

- Diagnosis is made by **needle aspiration of pleural fluid[Q]**.
- **Chest X-ray:** To assess the presence and extent of pleural cavity collection[Q]

> - A **supine position** with horizontal X-ray beam (decubitus position) is **better than erect film**, as about 400-500 ml of blood may be **hidden by diaphragm** on **upright chest X-ray[Q]**.

Management

- **Most patients** with hemothorax should be treated with **tube thoracostomy**, which allows **continuous quantification of bleeding[Q]**.
- In **most** of the **cases bleeding stops** as the **lung re-expands[Q]**.
- **Thoracoscopy** or thoracotomy: Pleural hemorrhage >200 mL/hour[Q]

Indications of Thoracotomy	
• Initial tube thoracostomy drainage of **>1000 mL (penetrating injury)[Q]** or **>1500 ml (blunt injury)[Q]** • Ongoing tube thoracostomy drainage of **>200 ml/hr** for **3 consecutive hours[Q]** in non-coagulopathic patients • **Caked hemothorax[Q]** despite of placement of two chest tubes • **Tracheo-bronchial injury[Q]**	• Selected **descending torn aorta** or **great vessel injury[Q]** • **Pericardial tamponade[Q]** • **Cardiac herniation[Q]** • **Massive air leak[Q]** from chest tube with inadequate ventilation • **Open pneumothorax[Q]** • **Esophageal perforation[Q]**

■ LUNG ABSCESS

LUNG ABSCESS

- **Lung abscess** refers to a **microbial infection** of the **lung** that results in necrosis of the pulmonary parenchyma.
- **MC cause** of **primary lung abscess:** Anaerobic bacteria[Q]
- **Etiology** of anaerobic lung abscess: **Aspiration[Q]**

Routes of Infection

- **Aspiration of organisms** that colonize oropharynx (MC)[Q]
- **Inhalation** of infection or aerosols
- **Hematogenous** dissemination from extrapulmonary site
- **Direct inoculation** (as in tracheal intubation or stab wounds)
- **Contiguous spread** from an adjacent site of infection

Clinical Features

- **Classic presentation:** An **indolent infection** that **evolves over several days or weeks**, usually in a host who has a **predisposition to aspiration[Q]**.
- A **common feature** is **periodontal infection** with **pyorrhea** or **gingivitis.**
- **Symptoms:** Fatigue, cough, sputum production, and fever[Q] Chills are uncommon.

Diagnosis

- Lung abscess can be detected by **chest X-ray** and **CT**
- **CT scan: Investigation of choice** for lung abscess[Q]

Treatment

- **Treatment** depends on the **presumed** or **established etiology.**
- Infections caused by **anaerobic bacteria:** Clindamycin[Q]

> - **Persistence of fever beyond 5–7 days** or **progression of the infiltrate** suggests **failure of therapy** and a need to **exclude** factors such as obstruction, complicating empyema, and **involvement of antibiotic-resistant bacteria[Q]**.

- Lung abscess due to **S. aureus:** Vancomycin[Q]
- **Indications for surgery: Failure to respond** to medical management, **suspected neoplasm**, and **hemorrhage[Q]**.

Causes of Failures of Medical Management	
• **Failure to drain** pleural collections[Q]	• **Giant abscess[Q]**
• **Inappropriate antimicrobial therapy[Q]**	• **Resistant pathogen[Q]**
• **Obstructed bronchus[Q]**	• **Refractory lesions[Q]**

■ POSTOPERATIVE LUNG COLLAPSE (ATELECTASIS)

POSTOPERATIVE LUNG COLLAPSE (ATELECTASIS)

- MC postoperative respiratory complication: Atelectasis[Q]
- As a result of the **anesthetic, abdominal incision,** and **postoperative narcotics,** the **alveoli in** the **periphery collapse** and a pulmonary shunt may occur.
- **Aggressive pulmonary toilet** to prevent buildup of secretions and secondary infection **High risk** in **heavy smokers, obese** patients[Q]

Clinical Features

- MC cause of a **postoperative fever** in the **first 48 hours:** Atelectasis[Q]
- **Symptoms: Low-grade fever, malaise** and **diminished breath sounds** in the lower lung fields.

Management

- **Prevention of atelectasis: Pain control, deep breaths (spirometry)** & cough[Q]
- Rarely, intermittent positive pressure breathing and **chest physiotherapy** may be required.

> - **Encouraging** the patient **to breathe deeply** and **cough** is the **single most valuable management** approach **in preventing** and **resolving atelectasis** and **pneumonia**[Q].

- **Pneumonia:** Managed with **aggressive pulmonary toilet,** induced **sputum for culture** and **sensitivity** testing, **IV antibiotic therapy.**

■ PULMONARY EMBOLISM

PULMONARY EMBOLISM

- Risk factors for pulmonary embolism are the **risk factors for thrombi formation** within **venous circulation.**
- **Calf venous thrombosis: Low risk** for embolism
- **MC form of thromboembolic disease**
- **Thrombosis of larger veins: High risk** for **embolism** (due to **loosely attached thrombus** to **venous wall**)

> - **MC site for DVT: Calf veins**[Q]
> - **MC source for pulmonary emboli: Proximal vein of lower extremity**[Q] (femoro-popliteal and iliac vein)

Risk Factors for Pulmonary Thromboembolism	
• **Age (Increasing age)**[Q]	• **Nephrotic syndrome**[Q]
• **Obesity**[Q]	• Inflammatory bowel disease[Q]
• **Immobility (bed rest >4 days)**[Q]	• **Polycythemia**[Q]
• **Pregnancy**[Q] and **Puerperium**[Q]	• **PNHQ** or **Lupus anticoagulant**
• **High dose estrogen therapy**[Q]	• **Behcet's syndrome**[Q]
• **Surgery/trauma** (especially of **pelvis, hip or lower limb**)[Q]	• **Homocystinuria**[Q]
• Malignancy (especially **pelvis, abdominal, metastatic**)	• **Paralysis** of lower limb
• Heart failure/Recent MI[Q]	• Varicose veins, **Infection**

Clinical Features

- Most (60–80%) are **clinically silent** beause they are **small** and there is **dual circulation** in **lungs.**
- **Symptoms: Dyspnea (MC)**[Q], chest pain, hemoptysis and cough
- **Signs: Tachypnea (MC)**[Q], fever, unilateral leg swelling, wheeze, pleural friction rub
- More than **60% obstruction** occurs in **pulmonary circulation** leading to sudden death, COR pulmonale or cardiovascular collapse.
- Multiple emboli over time may cause pulmonary hypertension and right ventricular failure.
- Paradoxical embolus can pass through an inter-atrial or inter ventricular defect. There by entering the systemic circulation.

> - Any patient with **high likelihood** of pulmonary embolism on clinical evaluation **straightaway undergoes** imaging **tests,** while a patient with **low clinical likelihood** should **first undergo D-dimer test.**

Factors for Clinical Assessment of Pulmonary Embolism	
• Clinical **signs** and **symptoms of DVT**[Q]	• **Immobilization** or **previous surgery in 4 weeks**[Q]
• An alternative diagnosis is less likely than pulmonary embolism	• **Previous DVT/PE**[Q]
• **Heart rate > 100/min**[Q]	• **Malignancy**[Q] (on treatment, treatment in past 6 months)
• **Hemoptysis**[Q]	

ECG Changes in Pulmonary Embolism (Sinus tachycardia: MC and non-specific finding on ECG[Q])	
Features of Acute Right Heart Strain	**Highly predictive of PE**
• Acute **right axis deviation**	• $S_1Q_3T_3$[Q]: Seen in **<12%** patients
• **P pulmonale**	– **S** wave in lead **I**
• **Right bundle branch block**	– **Q** wave in lead **III**
• **Inverted T waves**	– Inverted **T** wave in lead **III**
• ST segment change	– S wave in lead I, II, and III ($S_1S_2S_3$)

Contd…

Contd…

Diagnosis

- **D-dimer: Excellent screening test** for the diagnosis of PE[Q].
- **Best investigation in clinical suspicion of PE: Multidetector CT**[Q]
- Lung scanning is now a 2nd line diagnostic test for PE.
- **Pulmonary angiography: Gold standard for diagnosis of PE**[Q] (but expensive and cumbersome)
- **Modified Well's criteria: Used for predicting PE**[Q]

Treatment

- Most pulmonary emboli can be treated by **anticoagulation & observation**[Q]
- In cases of **severe right heart strain & shortness of breath, fibrinolytic treatment**[Q] or **radiologically guided catheter embolectomy**[Q] should be performed.

Prophylaxis Against PE

- **IVC filter** in patients with **high risk** of embolism **when anticoagulants are contraindicated**[Q]

■ FAT EMBOLISM SYNDROME

FAT EMBOLISM SYNDROME

Pathophysiology

- Fat embolism is a common phenomenon, more commonly seen in **multiple fracture and in fractures involving lower limbs especially femur**[Q].
- Circulating **fat globules>10 micron**[Q] in diameter occur in most adults after **close fracture of long bones**[Q] and histological traces of fat can be found in the lungs and other internal organs.

Clinical Presentation

- Usually manifests itself **within 24-48 hours**[Q].
- Early **warning signs** (within 72 hours of injury): Slight rise in temperature (**pyrexia**) and pulse rate (**tachycardia**)[Q]

> - In more pronounced cases there is **breathlessness**, mild mental confusion or restlessness, **petechiae on chest, axillae, retina and conjunctival folds**[Q]; progressive to **marked respiratory distress** and coma in severe cases.

Diagnosis

- In addition to the classic clinical features, signs of **retinal artery emboli (Striate hemorrhage** and **exudates**[Q]) may be present.
- **Sputum and urine: Presence of fat globules**[Q].
- Chest X-ray: **Patchy pulmonary infiltration (Snow storm appearance)**[Q]

Laboratory Tests	
No characteristic laboratory test, suggestive findings are:	
• **Thrombocytopenia**[Q]　•　(platelets <1.5 lacks)	• **Tachycardia**[Q]　　•　**Pyrexia**[Q]
• **PO$_2$ <60 mm Hg**[Q]	• **Fall in hemoglobin value**[Q]

Management

- **Supportive pulmonary care, definitive fracture management** and **effective treatment of shock** are the **corner stones** of current fat embolism management.

Respiratory support	Treatment of shock	Fracture stabilization
• Ranges from **oxygen administration** to **full respiratory support** with mechanical ventilation • **Oxygen** is the **only therapeutic tool** of **proven use**[Q]	• Maintain adequate intravascular volume • **Aggressive fluid resuscitation** • **Appropriate CVP monitoring** to avoid fluid overload. • **Albumin** for **fluid resuscitation** along **with** a **balanced electrolyte solution** because it not only restores blood volume but also binds free fatty acids.	• **Maintain adequate intravascular volume** • Since **movement at** the **fracture site** has been shown to **increase** the **fat emboli** in circulation, **early immobilization of lower extremity fractures**[Q] is advocated

Additional Therapies	
• **Steroids**: Prophylactic corticosteroids **benefit high risk patients** • **Heparin: Increase** serum **lipase activity** and decrease number of circulating fat globules • **Hypertonic glucose**: Metabolically **decrease production** of **free fatty acids**	• **Dextran**[Q]: To **reduce red cell aggregation, expand plasma volume, decrease blood viscosity** and **reduce platelet adherence** • **Aprotinin**: Decrease platelet aggregation and serotonin release • **Alcohol**: Reduces serum lipase activity

■ TRACHEOBRONCHIAL FOREIGN BODY

TRACHEOBRONCHIAL FOREIGN BODY

- **Aspiration of foreign bodies most commonly** occurs **in** the **toddler age**[Q] group.
- **Peanuts** are the object **most frequently aspirated**[Q].
- **MC anatomic location** for a foreign body is the **right main stem bronchus** or the **right lower lobe**[Q].

Clinical Features

- The child usually will **cough** or **choke while eating** but **may then become asymptomatic**.
- **Total respiratory obstruction** may occur **with a tracheal foreign body**; however, respiratory distress is usually mild if present at all.
- **A unilateral wheeze** is often heard **on auscultation**[Q].

Diagnosis

- **Chest X-ray: Radiopaque foreign body**

> - **Bronchoscopy (rigid) confirms** the **diagnosis** and **allows removal of** the **foreign body**[Q].

Complications

- A **solid foreign body** often will cause **air trapping**, with **hyperlucency** of the affected lobe or lung seen especially on expiration.
- **Delay in diagnosis** can lead to **atelectasis** and **infection**[Q].

■ MASSIVE HEMOPTYSIS

MASSIVE HEMOPTYSIS

- Hemoptysis of **>200-600 cc in 24 hours**[Q]
- Massive hemoptysis should be considered a **medical emergency**.

Diagnostic Evaluation

- For most patients, the **next step in evaluation of hemoptysis** should be a **standard chest radiograph**[Q].
- If a **source of bleeding** is **not identified** on plain film, a **CT of the chest**[Q] should be obtained.

> - If all of these studies are unrevealing, **bronchoscopy should be considered.**
> - **Rigid bronchoscopy** with an 8.5 mm or larger bronchoscope is needed.

Treatment

- Large-volume, life-threatening hemoptysis generally requires **immediate intervention regardless of the cause**[Q].
- The first step is to establish a **patent airway** usually by endotracheal intubation and subsequent **mechanical ventilation**[Q].

> - As most **large-volume hemoptysis arises from an airway lesion**, it is ideal if the site of the bleeding can be identified either by **chest imaging or bronchoscopy (more commonly rigid than flexible)**[Q].

> - If the bleeding does not stop with therapies of the underlying cause and passage of time, **severe hemoptysis from bronchial arteries can be treated with angiographic embolization of the culprit bronchial artery**[Q].

■ PULMONARY HAMARTOMA

PULMONARY HAMARTOMA

- **MC benign tumor of lung: Hamartoma**[Q]
- Most commonly, **hamartomas** are manifested by **overgrowth of cartilage**[Q].

Clinical Features

- Typically seen in **40–60 years** of age, **more common in males**[Q].
- **Usually peripheral, grow slowly** in the lung[Q].

Diagnosis

- **Chest X-ray: Popcorn calcification** is **diagnostic**[Q].
- **CT scan: Coin lesion**[Q]

Treatment

- **Definitive treatment: Excision of lesion**[Q]

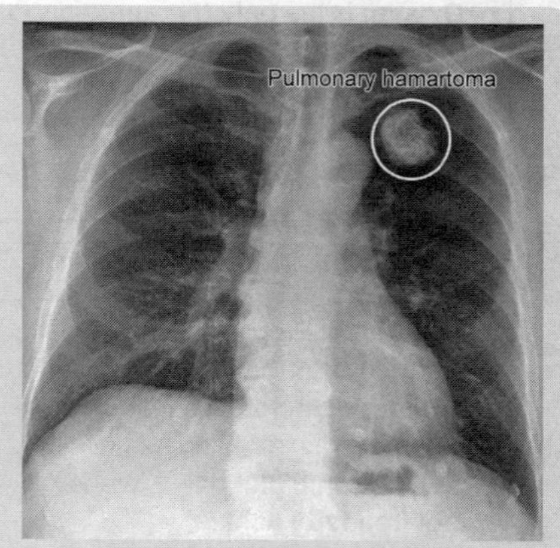

■ BRONCHIAL ADENOMA

BRONCHIAL ADENOMA

- Centrally located slow-growing endobronchial lesions that are **generally carcinoid tumors** (80%), **adenocystic tumors** (so called cylindromas, 10–15%), or **mucoepidermoid tumors** (2–3%).
- **Mean age at presentation** is **45 years** (range 15–60).

Clinical Features

- MC symptom: Recurrent Hemoptysis[Q]
- History of **chronic cough, intermittent hemoptysis**[Q], or **repeated episodes of airway obstruction** with **atelectasis**, or **pneumonias with abscess formation** due to endobronchial lesions obstructing the airway.

Diagnosis

- Usually **visible at bronchoscopy** but are **highly vascular** and may **bleed profusely after a bronchoscopic biopsy**[Q].

Treatment

- They are **largely curable by surgical resection (local excision)**, but they **may recur locally** or **become invasive** and **metastasize**[Q].
- **Five-year survival after resection** is 95% for localized **disease**.

■ BRONCHIAL CARCINOID

BRONCHIAL CARCINOID

- **Bronchial carcinoids (least malignant)** are the **most indolent** of the spectrum of pulmonary **neuroendocrine tumors**
- Most patients are **<40 years; Not related to smoking**[Q]

> - **Lower respiratory tract (Bronchus, lung, trachea)** is the **MC site of carcinoid tumor**[Q]
> - **Carcinoid syndrome** is **uncommon**[Q]

Pathology

- **Most tumors** are **confined to main stem bronchus**, commonly **projects into** the **lumen**[Q]
- Some tumors penetrate the bronchial wall to fan out in the peribronchial tissue producing the **collar-button lesion**[Q]

Most bronchial carcinoids
• **Do not have secretary activity**[Q]
• **Do not metastasize** to distant sites[Q]
• Are **amenable to resection**[Q]

■ MALIGNANT MESOTHELIOMA

MALIGNANT MESOTHELIOMA

- **Malignant mesothelioma** is MC **tumor of** the **pleura**[Q]
- In **20%** of malignant mesotheliomas, the **tumor arises from peritoneum**[Q]
- **Exposure to asbestos**[Q] is the **major known risk factor**
- More common in **males**[Q], most common **after 40 years** of age.

> - Three types: **Epithelial, sarcomatous**, and **biphasic**[Q]
> - **Epithelial types** are **associated with** a more **favorable prognosis**[Q]

Pathophysiology

- Physical characteristics of **specific fibers** (referred to as **serpentine** or **amphibole**) have been shown to be important.

> - **Serpentine fibers:** Large and curly, **not able to travel beyond larger airways**.
> - **Straight amphibole fibers:** In particular the **crocidolite**[Q] fibers **navigate distally** into the pulmonary parenchyma, **most clearly associated with mesotheliomas**.

- **Latency period** between asbestos exposure and the development of mesothelioma is **at least 20 years**.

> • **Multicentric tumor** with **multiple pleura-based nodules** coalescing to form sheets of tumor (but **not bilaterally symmetrical**[Q])

- Natural history of the disease in **untreated patients culminates in death** due to **local extension**.

Clinical Features

- Most patients present with **dyspnea** and **chest pain**[Q].
- Over **90%** have a **pleural effusion**[Q].

Contd…

Contd…

Diagnosis

- Results of **thoracentesis** are **diagnostic in <10%** of patients.
- **Chest X-ray: Pleural effusion**, generalized **pleural thickening** and **shrunken hemithorax**[Q].
- **Thoracoscopy** or **open pleural biopsy** with **special staining** of tumor samples is **required to differentiate mesotheliomas from adenocarcinomas**[Q].
- **Butchart**[Q] staging is used for **mesothelioma**

Management

- **No effective therapy**[Q]
- **Treatment option**s: Supportive care only, surgical resection, and multimodality approaches (using a combination of surgery, chemotherapy, and radiation therapy).

Differentiation of Mesothelioma from Adenocarcinoma		
	Mesothelioma	**Adenocarcinoma**
CEA	Negative	**Positive**[Q]
Cytokeratins (Low molecular weight)	**Positive**[Q]	Negative
Vimentin	**Positive**[Q]	Negative
Electron microscopic features	**Long, sinuous villi**	**Short, straight villi with fuzzy glycocalyx**

■ CARCINOMA LUNG (BRONCHOGENIC CARCINOMA)

CARCINOMA LUNG (BRONCHOGENIC CARCINOMA)

- **MC type** of lung neoplasm[Q]
- **Arises from respiratory epithelium** of bronchi, bronchioles and alveoli

• **MC visceral malignancy** and leading cancer **causing death: CA lung**[Q]

- **Mostly arise from lung hilum** except bronchoalveolar carcinoma and some adenocarcinoma[Q].
- **Mucinous bronchoalveolar carcinoma** tends to **spread aerogenously** forming **satellite tumors**[Q].

Etiology and Risk factors	
• **Smoking**[Q] (both active and passive)	• **Old infarct** and **lung scars** (most progress to **adenocarcinoma**[Q])
• Air pollution (**Radon**[Q])	• Ionizing **radiation** exposure[Q]
• Exposure to **asbestos**, **uranium** and **nickel**[Q]	

Oncogenic abnormality	
Small Cell Carcinoma	**Non-small Cell Carcinoma**
• Over expression of **bcl-2**, **myc** and **telomerase**[Q]	• Over expression of **bcl-2** and **telomerase** with abnormal **ras** gene[Q]
	• **K-ras** mutation is **MC mutation** (90%) in **adenocarcinoma**[Q]

Clinical Features

- **MC symptoms** are **cough**[Q] (MC) > dyspnea > chest pain>hemoptysis.
- Slightly **more common** on **right side,** more frequently occurs in **upper lobes**[Q]
- **Major source** of **hemoptysis** are **bronchial arteries**[Q]
- Endobronchial growth of central tumors cause cough, stridor, wheeze and dyspnoea
- **Peripheral tumors** present as **pain** due to pleural or chest wall involvement

Symptoms due to regional spread	
• Tracheal obstruction, esophageal compression, **RLN paralysis**[Q]	• Horner's syndrome
• **Pancoast syndrome**[Q] (involvement of **C8T1 nerves** by pancoast tumor causing pain in **ipsilateral shoulder** and **arm**[Q])	• **SVC syndrome** (MC cause is **small cell carcinoma** >SCC)[Q]
	• **Malignant pleural effusion**[Q]

Metastases

- **MC Site of metastasis:** <u>Brain</u>[Q] > <u>Bone</u>[Q] > <u>Liver</u>[Q] > <u>Adrenal</u>[Q] > <u>Lung</u>[Q] (BBLAL)
- **CA lung is MC primary for metastasis** to Kidney, Esophagus, Pancreas, Adrenal, Brain & Skin (KEPABS).

Paraneoplastic syndromes	
• **CVS:** Thrombophlebitis, non-bacterial thrombotic endocarditis	• **GIT:** Carcinoid syndrome
• **Metabolic:**	• Erythrocytosis
– Inappropriate **ACTH** and **ADH** secretion (**small cell**)[Q]	• **Neuromuscular:**
– **Hypercalcemia (SCC)**[Q]	– Dementia, optic neuritis, retinopathy, limbic encephalitis
• Acanthosis nigricans (adenocarcinoma), dermatomyositis, icthyosis, erythema gyretum repens	– **Autonomic neuropathy (small cell)**[Q]
	– **Lambert-Eaton syndrome**[Q] (small cell)
	– Polymyositis, **cerebellar degeneration**[Q]

Contd…

Contd…

Diagnosis and Staging

- **Tissue diagnosis**: Tumor tissue can be obtained by **bronchial** or **transbronchial biopsy**[Q] through **fiberoptic bronchoscopy**[Q]; by percutaneous biopsy of enlarge node
- **Integrated PET-CT** scan is the **best imaging modality**[Q] for diagnosis and staging

■ 8TH AJCC TNM CLASSIFICATION OF LUNG CANCER

8th AJCC (2017) TNM Classification of Lung Cancer
Tis: Carcinoma in situ
T1a: Tumor ≤1 cm in greatest dimension[Q]
T1b: Tumor >1 cm but ≤2 cm in greatest dimension[Q]
T1c: Tumor >2 cm but ≤3 cm in greatest dimension[Q]
T2: Tumor >3 cm but ≤5cm or tumor with any of the following features: Involves **main bronchus**, regardless of **distance to the carina** but **without involvement of carina**[Q] Invades **visceral pleura**[Q] Associated with **atelectasis** or **obstructive pneumonitis** that extends to the hilar region either involving part of or the entire lung[Q] **T2a**: Tumor >3 cm but ≤4 cm in greatest dimension[Q] **T2b**: Tumor >4 cm but ≤5 cm in greatest dimension[Q]
T3: **Tumor >5 cm but ≤7 cm** in greatest dimension or one that **directly invades any of the following**: parietal pleura, **chest wall** (including superior sulcus tumors), **phrenic nerve, parietal pericardium**; or separate tumor nodule(s) in the same lobe as the primary[Q]
T4: Tumor **>7 cm or of any size** that **invades any** of the following: **diaphragm, mediastinum, heart, great vessels, trachea, recurrent laryngeal nerve, esophagus, vertebral body, carina**; or **Separate tumor nodule(s)** in a **different ipsilateral lobe to that of primary**[Q]
N1: Metastasis in **ipsilateral peribronchial** and/or **ipsilateral hilar lymph nodes** and **intrapulmonary nodes**, including involvement by direct extension[Q]
N2: Metastasis in **ipsilateral mediastinal** and/or **subcarinal lymph node(s)**[Q]
N3: Metastasis in **contralateral mediastinal, contralateral hilar, ipsilateral or contralateral scalene**, or **supraclavicular lymph node(s)**[Q]
M1a: **Separate tumor nodule(s)** in a **contralateral lobe**; tumor with **pleural or pericardial nodules** or **malignant pleural (or pericardial) effusion**[Q] **M1b**: Single extra-thoracic metastasis in a single or multiple organs[Q] **M1c**: Multiple extra-thoracic metastasis in single or multiple organs[Q]

8th AJCC (2017) TNM Stage Groupings			
Stage	**T**	**N**	**M**
Occult cancer	TX	N0	M0
0	**Tis**	N0	M0
IA	**T1**	N0	M0
IA1	T1mi-T1a	N0	M0
IA2	T1b	N0	M0
IA3	T1c	N0	M0
IB	T2a	N0	M0
IIA	T2b	N0	M0
IIB	T1a-c, T2a-b	**N1**	M0
	T3	N0	M0
IIIA	T1a-c, T2a-b	**N2**	M0
	T3	**N1**	M0
	T4	**N0-1**	M0
IIIB	T1a-c, T2a-b	N3	M0
	T3, T4	N2	M0
IIIC	**T3, T4**	N3	M0
IVA	Any T	Any N	**M1a/b**
IVB	Any T	Any N	**M1c**

Contd…

Contd…

Treatment of Operable NSCCL
- Stage IA, IB, IIA, IIB: **Surgical resection**[Q]
- **Adjuvant chemotherapy** is given in **stage II**[Q]
- Stage IIIA with **minimal N2 involvement**: Neoadjuvant chemotherapy followed by **surgical resection** with **complete mediastinal LN dissection**[Q]
- **Postoperative radiotherapy** for patients found to have **N2 disease**[Q]

WHO Classification of Carcinoma Lung			
Adenocarcinoma	**Squamous Cell Carcinoma**	**Small Cell Carcinoma**	**Large Cell Carcinoma**
• **MC** histological **type**[Q] • MC in **non-smokers, young** patients, **females**[Q] • Located **peripherally**[Q] • **Slow growth** and propensity to **metastasize** to **opposite lung**[Q] • **Metastasize** more frequently to **CNS**[Q] • Most cells contain **mucin**[Q] • **Noguchi classification**[Q] is used for adenocarcinoma	• **MC** in **smokers**[Q] • MC type in **India** • MC variety associated with **hypercalcemia** (produces **PTH-rp**)[Q] • **Central**[Q] in distribution • Prone to undergo **central necrosis & cavitation**[Q] • **Pancoast** tumor is histologically **SCC**[Q] • Associated with **best prognosis**[Q]	• **Most malignant, central**[Q] in distribution, strongly related to **smoking**[Q] • Cells are small with little cytoplasm called "**oat cell**"[Q] • Associated with **massive hilar** or **mediastinal lymphadenopathy, mediastinal invasion** and **perihilar mass**[Q] • **MC variety** associated with **paraneoplastic syndrome, hypokalemia** and **SVC syndrome**[Q] • Most responsive to **chemotherapy** (cisplatin + etoposide) • Shows response to **radiotherapy**[Q] • Hormones produced by small cell carcinoma: **ACTH, AVP** (vasopressin), **calcitonin, ANF**, gastrin releasing peptide[Q]	• Highly **undifferentiated** with **cavitating nature** • **Metastasize early** with **poor prognosis**

■ PANCOAST TUMOR (SUPERIOR SULCUS TUMOR)

PANCOAST TUMOR (SUPERIOR SULCUS TUMOR)

- Pancoast's (or superior sulcus tumor) syndrome results **from local extension of** a **tumor growing in the apex of the lung** with **involvement of eighth cervical and 1st and 2nd thoracic nerves**, with **shoulder pain characteristically radiates in the ulnar distribution of** the arm, often with **radiologic destruction of 1st and 2nd ribs**[Q].
- Often **Horner's syndrome** and Pancoast's syndrome co-exist
- **IOC for diagnosis: MRI**[Q]

Treatment
- **Preoperative RT** followed by **En bloc resection** of lung and **chest wall** with consideration of **postoperative RT** or **intra-operative brachytherapy**[Q].

■ CARDIAC TUMORS

CARDIAC TUMORS

- MC primary cardiac tumor: **Myxoma**[Q]
- MC malignant tumor of heart in adults: **Angiosarcoma**[Q]
- MC benign tumor of heart in children: **Rhabdomyoma**[Q]
- MC malignant tumor of heart in children: **Rhabdomyosarcoma**[Q]
- MC tumor of **cardiac valves**: Papillary fibroelastoma[Q]
- MC site of involvement in cardiac metastasis: **Pericardium**[Q]

■ CHEST WALL TUMORS

CHEST WALL TUMORS

- MC chest wall tumor: **Metastasis**[Q]
- MC benign primary chest wall neoplasm: **Osteochondroma**[Q]
- MC **malignant** primary chest wall neoplasm: **Chondrosarcoma**[Q]

■ MEDIASTINAL TUMORS

1. **Which of the following is not an anterior mediastinal mass?**
   (Recent Question 2018)
   - a. Thymoma
   - b. Neurogenic tumor
   - c. Thyroid mass
   - d. Lymphoma

2. **Common location of thoracic pheochromocytoma:**
   (Recent Question 2017)
   - a. Anterior mediastinum
   - b. Posterior mediastinum
   - c. Middle mediastinum
   - d. Superior mediastinum

3. **The commonest anterior mediastinal tumors is:**
   (MCI June 2018, Recent Question 2017, WBPG 2015, Recent Question 2015, COMEDK 2008)
   - a. Aneurysm of descending aorta
   - b. Neurogenic tumour
   - c. Thymoma
   - d. Bronchogenic cyst

4. **During exploration, a patient is found to have a tumor in the thymus that is invading the pericardium and surrounding the left and right phrenic nerves. The pathologist says that appears on frozen section to be a benign thymoma. The surgeon now should:** *(Recent Question 2018)*
   - a. Repeat frozen section
   - b. Attempt as complete a resection as possible
   - c. Close the chest and plan irradiation therapy
   - d. Close the chest and await permanent sections

5. **Posterior mediastinal tumors:** *(PGI June 2003)*
   - a. Neuroblastoma
   - b. Bronchogenic cyst
   - c. Neuroenteric cyst
   - d. Lymphoma
   - e. Anterior thoracic meningioma

6. **Most common tumor in the posterior mediastinum is:**
   (Recent Question 2016, DNB 2005, 2000, All India 2008, DPG 2008)
   - a. Neurofibroma
   - b. Teratoma
   - c. Lymphoma
   - d. Bronchogenic cyst

7. **The most common primary tumor of mediastinum:**
   - a. Lymphoma
   - b. Teratoma
   - c. Neurogenic tumor
   - d. Thymoma

8. **Most common tumour of mediastinum:** *(MCI Dec 2019)*
   - a. Thymoma
   - b. Lymphoma
   - c. Neurogenic tumor
   - d. Neuroblastic tumor

■ PLEURAL EFFUSION

9. **Most common site for putting chest drain in case of pleural effusion:** *(Bihar PG 2014, AIIMS June 2000, All India 2002)*
   - a. 2nd intercostal space mid-clavicular line
   - b. 7th intercostal space mid-axillary line
   - c. 5th intercostal space mid clavicular line
   - d. 5th intercostal space just lateral to vertebral column

10. **Pseudochylous pleural effusion is most often seen in:**
    - a. TB
    - b. Lymphoma
    - c. CA lung
    - d. Filariasis

11. **A rapidly filling hemorrhagic pleural effusion is suggestive of:** *(COMEDK 2004)*
    - a. Pneumococcal infection
    - b. Tuberculosis
    - c. Bronchiectasis
    - d. Bronchogenic carcinoma

■ PNEUMOTHORAX

12. **In a patient with one episode of spontaneous pneumothorax, which is advised?** *(Jharkhand 2003)*
    - a. Stop diving
    - b. Stop smoking
    - c. Stop flying
    - d. All

13. **A case of spontaneous pneumothorax comes to you. What will be earliest treatment of choice?** *(AIIMS June 97)*
    - a. IPPV
    - b. Needle aspiration
    - c. ICD
    - d. Wait and watch

14. **While inserting a central venous catheter, a patient develops respiratory distress. The most likely cause is:**
    (Bihar PG 2014, All India 2002)
    - a. Hemothorax
    - b. Pneumothorax
    - c. Pleural effusion
    - d. Hypovolemia

■ TENSION PNEUMOTHORAX

15. **A patient after road traffic accident presented with tension pneumothorax. What is the first line of management?**
    - a. Insert wide bore needle in 2nd intercostal space
    - b. Immediate chest X-ray *(MCI June 2019, AIIMS Nov 2013)*
    - c. CT scan
    - d. Emergency thoracotomy

16. **Condition which builds within hemithorax resulting in collapsed lung, flattened diaphragm, contralateral mediastinal shift and compromised venous return to right side of heart is known as:** *(MCI Dec 2019, Sept 2007)*
    - a. Open pneumothorax
    - b. Flail chest
    - c. Massive pulmonary hemorrhage
    - d. Tension pneumothorax

17. **What is the emergent management of tension pneumothorax?**
    - a. Chest X-ray *(AIIMS Nov 2014)*
    - b. Emergency room thoracotomy in unstable patients
    - c. Insert needle in 2nd intercostal space
    - d. Tube thoracostomy in 5th intercostal space

18. **A person met with road traffic accident and came to casualty with contusion on anterior chest wall with Pulse rate-90/minute, BP-120/80 mm Hg, respiratory rate-16/minute. Normal heart sounds are heard but breath sounds were decreased on the left side and trachea was deviated towards right. Which of the following is the first line management?**
    - a. Needle thoracostomy *(AIIMS May 2017)*
    - b. Pericardiocentesis
    - c. Chest tube insertion and drainage
    - d. Immediate exploratory thoracotomy

■ HEMOTHORAX

19. **Decision regarding surgery in a case of hemothorax due to blunt trauma chest should be based on:** *(All India 2008)*
    - a. Chest symptoms
    - b. Hemodynamic status
    - c. Nature of chest tube output
    - d. X-ray finding

20. **Excessive bleeding during hemothorax is caused usually by:**
    (AIIMS June 94)
    - a. Vena cava
    - b. Internal mammary artery
    - c. Heart
    - d. Major artery

21. **Which of the following vessel is injured in hemothorax patient?** *(Recent Question 2017)*
    a. Pulmonary artery
    b. Pulmonary vein
    c. Bronchial artery
    d. Intercostal arteries

■ LUNG ABSCESS

22. **A 80-year-old male presented with lung abscess in left upper zone. Best treatment modality is:** *(UPPG 2008)*
    a. Antibiotics according to organisms
    b. Surgical drainage
    c. Tube thoracostomy
    d. Wait and Watch

23. **Empyema can be caused by the following parasites except:** *(MHSSMCET 2008)*
    a. E. granulosus
    b. Entamoeba coli
    c. Paragonimus westermani
    d. Strongyloides stercoralis

■ PLEURAL COLLECTIONS

24. **True about chylothorax:** *(DPG 2007)*
    a. Left side more common
    b. Clear fluid
    c. Immediate thoracotomy should be done
    d. TOC is excision and ligation of thoracic duct

25. **Chyluria is caused by all except:** *(MCI Sept 2009)*
    a. Pregnancy
    b. Childbirth
    c. Filariasis
    d. Bile duct stones

■ SEQUESTRATION OF LUNGS

26. **Intralobar sequestration of lungs takes its blood supply from:** *(Recent Question 2014, AIIMS Nov 94)*
    a. Internal mammary artery
    b. Descending abdominal aorta
    c. Pulmonary artery
    d. None of the above

27. **Intralobar sequestration of lung is commonest in the:**
    a. Apical segment of upper lobe   *(Recent Question 2016)*
    b. Medial segment of middle lobe
    c. Lateral basal segment of lower lobe
    d. Posterior basal segment of lower lobe

28. **Diagnosis of lung sequestration by:** *(JIPMER 2000)*
    a. CT
    b. Angiography
    c. MRI
    d. X-ray

■ TRACHEOBRONCHIAL FOREIGN BODY

29. **In erect posture, commonest site of foreign body in bronchus:** *(AIIMS June 99)*
    a. Right posterior basal
    b. Right anterior basal
    c. Lateral basal
    d. Medial basal

30. **Foreign body aspiration in supine position causes which of the following parts of the lung commonly to be affected?**
    a. Apical left lobe   *(Recent Question 2014, AIIMS June 2002)*
    b. Apical lobe of right lung
    c. Apical part of the lower lobe
    d. Posterobasal segment of left lung

■ VATS

31. **In Video assisted thoracoscooic surgery for better vision, the space in the operative field is created by:** *(AIIMS June 2002)*
    a. Self retaining retractor
    b. CO_2 insufflations
    c. Collapse of ipsilateral lung
    d. Rib spacing

32. **VATS refers to:** *(Orissa 2011)*
    a. Vacuum assisted thoracic surgery
    b. Video assisted thoracoscopic surgery
    c. Video assisted transplant surgery
    d. None of the above

■ THORACOTOMY

33. **Thoracotomy is indicated in all the following except:**
    a. Penetrating chest injuries   *(MHPGMCET 2003)*
    b. Rapidly accumulating hemothorax
    c. Massive air leak
    d. Pulmonary contusion

34. **During emergency thoracotomy, the incision is made > 1 cm lateral to sternal margin to preserve:** *(All India 2012)*
    a. Intercoastal artery
    b. Superior epigastric artery
    c. Internal mammary artery
    d. Intercostal vein

■ BENIGN LUNG TUMORS

35. **The most common benign tumor of the lung is:** *(COMEDK 2008)*
    a. Hamartoma
    b. Alveolar adenoma
    c. Teratoma
    d. Fibroma

36. **The following is true about bronchial carcinoids:**
    a. Highly radiosensitive   *(JIPMER 2011)*
    b. Metastasis common
    c. Carcinoid syndrome does not manifest
    d. Commonly arises from terminal bronchioles

37. **Blood stained sputum may be the only symptom in:** *(Kerala 90)*
    a. Bronchiectasis
    b. Carcinoma bronchus
    c. Adenoma bronchus
    d. Pulmonary T.b.

■ MESOTHELIOMA

38. **All are true regarding mesothelioma except:**
    a. Bilaterally symmetrical   *(AIIMS May 2011)*
    b. Associated with asbestos exposure
    c. Histopathology shows biphasic pattern
    d. Occurs in late middle age

39. **Which of the following is true about Mesothelioma?**
    a. Pleural effusion is exudative   *(Recent Question 2017, 2016)*
    b. Butchart staging is used
    c. Manganese exposure is a predisposing factor
    d. Cough and dyspnoea are common late features

■ SQUAMOUS CELL CARCINOMA

40. **Cavity formation in bronchogenic carcinoma occurs in:** *(Recent Question 2016)*
    a. Oat cell carcinoma
    b. Squamous cell carcinoma
    c. Adenocarcinoma
    d. Bronchoalveolar

■ ADENOCARCINOMA

41. **A patient presented with 1cm coin lesion over right upper lobe of lung on X-ray not suggestive of metastasis. FNAC revealed adenocarcinoma, no lymphadenopathy. Treatment is:**
    a. Surgery   *(JIPMER 2010)*
    b. Surgery + chemotherapy
    c. Surgery + Radiotherapy
    d. Surgery + chemoradio therapy

42. **Commonest type of lung carcinoma in nonsmokers is:** *(Kerala PG 2015, AIIMS Dec 94)*
    a. Squamous cell carcinoma
    b. Adenocarcinoma
    c. Alveolar cell carcinoma
    d. Small cell carcinoma

43. **Lung to lung metastasis is seen in:**
    a. Adenocarcinoma of lung
    b. Squamous cell carcinoma
    c. Small cell carcinoma
    d. Neuroendocrine tumor of lung

■ SMALL CELL CARCINOMA

44. **Which of the following statements about small cell carcinoma is true?**   *(All India 2009)*
    a. Bone metastasis is uncommon
    b. Peripheral in location
    c. Chemosensitive tumor
    d. Paraneoplastic syndrome with PTH is common

45. **Poorest prognosis in lung cancer is associated with:**   *(COMEDK 2005)*
    a. Small cell carcinoma   b. Adenocarcinoma
    c. Squamous cell carcinoma   d. Adenosquamous cancer

46. **Marker of small cell cancer of lung is:**   *(DNB 2011)*
    a. Synaptobrevin   b. Chromogranin
    c. Cytokeratin   d. Vimentin

47. **In a chronic smoker, a highly malignant aggressive and metastatic lung carcinoma is:**   *(AIIMS May 2001)*
    a. Squamous cell carcinoma   b. Small cell carcinoma
    c. Adenocarcinoma   d. Large cell carcinoma

48. **Carcinoma lung responding best to chemotherapy:**
    a. Squamous cell carcinoma   b. Oat cell type
    c. Adenocarcinoma   d. All respond equally

■ CARCINOMA LUNG

49. **A 60-year-old male presented to the emergency with breathlessness, facial swelling and dilated veins on the chest wall. The most common cause is:**   *(All India 2003)*
    a. Thymoma
    b. Lung cancer
    c. Hodgkin's lymphoma
    d. Superior vena caval obstruction

50. **Which of the following tumor is most commonly associated with superior vena cava syndrome?**   *(All India 2011)*
    a. Lymphoma
    b. Small cell carcinoma
    c. Non small cell carcinoma
    d. Metastasis

51. **Which of the following has no infectious etiology?**
    a. Nasopharyngeal carcinoma   *(AIIMS Nov 2009)*
    b. Hepatocellular carcinoma
    c. Non-small cell lung carcinoma
    d. Gastric carcinoma

52. **Most common site of metastasis in lung carcinoma:**
    a. Liver   b. Adrenal   *(AIIMS May 2007)*
    c. Bone   d. Brain

53. **Superior sulcus tumor of the lungs characteristically present with:**   *(JIPMER 2011)*
    a. Horner syndrome   b. Breathlessness
    c. Hemoptysis   d. Pancoast syndrome

54. **Superior vena cava syndrome is caused most commonly by:**   *(MCI Sept 2009, AIIMS Nov 95)*
    a. Adenocarcinoma   b. Squamous cell carcinoma
    c. Small cell carcinoma   d. Large cell carcinoma

55. **Hoarseness secondary to bronchogenic carcinoma is usually due to extension of the tumor into:**   *(UPSC 2002)*
    a. Vocal cord
    b. Superior laryngeal nerve
    c. Left recurrent laryngeal nerve
    d. Right vagus nerve

56. **Most common site of metastasis of carcinoma bronchi:**
    a. Liver + Bones   b. Prostate   *(HPU 2005)*
    c. Kidney   d. Breast

57. **The site of temporal bone metastasis is most commonly seen with:**   *(UPPG 2010)*
    a. Carcinoma breast   b. Carcinoma bronchus
    c. Carcinoma kidney   d. Carcinoma prostate

58. **Carcinoma responding maximally to radiotherapy is:**   *(MCI Sept 2006)*
    a. Squamous cell carcinoma   b. Adenocarcinoma
    c. Small cell carcinoma   d. Large cell carcinoma

59. **Most common type of carcinoma lung is:**   *(AIIMS May 93)*
    a. Small cell carcinoma   b. Adenocarcinoma
    c. Squamous cell carcinoma   d. Large cell carcinoma

60. **All of the following are true regarding oat cell carcinoma of lung, except:**   *(AIIMS June 99)*
    a. Variant of large cell anaplastic carcinoma
    b. Chemotherapy is effective
    c. Paraneoplastic syndrome may be present
    d. Causes SIADH

61. **Pancoast's syndrome is due to:**   *(Recent Question 2017)*
    a. C4-5 invasion   b. C8-T1 invasion
    c. Lower trunk involvement   d. C5-6 invasion

62. **In case of CA lung, which among the following will be contraindication for surgical resection?**   *(AIIMS Nov 2000)*
    a. Malignant pleural effusion
    b. Hilar lymphadenopathy
    c. Consolidation of one lobe
    d. Involvement of visceral pleura

63. **A patient presents with secondaries to the adrenals. The most common site of primary is:**   *(WBPG 2012, All India 2000)*
    a. Lung   b. Kidney
    c. Breast   d. Stomach

64. **Most common symptom of lung carcinoma:**   *(AIIMS 90)*
    a. Cough   b. Dyspnea
    c. Weight loss   d. Chest pain

65. **The commonest intrabronchial cause of hemoptysis is:**   *(AIIMS May 95)*
    a. Carcinoma lung   b. Adenoma lung
    c. Emphysema   d. Bronchiectasis

66. **A patient presents with a cavitatory lesion in right upper lobe of lung. The best investigation is:**   *(All India 2000)*
    a. Bronchoscopy, lavage and brushing
    b. CT scan
    c. X-ray
    d. FNAC

■ PULMONARY EMBOLISM

67. **All of the following conditions may predispose to pulmonary embolism except:**   *(All India 2003)*
    a. Protein S deficiency   b. Malignancy
    c. Obesity   d. Progesterone therapy

68. **A patient had a femur fracture for which internal fixation was done. Two days later, the patient developed sudden onset shortness of breath with low-grade fever. What is the likely cause?**   *(AIIMS May 2017)*
    a. Pneumothorax   b. Fat embolism
    c. Pleural effusion   d. Congestive heart failure

69. **In acute pulmonary embolism, the most frequent ECG finding is:**   *(AIIMS May 2006)*
    a. S1Q3T3 pattern   b. 'P' pulmonale
    c. Sinus tachycardia   d. Right axis deviation

70. **Most common symptom in pulmonary embolism:**
    (MCI Sept 2007)
    a. Dyspnea b. Pleuritic chest pain
    c. Cyanosis d. Hemoptysis

71. **Gold standard to diagnose pulmonary embolism is:**
    a. Chest X-ray *(MHCET 2016)*
    b. Pulmonary angiography
    c. Ventilation purfusion scintiscan
    d. CT chest

72. **Investigation of choice in pulmonary embolism:** *(JIPMER 2010)*
    a. Ventilation perfusion scan
    b. MRI
    c. CECT
    d. X-ray

73. **D-Dimer is the most sensitive diagnostic test for:** *(DPG 2011)*
    a. Pulmonary embolism
    b. Acute pulmonary edema
    c. Cardiac tamponade
    d. Acute myocardial infarction

74. **The sequence of symptoms in pulmonary embolism is:**
    a. Fever, pain, dyspnea *(DNB 90)*
    b. Fever, dyspnea
    c. Dyspnea, pain, hemoptysis
    d. Dyspnea, cough, purulent sputum

■ THORACIC INJURY

75. **True about chest trauma:** *(PGI June 2008)*
    a. ECG done in all cases associated with sternal fracture
    b. Under water seal drainage if associated with pneumo-thorax
    c. X-ray chest investigation of choice
    d. Urgent surgery needed in all cases

76. **Interstitial emphysema may be found in the following conditions:** *(Kerala 98)*
    a. Chest injury b. Tracheostomy
    c. Surgical wound d. All

■ ADULT RESPIRATORY DISTRESS SYNDROME

77. **Most common abnormality associated with ARDS:**
    a. Hypoxemia *(JIPMER 2011)*
    b. Hypercapnea
    c. Diffuse alveolar damage
    d. Bilateral alveolar infiltrates

78. **Which of the following is most characteristic feature of ARDS?**
    a. Diffuse alveolar damage *(All India 2012)*
    b. Hypoxia and hypoxemia
    c. Surfactant deficiency
    d. Hypocapnia

79. **All are seen in ARDS, except:** *(AIIMS May 95)*
    a. Pulmonary edema
    b. Decreased tidal volume
    c. Hypercapnia
    d. Decreased compliance

■ PULMONARY TUBERCULOSIS

80. **A young man with pulmonary tuberculosis presents with massive recurrent hemoptysis. For angiographic treatment, which vascular structure should be evaluated first?**
    (All India 2004)
    a. Pulmonary artery b. Bronchial artery
    c. Pulmonary vein d. Superior vena cava

■ CARDIAC TUMORS

81. **The most common primary cardiac tumor is:**
    (Recent Question 2016, COMEDK 2004)
    a. Rhabdomyoma b. Myxoma
    c. Leiomyoma d. Lipoma

■ PECTUS EXCAVATUM AND CARINATUM

82. **Regarding pectus excavatum all are true except:**
    a. Gross CVS dysfunction *(PGI Dec 97)*
    b. Decrease in lung capacity
    c. Cosmetic deformity
    d. Depression in chest

■ MISCELLANEOUS

83. **Treatment of choice in postoperative lung collapse is all except:** *(AIIMS June 95)*
    a. Needle drainage b. Corticosteroids
    c. Pulmonary resection d. Endoscopic suction

84. **Following is true of eventration of diaphragm:**
    a. It is a development defect *(Recent Question 2016)*
    b. Early surgery is treatment
    c. Defect is usually muscular
    d. Diagnosed mostly clinically

85. **Which needle is used for pleural biopsy?** *(COMEDK 2007)*
    a. Vin silvermann's b. Abram's
    c. Abraham's d. Osgood's

86. **Heimlich valve is used for drainage of:** *(COMEDK 2008)*
    a. Pneumothorax b. Hemothorax
    c. Emphysema d. Malignant pleural effusion

87. **The organism most frequently related to mediastinal fibrosis is:** *(DPG 2010)*
    a. Actinomycosis b. Histoplasma
    c. Hansen's bacillus d. Staphylococcus

88. **Coronary graft is most commonly taken from:** *(DNB 2012)*
    a. Femoral vein b. Saphenous vein
    c. Axillary vein d. Cubital vein

89. **Hamman's sign is seen in:** *(APPG 2016)*
    a. Pneumomediastinum b. Diaphragmatic paralysis
    c. Empyema thoracis d. Subphrenic abscess

90. **Pulmonary infiltrates and respiratory distress in a 40 years old patient with femur fracture suggest the diagnosis of:**
    (MCI Dec 2019)
    a. Fat embolism b. Pulmonary embolism
    c. Air embolism d. Obstruction

Explanations

■ MEDIASTINAL TUMORS

1. **Ans. b. Neurogenic tumor** *(Ref: Sabiston 20/e p1608; Schwartz 11/e p728-729, 10/e p673; Bailey 27/e p936)*
2. **Ans. b. Posterior mediastinum** *(Ref: Imaging in Oncology by Michael A. Blake (2008)/p165)*

   - "The posterior mediastinum is the usual site of intrathoracic pheochromocytoma. They have also rarely been reported to occur in the middle mediastinum, with involvement of the left atrial wall or interatrial septum and aortic arch." –*Imaging in Oncology by Michael A. Blake (2008)/p165*

3. **Ans. c. Thymoma**
4. **Ans. b. Attempt as complete a resection as possible**
5. **Ans. a. Neuroblastoma, b. Bronchogenic cyst, c. Neuroenteric cyst, d. Lymphoma**
6. **Ans. a. Neurofibroma**
7. **Ans. c. Neurogenic tumor**
8. **Ans. c. Neurogenic tumor** *(Ref: Schwartz 11/e p728-729)*

■ PLEURAL EFFUSION

9. **Ans. None >b. 7th intercostal space mid-axillary line** *(Ref: Sabiston 20/e p1605; PJ Mehta 13th/361)*
10. **Ans. a. TB** *(Ref: http://radiology.rsna.org/content/216/2/478.long)*

    Most common cause of **pseudochylous pleural effusion** is **tuberculous pleurisy.**

    #### CHYLIFORM PLEURAL EFFUSION (PSEUDOCHYLOUS OR CHOLESTEROL EFFUSION)
    - Chyliform pleural effusion, often called **pseudochylous** or cholesterol effusion, is a **high-lipid effusion** that is not chylous.
    - The **most common cause** of this pleural reaction is **tuberculous pleurisy**[Q], but it has **also been described in** association with **rheumatoid arthritis.**
    - The presence of a **fat-fluid level within the pleural space** is **unique to pseudochylous effusion**[Q].

11. **Ans. d. Bronchogenic carcinoma** *(Ref: Sabiston 20/e p1605; Schwartz 11/e p739, 10/e p680; Bailey 27/e p921)*

    A **rapidly filling hemorrhagic pleural effusion** is suggestive of **malignancy,** most commonly **bronchogenic carcinoma.**

    #### MALIGNANT PLEURAL EFFUSION
    - Malignancy is a common cause of pleural effusion.
    - **Most malignant pleural effusions** are **exudative**[Q].
    - They are the **second most common exudative effusive process**.
    - **Metastatic breast** and **lung cancers** are the **most common malignancies**[Q] that cause malignant effusions.

■ PNEUMOTHORAX

12. **Ans. d. All**

    #### AFTERCARE OF PNEUMOTHORAX
    - **Smoking cessation**[Q]
    - **Air travel** is **discouraged for** up to **7 days**[Q] after complete resolution of a pneumothorax if recurrence does not occur.
    - **Underwater diving** is **considered unsafe**[Q] after an episode of pneumothorax unless a preventative procedure has been performed.

13. **Ans. b. Needle aspiration**
14. **Ans. b. Pneumothorax**

■ TENSION PNEUMOTHORAX

15. **Ans. a. Insert wide bore needle in 2nd intercostal space** *(Ref: Sabiston 20/e p428; Schwartz 11/e p185-186, 10/e p164; Bailey 27/e p367)*

    - First line of management in tension pneumothorax: Insert wide bore needle in 2nd intercostal space.
    - "Treatment of tension pneumothorax consists of immediate decompression by rapid insertion of a large-bore needle into the 2nd intercostal space in the mid-clavicular line[Q] of the affected hemithorax."

16. **Ans. d. Tension pneumothorax**
17. **Ans. c. Insert needle in 2nd intercostal space**
18. **Ans. c. Chest tube insertion and drainage** *(Ref: Sabiston 20/e p230-231; Schwartz 11/e p185-186, 10/e p164; Harrison 20/e p2009)*

■ HEMOTHORAX

19. **Ans. b. Hemodynamic status, c. Nature of chest tube output** *(Ref: Bailey 27/e p366, 368; Trauma Manual: Companion to trauma 4/e p165)*

- Nature of chest tube drainage and Hemodynamic status both provide vital clues that may form an indication of surgery (Thoracotomy). However a deteriorating **hemodynamic status despite adequate volume resuscitation** should form the **most important guide, for urgent emergency thoracotomy** and is the **single best answer of choice.**

  - Bailey says "If the patient is **in extremis** with a **falling systolic blood pressure**, despite volume resuscitation, there is no choice but to proceed **immediately with** a **left anterolateral thoracotomy**".

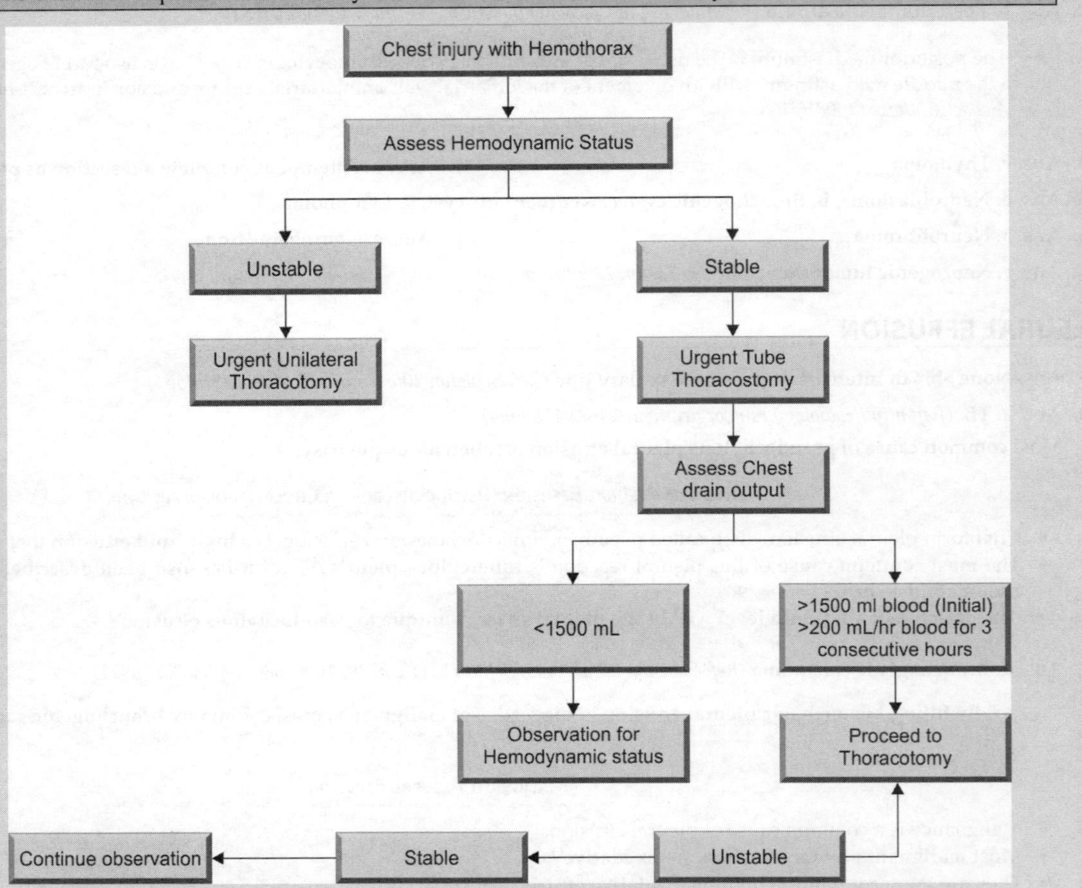

20. **Ans. d. Major artery**

21. **Ans. d. Intercostal arteries** *(Ref: Schwartz 11/e p222, 10/e p166; Bailey 27/e p368)*

"The most common cause of massive haemothorax in blunt injury is continuing bleeding from torn intercostal vessels or occasionally from the internal mammary artery secondary to the fracture of ribs." –Bailey 27/e p368

"After blunt trauma, a major hemothorax usually is due to multiple rib fractures with severed intercostal arteries, but occasionally bleeding is from lacerated lung parenchyma which is usually associated with an air leak. After penetrating trauma, a great vessel or pulmonary hilar vessel injury should be presumed." –Schwartz 11/e p222, 10/e p166

*"**Hemothorax** usually derives from bleeding of intercostal and internal mammary arteries and is caused by **vessel wall injury** from fractured ribs. **Very rarely, hemothorax** can be caused by traumatic laceration of diaphragmatic **vessels** from broken ribs." –Emergency Radiology: Imaging and Intervention edited by Borut Marincek, Robert F. Dondelinger (2007)/p187*

■ LUNG ABSCESS

22. **Ans. a. Antibiotics according to organisms** *(Ref: Harrison 20/e p921; Sabiston 20/e p1595; Schwartz 11/e p708, 10/e p650-651; Bailey 27/e p937)*

23. **Ans. d. Strongyloides strecoralis** *(Ref: Bailey 24/e p117)*

Parasitic Causes of Empyema	
• Paragonimus wetermani[Q] • E. granulosus[Q]	• Entamoeba coli[Q]

■ PLEURAL COLLECTIONS

24. **Ans. d. TOC is excision and ligation of thoracic duct** *(Ref: Sabiston 20/e p1606; Schwartz 11/e p742, 10/e p685-687; Bailey 27/e p1013)*

25. **Ans. d. Bile duct stones** *(Ref: Bailey 27/e p1003, 1004, 1013)*

■ SEQUESTRATION OF LUNGS

26. **Ans. b. Descending abdominal aorta** *(Ref: Sabiston 20/e p1581; Schwartz 11/e p1715-1716, 10/e p1607; Bailey 27/e p937)*

27. **Ans. d. Posterior basal segment of lower lobe**   28. **Ans. a. CT**

■ TRACHEOBRONCHIAL FOREIGN BODY

29. **Ans. a. Right posterior basal** *(Ref: Schwartz 11/e p1716-1717, 10/e p1607-1608; Bailey 27/e p924)*

30. **Ans. c. Apical part of the lower lobe**

■ VATS

31. **Ans. c. Collapse of ipsilateral lung** *(Ref: Sabiston 20/e p355; Schwartz 11/e p701, 10/e p704; Bailey 27/e p370, 922-923, 931, 934)*

> **VIDEO ASSISTED THORACOSCOPIC SURGERY (VATS)**
>
> - In contrast to most laparoscopic techniques, the **working space for VATS is created not by adding an insufflating gas but rather by removing air from the ipsilateral lung parenchyma** causing **collapse of the ipsilateral lung**[Q].
> - **Used for pulmonary decortication, pleurodesis, and lung or pleural biopsies**

32. **Ans. b. Video assisted thoracoscopic surgery**

■ THORACOTOMY

33. **Ans. d. Pulmonary contusion**   34. **Ans. c. Internal mammary artery**

■ BENIGN LUNG TUMORS

35. **Ans. a. Hamartoma** *(Ref: Schwartz 11/e p677, 10/e p622, 9/e p526; Bailey 27/e p934)*

36. **Ans. c. Carcinoid syndrome does not manifest** *(Ref: Robbins 9/e p719; Harrison 20/e p602)*   37. **Ans. c. Adenoma bronchus**

■ MESOTHELIOMA

38. **Ans. a. Bilaterally symmetrical** *(Ref: Sabiston 20/e p1607; Schwartz 11/e p744, 10/e p688; Bailey 27/e p146, 922)*

39. **Ans. b. Butchart staging is used**

■ SQUAMOUS CELL CARCINOMA

40. **Ans. b. Squamous cell carcinoma**

■ ADENOCARCINOMA

41. **Ans. a. Surgery** *(Ref: Harrison 20/e p547; Sabiston 20/e p1590)*

42. **Ans. b. Adenocarcinoma**   43. **Ans. a. Adenocarcinoma of lung**

■ SMALL CELL CARCINOMA

44. **Ans. c. Chemosensitive tumor** *(Ref: Harrison 20/e p538)*

Small cell carcinomas are **highly chemosensitive** with an overall **90% regression rate with chemotherapy.**

Property	Small cell carcinoma		Non small cell carcinoma
Location	• **Central** location[Q]		• **Peripheral** location[Q]
Metastasis	• **Highly metastatic** lesion with widespread metastasis at time of diagnosis. • **Common site** of metastasis include **brain, bone, liver** and **adrenals**[Q]		• Less metastatic than small cell carcinoma
Paraneo-plastic syndrome	• **ACTH**[Q] • **Calcitonin**[Q] • Gastrin Releasing peptide	• **AVP** (Vasopression)[Q] • **ANF**[Q]	• **PTH-rp**[Q]
Response to chemo-therapy	• **Superior response**[Q] • Overall **regression rate 90%**[Q] • Rate complete regression in 30%		• **Inferior response** • Objective shrinkage in 30-50% • Complete response: uncommon

45. Ans. a. Small cell carcinoma

46. Ans. b. Chromagranin

47. Ans. b. Small cell carcinoma

48. Ans. b. Oat cell type

■ CARCINOMA LUNG

49. Ans. d. Superior vena caval obstruction *(Ref: Harrison 20/e p541)*

50. Ans. b. Small cell carcinoma

51. Ans. c. Non-small cell lung carcinoma

52. Ans. b. Adrenal

53. Ans. d. Pancoast syndrome *(Ref: Harrison 19/e p519; Sabiston 20/e p583; Schwartz 11/e p680, 10/e p623, 641-642; Bailey 27/e p926)*

54. Ans. c. Small cell carcinoma

55. Ans. c. Left recurrent laryngeal nerve

56. Ans. a. Liver + Bones

57. Ans. a. Carcinoma breast *(Ref: www.ncbi.nlm.nih.gov v.63(Suppl 1); Jul 2011)*

TEMPORAL BONE METASTASIS

- **Metastatic tumors** to the temporal bone are **uncommon**
- **Usually** seeded by the **hematogenous route**

> - **MC metastatic lesion** in the temporal bone: **CA Breast**[Q]

- **Lung, prostate** and **renal carcinomas** are all well **documented for** their **metastatic potential to** the **temporal bone**[Q].

58. Ans. c. Small cell carcinoma

59. Ans. b. Adenocarcinoma

Adenocarcinoma	
• **MC** histological **type**, MC in **non-smokers, young** patients, **females**[Q] • Located **peripherally** with slow growth and propensity to **metastasize** to **opposite lung**[Q]	• **Metastasize** more frequently to **CNS** • Most cells contain **mucin**[Q] • **Noguchi classification** is used for **adenocarcinoma**[Q]

60. Ans. a. Variant of large cell anaplastic carcinoma

61. Ans. b. C8-T1 invasion *(Ref: Sabiston 20/e p355; Schwartz 11/e p680, 10/e p623)*

62. Ans. a. Malignant pleural effusion

63. Ans. a. Lung

64. Ans. a. Cough

65. Ans. a. Carcinoma lung

66. Ans. a. Bronchoscopy, lavage and brushing *(Ref: Bailey 27/e p923)*

Uses of Bronchoscopy	
Diagnostic	Confirmation of disease: • **Carcinoma** of the **bronchus**[Q] • Inflammatory and Infective process
Investigative	• **Tissue biopsy**[Q]
Preoperative assessment	• **Before lung resection**[Q] • Before esophageal resection • **Persistent hemoptysis**[Q]
Therapeutic	• Removal of secretions • **Removal of foreign bodies**[Q] • Stent placement, endobronchial resection

■ PULMONARY EMBOLISM

67. Ans. d. Progesterone therapy *(Ref: Harrison 20/e p1910; Sabiston 20/e p294-296; Schwartz 11/e p2118, 10/e p924-925; Bailey 27/e p987)*

> - **Estrogen, not the progesterone** therapy **predisposes to thrombosis** and **pulmonary embolism**.

68. Ans. b. Fat embolism *(Ref: Harrison 20/e p1910; Robbins 9/e p128; Apley's 9/e p681; Rockwood 6/e p553)*

69. Ans. c. Sinus tachycardia

70. Ans. a. Dyspnea

71. Ans. b. Pulmonary angiography

72. Ans. c. CECT

73. Ans. a. Pulmonary embolism

74. Ans. c. Dyspnea, pain, hemoptysis

■ THORACIC INJURY

75. Ans. a. ECG done in all cases associated with sternal fracture, b. Under water seal drainage if associated with pneumothorax, c. X-ray chest investigation of choice *(Ref: Bailey 27/e p366, 938)*

CHEST TRAUMA

- **Sternal fracture** also constitute a **marker for serious associated injuries**, including **myocardial contusion, myocardial rupture,** esophageal perforation, airway injuries and thoracic aortic rupture.
- In **blunt cardiac injuries**, ECG is the **first diagnostic test**[Q].
- **Routine investigation** in the **emergency department** of **injury to** the **chest** is based on **clinical examination, supplemented by chest radiography.**
- In the **unstable patient, chest radiography** is the **investigation of first choice**[Q], provided that it does not interfere with resuscitation.

76. Ans. d. All

ADULT RESPIRATORY DISTRESS SYNDROME

77. Ans. a. Hypoxemia *(Ref: Harrison 20/e p2031; Sabiston 20/e p1599)*

78. Ans. a. Diffuse alveolar damage   **79. Ans. c. Hypercapnia**

PULMONARY TUBERCULOSIS

80. Ans. b. Bronchial artery *(Ref: Grainger Radiology 4/e p609)*

Brochial arteries are the major source of hemoptysis.

CARDIAC TUMORS

81. Ans. b. Myxoma *(Ref: Harrison 20/e p1847)*

PECTUS EXCAVATUM AND CARINATUM

82. Ans. a. Gross CVS dysfunction *(Ref: Sabiston 20/e p1601; Bailey 27/e p939, 940)*

MISCELLANEOUS

83. Ans. d. Endoscopic suction *(Ref: Sabiston 20/e p291-292)*

Endoscopic suction is not used in postoperative level collapse.

84. Ans. a. It is a development defect, c. Defect is usually muscular *(Ref: www.ncbi.nlm.nih.gov › ... Lung India › v.26(2); Apr-Jun 2009 by AP Kansal)*

85. Ans. b. Abram's *(Ref: Bailey 27/e p922)*

NEEDLES FOR PLEURAL BIOPSY

- **Abrams' needle**
- **Cope's needle**

86. Ans. a. Pneumothorax *(Ref: thorax.bmj.com ›Volume 58, Issue suppl 2)*

HEIMLICH VALVE

- **Heimlich chest drain valve** is a specially designed flutter valve used to replace underwater bottles in chest drainage.
- The valve allows **unidirectional flow**[Q].
- In clinical situations like **spontaneous pneumothorax, open thoracotomy, recurrent pleural effusion**[Q], chest drainage can be simplified with Heimlich chest drain valve.

87. Ans. b. Histoplasma *(Ref: Sabiston 20/e p1596; Schwartz 11/e p715, 10/e p679-680)*

The organism most frequently related to mediastinal fibrosis is Histoplasma.

88. Ans. b. Saphenous vein *(Ref: Bailey 27/e p890)*

- **Saphenous vein** are the **most commonly employed conduits in coronary vascularization.**
- **Most preferred graft for CABG: LIMA (left internal mammary artery) > Long saphenous vein**[Q]

89. Ans. a. Pneumomediastinum

90. Ans. a. Fat embolism *(Ref: Bailey 27/e p956)*

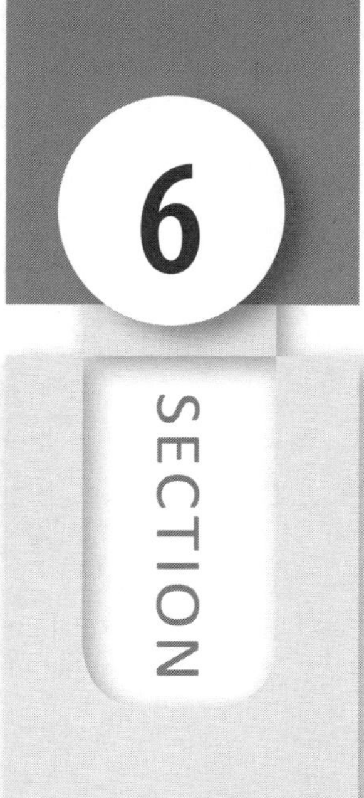

Plastic Surgery

- ❍ Burns
- ❍ Plastic Surgery and Skin Lesions
- ❍ Wound Healing, Tissue Repair and Scar

Burns

■ PATIENTS WITH THE FOLLOWING CRITERIA ARE REFERRED TO A DESIGNATED BURN CENTER

PATIENTS WITH THE FOLLOWING CRITERIA ARE REFERRED TO A DESIGNATED BURN CENTER

- Partial-thickness **burns >10% TBSA**[Q]
- Burns involving the **face, hands, feet, genitalia, perineum,** or **major joints**[Q]
- Any **full-thickness burn**[Q]
- **Electrical burns,** including **lightning injury**[Q]
- **Chemical burns**[Q]
- **Inhalation injury**[Q]
- Burns in patients with **preexisting medical disorders**[Q] that could complicate management, prolong recovery, or affect outcome
- Any patient with burns and **concomitant trauma**[Q] (e.g., **fractures**) in which the burn injury poses the greater immediate risk for morbidity and mortality.
- **Burned children in hospitals without qualified personnel** or equipment to care for children
- Burns in patients who will **require special social, emotional,** or long-term rehabilitative intervention

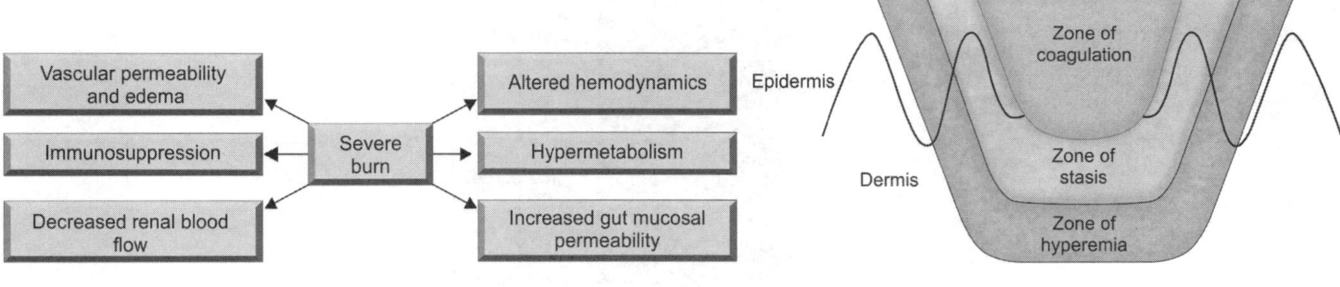

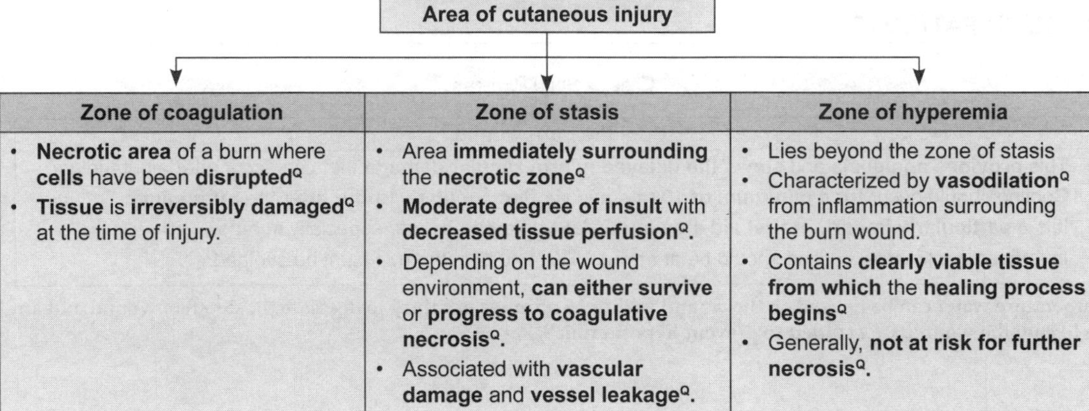

Pathophysiology of burns		
Area of cutaneous injury		
Zone of coagulation	**Zone of stasis**	**Zone of hyperemia**
• **Necrotic area** of a burn where **cells** have been **disrupted**[Q] • **Tissue** is **irreversibly damaged**[Q] at the time of injury.	• Area **immediately surrounding** the **necrotic zone**[Q] • **Moderate degree of insult** with **decreased tissue perfusion**[Q]. • Depending on the wound environment, **can either survive** or **progress to coagulative necrosis**[Q]. • Associated with **vascular damage** and **vessel leakage**[Q].	• Lies beyond the zone of stasis • Characterized by **vasodilation**[Q] from inflammation surrounding the burn wound. • Contains **clearly viable tissue from which** the **healing process begins**[Q] • Generally, **not at risk for further necrosis**[Q].

■ BURN CLASSIFICATION

Burns depth			
First Degree	**Second Degree**	**Third Degree**	**Fourth Degree**
• Epidermal burn[Q] • Involve **only epidermis**[Q] • **Do not blister**[Q] • **Erythematous**[Q] because of dermal vasodilatation • **Painful**[Q] • **Heal without scarring** in **5-10 days**[Q]	• **Partial thickness**[Q] burn • Involve **epidermis** and some **part of dermis**[Q] • **Divided into: Superficial and Deep** second degree	• **Full thickness burn**[Q] • Involve **all layers of dermis**[Q] • Characterized by **hard leathery eschar,** that is painless and **black, white** or **cherry red**[Q] • **No capillary refilling** or **pin-prick sensation**[Q] • **All dermal and epidermal components are lost**[Q] • **Heals** only by **wound contracture**[Q] • Require **excision with skin grafting** to heal[Q]	• Involve **other organs** beneath the skin, such as **muscle, bone** and **brain**[Q].

Superficial second degree	Deep second degree
• Involve **upper layer of dermis (papillary dermis)**[Q] • **Erythematous**[Q] • **Blisters are seen**[Q] • **Blanch to touch**[Q] • **Painful**[Q] • **Heals without scarring in 7-14 days**[Q]	• Also known as **deep partial thickness burn**[Q] • Injury extends to **reticular layer of dermis**[Q] • **Don't blanch**[Q] • **Mottled pink** and **white color** of wound surface[Q] • **Capillary refilling** is **absent** or occurs slowly[Q] • **Pain is absent**[Q] • **Pin-prick sensation is preserved**[Q] • **Heals in 3-9 weeks** with **scar formation**[Q]

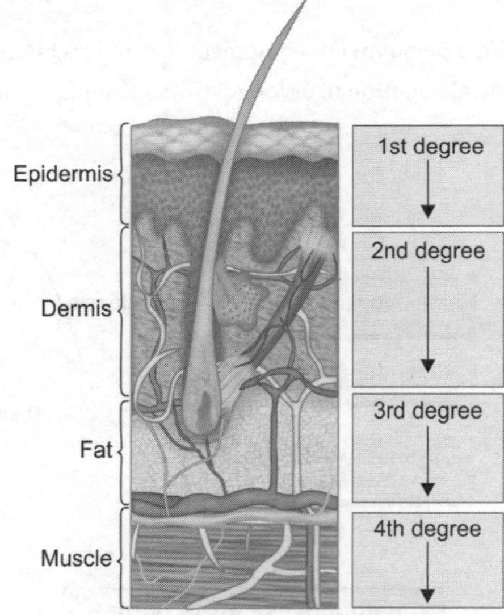

■ CARE OF BURN PATIENTS

Care of Burn Patients
Cool the burn wound
• This **provides analgesia** and **slows the delayed microvascular damage** that can occur after a burn injury. • Cooling should occur **for a minimum of 10 min** and is **effective up to 1 hour after** the **burn injury.** • It is a **particularly important first aid step in partial-thickness burns,** especially **scalds.** • In temperate climates, cooling should be at **about 15°C,** and hypothermia must be avoided.

• **Room temperature water** can be **poured** on the wound **within 15 minutes of injury** to decrease the depth of wound, but **any subsequent measures to cool** the **wound** are **avoided to prevent hypothermia**[Q].

Contd...

Contd...

> • Iced water should never be used, even on the smallest of burns[Q].
> • If ice or cold water is used on larger burns, systemic hypothermia often follows, and the associated cutaneous vasoconstriction can extend the thermal damage.

- The **entire constricting eschar** must be **incised longitudinally**[Q] to completely relieve the impediment to blood flow.
- **Superficial partial thickness burn** with blisters **heals without residual scarring in 2 weeks** irrespective of the dressing. Treatment is **non-surgical**. The simplest method of **treating superficial burn** is **by exposure**[Q].

■ BURN SIZE (% BSA)

BURN SIZE (% BSA)

- Determination of **burn size estimates** the **extent of injury**.
- **Burn size** is assessed by **Wallace rule of nines** (By **Alfred Russel Wallace**[Q])

Wallace rule of nines
• **In adults:**
– Each **upper extremity: 9%**[Q]
– **Head and neck: 9%**[Q]
– **Lower extremities: 18%**[Q]
– **Anterior** and **posterior** aspects of the **trunk: 18%**[Q]
– **Perineum** and genitalia: **1%**[Q]

- **Children** have a relatively **larger proportion** of body surface area **in** their **head** and **neck**, which is compensated for by a relatively smaller surface area in the lower extremities.
  - **In infants: Head** and **neck- 21%**[Q] ; **Each leg- 13%**[Q]
- **Berkow formula**[Q] is used to **accurately determine burn size** in **children**.
- **For estimating smaller burns: Area of open hand**[Q] (including palm and extended fingers) of the patient is approximately **1%**[Q] of TBSA
- This method is helpful in **evaluating splash burns** and burns of **mixed distribution**.

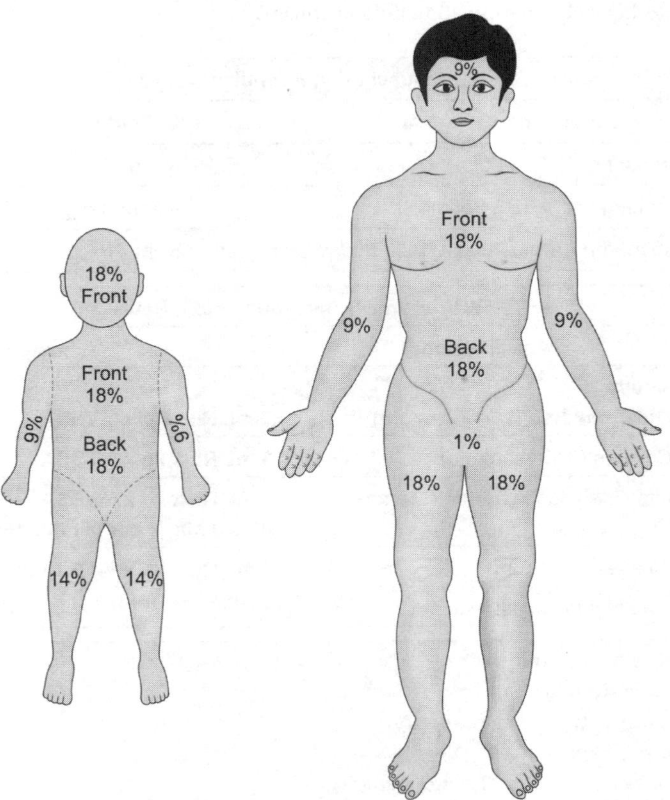

Estimation of burn size using the rule of nine

■ FLUID RESUSCITATION

FLUID RESUSCITATION

- **IV fluid resuscitation:** In **children** with burn **>10%**[Q] TBSA & **adult** with burn **>15%**[Q] TBSA
- **Regimen** of **fluid resuscitation follows** the **fluid loss**, which is at its **maximum in first 8 hours** and slows such that by 2-36 hours the patient can be maintained on her/his normal daily requirement.

Fluids used in resuscitation
• **Ringer Lactate** is **most commonly used**[Q].
• Some centers use **human albumin, FFP** or **hypertonic saline**[Q]

- If **oral resuscitation** is to be commenced, it is important that the **water given is not salt free. Hyponatremia** and **water intoxication can be fatal**[Q].
- In **children, maintenance fluid** must be given, usually **dextrose-saline.**[Q]
- **Simplest** and **most widely used formula: Parkland formula**[Q]

• **Hypertonic saline** has been **effective in treating burn shock**[Q].
• It produces **hyperosmolality** and **hypernatremia.**
• This reduces the shift of intracellular water to the extracellular space.
• Advantage includes **less tissue edema** and a resultant **decrease in escharotomies** and **intubation**[Q].

- **Protein** should be given **after the first 12 hours** of burn.
- The commonest **colloid based formula** is **Muir** and **Barclay formula**[Q].

Monitoring of Resuscitation

- The key to monitoring is **urine output**[Q].

• **Urine output** should be **0.5-1.0 mL/kg/hour**[Q] (i.e. 30-60 ml per hour[Q]).

- **Other measures for monitoring:**
  - Acid base balance and Hematocrit
  - In **cardiac dysfunction: Transesophageal USG** and **Central line**[Q]

Venous Access for Infusion

- In **adults:** Ideal sites are **veins in hand, antecubital fossa** or **neck.**
- **Saphenous vein cut down** is useful **in patient with difficult access** and is **used in preference to central venous cannulation.**
- **CVP line** is used for **CVP monitoring,** helps in **estimating fluid overload**[Q].

Resuscitation Formulas			
Formula	**Crystalloid Volume**	**Colloid Volume**	**Free water**
Parkland[Q]	**4 mL/kg** per % TBSA burn	None	None
Brooke[Q]	**1.5 mL/kg** per % TBSA burn	**0.5 mL/kg** per % TBSA burn	**2.0 L**
Galveston[Q] **(pediatric)**	**5000 mL/m² burned** area + **1500 mL/m² total** area	None	None

ATLS (2018) Burn Resuscitation Fluid Rates		
Category of Burn	**Age & Weight**	**Adjusted Fluid Rates**
Flame or scald	**Adults** **Older children (≥14 years old)**	**2 mL RL x kg x %TBSA**
	Children (**<14 years** old)	**3 mL RL x kg x %TBSA**
	Infants & young children (**≤30 kg**)	**3 mL RL x kg x %TBSA** **plus a sugar containing solution at maintenance rate**
Electrical injury	All ages	**4 mL RL x kg x %TBSA until urine clears**
RL: Ringer lactate; TBSA: Total burnt surface area		

• **MC cause** of **death** at the site of **burn:** Asphyxia
• **MC cause** of **death in burns:** Septicemia[Q]
• **MC cause** of **early death in burns:** Hypovolemic shock[Q]
• **MC cause** of **late death in burns:** Septicemia[Q]
• **MC organism** responsible for **sepsis in burns:** Pseudomonas[Q]

BURNS: % BSA

1. According to "rule of nines", burns involving perineum are:
a. 1%   b. 9%   *(MCI March 2009)*
c. 18%   d. 27%

2. A five years old child presents to the emergency department with burns. The burn area corresponding to the size of his palm is equal to: *(All India 2011)*
a. 1% BSA   b. 5% BSA
c. 10% BSA   d. 20%

3. Rule of nine of estimate surface area of a burnt patient was introduced by: *(Recent Question 2016)*
a. Mortix Kaposi   b. Wallace
c. Joseph Lister   d. Thomas Barclay

4. Best method to assess burns in 5 years old child caused by boiling water: *(AIIMS May 2013)*
a. Palm method   b. Rule of 9
c. Lund and Browder chart   d. Rule of one

5. Head and face burn in infant is: *(Recent Question 2014, 2013)*
a. 15%   b. 18%
c. 12%   d. 32%

6. Percentage of burn in children is best assessed by:
a. Rule of 9   *(DNB 2014)*
b. Rule of palm = 1%
c. Lund and Browder chart
d. Wallace rule

BURNS

7. Undue restlessness in a patient during the immediate post burn period is often a manifestation of: *(Karnataka 95)*
a. Hypoxia   b. Hypovolemia
c. Hyperkalemia   d. Anxiety

8. All require hospitalization except: *(DNB 2002, All India 91)*
a. 5% burns in children   b. 10% scalds in children
c. Electrocution   d. 15% deep burns in adults

BURNS DEPTH

9. Which of the following is not seen in 3rd degree burns?   *(MCI March 2009)*
a. Loss of skin appendages   b. No vesicles
c. Red color   d. Extremely painful

10. In second degree burns, re-epithelialisation occurs around:
a. 1 week   b. 2 weeks   *(MCI Sept 2009)*
c. 3 weeks   d. 4 weeks

11. Which of the following is false regarding deep 2nd degree burns?   *(MCI Sept 2009)*
a. Heal by scar deposition   b. Painless
c. Damage to deeper dermis   d. Less blanching

12. Blisters are seen in which type of burns?   *(DNB 2009)*
a. Superficial first degree   b. Superficial second degree
c. Third degree   d. Deep first degree

13. 2nd degree burns indicate involvement of: *(JIPMER 2013)*
a. Epidermis   b. Dermis
c. Subcutaneous tissue   d. Deep fascia

14. False regarding deep second-degree burns: *(MCI June 2018)*
a. Heal by scar deposition   b. Painless
c. Damage to deeper dermis   d. Less blanching

15. Which layer is involved in blister formation in a superficial partial thickness burn?   *(AIIMS Nov 2017)*
a. Epidermis   b. Dermis
c. Papillary dermis   d. Reticular dermis

16. A lady with 50% burns of dermis and subcutaneous tissue came to emergency department. Burns will be classified as: *(MCI Dec 2019)*
a. 1st degree   b. 2nd degree superficial
c. 2nd degree deep   d. 3rd degree burn

TREATMENT OF BURNS

17. In a 50 kg adult, how much of fluid should be given in first 8 hours in burns of 40%?   *(Recent Question 2018, MCI Nov 2017)*
a. 2 litres   b. 4 litres
c. 8 litres   d. 6 litres

18. During fluid resuscitation in a burns patient using Parkland's formula, volume of fluid given in first 8 hours:
a. 25%   b. 50% *(Recent Question 2017)*
c. 75%   d. 100%

19. IV formula for burn is: *(Recent Question 2015, UPPG 2009)*
a. Total % body surface area x weight x 4 = volume in mL
b. Total % body surface area x weight x 5 = volume in mL
c. Total % body surface area x weight x 6 = volume in mL
d. Total % body surface area x weight x 7 = volume in mL

20. Safest strategy of treatment for a patient of inhalational burn injury who has presented within 4-5 hours: *(MCI Nov 2017, MHPGMCET 2007)*
a. Binasal catheter O_2 inhalation
b. O_2 therapy with well-fitting face mask
c. Elective cricothyroidotomy
d. Elective endotracheal intubation

21. In burns management, which of the following is the fluid of choice?   *(Recent Question 2014, DNB 2012, 2005)*
a. Dextrose 5%   b. Normal saline
c. Ringer lactate   d. Isolyte-M

22. All of the following are true regarding fluid resuscitation in burn patients except: *(MCI March 2008)*
a. Consider intravenous resuscitation in children with burns greater than 15% TBSA
b. Oral fluids must contain salts
c. Most preferred fluid is Ringer's lactate
d. Half of the calculated volume of fluid should be given in first 8 hours

23. Which of the following is effected against Pseudomonas and is used in burns patients?   *(DNB 2009)*
a. Silver sulphadiazine   b. Silver sulphazine
c. Sulphamethoxazole   d. Sulphadoxine

24. In children with burns, maintenance IV fluid normally given is: *(MHCET 2006)*
a. Ringer lactate   b. 5% dextrose
c. Normal saline   d. Dextrose saline

25. **Which is the best method to administrator oxygen in case of airway burns?** *(MCI Nov 2017)*
    a. Elective intubation
    b. Mask
    c. Nasal prongs
    d. Tracheostomy

■ COMPLICATIONS OF BURNS

26. **Most common cause of death due to burns in early period is:**
    a. Sepsis
    b. Hypovolemic shock
    c. Both
    d. None *(APPG 2008)*

27. **Most common carcinoma after burns is:** *(DPG 2008)*
    a. Squamous cell carcinoma
    b. Adenocarcinoma
    c. Melanoma
    d. Mucoid carcinoma

28. **Most common cause of death in burns is:** *(Punjab 2008)*
    a. Primary shock
    b. Secondary shock
    c. Hemorrhagic shock
    d. Septicemic shock

29. **Burns shock is:** *(Punjab 2011)*
    a. Hypovolemic
    b. Neurogenic
    c. Endotoxic
    d. Cardiogenic

30. **Death from burns in first 10 days is due to all except:**
    a. Shock
    b. Infection *(DNB 2005)*
    c. Renal failure
    d. Respiratory distress

■ MISCELLANEOUS

31. **Domestic low-voltage electric supply can cause all the following except:** *(MHPGMCET 2007)*
    a. Contact wound
    b. Cardiac arrest
    c. Cardiac fibrillation
    d. Deep subcutaneous tissue damage

32. **Main danger with low tension (Domestic) electric AC current:** *(MHPGMCET 2009)*
    a. Renal injury (ARF)
    b. Cardiac arrest
    c. Muscle necrosis
    d. Paralysis

33. **Operation theatre fire is most commonly due to:** *(DNB 2010)*
    a. Argon beam coagulators
    b. Lasers
    c. Fibre optic illumination
    d. Electrosurgical equipment

34. **Myoglobinuria is seen in which type of burn?** *(DNB 2012)*
    a. Flame burn
    b. Scald burn
    c. Electric burn
    d. Contact burn

■ BURNS: % BSA

1. **Ans. a. 1%** *(Ref: Sabiston 20/e p507; Schwartz 11/e p1958, 10/e p227-236, 1820-1822; Bailey 27/e p621)*

2. **Ans. a. 1% BSA**

3. **Ans. b. Wallace**

4. **Ans. c. Lund and Browder chart** *(Ref: Schwartz 11/e p252, 10/e p199-200)*

"In children younger than 3 years old, the head accounts for a larger relative surface area and should be taken into account when estimating burn size. Diagrams such as the **Lund and Browder chart** give a **more accurate accounting of the true burn size in children**."- *Schwartz 10/e p199*

"For children and infants, the Lund-Browder chart is used to assess the burned body surface area. Different percentages are used because the ratio of the combined surface area of the head and neck to the surface area of the limbs is typically larger in children than that of an adult." *http://en.wikipedia.org/wiki/Total_body_surface_area*

5. **Ans. b. 18%** *(Ref: Sabiston 20/e p508)*

   A Child Has
   - **Circumferential burn of both of thighs = 6.5 + 6.5 = 13**
   - **Buttocks = 2.5 + 2.5 = 5**
   - **Face and scalp with singeing of hairs = 17**

   Total burn = 13 + 5 + 17 = 35%

Berkow Diagram to Estimate Burn Size (%) Based on Area of Burn in an Isolated Body Part						
Body Part	**0-1 yr**	**1-4 yr**	**5-9 yr**	**10-14 yr**	**15-18 yr**	**Adult**
Head	19	**17**	**13**	11	9	7
Neck	2	2	2	2	2	2
Anterior trunk	13	13	13	13	13	13
Posterior trunk	13	13	13	13	13	13
Right buttock	2.5	**2.5**	**2.5**	2.5	2.5	2.5
Left buttock	2.5	**2.5**	**2.5**	2.5	2.5	2.5
Genitalia	1	1	1	1	1	1
Right upper arm	4	4	4	4	4	4
Left upper arm	4	4	4	4	4	4
Right lower arm	3	3	3	3	3	3
Left lower arm	3	3	3	3	3	3
Right hand	2.5	2.5	2.5	2.5	2.5	2.5
Left hand	2.5	2.5	2.5	2.5	2.5	2.5
Right thigh	5.5	**6.5**	**8**	8.5	9	9.5
Left thigh	5.5	**6.5**	**8**	8.5	9	9.5
Right leg	5	5	5.5	6	6.5	7
Left leg	5	5	5.5	6	6.5	7
Right foot	3.5	3.5	3.5	3.5	3.5	3.5
Left foot	3.5	3.5	3.5	3.5	3.5	3.5

6. **Ans. c. Lund and Browder chart**

■ BURNS

7. **Ans. d. Anxiety**

8. **Ans. a. 5% burns in children**

■ BURNS DEPTH

9. **Ans. d. Extremely painful**

10. **Ans. b. 2 weeks**

11. **Ans. d. Less blanching**

12. **Ans. b. Superficial second degree**

13. Ans. b. Dermis

14. Ans. b. Painless

15. Ans. c. Papillary dermis *(Ref: Sabiston 20/e p506; Schwartz 11/e p252-253, 10/e p229; Bailey 27/e p622)*

16. Ans. d. 3rd degree burn *(Ref: Bailey 27/e p622)*

■ TREATMENT OF BURNS

17. Ans. b. 4 litres *(Ref: Sabiston 20/e p514; Schwartz 11/e p254, 10/e p230; Bailey 27/e p624)*

18. Ans. b. 50% *(Ref: Sabiston 20/e p514; Schwartz 11/e p254, 10/e p230; Bailey 27/e p624)*

19. Ans. a. Total % body surface area x weight x 4 = volume in mL

20. Ans. d. Elective endotracheal intubation *(Ref: Bailey 27/e p620)*

Initial Management of the Burned Airway

- Early elective intubation is safest[Q]
- Delay can make intubation very difficult because of swelling[Q]
- Be ready to perform an emergency cricothyroidotomy if intubation is delayed[Q]

21. Ans. c. Ringer lactate

22. Ans. a. Consider intravenous resuscitation in children with burns greater than 15% TBSA

- IV fluid resuscitation: In children with burn >10% TBSA and adult with burn >15% TBSA

23. Ans. a. Silver sulphadiazine

24. Ans. d. Dextrose saline

25. Ans. a. Elective intubation *(Ref: Bailey 27/e p620)*

"The burned airway creates problems for the patient by swelling and, if not managed proactively, can completely occlude the upper airway. The treatment is to secure the airway with an endotracheal tube until the swelling has subsided, which is usually after about 48 hours."
- Bailey 27/e p620

■ COMPLICATIONS OF BURNS

26. Ans. b. Hypovolemic shock

27. Ans. a. Squamous cell carcinoma

28. Ans. d. Septicemic shock

Carcinoma in Burns

- Squamous cell carcinoma is MC carcinoma in burns[Q].
- SCC commonly occurs in long standing (Marjolin's ulcer), old scar or keloid[Q].
- Both Marjolin's ulcer and keloid are complications that arise after burns[Q].

29. Ans. a. Hypovolemic *(Ref: Sabiston 20e p514; Schwartz 11/e p254, 10/e p204; Bailey 27/e p618-619)*

- Proper fluid management is critical to survival[Q] in burn patient.
- The hypovolemic shock[Q] in burn patient is special in the sense that total body water remains unchanged in a burn patient.
- The thermal injury leads to a massive shift from the intravascular compartment to the extravascular compartment leading to edema formation[Q].

30. Ans. c. Renal failure

■ MISCELLANEOUS

31. Ans. d. Deep subcutaneous tissue damage *(Ref: Bailey 27/e p631)*

32. Ans. b. Cardiac arrest

33. Ans. d. Electrosurgical equipment *(Ref: British Journal of Anesthesia, vol 50, Issue 7, Page 659-664)*

Operation Theatre Fire

- The two most common source of operation theatre fire is electrosurgical unit (ESU) and lasers.
- ECRI's analysis of case reports show that the most common ignition sources are electrosurgical instruments (68%) and lasers (13%).
- Most common fire location is airway (35%), head or face (28%), and elsewhere on or inside the patient (38%).
- An oxygen-enriched atmosphere was a contribution factor in 74% of all cases.

34. Ans. c. Electric burn

Plastic Surgery and Skin Lesions

■ GRAFT TAKE

GRAFT TAKE

- Skin graft take occurs in three phases, imbibition, inosculation, & revascularization.

Plasma Imbibition	Inosculation	Revascularization
• Graft survives up to **first 48 hours**[Q] because of plasma imbibition • Involves **free absorption of nutrients** into the graft	• **Donor** and **recipient capillaries are aligned** during inosculation[Q] • Inosculation **completes by 4–5 days**[Q]	• **After 5 days**[Q], revascularization occurs • Graft demonstrates **both arterial and venous outflow**[Q]

- During these initial few days the graft is most susceptible to deleterious factors such as **infection, mechanical shear forces and hematoma or seroma**[Q].

■ SKIN GRAFT

PARTIAL THICKNESS (THIERSCH) OR SPLIT SKIN GRAFT

- Consist of **epidermis & variable portion of dermis**[Q]
- **Large size of graft can be taken**[Q]
- **Site: Thigh (MC)**[Q] upper arm, flexor aspect of forearm and abdominal wall
- Grafts are **hairless** and **do not sweat**[Q] (these structures are not transferred)

> • Skin graft must be **applied to a well-vascularized recipient wound bed**. It will **not adhere to exposed bone, cartilage, or tendon** devoid of periosteum, perichondrium, or peritenon, respectively, or devoid of its vascularized perimembranous envelope.

- **MC causes** of **skin graft failure**: Hematoma (or seroma), infection, & movement (shear).
- **Pie crusting: Stab incisions** in the graft preemptively **to create small outlets for fluid to drain** from beneath the graft

> • **Beta hemolytic Streptococci** can **destroy split skin grafts completely, presence** of this organism is a **contraindication** to grafting[Q].

- **Graft immobilization** is **critical to the graft take** and can be accomplished with bolster dressing, light compression wraps or a vacuum assisted closure device.

SKIN GRAFTS

Partial Thickness (Thiersch) Graft	Full Thickness (Wolfes) Graft
• It includes **all epidermis & part of dermis**[Q]. • Partial thickness **grafts are thin, uptake of graft is easy (easy survival)**[Q]. • **Large grafts could be taken** as the donor site is left with a **part of dermis** which will cause **easy regeneration of epidermis**[Q]. • **Contract upto 40%, not useful for cosmetic surgeries**[Q]. • **Donor site** will **heal well**[Q] without any contraction, and is reusable.	• It includes **all epidermis & dermis**[Q]. • **Uptake** is **difficult** because of thickness • Less chances of survival • **Small grafts** could be **taken**[Q] as the donor site does not have epidermal or dermal remnants to allow epithelialization • **Very minimal contraction** making it **suitable for cosmetic surgeries on face**[Q]. • **Donor site** will have to be **closed primarily** or **left open to granulate** and contract[Q].

Contraction of Graft

- **Primary :** Occurs when the graft is harvested, **depends upon** amount of **dermis** present, **more in full thickness graft**
- **Secondary :** Occurs after the surgery, **more in partial thickness graft**

■ MESHED SKIN GRAFTS

MESHED SKIN GRAFTS

- **Split grafts** may be **meshed to expand** the **surface area** that can be covered[Q].
- This technique is **particularly useful** when a **large area must be resurfaced**, as **in major burns**.

  - **Meshed grafts** usually also have **enhanced reliability of engraftment**, because the **fenestrations allow for egress of wound fluid** and **excellent contour matching** of the wound bed by the graft[Q].

- **Fenestrations** in meshed grafts **re-epithelialize by secondary intention** from the surrounding graft skin.

  - **Major drawbacks** of meshed grafts are **poor cosmetic appearance** and **high secondary contraction[Q]**.

- **Meshing ratios** used usually range from **1:1.5 to 1:6**, with higher ratios associated with magnified drawbacks.

■ PEDICEL GRAFT OR FLAP

PEDICEL GRAFT OR FLAP

- Flap: **Partially** or **completely isolated segment** of tissue with its **own blood supply**[Q]

Absolute Indications for Flaps	
• **Exposed bone**[Q]	• **Open joint** or **non-biological**[Q] **implant materials**[Q]
• **Radiated vessel**[Q]	• **Pressure sores** at bony prominences
• **Brain**[Q]	

For **critical** and **small areas** such as an **eyelid**, a **full thickness graft** is selected, so that contraction of the grafted material is minimum.

Type of Flaps on the basis of source of Vascular Supply

Random	Axial	Free
• Random flaps **rely on** the **low perfusion pressures** found in **subdermal plexus**[Q] to sustain the flap • Used to **reconstruct relatively small, full-thickness defects** that are not amenable to skin grafting.	• Axial flap is **based on** a **named blood vessel**[Q] • Provide a **reproducible** and **stable skin** or **skin-muscle (myocutaneous) flap**[Q]. • Can be used to provide much needed length and bulk • **Axial flap** that **remains attached to its proximal blood supply** and **transposed to a defect** is known as a **pedicled flap**[Q].	• **Autogenous transplantation**[Q] of vascularized tissues. • **Complete detachment** of the flap, with **devascularization, from the donor site**[Q] • **Revascularization** of the flap with **anastomoses to blood vessels** in the **recipient site**[Q]

■ MARJOLIN'S ULCER

MARJOLIN'S ULCER

- **Low grade SCC**[Q], which develops on a **chronic benign ulcer** or a **long standing scar** tissue.
- **Arises from** the **edge**[Q] of the ulcer

Marjolin's ulcer may develop in	
• **Post burn scar**[Q]	• Chronically **discharging osteomyelitis sinus**[Q]
• Long standing **venous ulcer**[Q]	
• **Chronic ulcer**[Q] due to trauma	• **Post-radiation ulcer**

Characteristic Features

- **Slow growing**[Q] as scar tissue is **relatively avascular**
- **Painless** as there **no nerves in** the **scar tissue**[Q]
- **No secondary deposits**[Q] in regional lymph node, as there are **no lymphatic vessels** in scar tissue
- If the ulcer invades the normal tissue, then only lymph node may be involved by lymphatic spread
- **Radioresistant**[Q] due to **avascularity**

Diagnosis

- **IOC for diagnosis: Biopsy**[Q]

Treatment

- **Wide local excision** followed by **flap cover**[Q]
- **Radiotherapy is avoided**[Q]

■ BOWEN'S DISEASE

BOWEN'S DISEASE

- This is an **SCC in situ**[Q], of which 3–11% progress to SCC.
- **Etiological agents: Chronic solar damage, inorganic arsenic** and **HPV16**[Q]
- This is rare, **slow-growing intraepidermal SCC** that often **mimics a chronic dermatosis**[Q].
- It should now be considered as a **form of AIN III** (Anal intraepithelial neoplasia).

Clinical Features

- It usually **presents with pruritus**[Q] and on examination looks like **psoriasis** or **senile keratosis**.
- Presents as a **slowly enlarging, erythematous, scaly patch** or **plaque**[Q].

Treatment

- **Topical therapy** with **5-fluorouracil** or **imiquimod** is an effective treatment[Q].
- Alternatives: **Surgical excision** with a 4-mm margin or **Mohs' micrographic surgery**[Q] for larger or recurrent lesions.

■ BASAL CELL CARCINOMA (RODENT ULCER)

BASAL CELL CARCINOMA (RODENT ULCER)

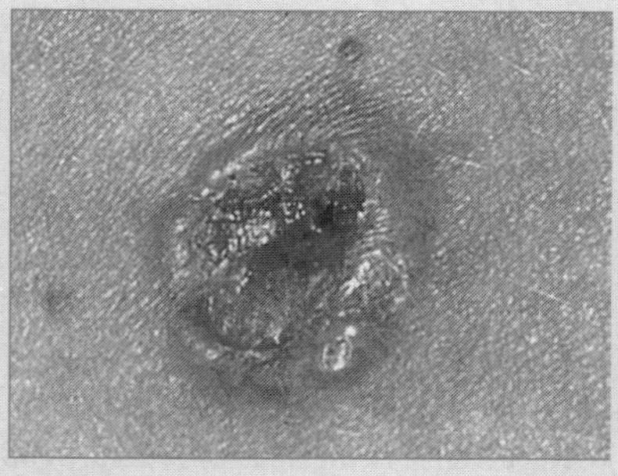

- **Locally invasive** carcinoma, **arises from** the **basal layer**[Q] of the epidermis
- **MC type of skin cancer**[Q]
- **90% of BCC** are seen **in the face**[Q], above a **line from** the **corner of mouth to lobule of ear**.
- **MC site: Nose >Inner canthus**[Q] of the eye, also known as **Tear cancer**[Q].

Types of BCC

- **Nodular: MC type of BCC**[Q], characterized by small slow growing **pearly nodules**, often with **telangiectatic vessels** on its surface. **Central depression** with **umbilication**[Q] is a classic sign.
- **Pigmented:** Mimic malignant melanoma
- **Cystic**
- **Superficial**

Characteristic Features of BCC	
• **Low grade malignancy**[Q] • **More common in fair** and **dry skinned** people • **Nuclear palisading**[Q] on histology	• **Exposure to sunlight**[Q] is an important etiological factor • Has been seen following prolonged administration of **Arsenic**[Q]

Spread

- BCC usually spreads by **local invasion**[Q], rarely metastasizes
- **Rodent ulcer:** It gradually **destroys the tissues**, it comes **in contact with**.
- **Lymphatic spread** is **not seen**[Q] (Regional lymph nodes are not enlarged)
- Blood spread is extremely rare.

Diagnosis

- Diagnostic procedure for BCC is **wedge biopsy**[Q].

Treatment

- **Non-aggressive tumor** on **trunk** or **extremities:** Excision or **electrodissection and curettage**[Q]
- **Large, aggressive,** located at **vital areas** or recurrent: **Moh's micrographic surgery**[Q]

■ SQUAMOUS CELL CARCINOMA (EPITHELIOMA OR EPIDERMOID CARCINOMA)

SQUAMOUS CELL CARCINOMA (EPITHELIOMA OR EPIDERMOID CARCINOMA)

- It is a carcinoma of the cells of epidermis that usually migrate outwards to the surface.
- Originate from **prickle cell layer**[Q]; **Seen in > 40 years of** age

- **MC skin cancer** in **darkly pigmented races**[Q]
- 2nd MC skin cancer in light skinned races[Q]
- **MC causative factor: Sunlight**[Q]
- **MC site:** Ears, cheeks, lower lip and back of hands[Q]

Predisposing Factors for SCC	
• **Senile** or **actinic keratosis**[Q] • **Chronic skin lesions** (lupus vulgaris[Q], cutaneous TB) • **Sunlight** or **irradiation**[Q] • **Chronic irritation; HIV, HPV-16**[Q]	• Contact with **tars** and **hydrocarbons**[Q] • **Erythroplasia of Queyrat**[Q] • **Immunosuppression**[Q] • **Psoralens, Arsenic exposure**[Q]

Contd…

Contd...

Pathology
- Microscopically mass of keratin is surrounded by normal looking squamous cells, presenting with characteristic **prickle cell appearance**[Q], which are arranged in concentric manner as seen in **'onion skin'**. This whole appearance is called "**cell nest** or **epithelial pearl**[Q]".
- **MC type of SCC: Ulcerative** type[Q]

Clinical Features
- **MC symptom: Nodule** or **ulcer**[Q]
- **Edge** of ulcer: **Raised** and **everted** with **indurated base (pathognomonic)**[Q]

Diagnosis
- **Diagnosis** is made by **wedge biopsy**[Q] (taken from **edge of ulcer**)

Treatment
- **Small (< 1 cm)** or **non-invasive SCC: Excision** with **1 cm margin**[Q]
- **Large, aggressive**, located at **vital areas** or **recurrent: Moh's micrographic surgery**[Q]

■ MOH'S MICROGRAPHIC SURGERY FOR SCC AND BCC

MOH'S MICROGRAPHIC SURGERY FOR SCC AND BCC

- **Mohs' technique** uses **serial excision** in small increments coupled with **immediate microscopic analysis to ensure tumor removal**, yet limit resection of aesthetically valuable tissue[Q].
- **Advantage: All specimen margins** are **evaluated**[Q].

> - **Major benefit**: Ability to remove a tumor with **minimal sacrifice** of **uninvolved tissue**[Q].
> - **Particular value** in managing tumors of the **eyelid, nose, or cheek**[Q]
> - **Indicated in large, aggressive tumors** located at **vital areas** or **recurrent tumors**[Q]

- **Major drawback: Procedure length** (Total lesion excision may require multiple attempts at resection, and many procedures may be carried out over several days)
- **Recurrence & metastases rates** are **comparable to** those of **wide local excision**[Q].

■ MALIGNANT MELANOMA

MALIGNANT MELANOMA

- Melanoma is neoplastic disorder produced by **malignant transformation of normal melanocytes**[Q].

> - **Site most commonly associated** with melanocytic transformation in the skin, where **melanocytes** reside **at the dermo-epidermal junction (Junctional melanocytes)**[Q].
> - **MC site** of MM **in men: Back & trunk**[Q]
> - **MC site** of MM **in women: Lower extremity**[Q]

- **Most susceptible individuals: Fair** complexions, **red** or **blonde hair, blue eyes** and **freckles** and who **tan poorly** and **sunburn easily**.
- **MM is positive for S-100, HMB-45, vimentin** but **negative for cytokeratin-20**[Q].

Risk factors for Malignant Melanoma	
• **Xeroderma pigmentosum**[Q]	• **Giant** congenital melanocytic nevus
• **Actinic damage (UVR)**[Q]	• **Increased number** of **ordinary melanocytic naevi**
• **Family history** of melanoma[Q]	
• Presence of **dysplastic naevus**[Q]	• **History** of **sunburn**[Q]

Types of Malignant Melanoma: (In order of decreasing frequency)	
Superficial spreading	• **MC type** of MM[Q] • **MC site: Torso**
Nodular	• **Most malignant**[Q] • **MC site: Head, neck** and **trunk** • Vertical growth phase only
Lentigo maligna	• **Least malignant**[Q] • **MC site: Face**
Acral lentiginous	• **Least common, worst prognosis**[Q], • **MC site: Sole, under great toe nail**

Contd...

Contd…

Characteristic Features

- **Classic appearance of melanoma:** ABCDE (Asymmetry, Border irregularity, Color variation, Diameter >6 mm) Evolving size, shape or color[Q]
- **MC route** of **metastasis:** Through **Lymphatics**[Q]
- **MC site** of **systemic metastasis:** Liver[Q]
- Other common visceral sites of metastasis: Lung, brain, GIT (small intestine), bone, adrenal.

> - **Microsatellites:** Discrete tumor nests > **0.05 mm** in diameter, **separated from main body** of tumor **by normal dermal collagen** or **subcutaneous fat**[Q].
> - **Microsatellites** are associated with **increased risk** of **regional LN metastasis**[Q].

Diagnosis

- Confirmed by **'full thickness excisional biopsy'**[Q]
- Incisional biopsy for large lesions and lesions in proximity to important structures (eye, nose, ear)

Treatment

- Treatment: **Surgical excision**[Q] with **sentinel LN biopsy** (Margin: **1 cm** for **< 1 mm** thickness, **2 cm** for **1–4 mm** thickness, **2–3 cm** for **> 4 mm** thickness)
- **LN dissection** if LN is palpable or positive on sentinel LN biopsy
- MM is **radioresistant tumor; Chemotherapy: IFN-alpha 2b**

Clark's levels[Q] (on the basis of **depth of invasion**): EPIRS	
I	• Melanoma restricting to **Epidermis** and appendages[Q]
II	• Invading **Papillary dermis** without filling it[Q]
III	• Reach **Interface** of papillary and reticular dermis[Q]
IV	• **Invading reticular dermis**[Q]
V	• **Invading subcutaneous tissue**[Q]

- MM is **sub-classified into 5 Clark levels,** to indicate their **depth of invasion** and **prognosis**[Q].
- **Breslow's depth of invasion:** Actual measurement of the **deepest invasion** from the **granular layer**[Q].

Breslow's Thickness	
Stage I	• **< 0.75 mm**[Q]
Stage II	• **0.75–1.5 mm**[Q]
Stage III	• **1.6–4.0 mm**[Q]
Stage IV	• **> 4.0 mm**[Q]

Prognostic Factors (**Depends** most importantly **on staging**[Q])	
• **Depth of invasion (most important prognostic factor)**[Q] • **Ulceration**[Q] (presence of ulceration carries worst prognosis)	• **Lymph node status**[Q] • **Satellite lesion**[Q] • **Distant metastasis**[Q]

■ VASCULAR ANOMALIES

Vascular Anomalies		
Port-wine Stain	**Strawberry Angiomas**	**Salmon Patch**
• A vascular malformation • **Present at birth**[Q] • **Grows along with** the **child**[Q] • **Do not regress**[Q] • **Face involvement** in areas supplied by **5th cranial nerve**[Q]	• Type of **capillary hemangioma** • **Baby** is **normal at birth**[Q] • **Appears at** the age of **1–3 weeks**[Q] • **Grows with** the **child upto 1 year** of age and then cease to grow[Q] • By the age of **9 years, 90%** demonstrate **complete involution**[Q] • **Emptying sign**[Q] is demonstrable	• Also known as **Macular stain** or **stork bite**[Q] • **Present at birth**[Q] • Seen over **forehead in** the **midline** and **over** the **occiput**[Q] • **Disappears by** the age **1 year**[Q]

■ EPIDERMOID CYST (SEBACEOUS OR EPIDERMAL CYST)

EPIDERMOID CYST (SEBACEOUS OR EPIDERMAL CYST)

- Epidermoid cyst results from **proliferation of epidermal cells** within a circumscribed space of dermis (which had got **implanted within** the **dermis**[Q])
- **Sebaceous cyst** is a **misnomer** as the cysts are **not of sebaceous origin** and the **white creamy material** filled within is not sebum, but is **keratin (desquamated epithelial cells**[Q])
- **Type of retention cyst** (secretions are pent up in a gland owing to blockage of the duct)

Pathology

- **Cyst wall** consist of a **layer of epidermis** oriented with the basal layer superficial and more matured layers are deep.
- **Desquamated cells (keratin)** collect in the centre and form creamy substance of the cyst.

Clinical Features

- Usually **asymptomatic**[Q], unless get infected or inflamed and become painful
- **Firm, round, flesh colored** to yellow or white subcutaneous nodules of variable size.
- **Central punctum**[Q] may teether the cyst to the overlying epidermis, from which the white creamy material can be expressed.
- Rarely **malignancies**[Q] **(BCC, SCC)** can develop in epidermoid cyst.

> - **No punctum** in **scrotal** and **scalp sebaceous cyst**[Q].

Treatment

- **Excision with** the **wall** is treatment of choice[Q].
- **Infected cyst: Incision and drainage** (After resolution of the abscess, **cyst wall** must be **excised to prevent recurrence**)[Q]

Cocks Peculiar Tumour	• **Infected or ulcerated sebaceous cyst of** the scalp[Q] • **Resembles fungating epithelioma**[Q]
Potts Puffy Tumour	• **Osteomyelitis** of the **Frontal bone of skull**[Q] • Associated with **subperiosteal swelling & edema**[Q]
Pilomatrixoma	• Also known as **Calcifying epithelioma of Malherbe**[Q] • **Benign hair follicle derived tumor**[Q]
Cylindroma	• A **malignant epithelial tumour** also known as **Turban tumor**[Q] • Known as cylindroma because of histological appearance

Multiple Choice Questions

■ SKIN GRAFTING

1. Thiersch graft is which type of graft?
(JIPMER 2012, MHPGMCET 2008, 2001, DPG 2005)
a. Partial thickness
b. Full thickness
c. Pedicle
d. Patch

2. Who said: "Skin is the best dressing"? *(Karnataka 2004)*
a. Joseph Lister
b. John Hunter
c. James Paget
d. Mc Neill Love

3. Within 48 hours of transplantation, skin graft survives due to: *(AIIMS Nov 2000, AIIMS Nov 99)*
a. Amount of saline in graft
b. Plasma imbibition
c. New vessels growing from the donor tissue
d. Connection between donor and recipient capillaries

4. Ideal graft for leg injury with 10 × 10 cm exposed bone:
(AIIMS Nov 99)
a. Amniotic membrane graft
b. Pedicle graft
c. Full thickness graft
d. Split thickness skin graft

5. Wolfe Graft is: *(APPG 2015)*
a. Thin split thickness graft
b. Thick split thickness skin graft
c. Medium thickness split thickness skin graft
d. Full thickness skin graft

6. Skin grafting is absolutely contraindicated in which skin infection? *(AIIMS June 97)*
a. Staphylococcus
b. Pseudomonas
c. Streptococcus
d. Proteus

7. All can take split thickness graft except:
(MCI June 2018, March 2005, AIIMS Sept 96)
a. Fat
b. Muscle
c. Skull bone
d. Deep fascia

8. The given instrument is used for harvesting the graft from healthy area in split skin thickness graft:

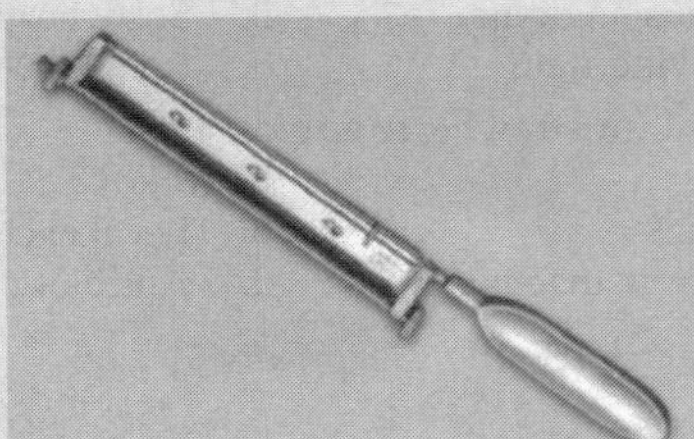

a. Dermatome
b. Silver's knife
c. Catlin amputating knife
d. Humby knife

9. Skin graft stored at 4°C can survive up to: *(DNB 2009)*
a. 1 week
b. 2 weeks
c. 3 weeks
d. 4 weeks

10. All are advantages of split thickness skin grafting except:
a. Good uptake
b. Reusable donor site
c. Less contraction
d. Large grafts can be harvested
(Recent Question 2013)

■ FLAPS

11. True statement for axial flap is: *(All India 97)*
a. Carries its own vessels within it
b. Kept in limb
c. Transverse flap
d. Carries its own nerve in it

12. The subdermal plexus forms the vascular basis for:
(JIPMER 2002)
a. Randomised flaps
b. Axial flaps
c. Mucocutaneous flaps
d. Fasciocutaneous flaps

13. Myocutaneous flap includes which tissues? *(DPG 2007)*
a. Muscle only
b. Muscle and vascular pedicle
c. Muscle and skin
d. Skin, muscle and vascular pedicle

14. Split thickness skin graft is not taken up by: *(MCI June 2018)*
a. Fat
b. Muscle
c. Deep fascia
d. Skull bone

■ MARJOLIN'S ULCER

15. The most common malignancy found in Marjolin's ulcer is:
a. Basal cell carcinoma *(MCI June 2018, DPG 2009 Feb)*
b. Squamous cell carcinoma
c. Malignant fibrous histiocytoma
d. Neutrophic malignant melanoma

16. Which ulcer is likely to develop in a long-standing chronic venous ulcer? *(MCI June 2019)*
a. Marjolin's ulcer
b. Aphthous ulcer
c. Bazin ulcer
d. Arterial ulcer

17. A tumour arising in a burns scar is likely to be:
(Recent Question 2014, COMEDK 2009, PGI June 2006, June 97)
a. Basal cell carcinoma
b. Squamous cell carcinoma
c. Malignant melanoma
d. Fibrosarcoma

■ PREMALIGNANT LESIONS OF SKIN

18. Bowen's disease is: *(DPG 2005)*
a. Mimics chronic dermatosis
b. Premalignant condition
c. Presents with pruritus
d. All of the above

■ SQUAMOUS CELL CARCINOMA

19. Margins of squamous cell carcinoma is: *(Recent Question 2016)*
a. Inverted
b. Everted
c. Rolled
d. Undermined

20. Moh's micrographic surgery is done for:
a. Cutaneous melanoma *(Recent Question 2016)*
b. Dermatofibrosarcoma protuberans
c. Squamous cell carcinoma
d. None of the above

■ BASAL CELL CARCINOMA

21. The commonest clinical pattern of basal cell carcinoma is:
(MCI Dec 2018, COMEDK 2008, MCI March 2005)
a. Nodular
b. Morpheaform
c. Superficial
d. Keratotic

22. Most common site of basal cell carcinoma is:
(All India 94, MHPGMCET 2001)

a. Face b. Trunk
c. Neck d. Extremities

23. **What is the most probable diagnosis based on the given image?** *(AIIMS Nov 2017)*

a. Basal cell carcinoma b. Malignant melanoma
c. Squamous cell carcinoma d. Marjolin's ulcer

24. **All of the following are true about basal cell carcinoma except:**
a. Most common site is upper eyelid *(DNB 2009)*
b. Locally invasive
c. Rarely metastasizes
d. Associated with exposure to sun

25. **Moh's micrographic excision for basal cell carcinoma is used for all of the following except:** *(Karnataka 2006)*
a. Recurrent Tumor
b. Tumor less than 2 cm in diameter
c. Tumors with aggressive histology
d. Tumors with perineural invasion

26. **Characteristic feature of basal cell carcinoma is:**
(AIIMS May 2012)
a. Keratin pearls b. Foam cells
c. Nuclear palisading d. Psammoma bodies

27. **Reconstruction of tip of nose after excision of basal cell carcinoma is done by:** *(DNB 2014)*
a. Bipedicled flap b. Bilobed flap
c. Full thickness skin graft d. Split skin graft

28. **Rodent ulcer is:** *(MCI Dec 2019)*
a. Basal cell carcinoma
b. Squamous cell carcinoma
c. Rhinophyma
d. Adenocarcinoma

■ MALIGNANT MELANOMA

29. **In malignant melanoma, change seen is all except:**
a. Ulceration b. Bleeding *(DPG 2006)*
c. Satellite lesions d. Hair in mole

30. **Treatment of choice for melanoma is:** *(DPG 2006)*
a. Chemotherapy b. Surgical excision
c. Radiotherapy d. Surgery and chemotherapy

31. **Most common origin of melanoma is from:**
(Bihar PG 2014, AIIMS Nov 2001)
a. Junctional melanocytes b. Epidermal cells
c. Basal cells d. Follicular cells

32. **Most common type of malignant melanoma is:**
a. Superficial spreading *(AIIMS Nov 2001, UPPG 2009)*
b. Lentigo maligna melanoma *(JIPMER 2014, 2012)*
c. Nodular
d. Acral lentiginous

33. **Most common site of lentigo maligna melanoma is:**
(DNB 2013, AIIMS Nov 2001)
a. Face b. Legs
c. Trunks d. Soles

34. **All of the following statements about malignant melanoma are true except:** *(All India 97)*

a. Prognosis is better in female than in male
b. Acral lentiginous melanoma carries a good prognosis
c. Stage IIa shows satellite deposits
d. Most common type is superficial spreading melanoma

35. **Melanoma staging is based on which classification?**
a. Breslow b. Clark's *(DNB 2009)*
c. Both a and b d. Bethesda

36. **Least common site for spread of melanomas:** *(DNB 2012)*
a. GIT b. Lungs
c. Liver d. Renal

37. **Inguinal lymph node enlargement is seen in:** *(MPPG 97)*
a. Seminoma testis b. Malignant melanoma foot
c. CA cervix d. None

38. **Risk factor for malignant melanoma all the following are risk factors for malignant melanoma except:** *(DNB 2014)*
a. Giant congenital nevi b. Family history melanoma
c. Exposure to UV light d. HPV infection

39. **All of the following are marker of melanoma except:**
(Recent Question 2016)
a. S-100 b. Cytokeratin-20
c. HMB-45 d. Vimentin

40. **Immunotherapy is effective in:** *(Recent Question 2016)*
a. SCC b. BCC
c. Malignant melanoma d. None

41. **Pigmented lesion suspicious of melanoma of size 1 cm with ulceration and features of ABCD. What is the next step?**
a. Wide local excision with 1 cm margin
b. Excision biopsy with 1-2 mm margin
c. Punch biopsy at the edge of the lesion
d. Incisional biopsy *(Recent Question 2017)*

■ SKIN PATCH/STAIN/HEMANGIOMA

42. **Which of the following is a regressing tumor?** *(DPG 2011)*
a. Portwine stain b. Strawberry angioma
c. Venous angioma d. Plexiform angioma

43. **Following is regressive tumor:** *(MHPGMCET 2007)*
a. Venous angioma b. Strawberry angioma
c. Portwine stain d. Juvenile angioma

44. **Treatment for strawberry angioma:**
(MHSSMCET 2006, JIPMER 95)
a. Steroids b. Local excision
c. Masterly inactivity d. Antibiotic coverage

45. **Salmon patch usually disappears by age:**
(Recent Question 2016)
a. One month b. One year
c. Puberty d. None of the above

46. **Best method to treat a large portwine hemangiomas:**
a. Radiotherapy *(DNB 2010)*
b. Tattooing
c. Excision with skin grafting
d. Pulsed eye laser

47. **Which of these does not change or remains same throughout life?** *(AIIMS Nov 2001)*
a. Salmon patch b. Strawberry angiomas
c. Portwine stain d. Capillary hemangiomas

48. **Spontaneous regression is seen in:** *(Recent Question 2016)*
a. Portwine hemangioma
b. Strawberry hemangioma
c. Cavernous hemangioma
d. Arterial angioma

49. **Identify the condition as shown in image:**
    (MCI Dec 2019)

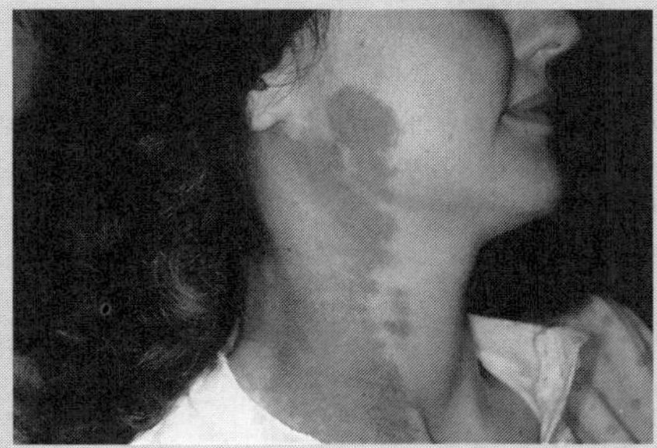

    a. Portwine stain   b. Strawberry nevus
    c. Erythema multiforme   d. Exanthem subitum

■ SEBACEOUS CYST

50. **Sebaceous cyst does not occur in the:**   *(MCI Dec 2018)*
    a. Scalp   b. Scrotum
    c. Back   d. Sole

51. **What is the most probable diagnosis based on the given image?**   *(Recent Question 2017)*

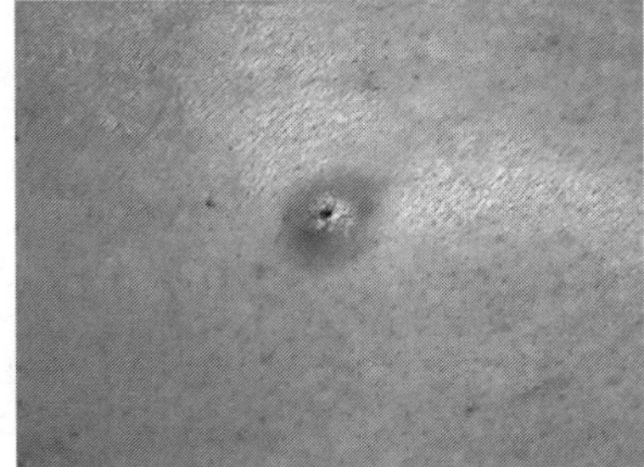

    a. Dermoid cyst   b. Sebaceous cyst
    c. Lipoma   d. Hemangioma

52. **Cystic lesion over scalp as shown in the image:**
    (MCI June 2019, Recent Question 2019)

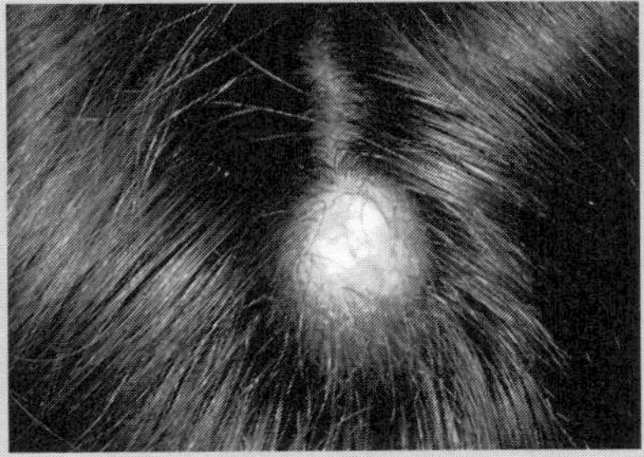

    a. Sebaceous cyst   b. Dermoid cyst
    c. Neural tumor   d. Meningioma

53. **Sebaceous cyst is:**   *(DNB 2004)*
    a. Distention cyst   b. Retention cyst
    c. Implantation dermoid   d. Mucous cyst

54. **Cock's peculiar tumor is:**
    (MCI June 2018, Recent Question 2014, AIIMS Nov 2010)
    a. Basal cell carcinoma   b. Squamous cell carcinoma
    c. Ulcerated sebaceous cyst   d. Cylindroma

■ LIPOMA

55. **The term universal tumor refers to:**
    a. Adenoma   b. Papilloma
    c. Fibroma   d. Lipoma

56. **Dercum's disease is commonest in the:** *(Recent Question 2016)*
    a. Face   b. Arm
    c. Back   d. Thigh

57. **Lipoma becomes malignant commonly at which site:**
    a. Subcutaneous   b. Retro-pertioneal
    c. Sub-aponeurotic   d. Intermuscular

58. **Dercum's disease is characterized by:**   *(DNB 2008)*
    a. Lipodermatosclerosis
    b. Tender subcutaneous lipoma
    c. Morbid obesity
    d. None

■ HIDRADENITIS SUPPURATIVA

59. **Hidradenitis suppurativa is found to occur in:**
    (Recent Question 2016)
    a. Axilla   b. Circumanal
    c. Scalp   d. Groin

■ KERATOACANTHOMA

60. **Keratoacanthoma is:**
    a. A type of basal cell carcinoma
    b. Infected sebaceous cyst
    c. Self healing nodular lesion with central ulceration
    d. Pre-malignant disease

■ MISCELLANEOUS

61. **Calcifying epithelioma is seen in:**   *(JIPMER 95)*
    a. Dermatofibroma   b. Adenoma sebaceum
    c. Pyogenic granuloma   d. Pilomatrixoma

62. **Frostbite is treated by:**   *(AMC 2000)*
    a. Rapid rewarming   b. Slow rewarming
    c. IV pentoxyphylline   d. Amputation

63. **Treatment for pyoderma gangrenosum is:**   *(Jharkhand 2003)*
    a. Steroids   b. IV antibiotics
    c. Surgery + antibiotics   d. Surgery alone

64. **Cylindroma is:**   *(DPG 2007)*
    a. Appendage tumor   b. Acinic cell carcinoma
    c. Pleomorphic adenoma   d. Warthin's tumor

65. **Bedsore is an example of:**   *(All India 99)*
    a. Tropical ulcer   b. Trophic ulcer
    c. Venous ulcer   d. Post-thrombotic ulcer

66. **Ainhum is seen in:**   *(Recent Question 2014, All India 99)*
    a. Base of great toe   b. Base of fingers tips
    c. Base of toe   d. Ankle

67. **The given condition is most commonly seen in:**

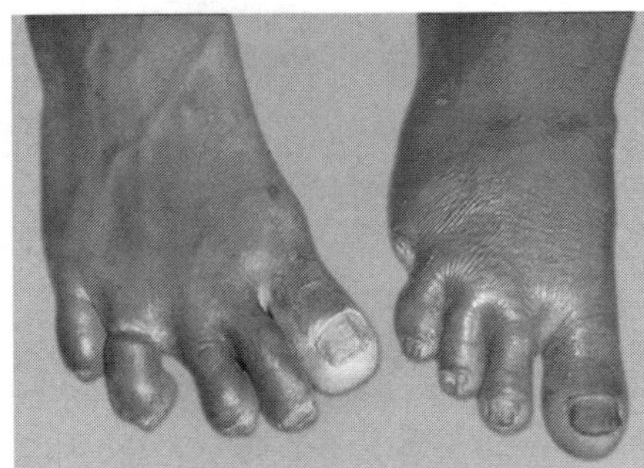

a. Great toe
b. Little toe
c. Third toe
d. Fourth toe

68. **Ulcer with undermined edges is seen in:** *(MHPGMET 2005)*
    a. Malignant ulcer
    b. Tubercular ulcer
    c. Venous ulcer
    d. Trophic ulcer

69. **Which of the following is not a true cyst?**
    (MHPGMCET 2006)

    a. Sebaceous cyst
    b. Dermoid cyst
    c. Bone cyst
    d. Apoplectic cyst

70. **Pilomatrixoma is:** *(MHPGMCET 2006)*
    a. A fleshy skin mass
    b. A type of skin tag
    c. A benign epithelial tumor
    d. A malignant skin neoplasm

71. **Sinus is lined by:** *(MHPGMCET 2007)*
    a. Simple squamous epithelium
    b. Columnar epithelium
    c. Granulation tissue
    d. Fibrous tissue

72. **A swelling which is variable in consistency with diffuse margins is likely to be:** *(MHSSMCET 2005)*
    a. Inflammatory
    b. Benign
    c. Malignant
    d. Non-specific

73. **Which of the following is a compressible swelling:**
    a. Lipoma
    b. Hernia *(DNB 2013, 2010)*
    c. Hemangioma
    d. Sebaceous cyst

74. **Potts puffy tumor is:** *(Recent Question 2019, 2018)*
    a. Subperiosteal abscess of ethmoid bone
    b. Subperiosteal abscess of frontal bone
    c. Mucocele of ethmoid bone
    d. Mucocele of frontal bone

■ SKIN GRAFTING

1. **Ans. a. Partial thickness** *(Ref: Sabiston 20/e p1939; Schwartz 11/e p296, 10/e p264-265, 266; Bailey 27/e p639)*

2. **Ans. a. Joseph Lister**

   - **Joseph Lister said "Skin is the best dressing".**

3. **Ans. b. Plasma imbibition**

4. **Ans. b. Pedicle graft** *(Ref: Sabiston 20/e p1939; Schwartz 11/e p296, 9/e p1651; Bailey 27/e p635, 637)*

   - Skin graft must be **applied to a well-vascularized recipient wound bed**. It will **not adhere to exposed bone[Q], cartilage[Q], or tendon[Q]** devoid of periosteum, perichondrium, or peritenon, respectively, or devoid of its vascularized perimembranous envelope.
   - Radiation damaged tissues are poor recipient sites.
   - So an exposed bone surface is covered by a graft which has its own blood supply. Such grafts are known as flaps or pedicle grafts.

5. **Ans. d. Full thickness skin graft**

6. **Ans. c. Streptococcus**

7. **Ans. c. Skull bone**

8. **Ans. d. Humby knife**

9. **Ans. b. 2 weeks** *(Ref: Facial Plastic and Reconstructive Surgery by Ira D. Papel/44)*

   Excess split-skin autografts harvested and meshed during a surgical session are often stored at short-term for later burn surgery or graft failure.

   The current procedure in **skin storage involves wrapping the meshed autograft** on a piece of **ringer lactate** or **normal saline moistened gauze**, transferring it into a sterile container and **storing it in a 40°C for 2 weeks.** The graft should never be totally immersed in saline because it will become macerated. After 14 days of storage the respiratory activity of skin graft reduced by 50%.

10. **Ans. c. Less contraction**

■ FLAPS

11. **Ans. a. Carries its own vessels within it** *(Ref: Sabiston 19/e p1917-1919; Schwartz 11/e p1997, 9/e p1651-1654; Bailey 27/e p637)*

12. **Ans. a. Randomised flaps**

13. **Ans. d. Skin, muscle and vascular pedicle**

14. **Ans. d. Skull bone**

■ MARJOLIN'S ULCER

15. **Ans. b. Squamous cell carcinoma** *(Ref: Schwartz 11/e p1955, 10/e p259, 1817; Bailey 27/e p605)*

16. **Ans. a. Marjolin's ulcer** *(Ref: Bailey 27/e p605)*

17. **Ans. b. Squamous cell carcinoma**

■ PREMALIGNANT LESIONS OF SKIN

18. **Ans. d. All of the above** *(Ref: Sabiston 20/e p748; Schwartz 11/e p526-528, 10/e p847, 1217-1218; Bailey 27/e p606, 607)*

■ SQUAMOUS CELL CARCINOMA

19. **Ans. b. Everted**

20. **Ans. c. Squamous cell carcinoma**

■ BASAL CELL CARCINOMA

21. **Ans. a. Nodular** *(Ref: Sabiston 20/e p748; Schwartz 11/e p528, 10/e p486-487; Bailey 27/e p604-605)*

22. **Ans. a. Face**

23. **Ans. a. Basal cell carcinoma** *(Ref: Harrison 19/e p500; Robbins 9/e p1157)*

   Lesion near inner canthus with raised, pearly borders and central crust and with telangiectasia on surface of the lesion is highly suggestive of basal cell carcinoma.

24. Ans. a. Most common site is upper eyelid
25. Ans. b. Tumor less than 2 cm in diameter *(Ref: Sabiston 20/e p735; Schwartz 11/e p529, 10/e p486-487; Bailey 27/e p605)*
26. Ans. c. Nuclear palisading
27. Ans. b. Bilobed flap *(Ref: Bailey 27/e p641)*

> Bilobed flap is used to cover a convex defect as on tip of nose. The bilobed flap is widely used for small nasal defects because it allows one to distribute tensions further from he primary defect, thus controlling the degree of tension along the alar margin.

28. Ans. a. Basal cell carcinoma *(Ref: Bailey 27/e p674)*

■ MALIGNANT MELANOMA

29. Ans. d. Hair in mole
30. Ans. b. Surgical excision
31. Ans. a. Junctional melanocytes
32. Ans. a. Superficial spreading
33. Ans. a. Face
34. Ans. b. Acral lentiginous melanoma carries a good prognosis, c. Stage IIa shows satellite deposits
According to latest staging, presence of satellites is included in stage III.
35. Ans. c. Both a and b
36. Ans. d. Renal
37. Ans. b. Malignant melanoma foot
38. Ans. d. HPV infection
39. Ans. b. Cytokeratin-20
40. Ans. c. Malignant melanoma
41. Ans. b. Excision biopsy with 1–2 mm margin *(Ref: Devita 10/e p1354; Sabiston 20/e p734; Schwartz 11/e p531, 10/e p490)*

■ SKIN PATCH/STAIN/HEMANGIOMA

42. Ans. b. Strawberry angioma *(Ref: Schwartz 11/e p527, 10/e p485; Bailey 27/e p613)*
43. Ans. b. Strawberry angioma
44. Ans. c. Masterly inactivity
45. Ans. b. One year
46. Ans. d. Pulsed eye laser *(Ref: (Roxburgh 17/e p194, 205)*

> Selective photothermolysis or pulsed eye laser is the treatment of choice for portwine hemangioma.
>
> Excellent results have been obtained with careful and time-consuming treatment with a 585-nm flash lamp-pumped pulsed eye laser. Treatment sessions can begin in babies and anesthesia is not always necessary.

47. Ans. c. Portwine stain
48. Ans. b. Strawberry hemangioma
49. Ans. a. Portwine stain

■ SEBACEOUS CYST

50. Ans. d. Sole *(Ref: Schwartz 11/e p527, 10/e p1218; Bailey 27/e p598-599)*
51. Ans. b. Sebaceous cyst *(Ref: Sabiston 20/e p1860; Schwartz 11/e p527, 10/e p486; Bailey 27/e p598)*
52. Ans. a. Sebaceous cyst
53. Ans. b. Retention cyst
54. Ans. c. Ulcerated sebaceous cyst

■ LIPOMA

55. Ans. d. Lipoma *(Ref: Sabiston 20/e p2011; Schwartz 11/e p528, 10/e p486; Bailey 27/e p544, 936)*
56. Ans. c. Back
57. Ans. b. Retro-pertioneal *(Ref: Sabiston 20/e p2011-2012; Schwartz 11/e p528, 9/e p413; Bailey 27/e p1065)*
58. Ans. b. Tender subcutaneous lipomas

■ HIDRADENITIS SUPPURATIVA

59. Ans. a. Axilla, b. Circumanal, d. Groin *(Ref: Sabiston 20/e p1410; Schwartz 11/e p517, 10/e p476,506,1233; Bailey 27/e p595-596,1367-1368)*

■ KERATOACANTHOMA

60. **Ans. c. Self healing nodular lesion with central ulceration** *(Ref: Bailey 27/e p606)*

■ MISCELLANEOUS

61. **Ans. d. Pilomatrixoma**

62. **Ans. b. Slow rewarming** *(Ref: Bailey 27/e p953, 422)*

> ### FROSTBITE
>
> - **Frostbite** injuries **affect** the **peripheries in cold climates.**
> - **The initial treatment** is with **slow rewarming**[Q] **in a bath at 42°C.**
> - The cold injury produces **delayed microvascular damage.**
> - Level of damage is difficult to assess.
> - **Surgery** usually **does not play a role** in its management, until there is absolute demarcation of the level of injury.

63. **Ans. a. Steroids** *(Ref: Bailey 27/e p596)*

> ### PYODERMA GANGRENOSUM
>
> - Relatively uncommon **destructive cutaneous lesion.**
> - Clinically, a **rapidly enlarging, necrotic lesion** with **undermined border** and **surrounding erythema** characterize this disease.
> - Commonly associated with **IBD, rheumatoid arthritis, hematologic malignancy** and **monoclonal immunoglobulin A gammapathy.**
>
> **Treatment**
>
> - **First-line therapy:** Systemic treatment by **corticosteroids and cyclosporine**[Q].
> - **If ineffective, alternative therapeutic procedures** include systemic treatment with **corticosteroids** and **mycophenolate mofetil;** mycophenolate mofetil and cyclosporine.

64. **Ans. a. Appendage tumor**   65. **Ans. b. Trophic ulcer**

66. **Ans. c. Base of toe** *(Ref: Bailey 25/e p914)*

> ### AINHUM
>
> - Ainhum is a disease of **unknown etiology**
> - Usually **affects black men**[Q] (and occasionally women) who have **run barefoot in childhood**[Q].
> - It is recorded in **central Africa, central America** and the **Orient.**
> - A **fissure appears** at the level of the **interphalangeal joint of a toe,** usually of the **little toe**[Q].
> - **Fissure is followed by a fibrous band** that **encircles** the **digit** and **causes necrosis**[Q].
>
> **Treatment**
>
> - **Early stage: Z-plasty**[Q]**; Later stage: Amputation**[Q]

67. **Ans. b. Little toe**   68. **Ans. b. Tubercular ulcer**

69. **Ans. d. Apoplectic cyst** *(Ref: Bailey 24/e p209)*

> ### CYST
>
> - Cyst is a sac that is filled with a fluid or semi-fluid material.
> - Two of the most common types of cyst that occur under the skin surface are **sebaceous cyst** and **dermoid cyst**. These are **true cyst, line by epithelium.**
> - **Pseudocyst of pancreas** and **apoplectic cyst** are **not lined by epithelium,** and are **not true cyst**[Q].

70. **Ans. c. A benign epithelial tumor**

71. **Ans. c. Granulation tissue** *(Ref: Bailey 27/e p616)*

> - A **sinus** is **a blind-ending tract** that **connects a cavity lined with granulation tissue** (often an abscess cavity) with an epithelial surface.

72. **Ans. c. Malignant**

73. **Ans. c. Hemangioma**

74. **Ans. b. Subperiosteal abscess of frontal bone**

Wound Healing, Tissue Repair and Scar

■ WOUND

WOUND

- **Wound**: Breach in continuity of skin or surface epithelium
- **Simple wound**: Only **skin & subcutaneous tissue** is involved[Q]
- **Complex wound**: Involves underlying **nerves, vessels, tendons** with **devitalized tissue**[Q]

■ WOUND HEALING

WOUND HEALING

- Mechanism by which body attempts to restore the integrity of injured part

Phases of Wound Healing		
Inflammatory Phase	**Proliferative Phase**	**Remodeling Phase**
• Begins **immediately after wounding**[Q] • Last for **2-3 days**[Q] • **Bleeding → Vasoconstriction & thrombus formation** to limit blood loss → **Platelets stick** to damaged **endothelial linings**[Q]	• Last from **3rd day to 3rd week**[Q] • Consist of **fibroblast activity** with **production of collagen, glycosaminoglycans & proteoglycans**[Q] • **Angioneogenesis**[Q]: Growth of new vessels as capillary loops • **Re-epithelialization**[Q] of wound surface • **Increase in tensile strength** of wound due to **increased type III collagen**, deposited in random fashion[Q] • **Wound contraction**[Q]: Reduces the surface area of wound	• Characterized by **maturation of collagen**[Q] • **Type I collagen replacing type III** until a ratio of 4:1 is achieved[Q] • **Realignment of collagen fibers** along the line of tension[Q] • **Decreased wound vascularity**[Q] • **Wound contraction**[Q] • **Maturation of collagen**: Increased tensile strength of wound[Q] • **Wound strength is maximum at 12th week post injury**[Q] (represents approximately **80% of uninjured skin strength**[Q])

■ FACTORS ADVERSELY AFFECTING WOUND HEALING

Factors that Inhibit Wound Healing

Local Factors	Systemic Factors
• **Infection**[Q] • **Ischemia**[Q] • **Foreign body**[Q] • **Hematoma**[Q] • Movement • Mechanical stress • Necrotic tissue	• **Diabetes mellitus**[Q] • **Ionizing radiation**[Q], **temperature**[Q] • **Advanced age**[Q], **Malnutrition**[Q] • Vitamin **C** and **A** deficiency[Q] • Mineral (**Zinc** and **Iron**[Q]) deficiencies • Drugs (**Steroids**[Q], **Doxorubicin**) • **Jaundice**[Q], **Uremia**[Q], **Malignancy**[Q]

■ CLASSIFICATION OF SURGICAL WOUNDS

Classification of Surgical Wounds	
Wounds Class	**Definition**
I: Clean	• **Uninfected operative wound without inflammation**[Q] • **Respiratory, alimentary, genital or infected urinary tract is not entered**[Q] • **Wounds** are **closed primarily**[Q], if necessary **drained with closed drainage**[Q] **Examples of Clean Wound** • **Inguinal hernia**[Q] • **Mastectomy**[Q] • **Joint replacement**[Q] • Abdominal aortic aneurysm (**AAA**) repair[Q] • **Thyroidectomy**[Q]
II: Clean contaminated	• Operative wound in which **respiratory tract, GIT or genitourinary tract is entered under controlled condition without unusual contamination**[Q] **Examples of Clean Contaminated Wound** • **Cholecystectomy**[Q] • **Elective GI surgeries (elective colonic resection**[Q], **gastrectomy**[Q]**)** • **CBD exploration**[Q]
III: Contaminated	• **Open, fresh accidental wounds**[Q] • **Operations with major break in sterile techniques**[Q] • **Gross spillage from GIT**[Q] • Incision in which **acute non-purulent inflammation is encountered**[Q] **Examples of Contaminated Wound** • **Spill during elective GI surgery**[Q] • **Enterotomy during bowel obstruction**[Q] • **Perforated gastric ulcer**[Q] • **Human bite**[Q] • **Appendicular perforation**[Q] • **Open fracture**[Q] • **Penetrating abdominal trauma**[Q]
IV: Dirty	• **Old traumatic wound with retained devitalized tissue**[Q] • Wound with **clinical infection** or **perforated viscera with high degree of contamination**[Q] • **Organism causing post-op infection is already present**[Q] in the wound before operation • Associated with **severe inflammation**[Q] **Examples of Dirty Wound** • **Perforated diverticulitis**[Q] • **Fecal peritonitis**[Q] • **Frank pus**[Q] • **Necrotizing soft tissue infection**[Q]

Wounds Class	Risk of Infection	Need for Prophylaxis
Clean	5%[Q]	• Usually **not required**[Q]
Clean-contaminated	10%[Q]	• Usually **required**[Q]
Contaminated	20–30%[Q]	• **Required**[Q]
Dirty	30–40%[Q]	• **Treatment required**[Q] (not the prophylaxis)

■ CLASSIFICATION OF WOUND CLOSURE & HEALING

Classification of Wound Closure & Healing		
Healing by Primary Intention	**Healing by Secondary Intention**	**Healing by Tertiary Intention**

• Also known as **healing by first intention**[Q]
 • Occurs when there is:
    – **Apposition of wound edges**[Q]
    – **Minimal surrounding tissue trauma & least inflammation**[Q]
    – Associated with **best scar**[Q]
	• Occurs in the wounds that are:
	    – **Left open**[Q]
	    – Allowed to **heal by granulation, contraction & epithelialization**[Q]
		• Also known as **"delayed primary intention healing"**[Q]
		 • Occurs when **wound edges are not opposed immediately**, in contaminated or **untidy wounds**[Q]
		 • **Delayed closure of wound**[Q] is done when inflammatory & proliferative phase of healing is well established
		 • Results in **less satisfactory scar**[Q] as compared to healing by primary intention

■ CHRONIC WOUND

CHRONIC WOUND

- Wounds that **do not heal within 3 months**[Q]
- **Delay in healing** can occur at any phase but **most often occur in inflammatory phase**[Q]

Treatment

- **Surgical treatment** is only indicated if **non-operative treatment has failed** or patient suffers from **intractable pain**[Q]

■ DEGLOVING INJURY

DEGLOVING

- **Skin & subcutaneous fat** are **stripped by avulsion from the underlying fascia**[Q]
- **Leaving neurovascular structures, tendon or bone exposed**[Q]

■ COMPARTMENT SYNDROME

COMPARTMENT SYNDROME

- Typically occur in **closed lower limb injuries**[Q]

Clinical Features

- Characterized by **severe pain**[Q]; **Pain on passive movement** of affected compartment muscle[Q]
- **Distal sensory disturbance**[Q]
- Finally by **absence of pulses distally**[Q] **(a late sign**[Q]**)**

Diagnosis

- **Compartment pressure** is measured by using a **pressure monitor & catheter placed in muscle compartment**[Q]

Treatment

- **Fasciotomy if pressure is constantly > 30 mm Hg** or presence of **clinical signs of compartment syndrome**[Q]
- **In fasciotomy: Longitudinal incision** is given over **skin, subcutaneous fat & fascia; muscle** should **bulge through fasciotomy opening**[Q]

■ PRESSURE SORE

PRESSURE SORE

- Also known as **Bed sores/Pressure ulcer/Decubitus ulcer/Pressure sore/Trophic ulcer/Penetrating ulcer**[Q]
- **Definition: Tissue necrosis with ulceration due to prolonged pressure**[Q]
- **Preventable**
- Incidence: **5% of hospitalized patients; Higher incidence** in: **Paraplegic**[Q] patients, **elderly & severely ill**[Q] patients
- MC site: **I**schium[Q] > **G**reater trochanter[Q] > **S**acrum[Q] > **H**eel[Q] > **M**alleolus[Q] > **O**cciput[Q] (Indira Gandhi Stadium inauguration by **HM Office**)
- Mechanism: **External pressure exceeds the capillary occlusive pressure (>30 mm Hg)** → Blood flow to the skin stops → **Tissue hypoxia, necrosis & ulceration**[Q]
- Other mechanisms: Due to **impaired nutrition, defective blood supply, neurological deficit**[Q]

Neurological Causes (SPL DPT)	
• **S**yringomyelia, **S**pina bifida, **S**pinal injury[Q]	• **D**iabetic neuropathy[Q]
• **P**eripheral neuritis, **P**eripheral nerve injury[Q]	• **P**araplegia[Q]
• **L**eprosy[Q]	• **T**abes dorsalis[Q]

Clinical Features

- **Painless punched out ulcer**[Q]; **Base formed by bone**[Q]

Staging of Pressure Sore	
Stage	**Description**
1	• **Non-blanchable erythema without a breach** in epidermis **(early superficial ulcer**[Q]**)**
2	• **Partial thickness skin loss** involving **epidermis & dermis (Late superficial ulcer**[Q]**)**
3	• **Full thickness skin loss extending into subcutaneous tissue** but not through underlying fascia **(Early deep ulcer**[Q]**)**
4	• **Full thickness skin loss through fascia with extensive tissue destruction**, maybe **involving muscle, bone, tendon or joint (Late deep ulcer**[Q]**)**

Contd…

Contd…

Management

- **Prevention is the best treatment**[Q] with: Good skin care; special **pressure dispersion cushions or foams**; Use of **low air-loss & air-fluidized beds**[Q]; Urinary or fecal diversion in selected case
- **Bed bound patients: Turned** at least **every 2 hours**[Q]
- **Wheel chair bound patients: Lift** themselves **off** their seat for **10 second every 10 minutes**[Q]
- **Surgical treatment:** Reserved for the patient with **no improvement after conservative management**; includes **adequate debridement, vacuum assisted closure** or **Flap closure**

> - **Large skin flaps with muscle & intact sensory innervations is preferred**[Q] (Example: Extensor fascia lata with lateral cutaneous nerve of thigh[Q])

■ VACUUM ASSISTED CLOSURE/ NEGATIVE PRESSURE WOUND THERAPY

VACUUM ASSISTED CLOSURE/NEGATIVE PRESSURE WOUND THERAPY (NPWT)

- NPWT promotes wound healing by **applying a vacuum through a special sealed dressing.**
- Continued **vacuum draws out the fluid** from wound & **increases blood flow** to the area.
- **Vacuum** may be **applied continuously or intermittently**, depending upon the types of wound being treated & clinical objectives.
- **Negative pressure** of **–125 mm Hg**[Q] is used.
- **Dressing** should be **changed 2-3 times/week**[Q]

Primary Effects of NPWT on Wound Healing	
Macrodeformation[Q]	Drawing the wound edges together leading to contraction
Stabilization of wound environment[Q]	Wound protected from outside micro-organisms in a warm & moist environment
Reduced edema[Q]	With removal of soft tissue exudates
Microdeformation[Q]	Leading to cellular proliferation on the wound surface

Contraindications for NPWT Use	
• **Malignancy in the wound**[Q]	• **Non-enteric & unexplored fistula**[Q]
• **Untreated osteomyelitis**[Q]	• **Necrotic tissue with eschar**[Q]

■ SCAR

SCAR

- **Maturation phase** of wound healing **leads to formation of scar**[Q]
- **Immature scar (Pink, raised, hard & itchy**[Q]) → As the **collagen matures & becomes denser, scar** becomes almost **acellular**, as fibroblast & blood vessels reduce → Scar becomes **paler, flattens, softer & itching diminishes**[Q] → Tensile strength of scar increases; maximum at **12th week**[Q] **(after 3 months) post-injury**; represent approx. **80%** of uninjured skin strength[Q]
- **Types of scar:** Atrophic scar, hypertrophic scar & keloid

■ ATROPHIC SCAR

ATROPHIC SCAR

- **Pale, flat & stretched in appearance**; Appear on the **back** & in **areas of tension**[Q]
- **Easily traumatized** as epidermis & dermis are thinned; **Excision & resuturing rarely improves such scar**[Q]

■ HYPERTROPHIC SCAR

HYPERTROPHIC SCAR

- **Excessive scar tissue** that **does not extend beyond the boundaries of original incision or wound**[Q]
- Results from **prolonged inflammatory phase**[Q] of wound healing and/or **unfavorable scar citing**[Q] (across the lines of skin tension)

Contd…

Histology

- Excess collagen & hypervascularity[Q] **(more marked in keloid** with more type III collagen)
- Contains **well organized type III collagen; Improves spontaneously with time**[Q]

Treatment

- **Linear hypertrophic scar:** Treated with **pressure therapy** or **silicone gel sheet application**[Q]
- **Ongoing hypertrophy:** Treated with **intralesional steroids (Triamcinolone**[Q]**)**
- **Scars persist after 1 year:** Surgical **excision + primary closure** of wound[Q]

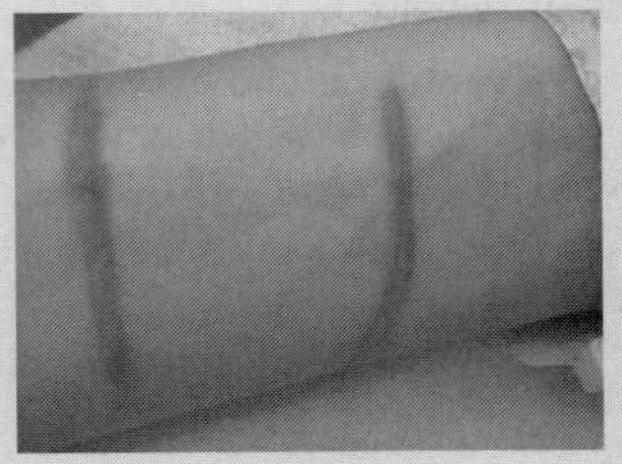

■ KELOID

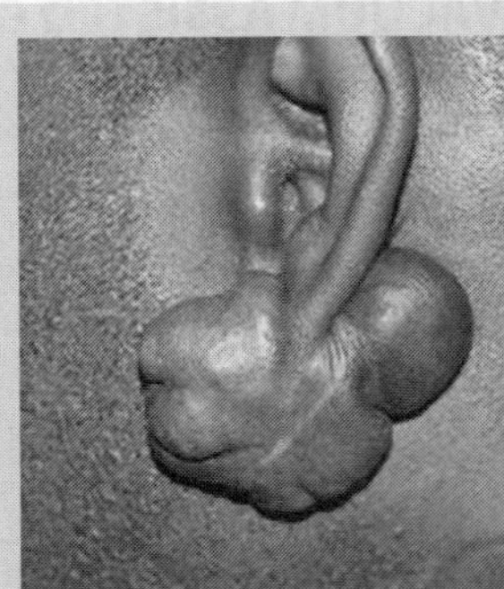

- **Excessive scar tissue** that **extends beyond the boundaries of original incision or wound**[Q]
- **Etiology:** Unknown; **Genetic predisposition, more common in blacks**[Q]
- Associated with: **Elevated levels of growth factors; deeply pigmented skin**[Q]
- **Common** in certain areas of body: **Above clavicle**[Q]**, upper extremities**[Q]**, on the trunk**[Q]**, face**[Q] (Especially seen in **triangle** whose boundaries are **xiphisternum & each shoulder tip**[Q])

Histology

- **Excess collagen & hypervascularity;** Contain **disorganized type I & III collagen**[Q]
- **Thicker collagen bundles**[Q] form acellular node like structures

Treatment

- **Keloids rarely regress with time**, often **refractory to medical & surgical intervention**[Q]
- **First line treatment: Silicones** in combination with **pressure therapy & intralesional corticosteroid** injection[Q]
- **Refractory cases** (after 12 months of therapy): **Excision + Post-op radiotherapy**[Q] (external beam or brachytherapy)
- **New treatment modalities: Internal cryotherapy**[Q] **& 5% Imiquimod**[Q]

Feature	Hypertrophic Scar	Keloid
Genetic	Not familial[Q]	May be **familial**[Q]
Race	Not race related[Q]	**Black**[Q] >white
Sex	Female = male	**Female**[Q] >male
Age	Children[Q]	10-30 years[Q]
Border	Remains **within wound**[Q]	**Outgrows** wound area
Natural history	**Subsides** with time	Rarely subsides
Site	Flexor surfaces[Q]	**Sternum (MC**[Q]**),** shoulder, face
Etiology	Related to **tension**[Q]	Unknown
Develop	Within 4 weeks	3 months to year after trauma
Symptoms	**Raised**, some pruritus **Respect wound confines**	**Pain, pruritus, hyperesthesia** **Growth beyond wound margins**
Histology	**Parallel orientation** of collagen fibers	**Thick wavy** collagen fibers in **random orientation**

■ WOUND HEALING

1. Management of an open wound seen 12 hours after the injury: *(DPG 2011)*
   a. Suturing
   b. Debridement and suture
   c. Secondary suturing
   d. Heal by granulation

2. The tensile strength of the wound starts and increases after: *(WBPG 2012, MAHE 2005)*
   a. Immediate suture of the wound
   b. 3–4 days
   c. 7–10 days
   d. 6 months

3. In a sutured surgical wound, the process of epithelialization is completed within: *(UPSC 2007)*
   a. 24 hours
   b. 48 hours
   c. 72 hours
   d. 96 hours

4. Patient has lacerated untidy wound of the leg and attended the casualty after 2 hours. His wound should be: *(Recent Question 2016)*
   a. Sutured immediately
   b. Debrided and sutured immediately
   c. Debrided and sutured secondarily
   d. Cleaned and dressed

5. In the healing of clean wound the maximum immediate strength of the wound is reached by:
   a. 2–3 days
   b. 4–7 days
   c. 10–12 days
   d. 13–18 days

6. Tensile strength of wound becomes normal after: *(Recent Question 2013)*
   a. 6 weeks
   b. Never
   c. 4 months
   d. 6 months

■ KELOID AND HYPERTROPHIC SCAR

7. True statement regarding hypertrophic scar: *(JIPMER May 2018)*
   a. Usually occurs across the flexural areas
   b. Does not improve with time
   c. Overgrows its boundaries
   d. Develops months after surgery

8. Which of the following is true about keloid? *(Recent Question 2018, 2017)*
   a. Wide local excision is treatment of choice
   b. Collagen is same but arranged haphazardly
   c. Will not spread beyond wound site
   d. More amount of growth factors

9. The following statement about keloid is true: *(Recent Question 2018)*
   a. Elevated levels of growth factor is not seen
   b. Extended excision is the treatment of choice
   c. It do not extend beyond the wound
   d. It will have more collagen and vascularity

10. First line treatment for keloid is:
    a. Intralesional injection of keloid
    b. Local steroid *(Recent Question 2015, AIIMS Dec 94)*
    c. Radiotherapy
    d. Wide excisio

11. Keloid scar is made up: *(Recent Question 2016)*
    a. Dense collagen
    b. Loose fibrous tissue
    c. Granulomatous tissue
    d. Loose areolar tissue

12. The following statement about keloid is true: *(Recent Question 2016)*
    a. They do not extend into normal skin
    b. Local recurrence is common after excision
    c. They often undergo malignant change
    d. They are more common in whites than in blacks

13. Keloid formation is not seen over: *(Recent Question 2016)*
    a. Ear
    b. Face
    c. Eyelids
    d. Neck

14. Most appropriate management of recurrent keloid is: *(MCI June 2019)*
    a. Excisional surgery
    b. Intramarginal excision followed by radiation
    c. Cryosurgery
    d. Silicone gel sheeting

■ VACUUM ASSISTED CLOSURE

15. Vacuum assisted closure is contraindicated in:
    a. Chronic osteomyelitis *(Recent Question 2017)*
    b. Large amount of necrotic tissue with eschar
    c. Abdominal wound
    d. Surgical wound dehiscence

16. All of the following are principles of negative pressure wound therapy except: *(Recent Question 2017)*
    a. Stabilization of wound environment
    b. Clearance of infection
    c. Macrodeformation of the wound
    d. Decreased edema

17. Negative pressure wound therapy (NPWT) is used in:
    a. Bedsore in sacrum after debridement
    b. After amputation negative suction
    c. Osteomyelitis
    d. Unexplored fistulas *(Recent Question 2018)*

■ MISCELLANEOUS

18. In treatment of hand injuries, the greatest priority is: *(All India 96)*
    a. Repair of tendons
    b. Restoration of skin cover
    c. Repair of nerves
    d. Repair of blood vessels

19. Criteria for viability of muscle are all except: *(Recent Question 2014)*
    a. Colour
    b. Intact fascia
    c. Contractibility
    d. Bleeding on cutting

20. Degloving injury: *(Recent Question 2019, 2018)*
    a. Separation of skin only
    b. Separation of skin + subcutaneous tissue
    c. Separation of skin + subcutaneous tissue + fascia exposing tendons
    d. Separation of tendon exposing the bone

Explanations

■ WOUND HEALING

1. **Ans. b. Debridement and suture** *(Ref: Sabiston 19/e p245; Schwartz 11/e p274, 10/e p234,1820; Bailey 27/e p24-26, 89; Robbins 9/e p109)*

- If the **blood supply to the wound** is **adequate** and **bacterial invasion** is **absent**, wound can be **safely closed anytime following proper debridement** and **irrigation**[Q].
  - If there is **established infection** and **tissue** is of **doubtful viability** has been left in-situ, then the **wound is left open** and **re-explored after 48 hours**[Q].
  - If there is **infection**, and the **doubtful viable tissue** is **now healthy**, the **deep tissues can be repaired** and the **wound is closed**[Q].
  - If however there is **further necrosis** and **infection**, the wound is **again debrided** and **left open**[Q].

2. **Ans. b. 3–4 days**

3. **Ans. b. 48 hours**

4. **Ans. b. Debrided and sutured immediately**

5. **Ans. d. 13–18 days**

6. **Ans. b. Never**

■ KELOID AND HYPERTROPHIC SCAR

7. **Ans. a. Usually occurs across the flexural areas**

8. **Ans. d. More amount of growth factors** *(Ref: Bailey 27/e p31)*

"A keloid scar is defined as excessive scar tissue that extends beyond the boundaries of the original incision or wound. Its aetiology is unknown, but it is associated with elevated levels of growth factor, deeply pigmented skin, an inherited tendency and certain areas of the body (e.g. a triangle whose points are the xiphisternum and each shoulder tip). The histology of both hypertrophic and keloid scars shows excess collagen with hypervascularity, but this is more marked in keloids where there is more type III collagen."
-Bailey 27/e p31

9. **Ans. d. It will have more collagen and vascularity**

10. **Ans. a. Intralesional injection of keloid** *(Ref: Bailey 27/e p31)*

11. **Ans. a. Dense collagen**

12. **Ans. b. Local recurrence is common after excision**

13. **Ans. c. Eyelids**

14. **Ans. b. Intramarginal excision followed by radiation** *(Ref: Bailey 27/e p31)*

■ VACUUM ASSISTED CLOSURE

15. **Ans. b. Large amount of necrotic tissue with eschar** *(Ref: Long, Mary Arnold; Blevins, Anne (2009). "Options in negative pressure wound therapy". Journal of wound, ostomy and continence nursing 36 (2): 202-11)*

16. **Ans. b. Clearance of infection**

17. **Ans. a. Bedsore in sacrum after debridement**

■ MISCELLANEOUS

18. **Ans. d. Repair of blood vessels**

19. **Ans. b. Intact fascia**

20. **Ans. b. Separation of skin + subcutaneous tissue** *(Ref: Bailey 27/e p27)*

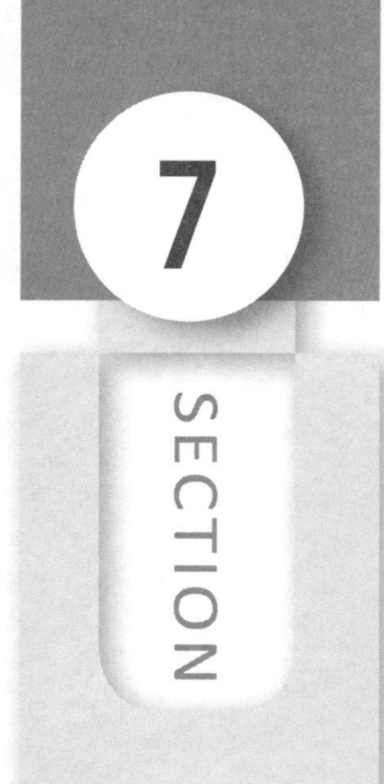

Neurosurgery

- Cerebrovascular Diseases
- CNS Tumors

Cerebrovascular Diseases

■ ARNOLD-CHIARI MALFORMATION

Arnold-Chiari malformation

Type I Chiari malformation	Type II Chiari malformation
• Displacment of **cerebellar tonsil into cervical canal**[Q] • Associated with **syringomyelia** of cervical canal • Typically produces symptoms **during adolescence or adult life**[Q] • **Not associated with hydrocephalus.**[Q] • Patients complain of **recurrent headache, neck pain, urinary frequency**, and **progressive lower extremity spasticity**[Q].	• Lesion represents an **anomaly** of the **hindbrain** • Characterized by **elongation of** the **4th ventricle** and **kinking** of the **brainstem**, with **displacement** of the **inferior vermis, pons**, and **medulla** into the cervical canal[Q]. • **Type II Chiari** malformation is characterized by **progressive hydrocephalus** with a **myelomeningocele**[Q]. • Plain skull radiographs show a **small posterior fossa** and a **widened cervical canal**[Q]. • CT scanning with contrast and MRI display the **cerebellar tonsils protruding downward** into the **cervical canal** and the **hindbrain abnormalities**. • The anomaly is treated by **surgical decompression**[Q].

■ VERTEBRAL BODY ANOMALIES

Vertebral Body Anomalies

Spina Bifida Occulta	Spina Bifida Aperta
	• Meningocele • Myelomeningocele • Myeloschisis

■ MENINGOCELE

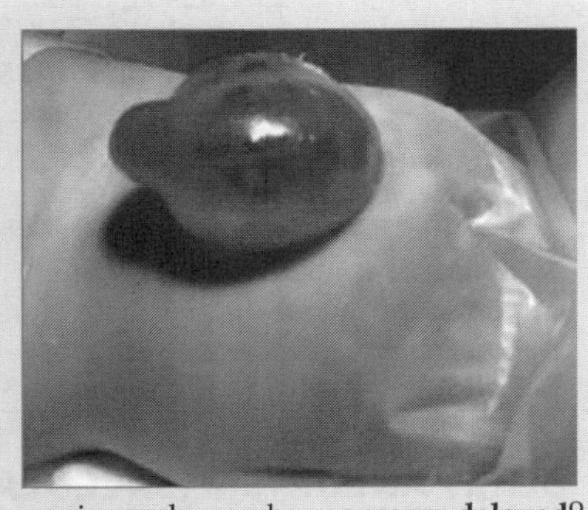

MENINGOCELE

• **Herniation** of **meninges** through a **defect** in the **posterior vertebral arches**[Q].
• **Spinal cord** is **usually normal** and assumes a **normal position** in the spinal canal
• There may be tethering, syringomyelia, or diastematomyelia.

Clinical Features

• A **fluctuant midline mass,** that may transilluminate occurs along the vertebral column, in the lower back[Q].
• Most meningoceles are **well-covered with skin** and pose no threat to the patient.

Diagnosis

• **Plain roentgenograms** demonstrate a defect[Q].

Treatment

• **Asymptomatic children** with **normal neurologic findings** and **full-thickness skin** covering the meningocele may have **surgery delayed**[Q].
• Patients with **leaking CSF** or a **thin skin** covering should undergo **immediate surgical treatment** to prevent meningitis[Q].

■ MYELOMENINGOCELE

MYELOMENINGOCELE

• **Most severe form of dysraphism** involving the vertebral column
• **Incidence: 1/4,000** live births[Q]
• **MC site** of myelomeningocele: **Lumbosacral region (75%)**[Q]

Contd…

Contd...

Etiology

- **Genetic predisposition** exists; the risk of recurrence after **one affected child** increases to **3-4%** and increases to **10%** with **two** previous abnormal pregnancies.

  - **Nutritional** and **environmental factors: Folate**[Q] is intricately involved in the prevention and etiology of NTDs.
  - **Maternal peri-conceptional use** of folic acid supplementation **reduces** the **incidence** of **neural tube defects** in pregnancies at risk by at least **50%**[Q].
  - To be effective, folic acid supplementation should be **initiated before conception** and **continued until** at least the **12th week of gestation** when neurulation is complete[Q].

Prevention

- All women of childbearing age and who are capable of becoming pregnant take 0.4 mg of folic acid daily.

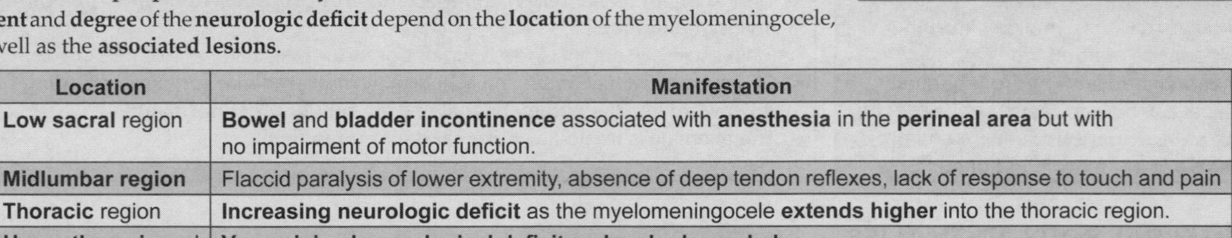

Drugs increasing the risk of myelomeningocele	
• Trimethoprim[Q]	• Phenobarbital[Q]
• Carbamazepine[Q]	• Primidone[Q]
• Phenytoin[Q]	• Valproic acid[Q]

Clinical Features

- Produces **dysfunction of skeleton, skin, gastrointestinal** and **genitourinary tracts**, in addition to the **peripheral nervous system** and **CNS**[Q].
- **Extent** and **degree** of the **neurologic deficit** depend on the **location** of the myelomeningocele, as well as the **associated lesions**.

Location	Manifestation
Low sacral region	**Bowel** and **bladder incontinence** associated with **anesthesia** in the **perineal area** but with no impairment of motor function.
Midlumbar region	Flaccid paralysis of lower extremity, absence of deep tendon reflexes, lack of response to touch and pain
Thoracic region	**Increasing neurologic deficit** as the myelomeningocele **extends higher** into the thoracic region.
Upper thoracic and **cervical region**	**Very minimal neurological deficit and no hydrocephalus**

■ CAUSES OF CEREBROVASCULAR ACCIDENTS

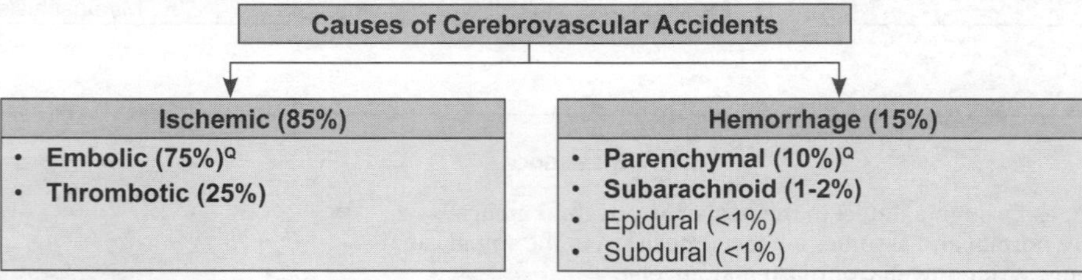

Intracerebral (Parenchymal) Hemorrhage	Subarachnoid Hemorrhage
• **MC type** of **intracranial hemorrhage**[Q] • **MC cause is hypertension**[Q], causing rupture of small perforating arteries or arterioles[Q] • **MC site: Basal ganglia (Putamen**[Q]**)**	• **2nd MC cause** of intracranial hemorrhage[Q] • **MC cause: Trauma >** Spontaneous rupture of **Berry aneurysm**[Q] • **MC site** of Berry aneurysm is **anterior circulation** of **"circle of willis"**[Q]

■ BERRY ANEURYSM (SACCULAR OR CONGENITAL ANEURYSM)

Berry Aneurysm (Saccular or Congenital Aneurysm)

- **Berry aneurysms: MC intracranial aneurysm**[Q], **saccular** in appearance, arising at the **bifurcation of intracranial arteries**.
- About **85%** aneurysms occur in the **anterior circulation**, on the **circle of willis**[Q].

Occurrence of Berry aneurysm in order of frequency	
• **Anterior communicating artery-Anterior Cerebral junction (29%)**[Q]	
• Posterior communicating artery-Internal carotid junction (28%)	
• Middle cerebral bifurcation (18%)	
• Intracranial carotid bifurcation (8%)	• Vertebrobasilar or basilar bifurcation (3%)

Contd…

- **MC type of intracranial aneurysm**[Q]; **Multiple** in **20-30%** cases
- **Predisposing factors: Smoking** and **hypertension**[Q]
- **Wall of Berry aneurysm** is made up of **thickened hyalinized intima**[Q]. The adventitia covering the sac is continuous with that of parent artery.

Increased Risk of Berry Aneurysm in (FM)	
• ADPKD[Q]	• Marfan's syndrome
• Ehlers-Danlos syndrome	• Fibromuscular dysplasia
• NF-1[Q]	• Coarctation of aorta

- **Rupture of aneurysm** usually occurs **at the apex**[Q] **(dome)** resulting in **subarachnoid hemorrhage**[Q] or **intraparenchymal hemorrhage** or **both**[Q].
- Unruptured aneurysms are **usually completely asymptomatic**[Q].

Treatment

- Treatment consists of **coiling, coiling through a stent, or surgical clipping**
- **Endovascular coil occlusion** is preferred over surgical clipping[Q]
- **Open craniotomy & clipping** is reserved for lesions not to be amenable to endovascular coiling[Q].

■ EXTRADURAL HEMATOMA AND SUBDURAL HEMATOMA

Extradural Hematoma	Subdural Hematoma (Acute)
• EDH is a **neurosurgical emergency**[Q]. • Nearly always **associated with** a **skull fracture**[Q] • More common in **young male patients**[Q]. • Associated with **tearing of a meningeal artery**[Q] • Hematoma accumulates in the space between **bone & dura**. • **MC site: Temporal**[Q] (**pterion** is **thinnest part** of skull & **overlies middle meningeal artery**) • **Not always arterial**: disruption of a major dural venous sinus can result in an EDH. • Force required to sustain a skull fracture can be surprisingly small[Q] – a fall from standing or a single blow to the head. • **Classical presentation**: Initial injury followed by a **lucid interval**[Q] (occurring in <1/3rd of cases) • **Early recognition & treatment** is likely to result in **full recovery** • Delays in diagnosis and treatment can result in **death** from secondary brain injury. • **EDH on CT scan**: Lentiform (**lens shaped** or **biconvex**[Q]) **hyperdense lesion** between the skull and brain. • **Treatment of EDH**: Immediate surgical evacuation[Q] via a craniotomy. • **Overall mortality** for all cases of EDH is about **18%** but for **isolated EDH** it is about **2%**.	• **SDH** accumulates in the space **between dura** and **arachnoid**[Q]. • **Disruption of** a **cortical vessel** or **brain laceration**[Q] • Nearly **always associated with** a **significant primary brain injury**[Q]. • Patients present with an **impaired conscious level** from the time of injury, but further deterioration can occur as the hematoma expands. • **CT appearance** of SDH: **Hyperdense** (acute blood) **concavo-convex appearance**[Q]. • **Treatment** of SDH: **Evacuation** via craniotomy. • **Small hematomas** with little mass effect may be **managed conservatively** in neurosurgical centers. • **Mortality rate** from **SDH** is **much higher** than for EDH and is as high as **40%** in some series[Q].

■ CLASSIFICATION OF SDH

Classification of SDH		
• **Acute SDH:** < 3 days[Q]	• **Subacute SDH: 4-21 days**[Q]	• **Chronic SDH: >21 days**[Q]

■ SUBARACHNOID HEMORRHAGE

Subarachnoid Hemorrhage

- **MC cause: Trauma** >Spontaneous rupture of **Berry aneurysm**[Q]

Clinical Features

- **Sudden transient loss of consciousness**[Q] (occurs in nearly half of the patients)
- **Excruciating severe headache**[Q]: presenting complaint in 45% of cases (worst headache of patients life) more common upon regaining consciousness when loss of consciousness is associated

Contd…

Contd...

> - **Neck stiffness** and **vomiting**[Q]: are common associations
> - **Focal neurological deficit**: uncommon.
> - **Sudden headache** in the **absence of focal neurological deficit** is the **hallmark of aneurysmal rupture.**[Q]

- Associated prodromal symptoms (suggest **location** of progressively enlarging unruptured aneurysm):
  - **Third cranial nerve palsy**[Q]: Aneurysm at junction of **PCA** and **ICA**
  - **Sixth nerve palsy**[Q]: Aneurysm in **cavernous sinus**
  - Occipital and posterior cervical pain: **Inferior cerebellar artery aneurysm**
  - **Pain** in or **behind the eye**[Q]: MCA aneurysm

Diagnosis

- **Noncontrast CT scan: Investigation of choice** (Lumbar puncture is not indicated prior to an imaging procedure)
- **CSF picture: Hallmark** of aneurysmal rupture is **blood in CSF (Xanthochromic spinal fluid**[Q]**)**

> - **Lumbar puncture** should be performed, **if the CT scan fails to establish the diagnosis of SAH** and **no mass lesion** or **obstructive hydrocephalus** is found to establish the presence of subarachnoid blood.[Q]

Treatment

- **Traumatic subarachnoid hemorrhage** is **managed conservatively**[Q].

■ DIFFUSE AXONAL INJURIES (DAI)

DIFFUSE AXONAL INJURIES (DAI)

- **DAI** represents the **presence of widespread axonal damage (white matter) in** both **hemispheres secondary to severe head injury**[Q].
- Results from application of **severe acceleration/deceleration** or **angular strain** to the brain (**injuries to axons by shearing force**[Q])
- **MC location: Lobar white matter** at the **junction of grey and white matter**[Q] > **Corpus callosum** > **Brain stem**

Pathology

- **Hemorrhagic** or **non-hemorrhagic white matter tears** in both hemispheres.

Clinical Features

- Clinical presentation vary from concussion to coma
- **Loss of consciousness** is a common finding[Q]
- **DAI: MC cause** of **post-traumatic vegetative state**[Q]
- **Raised ICT may** or **may not be associated**[Q]

Diagnosis

- **MRI is IOC for DAI**[Q] (better than CT scan).

Prognosis

- **DAI** carries an **extremely poor prognosis**[Q].

Brain Injury	
Primary Brain Injury	**Secondary Brain Injury**

• Primary brain injury occurs **at the time of impact**
• Includes injuries such as:
  – **Brainstem** and **hemispheric contusions**[Q]
  – **Diffuse axonal injury**[Q]
  – **Cortical lacerations**[Q]
	• Secondary brain injury occurs at **some time after** the **moment of impact**[Q]
	• **Preventable**[Q]
	• **Principle causes: Hypoxia, hypotension, raised ICP, reduced cerebral perfusion pressure** and **pyrexia**[Q]

■ CEREBRAL CONTUSIONS

CEREBRAL CONTUSIONS

- **Cerebral contusions** result from the **brain being damaged by:**
  - **Impacting against** the **skull** either at the **point of impact** (the 'coup') or on the **other side of** the head ('contre-coup')[Q]
  - As the **brain slides forwards** and **backwards over** the ridged cranial fossa floor (most often affecting the **inferior frontal lobes** and **temporal poles**)[Q]

Diagnosis

- **CT scan: Heterogeneous** with **mixed areas of high** and **low density**[Q].
  - There may be an associated mass effect. Contusion appears uniformly hyperdense.

Contd...

Contd…

Treatment

- Cerebral contusions **rarely require immediate surgical treatment**.

> - Patient with **cerebral contusions** must be **admitted for observation** as these lesions will **tend to mature** and **expand for 48–72 hours** following injury[Q].

- **Small proportion** of cerebral contusions will require **delayed surgical evacuation to reduce** the **mass effect**[Q].

■ SKULL BASE FRACTURES

Skull Base		
Anterior Cranial Fossa	**Middle Cranial Fossa**	**Posterior Cranial Fossa**
• Formed by frontal bone[Q]	• Formed by temporal & sphenoid bone[Q]	• Formed by occipital bone[Q]
Cribriform plate: Sieve like structure between anterior cranial fossa & nasal cavity		

Anterior Cranial Fossa Fracture	**Middle Cranial Fossa Fracture**	**Posterior Cranial Fossa Fracture**

• **MC type** of skull base fracture[Q]
• Caused by **fracture of cribriform plate**[Q]
• **Clinical features**:
  – Subconjunctival hematoma[Q]
  – **CSF rhinorrhea**[Q]
  – **Epistaxis**[Q]
  – **Anosmia**[Q]
  – Periorbital hematoma or **"Raccoon eyes"**[Q]
  – **Carotico cavernous fistula**[Q]
  – **Frontal lobe contusion**[Q]
	• Caused by **fracture of petrous part of temporal bone**[Q]
	• **Clinical features**:
	  – **CSF otorrhea**[Q]
	  – **Paradoxical rhinorrhea**[Q]
	  – **Hemotympanum**[Q]
	  – **Battle sign**[Q]: Bruising or ecchymosis behind ear
	  – **Ossicular disruption**[Q]
	    VII & VIII cranial nerve palsies[Q]
	  – **Temporal lobe contusion**[Q]
		• Caused by **fracture of occipital bone**[Q]
		• **Clinical features**:
		  – **Visual disturbances**[Q]
		  – **VI cranial nerve injury**[Q]
		  – **Jugular foramen syndrome (Vernet syndrome**[Q]**): Paresis of IX, X, XI cranial nerves**[Q]
		  – **Basilar artery injury**[Q]
		  – **Occipital contusion**[Q]

■ BRAIN ABSCESS

BRAIN ABSCESS

- Intracerebral abscess may occur as a result of **direct spread from air sinus infection**, following **surgery** or from **hematogenous spread** especially associated with **respiratory infection, endocarditis** or **dental infection**[Q].
- **Increased risk** of abscess in: **Cyanotic heart disease, immunocompromised** (diabetes, solid organ transplant, hematological malignancy or long-term steroids)[Q]

Etiology	Location
Otitis media, mastoiditis	Temporal lobe[Q] >Cerebellum
Paranasal sinusitis, dental infections	Frontal lobes[Q]
Hematogenous	Parietal lobe[Q]

Clinical Features

- Presentation is with **focal signs, seizures** and **raised ICP**, as with other mass lesions, but the **time course is often short**[Q]
- Patients may be febrile or have a raised peripheral white cell count or inflammatory markers.

Diagnosis

- **IOC for diagnosis: MRI**[Q]
- **CT scan: Ring-enhancing mass lesion** (may be **multiple** in case of **hematogenous spread**)[Q]

Treatment

- **Surgical drainage + IV antibiotics** for at least 6 weeks[Q].
- **Multiple small abscesses** may be **treated medically** with antibiotics targeted against organisms
- **Steroids** are **reserved for** cases with **significant edema** or **mass effect**[Q]
- Owing to the **high risk of seizures**, patients should also be **treated with anticonvulsants**.

Multiple Choice Questions

■ BERRY ANEURYSM

1. The most common site of Berry aneurysm is: *(All India 94)*
   a. Junction of anterior communication artery with anterior cerebral artery
   b. Junction of posterior communicating artery with internal carotid artery
   c. Bifurcation of middle cerebral artery
   d. Vertebral artery

2. Which is least common site of Berry aneurysm? *(AIIMS Dec 95)*
   a. Basilar artery
   b. Vertebral artery
   c. Anterior cerebral artery
   d. Posterior cerebral artery

■ CEREBROVASCULAR ACCIDENTS

3. The most common site of hypertensive intracranial hemorrhage is: *(ComedK 2010)*
   a. Putamen
   b. Midbrain
   c. Medulla
   d. Cerebrum

4. Which of the following is the most common location of hypertensive hemorrhage?
   (KERALA PG 2015; All Indian 2003, 94, AIIMS Nov 2002)
   a. Pons
   b. Thalamus
   c. Putamen/external capsule
   d. Subcortical white matter

5. Which of the following is the most common cause of late neurological deterioration in case of cerebrovascular accident? *(AIIMS Nov 2000)*
   a. Rebleeding
   b. Vasospasm
   c. Embolism
   d. Hydrocephalus

6. 'Duret hemorrhages' are seen in: *(AIIMS May 2008)*
   a. Brain
   b. Kidney
   c. Heart
   d. Lung

■ EDH AND SDH

7. Subdural hematoma is caused by injury of:
   (Recent Question 2017)
   a. Cortical vessels
   b. Venous sinus
   c. Middle cerebral artery
   d. Middle meningeal artery

8. Lucid interval is classically seen in: *(MCI June 2018, DNB 2010, ComedK 2007, PGI Dec 97)*
   a. Intracerebral hematoma
   b. Acute subdural hematoma
   c. Chronic subdural hematoma
   d. Extradural hematoma

9. Middle meningeal vessel damage results in: *(ComedK 2011)*
   a. Subdural hemorrhage
   b. Subarachnoid hemorrhage
   c. Intracerebral hemorrhage
   d. Epidural hemorrhage

10. Common site for extradural hemorrhage: *(DNB 2012)*
    a. Frontal
    b. Temporoparietal
    c. Occipital
    d. Brainstem

11. Subdural hematoma most commonly results from:
    a. Rupture of intracranial aneurysm *(AIIMS May 2004)*
    b. Rupture of cerebral AVM
    c. Injury to cortical bridging veins
    d. Hemophilia

■ SUBARACHNOID AND INTRACRANIAL HEMORRHAGE

12. The common cause of subarachnoid hemorrhage is:
    a. Arteriovenous malformation *(All India 2006)*
    b. Cavernous angioma
    c. Aneurysm
    d. Hippocampus

13. A patient comes to ER with headache describing it as worst headache in his life. What is the next step?
    a. CT brain
    b. Lumbar puncture
    c. MRI brain *(AIIMS Nov 2017)*
    d. Observation and analgesics

14. Most common cause of subarachnoid hemorrhage is:
    (Recent Question 2016, 2014, AIIMS Nov 98, All India 1999)
    a. Hypertension
    b. AV malformation
    c. Berry aneurysm
    d. Tumors

15. Identify the condition shown in the CT scan below:
    a. Extradural hemorrhage *(Recent Question 2018)*
    b. Subdural hemorrhage
    c. Subarachnoid hemorrhage
    d. Intraventricular hemorrhage

16. An adult hypertensive male presented with sudden onset severe headache and vomiting. On examination, their is marked neck rigidity and no neurological deficit was found. The symptoms are most likely due to:
    a. Intracranial parenchymal hemorrhage
    b. Ischemic stroke *(AIIMS May 2013, AIIMS May 2012)*
    c. Meningitis
    d. Subarachnoid hemorrhage

■ HEAD INJURY

17. Which of the following is not correct about head injury?
    a. MRI needed to assess hemorrhage
    b. GCS assessment helps in prognosis
    c. Hematoma must be operated
    d. All of the above *(Recent Question 2018)*

18. A man was presented to emergency department with head injury after an accident with vehicle. Investigation of choice should be: *(MCI Dec 2019)*
    a. CECT
    b. MRI
    c. NCCT
    d. EEG

19. Not a primary brain injury: *(Punjab 2011)*
    a. Diffuse axonal injury
    b. Contusion
    c. Concussion
    d. Intracerebral hematoma

20. Which among the following is a not a primary brain injury? *(JIPMER 2010)*
    a. Cortical lacerations
    b. Brainstem herniation
    c. Diffuse axonal injury
    d. Brainstem contusion

21. A 25 years old male of head injury was brought to emergency in unconscious state. What is the name of sign seen in this image?

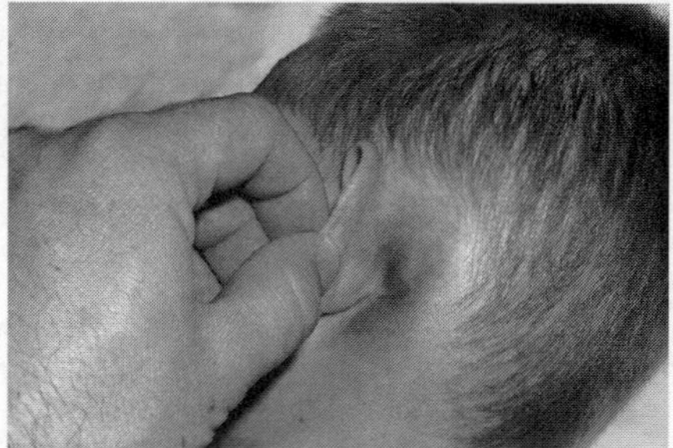

    a.   Duret hemorrhage   b.   Battle sign
    c.   Kernohan's phenomenon   d.   Raccoon sign

22. **In a vehicular accident, extensive contusions of brain due to acceleration and deceleration injury indicate what kind of injury?** *(MHSSMCET 2006)*
    a.   Penetrating injury   b.   Coup-Countercoup injury
    c.   Second impact syndrome   d.   Crush injury

23. **Raised intracranial pressure will cause:** *(MCI March 2007)*
    a.   Tachycardia   b.   Hypotension
    c.   Papilloedema
    d.   Normal looking anterior fontenalle in infants

24. **Best prognostic factor for head injury is:** *(All India 2007)*
    a.   Glasgow coma scale   b.   Age
    c.   Mode of injury   d.   CT

25. **Identify the following condition:** *(MCI Dec 2019)*

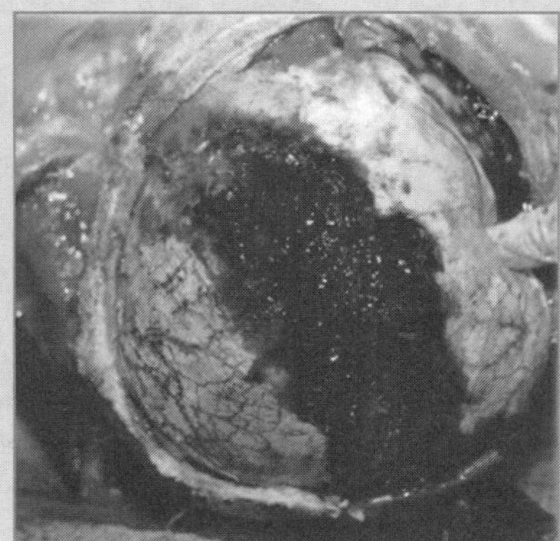

    a.   Subdural hemorrhage
    b.   Extradural hemorrhage
    c.   Subarachnoid hemorrhage
    d.   Intracranial hemorrhage

26. **A 25 years old male was brought to casualty with history of RTA. NCCT was done. What is the diagnosis?**
    a.   EDH   *(MCI Dec 2019, Recent Question 2017)*
    b.   SDH
    c.   Subarachnoid hemorrhage
    d.   None of the above

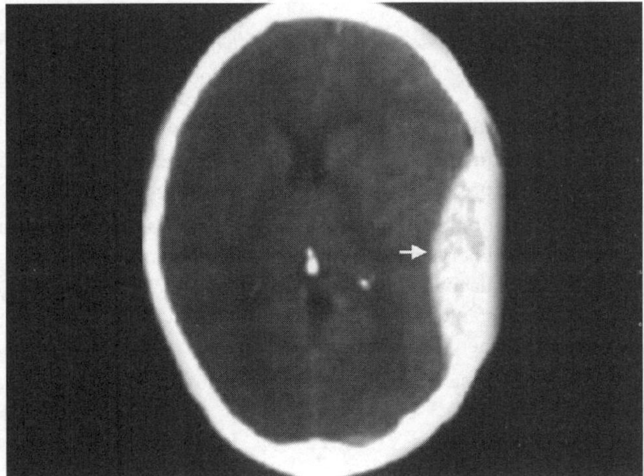

27. **A 65 years old male was brought to casualty with history of RTA. NCCT was done. What is the diagnosis?**
    a.   EDH   *(Recent Question 2017)*
    b.   SDH
    c.   Subarachnoid hemorrhage
    d.   None of the above

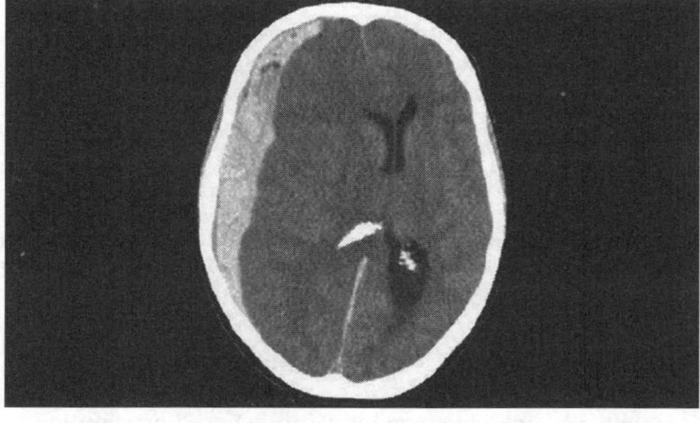

28. **False statement regarding subdural hematoma:** *(JIPMER May 2018)*
    a.   Occurs on both sides   b.   Not visible on X-ray
    c.   Surgery can be done   d.   Unilateral surgery

29. **All of the following statements about Diffuse Axonal Injury (DAI) are true except:** *(All India 2008)*
    a.   Caused by shearing force
    b.   Predominant white matter hemorrhages, in basal ganglion and corpus callosum
    c.   Increased intracranial tension is seen in all cases
    d.   Most common at junction of grey and white matter

30. **Neurosurgery is indicated for all except:** *(Recent Question 2013)*
    a.   SDH   b.   EDH
    c.   Depressed fracture   d.   Diffuse axonal injury

31. **Patient with a history of fall presents weeks later with headache and progressive neurological deterioration. The diagnosis is:** *(Recent Question 2016)*
    a.   Acute subdural hemorrhage
    b.   Extradural hemorrhage
    c.   Chronic subdural hemorrhage
    d.   Fracture skull

32. **Signs of cerebral compression are all except:** *(Recent Question 2016)*
    a.   Bradycardia   b.   Hypotension
    c.   Papilloedma   d.   Vomiting

33. **All of the following are indications of CT scan in head injured patient except:** *(DNB 2014)*
    a.   GCS < 13   b.   Vomiting 1 episode
    c.   Focal neurological deficit
    d.   Mild head injury in patient Age > 65 years

34. **All of the following are the components of Cushing triad except:** *(Recent Question 2017)*
    a.   Bradycardia   b.   Hypertension
    c.   Pupillary dilatation   d.   Respiratory irregularity

35. **Management of raised ICP are all except:** *(Recent Question 2017)*
    a.   Hypothermia
    b.   Hypercapnia
    c.   Decompressive craniectomy
    d.   Barbiturate

■ GLASGOW COMA SCALE

36. **True about Glasgow coma scale:** *(JIPMER 2011)*
    a.   Includes verbal response
    b.   Includes papillary reflex
    c.   High score means poor prognosis
    d.   Includes measurement of intracranial pressure

37. **Glasgow outcome score of vegetative state:** *(Recent Question 2017)*
    a.   2   b.   3
    c.   5   d.   8

38. Best predictor in the GCS: *(Recent Question 2017)*
    - a. Eye opening
    - b. Motor response
    - c. Verbal response
    - d. All

39. Minimal Glasgow coma scale is:
    (Recent Question 2015, DNB 2012, UPPG 2010, MCI March 2007)
    - a. 0
    - b. 1
    - c. 2
    - d. 3
    - e. 4

40. Which of the following is not a component of Glasgow coma scale?   *(DNB 2009, All India 2006)*
    - a. Eye opening
    - b. Motor response
    - c. Pupil size
    - d. Verbal response

41. Glasgow coma scale of a patient with head injury, who is confused, able to localize on right side and does flexion on left side and opens eye for painful stimuli on sternum:
    - a. 6
    - b. 11   *(Recent Question 2018)*
    - c. 12
    - d. 7

42. Calculate the GCS of a patient exhibiting eye opening on pain, conscious but confused and cannot tell time and exhibits flexion on painful noxious stimuli to the arm:
    - a. 8
    - b. 9   *(MCI June 2019)*
    - c. 10
    - d. 11

43. According to GCS, a verbal score of 1 indicates:
    (MCI June 2018)
    - a. No response
    - b. Inappropriate words
    - c. Incomprehensible sounds
    - d. Disoriented response

■ BRAIN ABSCESS

44. Management of epidural abscess is: *(DNB 2011)*
    - a. Immediate surgical evacuation
    - b. Conservative management
    - c. Antibiotics
    - d. Aggressive debridement

45. Brain abscess in cyanotic heart disease is commonly located in: *(All India 2006)*
    - a. Cerebellar hemisphere
    - b. Thalamus
    - c. Temporal lobe
    - d. Parietal lobe

46. Subdural collection of pus in a head injury patients after 3 days, the responsible organism is: *(UPPG 2009)*
    - a. Staph aureus
    - b. B hemolytic streptococcus
    - c. H. influenza
    - d. Pneumococcus

■ CNS CONGENITAL ANOMALIES

47. Commonest site of meningocele is:
    (BIHAR PG 2014, DNB 2005, 2001, All India 89)
    - a. Lumbosacral
    - b. Occipital
    - c. Frontal
    - d. Thoracic

48. Which of the following statement is correct?

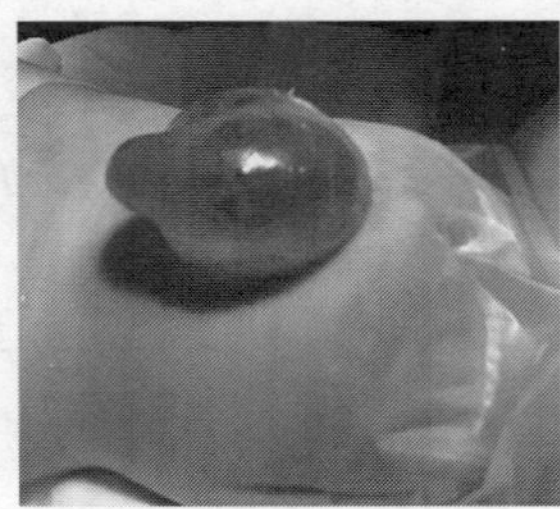 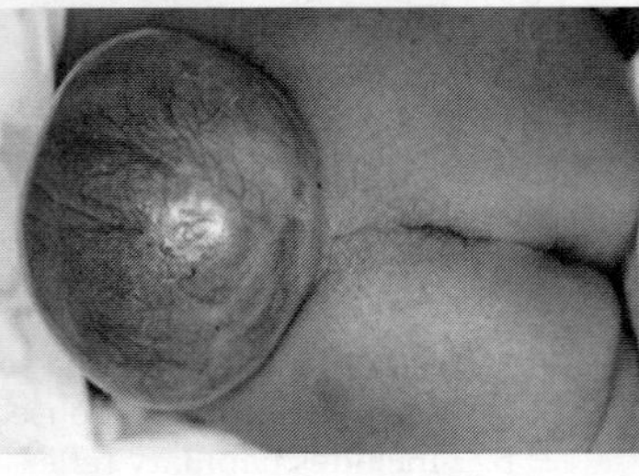

- a. 1-Meningocele, 2-Meningomyelocele
- b. 1-Meningocele, 2-Encephalocele
- c. 1- Encephalocele, 2-Meningomyelocele
- d. 1- Encephalocele, 2- Meningocele

49. A new born with meningomyelocele has been posted for surgery. The defect should be immediately covered with:
    - a. Normal saline guaze   *(AIIMS May 2013, All India 2012)*
    - b. Povidone iodine guaze
    - c. Tincture benzoin guaze
    - d. Methylene blue guaze

50. Comment on the diagnosis:

- a. Lipoma
- b. Encephalocele
- c. Cystic hygroma
- d. Lymphadenopathy

■ HYDROCEPHALUS

51. Most commonly performed shunt for hydrocephalus is:
    (AIIMS May 2015)
    - a. Ventriculoperitoneal
    - b. Ventriculopericardial
    - c. Ventriculopleural
    - d. Lumboperitoneal

■ MISCELLANEOUS

52. A dome shaped skull with a high forehead in the infant with slight hydrocephalus (Olympian brow) is seen in:
    (Recent Question 2016)
    - a. Marasmus
    - b. Congenital syphilis
    - c. Rickets
    - d. Arnold Chiari syndrome

53. Blow out fracture refers to: *(JIPMER 2011)*
    - a. Fracture of orbit
    - b. Fracture of nasal septum
    - c. Fracture base of skull
    - d. Fracture of mandible

54. The 'Phenomenon of Kernohan's notch' is associated with:
    - a. Third nerve palsy with contralateral hemiplegia
    - b. Subfalacine herniation   *(MHSSMCET 2006)*
    - c. Transtentorial herniation
    - d. Foramen magnum fracture

55. Signs of base of skull fracture are following except:
    (MHSSMCET 2011)
    - a. Raccoon eyes
    - b. Battle's sign
    - c. Constricted pupil
    - d. Hemotympanum

■ BERRY ANEURYSM

1. **Ans. a. Junction of anterior communication artery with anterior cerebral artery** *(Ref: Harrison 20/e p1904; Sabiston 20/e p1904; Schwartz 11/e p1852, 9/e p1534; Bailey 26/e p311)*

2. **Ans. b. Vertebral artery**

■ CEREBROVASCULAR ACCIDENTS

3. **Ans. a. Putamen** *(Ref: Harrison 20/e p3092)*

4. **Ans. c. Putamen/external capsule**

5. **Ans. b. Vasospasm** *(Ref: Harrison 20/e p2086)*

VASOSPASM

- **Narrowing of** the **arteries** at the **base of** the **brain following SAH** occurs regularly.
- This **vasospasm** causes **symptomatic ischemia** and **infarction in** approximately **30%** patients and is the **major cause of delayed morbidity** or **death**[Q].
- **Sign of ischemia** appear 4-14 days after the hemorrhage, **most frequently at** about **7 days**[Q].

Major Causes of Delayed Neurological Deficit after CVA	
Re-rupture[Q]	Vasospasm[Q]
Hydrocephalus[Q]	Hyponatremia[Q]

6. **Ans. a. Brain** *(Ref: Robbins 9/e p1255)*

DURET HEMORRHAGE

- In case of **increased ICP down ward herniation of brainstem** occur, which cause **stretching of perforators** of **basilar artery** and may results in **bleed (Duret hemorrhage)**[Q].
- Duret hemorrhage is **small area of bleeding** in **ventral** and **paramedian part** of **upper brainstem** (midbrain and pons)[Q].
- It usually indicates a fatal outcome, however survival has been reported.
- Diagnosis is made on **CT** or **MRI**.

■ EDH AND SDH

7. **Ans. a. Cortical vessels** *(Ref: Sabiston 20/e p1916; Schwartz 11/e p1838, 10/e p1719; Bailey 27/e p334)*

8. **Ans. d. Extradural hematoma**

9. **Ans. d. Epidural hemorrhage**

10. **Ans. b. Temporoparietal**

11. **Ans. c. Injury to cortical bridging veins**

■ SUBARACHNOID AND INTRACRANIAL HEMORRHAGE

12. **Ans. c. Aneurysm**

13. **Ans. a. CT brain** *(Ref: Harrison 20/e p2084)*

14. **Ans. c. Berry aneurysm**

15. **Ans. c. Subarachnoid hemorrhage**

16. **Ans. d. Subarachnoid hemorrhage**

■ HEAD INJURY

17. **Ans. c. Hematoma must be operated**

18. **Ans. c. NCCT**

19. **Ans. d. Intracerebral hematoma** *(Ref: Bailey 27/e p331-332)*

20. **Ans. b. Brainstem herniation**

21. **Ans. b. Battle sign** *(Ref: Schwartz 11/e p196, 1835, 10/e p174; Bailey 27/e p332)*

"Battle's sign: A skull base fracture may be associated with bruising over the mastoid process."-Bailey 27/e p332

22. **Ans. b. Coup-Countercoup injury** *(Ref: Bailey 27/e p336)*

23. Ans. c. Papilloedema

24. Ans. a. Glasgow coma scale

25. Ans. b. Extradural hemorrhage *(Ref: Bailey 27/e p333)*   26. Ans. a. EDH

27. Ans. b. SDH   28. Ans. a. Occurs on both sides

29. Ans. c. Increased intracranial tension is seen in all cases *(Ref: Harrison 20/e p2077; Sabiston 20/e p1916-1916)*

30. Ans. d. Diffuse axonal injury

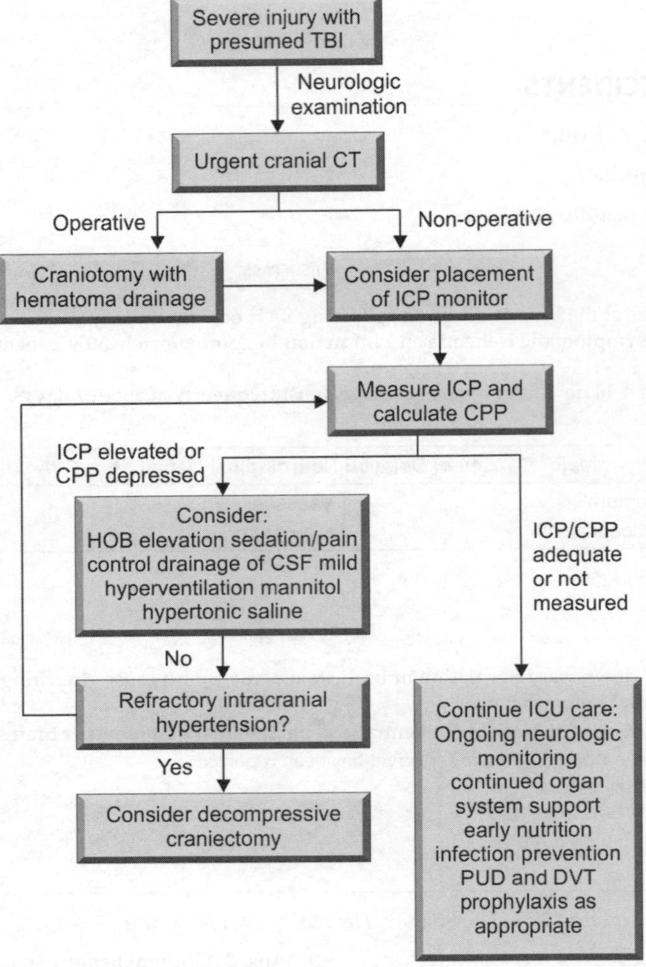

Traumatic brain injury (TBI)

31. Ans. c. Chronic subdural hemorrhage   32. Ans. b. Hypotension

33. Ans. b. Vomiting 1 episode *(Ref: Bailey 27/e p330)*

NICE Guidelines for CT Imaging within 1 Hour	
1. GCS < 13 at any point	1. Suspected open, depressed or basal skull fracture
2. GCS 13 or 14 at 2 hours	2. Seizures
3. Focal neurological deficit	3. Vomiting > one episode

Indications for CT Imaging within 8 Hours	
1. Age > 65 years	3. Dangerous mechanism of injury (CT within 8 hours)
2. Coagulopathy (e.g. on warfarin)	4. Retrograde amnesia > 30 min

34. Ans. c. Pupillary dilatation *(Ref: Schwartz 11/e p1832, 10/e p1713; Bailey 27/e p328)*

> *"Cushing's triad is the classic presentation of intracranial hypertension, bradycardia, and irregular respirations."- Schwartz 11/e p1832, 10/e p1713*

35. Ans. b. Hypercapnia *(Ref: Sabiston 20/e p1919; Bailey 27/e p336)*

■ GLASGOW COMA SCALE

36. Ans. a. Includes verbal response *(Ref: Harrison 20/e p3183; Sabiston 20/e p1918; Schwartz 11/e p1830, 10/e p168,1711; Bailey 27/e p331, 26/e p312)*

REVISED GLASGOW COMA SCALE 2014

Revised GCS (2014)					
Eye Opening (E)		*Verbal Response (V)*		*Best Motor Response (M)*	
Spontaneous	4	Oriented	5	Obeying commands	6
To **Speech**[Q]	3	Confused	4	Localizing	5
To **Pressure**[Q]	2	**Words**[Q]	3	Normal flexion (withdrawal)	4
None	1	**Sounds**[Q]	2	Abnormal flexion	3
		None	1	Extension	2
				None	1

- **GCS** specifically **recommends avoiding sternal rubs**[Q] as it causes bruising & responses can be difficult to interpret. They also **do not recommend routine use of retromandibular pressure**[Q].
- **Revised GCS (2014)** changes are highlighted in the above table.
- **Maximum score-15**[Q], **minimum score-3**[Q].
- **Best predictor of outcome: Motor response**[Q]

- Reporting of Non-testable Score Aspects: In cases of a non-testable aspect, the new GCS should only be noted in its components. Any element that cannot be tested should be marked as NT, for "not testable".
- For intubated patients or patients with tracheostomy, VNT is used. It is no longer recommend to assign 1 point to non-testable elements, therefore a combined score should not be used.

GCS-P	**GCS-PA CT**
<ul><li>**GCS-P** is calculated by **subtracting the Pupil Reactivity Score (PRS) from the Glasgow Coma Scale (GCS) total score: GCS-P = GCS – PRS**[Q]</li><li>**Pupil reactivity score** represents the **number of nonreactive pupils (0, 1, or 2)**[Q].</li><li>This **number is subtracted from the GCS score (3–15)**, resulting in the **GCS-P (1-15)**[Q].</li></ul>	<ul><li>**GCS-PA CT: GCS, Pupils, Age & CT findings**[Q]</li><li>**Probability of mortality 6 months after head injury based on** the patient's admission **GCS-P** and **age with no CT abnormality (A), exactly 1 CT abnormality (B),** and **2 or more CT abnormalities (C).**</li><li>**Potential CT abnormalities** include **intracranial hematoma, absent cisterns & SAH**[Q].</li></ul>

Pupils Unreactive to Light	PRS
Both pupils	2
One pupil	1
Neither pupil	0
Note: Higher score is assigned to non-reactive pupils.	

37. Ans. b. 3 *(Ref: Sabiston 20/e p1918; Schwartz 11/e p1830, 10/e p1712; Bailey 27/e p331)*

38. Ans. b. Motor response *(Ref: Sabiston 20/e p1918; Schwartz 11/e p1830, 10/e p1712; Bailey 27/e p331)*

39. Ans. d. 3

40. Ans. c. Pupil size

41. Ans. b. 11

42. Ans. c. 10

43. Ans. a. No response *(Ref: Bailey 27/e p331)*

■ BRAIN ABSCESS

44. Ans. a. Immediate surgical evacuation *(Ref: Bailey 27/e p656-657)*

45. Ans. d. Parietal lobe *(Ref: Harrison 20/e p1014; Sabiston 20/e p1934-1935; Schwartz 11/e p1868, 10/e p1745; Bailey 26/e p609-610)*

Brain abscess in congenital heart diseases occur due to hematogenous seeding of blood borne bacteria. These blood borne bacteria bypass the capillary bed due to right to left shunt. They commonly infect parietal and frontal lobes (territory of middle cerebral artery).

46. Ans. a. Staph aureus

■ CNS CONGENITAL ANOMALIES

47. Ans. a. Lumbosacral *(Ref: Sabiston 20/e p1932; Schwartz 11/e p1872, 10/e p1750; Bailey 27/e p484, 667)*

48. Ans. a. 1-Meningocele, 2-Meningomyelocele *(Ref: Sabiston 20/e p1931-1932; Schwartz 11/e p1872, 10/e p1750; Bailey 27/e p667)*

49. **Ans. a. Normal saline guaze** *(Ref: Sabiston 20/e p1931-1932; Schwartz 11/e p1872, 10/e p1645; Bailey 27/e p484, 667)*

    Meningomyelocele should be covered with a non-sticking sterile saline soaked guaze and plastic shield wrap to maintain moisture.

50. **Ans. b. Encephalocele** *(Ref: Bailey 27/e p667)*

■ HYDROCEPHALUS

51. **Ans. a. Ventriculoperitoneal** *(Ref: Bailey 27/e p653-656; Nelson 19/e p2008-2011)*

    Most common shunt used for hydrocephalus is ventriculoperitoneal shunt.

    > *"Therapy for hydrocephalus depends on the cause. Medical management, including the use of acetazolamide and furosemide, can provide temporary relief by reducing the rate of CSF production, but long-term results have been disappointing. Most cases of hydrocephalus require extracranial shunts, particularly a ventriculoperitoneal shunt. Endoscopic third ventriculostomy (ETV) has evolved as a viable approach and criteria have been developed for its use, but the procedure might need to be repeated to be effective." - Nelson 19/e p2011*

■ MISCELLANEOUS

52. **Ans. b. Congenital syphilis**

53. **Ans. a. Fracture of orbit**

54. **Ans. c. Transtentorial herniation** *(Ref: Harrison 19/e p1772; Bailey 25/e p624)*

    #### KERNOHAN'S NOTCH PHENOMENON

    - **Kernohan's notch** is a **cerebral peduncle indentation** associated with some forms of **transtentorial herniation (uncal herniation)**[Q].
    - **Compression of** the **contralateral cerebral peduncle** against the **free edge of** the **tentorium (Kernohan's notch)** causes an **ipsilateral hemiparesis** with **ipsilateral 3rd nerve palsy**[Q].

    #### KERNOHAN-WOLTMAN SIGN

    - **Lateral displacement of** the **midbrain** may **compress** the **opposite cerebral peduncle**, producing a **Babinski's sign** and **hemiparesis contralateral to** the **original hemiparesis** (the **Kernohan-Woltman sign**[Q]).

55. **Ans. c. Constricted pupil**

CNS Tumors

■ WHO CLASSIFICATION OF BRAIN TUMORS

WHO Classification of Brain Tumors

1. **Neuroepithelial tumours**:
  – **Glioma**: Astrocytomas, Oligodendrogliomas, Ependymoma, Choroid plexus tumour
  – **Pineal tumours**
  – **Neuronal tumours**: Ganglioglioma, Gangliocytoma, Neuroblastoma
  – **Medulloblastoma**

2. **Nerve sheath tumours**: Vestibular schwannoma
3. **Meningeal tumours**: Meningioma
4. **Pituitary tumours**
5. **Germ cell tumours**: Germinoma, Teratoma
6. **Lymphomas**
7. **Tumour-like malformations**: Craniopharyngioma, Epidermoid tumours, Dermoid tumour, Colloid cyst
8. **Metastatic tumours**
9. **Contiguous extension from regional tumours**: Glomus tumour

■ BRAIN TUMOR

• **MC primary brain tumor**	• **Meningioma**[Q] (35%) > **glial tumors**[Q] (30%)
• **MC brain tumor**	• **Metastasis**[Q]
• **MC malignant BT of childhood** • **Most radiosensitive BT**	• **Medulloblastoma**[Q]
• **BT associated with calcification (COM)**	• **Craniopharyngioma**[Q] (most) > **ODG**[Q] (90%) > **Meningioma**[Q] (20–25%)

BRAIN TUMOR

- Most brain tumors occur **sporadically**[Q]
- **Radiation exposure** & **genetic abnormalities** are the risk factors[Q]

Genetic abnormalities associated with brain tumors (RL not in MTV GT)	
• **R**etinoblastoma[Q]	• **T**urcot's syndrome[Q]
• **L**i-Fraumeni[Q]	• **V**HL syndrome[Q]
• **N**F-1 & 2[Q]	• **G**orlin syndrome[Q]
• **M**EN 1[Q]	• **T**uberous sclerosis[Q]

Clinical Features

- **Three cardinal symptoms: Seizures, Raised ICT & focal neurological deficit**[Q] (FND)
- **Raised ICT** leads to **headache (worse in morning & straining**[Q], associated with nausea & vomiting)
- **FND: Progressive over time, characteristic of location**[Q]
- **Pituitary adenoma** may also present with **endocrine abnormalities**[Q]

Diagnosis

- **IOC for diagnosis: MRI**[Q]

Contd…

Contd…

Treatment:

- **Dexamethasone: Reduces peritumoral edema**[Q]
- **Anti-epileptics: For tumors close to sensorimotor strip**[Q]
- **Mannitol:** Administered before dural opening & operative resection[Q]
- **Surgery:** Primary goals of surgery includes **histologic diagnosis & reduction of mass effect** by removal of as much as tumor with preservation of neurological function[Q]
- **Radiotherapy:** In cases of **positive margins & tumor infiltrating surrounding brain**[Q]
- **Craniospinal irradiation:** For tumors associated with **CSF spread**

■ ASTROCYTOMA

ASTROCYTOMA

- **Astrocytomas** arise from **astrocytes**[Q]
- **Mostly supratentorial in adults & infratentorial in children**[Q]
- **Astrocytoma is MC posterior fossa tumor in children**[Q]
- **Majority** of astrocytoma are **low grade in children & high grade in adults**[Q]
- **MC astrocytoma in children: Pilocytic astrocytoma**[Q]
- **MC astrocytoma in adults: Glioblastoma multiforme**[Q] **(GBM)**

Pathology

- Majority of **astrocytomas infiltrate** adjacent **brain. Juvenile pilocytic astrocytomas & pleomorphic xanthoastrocytomas are exceptions**[Q]
- Histologic features associated with higher grade tumors: Hypercellularity, nuclear atypia & endovascular hyperplasia[Q].
- **Necrosis**[Q] is present **only with GBMs**; it is required for the diagnosis.

WHO Classification of Astrocytoma			
Grade I or Pilocytic Astrocytoma	**Low-grade, or grade II Astrocytomas**	**Grade III or Anaplastic**	**Grade IV or Glioblastoma Multiforme**
• **Discrete** appearing, **contrast enhancing** and often **cystic** with a **mural nodule**[Q]. • **Mean age: First two decades** of life. • Curable by **radical resection**[Q] (no infiltration of surrounding brain) • **Radiation therapy** and **chemotherapy** have **no role** • **Median survival** time: **8-10 years**.	• Occur in **children** and **young adults**[Q]. • Most patients present with **seizures**[Q]. • Typically demonstrate **nuclear atypia**; have a **low degree of cellularity** • **Treatment: Observation** and follow-up, **radiation** with or without **chemotherapy**, and **surgery**. • **Surgery** is **not curative** because most of these tumors are **infiltrative** with **no clear margins**[Q]. • **Median survival** time: **7–8 years**.	• **Irregular enhancement** on **MRI** • **Treatment: Cytoreductive surgery** followed by **EBRT**[Q]. • **Median survival** time: **2–3 years**	• **Endothelial proliferation** or **necrosis**[Q] on histology makes the tumor **grade IV**. • Know as **butterfly tumor** as it crosses midline[Q] • Seen in **older patients (>50 years)**. • GBMs: **Ring enhancement** with **central necrosis** on **MRI**[Q]. • **Treatment: Cytoreductive surgery** followed by **EBRT**[Q]. • **Extent of tumor resection** has a **significant effect** on time to tumor **progression** & median **survival**[Q]. • **Carmustine & cisplatin** have been the primary agents used against **malignant gliomas**[Q]. • **Temozolomide**[Q] has shown some promise in the management of **newly diagnosed & recurrent GBM**. • **Median survival** time for **GBM** is **<1 year**.

■ OLIGODENDROGLIOMA (ODG)

OLIGODENDROGLIOMA (ODG)

- **ODG** accounts for approximately **10% of gliomas**
- Predilection for **cortex & white matter of cerebral hemispheres (frontal lobe in 50–65%)**
- **MC genetic alterations** include **loss of heterozygosity** on chromosome **19q >1p**[Q]. These alterations are usually associated with a **better prognosis**.

> - **Characterized by** classic histologic feature of **"fried egg" cytoplasm, "chicken wire" vasculature, & microscopic calcifications**[Q].

Clinical Feature

- This tumor frequently presents with **seizures**

Diagnosis

- **Calcifications** and **hemorrhage** on CT or MRI **suggest** the **diagnosis**[Q].
- **Calcifications** is seen in **28-60%** in ODGs on **plain radiographs**, and on **90% of CT**[Q].

Contd…

Treatment
- Primary modality of treatment: **Surgical resection + Chemotherapy**[Q]
- Respond to procarbazine, lomustine (**CCNU**), vincristine (**PCV**) **chemotherapy.**
- Chromosomal deletion, **1p** and **19q**, has been associated with **robust response** to temozolomide[Q].

Prognosis
- **Median survival time** ranges from **3 to 5 years**

■ EPENDYMOMA

EPENDYMOMA

- Arise from **ependymal lining** of **cerebral hemispheres** & remnants of **central canal** of **spinal cord.**
- Manifest predominantly in **children** (within the **fourth ventricle**) and **young adults.**
- **MC histologic type** in **adults:** Myxopapillary ependymoma[Q], which typically **arises from filum terminale**[Q] of spinal cord and appears in **lumbosacral region**[Q].

Diagnosis
- **On CT or MRI**, ependymomas typically appear as **diffusely enhancing masses**[Q] relatively well demarcated from adjacent neural tissue.
- **MRI findings** include a **well-circumscribed** lesion with varying degrees of enhancement. **Ventricular** or **brainstem displacement** and **hydrocephalus** are frequent features.

Treatment
- Optimal treatment includes **maximal possible resection** without causing neurological deficits followed by **EBRT.**
- Ependymomas have the potential to **spread through** the **neuraxis** by **seeding** of **CSF**; **craniospinal radiation**[Q] is recommended in this case.

■ MEDULLOBLASTOMA

MEDULLOBLASTOMA

- **MC malignant brain tumor of childhood:** Medulloblastoma
- **Turcot syndrome (A variant of FAP) is associated with increased incidence of medulloblastoma**
- **Highly malignant tumor** found in **cerebellum**[Q] and **infratentorial** location
- Occur predominantly in **children**[Q] (peak incidence at **3-4 years**[Q])
- **Medulloblastoma** is **most radiosensitive brain tumor**[Q]

• **MC site: Vermis (75%)**	• **MC site** in **adults: Lateral cerebellar hemisphere**

Clinical Characteristics
- **Child** usually presents with features of **increased intracranial tension**[Q].
- **Adults** present with **ataxia** and **unilateral dysmetria** as lateral origin is more common[Q].

Metastasis
- **Dissemination through CSF** is common leading to **drop metastasis**[Q].
- **Metastasis outside CNS**[Q] affects **bone, lymph node** and **liver.**
- **Tumor dissemination** is **most important prognostic factor**[Q].

Treatment
- Despite of extreme radiosensitivity, it should be **surgically excised**[Q].
- Surgical excision should be **followed by radiotherapy** and **chemotherapy**[Q].

■ MENINGIOMA

MENINGIOMA

- **MC primary brain tumor: Meningioma (35%) >Glial tumors (30%)**
- **MC intracranial, extra-axial dural-based neoplasm**[Q].
- Predominantly benign tumors of **adults**[Q], **more common** in **women**[Q].

• Derived from **meningomesothelial cells of arachnoid**[Q]
• Mostly occur **along the superior sagittal sinus**[Q]
• **Most** are **slow growing & encapsulated**[Q]

Contd…

Pathology

- **Round encapsulated mass** showing characteristic **enplaque pattern of growth**[Q]
- Tumor may show extreme **calcification & psammoma bodies**[Q]

Clinical Presentation

- **Motor deficit** in **90%** (spasticity & lower limb weakness), **sensory deficit** in **60%** or **sphincter dysfunction** of **bladder**[Q].

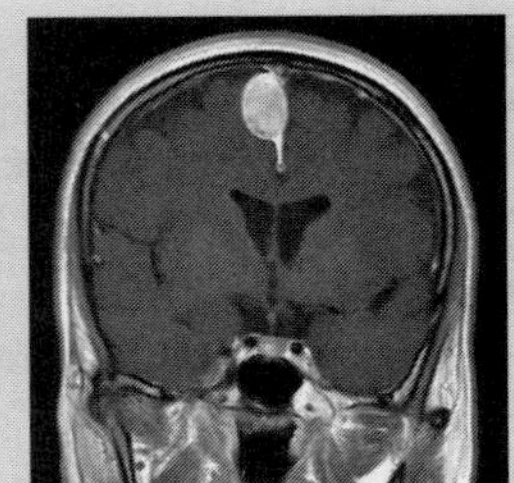

Radiological findings in Meningioma	
• Nearly all meningiomas **enhance intensely**[Q] following contrast administration. • **Abnormal vascular markings**[Q] • **Enlarged foramen spinosum**[Q] on the side of lesion • **Dural tail** • **Calcification (20-25%)** in the tumor[Q]	• Invasion of bone cause localized **bony hyperostosis**/mixed osteoblastic & osteolytic response less commonly. It may show **'sun ray spicules'** & local bone expansion with pneumatization so called **'blistering'** • **Signs of increased intracranial tension**[Q]

Treatment

- **Surgery** is the **treatment of choice** for symptomatic meningiomas.
- **Extent of resection** is the **most important factor** in the prevention of **recurrence**.

CNS Tumors	
Intra-axial (LANe)	**Extra-axial (PSM)**
• **Neuronal** • **Astrocytoma (Glioma)**[Q] • **Lymphoma**	• **Pituitary**[Q] • **Schwannoma**[Q] • **Meningioma**[Q]

■ PITUITARY ADENOMA

PITUITARY ADENOMA

- Pituitary adenomas arise primarily from **anterior pituitary gland**[Q]
- **MC cause** of **hyperpituitarism: Pituitary adenoma**[Q]
- Classified as either **functional** (secreting) or **nonfunctional** (nonsecreting) tumors
- Former presenting **earlier with symptoms** caused **by physiologic effects** and the latter presenting when of **sufficient size** to cause **neurologic deficits** by **mass effect** on the **chiasm** with consequent **bitemporal hemianopsia**[Q].
- Incidence is increased in **MEN-1**[Q]

> - **Pituitary adenoma** can be **differentiated from hyperplasia by reticulin stain**[Q]
> - **Absence of reticulin stain in pituitary adenoma**[Q]

Clinical Features

- Occur commonly in **third & fourth decades** and affect **both sexes equally**[Q].
- **MC functional tumor** is **prolactinoma**[Q], which causes **amenorrhea & galactorrhea** in women[Q].

Diagnosis

- **MRI** is **IOC for pituitary tumors**[Q]
- Diagnostic workup includes a **full endocrinologic profile** and a **formal visual fields test**[Q].

Treatment

- **Dopamine agonist, bromocriptine**[Q], can **shrink prolactinomas** in **75%** of patients with **macroadenomas** in **6-8 weeks**, but only as long as therapy is maintained.
- Bromocriptine may also work on **GH-secreting tumors** with tumor **shrinkage** in **<20%**.
- **Octreotide**[Q] can **reduce GH levels** in 71% of patients, with a **significant reduction** in tumor **volume** in **30%** of cases.

Indications of Surgery as an Initial Treatment	
• **GH-secreting tumors**[Q] • **Primary Cushing's disease**[Q] • Any **adenoma** causing **acute visual deterioration**[Q]	• **Nonprolactin-secreting macroadenomas** causing symptoms by **mass effect**[Q]

- **Surgical approach of choice:** **Sublabial** or **intranasal trans-sphenoidal**[Q] approach
- **Radiosurgery** can also be used either as **primary therapy**, as an **adjuvant therapy** after subtotal resection, or **for recurrent disease**.

> - **MC suprasellar mass in children: Craniopharyngioma**[Q]
> - **MC suprasellar mass in adults: Pituitary adenoma**[Q]

■ CRANIOPHARYNGIOMA

CRANIOPHARYNGIOMA

- Craniopharyngiomas are **benign cystic lesions** that occur **most frequently** in **children**[Q].
- There is a **second peak** of incidence around **50 years** of age.
- Derived from **Rathke's pouch**[Q] and arise near the pituitary stalk, commonly extending into the suprasellar cistern.

> - Craniopharyngiomas are often **large, cystic,** and **locally invasive**[Q].

Clinical Features

- **More than half** of all patients present **before 20 years**[Q]
- Presents with signs of **increased intracranial pressure**[Q], including headache, vomiting, papilledema, and hydrocephalus.
- Associated symptoms include **visual field abnormalities**[Q], personality changes and cognitive deterioration, cranial nerve damage, sleep difficulties, and weight gain.

> - Associated with **hypopituitarism (90%), diabetes insipidus (10%) & growth retardation (50%)**[Q]

Diagnosis

- **Calcification** occurs in **all pediatric** and roughly **half** of **adult** craniopharyngiomas[Q].
- **MRI** is superior to CT for **evaluating cystic structure** and **tissue components** of craniopharyngiomas[Q].
- **CT** is useful to define **calcifications** and evaluate **invasion** into surrounding **bony structures & sinuses.**

Treatment

- Treatment involves transcranial or **transsphenoidal**[Q] **surgical resection** followed by **postoperative radiation** of residual tumor.
- Most patients require **lifelong pituitary hormone replacement**[Q].

> - **Cortisol (hydrocortisone)** is the **first hormone to be replaced**[Q] in patients with **panhypopituitarism after craniopharyngioma surgery.**

■ PRIMARY CNS LYMPHOMA

PRIMARY CNS LYMPHOMA

- PCNSL is a rare **non-Hodgkin's lymphoma**[Q] accounting for **<3%** of primary brain tumors.
- The **incidence** is **rising** due to the **high frequency** of CNS lymphoma in **AIDS** patients and **transplant recipients**[Q].

> - PCNSL in **immunocompetent patients** usually consists of **diffuse large B-cell lymphomas**[Q].
> - PCNSL in **immunocompromised patients** is typically **large cell** with **immunoblastic** and more **aggressive features**[Q].
> - Also known as **ghost-cell tumor** because of its tendency for **partial to complete resolution on CT** after the administration of **steroids**[Q].

- **Epstein-Barr virus** frequently plays an **important role** in the pathogenesis of **HIV-related PCNSL**[Q].

Clinical Features

- PCNSL usually presents as a **mass lesion**, with **neuropsychiatric symptoms**, symptoms of **increased intracranial pressure**, lateralizing signs, or **seizures**[Q].
- Median age at diagnosis: **52 years** (younger in the immunocompromised).

Diagnosis

- On **contrast-enhanced MRI: Densely enhancing tumor**[Q]
- **Immunocompetent** patients have **solitary lesions** more often than immunosuppressed patients.
- Frequent **involvement** of the **basal ganglia, corpus callosum,** or **periventricular region**[Q].
- **Stereotactic biopsy** is necessary for **histologic diagnosis**[Q].

> - **Glucocorticoids** should be **withheld** before **biopsy** due to **cytolytic effect** on **lymphoma cells** leading to nondiagnostic tissue (**Ghost cell tumor**)[Q]

Treatment

- PCNSL is relatively sensitive to glucocorticoids, chemotherapy and radiotherapy.
- **High-dose methotrexate**[Q] produces **response rates** of **35-80%** and median survival up to 50 months.

> - In **non-AIDS cases**, chemotherapy + **EBRT** prolongs survival compared with EBRT alone.
> - **AIDS patients** are treated with **whole-brain radiotherapy, high-dose methotrexate,** and initiation of **highly active antiretroviral therapy**[Q].

■ SPINAL TUMORS

<table>
<tr><td colspan="2" align="center">SPINAL TUMORS</td></tr>
<tr><td>

- MC spinal tumor: Metastasis[Q]
- MC primary spinal tumor: Nerve sheath tumor[Q]

</td><td>

- MC intramedullary tumor: Astrocytoma[Q]
- MC site of primary spinal tumor: Intradural extramedullary[Q]

</td></tr>
</table>

Tumors that spread through CSF (CPM germ CAP)	
• **C**NS Lymphomas[Q]	• **C**horoid plexus carcinoma
• **P**inealoblastomas[Q]	• **A**naplastic ependymomas
• **M**edulloblastoma[Q]	• **P**rimitive neuroectodermal tumors
• **G**erm cell tumors[Q]	

■ STEREOTACTIC RADIOSURGERY

<table>
<tr><td align="center">STEREOTACTIC RADIOSURGERY</td></tr>
</table>

- SRS is a **non-surgical radiation therapy used to treat functional abnormalities & small tumors** of brain[Q].
- **Deliver precisely-targeted concentrated dose of radiation in fewer high-dose treatments to a defined volume** in the brain[Q]
- When **SRS** is **used to treat body tumors**, it's called **stereotactic body radiotherapy**[Q] (SBRT).

Two methods of frame-based stereotactic radiosurgery are currently widely used
• **Gamma knife uses cobalt-201**[Q] radiation sources focused on one point.
• **Modified linear accelerators**[Q] deliver **high-energy x-rays (photons)** in multiple arcs, thereby minimizing the effect on surrounding brain tissue.

- **Primary risks** of stereotactic radiosurgery are **radiation necrosis & radiation injury** to surrounding structures.

Common uses of Stereotactic Radiosurgery (BAT)	
• **B**rain tumor[Q] (Benign, malignant, primary & metastatic tumors, single & multiple)	• **A**rteriovenous malformations[Q]
• **B**enign lesions of cranial nerves[Q]	• **T**rigeminal neuralgia[Q]

■ METASTATIC BRAIN TUMORS

<table>
<tr><td align="center">METASTATIC BRAIN TUMORS</td></tr>
</table>

- **Metastatic brain tumors** are the **MC tumors** of the **brain**[Q].
- They outnumber primary brain tumors by **10 to 1.**

• **Location: Cerebral hemispheres** (80%) mainly the **frontal lobes**[Q], cerebellum (15%) and brainstem (5%).
• **MC primary sites: CA lung**[Q] (50%) > **breast cancer**[Q] (15-20%)

- Metastases to the brain are **multiple in >70%** of cases.

Diagnosis

- **IOC: MRI** with **gadolinium** enhancement[Q]
- Lesions are at the **gray-matter** and **white-matter junction, well circumscribed**, surrounded by **edema**[Q].

Treatment

- **Surgery** is recommended for accessible lesions (**up to 3**) causing mass effect followed by **whole-brain radiation therapy (WBRT) to eradicate micrometastases**[Q].
- **Stereotactic radiosurgery** followed by **WBRT** has also been shown to be as effective as surgery in the management of metastatic brain tumors (**< 3 cm**).
- **Chemotherapy** is not useful in most brain metastases except **small cell lung cancer** and **seminomas**.

Prognosis

- **Median survival time** with optimal treatment: **7–12 months**

Multiple Choice Questions

■ CNS TUMORS PREDISPOSING FACTORS

1. All of the following statements about Neurofibromatosis are true, except: *(All India 2009)*
   a. Autosomal recessive inheritance
   b. Cutaneous neurofibromas
   c. Cataract
   d. Scoliosis

2. All of the following may be associated with Von-Hippel Lindau syndrome, except: *(All India 2009)*
   a. Retinal and cerebella hemangioblastomas
   b. Gastric carcinoma
   c. Pheochromocytoma
   d. Renal cell carcinoma

3. Which of the following statement about VHL syndrome is true? *(All India 2012)*
   a. Multiple tumors are rarely seen
   b. Craniospinal hemangioblastoma are common
   c. Supratentorial tumors are common
   d. Tumors of Schwann cells are common

4. Triad of tuberous sclerosis includes all, except: *(All India 2009)*
   a. Epilepsy
   b. Adenoma sebacium
   c. Low intelligence
   d. Hydrocephalus

■ CNS TUMORS: CLINICAL FEATURES AND TREATMENT

5. All of the following are features of brain tumor except: *(Recent Question 2017)*
   a. Pin point pupil
   b. Seizures
   c. Headache
   d. Focal neurological deficit

6. Most common brain tumour: *(Recent Question 2017)*
   a. Meningioma
   b. Glioma
   c. Metastasis
   d. Astrocytoma

7. Which of the following tumor is not known to increase in pregnancy? *(All India 2006)*
   a. Glioma
   b. Pituitary adenoma
   c. Meningioma
   d. Neurofibroma

8. Which one of the following tumors shows calcification on CT scan? *(All India 2005)*
   a. Ependymoma
   b. Medulloblastoma
   c. Meningioma
   d. CNS lymphoma

9. Stereotactic radiosurgery is done for: *(JIPMER 2002)*
   a. Glioblastoma multiforme
   b. Medulloblastoma spinal cord
   c. Ependymoma
   d. AV malformation of brain

10. Which of the following brain tumors doesn't spread via CSF? *(DPG 2011, All India 2004)*
    a. Germ cell tumor
    b. Medulloblastoma
    c. CNS Lymphoma
    d. Craniopharyngioma

11. Cerebellar hemangioblastoma and retinal tumours are seen in: *(JIMPER 2012)*
    a. VHL syndrome
    b. NF-1
    c. Tuberous selerosis
    d. NF-2

■ BRAIN METASTASIS

12. Which of the following carcinoma most frequently metastasizes to brain? *(MCI June 2018; AIIMS 2005)*
    a. Small cell carcinoma lung
    b. Prostate cancer
    c. Rectal carcinoma
    d. Endometrial cancer

13. Most common site of brain metastasis: *(DNB 2011)*
    a. Brainstem
    b. Cerebellum
    c. Cerebral cortex
    d. Thalamous

■ ASTROCYTOMA

14. Which of the following is the most common type of glial tumors? *(All India 2006)*
    a. Astrocytomas
    b. Medulloblastomas
    c. Neurofibromas
    d. Ependymomas

15. Which of the following brain tumors is highly vascular in nature? *(AIIMS May 2006)*
    a. Glioblastoma
    b. Meningiomas
    c. CP angle epidermoid
    d. Pituitary adenomas

16. What is the most probable diagnosis based on the given MRI image? *(Recent Question 2016)*
    a. Pilocytic astrocytoma
    b. Glioblastoma multiforme
    c. Oligodendroglioma
    d. Meningioma

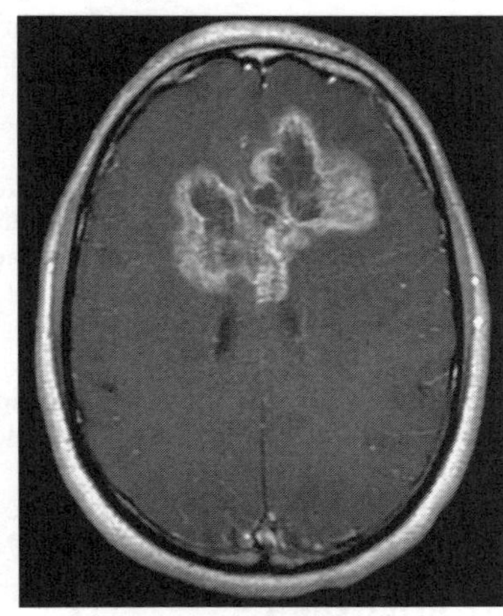

17. Which of the following statements about cerebellar astrocytomas in pediatric age group is false? *(All India 2008)*
    a. These are usually low grade tumors
    b. These are more commonly seen in the 1st and 2nd decades
    c. These tumors have a good prognosis
    d. These tumors are more common in females

18. Most common site of sub ependymal astrocytoma (Giant cell): *(AIIMS Nov 2007)*
    a. Trigone of lateral ventricle
    b. Foramen of Monro
    c. Temporal horn of lateral ventricle
    d. 4th ventricle

19. All are true regarding pilocytic astrocytoma, except:
    a. Seen in elderly above 80 years *(AIIMS May 2009)*
    b. Seen in posterior fossa
    c. Good prognosis
    d. Most common primary brain tumor in children

20. A child present with raised ICT. On CT scan, a lesion is seen around foramen of Monroe and multiple periventricular calcific foci. What is the most probable diagnosis? *(AIIMS Nov 2011)*
    a. Central neurocytoma
    b. Ependymoma
    c. Subependymal giant cell astrocytoma
    d. Ganglioglioma

■ MEDULLOBLASTOMA

21. Chang staging is used for? *(AIIMS May 2010)*
    a. Retinoblastoma
    b. Medulloblastoma
    c. Ewing's sarcoma
    d. Rhabdomyosarcoma

22. Long term effect of craniospinal irradiation for medulloblastoma is: *(JIPMER 2011)*
    a. Secondary malignancy
    b. Neuro endocrine abnormalities
    c. Neurocognitive effects
    d. Hearing loss

■ MENINGIOMA

23. A 45-years old female complains of progressive lower limb weakness, spasticity, urinary hesitancy. MRI shows intra-dural enhancing mass lesion. Most likely diagnosis is: *(AIIMS Nov 2011, Nov 2006, All India 2007)*
    a. Dermoid cyst
    b. Intradural lipoma
    c. Neuroepithelial cyst
    d. Meningioma

24. Best prognosis among following is seen in: *(DNB 2007)*
    a. Astrocytoma
    b. Oligodendroglioma
    c. Meningioma
    d. Medulloblastoma

25. Extra-axial intracranial lesion showing contrast enhancement on MRI: *(All India 2012)*
    a. Meningioma
    b. Ependymoma
    c. Arachnoid cyst
    d. Astrocytoma

■ CRANIOPHARYNGIOMA

26. A six year old child managed by complete surgical removal of craniopharyngioma developed multiple endocrinopathies. Which of following hormones should be replaced first? *(All India 2011)*
    a. Hydrocortisone
    b. Growth Hormone
    c. Thyroxine
    d. Prolactin

27. Which of the following is the most common cause of a mixed cystic and solid suprasellar mass seen on cranial MR scan of a 10 years old child? *(AIIMS 2005)*
    a. Pituitary adenoma
    b. Craniopharyngioma
    c. Optic chiasmal glioma
    d. Germinoma

■ PITUITARY ADENOMA

28. The most preferred approach for pituitary surgery at the present time is: *(JIPMER Nov 2017; All India 2006)*
    a. Transcranial
    b. Transethmoidal
    c. Transphenoidal
    d. Transcallosal

29. A 30 years old male complains of loss of erection; he has low testosterone and high prolactin level in blood; what is the likely diagnosis? *(All India 2001)*
    a. Pituitary adenoma
    b. Testicular failure
    c. Craniopharyngioma
    d. Cushing's syndrome

30. Most common cause of hypersecreting pituitary tumour is: *(DNB 2009)*
    a. Pituitary adenoma
    b. Pituitary carcinoma
    c. Autoimmue disease of pituitary
    d. Transection of stalk

■ SPINAL TUMORS

31. The commonest extradural spinal tumor is:
    a. Neurofibroma
    b. Glioma
    c. Meningioma
    d. Metastasis

32. Commonest spinal tumour is: *(SCTIMS 98)*
    a. Meningioma
    b. Ependymoma
    c. Neurofibroma
    d. Neuroblastomas

33. Most common location of spinal tumors: *(AIIMS Nov 2007)*
    a. Intramedullary
    b. Intradural extramedullary
    c. Extradural
    d. Equally distributed

■ MISCELLANEOUS

34. Commonest orbital tumour causing exophthalmos is: *(Recent Question 2016)*
    a. Glioma
    b. Meningioma
    c. Hemangioma
    d. Neuroblastoma

35. Witzelsucht syndrome (i.e. "Pathological Joking") is seen in: *(All Inida 90)*
    a. Frontal lobe tumours
    b. Parietal lobe tumours
    c. Temporal lobe tumours
    d. Intra Ventricular tumours

36. MRI is the investigation of choice in all of the following except: *(COMEDK 2007, 2004)*
    a. Syringomyelia
    b. Brain stem tumors
    c. Skull bone tumors
    d. Multiple sclerosis

37. Imaging modality of choice for detecting radiation induced cerebral necrosis: *(AIIMS Nov 2009, 2005)*
    a. PET scan
    b. Biopsy
    c. MRI
    d. CT

38. Enlargement of pituitary tumour after adrenalectomy is called as: *(DNB 2009)*
    a. Nelson syndrome
    b. Steel-Richardson syndrome
    c. Hamman-Rich syndrome
    d. Job's syndrome

39. Highly vascular tumor of brain and spinal cord in adults: *(AIIMS May 2013)*
    a. Metastasis
    b. Pilocytic astrocytoma
    c. Hemangioblastoma
    d. Cavernous malformation

■ CNS TUMORS PREDISPOSING FACTORS

1. **Ans. a. Autosomal recessive inheritance** *(Ref: Harrison 20/e p649; Sabiston 20/e p754; Schwartz 11/e p733, 322, 10/e p677; Bailey 27/e p145)*

Neurofibromatosis	
Neurofibromatosis-1	**Neurofibromatosis-2**
• Also known as **peripheral** neurofibromatosis or **von-Recklinghausen's syndrome**[Q] • **Most prevalent** type (**90%**[Q]) • **NF-1 gene**: Chromosome **17**[Q] • **Autosomal dominant**[Q] • **Diagnostic Criteria for NF-1** (Diagnosed when **any two** of the following are present): 1. **≥6** *café-au-lait* **macules**[Q] >5 mm in greatest diameter in prepubertal individuals and >15mm in greatest diameter in post-pubertal individuals. 2. **Axillary** or **inguinal freckling**[Q] 3. **≥2 iris Lisch nodules**[Q] 4. **≥2 neurofibromas** or **one plexiform neurofibroma**[Q] 5. Sphenoid dysplasia or cortical thinning of long bone, with or without pseudoarthrosis 6. **Optic gliomas**[Q] 7. A **first degree relative** with NF-1 whose diagnosis was based on the aforementioned criteria.	• Also known as **central** neurofibromatosis or **bilateral acoustic neurofibromatosis**[Q] • Less prevalent (10%) • **NF-2 gene**: Chromosome **22**[Q] • **Autosomal dominant**[Q] • **Diagnostic Criteria for NF-2**[Q] (Diagnosed when **any one** of the following is present): 1. **Bilateral 8**[th] **nerve masses** consistent with **acoustic neuromas**[Q] 2. A parent, sibling, or child with NF-2 and either 3. **Unilateral 8**[th] **nerve mass** or **any two** of the following: – **Neurofibroma**[Q] – **Meningioma**[Q] – **Glioma**[Q] – **Schwannoma**[Q] • Bilateral acoustic neuromas are the most distinctive tumors in patients with NF-2[Q].

2. **Ans. b. Gastric carcinoma** *(Ref: Harrison 20/e p649; Sabiston 20/e p693; Bailey 27/e p145)*

Von Hippel Lindau Syndrome (AD)	
Characteristic Tumors/Cysts	**Other Tumors/Cysts**
• **Hemangioblastomas:** – **Cerebellar** hemangioblastoma[Q] – **Retinal** hemangioblastoma[Q] – **Spinal** hemangioblastoma[Q]	• **RCC**[Q] • **Pheochromocytoma**[Q] • Pancreatic endocrine tumors • Adrenal carcinomas • **Benign cysts** in **kidney, epididymis, liver** or **pancreas**[Q]

• **Polycythemia** is a **characteristic feature** in VHL due to **erythropoietin production** by **hemangioblastoma** and/or **RCC**[Q].

3. **Ans. b. Craniospinal hemangioblastoma are common**   4. **Ans. d. Hydrocephalus**

■ CNS TUMORS: CLINICAL FEATURES AND TREATMENT

5. **Ans. a. Pin point pupil** *(Ref: Sabiston 20/e p1909; Schwartz 11/e p1856, 10/e p1732; Bailey 27/e p662-663)*
6. **Ans. c. Metastasis** *(Ref: Sabiston 20/e p1915; Schwartz 11/e p1854, 10/e p1732; Bailey 27/e p663)*
7. **Ans. a. Glioma** *(Ref: CGDT 9/e p429)*

• Although brain tumors are not specifically related to gestation, **meningiomas**, **angiomas**, and **neurofibromas** are thought to **grow more rapidly with pregnancy**[Q].

8. **Ans. c. Meningioma** *(Ref: Sutton Radiology 7/e p1739)*

• **Meningioma** range from **firm** and **fibrous to finely gritty** or they may be **extremely calcified** with **Psammoma bodies**[Q].
• **Calcification** is also **seen in ependymoma**, but **more common in meningioma**[Q].

9. **Ans. d. AV malformation of brain** *(Ref: Sabiston 20/e p1923; Schwartz 11/e p1872, 10/e p1749)*
10. **Ans. d. Craniopharyngioma** *(Ref: Harrison 20/e p648)*   11. **Ans. a. VHL syndrome**

■ BRAIN METASTASIS

12. **Ans. a. Small cell carcinoma lung** *(Ref: Harrison 20/e p649)*
13. **Ans. c. Cerebral cortex**

■ ASTROCYTOMA

14. **Ans. a. Astrocytomas** *(Ref: Harrison 20/e p644; Sabiston 20/e p1911; Schwartz 11/e p1855, 10/e p1733, 1738-1739; Bailey 27/e p664)*

15. **Ans. a. Glioblastoma** *(Ref: Harrison 20/e p645; Osborn Neuroradiology (1994)/541, 591)*
    - Osborn says "**Glioblastoma** is **highly vascular**, sometimes so vascular that it **resembles an AV malformation on angiography**."

16. **Ans. b. Glioblastoma multiforme** *(Ref: Sabiston 20/e p1911; Harrison 20/e p645; Robbins 9/e p1307)*

17. **Ans. d. These tumors are more common in females** *(Ref: Nelsons 20/e p2455)*
    Cerebellar astrocytomas do not show any clear gender predilection and are **equally common** in **both males** and **females**.

18. **Ans. b. Foramen of Monro** *(Ref: Neurology in Clinical Practice 4/e p428; Sutton Radiology 7/e p1735)*

SUBEPENDYMAL GIANT CELL ASTROCYTOMA

- **Most common site** of **subependymal giant cell astrocytoma** is the **ependymal wall of lateral ventricle near** the **foramen of Monro**[Q].
- Causes **obstruction at** the **foramen of Monro** leading to **ventricular enlargement** and **raised ICT.**

> - Presence of **multiple periventricular calcific foci (calcified subependymal nodules)** suggest the diagnosis of **Tuberous sclerosis** with **subependymal giant cell astrocytoma**[Q]

19. **Ans. a. Seen in elderly above 80 years**

20. **Ans. c. Subependymal giant cell astrocytoma**

■ MEDULLOBLASTOMA

21. **Ans. b. Medulloblastoma**

22. **Ans. c. Neurocognitive effect** *(Ref: www.ncbi.nlm.nih.gov/pubmed/9121399)*

CRANIOSPINAL IRRADIATION (CSI)

- **Hypothyroidism:** One of the **earliest late side effects of CSI** and **2nd MC (after GH disturbance**[Q]**)**
- **Prevalence of hypothyroidism is 40–80% after CSI**[Q]
- Significantly increased risk of development of **benign thyroid nodules** and **papillary carcinoma of the thyroid** many years later[Q].

■ MENINGIOMA

23. **Ans. d. Meningioma** *(Ref: Harrison 20/e p648; Chapman 4/e p 431; Sabiston 20/e p1913; Schwartz 11/e p1857, 10/e p1735,1738; Bailey 27/e p665)*

24. **Ans. c. Meningioma**
    - Meningioma is slow growing and encapsulated tumor having best prognosis among the given options.

25. **Ans. a. Meningioma**

■ CRANIOPHARYNGIOMA

26. **Ans. a. Hydrocortisone**   27. **Ans. b. Craniopharyngioma**

■ PITUITARY ADENOMA

28. **Ans. c. Transphenoidal**

29. **Ans. a. Pituitary adenoma**

30. **Ans. a. Pituitary adenoma**

■ SPINAL TUMORS

31. **Ans. d. Metastasis** *(Ref: Scott Atlas, MRI of the Brain and Spine 3rd/1742; Sabiston 20/e p1913; Schwartz 11/e p1859, 10/e p1737-1739)*

32. **Ans. c. Neurofibroma**   33. **Ans. c. Extradural**

■ MISCELLANEOUS

34. **Ans. a. Glioma**

35. **Ans. a. Frontal lobe tumours**

36. Ans. c. Skull bone tumors *(Ref: Bailey 27/e p197-198,199)*

MAGNETIC RESONANCE IMAGING

- MRI was discovered by **Lauterbeur**[Q] in 1973.
- MRI is **best for soft tissues**[Q].

37. Ans. a. PET scan

38. Ans. a. Nelson syndrome *(Ref: Harrison 20/e p2682)*

NELSON SYNDROME

- Nelson syndrome refers to a spectrum of symptoms and signs arising from an **adrenocorticotropin (ACTH)–secreting pituitary macroadenoma after a therapeutic bilateral adrenalectomy.**
- The spectrum of clinical features observed relates to the **local effects of the tumor on surrounding structures**, the **secondary loss of other pituitary hormones**, and the **effects of the high serum concentrations of ACTH on the skin.**

39. Ans. c. Hemangioblastoma *(Ref: Harrison 20/e p2754; Sabiston 20/e p1913; Schwartz 11/e p1858, 10/e p1735-1736)*

- *Highly vascular tumor of brain and spinal cord in adults Hemangioblastoma.*

Head and Neck

- Oral Cavity
- Salivary Glands
- Neck
- Facial Injuries and Abnormalities

Oral Cavity

RISK FACTORS FOR CANCER OF ORAL CAVITY

Risk Factors for Cancer of Oral Cavity		
• **Tobacco**[Q] • **Alcohol**[Q] • **Areca nut/pan masala**[Q] • **Sharp** or **jagged tooth**[Q]	• **Ill-fitting dentures**[Q] • **Syphilitic glossitis**[Q] • **Human papilloma virus**[Q]	• **Epstein-Barr virus**[Q] • **Plummer-Vinson syndrome**[Q] • Poor nutrition

Conditions Associated with Malignant Transformation

High-risk Lesions	Medium-risk Lesions	Low-risk or Equivocal-risk Lesions
• **Erythroplakia**[Q] • **Speckled Erythroplakia**[Q] • **Chronic hyperplastic candidiasis**[Q]	• **Oral submucous fibrosis**[Q] • **Syphilitic glossitis**[Q] • **Sideropenic dysphagia**[Q] (Paterson-Kelly syndrome)	• Oral lichen planus • Discoid lupus erythematosus • Discoid keratosis congenita

ORAL SUBMUCOUS FIBROSIS

ORAL SUBMUCOUS FIBROSIS

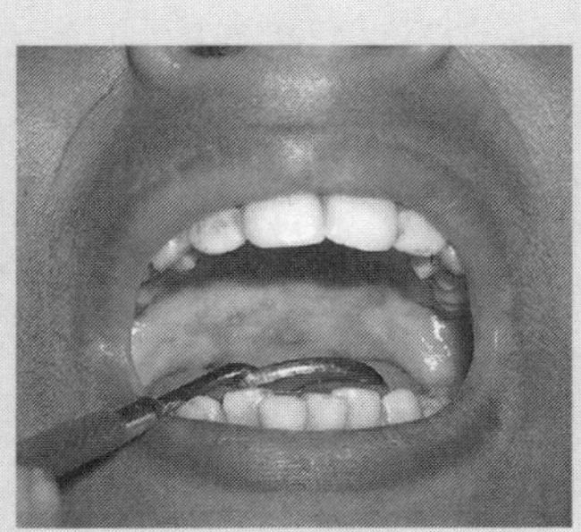

- Oral submucous fibrosis is a **progressive disease** in which **fibrous bands form beneath** the **oral mucosa**[Q].
- Almost **entirely confined to the Asian population**[Q]
- **Risk factor** for **oral cavity malignancies** (squamous cell carcinoma[Q])

Risk Factors
- Research strongly indicates that oral submucous fibrosis is **significantly associated with** the use of **pan masala areca nut, with or without concurrent alcohol use**[Q].
- **Tobacco smoking alone** is **not associated** with oral submucous fibrosis.

Pathology
- Characterised by **epithelial fibrosis** with **associated atrophy** & **hyperplasia** of overlying **epithelium**[Q].
- **Epithelium** shows changes of **epithelial dysplasia**[Q].

Clinical Features
- **Scarring produces contracture**, resulting in **limited mouth opening** & **restricted tongue movement**[Q].

Treatment
- **Restricted mouth opening** can be treated with either **intralesional steroids** or **surgical excision** & **skin grafts**[Q].

IMPORTANT POINTS ABOUT CARCINOMA ORAL CAVITY

- MC gene mutated in CA oral cavity: p53[Q]
- MC site of CA oral cavity: Tongue >Lip[Q]
- MC histological type of CA oral cavity: Squamous cell carcinoma[Q]
- MC type of cancer in India: CA oral cavity[Q]
- MC site of CA oral cavity in India: Buccal mucosa[Q] (38%) > Anterior tongue (16%) > Lower alveolus (15.7%)
- MC pattern of spread: Local extension & regional lymphatic spread[Q]
- LN metastasis is most common in: CA tongue[Q] > Floor of mouth > Lower alveolus > Buccal mucosa > Upper alveolus > **Hard palate > Lip**[Q].

Contd...

Contd…

- **Bilateral lymphatic spread** is common in: Lower lip[Q], supraglottis[Q] & soft palate[Q].
- **MC site of metastasis:** Lung[Q]
- **Edge biopsy** is recommended for **diagnosis** of oral cavity malignancies[Q].
- **MRI: IOC** for **staging of head & neck malignancies**[Q].
- **MC flap used** for reconstruction of **head & neck malignancies:** PMMC (pectoralis major myocutaneous) flap based on pectoral branch of Thoracoacromial vessels[Q]

8th AJCC (2017) TNM Classification of Carcinoma Lip & Oral Cavity				
Primary Tumor (T)			**Regional Lymph Nodes (N)**	
Tis	Carcinoma in situ.		N1	Metastasis in a **single ipsilateral LN**, **≤3 cm** in greatest dimension without extranodal extension[Q]
T1	Tumor **≤2 cm** in greatest dimension & **≤5 mm depth of invasion**[Q]		N2a	Metastasis in **single ipsilateral LN, >3 cm** but **≤6 cm** in greatest dimension without extranodal extension[Q]
T2	Tumor **≤2 cm** in greatest dimension & **>5 mm but ≤10 mm depth of invasion** or tumor **>2 cm but ≤4 cm** in greatest dimension & **depth of invasion ≤10 mm**[Q]		N2b	Metastases in **multiple ipsilateral LN**, none >6 cm in greatest dimension without extranodal extension[Q]
T3	Tumor **>4 cm** in greatest dimension **>10 mm depth of invasion**[Q]		N2c	Metastases in **bilateral** or **contralateral LN,** none >6 cm in greatest dimension without extranodal extension[Q]
T4a	**Lip:** Tumor invades through **cortical bone, inferior alveolar nerve, floor** of mouth, or **skin (of chin or nose)**[Q]		N3a	Metastasis in a **LN >6 cm** in greatest dimension without extranodal extension[Q]
			N3b	Metastasis in **a single or multiple LNs with clinical extranodal extension**[Q]
	Oral cavity: Tumor invades through **cortical bone** mandible or maxillary sinus or invades the **skin of face**[Q].		**Distant Metastasis**	
T4b	Tumor invades **masticator space, pterygoid plates,** or **skull base** and/or encases **internal carotid artery**[Q].		M0	No distant metastasis.
			M1	Distant metastasis.

Stage Grouping						
0	**I**	**II**	**III**	**IVA**	**IVB**	**IVC**
Tis N0M0	T1 N0M0	T2 N0M0	T3 N0M0 T1-3 N1 M0	**T4a N0-1** M0 **T1-4a N2** M0	Any T **N3** M0 **T4b** Any N M0	Any N Any T **M1**

■ CARCINOMA LIP

Carcinoma Lip

- **MC site of CA lip: Vermillion of lower lip**[Q]
- Typically seen in **males of 40-70 years**[Q]
- Definite correlation between **CA lip** and **exposure to sunlight** (UV radiations[Q])
- **MC presentation: Non-healing ulcer** or growth[Q]
- **LN metastasis** is **rare** and **develops late**, mainly to **submental** and **submandibular** LNs[Q].
- **Bilateral lymphatic spread** is seen in **CA lower lip**[Q].

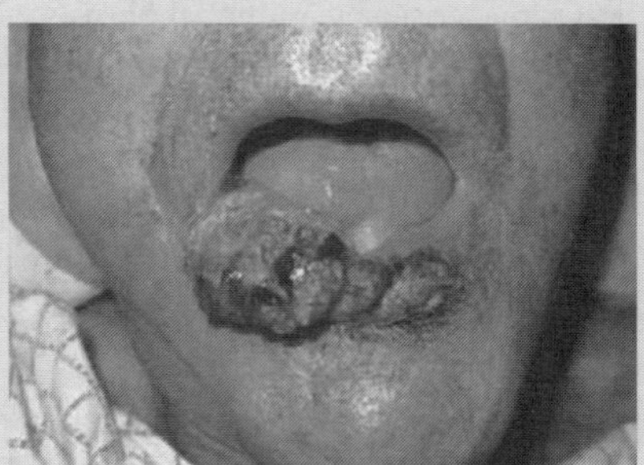

Treatment of Carcinoma Lip	
• **T1 and T2**	• **Surgery is TOC**[Q] • If **1/3rd or less** of lip is involved: 'V' or 'W' shaped **full thickness excision** with lateral margin of 5 mm + **Primary closure**[Q] • If **more than 1/3rd of lip is involved:** Flap reconstruction (**Abbe-Estlander** flap)[Q]
• **T3 and T4**	• **Combined radiation** and **surgery**[Q] (vermilonectomy or lip shave)

Prognosis

- CA lip has the **best prognosis**[Q] in CA oral cavity.

Lip Reconstruction	
Cross-lip Flaps	**Circumoral Advancement Flaps**
• **Lip-Switch (Abbe-Estlander) flap**[Q] used to repair defects of either upper or lower lip, based on **superior labial artery**[Q]	• **Karapandzic flap**[Q]: Uses a sensate, **neuromuscular flap** based on **labial artery**[Q]. • **Webster-Bernard repair**[Q]: Use lateral nasolabial flap with buccal advancement

■ CARCINOMA BUCCAL MUCOSA (CHEEK)

CARCINOMA BUCCAL MUCOSA (CHEEK)

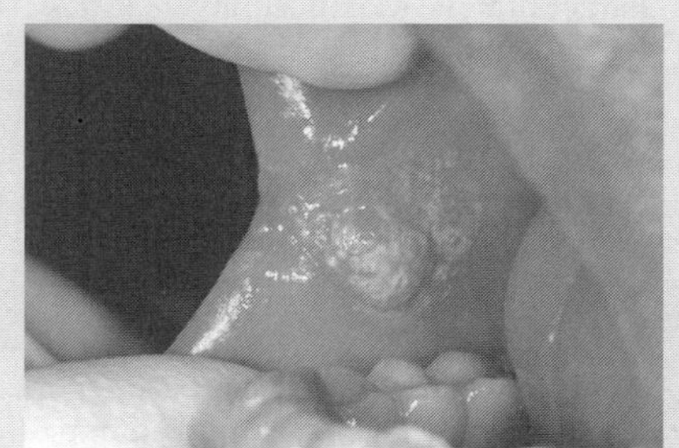

- **MC site** of CA oral cavity in India: Buccal mucosa[Q]
- Related to chewing a combination of **tobacco mixed with betel leaves**, **areca nut** and **lime shell**[Q]
- Most malignant tumors are **low grade SCC**[Q]
- Frequently appearing on background of leukoplakia
- **Lymphatic spread** is first to **level I and II LNs**[Q].

Clinical Feature

- **Pain is minimal**, obstruction of Stenson's duct can lead to parotid enlargement.

Treatment

- **T1: Excision** with primary closure[Q]
- **T2: Surgery ± Radiotherapy**[Q]
- **T3 and T4: Surgery + Radiotherapy** or **chemoradiation**[Q]

■ CARCINOMA TONGUE

CARCINOMA TONGUE

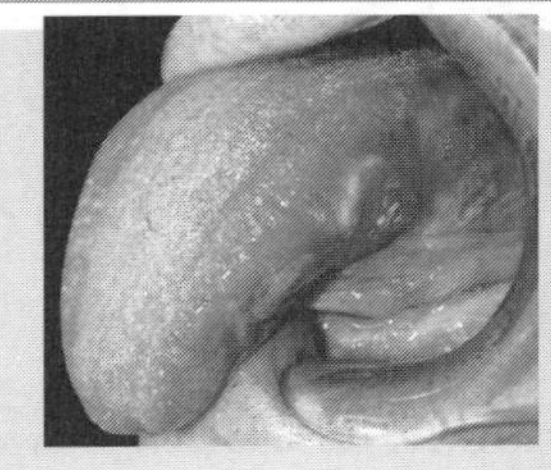

- **MC site** is **middle of lateral border**[Q] or ventral aspect of the tongue.
- **MC histological type** is **squamous cell carcinoma**[Q].
- **MC associated risk factors** are **tobacco** and **alcohol**[Q].
- **MC variety** is **ulcerative**[Q].
- **30% patients** presents with **cervical node metastasis**[Q].

■ CARCINOMA ORAL TONGUE

CARCINOMA ORAL TONGUE

- The intrinsic tongue musculature provide little restriction to tumour growth, thus it may enlarge considerably before producing symptoms.
- Presents as **painless mass** or **ulcer** that **fails to heal** after minor trauma[Q]
- **MC complaint: Mid-irritation of tongue**[Q].
- **MC site: Lateral border** of the **junction of middle & posterior third**[Q].
- **Primary basin** for **cervical metastasis** is **superior deep jugular nodes (Level II)**[Q].
- For diagnosis, **wedge biopsy** is taken **from the edge of ulcer** but in **proliferative growth, punch biopsy** is taken[Q].

Treatment of Carcinoma Oral Tongue	
T1	• **Partial glossectomy** with primary closure[Q]
T2	• **Hemiglossectomy** for **small well-circumscribed** and **well differentiated** lesion[Q] • **Radiotherapy** for **large, poorly differentiated lesion**[Q]
T3	• **Total glossectomy** followed by **radiation**[Q]
T4	• **Surgery** (Total glossectomy, **mandibulectomy**, MRND, laryngectomy) + **Postoperative radiation**[Q]

Management of Recurrence

- **Most recurrences** occur within **2 years.**
- **Radiation failure** is managed by **glossectomy**[Q].
- **Surgical failure** is managed by **radiation**[Q].
- If **recurrence is limited to mucosa**, it is best managed by **surgery**
- If **recurrence is in the soft tissue of the neck, palliation** is indicated.

■ CANCER OF HARD PALATE

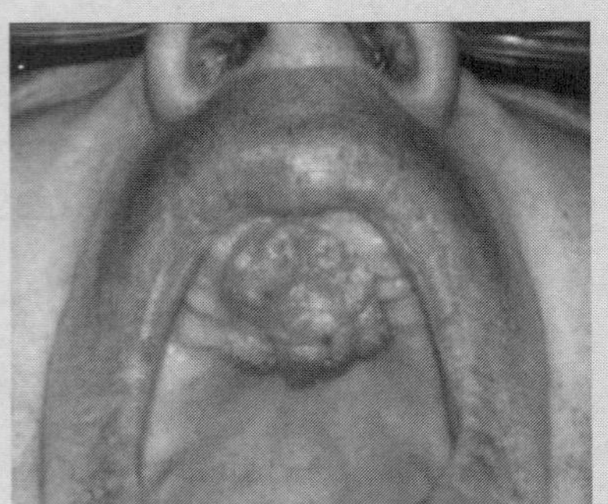

CANCER OF HARD PALATE

- SCC of hard palate is **rare, Associated with reverse smoking**
- Minor salivary gland tumors occur in the hard palate.
- Most cancers are **well differentiated** and of **ulcerative variety**[Q].

Clinical Features

- Presents as painless mass[Q] in the roof of the mouth
- **Lymphatic metastasis** is **uncommon**, mainly to level I and II.

Treatment

- **Smaller tumors: Excision** with underlying bone.
- **Larger tumors: Maxillectomy**
- **Radiotherapy** is used in advanced lesions.

■ CHEMOTHERAPY IN CANCERS OF ORAL CAVITY, HEAD AND NECK

CHEMOTHERAPY IN CANCERS OF ORAL CAVITY, HEAD AND NECK

- Adjuvant **chemotherapy** has been reported to **improve the rate of organ preservation** with **no change in overall survival**[Q].
- Chemotherapy is often **employed in palliative setting** in patients with **recurrent, unresectable** or **distant metastases**[Q].
- **Drugs used: Cisplatin**[Q], **Methotrexate**, 5-FU, Docetaxel and Paclitaxel

> - **Cisplatin** is the **cornerstone drug** in the modern management of head & neck cancer[Q].
> - **Most beneficial** is **concurrent chemotherapy**[Q].

- The addition of **concurrent chemotherapy (cisplatin)** to conventional radiation **significantly improved survival over radiation alone**[Q].
- **Concurrent chemoradiation** protocols have **improved locoregional control** and **reduce** the **development of distant disease**[Q].

■ RADIOTHERAPY IN CANCERS OF ORAL CAVITY

RADIOTHERAPY IN CANCERS OF ORAL CAVITY

- **SCC** is **vascularized** and **well-oxygenated** tends to be **most radiosensitive**[Q].
- **Large cervical metastatic nodes** are **best managed by** a combination of surgery and **radiation therapy** rather than by radiation alone[Q].
- Mostly given as **EBRT** (External Beam Radiotherapy), **60 Gray** over **6 weeks**[Q].

Complications of Radiotherapy
1. **Xerostomia (MC)**[Q]
2. **Mucositis**[Q]
3. Temporary or permanent dysgeusia
4. **Osteoradionecrosis (ORN)**[Q]:
– Related to **carries tooth** in the radiation field[Q]
– Results from **decreased production of saliva** and **damage to microvasculature** of mandible and maxilla[Q]
– Best managed with **prophylactic dental care**[Q]
– ORN may require daily **hyperbaric oxygen treatments** for 4-6 weeks, either alone or in conjunction with surgical intervention[Q]

■ MANDIBULECTOMY

Mandibulectomy	
Marginal Mandibulectomy	**Segmental Mandibulectomy**

- **Conservative mandibulectomy**[Q]
- Refers to **partial excision** of the **superior portion** of mandible in vertical phase[Q]
- **Inner cortical surface** and a portion of **underlying medullary cavity** is excised[Q]
- **Preserve mandibular continuity**[Q]
- Indicated **when tumor lies within 1 cm** of the mandible or **abuts the periosteum** without evidence of direct bony invasion[Q]
	- **Entire through and through segment of mandible is resected.**
	- Results in **mandibular discontinuity**[Q]
	- Requires **major reconstructive procedure** for cosmetic and functional purposes[Q]
	- **Indications:**
	  1. **Invasion of medullary space** of mandible[Q]
	  2. **Tumor fixation to occlusal surface** of mandible in **edentulous patient**[Q]
	  3. **Invasion** of tumor into the mandible **via mandibular** or **mental foramen**[Q]
	  4. **Tumor fixed** to the mandible[Q]

Multiple Choice Questions

■ CARCINOMA ORAL CAVITY PREDISPOSING FACTORS

1. **Regarding premalignant oral lesions:** *(COMEDK 2005)*
   a. Leukoplakia should be proved by biopsy
   b. Leukoplakia does not disappear after cessation of smoking
   c. Erythroplakia has a higher risk for malignancy
   d. Oral submucous fibrosis is seen in all parts of the world

2. **All of the following are precancerous lesions for carcinoma oral cavity except:** *(Recent Question 2017)*
   a. Erythroplakia
   b. Speckled erythroplakia
   c. Discoid lupus erythematosus
   d. Chronic hyperplastic candidiasis

3. **Treatment of leukoplakia:** *(JIPMER 2011)*
   a. Local excision
   b. Excision and radiotherapy
   c. Topical chemotherapy
   d. Repositioning of ill fitting dentures

4. **All are premalignant conditions of the oral cavity except:** *(MCI Dec 2018)*
   a. Chronic hyperplastic candidiasis
   b. Oral submucosal fibrosis
   c. Oral lichen planus
   d. Leucoplakia

5. **Treatment of erythroplakia:** *(MHSSMCET 2007)*
   a. Excision
   b. Stoppage of alcohol and tobacco
   c. Vitamin supplementation
   d. Laser ablation

6. **The pre-malignant condition with the highest probability of progression to malignancy is:** *(Bihar PG 2014, All India 2002)*
   a. Dysplasia
   b. Hyperplasia
   c. Leukoplakia
   d. Erythroleukoplakia

7. **The commonest pre-malignant condition of oral cancer is:** *(All India 95)*
   a. Leukoplakia
   b. Aphthous ulcer
   c. Lichen planus
   d. Erthro-leukoplakia

8. **Which of the following is the cause of submucosal fibrosis?** *(MCI Nov 2017)*
   a. Alcohol
   b. Candidiasis
   c. Betel nut chewing
   d. Pan leaf chewing

■ CARCINOMA ORAL CAVITY

9. **The commonest site of oral cancer among Indian population is:** *(Kerala PG 2015, All India 2004)*
   a. Tongue
   b. Floor of mouth
   c. Alveobuccal complex
   d. Lip

10. **Most common type of oral cancer:** *(MCI Dec 2019)*
    a. Squamous cell carcinoma
    b. Adenocarcinoma
    c. Transitional cell carcinoma
    d. Mucoepidermoid carcinoma

11. **Areas of carcinoma of oral mucosa can be identified by staining with:** *(Recent Question 2016)*
    a. 1% zinc chloride
    b. 2% silver nitrate
    c. Gentian violet
    d. 2% toluidine blue

12. **Most common site of oral cancer:** *(Recent Question 2017)*
    a. Lips
    b. Tongue
    c. Buccal mucosa
    d. Alveolus of teeth

13. **All of the following are indications for adjuvant radiotherapy in head and neck cancers except:** *(Recent Question 2017)*
    a. Multiple lymph node disease
    b. Extranodal involvement
    c. Lymphovascular invasion
    d. Lymph node >3 cm

■ CARCINOMA LIP

14. **Abbe-Estlander flap is used for:** *(All India 2008)*
    a. Lip
    b. Tongue
    c. Eyelid
    d. Ears

15. **What is the diagnosis of this 60 years old man, whose picture is given below?** *(MCI Dec 2018)*

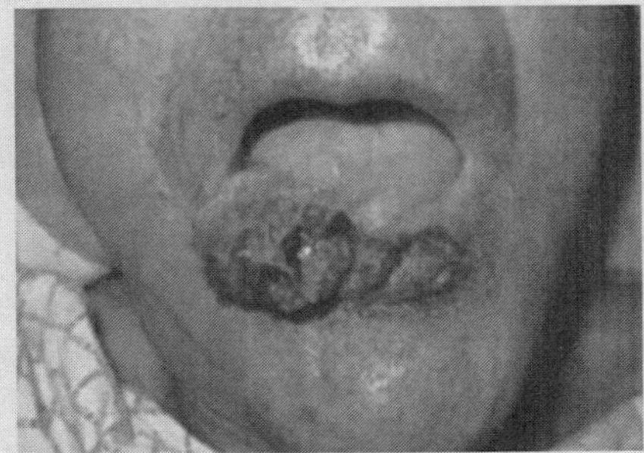

    a. Basal cell carcinoma
    b. Plunging ranula
    c. Epulis
    d. SCC of lip

16. **Abbey Estlander flap is based on:** *(AIIMS May 2008)*
    a. Lingual artery
    b. Facial artery
    c. Labial artery
    d. Internal maxillary artery

17. **Stain used to diagnose premalignant lesions of lip is:** *(DNB 2011, 2006)*
    a. Crystal violet
    b. H and E
    c. Toluidine blue
    d. Giemsa

18. **Treatment of choice for carcinoma of lip of less than 1 cm is:**
    a. Radiation
    b. Chemotherapy
    c. Excision *(All India 90)*
    d. Radiation and chemotherapy

19. **Neuromuscular preserving flap in lip:** *(Recent Question 2017)*
    a. Abbe flap
    b. Webster flap
    c. Karpandzic flap
    d. Johansen flap

■ CARCINOMA BUCCAL MUCOSA AND CHEEK

20. **Metastasis of CA buccal mucosa goes to:** *(AIIMS Nov 96, All India 97)*
    a. Regional lymph node
    b. Liver
    c. Heart
    d. Brain

21. In carcinoma cheek, what is the best drug for single drug chemotherapy? *(AIIMS June 93)*
    a. Vincristine
    b. Cyclophosphamide
    c. Cisplatin
    d. Daunorubicin

22. A patient with cheek cancer has a tumour of 2.5 cm located close to and involving the lower alveolus. A single mobile ipsilateral lymph node measuring 6 cm is palpable. The TNM stage is: *(Recent Question 2013, COMEDK 2008)*
    a. T1N1M0
    b. T2N2M0
    c. T2N1M0
    d. T4N2M0

■ CARCINOMA PALATE

23. All are true about carcinoma palate, except:
    (AIIMS June 94, Nov 93)
    a. Slow growing
    b. Bilateral lymphatic spread
    c. Adenocarcinoma
    d. Presents with pain

■ CARCINOMA TONGUE

24. A patient presented with a 1 X 1.5 cms growth on the lateral border of the tongue. The treatment indicated would be:
    a. Laser ablation *(Recent Question 2014, AIIMS June 2002)*
    b. Interstitial brachytherapy
    c. External beam radiotherapy
    d. Chemotherapy

25. Carcinoma of tongue most commonly occur at:
    a. Dorsum *(Recent Question 2013 MCI March 2009)*
    b. Lateral border of anterior 2/3rd
    c. Lateral border of posterior 1/3rd
    d. Tip

26. Tongue ulcer with everted edges is: *(MHPGMCET 2005, 2001)*
    a. Aphthous ulcer
    b. Tubercular
    c. Malignant
    d. Dental

27. The commando operation is: *(Recent Question 2016)*
    a. Abdomino-perineal resection of the rectum for carcinoma
    b. Disarticulation of the hip for gas gangrene of the leg
    c. Extended radical mastectomy
    d. Excision of carcinoma of the jaw and lymph nodes enbloc

■ CARCINOMA MAXILLA

28. Treatment for stage T3N1 of carcinoma maxilla is:
    (DNB 2012, AIIMS June 96)
    a. Radiation therapy only
    b. Chemotherapy only
    c. Surgery and radiation
    d. Chemotherapy and radiation

29. The lymph not to be involved first in maxillary carcinoma:
    a. Superior deep cervical nodes *(DNB 2007)*
    b. Jugulodigastric nodes
    c. Submandibular
    d. Subdigastric nodes

■ MANDIBLE AND MANDIBULECTOMY

30. A 80-year-old patient presents with a midline tumor of the lower jaw, involving the alveolar margin. He is edentulous. Treatment of choice is: *(All India 2001)*
    a. Hemimandibulectomy
    b. Commando operation
    c. Segmental mandibulectomy
    d. Marginal mandibulectomy

■ TRISMUS

31. Trismus in oral cancer patients is severe in those treated with: *(Karnataka 99)*
    a. Surgery and Radiotherapy
    b. Chemotherapy alone
    c. Surgery alone
    d. Not related to treatment

■ DENTAL CYST AND ABNORMALITIES

32. The most frequent tooth to be impacted is:
    (UPSC 2007, Karnataka 98)
    a. Lower third molar
    b. Lower canine
    c. Upper third molar
    d. Upper premolar

33. Impacted wisdom teeth may produce referred pain via:
    a. Lingual nerve *(Orissa 99)*
    b. Facial nerve
    c. Branch of the auriculotemporal nerve
    d. None of the above

34. The most common cyst of the oral region is: *(DPG 2008)*
    a. Dentigerous cyst
    b. Keratosis cyst
    c. Dermoid cyst
    d. Periapical cyst

35. Dentigerous cyst arises from:
    (DPG 2009 Feb, MHPGMCET 2003)
    a. The root of a caries tooth
    b. The periosteum of the fractured mandible
    c. An unerupted permanent tooth
    d. The sequestrum of osteomyelitis of mandible

36. Which of the following is correct about ameloblastoma?
    a. Highly malignant *(Recent Question 2016)*
    b. Occurs in children <5 years
    c. Most common odontogenic tumour
    d. Mandible is not the most common site

■ EPULIS

37. Epulis arises from: *(Recent Question 2013, PGI Dec 99)*
    a. Enamel
    b. Root of teeth
    c. Gingiva
    d. Pulp

38. Epulis is: *(DNB 2014)*
    a. Benign
    b. Malignant
    c. Reactive process
    d. Precancerous

■ MISCELLANEOUS

39. Multiple painful ulcers on tongue are seen in all except:
    (All India 96)
    a. Aphthous ulcer
    b. Tuberculous ulcers
    c. Herpes ulcers
    d. Carcinomatous ulcers

40. Reparative granuloma of jaw is treated by: *(DPG 2009 Feb)*
    a. Antibiotics
    b. Wedge resection
    c. Resection and bone grafting
    d. Curettage

41. N-3 TNM staging of head and neck tumors shows:
    (Recent Question 2018)
    a. Metastasis in lymph nodes >2 cm
    b. Metastasis in lymph nodes >5 cm
    c. Metastasis in a lymph node >6 cm
    d. None

■ CARCINOMA ORAL CAVITY PREDISPOSING FACTORS

1. **Ans. c. Erythroplakia has a higher risk for malignancy** *(Ref: Bailey 27/e p761-762; Devita 9/e p564; Cancer of the Head and Neck by Suen and Myer 4/e p284-285)*

   - **Oral submucous fibrosis** is almost **entirely confined to** the **Asian population** and is characterized pathologically by **epithelial fibrosis** with associated **atrophy** and **hyperplasia** of the overlying **epithelium.**

Leukoplakia	Erythroplakia
• **White keratotic plaque** or patch that **cannot be rubbed off**[Q] and cannot be given another diagnostic name • **Risk factors: Smoking, alcohol, ill-fitting dentures, jagged tooth**[Q] • **Key pathologic features: Hyperkeratosis, parakeratosis, acanthosis**[Q] • In **most cases,** lesions **regress spontaneously** after stopping alcohol or tobacco consumption or correction of underlying cause[Q]. • **Baseline biopsy** should be done[Q] • Lesions with **moderate to severe dysplasia** should be **excised**[Q]. • Oral leukoplakia has **low potential for malignancy**[Q].	• **Red mucosal plaque,** most commonly found on the **soft palate** and **tonsillar pillars**[Q] • Does not arise from an obvious mechanical or inflammatory cause • Cannot be ascribed to another clinical or pathological condition • **Key pathologic features: severe cellular dysplasia**[Q] • Because of **increased malignant potential, all erythoplakic lesions** must be **biopsied**[Q]. • **Higher risk (17 times)** of malignant transformation than leukoplakia[Q].

2. **Ans. c. Discoid lupus erythematosus** *(Ref: Sabiston 20/e p789; Schwartz 11/e p630, 10/e p580; Bailey 27/e p761)*

3. **Ans. d. Repositioning of ill fitting dentures**

> **LEUKOPLAKIA**
>
> - In **most cases,** lesions **regress spontaneously after stopping alcohol or tobacco** consumption or **correction of underlying cause**[Q].

4. **Ans. c. Oral lichen planus** *(Ref: Bailey 27/e p761-763)*

5. **Ans. a. Excision**

6. **Ans. d. Erythroleukoplakia**

7. **Ans. a. Leukoplakia**

8. **Ans. c. Betel nut chewing**

■ CARCINOMA ORAL CAVITY

9. **Ans. c. Alveobuccal complex** *(Ref: Bailey 26/e p709-710; Devita 9/e p729; Cancer of the Head and Neck by Suen and Myer 4/e p297-304)*

10. **Ans. a. Squamous cell carcinoma** *(Ref: Bailey 27/e p761)*

11. **Ans. d. 2% toluidine blue** *(Ref: www.headandneckoncology.org/content/1/1/5)*

> **TOLUIDINE BLUE**
>
> - Toluidine blue is a **basic metachromatic dye** with **high affinity for acidic tissue** components, thereby **staining tissues rich in DNA** and **RNA**[Q].
> - **Wide applications** both as **vital staining in living tissues** and as a **special stain** used in vivo to **identify dysplasia** and **carcinoma of** the **oral cavity**[Q].

12. **Ans. b. Tongue** *(Ref: Sabiston 20/e p796; Schwartz 11/e p630, 10/e p582; Bailey 27/e p765)*

13. **Ans. d. Lymph node >3 cm** *(Ref: Devita 10/e p430)*

■ CARCINOMA LIP

14. **Ans. a Lip** *(Ref: Bailey 27/e p769; Devita 9/e p744-745; Cancer of the Head and Neck by Suen and Myer 4/e p301-302)*

15. **Ans. d. SCC of lip** *(Ref: Bailey 27/e p765, 769)*

16. **Ans. c. Labial artery** (*Ref: Bailey 27/e p769; Devita 9/e p744; Cancer of the Head and Neck by Suen and Myer 4/e p301-302*)

Lip Reconstruction	
Cross-lip Flaps	**Circumoral Advancement Flaps**
• **Lip-Switch (Abbe-Estlander) flap**[Q] used to repair defects of either upper or lower lip, based on superior **labial artery**[Q]	• **Karapandzic flap**[Q]: Uses a sensate, **neuromuscular flap** based on **labial artery**[Q]. • **Webster-Bernard repair**[Q]: Use lateral nasolabial flap with buccal advancement

17. **Ans. c. Toluidine blue** (*Ref: Indian Journal od Dental Research 2007; vol-18; Issue 3; p103-105*)

   • **Toluidine blue detects efficiently and rapidly mitotic figures** in sections of paraffin embedded human tissues **especially in oral cavity.**

18. **Ans. c. Excision**

19. **Ans. c. Karpandzic flap** (*Ref: Grabb & Smith /p378*)

■ CARCINOMA BUCCAL MUCOSA AND CHEEK

20. **Ans. a. Regional lymph node**

21. **Ans. c. Cisplatin** (*Ref: Bailey 27/e p155; Devita 9/e p749; Cancer of the Head and Neck by Suen and Myer 4/e p291-292*)

22. **Ans. d. T4N2M0**

■ CARCINOMA PALATE

23. **Ans. d. Presents with pain** (*Ref: Bailey 27/e p774; Devita 9/e p750; Cancer of the Head and Neck by Suen and Myer 4/e p311-313*)

■ CARCINOMA TONGUE

24. **Ans. b. Interstitial brachytherapy** (*Ref: Bailey 27/e p769; Devita 9/e p747-749, 752-754; Cancer of the Head and Neck by Suen and Myer 4/e p297-301*)
   • Suen and Myer says "**Radiation therapy** may be **curative in early cancer (T1** and some **T2)** and may **preserve maximal normal anatomy** and **function. Brachytherapy** allows delivery of a **large radiation boost** to the **primary tumor bed.**"

25. **Ans. b. Lateral border of anterior 2/3rd**

26. **Ans. c. Malignant** (*Ref: Bailey 27/e p616*)

Type of Ulcer	Edge
• Septic ulcer	• **Sloping** edges[Q]
• Tuberculous ulcer	• **Undermined** edges[Q]
• Carcinomatous ulcer	• **Everted hard** edges[Q]
• Rodent ulcer	• Barely visible **pearly edges**[Q]
• Syphilitic ulcer	• **Punched-out** appearance with **raised indurated edges**[Q]

27. **Ans. d. Excision of carcinoma of the jaw and lymph nodes en-bloc** (*Ref: Cancer of the Head and Neck by Suen and Myer 4/e p291*)

COMMANDO'S OPERATION (COMBINED MANDIBULECTOMY AND NECK DISSECTION OPERATION)

   • **Commando's operation:** Total glossectomy hemimandibulectomy + Removal of floor of mouth + Radical lymph node dissection[Q]
   • Indicated when **carcinoma** is **fixed to mandible** with **infiltration of floor of mouth**[Q].

■ CARCINOMA MAXILLA

28. **Ans. c. Surgery and radiation** (*Bailey 27/e p774; Devita 9/e p768-771; Cancer of the Head and Neck by Suen and Myer 4/e p179*)

29. **Ans. c. Submandibular nodes** (*Ref: Grays 39/e p577*)

■ MANDIBLE AND MANDIBULECTOMY

30. **Ans. c. Segmental mandibulectomy** (*Ref: Devita 9/e p746; Cancer of the Head and Neck by Suen and Myer 4/e p293-294*)

■ TRISMUS

31. **Ans. a. Surgery and Radiotherapy** *(Ref: Bailey 25/e p750)*

■ DENTAL CYST AND ABNORMALITIES

32. **Ans. a. Lower third molar** *(Ref: Scott-Brown's Otorhinolaryngology 7/e p1924-1925)*

IMPACTED TOOTH

- Tooth that has failed to erupt completely or partially to its correct position in the dental arch and its eruption potential has been lost.
- **MC affected tooth: Lower 3rd molar^Q >Upper 3rd molar >**Upper canine

33. **Ans. c. Branch of the auriculotemporal nerve** *(Ref: Scott-Brown's Otorhinolaryngology 7/e p1924-1925)*

- **Unerupted wisdom teeth, erupting teeth,** and **malocclusion** can cause **ear pain** secondary to direct impingement of the **auriculotemporal nerve^Q.**

34. **Ans. d. Periapical cyst** *(Ref: Scott-Brown's Otorhinolaryngology 7/e p1924-1925)*

PERIAPICAL CYST (RADICULAR CYST)

- MC type of jaw cyst^Q
- Periapical cyst is **inflammatory in origin^Q.**
- Extremely common lesions found at the **apex of teeth^Q.**
- Develop as a result of **long-standing pulpitis,** caused by advanced carious lesions or by trauma to the tooth.
- **Periapical inflammatory lesions** persist as a result of the **continued presence** of **bacteria** or other offensive agents in the area.
- **Treatment:** Complete removal of offending material and appropriate restoration of the tooth or extraction.

35. **Ans. c. An unerupted permanent tooth** *(Ref: Scott-Brown's Otorhinolaryngology 7/e p1924-1925)*

- Dentigerous cyst arises from an unerupted permanent tooth.

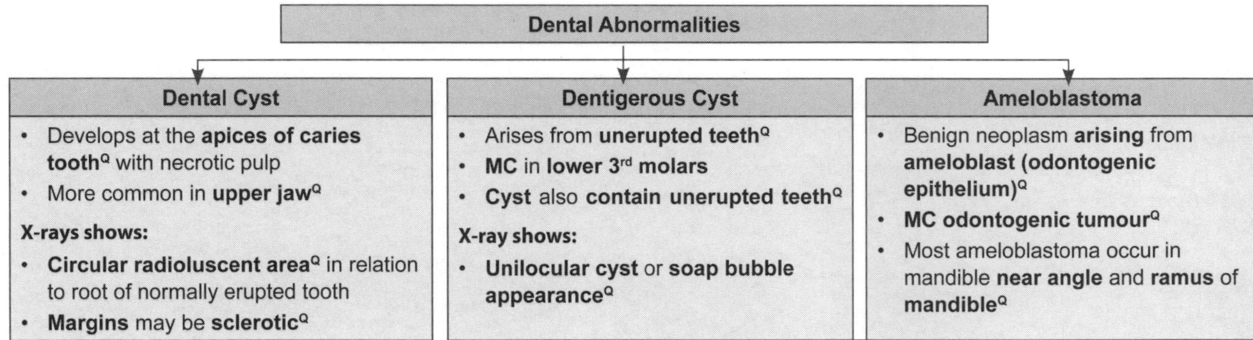

Dental Abnormalities

Dental Cyst	Dentigerous Cyst	Ameloblastoma
• Develops at the **apices of caries tooth^Q** with necrotic pulp • More common in **upper jaw^Q** **X-rays shows:** • **Circular radioluscent area^Q** in relation to root of normally erupted tooth • **Margins** may be **sclerotic^Q**	• Arises from **unerupted teeth^Q** • **MC** in **lower 3rd molars** • **Cyst** also **contain unerupted teeth^Q** **X-ray shows:** • **Unilocular cyst** or **soap bubble appearance^Q**	• Benign neoplasm **arising** from **ameloblast (odontogenic epithelium)^Q** • **MC odontogenic tumour^Q** • Most ameloblastoma occur in mandible **near angle** and **ramus** of **mandible^Q**

36. **Ans. c. Most common odontogenic tumour**

■ EPULIS

37. **Ans. c. Gingiva**

EPULIS

- **Epulis** is any **benign lesion** situated on the **gingiva.**
- Three types: fibromatous, ossifying and acanthomatous.

38. **Ans. a. Benign**

■ MISCELLANEOUS

39. **Ans. d. Carcinomatous ulcers**
    Aphthous ulcers, tubercular and herpetic ulcers are painful.

CARCINOMATOUS ULCER

- Carcinomatous ulcers are **painless** but may become painful in advanced stages, with extension into surrounding tissues.

40. Ans. d. Curettage *(Ref: medind.nic.in/ibn/t06/i4/ibnt06i4p677)*

- Reparative granuloma of Jaw is treated by curettage.

GIANT CELL REPARATIVE GRANULOMA

- Giant cell reparative granuloma is an apparently **reactive intraosseous lesion** of the **mandible** and **maxilla** following **trauma induced intraosseous hemorrhage**[Q] and containing prominent giant cells.
- Also known as **Central giant cell granuloma**[Q]
- **MC site: Anterior part** of **mandible**[Q] (2/3rd of cases) between the **2nd premolar** and **2nd molar**[Q] with extension across the midline.
- **2nd MC site: Small bones** of **hands** and **feet**[Q]

Clinical Features

- It is a **disease of the young** presenting as a **painless swelling** in the anterior jaw and
- Radiographically appearing as a **lytic expansile lesion** with a characteristic **tendency of resorbing the root tips** of adjacent unerupted teeth.

Treatment

- **Curettage** or **local excision**[Q]
- **Recurrence rate: 22-50%**
- Lesion eradication typically **does not require >2 excisions**.
- **Chemical cautery, electrocautery, cryotherapy**, calcitonin, Interferon alpha and intralesional steroids are used **for more aggressive** and **recurrent lesions**.

41. Ans. c. Metastasis in a lymph node >6 cm

Salivary Glands

■ ETIOLOGY OF SALIVARY GLAND TUMORS

ETIOLOGY OF SALIVARY GLAND TUMORS

- **Radiotherapy** to head and neck (for mucoepidermoid carcinoma)[Q]
- **EBV** infection (for lymphoepithelial carcinoma)[Q]
- Exposure to **silica dust, nitrosamines**[Q]
- Increased risk in females with **early menarche** and **nulliparity**[Q]
- **Trisomy 5** in primary mucoepidermoid carcinoma of **minor** salivary glands
- Polysomy of **3 and 17** especially in **adenoid cystic carcinoma**
- **Translocation** involving chromosome **11** in mucoepidermoid carcinoma

  - **MC neoplasm of salivary gland: Pleomorphic adenoma**[Q]
  - **MC malignant tumor** of salivary gland: **Mucoepidermoid carcinoma**[Q]
  - **MC neoplasm of salivary gland in children: Hemangioma**[Q]
  - **MC malignant tumor** of salivary gland **in children: Mucoepidermoid carcinoma**[Q]
  - **MC malignant tumor of minor salivary glands: Adenoid cystic carcinoma**[Q]
  - **Best diagnostic modality for parotid swelling: FNAC**[Q]
  - **Open incisional biopsy is contraindicated**[Q] due to **tumor cell implantation** and formation of **parotid fistula**[Q].
  - **Best imaging investigation** for **salivary gland neoplasms: MRI**[Q]

■ IN SALIVARY GLAND TUMORS

IN SALIVARY GLAND TUMORS

- **MC site** of **minor salivary gland tumors** are oral cavity (**hard palate**)[Q]
- There are no minor salivary glands in the anterior half of the palate, so tumors arise on **posterolateral hard palate** and all of the **soft palate**[Q]
- **Malignancy varies inversely with** the **size of gland**[Q] (most of minor salivary gland tumors are malignant)

  - **Parotid** gland: **25%**[Q] malignant, **Submandibular and Sublingual gland: 50%**[Q] malignant, **Minor salivary glands: 75%**[Q] malignant

- **Open** surgical **biopsy is contraindicated**[Q], as it can cause **tumor seeding** of the track

  - Most salivary gland tumors are **radioresistant**[Q]
  - **Neutron therapy** has been used in the management of **unresectable** salivary gland **tumors**[Q]
  - Name of incision for parotidectomy: **Sistrunk incision**[Q]

Indications of Radiotherapy in Salivary Gland Tumors	
High grade tumors[Q]	**Bone invasion**[Q]
Large primary lesions[Q]	Cervical **LN metastasis**[Q]
Perineural invasion[Q]	**Positive surgical margins**[Q]

■ PLEOMORPHIC ADENOMA

PLEOMORPHIC ADENOMA

- It is **MC benign** salivary gland tumor and **MC tumor** of **major salivary glands**[Q].
- **MC site** is **parotid tail (superficial lobe)**[Q]
- Less common in the submandibular glands and sublingual glands, relatively rare in minor salivary glands.

Contd...

Contd...

> - Known as **mixed tumor**[Q] as it is composed of both **epithelial & mesenchymal** components
> - Encapsulated but sends **pseudopodia (finger-like projections)**[Q] into surrounding glands, **enucleation** is **not done** to avoid recurrence.

- Pleomorphic adenoma is **unicentric** but **recurrences are multicentric**[Q]
- Usually **not involve** the **facial nerve**.

Clinical Features

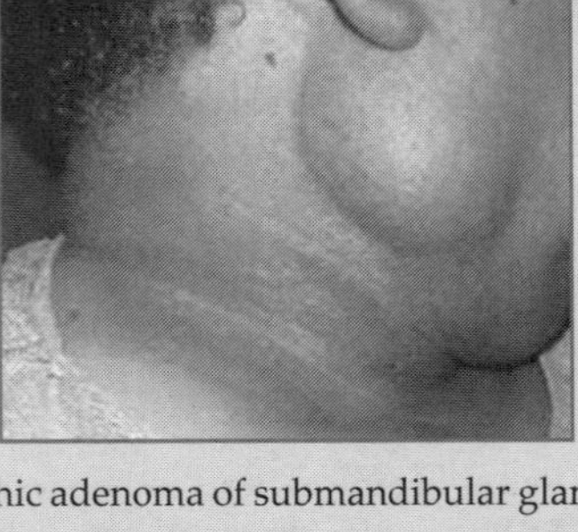

- Presents as **painless swelling** without any appreciable change in size, with typical site at **below, in front** and **behind** the **ear lobule**[Q].
- Slow growing lobular tumor affecting **women** around **40 years.**
- Pleomorphic adenoma involving deep lobe may push the tonsil and pillars of fauces towards midline and known as **dumbbell tumor**[Q] with component both in neck and oral cavity.

Diagnosis

- **FNAC** is diagnostic[Q]

Treatment

- Superficial parotidectomy (**Patey's operation**)[Q]   • Excision of whole gland in cases of pleomorphic adenoma of submandibular gland
- Name of incision for parotidectomy: **Lazy 'S', modified Blairs or Sistrunk incision**

Complications

- **Malignant change (3-5%)**
  - Known as **carcinoma ex pleomorphic adenoma** or **malignant mixed tumor**
  - **Rapid growth, pain,** paraesthesia, **enlarged cervical LN** and restriction of jaw movements, **facial weakness** or skin invasion and **fixation of mastoid tip** is suggestive of malignant transformation
  - Histological findings suggestive of malignant change are microscopic foci of **necrosis, hemorrhage, calcification** and **excessive hyalinization**[Q]
- **Recurrence**[Q], particularly after enucleation

■ WARTHIN'S TUMOR (PAPILLARY CYSTADENOMA LYMPHOMATOSUM)

WARTHIN'S TUMOR (PAPILLARY CYSTADENOMA LYMPHOMATOSUM)

- **Second MC benign tumor** of the **parotid gland**[Q]
- Derived from **salivary tissues inclusion** in **lymph nodes**[Q] (so can arise from cervical nodes)
- Occurs **exclusively in parotid gland**[Q] and almost always occur in the **lower portion of parotid**[Q] overlying the angle of mandible.

> - Consists of **both epithelial & lymphoid elements**[Q] thus known as **adenolymphoma** (probably arises from remnants of parotid tissue trapped in lymph nodes within the parotid gland)
> - More common in **males**[Q], in **5th to 7th decade**[Q].
> - Associated with **smoking**[Q], bilateral in **10%**[Q] cases, never involves facial nerve.
> - It is **well encapsulated, cystic**, extremely slow growing tumor, **never turns malignant**[Q].

- Peculiar feature of Warthin's tumor: **'hot' spot in 99mTc-pertechnate scan**[Q]. (Other tumors of the parotid show 'cold' spot)

Histopathology

- **Papillary cystic pattern** lined with columnar oncocytes and cuboidal cells with **marked lymphoid component**[Q]
- **Lined by a double layer of neoplastic epithelial cells**[Q] resting on a dense lymphoid stroma sometimes bearing germinal centers.

> - **The double layer of lining cells distinctive**[Q], with a surface palisade of columnar cells resting on a layer of cuboidal to polygonal cells

Diagnosis

- **FNAC** is **best diagnostic modality**

Treatment

- **Superficial parotidectomy**[Q]

■ MUCOEPIDERMOID CARCINOMA

MUCOEPIDERMOID CARCINOMA

- **MC malignant tumor** of **parotid, MC radiation induced neoplasm**[Q] of parotid
- **MC malignant** salivary gland tumor in children[Q]

Contd...

Contd...

- Consist of admixture of **squamous cells, mucous secreting cells, intermediate cells** and **clear** or **hydropic cells**[Q]
- Include two major elements- **mucin producing cells** and **epithelial cells**[Q] of epidermoid variety

- Greater the epidermoid content, more malignant is the behavior
- Usually **not causes facial paralysis**[Q]
- Of two types: Low grade and high grade

Low-grade Type	High-grade Type
• Well circumscribed mass having **cystic mucinous**[Q] material	• Grossly **infiltrative** and has less tendency to cyst formation (**hard tumor**)
• **Mucin producing**[Q] cells predominate	• **Squamous cells** predominate
• **Well differentiated**	• **Poorly differentiated**[Q]
• More common in **children**	• Less common
• **TOC: Superficial** or **total** parotidectomy[Q]	• **TOC: Total parotidectomy** +/- radical neck dissection

■ ADENOID CYSTIC CARCINOMA

ADENOID CYSTIC CARCINOMA

- **Second MC malignant tumor** after mucoepidermoid carcinoma[Q]
- **MC malignant tumor** in **submandibular, sublingual and minor salivary glands**[Q]

- **MC site of origin** is in **minor salivary glands** located in **oral cavity (hard palate)** followed by **sinonasal tract**[Q]
- MC type is **Cribriform pattern**[Q], and is characterized by "Swiss-Cheese" appearance[Q]
- It has **neurotropic properties**, MC involved nerves are **facial nerve**[Q], mandibular (V3) and maxillary branches of trigeminal nerve.

- **Skip lesions**[Q] along nerves are common.
- May grow along **Haversian system** of bone without showing bone destruction
- It is **traecherous tumor** as it appears benign even when it is malignant

Clinical Features

- Characterized by its **tendency to invade perineural tissues** and **lymphatics**, thus causes **pain**.
- High incidence of **distant metastasis** but **indolent growth**[Q]

- Incidence of **distant metastasis** is correlated with **stage of disease** (size of primary tumor and status of LNs)
- MC site of metastasis is **lung**, lung metastasis are **usually multiple** and **prolonged survival** without treatment is **not unusual**[Q]

Diagnosis

- Best diagnostic modality is **FNAC**[Q]
- **MRI** is **radiological IOC** as it detects **early perineural spread** and **intracranial extension**[Q]

Treatments

- **Radical excision** (irrespective of benign appearance) with **largest cuff of normal tissues** around the boundaries of tumor (poorly incapsulated with infiltrating nature)[Q].
- **Post-op radiotherapy** should be given if **margins are positive**[Q].

■ SIALOLITHIASIS

SIALOLITHIASIS

- **80% of all salivary gland stones occur in submandibular gland**[Q], 10% occur in parotid, 7% in sublingual and the remainder in minor salivary glands.

- **MC site is Wharton's duct**[Q] > submandibular gland substance

- **Composition of stone: Calcium and magnesium phosphate** or **carbonate**[Q]
- Due to deposition of **calcium salts**, 80% stones are **radio opaque**[Q]

Submandibular Salivary Gland Calculi are More Common than Parotid Because

- **Wharton's duct** has **long, curved and upward course** and is **hooked** by **lingual nerve** leading to **inadequate drainage**[Q]
- Secretion is **more viscid**[Q] than parotid gland secretion

Contd...

Contd...

Clinical Features
- **Pain** and **swelling**[Q] of submandibular region, aggregated by food, classically by sucking a lemon
- **Stone impacted** in the **duct** may produce the referred **pain** in the **tongue** due to irritation of **lingual nerve,** as it hooks around the submandibular duct[Q]

Diagnosis
- IOC for diagnosis of sialolithiasis: NCCT[Q]

Treatments
- Stone in the duct is removed by giving **incision directly over** the **stone**[Q] in long axis
- **Excision** of **submandibular gland**[Q] when stone is in the gland substance.

■ COMPLICATIONS OF PAROTIDECTOMY

COMPLICATIONS OF PAROTIDECTOMY

- **Facial nerve paresis or paralysis**[Q]
- **Frey's syndrome**[Q]
- **Sensory abnormalities (Numbness of Face)** associated with sacrifice of **greater auricular nerve**[Q]
- **Salivary fistula**[Q]

■ FREY'S SYNDROME OR AURICULOTEMPORAL SYNDROME (GUSTATORY SWEATING)

FREY'S SYNDROME OR AURICULOTEMPORAL SYNDROME (GUSTATORY SWEATING)

- It results from **damage** of **auriculotemporal**[Q] nerve during dissection in parotidectomy
- **Aberrant cross innervations** between **secretomotor parasympathetic fibers** of parotid gland and **sympathetic fibers** supplying the **sweat gland**[Q]

Clinical Feature
- **Sweating** and **erythema** over the region of parotid glands as a consequence of autonomic stimulation of salivation by smell or taste of food.

Diagnosis
- **Minor's starch iodine test**[Q]

Treatment
- **Antiperspirant (aluminium chloride)** application
- **Botulinum toxin** treatment is used for symptomatic **Frey's syndrome**
- **Surgical interruption** of secretary fibers by **tympanic neurectomy, in non-responding cases**

■ PAROTID FISTULA

PAROTID FISTULA

- Internal fistula opens inside the mouth and doesn't give rise to symptoms
- **External fistula:** gland fistula or duct fistula

Causes
- **Rupture of parotid abscess**[Q]
- Penetrating injury
- **Inadvertent incision** during **drainage of parotid abscess**[Q]
- After **superficial parotidectomy**[Q]

Clinical Presentation
- When the external fistula is **connected** to the **gland, external opening** is **pinpoint**, though discharge is present for several months, usually **closes spontaneously.**
- When external fistula is **connected** with **major duct**, there is **outpouring** of **parotid secretions** onto cheek during meals with **excoriation** of surrounding skin

Diagnosis
- **Sialograply** or **sialogram**

Treatment
- **Newman** and **Seabrock's operation**[Q] (in cases of fistula connected with main duct, this operation reconstructs the duct)

■ RANULA

RANULA

- A **cystic swelling in** the **floor of mouth** that resembles a **frog belly**[Q].
- Term ranula should only be applied to a **mucous extravasation cyst** that arises from the **sublingual gland**[Q]

Etiology

- **Commonly** the lesion is induced by **local trauma** and **duct rupture,** followed by mucin spillage into the surrounding soft tissues (**mucous extravasation phenomenon**)[Q]
- Uncommonly, it is due to **obstruction**, probably caused by mucous plug or a sialolith

Histopathology

- Mucin accumulation surrounded by granulation and fibrous tissue (**mucous extravasation phenomenon**)[Q]
- A cyst cavity, filled with mucin and lining by the ductal epithelium (mucous retention cyst)[Q]

Clinical Features

- **Exclusively** present on the **floor of mouth**[Q]
- **Usually unilateral**, lateral to midline[Q]
- **Smooth, dome shape, fluctuating** and **painless** swelling[Q]
- Color is usually **bluish.**

Diagnosis

- Diagnosis is usually made **clinically**[Q].

Treatment

- **Surgical removal** or **marsupialization**[Q].
- **MC structure injured during ranula surgery: Submandibular duct**[Q]

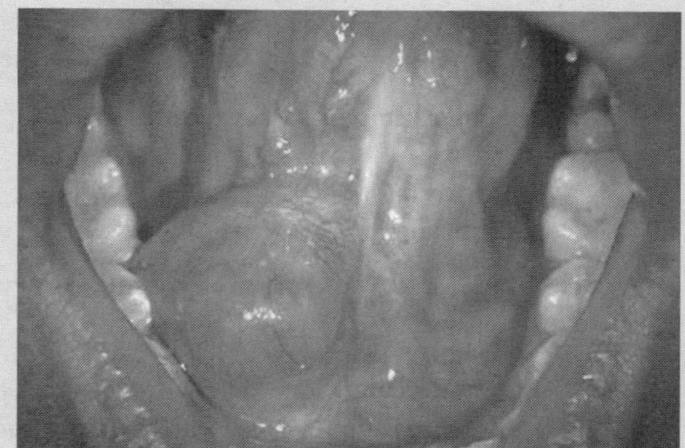

■ PLUNGING RANULA

PLUNGING RANULA

- **Intraoral ranula** with **cervical prolongation**[Q].
- Plunging ranula **extends from** the **floor** of the mouth below the mylohyoid **into** the **neck.**
- This is nearly always an **extravasation pseudocyst.**
- Presents as **soft painless, ballottable mass** with **cross fluctation**[Q].

■ SALIVARY GLAND TUMORS

1. Which among the following is most common neoplasm of salivary gland? *(Recent Question 2014, WBPG 2012, AIIMS June 98, All India 2002)*
   a. Pleomorphic adenoma
   b. Adenoid cystic carcinoma
   c. Mucoepidermoid carcinoma
   d. Mixed tumor

2. Most common tumor of parotid gland is: *(MCI June 2018, DNB 2008, 2000, AIIMS June 93)*
   a. Squamous cell carcinoma
   b. Pleomorphic adenoma
   c. Adenolymphoma
   d. None of the above

3. Best diagnostic modality for parotid swelling is: *(AIIMS Nov 94)*
   a. Enucleation
   b. FNAC
   c. Superficial parotidectomy
   d. Excisional biopsy

4. Swelling of deep lobe of parotid gland presents as swelling in: *(DNB 2001)*
   a. Parapharyngeal space
   b. Cheek
   c. Temporal region
   d. Below the ear

5. Open biopsy is done for salivary gland tumor unless they are arising from: *(Recent Question 2015)*
   a. Palate
   b. Buccal
   c. Sublingual
   d. Parotid

6. Surgical treatment of parotid tumor involving the deep lobe is: *(Recent Question 2016)*
   a. Total parotidectomy with facial nerve preservation
   b. Total parotidectomy with facial nerve sacrifice
   c. Subtotal parotidectomy
   d. Subtotal parotidectomy with facial nerve sacrifice

7. Treatment of pleomorphic adenoma without facial nerve infiltration and limited to superficial lobe:
   a. Superficial parotidectomy *(Recent Question 2016)*
   b. Total parotidectomy
   c. Parotidectomy followed by radiotherapy
   d. Observation

■ PLEOMORPHIC ADENOMA

8. A patient presented with gradually progressive painless mass since 10 years. It is firm to nodular & variable in consistency at each site. Most probable diagnosis is: *(Recent Question 2019)*

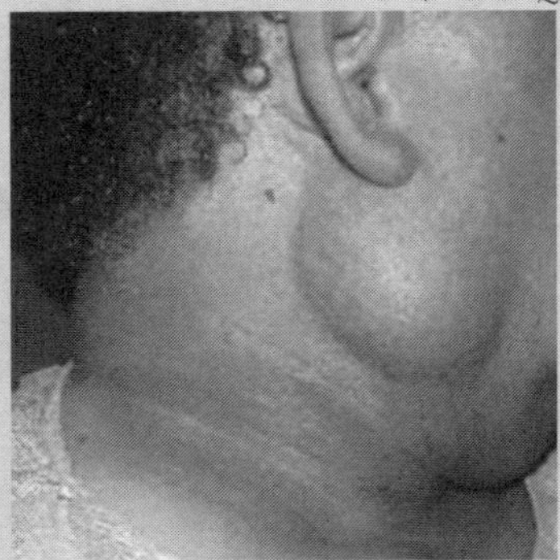

   a. Dermoid cyst
   b. Sebaceous cyst
   c. Pleomorphic adenoma
   d. Malignancy

9. True regarding benign mixed parotid tumour is: *(DNB 2005)*
   a. Slow growing and lobular
   b. Firm and capsulated
   c. 50% of parotid tumour
   d. All of the above

10. Most common tumor of parotid gland: *(MCI June 2018, MHPGMCET 2007)*
    a. Warthin's tumor
    b. Pleomorphic adenoma
    c. Adenocarcinoma
    d. Hemangioma

11. Treatment of choice for pleomorphic adenoma: *(Recent Question 2015, 2014, DNB 2008, DPG 2008, MCI Sept 2010, 2007, AIIMS Nov 2001, Nov 95, All India 97)*
    a. Superficial parotidectomy
    b. Radical parotidectomy
    c. Enucleation
    d. Radiotherapy

12. Which of the following is an indication of radiotherapy in pleomorphic adenoma of parotid? *(All India 2004)*
    a. Involvement of deep lobe
    b. 2nd histologically benign recurrence
    c. Microscopically positive margins
    d. Malignant transformation

■ WARTHIN'S TUMOR

13. True statement regarding Warthin's tumor:
    a. Common in females *(Recent Question 2016, JIPMER 2010)*
    b. Most malignant
    c. Hot spots on Tc-99 scan
    d. Most common tumor of minor salivary gland

14. Warthin's tumour is: *(DNB 2012, AIIMS May 2005, June 2003)*
    a. An adenolymphoma of parotid gland
    b. A pleomorphic adenoma of parotid
    c. A carcinoma of the parotid
    d. A carcinoma of submandibular salivary gland

15. Treatment of choice for Warthin's tumour: *(AIIMS Nov 2001, All India 98, 96)*
    a. Superficial parotidectomy
    b. Enucleation
    c. Radiotherapy
    d. Injection of a sclerosant agent

16. Hot spot on Tc-99 is seen in which parotid tumour? *(Recent Question 2016, JIPMER 2014, 2010; AIIMS May 2013)*
    a. Adenolymphoma
    b. Adenoid cystic carcinoma
    c. Acinic cell tumour
    d. Adenocarcinoma

■ MUCOEPIDERMOID CARCINOMA

17. Most common malignant tumour of parotid is: *(Recent Question 2016, DNB 2011, 2010, DPG 2008)*
    a. Epidermoid carcinoma
    b. Mucoepidermoid carcinoma
    c. Squamous cell carcinoma
    d. Adenocarcinoma

■ ADENOID CYSTIC CARCINOMA

18. The most common tumour of the minor salivary gland is: *(DNB 2013, WBPG 2012, COMEDK 2008)*
    a. Mucoepidermoid carcinoma
    b. Acinic cell carcinoma
    c. Adenoid cystic carcinoma
    d. Pleomorphic adenocarcinoma

19. **Tumor with perineural invasion:**
    (Recent Question 2015, DNB 2009, AIIMS Nov 2010, MHSSMCET 2007)
    a. Adenocarcinoma
    b. Adenoid cystic carcinoma
    c. Basal cell carcinoma
    d. Squamous cell carcinoma

20. **Which among the following parotid tumor spreads through neural sheath?**
    (Karnataka 2013, NEET Pattern, DNB 2013, AIIMS June 97, 96)
    a. Mixed parotid tumor
    b. Adenoid cystic carcinoma
    c. Squamous Cell carcinoma
    d. Oxyphilic lymphoma

■ ACINIC CELL CARCINOMA

21. **Acinic cell carcinomas of the salivary gland arise most often in the:**   *(All India 2006)*
    a. Parotid gland
    b. Minor salivary glands
    c. Submandibular gland
    d. Sublingual gland

■ CARCINOMA PAROTID

22. **All of the following statements about lymphoepithelioma of the parotid gland are true, except:**   *(All India 2009)*
    a. Parotid gland is the most common site of lymphoepithelioma in the head and neck region
    b. It is associated with EBV infection
    c. It is highly radiosensitive
    d. It is a type of squamous cell carcinoma

23. **Patient complains of painless swelling over the face with difficulty in swallowing. The appearance of the face is shown. The probable diagnosis is?**   *(MCI Dec 2018)*

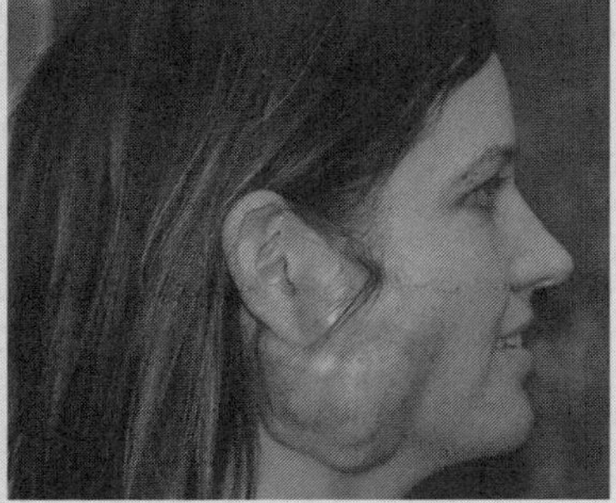

    a. Acute parotitis
    b. Cancer of parotid gland
    c. Angioedema of face
    d. Acute sialadenitis

24. **All of the following are true regarding malignant salivary gland tumours except:**   *(DNB 2010)*
    a. Painful
    b. Present with skin ulceration
    c. Cervical lymphadenopathy
    d. Simple enucleation is treatment of choice

■ SALIVARY GLAND STONES

25. **Commonest salivary gland to get stones:**   *(APPG 2015, Recent Question 2014, NEET 2013, DNB 2011, 2003, DPG 2006, MCI March 2005, 2007, AIIMS Nov 99, June 99)*
    a. Parotid
    b. Submandibular
    c. Minor salivary gland
    d. Sublingual

26. **All of the following statement regarding stones in the submandibular gland are true except:**   *(MCI March 2007)*
    a. 80% of stones occur in the submandibular gland
    b. Majority of submandibular stones are radiolucent
    c. Stones are the most common cause of obstruction within the submandibular gland
    d. Patient presents with acute swelling in the region of the submandibular gland

27. **Investigation using dye to find out stone in salivary gland:**   *(Recent Question 2013)*
    a. Sialography
    b. Mammography
    c. MR angiography
    d. USG

28. **What percent of submandibular salivary gland stones are radiopaque?**   *(MHCET 2016)*
    a. 10%
    b. 70%
    c. 80%
    d. 90%

■ PAROTIDECTOMY AND COMPLICATIONS

29. **Frey's syndrome occurs due to aberrant misdirection of fibers from salivary glands to sweat glands. These fibers come from which of the following?**   *(Recent Question 2019)*
    a. Facial nerve
    b. Trigeminal nerve
    c. Auriculotemporal nerve
    d. Glossopharyngeal nerve

30. **All of the following statements are true about Frey's syndrome except:**   *(Recent Question 2019)*
    a. Gustatory sweating
    b. Aberrant misdirection of sympathetic fibers of auriculotemporal nerve
    c. Botulinum toxin is one of the treatments suggested
    d. Less chances with enucleation than parotidectomy

31. **The 'Starch iodine test' is useful to diagnose:**   *(MHSSMCET 2011)*
    a. Wegener's granulomatosis
    b. Cat scratch disease
    c. Sarcoidosis
    d. Frey's syndrome

32. **The nerve sacrificed in parotid surgery:**   *(DNB 2013, APPG 98)*
    a. Auriculotemporal
    b. Facial
    c. Buccal
    d. Cervico facial

33. **Incision for superficial parotidectomy:**   *(WBPG 2015)*
    a. L-shaped
    b. Y-shaped
    c. S-shaped
    d. Z-shaped

■ PAROTID FISTULA

34. **Newman and Seabrook's operation is used for:**
    a. Repair of parotid fistula   *(Recent Question 2016)*
    b. For parotid calculi
    c. For carcinoma of tongue
    d. For treatment of recurrent chronic parotitis

■ RANULA

35. **Which of the following best represents 'ranula'?**
    a. A type of epulis   *(AIIMS May 2005)*
    b. A thyroglossal cyst
    c. Cystic swelling in the floor of mouth
    d. Forked uvula

36. What is the most probable diagnosis based on the given image?

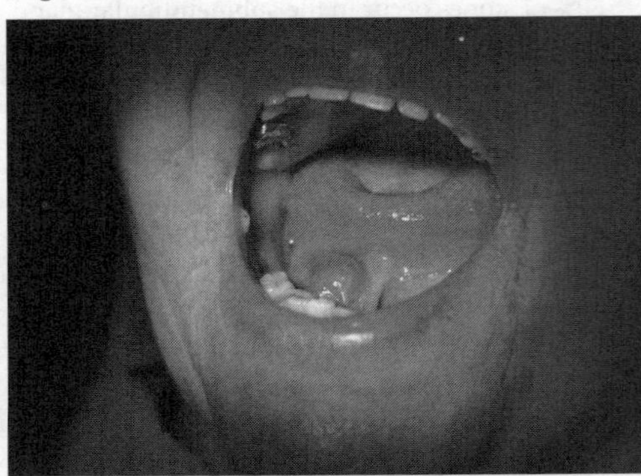

a. Pleomorphic adenoma   b. Ranula
c. Warthin's tumor   d. Adenoid cystic carcinoma

37. What is ranula?   *(DNB 2007, 2005)*
    a. Retention cyst of sublingual gland
    b. Retention cyst of submandibular gland
    c. Extravasation cyst of sublingual glands
    d. Extravasation cyst of submandibular glands

38. Excision of ranula is associated with injury to:
    (DNB 2010, MHSSMCET 2007, PGI 96)
    a. Lingual nerve
    b. Lingual artery
    c. Parotid gland
    d. Submandibular duct

39. Plunging ranula is: *(Recent Question 2015)*
    a. Cystic growth of sublingual gland
    b. Lymph node
    c. A tumor in floor of mouth
    d. None

40. Which procedure is done in case of ranula management?
    (MCI June 2019)
    a. Incision and drainage
    b. Aspiration
    c. Excision
    d. Sclerosant injection

■ SALIVARY GLANDS ANATOMY AND PHYSIOLOGY

41. In submandibular gland surgery, the nerve least likely to be injured is: *(DPG 2011, JIPMER 93)*
    a. Inferior alveolar nerve   b. Hypoglossal nerve
    c. Lingual nerve
    d. Mandibular branch of facial nerve

42. Most common location of ectopic submandibular salivary gland tissue is: *(MCI Sept 2009, UPPG 2002)*
    a. Cheek   b. Palate
    c. Angle of mandible   d. Tongue

43. In surgery of submandibular salivary gland, nerve often involved: *(PGI June 97)*
    a. Hypoglossal   b. Glossopharyngeal
    c. Facial   d. Lingual

■ SALIVARY GLAND TUMORS

1. **Ans. a. Pleomorphic adenoma** *(Ref: Bailey 27/e p787; Devita 9/e p774; Cancer of the Head and Neck by Suen and Myer 4/e p480-490)*

- **MC neoplasm** of **salivary gland: Pleomorphic adenoma**[Q]
- **MC malignant tumor** of salivary gland: **Mucoepidermoid carcinoma**[Q]
- **MC neoplasm** of salivary gland **in children: Hemangioma**[Q]
- **MC malignant tumor** of salivary gland **in children: Mucoepidermoid carcinoma**[Q]
- **MC malignant tumor** of **minor salivary glands: Adenoid cystic carcinoma**[Q]

ALL SALIVARY GLAND TUMORS ARE MOST COMMON IN PAROTID EXCEPT

- **Adenoid cystic carcinoma: MC malignant tumor** of **minor salivary glands**[Q]
- **Squamous cell carcinoma:** Mostly seen in **submandibular gland**[Q]

2. **Ans. b. Pleomorphic adenoma**
3. **Ans. b. FNAC**
4. **Ans. a. Parapharyngeal space**
5. **Ans. d. Parotid**
6. **Ans. a. Total parotidectomy with facial nerve preservation**
7. **Ans. a. Superficial parotidectomy**

■ PLEOMORPHIC ADENOMA

8. **Ans. c. Pleomorphic adenoma** *(Ref: Bailey 27/e p787)*
9. **Ans. d. All of the above**
10. **Ans. b. Pleomorphic adenoma**
11. **Ans. a. Superficial parotidectomy**
12. **Ans. c. Microscopically positive margins** *(Ref: Devita 9/e p776; Cancer of the Head and Neck by Suen and Myer 4/e p499-501)*

■ WARTHIN'S TUMOR

13. **Ans. c. Hot spots on Tc-99 scan** *(Ref: Bailey 27/e p789; Devita 9/e p774; Cancer of the Head and Neck by Suen and Myer 4/e p414)*
14. **Ans. a. An adenolymphoma of parotid gland**
15. **Ans. a. Superficial parotidectomy**
16. **Ans. a. Adenolymphoma**

■ MUCOEPIDERMOID CARCINOMA

17. **Ans. b. Mucoepidermoid carcinoma** *(Ref: Bailey 27/e p788; Devita 9/e p774-777; Cancer of the Head and Neck by Suen and Myer 4/e p489)*

■ ADENOID CYSTIC CARCINOMA

18. **Ans. c. Adenoid cystic carcinoma** *(Ref: Bailey 27/e p727,778; Devita 9/e p777-778; Cancer of the Head and Neck by Suen and Myer 4/e p487-489)*
19. **Ans. b. Adenoid cystic carcinoma**
20. **Ans. b. Adenoid cystic carcinoma**

■ ACINIC CELL CARCINOMA

21. **Ans. a. Parotid gland** *(Ref: Devita 9/e p774; Cancer of the Head and Neck by Suen and Myer 4/e p489-490)*

■ CARCINOMA PAROTID

22. **Ans. a. Parotid gland is the most common site of Lymphoepethelioma in the Head and Neck region** *(Ref: Devita 9/e p729, 752, 774)*
    - The **most common site** of **limphoepithelioma** is the **nasopharynx**[Q]. Limphoepithelioma occurs **rarely in** the **parotid** and **submandibular glands.**

LIMPHOEPITHELIOMA

- Lymphoepithelioma: Undifferentiated carcinoma of the nasopharyngeal type
- Lymphoepithelioma is a **variant of squamous cell carcinoma**[Q] that arises in lymphoid bearing areas
- Found **most commonly in** the **nasopharynx**[Q]
- **Rarely occur in parotid** and **submandibular glands**[Q]

Contd…

Contd...

Common sites of Lymphoepethelioma in Head and Neck		
• **Nasopharynx (MC site)**[Q]	• **Faucial tonsils**	• **Lingual tonsils (base of tongue)**

- Histologically the squamous component is highly undifferentiated while the lymphoid component is essentially benign (non-neoplastic lymphocytes)
- **EBV** is **commonly linked** when this tumor is located in the **nasopharynx**[Q]
- **High tendency to metastasize** and is **exquisitely radiosensitive**[Q]

Important characteristic features	
• **High tendency to metastasize**[Q]	• **Extreme radiosensitivity**[Q]

23. Ans. b. Cancer of parotid gland *(Ref: Bailey 27/e p786, 788, 795)*

24. Ans. d. Simple enucleation is treatment of choice

■ SALIVARY GLAND STONES

25. Ans. b. Submandibular *(Ref: Bailey 27/e p780)*   26. Ans. b. Majority of submandibular stones are radiolucent

27. Ans. a. Sialography *(Ref: Sutton's radiology 7/e p535, Bailey & Love 25/e p760)*

28. Ans. c. 80%

■ PAROTIDECTOMY AND COMPLICATIONS

29. Ans. c. Auriculotemporal nerve *(Ref: Bailey 27/e p792)*

30. Ans. b. Aberrant misdirection of sympathetic fibers of auriculotemporal nerve *(Ref: Bailey 27/e p792)*

31. Ans. d. Frey's syndrome   32. Ans. b. Facial   33. Ans. c. S-shaped

■ PAROTID FISTULA

34. Ans. a. Repair of parotid fistula

■ RANULA

35. Ans. c. Cystic swelling in the floor of mouth *(Ref: Bailey 27/e p779)*

36. Ans. b. Ranula *(Ref: Bailey 27/e p779)*   37. Ans. c. Extravasation cyst of sublingual glands

38. Ans. d. Submandibular duct *(Ref: Clinical Surgery by Rob's and Smith vol-9/56)*

> The **treatment of ranula** constitutes a problem, owing to technical **difficulty of complete excision without damage to adjacent structures such as submandibular duct.**

39. Ans. a. Cystic growth of sublingual gland

40. Ans. c. Excision *(Ref: Bailey 27/e p779)*

■ SALIVARY GLANDS ANATOMY AND PHYSIOLOGY

41. Ans. a. Inferior alveolar nerve *(Ref: Bailey 27/e p780)*

Important anatomical relationships of the submandibular glands	
• **Lingual nerve**[Q]	• **Facial artery**[Q]
• **Hypoglossal nerve**[Q]	• **Marginal mandibular branch** of the **facial nerve**
• Anterior **facial vein**[Q]	

42. Ans. c. Angle of mandible *(Ref: Bailey 27/e p780)*

Ectopic/Aberrant Salivary Gland Tissue

- **MC ectopic salivary tissue** is the **Stafne bone cyst.**
- This presents as an **asymptomatic, clearly demarcated radiolucency** of the **angle of the mandible,** characteristically **below the inferior dental neurovascular bundle**[Q].
- It is formed by **invagination into the bone** on the lingual aspect of the mandible **of an ectopic lobe** of the **juxtaposed submandibular gland**[Q].
- **No treatment** is required[Q].

43. Ans. a. Hypoglossal, c. Facial, d. Lingual

Neck

■ CAROTID BODY TUMOR

CAROTID BODY TUMOR (CHEMODECTOMA)

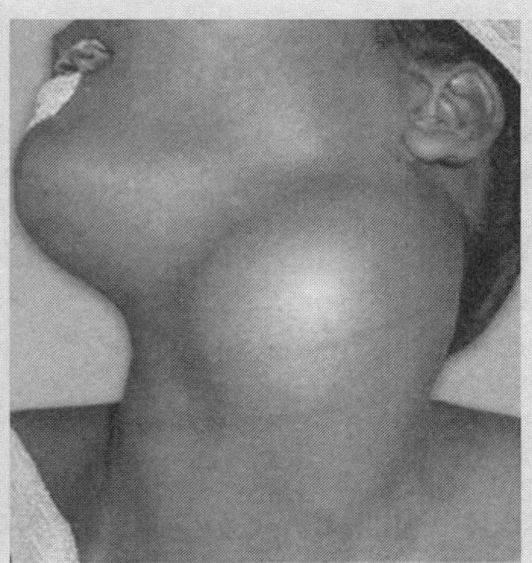

- Arises from **chemoreceptor cells**[Q] on the **medial side** of carotid bulb
- Histologically it is a **non-chromaffin paraganglioma**[Q]
- Usually **benign, unifocal** and **nonhereditary, Schamblin classification** is used for **carotid body tumour**
- Associated with **pheochromocytoma**[Q]

> - **Higher incidence** in areas where **people live at high altitudes** because of **chronic hypoxia** leading to **carotid body hyperplasia**.

Clinical Features

- Present most commonly in the **5th decade**[Q]
- Approximately **10%** have **family history**[Q].
- Patient presents with a **long history** of several years of a **slowly enlarging painless lump** at the **carotid bifurcation.**
- Mass is **firm, rubbery, pulsatile** and is **mobile from side to side** but not up and down
- A **bruit**[Q] may also be present

Diagnosis

- Doppler study
- **Carotid angiogram: Lyre sign**[Q] (**splaying** of **internal** & **external** carotid arteries)
- **FNAC** & **biopsy** are **contraindicated**[Q] because of their **highly vascular nature**

Treatment

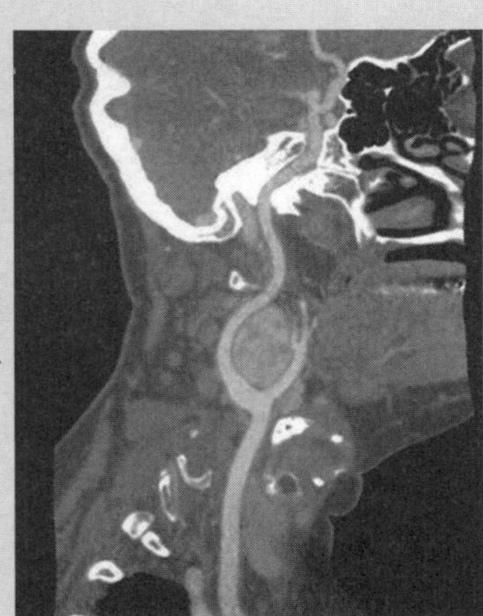

- Because these tumors **rarely metastasize**[Q] and their **overall rate of growth** is **slow**, the need for **surgical removal** must be **considered carefully** as complication of surgery are potentially serious.
- **Operation** is **best avoided in elderly patients**[Q].
- **Preoperative embolization** is performed for tumors **>3 cm.**
- Tumors **>5 cm** are associated with a need for **concurrent carotid artery replacement.**

Complications

- **Most frequent sequela from resection: Cranial nerve injury** (MC-**superior laryngeal nerve**[Q])
- **First-bite syndrome**[Q]: **Pain** with the **initiation of mastication**
- **Excision of bilateral carotid body tumors** may lead to **baroreceptor failure,** with **wide fluctuations in BP.**

■ CYSTIC HYGROMA

CYSTIC HYGROMA

- Cystic hygromas are **multiloculated cystic spaces**[Q] lined by endothelial cells
- It results due to **sequestration of** a portion of **jugular lymph sac** from the **lymphatic system**[Q].
- **Cysts are filled with clear lymph** and are **lined by endothelium**[Q].
- **Turner's syndrome** is associated with cystic hygroma[Q].
- **Most** cystic hygromas **involve** the **lymphatic jugular sacs**

Contd...

Contd...

> - MC site: Posterior neck region[Q] (Posterior triangle[Q])
> - Other **common sites**: Axilla, mediastinum, inguinal & retroperitoneal regions[Q]
> - Approximately **50%** of them **present at birth**[Q]
> - It may show **spontaneous regression**[Q]

Clinical Features

- Usually present as **soft cystic masses** that distort the surrounding anatomy, can result in acute airway obstruction.
- Usually **manifests in** the **neonates** or in **early infancy**[Q] (**50%** present **at birth**).
- Prone to **infection** & **hemorrhage** within the mass.
- Swelling is **soft** & **partially compressible** and invariably increases in size when the child coughs or cries.

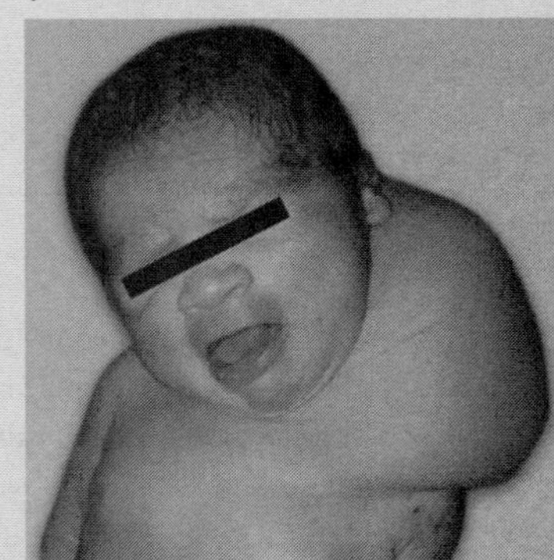

> - **Characteristic features: Brilliantly translucent**[Q]

Diagnosis

- **IOC for diagnosis: MRI**[Q]
- **MRI** play a **crucial role in preoperative planning**[Q]

Treatment

- **Complete surgical excision** is the **preferred treatment**[Q].
- **Injection of sclerosing agents**[Q] such as **bleomycin** or **OK-432 (Picibanil)**, derived from **Streptococcus pyogenes** may eradicate the cystic hygroma.

■ BRANCHIAL CLEFT REMNANTS

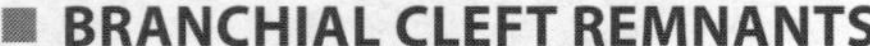

BRANCHIAL CLEFT REMNANTS

- **Branchial cleft remnants** typically present as a **lateral neck mass**[Q] on a toddler.
- Structures of the head & neck are derived from **6 pairs of branchial arches**, their intervening **clefts** & **pouches**.

> - **All branchial remnants** are **present at the time of birth**; however, they are **often not recognized** until later in life.
> - These lesions may present as **sinuses, fistulas, or cartilaginous rests in infants**[Q].
> - They occur **more commonly as cysts in older children** and **adolescents**[Q].

Branchial Cleft Remnants

First Branchial Cleft Remnants	Second Branchial Cleft Remnants	Third Branchial Cleft Remnants
- Typically located in the **front** or **back of** the **ear** or in the **upper neck near** the **mandible**[Q]. - **Fistulas** typically **course through** the **parotid gland**, deep or **through branches of the facial nerve**, and **end in** the **external auditory canal**[Q].	- **Most common**[Q] - **External ostium** is **located along** the **anterior border** of the **SCM muscle**, in the vicinity of the **upper half to lower third** of the muscle[Q]. - **Stepladder counterincisions** are **often necessary** to excise the **fistula completely**[Q]. - Typically, the **fistula penetrates platysma, ascends along** the **carotid sheath** to the level of **hyoid bone**, and **turns medially** to **extend between carotid artery bifurcation**[Q]. - The fistula then **courses behind** the **posterior belly of digastric** and **stylohyoid muscles** to end in the **tonsillar fossa**[Q].	- Third branchial cleft remnants usually **do not have associated sinuses** or **fistulas** - **Located in** the **suprasternal notch** or **clavicular region**[Q]. - **Most often contain cartilage**[Q] - **Present** clinically as a **firm mass** or **subcutaneous abscess**[Q].

■ BRANCHIAL ABNORMALITIES

Branchial Abnormalities

Branchial Cyst	Branchial Fistula
• Develops from **vestigial remnants of 2nd branchial cleft**[Q]	• Branchial fistula may be **unilateral** or **bilateral**[Q]
• Lined by **squamous epithelium**[Q]	• Thought to represent a **persistent 2nd branchial cleft**[Q].
• Contains **thick, turbid fluid** full of **cholesterol crystals**[Q].	• Tract is **lined by ciliated columnar epithelium**[Q]
• Cyst usually **presents in** the **upper neck** in **early** or **middle adulthood**[Q]	• There may be a small amount of **recurrent mucous** or **mucopurulent discharge** onto the neck[Q].
• Found at the **junction of upper third & middle third** of the **SCM muscle** at its **anterior border**[Q].	• **External orifice** is nearly **always situated** in the **lower third** of the **neck near** anterior border of SCM[Q]
• **Fluctuant swelling** that may transilluminate and is often **soft** in its early stages[Q].	• **Internal orifice** is located on the **anterior aspect** of **posterior faucial pillar** just **behind the tonsil**[Q].
• **USG** and **FNAC aid diagnosis**	• **Internal aspect** of the tract **may end blindly** at or close to the lateral pharyngeal wall, **constituting a sinus rather than a fistula.**
• **Treatment** is by **complete excision**[Q]	• The **tract follows the same path** as a branchial cyst and **requires complete excision**, often by **more than one transverse incision** in the neck[Q].

■ CERVICAL RIB

CERVICAL RIB

- **Rib arising from 7th cervical vertebra**[Q]
- **MC on right side**[Q]

Types

1. **Complete**: Reaches **up to 1st thoracic rib**[Q]
2. **Bulbous end**: Has a **bulbous end**
3. **Tapering end**: Rib **tapers**
4. **Fibrous band**: Rib is represented by thick fibrous band

Clinical Features

- Cervical rib with **local symptoms**: Lump & tenderness in supraclavicular fossa[Q]
- Cervical rib with **vascular symptoms**: Pain, pallor & pulselessness[Q]
- Cervical rib with **nerve pressure symptoms**: Pain & paraesthesia along **medial aspect of forearm & hand**[Q]

Diagnosis

- Diagnosed by **X-ray of neck**[Q]

Treatment

- **Mild cases**: Sling exercise
- **In severe cases**: Scalenotomy (resection of scalenus anterior muscles)
- **In troublesome cases**: Removal of cervical rib[Q]

■ CERVICAL LYMPH NODES

CERVICAL LYMPH NODES

- **Cervical lymphatic nodal basins** contain 50-70 lymph nodes per side
- **Virchow or left supraclavicular nodes** are included in **level IV**[Q].
- Divided into seven levels

Level	Lymph Node
IA	• **Submental**[Q]
IB	• **Submandibular**[Q]
II	• **Upper**[Q] jugular
III	• **Middle**[Q] jugular
IV	• **Lower**[Q] jugular
V	• **Posterior triangular**[Q]
VI	• **Anterior compartmental or central**[Q]
VII	• **Superior mediastinal**[Q]

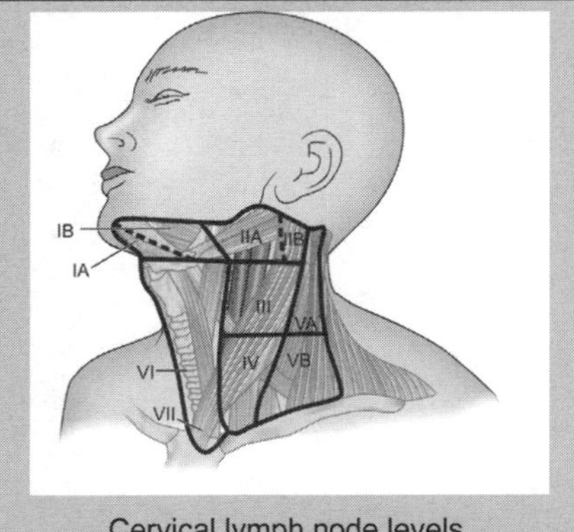

Cervical lymph node levels

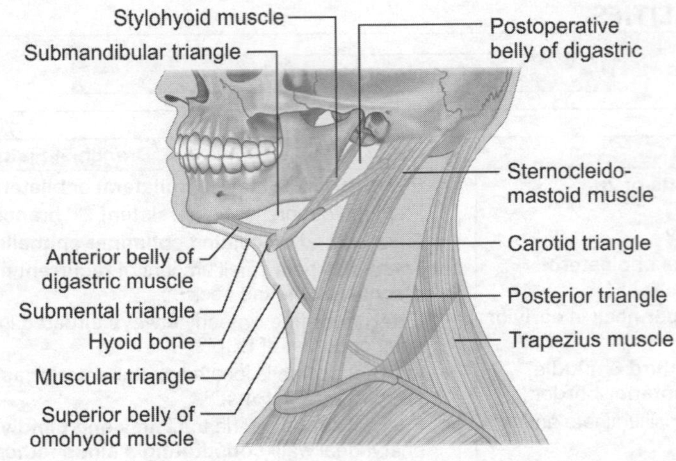

■ NECK DISSECTION

Neck Dissection

Comprehensive Neck Dissection

- **Radical Neck Dissection:** Removal of lymph nodes **I-V** + **spinal accessory nerve** + **internal jugular vein** + **sternocleidomastoid muscle**[Q]
- **Extended Radical Neck Dissection**: Radical Neck Dissection + removal of **one or more groups** of lymph nodes, **non-lymphatic structures** or both
- **Bilateral Radical Neck Dissection**
- **Modified Radical Neck Dissection**: Removal of level **I-V lymph nodes** with- (Mnemonic: **SISm**)
  - **Type I:** preserves only **spinal accessory nerve**[Q]
  - **Type II:** preserves both **spinal accessory nerve** and **internal jugular vein**[Q]
  - **Type III:** preserves **spinal accessory nerve, internal jugular vein and sternocleidomastoid muscle**[Q] (**Functional neck dissection**[Q])

Selective Neck Dissection

- **Supraomohyoid Neck Dissection:** Removal of level I-III LNs[Q]
- **Extended supraomohyoid Neck Dissection:** Removal of level I-IV LNs[Q]
- **Posterolateral Neck Dissection:** Removal of level II-V LNs + **suboccipital** LNs + **retroauricular** LNs
- **Lateral Neck Dissection:** Removal of level II-V LNs + **internal jugular vein**
- **Central Compartment Neck Dissection:** Removal of **level VI** LNs

Multiple Choice Questions

■ CAROTID BODY TUMOR

1. A 40-years old patient is suffering from carotid body tumor. Which of the following is the best choice of treatment for him? *(AIIMS Nov 2004)*
   a. Excision of tumor
   b. Radiotherapy
   c. Chemotherapy
   d. Carotid artery ligation both proximal and distal to the tumor

2. Which one is not true regarding carotid body tumour?
   a. Unilateral *(Recent Question 2016, AIIMS June 97)*
   b. Surgical resection is the treatment
   c. Non-chromaffin paraganglioma
   d. Middle age group is affected

■ CYSTIC HYGROMA

3. Cystic hygroma may be associated with: *(MCI March 2005)*
   a. Turner's syndrome
   b. Klinefelter's syndrome
   c. Down's syndrome
   d. All of the above

4. This is the image of a newborn baby. The swelling is:
   a. Transilluminant
   b. Brilliantly transilluminant
   c. Translucent
   d. Brilliantly translucent

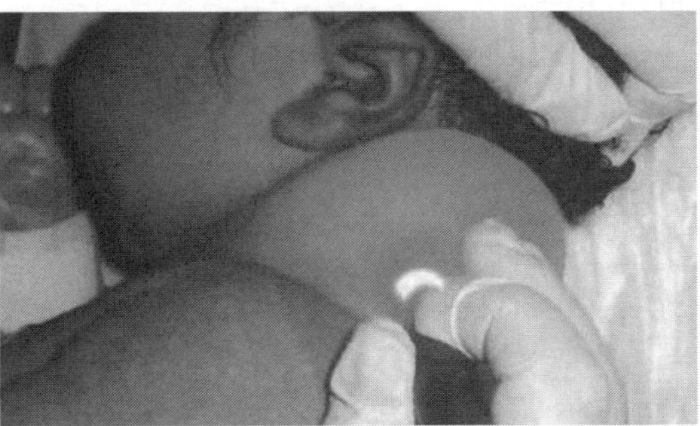

5. Cystic hygroma is known to occur in all except:
   (Karnataka 2005, MHPGMCET 2002)
   a. Calf
   b. Neck
   c. Axilla
   d. Mediastinum

6. Treatment of choice for cystic hygroma:
   (DNB 2013, MHPGMCET 2007)
   a. Percutaneous aspiration
   b. Intralesional sclerosant injection
   c. En-bloc resection
   d. Surgical excision

7. Cystic compressible, translucent swelling in the posterior triangle of neck: *(DNB 2008, All India 89)*
   a. Cystic hygroma
   b. Branchial cyst
   c. Thyroglossal cyst
   d. Dermoid cyst

8. The following are examples of Retention cysts due to blockade of excretory duct except one which is an example of Distension cyst due to exudation. Which is the one? *(APPG 2016)*
   a. Cystic hygroma
   b. Sebaceous cyst
   c. Bartholin's cyst
   d. Ranula

■ BRANCHIAL CYST AND FISTULA

9. True about branchial anomaly: *(AIIMS Nov 2006)*
   a. Cysts are more common than sinuses
   b. For sinuses surgery is not always indicated
   c. Cysts present with dysphagia and hoarseness of voice
   d. Most commonly due to 2nd branchial remnant

10. Branchial cyst arises from which branchial cleft?
    a. First
    b. Second *(MCI Sept 2009)*
    c. Third
    d. Fourth

11. The commonest site of branchial cysts is:
    (MCI June 2018, All India 94)
    a. Upper 1/3rd of the SCM
    b. Lower 1/3rd of the SCM
    c. Upper 2/3rd of the SCM
    d. Lower 2/3rd of the SCM

12. Commonest treatment of branchial cyst: *(HPU 2005)*
    a. Cystectomy
    b. Aspiration
    c. Excision
    d. Nothing done

13. Brachial cyst is lined by: *(Recent Question 2017)*
    a. Columnar epithelium
    b. Cuboidal epithelium
    c. Squamous epithelium
    d. Ciliated columnar epithelium

■ THYROGLOSSAL CYST AND FISTULA

14. Excision of the hyoid bone is done in: *(HPU 2005)*
    a. Branchial cyst
    b. Branchial fistula
    c. Thyroglossal cyst
    d. Sublingual dermoids

15. Thyroglossal fistula develops due to: *(Kerala 91)*
    a. Developmental anomaly
    b. Injury
    c. Incomplete removal of thyroglossal cyst
    d. Inflammatory disorder

■ CERVICAL RIB

16. Adson's test is positive in: *(Kerala 89)*
    a. Cervical rib
    b. Cervical spondylosis
    c. Cervical fracture
    d. Cervical dislocation

■ NECK DISSECTION

17. Structures preserved in radical neck dissection is:
    (Recent Question 2017, All India 2000)
    a. Vagus nerve
    b. Submandibular gland
    c. Sternocleidomastoid
    d. Internal Jugular Vein

18. Which structure is preserved during modified radical neck dissection? *(DNB 2004)*
    a. Phrenic nerve
    b. Submandibular gland
    c. Sternocleidomastoid
    d. Thoracic duct

19. Level V cervical nodes includes: *(MCI Sept 2007)*
    a. Upper jugular nodes
    b. Middle jugular nodes
    c. Lower jugular nodes
    d. Posterior triangle nodes

20. In radical neck dissection, which structure is not removed?
    a. Cervical group of lymph nodes *(MCI March 2005)*
    b. Sternocleidomastoid muscle
    c. Internal jugular vein
    d. None of the above

21. In extended supraomohyoid neck dissection, lymph lode dissection is done up to: *(Recent Question 2016)*
    a. 2   b. 3   *(MHSSMCET 2010)*
    c. 4   d. 5

22. Structures preserved in functional radical dissection of the neck: *(Recent Question 2017)*
    a. Internal jugular vein   b. Sternomastoid
    c. Lymph nodes   d. Accessory nerve

23. Radical dissection of neck includes all except: *(Recent Question 2017)*
    a. Cervical lymph nodes   b. Sternocleidomastoid
    c. Phrenic nerves   d. Internal jugular vein

24. A nerve injured in radical neck dissection leads to loss of sensation in medial side of the arm, nerve injured is:
    a. Long thoracic nerve   *(DNB 2014)*
    b. Thoracodorsal nerve
    c. Dorsal scapular nerve
    d. Medial cutaneous nerve of arm

25. Removal of level I, II, III, IV lymph node in neck is called: *(Recent Question 2016)*
    a. Extended supraomohyoid dissection
    b. Supraomohyoid dissection
    c. Anterolateral dissection
    d. Posterolateral dissection

Explanations

■ CAROTID BODY TUMOR

1. Ans. a. Excision of tumor
2. Ans. None

■ CYSTIC HYGROMA

3. Ans. a. Turner's syndrome *(Ref: Sabiston 20/e p1861; Schwartz 11/e p1711-1712, 10/e 598, 1852; Bailey 27/e p754)*
4. Ans. b. Brilliantly transilluminant
5. Ans. a. Calf
6. Ans. d. Surgical excision   7. Ans. a. Cystic hygroma   8. Ans. a. Cystic hygroma

■ BRANCHIAL CYST AND FISTULA

9. Ans. d. Most commonly due to 2nd branchial remnant *(Ref: Sabiston 20/e p1862; Schwartz 11/e p649, 10/e p598,1602; Bailey 27/e p753-754)*
10. Ans. b. Second
11. Ans. a. Upper 1/3rd of the SCM
12. Ans. c. Excision
13. Ans. c. Squamous epithelium *(Ref: Sabiston 20/e p1862; Schwartz 11/e p649, 10/e p598; Bailey 27/e p753)*

■ THYROGLOSSAL CYST AND FISTULA

14. Ans. c. Thyroglossal cyst
15. Ans. c. Incomplete removal of thyroglossal cyst

■ CERVICAL RIB

16. Ans. a. Cervical rib

■ NECK DISSECTION

17. Ans. a. Vagus nerve
18. Ans. c. Sternocleidomastoid
19. Ans. d. Posterior triangle nodes *(Ref: Sabiston 20/e p792; Schwartz 11/e p647, 10/e p595-597; Bailey 27/e p728,729,764,800,801)*
20. Ans. d. None of the above
21. Ans. c. 4 *(Ref: Sabiston 20/e p794; Schwartz 11/e p647, 10/e p595; Bailey 27/e p758-759; Cancer of the Head and Neck by Suen and Myer 4/e p416-418)*
22. Ans. a. Internal jugular vein; b. Sternomastoid; d. Accessory nerve
23. Ans. c. Phrenic nerves
24. Ans. d. Medial cutaneous nerve of arm *(Ref: Bailey 25/e p733)*
25. Ans. a. Extended supraomohyoid dissection

Facial Injuries and Abnormalities

■ CLEFT LIP AND CLEFT PALATE

CLEFT LIP AND PALATE

- **Clefts** of the **lip, alveolus & hard** and **soft palate** are the **MC congenital abnormalities** of the **orofacial structures**[Q].
- Frequently **occur as isolated deformities** but **can be associated with** other medical conditions, particularly **congenital heart disease**[Q].

> - **Incomplete clefts** affect only a portion of the lip and contain a **bridge of tissue connecting** the **central & lateral lip elements**, referred to as **Simonart's band**[Q].
> - **Cleft lip** is due to **non-fusion of maxillary process** with **medial nasal process**[Q].
> - **Unilateral cleft lip** is associated with **posterior displacement** of **alar cartilage**[Q]

Incidence

- **Highest incidence** reported for **cleft lip & palate** occurs in the **Indian tribes of Montana**, USA (1:276).
- **Cleft lip/palate** predominates **in males**[Q]
- **Cleft palate alone** appears to be **more common in females**[Q].

> | - **Incidence of cleft lip & palate is 1:600 live births**[Q] | - **Incidence of isolated cleft palate is 1:1000 live births**[Q]. |
> | --- | --- |

Distribution

- In **unilateral cleft lip** the deformity affects the **left side**[Q] **in 60%** of cases.

Typical Distribution of Cleft Types		
- Cleft lip alone: 15%	- Cleft lip & palate: 45% (MC)[Q]	- Isolated cleft palate: 40%

Etiology of cleft lip and palate

- **Etiology of cleft lip & palate:** Genetic predisposition & a contributory environmental component[Q].
- **Environmental factors:** Maternal epilepsy[Q] & drugs (**steroids, diazepam & phenytoin**[Q]).

Associated syndromes

- Although most clefts of the lip and palate occur as an isolated deformity, **Pierre Robin sequence** remains the **most common syndrome**[Q].
- Other associated syndromes: **Stickler's** (ophthalmic and musculoskeletal abnormalities), **Shprintzen's** (cardiac anomalies), **Down's, Apert's** and **Treacher-Collins' syndromes**.

Types of Cleft Lip	Types of Cleft Palate
- **Unilateral** cleft lip	- **Incomplete: Cleft of** the **hard palate** remains **attached to the nasal septum** and **vomer**[Q]
- **Bilateral** cleft lip	- **Complete: Nasal septum** and **vomer** are **completely separated** from the **palatine processes**[Q]

Antenatal diagnosis

- All but **isolated cleft palate** can be **diagnosed by ultrasound** after **18 weeks**[Q] gestation

Problems immediately after birth

- Some babies are able to feed normally but **some** will **need assistance**
- **Breathing problems** in **Pierre Robin sequence** may be **life threatening**

Contd…

Contd…

Management

- **Surgical techniques** are aimed at **restoring normal anatomy**.

•	Cleft lip	• Repaired between **3 and 6 months** of age[Q]
•	Cleft palate	• Repaired between **6 and 18 months** of age[Q]

Principles of Surgery

- **Cleft lip surgery attaches** and **reconnects** the **muscles around** the **oral sphincter**[Q]
- **Cleft palate surgery** aims to **bring together mucosa** and **muscles** with **minimal scarring**[Q]
- **Two-stage procedures** attempt to **minimize dissection**[Q]

Secondary Management

- Following primary surgery, **regular review by a multidisciplinary team** is essential[Q].
- Many aspects of cleft care require long-term review: **Hearing, speech, dental development, facial growth**[Q].

■ CLEFT LIP REPAIR TECHNIQUES

CLEFT LIP REPAIR TECHNIQUES

- Millard Rotation Advancement Technique: Most widely used[Q]
- Le Muserier[Q]
- Thompson[Q]
- Tennison-Rendall[Q]

■ TIMING OF PROCEDURES FOR CLEFT LIP AND CLEFT PALATE

Timing of Primary Cleft Lip and Palate Procedures (After Delaire)

Cleft lip alone	Cleft palate alone	Cleft lip and palate

• **Unilateral** (one side): One operation at **5-6 months**
• **Bilateral** (both sides): One operation at **4-5 months**
	• **Soft palate only**: One operation at **6 months**[Q]
	• **Soft and hard palate**: Two operations
	  – **Soft palate** at **6 months**[Q]
	  – **Hard palate** at **15-18** months
		• **Unilateral**: Two operations
		• **Cleft lip** and **soft palate** at **5-6 months**
		• **Hard palate and gum pad** with or without lip revision at **15-18 months**
		• **Bilateral:** Two operations
		  – **Cleft lip and soft palate** at **4-5 months**
		  – **Hard palate and gum pad** with or without lip revision at **15-18 months**

■ MANDIBULAR FRACTURE

FRACTURES OF THE MANDIBLE

- **Condylar neck**[Q] is the **weakest part** of the mandible and **MC site** of **fracture**[Q]

> - Mandible **may fracture directly** at the **point of** the **blow**[Q]
> - **Indirectly** where the **force from** the **blow is transmitted** and the **mandible fractures at a point of weakness** distant from the **original blow**, known as **'guardsman' fracture**[Q].

- **'Butterfly' fracture** of the mandible: A **segment of mandible** is **detached from** the **rest of** the **mandible** in the canine regions[Q].

Diagnosis

- Recommended radiographic evaluation of a **mandible fracture: Panoramic radiograph (Panorex)** and **Towne's view X-ray**[Q].

Treatment

- As in midface fractures, **restoration of dental occlusion forms** the **foundation for fracture management**[Q].

> - **Intermaxillary fixation before fracture exposure** and **plating is necessary**[Q].

- **Condylar** and **subcondylar mandible fractures** are most often **treated by IMF alone**[Q].
- **Medical management** of mandibular fractures involves a **purée-type diet, interdental fixation** for several weeks, **1% chlorhexidine** mouth rinses, and **antibiotics**[Q].

■ MIDFACE FRACTURE

MIDFACE FRACTURES

- **Midface fractures** involving the **maxilla** can be classified by fracture patterns know as **Le Fort I, II, and III.**

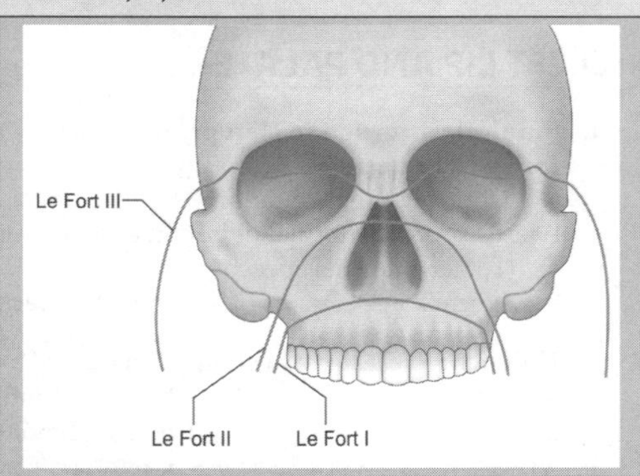

Le Fort I	• Fracture line runs above and parallel to palate[Q] • Effectively **separates alveolus** and **palate from** the **facial skeleton above**[Q]
Le Fort II	• **Pyramidal** in shape[Q] • Passes through the **root of nose, lacrimal bone, floor of orbit, upper part** of maxillary sinus and **pterygoid plate**[Q] • **Orbital floor** is **always involved**[Q]
Le Fort III	• **Complete disjunction** of the **facial skeleton from** the **skull base**[Q] • **Fracture line** runs high through the **nasal bridge, septum** and **ethmoids,** and through the **bones of orbit to** the **frontozygomatic suture**[Q].

Management

- Interdental or intermaxillary fixation is **necessary to reestablish** the **proper dentoskeletal relationships, immobilize the fractured bones,** and **ensure normal postoperative occlusion**[Q].

■ ZYGOMATIC BONE FRACTURE

ZYGOMATIC BONE FRACTURE

- **MC fracture** of the **middle third of the face: Nose > zygomatic bone**[Q]
- Also known as **Tripod fracture**[Q], because the zygoma is fractured at its 3 processes:
  1. **Zygomatico-frontal** fracture[Q]
  2. **Zygomatico-temporal** fracture[Q]
  3. **Infraorbital** fracture[Q]

Clinical Features of Zygomatic Bone Fracture

• **Flattening** of **malar prominence**[Q] • **Step-deformity** of infraorbital margin • **Epistaxis**[Q] • **Restricted ocular movements** due to entrapment of **inferior rectus muscle**[Q] (may lead to **diplopia**[Q])	• **Anesthesia** in the distribution of **infraorbital nerve**[Q] • **Oblique palpebral fissure**, due to entrapment of lateral palpebral ligament • **Periorbital emphysema** due to escape of air from the maxillary sinus

Diagnosis

- **X-ray Water's view**[Q]
- **CT scan:** Best for diagnosis of zygomatic bone fracture[Q]

Treatment

- Only **displaced fractures** require **treatment**[Q]
- **Treatment of choice:** Open reduction and internal fixation[Q]

■ BLOW OUT FRACTURE OF ORBIT

BLOW-OUT FRACTURES OF THE ORBIT

- **Direct trauma to** the **globe of the eye** may push it back within the orbit.
- Occur when a **blunt object strikes** the **globe**[Q].
- **Weakest plate of bone,** most commonly the **orbital floor, fractures,** and the **orbital contents herniate down into** the **maxillary antrum**[Q].
- **Tear-drop sign**[Q] is seen

• **Soft-tissue herniation** lead to **muscular dysfunction**, particularly the **inferior oblique** and **inferior rectus**, leading to **failure of** the **eye to rotate upwards**. • **Enophthalmos** and **diplopia** can follow[Q] • **Paraesthesia** in the distribution of the **infraorbital nerve** is an important clue to the blow-out fracture[Q].

Treatment

- Significant **delay in treatment** may be associated with **less success** than early diagnosis and planned treatment.
- **Orbital floor exploration** allows for **release of displaced** or **entrapped soft tissue, correcting** any **extra-ocular motility disturbances**[Q].

Section 8

Head and Neck

Multiple Choice Questions

■ CLEFT LIP AND PALATE

1. Surgical correction in cleft palate primarily aims at all of the following except: *(MCI March 2010)*
   a. Control of regurgitation
   b. To promote normal dentition and facial growth
   c. To get a normal speech
   d. Normal appearance of lips, nose and face

2. Unilateral cleft lip is best repaired at: *(Recent Question 2017)*
   a. 4-5 months
   b. 5-6 months
   c. 6-9 months
   d. 9-12 months

3. All are do about submucosal cleft palate except: *(DNB 2012)*
   a. Bifid uvula
   b. Notched hard palate
   c. Lip pits
   d. Zona pellucida

4. With respect to repair of cleft palate, the soft palate is first repaired, ideal time for which is? *(Recent Question 2016)*
   a. 12 months
   b. 9 months
   c. 6 months
   d. 3 months

5. In cleft lip operation all the stitches are removed on: *(Recent Question 2016)*
   a. 2nd day
   b. 4th day
   c. 10th day
   d. 14th day

6. The following is the method for operating cleft lip except: *(Recent Question 2016)*
   a. Le Muserier's method
   b. Tennison's method
   c. Millard's method
   d. Wardill's method

7. Most common congenital anomaly of the face is:
   a. Cleft lip alone *(MCI March 2008)*
   b. Isolated cleft palate
   c. Cleft lip and cleft palate
   d. All have equal incidence

8. Which of the following is the ideal time for the repair of cleft palate? *(Recent Question 2014, AIIMS Nov 2014)*
   a. 9-12 months
   b. 18-24 months
   c. 2-3 years
   d. 5-6 years

■ MAXILLOFACIAL INJURY

9. Fracture mandible with edentulous jaw is best treated with:
   a. External fixator *(UPPG 2004)*
   b. Minerva-plaster
   c. Interdental wiring
   d. Intermaxillary elastic traction

10. Most common site of mandible fracture: *(Recent Question 2017)*
    a. Condyle
    b. Angle
    c. Ramus
    d. Body

11. A man sustained injury and presented with fluid coming out through nose. What could be the possible fracture? *(MCI March 2007)*
    a. Fracture base of skull
    b. Fracture of mandible
    c. Fracture of maxilla
    d. None of the above

12. Mandible is commonly fractured: *(Recent Question 2016)*
    a. At the neck of the condyle
    b. Through the angle
    c. Through the cannine fossa
    d. At the middle

13. Le Forte II facial fracture implies: *(Recent Question 2016)*
    a. Fracture running through alveolar ridge
    b. Fracture running through midline of the palate and zygomatico maxillary suture
    c. Fracture running through zygomatic process of the maxilla, floor of orbit, root of nose on one side only
    d. Similar to C but on both sides

14. Le-Forte fracture is for: *(Recent Question 2017)*
    a. Facial skeleton
    b. Lower limb bone
    c. Spinal injury
    d. Pelvis fracture

15. Tripod fracture is seen in: *(DNB 2010)*
    a. Zygomatic bone
    b. Temporomandibular joint
    c. Maxilla
    d. Frontal bone

Explanations

■ CLEFT LIP AND PALATE

1. **Ans. d. Normal appearance of lips, nose and face** *(Ref. Sabiston 20/e p1947; Schwartz 11/e p1985-1987, 10/e p1840-1844; Bailey 27/e p692)*

OBJECTIVES OF THE CLEFT PALATE REPAIR

- To produce **anatomical closure** of the defect[Q].
- To create an apparatus for **development** and **production** of **normal speech**[Q].
- To **minimize** the **maxillary growth disturbances** and **dento-alveolar deformities**[Q].

2. **Ans. b. 5-6 months** *(Ref: Sabiston 20/e p1946; Schwartz 11/e p1987, 10/e p1844; Bailey 27/e p692)*
3. **Ans. c. Lip pits** *(Ref. Cleft Palate and Craniofacial abnormalities by Ann W. Kummer/51)*

SUBMUCOSAL CLEFT PALATE

- A congenital defect that affects the underlying structure of the palate, while the **oral surface mucosa is intact**
- Most children with submucosal cleft palate are asymptomatic and this is often not diagnosed until later
- Identification of submucosal cleft palate requires intraoral examination for:
    1. Bifid uvula
    2. **Zona pellucida** (submucosal absence of muscularis uvulae)
    3. **Notching of posterior border of hard palate**
    4. **Nasopharyngeal regurgitation during feeding** (only finding of occult submucosal cleft palate)

4. **Ans. c. 6 months** *(Ref. Bailey 27/e p692)*
5. **Ans. b. 4th day** *(Ref. Sabiston 18/e p2134)*

Guidelines for Day of Suture Removal by Area			
Body Regions	**Removal**	**Body Regions**	**Removal**
Eyelid	**3-4**	Chest, abdomen	8-10
Eyebrow	**3-5**	Ear	10-14
Nose	**3-5**	**Back**	**12-14**
Lip	**3-4**[Q]	**Extremities**	**12-14**
Face (other)	**3-4**[Q]	**Hand**	**10-14**
Scalp	6-8 days	**Foot, sole**	**12-14**

6. **Ans. d. Wardill's method** *(Ref. Sabiston 20/e p1947; Schwartz 11/e p1990-1992, 10/e p1840-1844; Bailey 27/e p692)*
7. **Ans. c. Cleft lip and cleft palate**   8. **Ans. a. 9-12 months**

■ MAXILLOFACIAL INJURY

9. **Ans. a. External fixator** *(Ref. Sabiston 20/e p422; Schwartz 11/e p2002, 10/e p197; Bailey 27/e p358)*
10. **Ans. a. Condyle** *(Ref: Sabiston 20/e p1949; Schwartz 11/e p2002, 10/e p1853; Bailey 27/e p358)*
11. **Ans. a. Fracture base of skull** *(Ref. Sabiston 20/e p420; Schwartz 11/e p2002, 10/e p576; Bailey 27/e p333)*

BASILAR SKULL FRACTURE

- **Fracture of the base of the skull**, typically involving the **temporal** bone, **occipital** bone, **sphenoid bone**, and/or **ethmoid** bone[Q].
- **Such fractures** can cause **tears in the** meninges, with resultant **leakage of** the CSF[Q].

  - **Leaking fluid** may accumulate in the **middle ear space**, and **dribble out through a perforated eardrum (CSF otorrhea**[Q]**)** or into the **nasopharynx via** the **eustachian tube**, causing a **salty taste**.
  - **CSF** may also **drip from the nose (CSF rhinorrhea**[Q]**)** in fractures of the **anterior skull base**, yielding a **halo sign**[Q].
  - These signs are **pathognomonic for basilar skull fracture**[Q].

12. **Ans. a. At the neck of the condyle**
13. **Ans. d. Similar to c but on both sides** *(Ref. Sabiston 20/e p422; Schwartz 11/e p628-629, 10/e p577; Bailey 27/e p360)*
14. **Ans. a. Facial skeleton** *(Ref: Schwartz 10/e p577; Bailey 27/e p360)*
15. **Ans. a. Zygomatic bone**

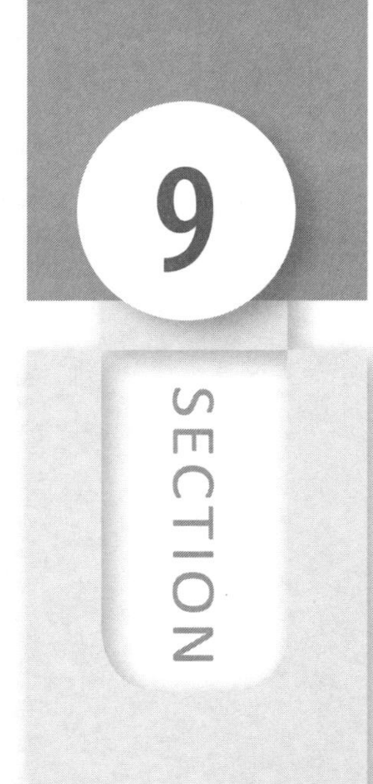

Oncology

Oncology

SCREENING IN MALIGNANCY

Well-established Benefit of Screening in			
• Colorectal cancer[Q]	• CA cervix[Q]	• CA oral cavity[Q]	• CA breast[Q]

American Cancer Society Recommendations for Early Detection of Cancer in Average-Risk, Asymptomatic Individuals			
Cancer Site	**Population**	**Test or Procedure**	**Frequency**
• **Breast**	Women aged ≥ 20 years	• Breast self-examination • Clinical breast examination • Mammography	• **Monthly**, starting at age **20** • **Every 3 years**, ages 20–39; **Annual,** starting at age **40**[Q] • **Annual,** starting at age **40**[Q]
• **Colorectal**	Men and women aged ≥ 50 years	• Fecal occult blood test (**FOBT**) or fecal immunochemical test (FIT) • **Flexible sigmoidoscopy**[Q] • **FOBT** and **flexible sigmoidoscopy**[Q] • Double-contrast barium enema (**DCBE**)[Q] • **Colonoscopy**[Q]	• **Annual,** starting at age **50**[Q] • **Every 5 years**, starting at age **50** • **Annual FOBT** (or FIT) and **flexible sigmoidoscopy** every **5 years**, starting at age 50[Q] • **DCBE every 5 years**, starting at age 50[Q] • **Colonoscopy every 10 years**[Q], starting at age 50
• **Prostate**	Men aged ≥50 years	• Digital rectal examination (**DRE**) and prostate-specific antigen (**PSA**) test[Q]	• Offer PSA test and DRE annually, starting at **age 50**, for men who have life expectancy of at least 10 years
• **Cervix**	Women aged ≥18 years	• **Pap test**[Q]	• Cervical cancer screening beginning **3 years after first vaginal intercourse**, but no later than age 21 years
• **Endometrial**	Women at **menopause**	—	• At the time of menopause, women at average risk should be informed about the risks and symptoms of endometrial cancer

SCREENING IMMUNOHISTOCHEMISTRY

SCREENING IMMUNOHISTOCHEMISTRY

- **Epithelial Markers:** Cytokeratin (positive in **carcinomas**)[Q]
- **Lymphoid Markers:** CD-45 (positive in **lymphoma**)[Q]
- **Melanocytic Markers:** S-100 (positive in **melanoma**)[Q]
- **Mesenchymal Markers:** Vimentin (positive in **sarcoma**)[Q]
- **Neuroendocrine Markers:** Chromagranin and **neuron specific enolase**[Q]

TUMOR MARKERS

TUMOR MARKERS

- Tumor markers are **indicators of cellular, biochemical, molecular, or genetic alterations** by which neoplasia can be recognized[Q].
- These **surrogate measures of** the **biology** of the cancer provide insight into the **clinical behavior** of the tumor[Q].
- This is particularly **useful when** the **cancer is not clinically detectable**[Q].
- **The information provided may:**
  - Be diagnostic and **distinguish benign from malignant disease**[Q]
  - **Correlate with** the amount of tumor present (so-called **tumor burden**[Q])
  - **Allow subtype classification** to more **accurately stage** patients[Q]
  - Be **prognostic,** either by the **presence or absence** of the marker or by its **concentration**[Q]
  - **Guide choice of therapy** and **predict response to therapy**[Q]

Markers	Associated Cancers	Non-neoplastic Conditions
Hormones		
• **Human chorionic gonadotropin** • **Calcitonin** • **Catecholamines**	• **Trophoblastic tumors**[Q], **nonseminomatous** testicular tumors • **Medullary carcinoma**[Q] of thyroid • **Pheochromocytoma**[Q]	• Pregnancy
Oncofetal Antigens		
• Alpha-Fetoprotein • **CEA**	• **Liver**[Q] cell cancer, **nonseminomatous**[Q] germ cell tumor of testis, **lung**[Q] cancer • Adenocarcinoma of the **colon**[Q], **pancreas**[Q], **lung**[Q], **breast**[Q], **ovary**[Q], **prostate**[Q]	• Cirrhosis, hepatitis • Pancreatitis, hepatitis, inflammatory bowel disease, smoking
Isoenzymes		
• Prostatic acid phosphatase • **Neuron-specific enolase** • Lactate dehydrogenase	• Prostate cancer • **Small cell** cancer of lung[Q], **Neuroblastoma**[Q] • Lymphoma, Ewing sarcoma	• Prostatitis, prostatic hypertrophy • Hepatitis, hemolytic anemia, many others
Specific Proteins		
• **Immunoglobulins** • PSA and prostate specific membrane antigen	• **Multiple myeloma**[Q] and other gammopathies • **Prostate cancer**[Q]	• Infection, MGUS • **Prostatitis, prostatic hypertrophy**[Q]
Mucins and Other Glycoproteins		
• CA-125 • CA-19-9 • CD30 • CD25	• **Cancer of ovary**[Q], fallopian tube, **endometrium**[Q], **cervix**, **breast**[Q], **lung**[Q], **pancreas**[Q] and **colon**[Q] • **Colon**[Q] cancer, **pancreatic**[Q] cancer • **Hodgkin's disease**[Q], anaplastic large cell lymphoma • **Hairy cell leukemia, adult T cell leukemia/lymphoma**[Q]	• **Pregnancy**[Q], **endometriosis**[Q], **PID**[Q], **uterine fibroids**[Q] • **Pancreatitis**, Ulcerative colitis

■ SENTINEL LYMPH NODE BIOPSY

SENTINEL LYMPH NODE BIOPSY

- **Sentinel LN: First LN** which **receives lymph directly from tumor**[Q]
- **Cabana** demonstrated the **concept of SLN first** in **carcinoma penis**[Q]
- **SLN biopsy in carcinoma penis is known as Cabana procedure**[Q]
- **SLN biopsy is usually done in: CA breast**[Q], **CA penis**[Q] & **Malignant melanoma**[Q]
- **SLN biopsy** is also **applied successfully** in **cancers of head & neck**[Q] and **vulva**[Q]
- **No special OT is required**[Q]
- **Indication of SLN biopsy in breast cancer: Clinically non-palpable axillary LN**[Q]
- **SLN biopsy** is usually **done intra-operatively** by using isosulphan blue dye[Q] (**1% lymphazurin**) or **radioactive (Tc-99 labeled sulphur**[Q]**) colloid. Accuracy of detection** of SLN biopsy is **best when both** of the methods **are combined**[Q].
- **Dye is injected around areola**[Q]
- When **radioactive colloid** is used, the **SLN is detected by gamma-camera**[Q]
- **Blue dye colors the afferent lymphatics & SLN**, hence **aids in the identification**[Q]
- Most of the times **>1 SLN in carcinoma breast**[Q]

Complications of SLN Biopsy in CA Breast		
• **Palpable lymphadenopathy**[Q]	• **Prior axillary surgery, chemotherapy** or **radiotherapy**[Q]	• **Multifocal breast cancer**[Q]
• **Skin tattooing**[Q] **(MC)** • **Necrosis**[Q]	• **Urine discoloration** • Anaphylaxis	• **Intercostobrachial nerve palsy**[Q] **(MC injured nerve** in SLN biopsy)

■ LYMPH NODE METASTASIS

Important Lymph Nodes	
Rotter's nodes[Q]	• **Interpectoral** nodes (**CA breast**)[Q]
Rouvier nodes[Q]	• **Retropharyngeal** nodes (**CA Nasopharynx**)[Q]
Delphian nodes[Q]	• **Pre-cricoid/Pre-tracheal/Pre-laryngeal** lymph nodes[Q]
Irish nodes[Q]	• Nodes in **left axilla (CA stomach)**[Q]
Sister Mary Joseph nodes[Q]	• **Periumbilical metastatic cutaneous** nodules
Virchow nodes[Q]	• **Left supraclavicular** node[Q]
Cloquet node[Q]	• **Femoral canal** node[Q]
LN of **Lund**[Q]	• **Cystic** lymph node[Q]
Krouse lymph node	• **Jugular fossa** lymph node[Q]

■ BONE METASTASIS

- MC site of primary for bone metastasis: CA Breast > CA prostate > RCC > CA lung > CA thyroid > CA bladder
- MC cause of osteoblastic secondaries in males: CA Prostate[Q]
- MC cause of osteoblastic secondaries in females: CA Breast[Q]
- MC tumor metastasize to bone in females: CA Breast[Q]
- Lytic expansile metastasis is seen in: RCC follicular carcinoma thyroid
- MC site of bone metastasis: Dorsal spine (Thoracic vertebra[Q])

BONE METASTASIS

- Metastatic tumors of bone are more common than primary bone tumors[Q].
- Tumors usually spread to bone hematogenously, axial skeleton is seeded more than appendicular skeleton partly due to persistence of red marrow[Q].

  - In order of decreasing frequency, the sites most often involved are vertebrae (most common)[Q] >proximal femur >pelvis >ribs > sternum >proximal humerus >skull.
  - Extremities distal to elbow and knee are least commonly involved sites[Q], but if distal extremity is involved there is high probability of myeloma[Q].
  - Metastasis to small bones originate from: Lung, kidney or colon[Q]

- Bone is a common site of metastasis for carcinoma of the prostate, breast, lung, kidney, bladder, thyroid, lymphomas and sarcomas[Q].
- Bateson's vertebral plexus allow cells to enter the vertebral circulation without first passing through the lungs and is responsible for high rate of prostate cancer metastasis to bone[Q].

Diagnosis

- Bone scan is investigation of choice for bone metastasis[Q].

  - Purely osteolytic lesions are best detected by plain radiography, but they are not apparent until they are >1 cm and have destroyed 30-50% of bone[Q].
  - These are associated with hypercalcemia and with the excretion of hydroxyproline containing peptides[Q].

Treatment

- Treatment options: Bisphosphonates, corticosteroids, radiotherapy (EBRT) and radionucleotides.
- EBRT is given in symptomatic bony metastasis[Q].
- Samarium-153, is a beta emitter, very effective in relieving pain of bone metastasis[Q].

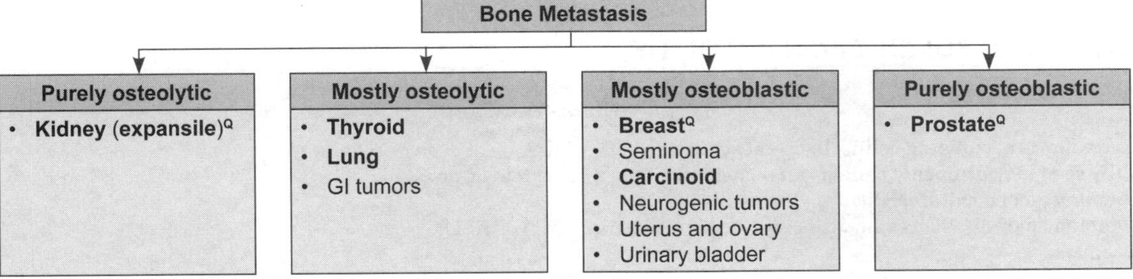

■ ONCOLOGICAL EMERGENCY

Oncologic Emergencies		
Structural-obstructive Oncologic Emergencies (Space Occupying Lesion) (PSM HAS Obstruction IN Urine)	Metabolic or Hormonal Emergencies (Paraneoplastic Syndromes) (HAS)	Treatment Related Emergencies (HT PNH)
• **P**ericardial tamponade[Q] • **S**VC syndrome[Q] • **M**alignant biliary obstruction • **H**emoptysis • **A**irway obstruction • **S**pinal cord compression[Q] • **O**bstruction — Intestinal **obstruction** • **I**ncreased intracranial pressure • Intracerebral leukocytostasis • **N**eoplastic meningitis • **U**rinary obstruction	• **H**ypercalcemia[Q] • **A**drenal insufficiency • **S**IADH	• **H**emolytic-Uremic syndrome • Human antibody infusion reactions • **T**umour lysis syndrome[Q] • Typhlitis[Q] • **P**ulmonary infiltrate • **N**eutropenia and infection • **H**emorrhagic cystitis

TUMOR LYSIS SYNDROME

TUMOR LYSIS SYNDROME

- Caused by **destruction of** large number of **rapidly proliferating neoplastic cells**[Q]
- Frequently, **acute renal failure** develops as a result of the syndrome[Q].
- **Most frequently associated with** the treatment of **Burkitt's lymphoma, ALL** and other **high grade lymphomas**[Q], **chronic leukemias** and rarely with solid tumors.

Pathophysiology

- **Hyperuricemia**: Due to destruction of malignant cells and rapid turnover of nucleic acid
- **Hyperkalemia:** Due to release of intracellular K leading to arrhythmia.
- **Hyperphosphatemia** and **Hypocalcemia:** Due to **release of intracellular phosphate,** which combines with calcium into bone, **calcium phosphate** gets **deposited in renal tubules** causing **renal failure**[Q].
- **Lactic acidosis**: Due to **deranged oxidative metabolism**[Q]

Characteristic Abnormalities of Tumor Lysis Syndrome	
• Hyperuricemia[Q] • Hyperkalemia[Q] • Hyperphosphatemia[Q]	• Lactic acidosis[Q] • Hypocalcemia[Q]

Treatment

- **Hydration, NaHCO$_3$, Allopurinol, Rasburicase** (recombinant urate oxidase), **Hemodialysis**[Q]

HYPERCALCEMIA OF MALIGNANCY

HYPERCALCEMIA OF MALIGNANCY

- **Main factor** leading to hypercalcemia is either **increased release of calcium form bone** or **increased calcium reabsorption** from DCT[Q].
- Mostly **underlying cause** is **secretion of PTH-rp**[Q].

Treatment

- **Mainstay of therapy: Rehydration** with a **0.9% saline** and diuresis with **furosemide**[Q]
- Other drugs used to lower serum calcium levels:
  - **Bisphosphonates (Zoledronic acid** is DOC), **Calcitonin**[Q]
  - **Mithramycin** (plicamycin), **Gallium nitrate**[Q]
  - **Glucocorticoids** (Hydrocortisone)[Q]

TYPHLITIS (NEUTROPENIC ENTEROCOLITIS)

TYPHLITIS (NEUTROPENIC COLITIS)

- Also referred to as **necrotizing colitis, ileocecal syndrome** and **cecitis**[Q]
- **Classically seen** in **neutropenic patients after chemotherapy**[Q] with cytotoxic drugs.
- **More common** among **children**[Q] than among adults
- **More common** among patients with **acute myelocytic leukemia** (AML) or **ALL**[Q]

Clinical Features

- Clinical syndrome of **fever** and **right-lower-quadrant tenderness** in an **immunosuppressed host**[Q].
- Associated **diarrhea (often bloody)** is common

Diagnosis

- Diagnosis can be confirmed by the finding of a **thickened cecal wall** on **CT** or **USG**[Q].

Treatment

- **Most cases resolve with medical therapy** alone[Q].
- **Surgical intervention:** If there is **no improvement by 24 hours** after start of antibiotic treatment and in **perforation**[Q]

SUPERIOR VENA CAVA SYNDROME

SUPERIOR VENA CAVA (SVC) SYNDROME

- Clinical manifestation of SVC obstruction, with severe reduction in venous return from head, neck and upper extremities.
- **MC cause** is **Lung cancer (small cell and squamous cell carcinoma)**[Q], alongwith **lymphoma** and **metastatic tumors** responsible for more than 90% of all SVC syndrome.
- **In young adults**, **malignant lymphoma** is the **leading cause** of SVC syndrome[Q].

Contd...

Contd...

Clinical Features
- Patients present with **neck and facial swelling** (especially around the eyes), **dyspnoea,** and **cough**[Q].
- Other symptoms include hoarseness, tongue swelling, headache, nasal congestion, epistaxis, dysphagia, pain, dizziness, syncope.
- **Characteristic physical findings are dilated neck veins, increased number of collateral veins covering the anterior chest wall, cyanosis, and edema of the face, arms and chest**[Q].

Diagnosis
- Most significant chest radiographic finding is **widening of the superior mediastinum (MC right side)**[Q]
- **CT scan: Investigation of choice**[Q].

Treatment
- Potentially life threatening complication of **superior mediastinal mass** is **tracheal obstruction**[Q].
- Diuretics with low salt diet, head elevation and oxygen may produce temporary symptomatic relief.

Treatment	Underlying cause
Radiation Therapy[Q]	**Non-small cell lung cancer,** Metastatic solid tumors
Chemotherapy[Q]	**Small cell carcinoma or lymphoma**
Surgery[Q]	All other cases

■ RADIOSENSITIVITY OF TUMORS

Most radiosensitive ovarian tumor	• **Dysgerminoma**[Q]
Most radiosensitive **brain** tumor	• **Medulloblastoma**[Q]
Most radiosensitive **testicular** tumor	• **Seminoma**[Q]
Most radiosensitive **lung** tumor	• **Small cell CA**[Q]
Most radiosensitive **kidney** tumor	• **Wilms tumor**[Q]
Most radiosensitive **bone** tumor	• **Ewing's Sarcoma**[Q] and **Multiple myeloma**[Q]

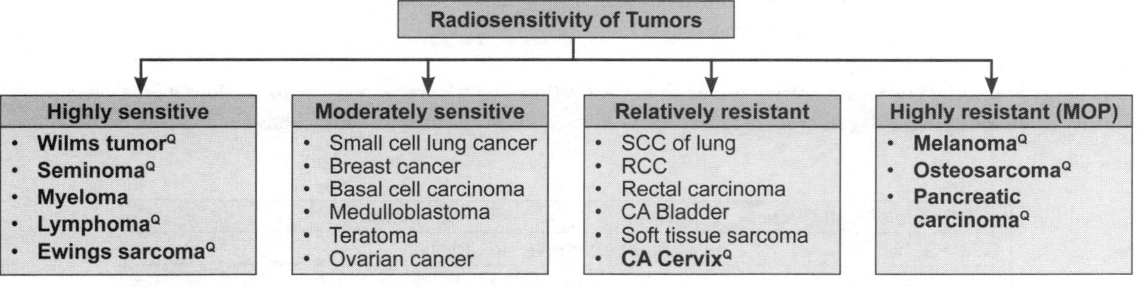

IN RADIOTHERAPY

- **Most radiosensitive tissue** of body: **Bone marrow**[Q]
- **Least** radiosensitive tissue of body: **Nervous tissue / Brain**[Q]
- **Most radiosensitive blood cell: Lymphocyte**[Q] (That's why Lymphocytic predominant Hodgkins lymphoma has best prognosis)
- **Least radiosensitive blood cell: Platelet**[Q]
- **Most common organ** to be affected by radiation: **Skin**[Q] (**Erythema earliest change, layer most commonly affected stratum basalis**)
- Sebaceous gland function does not recover after radiotherapy.
- **Pinna** and **axillae** are common sites of **radionecrosis** i.e. for skin doses.
- Most **radio resistant** organ: **Vagina**
- Most common **mucosa** to be affected by radiation: **Intestinal mucosa**[Q] (**Earliest symptom** is **diarrhea**)
- **Most sensitive abdominal organ: Kidney**

■ IONIZING RADIATIONS

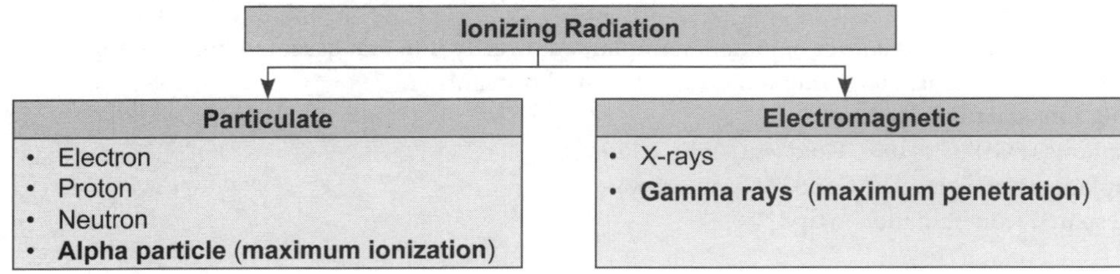

■ SYSTEMIC RADIONUCLIDES

SYSTEMIC RADIONUCLIDES

- **Systemic radionuclides** are **non-sealed** radionuclides which are administered orally, intravenously or intracavitary.
- Before administering it, **pregnancy** should be **ruled out**
- **Breastfeeding** should be **discontinued for 1–2 weeks**.

Types	T½ (Days)	Decay Particles	Use
Sodium iodide (I^{131})[Q]	8[Q]	Gamma, beta[Q]	**Hyperthyroidism** (diffuse toxic goiter, toxic multinodular goiter, or solitary toxic thyroid nodule), **thyroid carcinoma**[Q]
Sodium phosphate (P^{32}) Colloidal chromic Phosphate	14.3	Beta[Q]	Myeloproliferative disorders (**Polycythemia** and **thrombocytosis**[Q]) Intra-cavitary therapy of **malignant ascites**, **malignant pleural effusion** and **brain cyst**[Q]
Samarium-153 (Sm) chloride	1.9	Beta[Q]	**Painful bone metastases**[Q]
Strontium-89 (Sr) chloride	50.5	Beta[Q] Never gamma	**Painful bone metastases**[Q]
Rhenium (Re)	3.8	Beta and Gamma	**Painful bone metastases**[Q]

■ RADIOTHERAPY

RADIOTHERAPY

- **X-rays** and **gamma rays** are the **most common radiations used** to treat cancers.
- **X-rays** are **generated by linear accelerators**
- **Gamma rays** are generated **from decay of atomic nuclei** in radio-isotopes like **cobalt.**
- **Cobalt-60** is a synthetic radioactive isotope of cobalt with a **half-life** of 5.27 years
- **Cobalt-60** is **used only in teletherapy**
- **Radiation energy** is absorbed by tissue causing **ionization** or **excitation**[Q], which are responsible for various biological effects.
- **Susceptibility of various phases of cell cycle to radiation: G_2M[Q] >G_2>M >G_1>Early S >Late S Phase**[Q].

Phase of Cell Cycle	Comment
G_2M >G_2	• **Most sensitive**[Q] to radiation
End of S phase	• **Most resistant**[Q] to radiation
G_1	• Radiation exposure leads to **chromosomal aberration**
G_2	• Radiation exposure leads to **chromatid aberration**

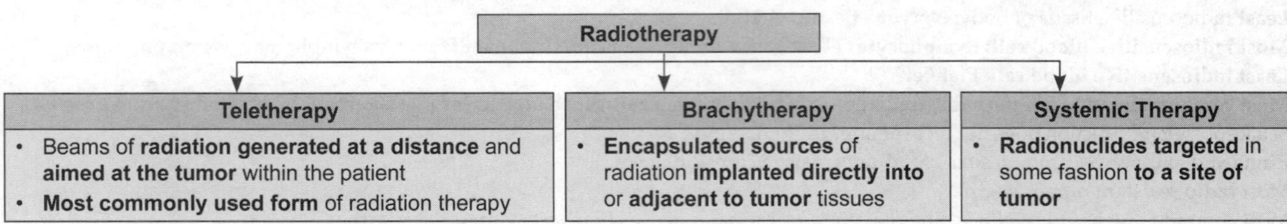

■ BRACHYTHERAPY

BRACHYTHERAPY

- **Radiation therapy with encapsulated source** of radiation **implanted directly into** or adjacent to **tumor tissue.**
- It is delivered in two ways (1) **Intracavitary implants**[Q] (2) **Interstitial implants**
- **Interstitial implantation** is of two types:
  1. **Permanent implants (PGI)**[Q]: Pd-103[Q], Gold (Au)-198[Q], I-125[Q]
  2. **Temporary implants (ICT)**[Q]: Ir-192[Q], Cs-137[Q] (Temporary)
- Normal tissues are spared from radiation injury[Q].

Interstitial implants

Permanent Interstitial Implants (PGI)	Temporary Interstitial Implants (ICT)

• Performed when the **tumor** to be treated **is inaccessible making** the **removal of radioisotope impossible** or impractical.
• These implants have usually **short half lives**.
• **Isotopes used (PGI):**
  – Palladium (**Pd**) 103[Q]
  – Gold (**Au**) 198[Q]
  – Iodine 125[Q]
• Used in deep seated lesion in **pelvis, abdomen, lung, colorectum**
	• Temporary **removable implants** are used in anatomic areas where there is **no body cavity** or **orifice to accept radioactive sources**.
	• **Isotopes used (ICT):**
	  – Iridium **192** (MC)[Q]
	  – Cesium **137**[Q] (ICT: Iridium cesium temporary)
	• Used in **breast** and **chest wall irradiation**, anterior, lateral and posterior wall of **vagina**

■ INTENSITY MODULATED RADIOTHERAPY

INTENSITY MODULATED RADIATION THERAPY (IMRT)

• The radiation dose is designed to **conform to the three dimensional (3-D) shape of** the **tumour** by modulation or controlling the intensity of the radiation beams to **focus a higher radiation dose to the tumour** while **minimizing radiation exposure to surrounding normal tissues**[Q].

Indications of IMRT	
• **Prostate cancer**[Q] • **Pancreatic tumors** • Head and neck cancers	• **Primary** and **metastatic brain tumors** • Liver tumors (HCC and metastasis)

Multiple Choice Questions

■ TUMOR MARKERS

1. **The following is a marker of Paget's disease of the mammary gland:** *(All India 2007)*
   a. S-100
   b. HMB-45
   c. CEA
   d. Neuron specific enolase

2. **In which of the following tumors alpha-feto protein is elevated?** *(AIIMS Nov 2005)*
   a. Choriocarcinoma
   b. Neuroblastoma
   c. Hepatocellular carcinoma
   d. Seminoma

3. **Which of the following is marker for carcinoma?**
   a. Cytokeratin
   b. Vimentin *(All India 2012)*
   c. Calcitonin
   d. CD-45

4. **CEA is increased in all except:** *(AIIMS May 2007)*
   a. Lung cancer
   b. Breast cancer
   c. Colon cancer
   d. Osteogenic sarcoma

■ SCREENING IN MALIGNANCY

5. **In which of the following diseases, the overall survival is increased by screening procedure?** *(All India 2005)*
   a. Prostate cancer
   b. Lung cancer
   c. Colon cancer
   d. Ovarian cancer

6. **Least amenable to screening is:** *(AIIMS June 94)*
   a. Breast
   b. Cervix
   c. Oral cavity
   d. Lung

■ LYMPH NODE METASTASIS

7. **Which one of the following is the most common tumor to produce metastasis to cervical lymph nodes?**
   a. Glottic carcinoma *(UPSC 2008, AIIMS June 2002)*
   b. Nasopharyngeal carcinoma
   c. Carcinoma base of tongue
   d. Carcinoma lip

8. **In which of the following head and neck cancers, is lymph node metastasis least common?** *(AIIMS May 2008)*
   a. Tongue
   b. Buccal mucosa
   c. Hard palate
   d. Lower alveolus

9. **Delphian nodes are:** *(COMEDK 2008)*
   a. Pretracheal
   b. Paratracheal
   c. Supraclavicular
   d. Posterior triangle

10. **Which carcinoma most commonly metastasizes to cervical lymph nodes?** *(AIIMS June 93)*
    a. Maxillary sinus
    b. Posterior tongue
    c. Cheek
    d. Hard palate

11. **Lymph node metastasis is a common feature with the following variant of soft tissue sarcoma:** *(All India 97)*
    a. Fibrosarcoma
    b. Angiosarcoma
    c. Liposarcoma
    d. Neurofibrosarcoma

■ BONE METASTASIS

12. **Most common cause of skeletal metastasis is:** *(UPPG 2009)*
    a. Kidney
    b. Prostate
    c. Breast
    d. Thyroid

13. **Treatment of bony metastasis is by:** *(JIPMER 2011)*
    a. Samarium-153
    b. I-131 with tositumumab
    c. P-32
    d. Yttrium

14. **Best investigation for bone metastasis is:**
    a. MRI
    b. CT *(All India 2012, 2011)*
    c. Bone scan
    d. X-ray

15. **Secondaries of all following cause osteolytic lesions except:**
    a. Prostate
    b. Kidney *(All India 95)*
    c. Bronchus
    d. Thyroid

16. **Expansile lytic osseous metastases are characteristic of primary malignancy of:**
    a. Kidney
    b. Bronchus
    c. Breast
    d. Prostate

17. **A malignant tumor of childhood, that metastasizes to bones most often is:** *(All India 2006)*
    a. Wilm's tumor
    b. Neuroblastoma
    c. Adrenal gland tumors
    d. Granulosa cell tumor of ovary

18. **All of the following produce osteoblastic secondaries except:** *(DNB 2012, All India 94)*
    a. CA Prostate
    b. Carcinoid tumors
    c. CA Breast
    d. Multiple myeloma

19. **Most common primary of metastatic bone tumor in a male is:**
    a. Lung
    b. Liver *(DNB 2009)*
    c. Bone
    d. Brain

■ ONCOLOGICAL EMERGENCIES

20. **Tumor lysis syndrome is associated with all of the following laboratory feature except:** *(DNB 2012, AIIMS Nov 2003)*
    a. Hyperkalemia
    b. Hypercalcemia
    c. Hyperuricemia
    d. Hyperphosphatemia

21. **Tumor lysis syndrome is characterized by all except:** *(AIIMS Nov 2017)*
    a. Hyperuricemia
    b. Hypercalcemia
    c. Hyperkalemia
    d. Hyperphosphatemia

22. **Hypercalcemia associated with malignancy is most often mediated by:** *(All India 2005)*
    a. PTH
    b. PTH-rp
    c. IL-6
    d. Calcitonin

23. **Which of the following tumor is most commonly associated with superior vena cava syndrome?** *(Recent Question 2014, WBPG 2012, All India 2011)*
    a. Lymphoma
    b. Small cell carcinoma
    c. Non-small cell carcinoma
    d. Metastasis

24. **Which of the following is not an oncological emergency?**
    a. Spinal cord compression *(AIIMS June 2003)*
    b. Superior vena cava syndrome
    c. Tumor lysis syndrome
    d. CA cervix stage IIIb with pyometra

■ LYMPHOMA

25. **The commonest site of lymphoma in the gastrointestinal system is:** *(COMEDK 2007)*
    a. Small bowel
    b. Stomach
    c. Large intestine
    d. Esophagus

26. **In neuroblastoma the most common presentation is:**
    a. Lytic lesion in skull with suture diastasis   *(All India 98)*
    b. Lung metastasis
    c. Renal invasion
    d. Secondaries in brain

27. **Commonest tumor of lumbar region in children is:**
    (AIIMS June 98)
    a. Dermoid cyst   b. Neuroblastoma
    c. Wilm's tumor   d. Appendix

■ SENTINEL LYMPH NODE BIOPSY

28. **Sentinel lymph node biopsy is an important part of the management of which of the following conditions?**
    (All India 2002)
    a. Carcinoma prostate   b. Carcinoma breast
    c. Carcinoma lung   d. Carcinoma nasopharynx

29. **The given image shows methylene blue being injected in the peritumoral region. Which of the given procedure is being performed?**   *(AIIMS May 2018)*

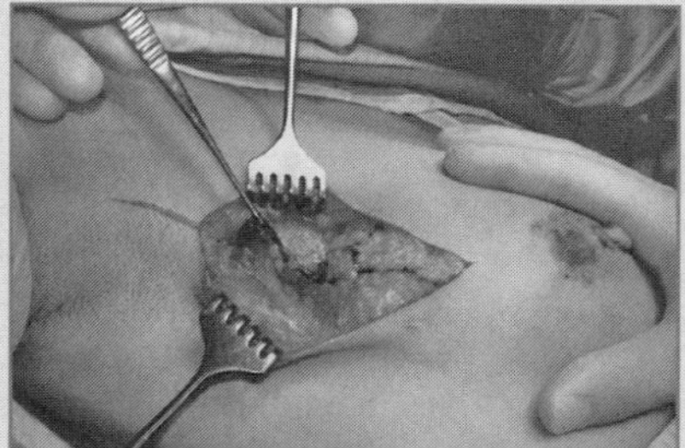

    a. Sentinel lymph node biopsy
    b. Tumor painting
    c. Breast tattooing
    d. Peritumor marking with dye

30. **Which of the following technique has been depicted in the image?**   *(AIIMS Nov 2018)*

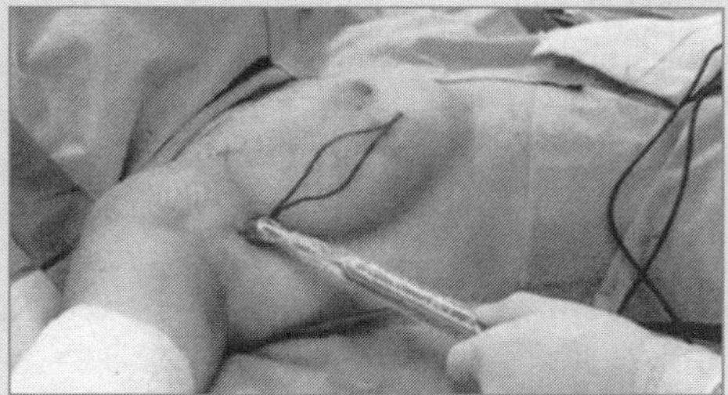

    a. Brachytherapy
    b. USG
    c. Sentinel lymph node biopsy
    d. Lateral pectoral nerve block

31. **Sentinel lymph node biopsy is most useful for:**
    (AIIMS Nov 2018)
    a. Carcinoma cervix   b. Carcinoma endometrium
    c. Carcinoma vulva   d. Carcinoma vagina

32. **Sentinel lymph node biopsy is done in all except:**
    a. CA breast   b. CA penis   *(DNB 2012)*
    c. Malignant melanoma   d. CA colon

■ GI MALIGNANCY

33. **By mucosal resection which carcinoma can be diagnosed early?**   *(AIIMS June 98)*
    a. Esophageal carcinoma   b. Anal carcinoma
    c. Colon carcinoma   d. Pancreatic carcinoma

34. **In which case immunoguided surgery is done?**
    (AIIMS June 98)
    a. CA colon   b. CA pancreas
    c. CA jejunum   d. CA anal canal

■ SPONTANEOUS REGRESSION

35. **In which case spontaneous regression is not seen?**
    (AIIMS Sept 96, All India 98)
    a. Malignant melanoma   b. Osteosarcoma
    c. Neuroblastoma   d. Choriocarcinoma

■ RADIOTHERAPY

36. **Most radio resistant phase in cell cycle:**
    (Recent Question 2014, JIPMER 2011)
    a. G_1 b. Early S
    c. Late S   d. G_2

37. **All of the following are pure beta emitters except:**
    (AIIMS May 2011)
    a. Yttrium-90   b. Phosphorus-32
    c. Strontium-90   d. Samarium-153

38. **All of the following radioisotopes are used as systemic radionuclide, except:**   *(All India 2006)*
    a. Phosphorus-32   b. Strontioum-89
    c. Iridium-192   d. Samarium

39. **Which of the following malignant tumors is radioresistant?**
    (All India 2006; AIIMS 2007)
    a. Ewing's sarcoma   b. Retinoblastoma
    c. Osteosarcoma   d. Neuroblastoma

40. **The most radiosensitive tumor among the following is:**
    (Recent Question 2014, All India 2006)
    a. Bronchogenic carcinoma   b. Carcinoma parotid
    c. Dysgerminoma   d. Osteogenic sarcoma

41. **Which of the following is the most radiosensitive phase of the cell cycle?**   *(MHCET 2016, AIIMS Nov 2012, All India 2008, PGI 2009, 2008)*
    a. G_2M b. G_2
    c. S   d. G_1

42. **Amifostine protects all of the following except:**
    (All India 2009)
    a. CNS   b. Salivary glands
    c. Kidneys   d. GIT

43. **Which of the following is the most radiosensitive tumor?**
    a. Ewing's sarcoma   *(Recent Question 2014, AIIMS Nov 2005)*
    b. Hodgkin's disease
    c. Carcinoma cervix
    d. Malignant fibrous histiocytoma

44. **Which of the following radioactive isotopes not used in brachytherapy?**   *(AIIMS 2005)*
    a. Iodine-125   b. Iodine-131
    c. Cobalt-60   d. Iridium-192

45. **Amifostine is:**   *(AIIMS May 2012)*
    a. Radiosensitiser   b. Radioprotector
    c. Radiomodifier   d. Radiomimetic

46. **Which of the following is radioprotective agent?**
    a. Cisplatin   *(Recent Question 2016, All India 2012)*
    b. Amifostine
    c. Methotrexate
    d. Colony stimulating factor

■ MISCELLANEOUS

47. Which of the following malignant disease of children has the best prognosis? *(AIIMS Nov 2003)*
    a. Wilm's tumor
    b. Neuroblastoma
    c. Rhabdomyosarcoma
    d. Primitive neuroectodermal tumor

48. Neoadjuvant chemotherapy is not used in: *(AIIMS Feb 97)*
    a. CA thyroid
    b. CA breast
    c. CA esophagus
    d. CA lung

49. Which of the following is the most beneficial technique of using chemotherapy with a course of radiotherapy in head and neck malignancies? *(AIIMS Nov 2004)*
    a. Neoadjuvant chemotherapy
    b. Adjuvant chemotherapy
    c. Concurrent chemotherapy
    d. Alternating chemotherapy and radiotherapy

50. What is the name of the given instrument?

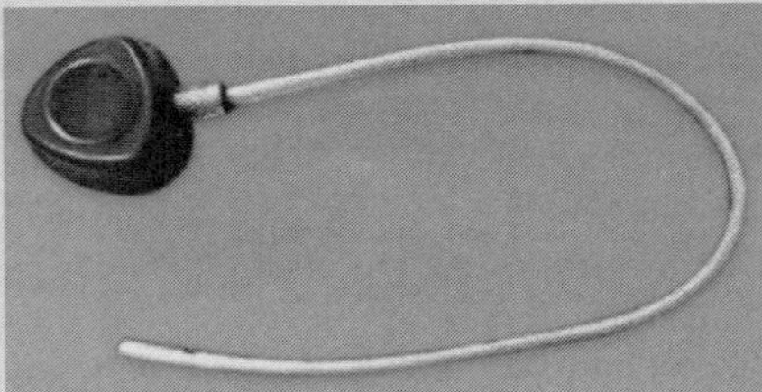

    a. Gamma camera
    b. Chemoport
    c. IVC filter
    d. Pacemaker

51. Drug of choice for chemotherapy induced vomiting: *(Recent Question 2019)*
    a. Granisetron
    b. Prazosin
    c. Clonidine
    d. Dimenhydrinate

52. Migratory thrombophlebitis is associated with the following malignancies except: *(AIIMS Nov 2004)*
    a. Lung cancer
    b. Prostate cancer
    c. Pancreas cancer
    d. Gastro-intestinal cancer

53. Small deposits of neuroendocrine cell hyperplasia in scarred lungs are known as: *(JIPMER 2014)*
    a. Teratoma
    b. Tumor let
    c. Carcinoid
    d. Hamartoma

54. Trousseau's sign is seen in all the following except: *(All India 94)*
    a. CA lung
    b. CA stomach
    c. CA pancreas
    d. Liposarcoma

55. Adjuvant chemotherapy is of definite value in: *(AIIMS Nov 2006)*
    a. CA colon
    b. CA pancreas
    c. CA gallbladder
    d. CA esophagus

56. Glomus tumor is seen in: *(Recent Question 2014, AIIMS Nov 2008)*
    a. Liver
    b. Adrenals
    c. Pituitary
    d. Finger

57. BRCA-1 gene is located on: *(Recent Question 2014, AIIMS May 2011)*
    a. Chromosome 13
    b. Chromosome 11
    c. Chromosome 17
    d. Chromosome 22

58. Octreotide is used in all except: *(AIIMS May 2011)*
    a. Insulinoma
    b. Glucagonoma
    c. Glioma
    d. Carcinoids

59. Most common site of carcinoma in India: *(MHPGMCET 2001)*
    a. Lung
    b. Oral cavity
    c. Breast
    d. Uterus

60. Acanthosis nigricans is seen in: *(DNB 2009)*
    a. GI malignancy
    b. Lung cancer
    c. Breast cancer
    d. All of the above

61. Smoking is a risk factor for all cancer except: *(DNB 2007)*
    a. Esophagus
    b. Urinary bladder
    c. Pancreas
    d. Gallbladder

62. Most common non-Hodgkin's lymphoma of orbit:
    a. B cell
    b. T cell *(AIIMS May 2013)*
    c. NK cell
    d. Plasma cell

63. Most common malignant chest wall tumor:
    a. Chondrosarcoma *(Recent Question 2017)*
    b. Osteosarcoma
    c. Synovial sarcoma
    d. Rhabdomyosarcoma

64. Reddish firm swelling which bleeds on touch in a 20 years old female is: *(Recent Question 2018)*
    a. Hemangioma'
    b. Fibroadenoma
    c. Pyogenic granuloma
    d. Lipoma

Explanations

■ TUMOR MARKERS

1. **Ans. c. CEA** *(Ref: Harrison 20/e p532; Schwartz 11/e p550, 565, 10/e p301-302; Sabiston 20/e p698-702)*
   Paget's disease of nipple is differentiated by superficial spreading melanoma by **CEA positivity[Q]**.

2. **Ans. c. Hepatocellular carcinoma**

3. **Ans. a. Cytokeratin** *(Ref: Robbins 9/e p334)*   4. **Ans. d. Osteogenic sarcoma**

■ SCREENING IN MALIGNANCY

5. **Ans. c. Colon cancer** *(Ref: Harrison 20/e p449; Schwartz 11/e p1293, 10/e p298, 9/e p252; Bailey 27/e p146-147)*

   Schwartz says "Because the **majority of colorectal cancers** are thought to **arise from adenomatous polyps**, preventive measures focus upon identification and removal of these premalignant lesions. In addition, **many cancers** are **asymptomatic** and **screening** may **detect** these **tumors at** an **early** and **curable stage.**

6. **Ans. d. Lung**

■ LYMPH NODE METASTASIS

7. **Ans. b. Nasopharyngeal carcinoma** *(Ref: Sabiston 20/e p803-805; Schwartz 11/e p644-645, 10/e 580, 593-594; Bailey 27/e p733-735; Devita 9/e p764-766)*

   ### NASOPHARYNGEAL CARCINOMA

   - **MC tumor** to produce **cervical LN metastasis[Q]**
   - **MC tumor** responsible for **secondaries in the neck** with **no obvious primary malignancy[Q]**

8. **Ans. c. Hard palate** *(Ref: Bailey 27/e p764-765; Devita 9/e p750; Cancer of the Head and Neck by Suen and Myer 4/e p288-289)*

   - **LN metastasis** is **most common in: CA tongue[Q]** >Floor of mouth >Lower alveolus >Buccal mucosa >Upper alveolus >**Hard palate >Lip[Q]**.

9. **Ans. a. Pretracheal** *(Ref: Bailey 27/e p800, 801)*   10. **Ans. b. Posterior tongue**

11. **Ans. b. Angiosarcoma** *(Ref: Harrison 20/e p654; Sabiston 20/e p766)*

■ BONE METASTASIS

12. **Ans. c. Breast** *(Ref: Harrison 20/e p471-472, 19/e p119e-4; Devita 9/e p2512-2513; CSDT 12/e p1202; Apley 9/e p216)*

13. **Ans. a. Samarium-153**   14. **Ans. c. Bone scan** *(Ref: Sutton 7/e p1251)*   15. **Ans. a. Prostate**

16. **Ans. a. Kidney**

   ### PULSATING SECONDARIES

   - **Follicular carcinoma thyroid[Q]**   - **RCC[Q]**

17. **Ans. b. Neuroblastoma** *(Ref: Schwartz 11/e p1748-1749, 10/e p678,1639-1640; Sabiston 20/e p1887-1888; Bailey 27/e p847; Harrison 20/e p454)*

   ### NEUROBLASTOMA

   - **Metastasis** is present in **60–70%** of patients **at the time of diagnosis[Q]**
   - **Common sites of metastasis: Long bones (MC)[Q]**, Liver, Lymph nodes and Skin
   - **Lung metastasis** is **rare** in **neuroblastoma[Q]**
   - **Neuroblastoma** is the **MC extracranial solid tumor** in **childhood[Q]**
   - **Neuroblastoma** is the **2nd MC solid malignancy** of childhood **after brain tumors[Q]**
   - **MC intra-abdominal solid tumor** in **childhood: Neuroblastoma[Q]**

18. **Ans. d. Multiple myeloma**

19. **Ans. a. Lung** *(Ref: Bailey 24/e p1330)*
    - "**Prostate, breast** and **lung primaries account for 80% of all bone metastasis.**"

■ ONCOLOGICAL EMERGENCIES

20. **Ans. b. Hypercalcemia**

21. **Ans. b. Hypercalcemia** *(Ref: Harrison 20/e p519; Sabiston 20/e p90; Schwartz 11/e p99, 10/e p81)*

> *"Tumor lysis syndrome (TLS) is characterized by hyperuricemia, hyperkalemia, hyperphosphatemia, and hypocalcemia and is caused by the destruction of a large number of rapidly proliferating neoplastic cells. Acidosis may also develop. Acute renal failure occurs frequently."-Harrison 20/e p519*

22. **Ans. b. PTH-rp** *(Ref: Harrison 20/e p663, 19/e p313, 609, 717, 2476, 2477)*

23. **Ans. b. Small cell carcinoma** *(Ref:Harrison 20/e p511, 19/e p1787)*

24. **Ans. d. CA cervix stage IIIb with pyometra** *(Ref: Harrison 20/e p511)*

■ LYMPHOMA

25. **Ans. b. Stomach** *(Ref: Sabiston 20/e p1278; Schwartz 11/e p1149, 10/e 1259; Bailey 27/e p1140-1141)*

> **GI LYMPHOMA**
>
> - **MC site** for **lymphoma**[Q] in the **GIT: Stomach >Ileum**
> - **MC site** of **gastric lymphoma: Antrum**[Q]
>> - **MC type** of **gastric lymphoma: Diffuse large B-cell lymphoma**[Q] (55%) > **MALToma** (40%)
>> - **DLBL** is **MC type of NHL, extranodal lymphoma** and **GI lymphoma.**

26. **Ans. a. Lytic lesion in skull with suture diastasis**   27. **Ans. b. Neuroblastoma**

■ SENTINEL LYMPH NODE BIOPSY

28. **Ans. b. Carcinoma breast** *(Ref: Harrison 20/e p559; Schwartz 11/e p590-591, 10/e 305-306, 545-547; Sabiston 20/e p849-851)*

29. **Ans. a. Sentinel lymph node biopsy** *(Ref: Harrison 20/e p559; Sabiston 20/e p849-851; Schwartz 11/e p590-591, 10/e p305-306)*

30. **Ans. c. Sentinel lymph node biopsy** *(Ref: Harrison 20/e p559; Sabiston 20/e p849-851; Schwartz 11/e p590-591, 10/e p305-306)*

31. **Ans. c. Carcinoma vulva** *(Ref: Harrison 20/e p559; Sabiston 20/e p849-851; Schwartz 11/e p1810, 10/e p306-306)*

32. **Ans. d. CA colon**

■ GI MALIGNANCY

33. **Ans. a. Esophageal carcinoma** *(Ref: Schwartz 11/e p1074, 10/e 1008-1009; Sabiston 20/e p1034-1035)*

> **ENDOSCOPIC MUCOSAL RESECTION (IN CA ESOPHAGUS)**
>
> - **EMR provides essential staging information** that **guides treatment**[Q].
> - It may also be used as a **therapeutic modality for premalignant** and **early malignant conditions**[Q].

34. **Ans. a. CA colon** *(Ref: www.ncbi.nlm.nih.gov/pubmed/11775180)*

> **RADIO-IMMUNOGUIDED SURGERY FOR COLORECTAL CANCER**
>
> - The **intra-operative detection** of **metastatic disease** in **colorectal cancer** depends on **tumor-associated antigen** and **antibodies** as well as **detection technology** (A **hand-held gamma detecting probe**)[Q].

■ SPONTANEOUS REGRESSION

35. **Ans. b. Osteosarcoma** *(Ref: Robbins 9/e p477, 1041, 955, 1339, 1149)*

Tumors with Spontaneous Regression (NCR MR)	
• **Neuroblastoma**[Q]	• **Malignant melanoma**[Q]
• **Choriocarcinoma**[Q]	• **Retinoblastoma**[Q]
• **Renal cell carcinoma**[Q]	

■ RADIOTHERAPY

36. **Ans. c. Late S** *(Ref: Harrison 19/e p103e-4; Schwartz 11/e p347, 10/e 313-314)*

37. **Ans. d. Samarium-153** *(Ref: Harrison 20/e p657)*

Pure Beta Emitters	
• **Strontium (Sr)-90**[Q]	• **H-3 (Tritium)** [Q]
• **Yttrium (Y)-90**[Q]	• **Phosphorus (P)-32**[Q]

38. **Ans. c. Iridium-192** *(Ref: Principle and Practice of Radiation Oncology (Lippincott) 4/e p637; Harrison 19/e p103e-4)*

39. **Ans. c. Osteosarcoma** *(Ref: Essentials of Radiology by Bhaduri/502)*

40. **Ans. c. Dysgerminoma**   41. **Ans. a. G_2M**

42. **Ans. a. CNS** *(Ref: Radiation Oncology 8/e p41; Harrison 19/e p839-840)*

AMIFOSTINE

- Amifostine offers **no protection to CNS**, as it **doesn't cross blood brain barrier**
- Amifostine is a radiation protector
- Amifostine provide **protection against hematologic** and **non-hematologic toxicity of cisplatin** also

Mechanism of action

- Amifostine **scavenge free radicals** produced by ionizing radiations

Tissue protected

- **Gut lining, hematopoietic system** and **salivary glands**

43. **Ans. a. Ewing's sarcoma**   44. **Ans. c. Cobalt-60** *(Ref: Text Book of Radiation Oncology by Leibel Philips 2nd/231)*

45. **Ans. b. Radioprotector** *(Ref: Radiation Oncology 8/e p41)*   46. **Ans. b. Amifostine**

■ MISCELLANEOUS

47. **Ans. a. Wilm's tumor** *(Ref: CSDT 11/e p1345; CPDT 16/e p807-809)*

- **5-year survival** in **localized Wilm's tumor** of **favorable histology: >97%**

48. **Ans. a. CA thyroid** *(Ref: Harrison 20/e p2716)*
- Thyroid carcinoma is poorly responsive to chemotherapy.

49. **Ans. c. Concurrent chemotherapy** *(Ref: Bailey 27/e p151, 155; Devita 9/e p749; Cancer of the Head and Neck by Suen and Myer 4/e p291-292)*

50. **Ans. b. Chemoport**

"Chemoports are totally implantable venous access devices used to facilitate chemotherapy administration. Internal jugular veins and subclavian veins are the commonly used venous access for port placement. These devices are usually retained over a period of 1 to 2 years or more after which the device is explanted. Some of the long-term complications include catheter embolism, catheter or port occlusion, catheter breakage, device rotation, and vascular thrombosis."

51. **Ans. a. Granisetron** *(Ref: Harrison 20/e p256)*

"5-HT3 antagonists like ondansetron and granisetron prevent postoperative vomiting, radiation therapy–induced symptoms, and cancer chemotherapy– induced emesis, but also are used for other causes of emesis."-Harrison 20/e p256

52. **Ans. b. Prostate cancer** *(Ref: Sabiston 20/e p1845; Schwartz 11/e p1485, 10/e p927; Bailey 27/e p990)*

Malignancies associated with Migratory Thrombophlebitis	
• **CA pancreas (MC)**[Q]	• **Prostate cancer**[Q]
• **CA lung**[Q]	• **Ovarian** cancer[Q]
• **GI malignancies**[Q]	• **Lymphoma**[Q]

- **Trousseau's syndrome**: Migratory thrombophlebitis[Q]
- **Trousseau's sign**: Carpopedal spasm in hypocalcemia[Q]
- **Troisier's sign**: Palpable left supraclavicular LN (Virchow's node)[Q]

53. **Ans. b. Tumor let**   54. **Ans. d. Liposarcoma**

55. **Ans. a. CA colon** *(Ref: Harrison 20/e p585)*

- Harrison says "**Chemotherapy** can be administered **as an adjuvant** (i.e. in addition to surgery or radiation) after all clinical apparent disease has been removed. This use of chemotherapy may have **curative potential in breast** and **colorectal neoplasms**, as it attempts to **eliminate clinically unapparaent tumor** that may have **already disseminated**."

56. Ans. d. Finger *(Ref: Bailey 27/e p614, 711, 712)*

GLOMUS TUMOUR

- These arise from **subcutaneous arteriovenous shunts** (Sucquet–Hoyer canals) especially in the **corium of** the **nail bed.**
- Typically, they are **small, purple nodules** measuring a few millimetres in size, which are **disproportionately painful in response to insignificant stimuli (including cold exposure).**
- **Subungual varieties** may be **invisible** causing **paroxysmal digital pain.**

57. Ans. c. Chromosome 17

TESTICULAR TUMORS

- **Testicular tumors** tend to **metastasize via** the **lymphatic system.**
- In general, the **testicular lymphatics** which **follow** the course of the **testicular vessels**, drain directly into the **lymph nodes in** or **near** the **renal hilus.**
- After involvement of these sentinel nodes, the **lumbar paraaortic nodes become involved** (unilaterally or bilaterally), followed by **spread to the mediastinal** and **supraclavicular nodes** or hematogenous dissemination to lungs, liver and brain.
- **Seminoma is c-kit positive tumor**[Q]

58. Ans. c. Glioma *(Ref: KDT 6/e p577)*

- **Somatostatin** is a 'universal switch off'. Somatostatin analogue **octreotide decreases secretion of** various **hormones.**

Uses of Octreotide	
• **Pancreatic neuroendocrine tumors (insulinoma, glucagonoma, VIPoma)**[Q]	• **Acromegaly**[Q]
	• **Bleeding varices**[Q]
• **Carcinoid tumors** and **syndrome**[Q]	• **Enterocutaneous fistula**[Q]

59. Ans. b. Oral cavity

60. Ans. d. All of the above

"**Acanthosis nigrican** can be a **reflection of an internal malignancy**, most commonly the **adenocarcinoma of GIT, lung, uterus and breast.**"

61. Ans. d. Gallbladder

62. Ans. a. B cell *(Ref: http://www.mdanderson.org/patient-and-cancer-information/cancer-information/cancer-types/eye-cancer/orbit.html)*

ORBITAL LYMPHOMA

- **MC type of cancer of** the **orbit in adults**[Q]
- Usually a form of **B-cell non-Hodgkin's lymphoma**[Q].

Clinical Features
- It may show up as a **nodule in the eyelid** or **around** the **eye**, or it may cause the **eye** to be **pushed out**[Q].
- This type of eye cancer **usually does not cause pain**[Q].

Diagnosis
- **First step in diagnosis** of orbital lymphoma may be a **CT scan of the orbit** followed by a **surgical biopsy**[Q].
- Making the correct diagnosis of the biopsy is very important.

Treatment
- **Radiation therapy, monoclonal antibody** therapy, **chemotherapy** or a combination of these, depending on type of lymphoma and the stage of the tumor.

63. Ans. a. Chondrosarcoma *(Ref: Sabiston 20/e p1602; Schwartz 11/e p722-723, 10/e p667)*

"Chondrosarcomas are the most common primary chest wall malignancy. As with chondromas, they usually arise anteriorly from the costochondral arches. CT scan shows a radiolucent lesion often with stippled calcifications pathognomonic for chondrosarcomas."-Schwartz 11/e p722-723, 10/e p667

64. Ans. c. Pyogenic granuloma *(Ref: Sabiston 20/e p2012; Bailey 27/e p614)*

"Pyogenic granuloma is a misnomer for an exuberant outburst of highly vascular granulation tissue at the site of previous relatively trivial trauma. These lesions are friable, bleed easily, and may grow rapidly. They respond to curettage or simple excision. They usually occur on the fingertips."-Sabiston 20/e p2012

Sarcoma

■ SOFT TISSUE SARCOMA

SOFT TISSUE SARCOMA

- Rare unusual neoplasm of soft tissues
- MC site: Extremity[Q] (lower >upper) > Trunk > Retroperitoneum >Head & Neck
- MC type: **Liposarcoma >Leiomyosarcoma** >Synovial sarcoma >Malignant peripheral nerve sheath tumor >**Malignant fibrous histiocytoma[Q] > GIST**
- **MC pediatric soft tissue sarcoma: Rhabdomyosarcoma[Q]**
- **Hematogenous spread** is **typical of sarcomas[Q]**

Histopathological Type of STS is Site Dependent	
• Extremity	• Malignant fibrous histiocytoma[Q] >Liposarcoma
• Retroperitoneum	• Liposarcoma[Q]
• Viscera	• GIST[Q]

Pathology

- **STS** tends to **grow along fascial planes[Q],** with the surrounding soft tissue compressed to **form a pseudocapsule[Q].**
- **Clinical behavior** of STS is determined by: **Anatomic location (depth), grade & size[Q]**
- **MC route of spread** in soft tissue sarcoma: **Hematogenous[Q]**
- **MC site of metastasis: Lung[Q]; Lymphatic metastasis is rare[Q]**

Clinical Features

- **MC symptom** of STS: **Painless mass[Q]**
- **Size at presentation** is **dependent on the location of tumor[Q].**

> - **Smaller tumors** are located **in distal extremities[Q]**
> - **Larger tumors** are detected **in proximal extremity** and **retroperitoneum[Q].**
> - **Retroperitoneal STS** almost always present as **large asymptomatic mass[Q]**

Diagnosis of Soft Tissue Sarcoma

- **Core-cut** or **true-cut biopsy (CT or USG guided)** is **diagnostic[Q]**
- **Incisional biopsy** is done if **core-cut biopsy** is **non-diagnostic[Q]**
- **FNAC: To confirm** or **rule out** presence of **metastatic focus** or **local recurrence[Q]**
- **MRI:** IOC for **assessing extremity STS[Q]**
- **CECT:** IOC for **assessing retroperitoneal sarcoma[Q]**

Treatment

- **Adequate excision + adjuvant radiotherapy** with or without adjuvant chemotherapy[Q].
- **Two most active chemotherapy agents** against STS: **Doxorubicin & ifosfamide[Q]**

Prognosis

- **Best prognostic factor** of soft tissue sarcoma:

Grade

- **Best prognosis** is seen in: **Extremity STS[Q]**
- **Most important predictor of metastasis in STS: Grade[Q]**
- **MC cause of death** in STS: **Metastasis[Q]; 5-year survival rate** for STS (all stages): **50–60%**

SARCOMAS WITH LN METASTASIS

- MC site of metastasis in sarcomas of extremity: Lungs[Q]
- MC site of metastasis in retroperitoneal sarcomas: Liver[Q] > Lungs[Q]
- LN metastasis is uncommon in soft tissue sarcoma[Q].

Sarcomas with Lymph Node Metastasis (MARCES)	
• **M**alignant fibrous histiocytoma[Q]	• **C**lear cell sarcoma[Q]
• **A**ngiosarcoma[Q]	• **E**pithelial sarcoma[Q]
• **R**habdomyosarcoma[Q]	• **S**ynovial sarcoma[Q]

RHABDOMYOSARCOMA

RHABDOMYOSARCOMA

- **Rhabdomyosarcoma** arises from **mesenchymal tissues.**
- **MC sites** of origin: Head & neck[Q] (parameningeal[Q])>Extremities >Genitourinary tract >Trunk
- **MC pediatric soft tissue sarcoma:** Rhabdomyosarcoma[Q]
- Associated with: **NF, Beckwith-Weidman syndrome, Li-fraumeni** and Fetal alcohol syndrome

Pathology

- **MC histological type:** Embryonal rhabdomyosarcoma[Q]; **MC type in adults: Pleomorphic variant[Q]**
- **Diagnostic cell:** Rhabdomyoblast[Q]
- May contain **tadpole cells** or **strap cells[Q]**
- **Embryonal type** consist of spindle cell variant and **sarcoma botryoides[Q]** (tumor cells resemble **tennis racket[Q]** and tumor cells form submucosal zone of hypercellularity known as **cambium layer[Q]**)
- **Best & most special marker for RMS: Myogenin[Q] > MYOD–1[Q] > Desmin[Q]**

Clinical Features

- **MC presenting symptom: Mass[Q]** (may or may not be painful)
- Bimodal, **first peak** between **2–5 years, second peak** between **15–19 years**
- **Extremity RMS** are **more common** in **lower extremity[Q]**
- **MC site of metastasis: Lung[Q]**

Diagnosis

- **Diagnosis** is **confirmed by biopsy[Q]**
- **MRI: IOC** for diagnosing **extent of disease[Q]**
- **CT:** Used to rule out **lung metastasis[Q]**

Treatment

- **Wide-local excision[Q]** of tumor with surrounding involved tissue
- Tumor **not amenable to primary excision: Neoadjuvant chemotherapy,** after the tumor has decreased in size, **resection of gross residual disease**
- **Radiation therapy:** When **microscopic** or **gross residual disease** exists after initial treatment.

Prognosis

- Prognosis is related to the **site of origin, resectability, presence of metastases, number of metastatic sites,** and **histopathologic features[Q].**
- **Embryonal variant** is a **favorable[Q]** and **alveolar type** has an **unfavorable prognosis[Q].**

Favorable Primary Sites	Unfavorable Primary Sites
• **Orbit[Q]**	• **Extremity[Q]**
• **Nonparameningeal head & neck[Q]**	• **Parameningeal[Q]**
• **Paratestis[Q]**	
• **Vagina[Q]**	

■ DERMATOFIBROSARCOMA PROTUBERANS

DERMATOFIBROSARCOMA PROTUBERANS (DFSP)

- **DFSP** is a **low-grade sarcoma** because it **may recur locally** but **rarely metastasizes**[Q].
- Monomorphous, mononuclear, **spindle cell lesion involving** both **dermis & subcutis**[Q].
- **MC site: Trunk**[Q] (50%) >Extremities (30%) >Head & neck (20%)

Pathology

- **Large lesions** often are associated with **satellite nodules; Positive** for **CD34**[Q]
- Have **unpredictable radial extensions**[Q] of tumor **permeating through** the **subcutaneous tissue** large distances from the primary nodule.
- **More than 75%** of DFSP have a **ring chromosome**[Q], composed of translocated portions of chromosomes **17 & 22**[Q]

Clinical Features

- Typically **presents in early** or **mid-adult life**, beginning as a **nodular cutaneous mass**[Q].
- **Pattern of growth: Slow** and **persistent**[Q]
- Lesion enlarges over many years, it **becomes protuberant**[Q]

Diagnosis

- **IOC for diagnosis: Incisional biopsy**

Treatment

- **Aggressive resection (2-4 cm margin) with** removal of **underlying fascia** with **special attention** to **radial margins** (local recurrence rate <5%)
- Up **to 50% recur after simple excision**[Q].
- **Imatinib: First line of treatment** for **advanced disease**[Q].
- **Neoadjuvant imatinib for unresectable tumors**[Q]

■ SOFT TISSUE SARCOMA

1. Most common sarcoma in a child is:
(Recent Question 2017, 2016, JIPMER 98)
- a. Fibrosarcoma
- b. Rhabdomyosarcoma
- c. Leiomyosarcoma
- d. Liposarcoma

2. The most common sarcoma in childhood:
- a. Malignant histiocytoma *(MHSSMCET 2008)*
- b. Rhabdomyosarcoma
- c. Osteosarcoma
- d. Liposarcoma

3. All of the following soft tissue sarcoma has propensity for lymphatic spread except: *(AIIMS Nov 2005)*
- a. Neurofibrosarcoma
- b. Synovial sarcoma
- c. Rhabdomyosarcoma
- d. Epitheloid sarcoma

4. MC retroperitoneal tumour is: *(DNB 2011, AIIMS June 98)*
- a. Fibrosarcoma
- b. Liposarcoma
- c. Dermoid cyst
- d. Rhabdomyosarcoma

5. Which of the following is best indicator of prognosis of soft tissue sarcoma? *(AIIMS Nov 2000, Feb 97, Nov 96, All India 98)*
- a. Tumor size
- b. Histological type
- c. Nodal metastasis
- d. Tumor grade

6. Most common site of rhabdomyosarcoma is: *(DNB 2011)*
- a. Orbit
- b. Nasopharynx
- c. Extremities
- d. Hypopharynx

7. Most common soft tissue tumour of adults is: *(DNB 2010)*
- a. Embryonal rhabdomyosarcoma
- b. Liposarcoma
- c. Synovial sarcoma
- d. Malignant fibrous histiocytoma

8. Blood borne spread is a feature of: *(DNB 2010)*
- a. Carcinoma
- b. Sarcoma
- c. Dysplasia
- d. Metaplasia

9. Malignant change in lipoma of retroperitoneum may present with: *(DNB 2009)*
- a. Asymptomatic
- b. Renal failure
- c. Abdominal pain
- d. All of the above

10. Commonly done surgery in sarcoma is: *(JIMPER 2012)*
- a. Wide excision
- b. Compartmental exlision/exenteration
- c. Excision
- d. Enucleation

11. In which of the following malignancies, histological grade is a good prognostic indicator? *(JIMPER 2011)*
- a. Soft tissue sarcoma
- b. RCC
- c. Malignant melanoma
- d. All

12. Most common site of metastasis in extremity sarcoma:
(Recent Question 2017, 2016)
- a. Lung
- b. Liver
- c. Kidney
- d. Lymph node

■ DERMATOFIBROSARCOMA PROTUBERANS

13. Maximum margin of excision is needed for:
- a. Malignant melanoma *(Recent Question 2016)*
- b. BCC
- c. SCC
- d. Dermatofibrosarcoma protuberans

■ KAPOSI SARCOMA

14. The tissue of origin of Kaposi sarcoma is: *(AIIMS 2005)*
- a. Lymphoid
- b. Neural
- c. Vascular
- d. Muscular

15. Commonest malignancy in HIV patient: *(AIIMS Nov 99)*
- a. Kaposi sarcoma
- b. Adenoma of stomach
- c. Astrocytoma
- d. CNS lymphoma

16. All are true regarding Kaposi sarcoma except:
- a. Predominant in male *(AIIMS Feb 97)*
- b. Multicentric origin
- c. Chemotherapy is treatment of choice
- d. Occurs in AIDS patients only

17. Kaposi sarcoma is caused by: *(Recent Question 2016)*
- a. HHV 17
- b. HHV 8
- c. HPV 16
- d. Human simian virus 40

Explanations

■ SOFT TISSUE SARCOMA

1. **Ans. b. Rhabdomyosarcoma** *(Ref: Devita 9/e p1780-1784; Sabiston 20/e p1890, 804, 805; Schwartz 11/e p1589, 10/e 1465,1470)*

2. **Ans. b. Rhabdomyosarcoma**

3. **Ans. a. Neurofibrosarcoma**

4. **Ans. b. Liposarcoma** *(Ref: Devita 10/e p1255)*

   - MC soft tissue sarcoma in adults: Liposarcoma > Leiomyosarcoma >Malignant fibrous histiocytoma
   - MC retroperitoneal tumor: Liposarcoma[Q]

5. **Ans. d. Tumor grade**

6. **Ans. a. Orbit**

7. **Ans. b. Liposarcoma**

8. **Ans. b. Sarcoma**

   Hematogenous spread is typical of sarcomas and lymphatic spread is typical of carcinoma.

9. **Ans. d. All of the above** *(Ref: Robbins 8/e p1318)*

   ### RETROPERITONEAL TUMORS

   - Deep seated mass **in abdomen**
   - When the tumor is **very large** do **symptoms of pain** or functional disturbances occur
   - Retroperitoneal tumors may present themselves with signs of weight loss, emaciation and abdominal pain
   - These tumors may also **compress the kidney** or **ureter** leading to **renal failure**

10. **Ans. a. Wide excision**

11. **Ans. a. Soft tissue sarcoma**

12. **Ans. a. Lung**

■ DERMATOFIBROSARCOMA PROTUBERANS

13. **Ans. d. Dermatofibrosarcoma protuberans** **(***Ref: Sabiston 20/e p750, 766)***)**

■ KAPOSI SARCOMA

14. **Ans. c. Vascular** *(Ref: Harrison 20/e p1448, 19/e p1242; Devita 9/e p2101-2104; Sabiston 20/e p750; Schwartz 11/e p527, 535, 10/e 485)*

15. **Ans. a. Kaposi sarcoma** *(Ref: Devita 9/e p2100)*

    - **Most common malignancy in HIV positive individuals: NHL>Kaposi sarcoma**[Q]

16. **Ans. d. Occurs in AIDS patients only**

17. **Ans. b. HHV 8**

Others

- Pediatric Surgery
- Trauma
- Transplantation
- Anesthesia and Perioperative Complications
- Robotics, Laparoscopy and Bariatric Surgery
- Sutures and Anastomoses
- Sterilization and Infection
- Fluid, Electrolyte and Nutrition
- Blood Transfusion
- Shock
- Miscellaneous

Pediatric Surgery

Multiple Choice Questions

1. The given tumor is embryological remnant of:

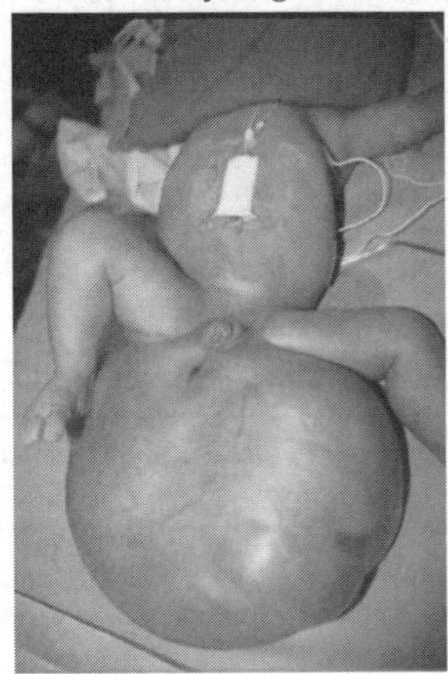

   a. Neural tube   b. Allantois
   c. Notochord   d. Primitive streak

2. Sacrococcygeal teratoma is embryological remnant of:
   (MHSSMCET 2007)
   a. Neural tube   b. Allantois
   c. Notochord   d. Primitive streak

3. Most common solid malignant tumor of infancy:
   a. Neuroblastoma   b. Nephroblastoma
   c. Germ cell tumor   d. Rhabdomyosarcoma

4. Most common posterior mediastinal mass in children is:
   a. Hodgkin's disease   *(Recent Question 2016)*
   b. Neuroblastoma
   c. Esophageal duplication cyst
   d. Bronchogenic cyst

5. Malignant tumor of childhood that metastasizes to bone most often is: *(Recent Question 2016)*
   a. Neuroblastoma   b. Nephroblastoma
   c. Adrenal gland tumors
   d. Ovarian granulose cell tumor

6. Which of the following is the most common tumor of newborn?   *(All India 2012)*
   a. Neuroblastoma   b. Wilm's tumors
   c. Leukemia   d. Sacrococcygeal teratoma

7. Primitive streaks remnants give rise to: *(DNB 2012)*
   a. Neuroblastoma   b. Wilm's tumour
   c. Sacrococcygeal teratoma   d. Hepatoblastoma

8. Most common renal tumor in children: *(Recent Question 2017)*
   a. Renal cyst
   b. Congenital mesoblastic nephroma
   c. Neuroblastoma   d. Nephroblastoma

9. Most common intra-abdominal tumor in infant:
   (Recent Question 2017)
   a. Neuroblastoma   b. Wilm's tumor
   c. HCC   d. Hypernephroma

Explanations

1. **Ans. d. Primitive streak** *(Ref: Sabiston 20/e p1893; Schwartz 11/e p1750, 10/e p1641)*

   Sacrococcygeal teratoma is thought to be a derivative of the primitive streak

2. **Ans. d. Primitive streak** *(Ref: Sabiston 20/e p1893-1894; Schwartz 11/e p1750-1751, 10/e p1641)*

   ### SACROCOCCYGEAL TERATOMA

   - Teratomas occur most frequently in the **neonatal period**, **sacrococcygeal region** is the **MC site**[Q].
   - More common in **females**[Q]

     - Thought to be a derivative of the **primitive streak**[Q]
     - Most often an obvious **external presacral mass**[Q]

   - **Most of** the **tumor** is **usually external**, with a **minimal intrapelvic presacral component**[Q]
   - These lesions should be **carefully followed** with **serial USG until delivery** because the **blood supply to the tumor** may grow to the point of **stealing a significant proportion of placental blood flow to the fetus**[Q].
   - The development of **hydrops** or **placentomegaly** is associated with a **poor prognosis**[Q].

     - **Most neonatal SCTs** are **benign**[Q].
     - **Incidence of malignancy** is **related to age at time of diagnosis** and is most frequently represented as **yolk sac tumors** or **embryonal carcinomas**[Q].

   Treatment
   - **Complete surgical excision**[Q] through a chevron-shaped buttock incision.

     - **Resection of** the coccyx is **critical**[Q] because **failure to remove** this structure **results in significantly higher local recurrence rates.**

3. **Ans. a. Neuroblastoma** *(Ref: Sabiston 20/e p1887-1888; Schwartz 11/e p1748-1749, 10/e p678,1639-1640; Bailey 27/e p138)*

4. **Ans. b. Neuroblastoma** *(Ref: Schwartz 11/e p1748-1749, 10/e p678)*

   Most common posterior mediastinal mass in children is neurogenic tumor (Neuroblastoma among the given options).

5. **Ans. a. Neuroblastoma**

6. **Ans. d. Sacrococcygeal teratoma** *(Ref: Surgery of Childhood Tumors (Springer) 2008/49)*

   - **Sacrococcygeal teratoma** is the **predominant teratoma** as well as the **most common neoplasm** in the **fetus** and **newborn**[Q] with an estimated incidence of 1:20,000 to 1:40,000 live births and a **female predominance**[Q] ranging from 2:1 to 4:1.

7. **Ans. c. Sacrococcygeal teratoma**

   - **Currarino triad:** Anorectal malformations + Sacrococcygeal osseous defect + Presacral mass

8. **Ans. b. Congenital mesoblastic nephroma** *(Ref: Campbell 11/e p2885)*

   "Although congenital mesoblastic nephroma (CMN) is a rare benign congenital renal tumor it is the most common solid renal tumor in the neonatal period." -Campbell 11/e p2885

9. **Ans. a. Neuroblastoma** *(Ref: Sabiston 20/e p1887; Schwartz 11/e p1748-1749, 10/e p1639; Bailey 27/e p847)*

Trauma

TRIMODAL MORTALITY MODEL FOR TRAUMA

Trimodal Mortality Model for Trauma		
Immediate Death (Within minutes of injury)	**Early Death** (Death within hours of arrival to hospital)	**Late Death** (Days to weeks after injury)

• **Declared dead at scene** or **die shortly after arrival to hospital**
• **Causes:**
  – **Irreversible brain injury**[Q]
  – **Hemorrhage** from injuries of heart, aorta, liver, lungs & pelvic fracture[Q]
	• **Intracranial hemorrhage**[Q]
	• **Internal hemorrhage** involving **respiratory system & abdominal organs**[Q]
	• Multiple injuries leading to **severe blood loss**[Q]
	• **Tension pneumothorax**[Q]
	• **Cardiac tamponade**[Q]
		• **Sepsis**[Q]
		• **Multiple organ failure**[Q]

TRIAGE

TRIAGE

- **Triage** means **to "sort"**, especially **used for mass-casualties**[Q]
- **Involves prioritizing** victims into categories based on: **Severity of injury**[Q], likelihood of survival[Q] & urgency of care[Q]
- **Triage tags: Colour codes** are **used to identify the patients**

Categorization of Triage Tags	
Red (immediate)	• **Most critically injured**[Q] • Includes patients with **major head injury**, injuries to **thorax or abdomen**[Q] • **Immediate care is required**[Q]
Yellow (delayed)	• **Less critically injured**[Q] • Require **in hospital treatment**[Q]
Green (ambulatory)	• **No life or limb threatening injuries**[Q]
Black (Expectant)	• **Dead or moribund patients**[Q]

PRIMARY, SECONDARY AND TERTIARY SURVEY

Primary Survey	Secondary Survey	Tertiary Survey
• Aimed at **detecting & simultaneously treating immediately life threatening injuries**[Q] • Identified by the mnemonic **'ABCDE'** • **A: Airway maintenance with cervical spine protection**[Q] • **B: Breathing (ventilation & oxygenation)**[Q] • **C: Circulation with hemorrhage control**[Q] • **D: Disability (Brief neurological examination)**[Q] • **E: Exposure /Environmental control**[Q]	• Consists of **head to toe systematic assessment** of abdominal, pelvic & thoracic areas[Q] • **Complete inspection of body surface** to find all injuries & **neurological examination**[Q] • Patients & surrogates should be queried to **obtain an AMPLE history** • **A**: Allergies[Q] • **M**: Medication[Q] • **P**: Past illness or pregnancy[Q] • **L**: Last meal[Q] • **E**: Events related to injury[Q]	• **Comprehensive** patient **evaluation after initial resuscitation period**[Q] • Usually performed about **24 hours after admission**[Q] • Include a **thorough physical examination** combined with **targeted radiographic imaging** (X-ray usage or CT) **based on examination finding**[Q] • **Decreases the delay in diagnosis** of **potentially life-threatening injuries**[Q]

■ PRIMARY SURVEY

A: Airway Maintenance with Cervical Spine Protection

- **Cervical spine injury** should be **suspected in all the patients**[Q]
- **All trauma patients** should have **cervical spine immobilization** & **protected through out**[Q]
- **First priority: Cervical spine followed by airway**[Q]
- **Asses the patency of airway: Elicit the verbal response**[Q] (simplest way: Ask the patients name; **ability to speak indicates adequate airway protection**[Q])
- In **patients, who cannot speak,** suspect **mental status depression** or **airway obstruction**. Both are **indication for airway management**[Q]
- **Other indications:** Noisy breathing[Q], facial trauma[Q] & GCS ≤ 8[Q]

Compromised Airway Require Stepwise Progression
• First **clearing the airway by suctioning** secretions or blood followed by **jaw thrust** or **chin lift**[Q]
• Insertion of **oropharyngeal or nasopharyngeal airway**[Q]
• **Definitive airway of choice** for most injured patients: **Oral endotracheal intubation** with **cuffed endotracheal tube**[Q]
• **ATLS updates (2018)** recommended **use of video laryngoscope for intubation**[Q]
• **In severe maxillofacial injuries:** Emergency airway (Needle cricothyroidotomy[Q]) & Definitive airway (Tracheostomy[Q])

In Severe Maxillofacial Injuries	
Emergency Airway	**Definitive Airway**
• **Emergency airway: Needle cricothyroidotomy**[Q] • Performed quickly; **High flow O_2** is given **via 4-6 mm tube**[Q] • **Advantage:** Provides time for **definitive airway**[Q] • **Disadvantage: CO_2 retention** occurs **within 20-30 minutes**[Q] • **Avoided in children <12 years** of age it can lead to **subglottic stenosis**[Q]	• **Tracheostomy**[Q]

Breathing (Ventilation & Oxygenation)

- **Asses breathing by:** Visualizing chest movements[Q]; Rate & depth of respiration[Q]; Percussion & Auscultation of breath sounds[Q]
- **Limited respiratory effort** or dyspnea requires **support of ventilation** & **further assessment of chest**[Q]
- **Ventilation problems** are secondary to tension pneumothorax, massive hemothorax or flail chest with pulmonary contusion[Q]

Condition	Management
Tension pneumothorax	• Insertion of **large bore needle in 2nd intercostal space in midclavicular line** followed by **ICD insertion in triangle of safety**[Q] • **ATLS updates (2018)** says "Recent evidences support insertion of wide bore needle in 5th intercostal space slightly anterior to mid axillary line in adults"[Q]
Massive hemothorax	• **ICD insertion**[Q] • **Optimal size of chest tube** required to drain a hemothorax: **28–32 F**[Q]
Severe pulmonary contusion	• **Aggressive mechanical ventilation**[Q]

Circulation with Hemorrhage Control

- **Assess circulation** to look for shock; **Primary goal** is to **rule out shock**[Q]
- **MC cause of shock in trauma:** Hemorrhage[Q]
- **Assess vitals:** Pulse rate & BP[Q]
- **In case of shock** (PR >100/min[Q], BP <100 mm Hg[Q]): Put two large bore IV cannula[Q] (Green cannula[Q] is preferred); Send **blood for cross match**[Q]

> - **ATLS updates (2018):** Give only 1 liter of warm isotonic crystalloids for adults[Q] (Old edition recommended 1-2 liters of warm crystalloid solution)
> - **ATLS updates (2018):** In **children <40 kg,** give **20 mL/kg of warm isotonic crystalloids**[Q]

- **Rapid screening** should be done **to identify the cause of life threatening blood loss**[Q]

> - The **source of hemorrhage** is often described as "on the floor, plus four more"[Q]
> - **Five major locations** responsible for exsanguination: 1. External blood loss[Q]; 2. Thorax; 3. Abdomen; 4. Retroperitoneum (pelvic fracture) 5. Multiple long bone fracture

- **Initial physical examination:** Identifies source of external blood loss & long bone fractures; Managed immediately with direct pressure[Q] or splinting[Q] respectively
- **Chest X-ray:** To evaluate **thoracic blood loss**[Q]; X-ray pelvis: To identify pelvis fracture[Q]; FAST: To evaluate abdomen
- **Two most important X-rays in patients of trauma:** Chest X-ray[Q] & X-ray pelvis (AP view[Q]) as patients is in supine position
- After **initial administration of IV fluid,** patients are **assessed for ongoing signs of shock**[Q]
- For **non-responding patients, manage ongoing bleeding + blood transfusion**[Q]

Contd…

Contd…

> - **For trauma resuscitation:** Packed cell, plasma & platelets are used in the **ratio 1:1:1**[Q]
> - **Best indicator of tissue perfusion in trauma:** Urine output[Q]
> - **Best indicator to determine amount of fluid required:** CVP[Q]

- **Pediatric mass transfusion protocol (ATLS updates 2018):** Initial **20 mL/kg bolus**[Q] of isotonic crystalloid followed by 10-20 mL/kg of packed cells, plasma & platelets in the ratio of 1:1:1[Q].

CRASH-2 Trial (ATLS updates 2018)

- **Use of tranexamic acid** in **hypotensive trauma patients**[Q]
- **Tranexamic acid reduces** the risk of **mortality from bleeding** in both **blunt & penetrating trauma**[Q]
- **Dose: 1 gm IV over 10 minutes followed by 1 gm over 8 hours**[Q]
- **Given to all trauma patients suspected to have significant hemorrhage including SBP <110 mm Hg or PR >110/min**[Q]
- Should be **administered within 3 hours of injury**[Q]

DISABILITY (BRIEF NEUROLOGICAL EXAMINATION)

- Assess GCS & assess pupils (Size/ equality/ reaction)[Q]

Revised Glasgow Coma Scale 2014

Revised GCS (2014)

Eye Opening (E)		Verbal Response (V)		Best Motor Response (M)	
Spontaneous	4	Oriented	5	Obeying commands	6
To **Speech**[Q]	3	Confused	4	Localizing	5
To **Pressure**[Q]	2	**Words**[Q]	3	Normal flexion (withdrawal)	4
None	1	**Sounds**[Q]	2	Abnormal flexion	3
		None	1	Extension	2
				None	1

- **GCS** specifically **recommends avoiding sternal rubs**[Q] as it causes bruising & responses can be difficult to interpret. They also **do not recommend routine use of retromandibular pressure**[Q].
- **Revised GCS (2014)** changes are highlighted in the above table.
- **Maximum score-15**[Q], **minimum score-3**[Q].
- **Best predictor of outcome: Motor response**[Q]

> - **Reporting of Non-testable Score Aspects: In cases of a non-testable aspect, the new GCS should only be noted in its components. Any element that cannot be tested should be marked as NT, for "not testable".**
> - For **intubated patients** or **patients with tracheostomy**, V_{NT} is used. It is **no longer recommended to assign 1 point to non-testable elements,** therefore a combined score should not be used.

GCS-P	GCS-PA CT
- **GCS-P** is calculated by **subtracting the Pupil Reactivity Score (PRS) from the Glasgow Coma Scale (GCS) total score: GCS-P = GCS – PRS**[Q] - **Pupil reactivity score** represents the **number of nonreactive pupils (0, 1, or 2)**[Q]. - This **number is subtracted from the GCS score (3-15)**, resulting in the **GCS-P (1-15)**[Q].	- **GCS-PA CT: GCS, Pupils, Age & CT findings**[Q] - **Probability of mortality 6 months after head injury based on** the patient's admission **GCS-P and age with no CT abnormality (A), exactly 1 CT abnormality (B), and 2 or more CT abnormalities (C).** - **Potential CT abnormalities** include **intracranial hematoma, absent cisterns & SAH**[Q].

Pupils Unreactive to Light	PRS
Both pupils	2
One pupil	1
Neither pupil	0
Note: Higher score is assigned to non-reactive pupils.	

EXPOSURE (ENVIRONMENTAL CONTROL)

- **All clothing are removed** for adequate examination
- Core body temperature is obtained & **patient is kept warm**
- **Environmental control** should be maintained with **warm blankets, increased room temperature, heated fluid administration & body warmers.**

■ ATLS UPDATES (2018) ABOUT LIFE THREATENING INJURIES DURING PRIMARY SURVEY

Life Threatening Injuries During Primary Survey		
Airway	**Breathing**	**Circulation**
• Airway obstruction[Q] • Tracheobronchial injuries[Q]	• Tension pneumothorax[Q] • Open pneumothorax[Q]	• Massive hemothorax[Q] • Cardiac tamponade[Q] • Traumatic circulatory arrest[Q]

■ SECONDARY SURVEY

SECONDARY SURVEY

1. **Head & face:** Rule out skull fracture & laceration
2. **Neck:** Rule out neck injuries
3. **Chest:** Rule out rib fracture
4. **Abdomen: Rule out abdominal pain**, tenderness, bruising; **NG tube insertion** is **contraindicated** in presence of **facial fracture (orogastric tube** should be **inserted)**, **urinary catheter** should be inserted **if no blood is present at meatus**[Q]
5. **Back: Log Roll – 5 people** are required for examination of back, **3 for body, one for head** & **one for** examining back; **PR is done** at this time[Q]
6. **Extremities:** Each limb should be examined for **tenderness, crepitation** or **abnormal movement.**[Q]
7. **Neurological examination:**
   - **Repeat GCS**, re-evaluate the pupils   – Look for any localising/lateralising signs   – Look for **signs of cord injury**

- For **log roll, ideal number of people** required: **5**[Q]
- **Minimum number** of people required for log roll: **4**[Q]

■ TRAUMA SCORING SYSTEM

Trauma Scoring System		
Revised Trauma Score	**Trauma and Injury Severity Score (TRISS)**	**Mangled Extremity Severity Score (MESS)**

• RTS combines: (GB Road)
  – **Glasgow coma scale**[Q]
  – Systolic **Blood pressure**[Q]
  – **Respiratory rate**[Q]
	• **TRISS combines:**
	  – **Injury Severity Score** (ISS)[Q]
	  – **R**evised Trauma Score (**RTS**)[Q]
	  – **Age**[Q]
	  – **Mechanism**[Q] of Injury (Blunt/Penetrating)
		• MESS combines: (ELISA)
		  – **Energy** that caused the injury[Q]
		  – **Limb Ischemia**[Q]
		  – **Shock**[Q]
		  – Patient's **Age**[Q]

■ ABDOMINAL TRAUMA

ABDOMINAL TRAUMA

- **MC injured organ in blunt trauma abdomen:** Spleen[Q] >Liver[Q]
- MC injured organ in **penetrating trauma abdomen (ATLS 2018 update):** Liver[Q] (26%) >**Stomach**[Q] (17%) >**SI**[Q] (12.9%)
- **MC injured organ in gunshot wound:** Small intestine[Q] **(SI)**
- **MC injured bowel in blunt trauma abdomen:** Jejunum[Q]
- **MC injured structure in seat belt injury:** Mesentery[Q]
- **MC injured site in deceleration injury:** Duodenojejunal junction[Q]
- **First investigation** done in **blunt trauma abdomen:** FAST[Q]
- **Gold standard investigation** in **stable patients of blunt trauma abdomen:** CECT[Q]

■ FAST

FAST (FOCUSED ASSESSMENT WITH SONOGRAPHY FOR TRAUMA)

- **FAST: Emergency USG** done very fast, **performed within 2-4 minutes**[Q]
- **Rapid diagnostic examination to assess patients with potential thoracoabdominal injuries**[Q]
- **FAST** is the **first investigation** done in **blunt trauma abdomen; FAST has replaced DPL**[Q]
- **4 'P's** are evaluated **in the sequence: Pericardial sac** → **Perihepatic** region → **Perisplenic** region → **Pelvis**[Q]

Contd…

Contd…

Traditional Four Views of FAST	
Subxiphoid transverse view[Q]	• Assess **pericardial sac**[Q]
Right upper quadrant (**RUQ**) longitudinal view[Q]	• Assess **perihepatic** region[Q]
Left upper quadrant (**LUQ**) longitudinal view[Q]	• Assess **perisplenic** region[Q]
Suprapubic longitudinal & transverse view[Q]	• Assess **pelvis**[Q]

- **e-FAST (extended FAST)** has **two additional views, right & left thoracic views to rule out pneumothorax or hemothorax**[Q].
- **Stratosphere sign or barcode sign** is seen on **e-FAST** in **pneumothorax**[Q].

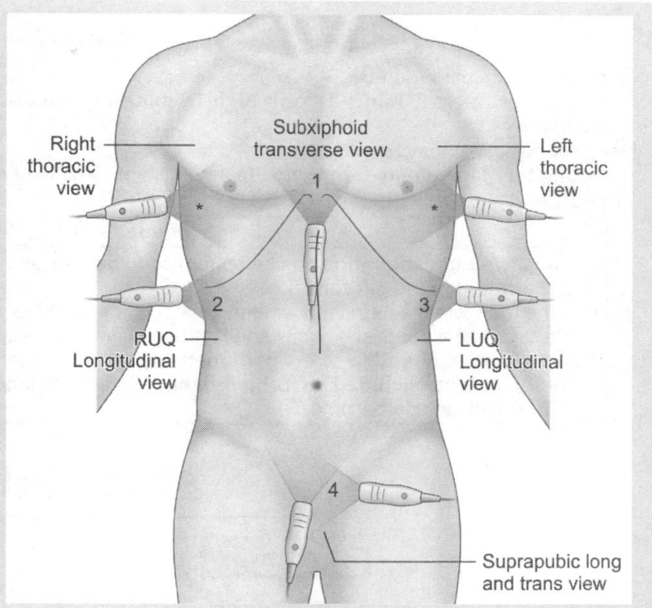

■ DIAGNOSTIC PERITONEAL LAVAGE

DIAGNOSTIC PERITONEAL LAVAGE

- Performed **for blunt trauma abdomen** patients
- DPL is performed through **vertical infra-umbilical midline incision** unless the patient has pelvic fracture or is pregnant[Q]
- Linea alba is sharply incised & **catheter is directed towards pelvis**[Q]
- **Abdominal contents** should initially be **aspirated using a 10-mL syringe**[Q].
- Through the catheter, **one liter of saline or RL** is **infused into peritoneal cavity**[Q].
- Lavage fluid is sent for assessment

Positive DPL	
• **>10 mL of gross blood** is **aspirated directly from peritoneal cavity**[Q]	• **Returned effluent contains:** – **RBCs >1 lac/mm³**[Q] – **WBCs >500/mm³**[Q] – **Demonstrable bacteria or bile**[Q] – **Amylase >174 IU/dL**[Q]

- **Sensitivity of DPL** for detecting significant intra-abdominal injury is **82-96%** & **specificity 87-99%**.

■ MANAGEMENT OF BLUNT TRAUMA ABDOMEN

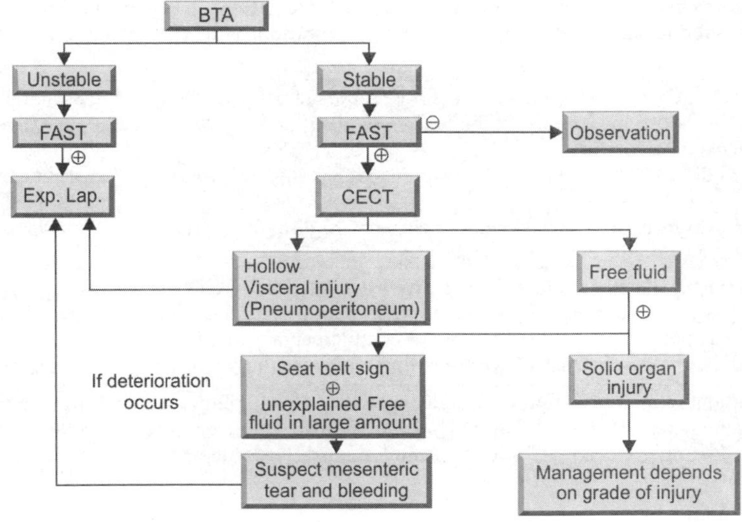

■ PENETRATING TRAUMA

PENETRATING ABDOMINAL INJURIES

- Gunshot Abdominal Wounds:
  - Chances of **internal injury** is **very high in gunshot wounds,** thus little preoperative evaluation is required and **laparotomy is mandatory**[Q].
- Stab Wounds to Abdomen:
  - **Exploratory laparotomy** is indicated in patients with isolated penetrating abdominal wound if **hypotensive** or **in shock** or **showing peritoneal signs**[Q].

Anterior Stab Wounds	Flank and Back Wounds
• **Local wound exploration** can be performed to determine **if there is any penetration of** the **peritoneal cavity**[Q]. • If the tract terminates without entering the peritoneum, the injury can be managed as a deep laceration[Q] and laparotomy is not needed. • Otherwise, **penetration of the peritoneum** is assumed and **significant injury** must be **excluded by further diagnostic evaluations**[Q] (FAST, CECT, DPL or laparoscopy)	• Risk of injury to **colon, kidney** and **ureter**[Q] • **Triple contrast CT**[Q] is advised **to detect colon** and **retroperitoneal injuries** and the **need for laparotomy.** • **Triple contrast: IV, Oral & Rectal contrast**

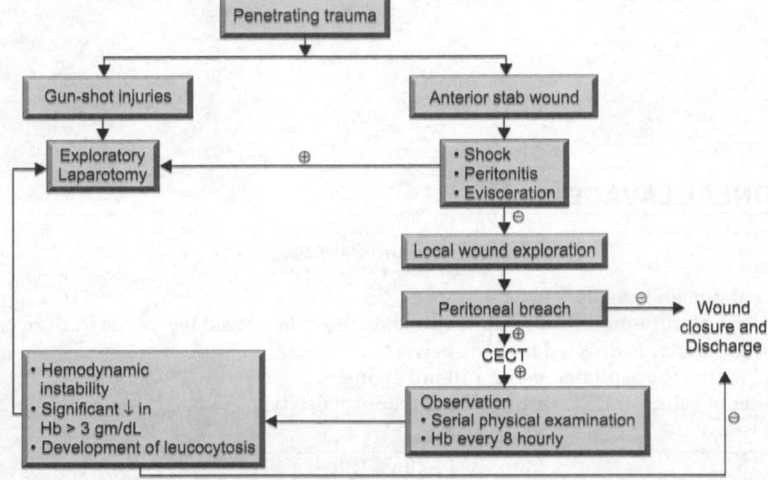

■ SPLENIC TRAUMA

SPLENIC INJURIES

- **MC organ injured in blunt trauma abdomen: Spleen**[Q]

Pathophysiology

- **Direct compression**[Q] of organ in the left upper quadrant of abdomen
- **Deceleration mechanism** that **tears the splenic capsule** or **parenchyma**[Q], mainly at areas fixed or tethered to the retroperitoneum

Diagnosis

- **Identification**[Q] **of splenic injuries** may occur **during laparotomy in unstable patients** taken **emergently to the operating room**[Q].
- **Unstable patients** with **intra-abdominal fluid on FAST** require **exploration,** with the **spleen** commonly being the **bleeding intra-abdominal organ**[Q].

> - In **stable patients,** abdominal CT performed with **IV contrast** is the **mainstay for diagnosing & characterizing splenic injuries**[Q].
> - **Images** are typically obtained with the contrast in the **portal venous phase** to enhance the splenic parenchyma maximally while still being able to visualize the vasculature.
> - **Splenic injuries** appear as **disruptions** in the **normal splenic parenchyma,** frequently with **surrounding hematoma & free intra-abdominal blood**[Q].
> - Occasionally, **active extravasation of contrast,** identified as a **high-density blush,** can be identified, **contained within a pseudoaneurysm** or **bleeding into** the **peritoneal space**[Q].

- **Angiography** has been used **for injuries that demonstrate active extravasation by CT**[Q].
- **Angiography** can **identify specific sites of bleeding** from the splenic parenchyma & underlying segmental or trabecular vessels; however, it cannot characterize the splenic parenchymal injury but can be complementary to CT.
- **Advantage of angiography:** Potential to **obstruct sites of bleeding endovascularly** using **angioembolization**[Q].

> - Patients who are candidates for **nonoperative management** of their splenic injury but **demonstrate a blush by CT,** indicating **active extravasation,** may **benefit from angiography with embolization** to eliminate the splenic pseudoaneurysm[Q].
> - **Angiographic embolization** is considered **only in hemodynamically stable patients**[Q].

Contd...

Contd…

Management
- With appropriate patient selection, **many patients with blunt splenic trauma** can be **managed without splenectomy**[Q].
- **No bleeding patient** should go **without splenectomy** or **splenic repair**, especially in an attempt to push the figurative nonoperative envelope[Q].

> - **Hemodynamic stability** is a **prerequisite for nonoperative management** and must be **present without ongoing intravascular volume support**[Q].
> - **Hemodynamic stability** is indicated by a **normal blood pressure** and **lack of tachycardia, no** physical examination findings indicating **shock**, and **absence of metabolic acidosis**[Q].

- **Nonoperative management is reserved** for grades I, II and **isolated** grade III injuries[Q].

Indications of Operative Management of Splenic Trauma
• **Instability** at admission[Q]   • **Exact location of bleeding is unknown**[Q]   • Failed nonoperative management[Q]

- **Best approach:** Midline incision with **packing of all four quadrants** in cases of hemodynamic **instability**[Q].
- **Drains should not be placed unless** there is concern that the **tail of the pancreas** was also **injured**[Q].

Splenic Injury Secondary to Penetrating Abdominal Trauma
• **Splenic injury** secondary to **penetrating abdominal trauma** is usually **identified during laparotomy** and should be **addressed based on** the presence or absence of **ongoing bleeding.**[Q]   • **Splenectomy** is performed **in cases of ongoing bleeding**[Q].

American Association for the Surgery of Trauma: Spleen Organ Injury Scale		
Grade	**Type**	**Description of Injury**
I	Hematoma	Subcapsular tear **<10%** surface area
	Laceration	**Capsular tear <1 cm** parenchymal depth
II	Hematoma	Subcapsular tear, **10–50%** surface area; intraparenchymal, **<5 cm in diameter**
	Laceration	Capsular tear, **1–3 cm** parenchymal depth that does not involve a trabecular vessel
III	Hematoma	Subcapsular tear **>50%** surface area or expanding; ruptured subcapsular or parenchymal hematoma; intraparenchymal hematoma **≥5 cm** or **expanding**
	Laceration	**>3 cm** parenchymal depth or **involving trabecular vessels**
IV	Laceration	Laceration involving **segmental** or **hilar vessels** producing **major devascularization (>25%** of spleen)
V	Hematoma	**Completely shattered spleen**
	Laceration	**Hilar vascular injury** devascularizes spleen

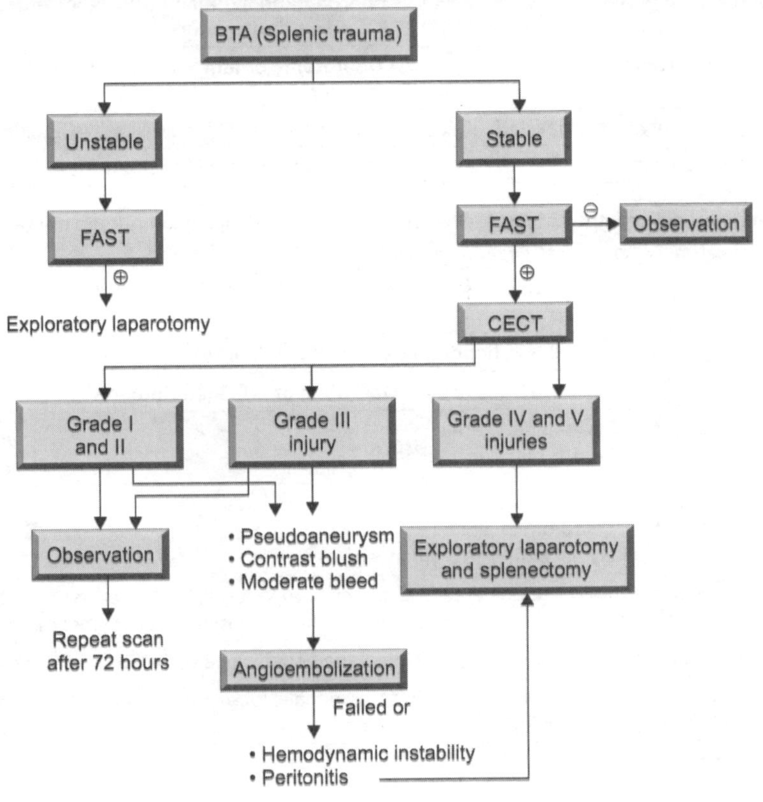

■ LIVER TRAUMA

HEPATIC INJURY

- MC organ injured in **blunt abdominal trauma**: Spleen > liver[Q]
- MC injured organ in penetrating trauma: Liver >Stomach >Small Intestine
- **Mechanisms** of blunt hepatic trauma: **Compression** with **direct parenchymal damage** and shearing forces, which tear hepatic tissue and disrupt vascular and ligamentous attachments.
- **Most liver injuries** (>85%) involve segments **6, 7** and **8** of the liver[Q].
- **Most liver injury bleeding** is **venous**[Q]; and therefore low pressure, tamponade is readily performed

Diagnosis

- Liver injuries are often **first diagnosed** on **entering the abdomen** in **unstable patient** explored for the finding of **free fluid on FAST examination**[Q].

> - **Stable patients** with suspected hepatic trauma should undergo **CECT abdomen**[Q].
> - Current **CT modalities** are **excellent** at providing **significant anatomic detail** that allows highly **accurate characterization of injuries.**

- **Contrast extravasation** visualized as a **high-density blush** is identified **indicating** the presence of a **pseudoaneurysm** or **active bleeding** external to the liver capsule[Q].
- **Beer claw laceration:** Multiple Linear laceration of liver on **CECT**
- Liver **injury grading** involves the **extent of parenchymal involvement** and presence of **vascular injury**[Q]

Management

- **Unstable patients: Immediate laparotomy**[Q]
  Conservative criteria for **non-operative management** require
  - Hemodynamically stable patient[Q]
  - No peritoneal signs on examination[Q]
  - Absence of other major injuries[Q]
- **Most treatment failures** occur **within** the **first 24 hours** of **admission**[Q].
- **Failure of nonoperative management** is defined as the development of **hemodynamic instability** or of liver-related **multiple transfusions** despite angiographic embolization, signs of **peritonitis,** or **abdominal compartment syndrome**[Q].

Deep Liver Laceration	• **Opening the liver wound** and **directly approaching** the **bleeding vessel**, a procedure known as **tractotomy**[Q].
Penetrating Liver Tracts	• **Tractotomy** or **tamponade** using a balloon catheter[Q]
Injuries in the **vicinity of retrohepatic IVC**	• **Packing alone**, without operative exploration [Q]
Retrohepatic IVC Injury	• **Atriocaval shunt (Shrock shunt)**[Q]

- **Liver parenchymal necrosis** is the **MC complication** of severe liver injury in patients who **undergo operation**[Q].
- **Rebleeding** is the **MC complication** of nonoperative management[Q].

Classification of Liver Injury (Moore)		
Grade	**Types**	**Operative or CT Scan findings**
I	Hematoma Laceration	Subcapsular, **<10%** of surface area Capsular tear, **<1 cm** in parenchymal depth
II	Hematoma Laceration	Subcapsular, **10-50%** of surface area Intraparenchymal, **<10 cm** in diameter **1-3 cm** in parenchymal depth, **<10 cm** in length
III	Hematoma Laceration	Subcapsular, >50% of surface area or expanding; ruptured subcapsular or parenchymal hematoma Intraparenchymal, hematoma **>10 cm** or **expanding >3 cm** in parenchymal depth
IV	Laceration	Parenchymal disruption involving **25-75%** of the hepatic lobe or **1-3 Couinauds segments** in a single lobe
V	Laceration Vascular	Parenchymal disruption involving **>75%** of the hepatic lobe or >3 **Couinauds segments** within a single lobe **Juxtahepatic venous injuries,** i.e. retrohepatic **vena cava**/ central **major hepatic veins**
VI	Vascular	**Hepatic avulsion**

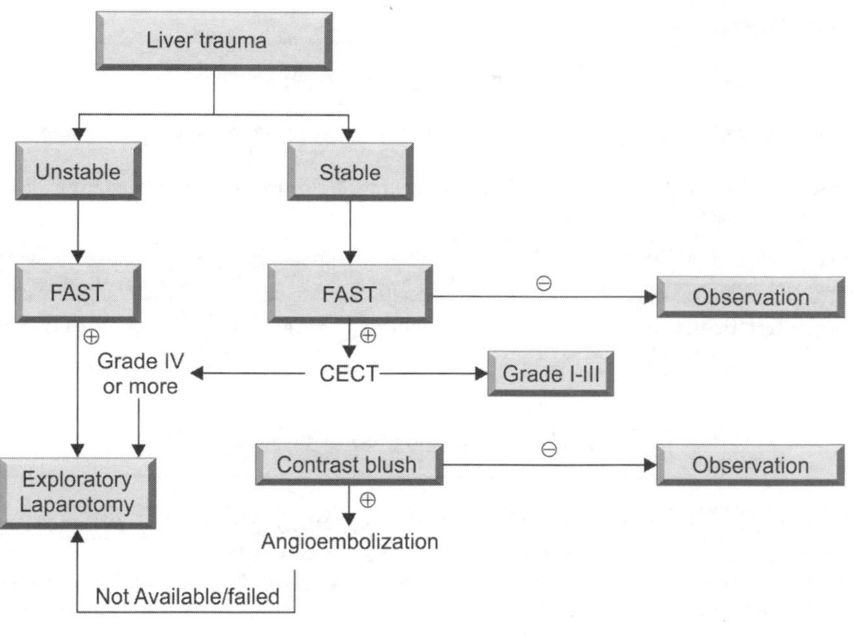

■ SEAT BELT INJURY

Seat Belt Injury

- Use of seat belt is associated with injury profile known as seat belt syndrome
- MC injured structure: Mesentery[Q]
- Classic seat belt sign: Skin abrasion of neck, chest & abdomen[Q]
- Classic seat belt sign is associated with high chances of internal organ injury[Q]
- Caused by sudden deceleration → Mesentery tear[Q]
- May compress pancreas over vertebral column → Pancreaticoduodenal injury[Q]

Longitudinal Tear	Transverse Tear
• Repair the tear as the bowel is perfused by adjacent tissues[Q]	• Leads to devascularization of bowel[Q] • Resection & anastomosis is done[Q]

■ TRAUMA TRIAD OF DEATH

Trauma Triad of Death

- Trauma triad of death: Hypothermia + Coagulopathy + Metabolic acidosis[Q]
- Coagulopathy is most commonly responsible for death[Q]

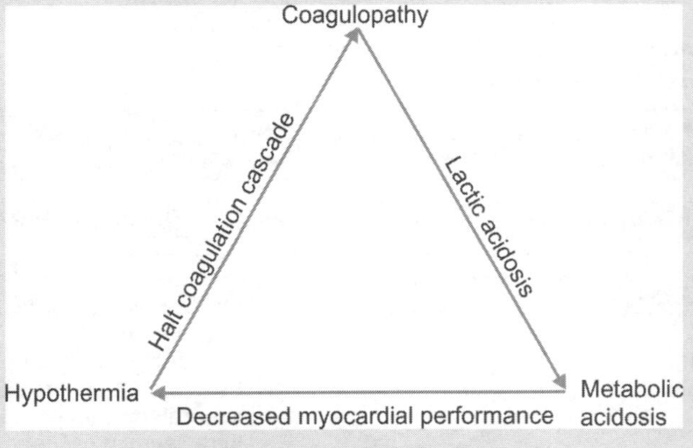

Trauma Triad of Death

■ DAMAGE CONTROL SURGERY

Damage Control Surgery (DCS)

- DCS centers on coordinating **staged operative interventions** with periods of **aggressive resuscitation** to salvage trauma patients sustaining major injuries[Q].
- **Damage control includes** an **abbreviated laparotomy, temporary packing, & closure of the abdomen** in an effort to **blunt the physiologic response to prolonged shock & massive hemorrhage**[Q].
  - These patients are often **at limits of their physiological reserve** when they present to operating room and **persistent operative efforts** result in exacerbation of their **underlying hypothermia, coagulopathy & acidosis**, initiating a **vicious cycle** that **culminates in death**[Q].
- In these situations, **abrupt termination of the procedure** after **control of surgical hemorrhage & contamination**, followed by **ICU resuscitation & staged reconstruction**, can be life saving[Q].

Phases of Damage Control Surgery

Phase I (Initial Exploration)	Phase II (Secondary Resuscitation)	Phase III (Definitive Operation)
• Consists of an **initial operative exploration** to attain rapid **control of active hemorrhage & contamination**[Q] • Abdomen is entered via a **midline incision** and if exsanguinating hemorrhage is encountered **four quadrant packing**[Q] should be performed • **Any violations of GI tract** should be treated with **suture closure** or **segmental stapled resection**[Q] • **External drains** are placed to control any major pancreatic or biliary injuries	• Following completion of initial exploration, the **critically ill patient** is **transferred to ICU**[Q]. • **Invasive monitoring & complete ventilator support**[Q] are often needed. • This phase focuses on **secondary resuscitation to correct hypothermia, coagulopathy & acidosis**[Q]	• It consists of **planned re-exploration & definitive repair**[Q] of injuries • This phase typically occurs **48 & 72 hours following initial** and **after successful secondary resuscitation**[Q] • Abdomen should be closed primarily if possible • **Risky GI anastomoses** or **complex reconstruction** should be **avoided**[Q]

Stages of DCS

Stage I	• **Patient selection**[Q]
Stage II	• **Operative control of hemorrhage & contamination**[Q]
Stage III	• **ICU resuscitation**[Q]
Stage IV	• **Definitive surgery**[Q]
Stage V	• **Abdominal closure**[Q]

■ ABDOMINAL COMPARTMENT SYNDROME

Abdominal Compartment Syndrome

- ACS is defined as increased intra-abdominal pressure (IAP >20 mm Hg) resulting in compression of abdominal structures[Q], producing **fatal complications** due to **pulmonary failure** and **mesenteric vascular compromise**.
- Normal IAP = 5-7 mm Hg; Intra-abdominal hypertension IAP ≥ 12 mm Hg
- ACS occurs **predominantly in:**
  - Patients in **profound shock**[Q]
  - Patients **requiring large amounts of resuscitation fluids & blood**[Q]
  - Those **with major visceral or vascular abdominal injuries**[Q]
  - **ACS is characterized by a sudden increase in IAP, increased peak inspiratory pressure, decreased urinary output, hypoxia, hypercapnia, & hypotension** secondary to decreased venous return to the heart[Q].

Physiologic Consequences of Increased Intra-abdominal Pressure

Decreased	Increased
• **Cardiac output**[Q] • **Central venous return**[Q] • **Visceral blood flow**[Q] • **Renal blood flow**[Q] • **Glomerular filtration**	• **Cardiac rate**[Q] • Pulmonary capillary wedge pressure[Q] • Peak inspiratory pressure[Q] • **Central venous pressure**[Q] • Intrapleural pressure • **Systemic vascular resistance**[Q]

Contd…

Diagnosis

- Diagnosis is confirmed by **measuring bladder pressure**, which ultimately represents IAP.
- A **urinary bladder catheter** is the **gold standard** indirect method used to measure IAP.

Abdominal Compartment Syndrome Grading System			
Grade	Bladder Pressure (mm Hg)	Clinical Features	Treatment
I	12–15	None	**Normovolemic** resuscitation
II	16–20	**Oliguria**[Q], splanchnic hypoperfusion	**Hypovolemic** resuscitation
III	21–25	**Anuria**, increased ventilation pressure	**Decompression**
IV	>25	**Anuria, increased ventilation pressure & decreased PO_2**[Q]	**Emergency re-exploration**

Treatment

- Treatment includes **rapid decompression** of elevated IAP **by opening the abdominal wound** & performing a **temporary closure** of abdominal wall with **mesh** or a **plastic bag (Bogota bag)**[Q].

■ NECK INJURIES

NECK INJURIES

- **Most severe neck injuries** are caused **by penetrating wounds** and may present an immediate threat to life as a result of **airway compromise** or **hemorrhage**[Q].

> - **Major vascular & aerodigestive structures** in the neck are **located in anterior triangle**, & all are deep to the platysma[Q].
> - **Platysma & SCM are useful anatomic boundaries**[Q].

- Injuries that **do not penetrate** the platysma can be **considered superficial**, and no further investigation is needed. Wounds that **penetrate the platysma** must be further evaluated.
- Injuries that are **anterior to SCM** present a **high likelihood of significant injury**, whereas those that track **posterior to SCM** are **unlikely to involve major vascular or aerodigestive structures.**
- **Penetrating injuries to** the **posterior triangle** should raise concern about **trauma to cervical spine & spinal cord**[Q].

Neck is divided into Three Horizontal Zones on craniocaudal location	
Zone I	• **At thoracic inlet**[Q] • Extends from **sternal notch to cricoid cartilage**[Q] • Injuries in this zone carry the **highest mortality** because of the **presence of great vessels**[Q] & difficult surgical approach.
Zone II	• **Midportion of** the **neck**[Q] • Extends from **cricoid cartilage to angle of mandible**[Q]
Zone III	• Extends from **angle of mandible to base of skull**[Q]

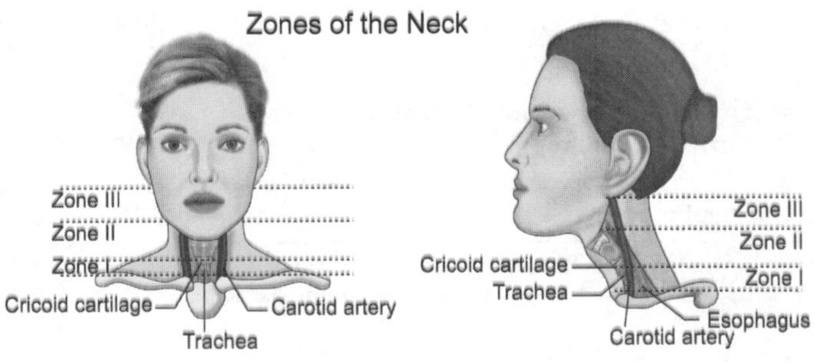

■ THORACIC INJURIES

THORACIC INJURIES

- **MC cause of mortality in blunt thoracic trauma:** Tracheobronchial injuries[Q]
- **MC cause of mortality in penetrating thoracic trauma:** Hemothorax[Q] (secondary to pulmonary laceration)
- **MC thoracic injuries:** Chest wall injuries[Q]

■ RIB FRACTURE

RIB FRACTURE

- Occurs secondary to compression of thoracic cage in anteroposterior direction or lateral direction
- **Uncommon** to have **fracture of floating ribs (11th & 12th ribs) & first rib fracture**[Q]
- High velocity impact can cause fracture of 1st rib & **10th-12th** ribs.

> - **MC rib fractured during CPR: 4th-6th rib**[Q]

- In cases of **1st rib fracture**, suspect injury of subclavian vessels, brachial plexus & apex of lung[Q]
- In cases of **10th-12th rib fracture**, on right side suspect injury to liver[Q] & on left side suspect injury to spleen[Q] (long axis of spleen is related to 10th rib)

Management

- Most rib fractures are **managed conservatively with adequate analgesia. Strapping should not be done**[Q]

■ PERICARDIAL TAMPONADE

PERICARDIAL TAMPONADE

- **Rapid accumulation of blood in pericardial space**[Q]
- **Quantity of fluid:** Even **200 mL fluid** which **collets rapidly** can lead to pericardial tamponade[Q]
- Caused by **penetrating trauma**[Q]

Clinical Features

- Characterized by **Beck's triad (MDH):** <u>M</u>uffled heart sounds + <u>D</u>istended neck veins + <u>H</u>ypotension[Q]

Diagnosis

- IOC for diagnosis: **Echocardiography**[Q]
- **Chest X-ray: Enlarged heart shadow**[Q]

Treatment

- **Emergency treatment: Needle pericardiocentesis**[Q]
- **TOC: Surgical pericardiotomy**[Q]

■ FLAIL CHEST

FLAIL CHEST

- A flail chest occurs when a **segment of** the **chest wall does not have bony continuity with** the **rest of** the **thoracic cage**[Q].
- This condition usually results from blunt trauma associated with multiple rib fractures, i.e. **two or more consequetive ribs fractured in two or more places**[Q].
- The blunt force required to disrupt the integrity of thoracic cage typically produces an **underlying pulmonary contusion** as well.

Clinical Features

- **On inspiration** the **loose segment** of chest wall is **displaced inwards** and less air therefore moves into the lungs (**Paradoxical respiration**)[Q]
- To confirm the diagnosis the chest wall can be observed for **paradoxical motion of a chest wall segment**[Q] for **several respiratory cycles** and **during coughing**.

> - **Voluntary splinting** as a result of pain, **mechanically impaired chest wall movement** and **associated lung contusion** are all **causes of hypoxia & respiratory failure**[Q].
> - The patient is also at high risk of developing a **pneumothorax** or **hemothorax**[Q].

Diagnosis

- **Diagnosis** is made **clinically**[Q], not by radiography.

Treatment

- **Chest strapping** or **splinting should be avoided**[Q].
- **Currently, treatment** consists of **oxygen administration, adequate analgesia** (including opiates) or **epidural analgesia & physiotherapy**[Q].
- **IPPV (Intermittent positive pressure ventilation)** is **reserved for** cases developing **respiratory failure** despite adequate analgesia & oxygen[Q].

■ DIAPHRAGMATIC INJURIES

DIAPHRAGMATIC INJURY

- Diaphragmatic injuries are often caused by penetrating injuries[Q].
- Patients sustaining penetrating injuries below the nipples and above the costal margins should be investigated to rule out diaphragmatic injury[Q].

Etiology

- Penetrating trauma (knife, bullet, repair of hiatus hernia)
- Blunt trauma (motor vehicle accident, fall from height, bout of hyperemesis):
  - Caused by compressive force applied to the pelvis and abdomen.
  - Rupture is usually large, with herniation of abdominal content into chest

Clinical Features

- Most diaphragmatic injuries are silent and the presenting features are those of injury to the surrounding organs[Q].
- Late complication: Herniation of abdominal contents in to the chest[Q].

> - Herniation of organ: Stomach[Q] >Colon >Small intestine >Omentum >Spleen >Kidney and pancreas.

Diagnosis

- There is no single standard investigation to diagnose diaphragmatic injuries[Q].
- Chest X-ray after placement of a nasogastric tune may be helpful (as this may show the stomach herniated into the chest)
- Contrast study of upper or lower GIT, CT scan and diagnostic peritoneal lavage all lack positive or negative predictive value.

> - Most accurate evaluation is by video assisted thoracoscopy (VATS) or laparoscopy[Q], offering the advantage of allowing the surgeon to proceed to repair and additional evaluation of abdominal organs.

Treatment

- Operative repair[Q] is recommended in all cases.
- All penetrating diaphragmatic injury must be repaired via the abdomen and not the chest, to rule out penetrating hollow viscus injury.

■ BLAST INJURIES

BLAST INJURIES

- Primary blast injuries result from the rapid overpressure or shock waves produced by an explosion
- These injuries result from the dramatic changes in barometric pressure projected from the point of detonation
- Primary blast injuries predominantly cause damage to air filled hollow organs of the body from rapid pressure change (barotraumas).

> - Damage to air filled organs includes middle ear, lungs & GIT.[Q]

- Most sensitive & most frequently injured hollow organ: Tympanic membrane[Q] > Lungs
- Blast damage to the lungs is the MC cause of life threatening injury[Q] following an explosion.

Most Severely Affected Organs	Most Commonly Affected Organs
- **Air Blast**: Lungs[Q]	- **Air**: Tympanic membrane[Q]
- **Underwater**: GIT[Q]	- **Underwater (Fully submerged)**: TM[Q]
	- **Underwater (Head is out)**: GIT[Q]

■ TRAUMA

1. First step in trauma: *(Recent Question 2013)*
a. Blood transfusion
b. IV fluids
c. Reconstruction
d. Maintenance of airways

2. In severe injury, first to be maintained is:
(Recent Question 2013, PGI June 97)
a. Hypotension
b. Dehydration
c. Airway
d. Cardiac status

3. A female with suspected child abuse was brought to the casualty with severe bleeding from perineum. What should be the first line of management? *(AIIMS Nov 2014)*
a. Airway maintenance
b. Internal iliac artery ligation
c. Whole blood transfusion
d. Inform police before starting the treatment

4. Back examination of poly-trauma patient is known as:
(Recent Question 2015)
a. Log roll
b. Barrel role
c. Chin lift
d. None

5. An unresponsive patient has been brought to you by the police. What is the first thing you will do?
(AIIMS Nov 2016)
a. Start chest compressions immediately
b. Check carotid pulse
c. Check for response and call help
d. Start rescue breaths

6. Balanced resuscitation in trauma management is:
(AIIMS Nov 2017)
a. Giving colloids and crystalloids ratio of 1:1
b. Maintaining pH by ensuring acid base are balanced
c. Maintaining permissible hypotension to avoid bleeding
d. Maintaining airway, breathing and circulation simultaneously

7. In trauma transfusion, ratio of RBCs, FFP and platelets is:
(Recent Question 2017)
a. 1:1:3
b. 1:1:1
c. 1:1:2
d. 1:1:4

8. Which of the following is an indicator of airway obstruction?
(Recent Question 2017)
a. Inability to speak
b. Poor air exchange
c. Throat pain
d. Surgical emphysema

9. Common cause of breathing difficulty in an unconscious patient:
(Recent Question 2017)
a. Foreign body
b. Tongue
c. Vomitus
d. Blood

10. Sequence of resuscitation in a trauma patient:
a. Circulation, airway and breathing *(Recent Question 2017)*
b. Airway, breathing and circulation
c. Airway, circulation and breathing
d. Breathing, airway and circulation

11. In an accident case, after the arrival of medical team, all should be done in early management except:
a. Stabilization of cervical spine *(MCI Dec 2019)*
b. Check BP and pulse
c. Check respiration
d. Glasgow coma scale

■ TRAUMA SCORING SYSTEM

12. Which one of the following is not a part of the Revised Trauma Score? *(UPSC 2001)*
a. Glasgow coma scale
b. Systolic blood pressure
c. Pulse rate
d. Respiratory rate

13. Trauma and injury severity score (TRISS) includes:
(Recent Question 2016, All India 2010)
a. GCS + BP + RR
b. RTS + ISS + age
c. RTS + ISS + GCS
d. RTS + GCS + BP

14. Mangled Extremity Severity Score (MESS) includes all of the following except: *(Recent Question 2016, AIIMS May 2011)*
a. Shock
b. Ischemia
c. Neurogenic injury
d. Energy of injury

■ TRIAGE

15. Which of the following is color code and explanantion is matched correctly as per the triage used in disaster management? *(AIIMS Nov 2017)*
a. Red-Deceased
b. Black-Minor injuries
c. Yellow- Stable patients, observation
d. Green-Need immediate intervention

16. Patients are categorized on the basis of chances of survival in disaster management by: *(MCI Dec 2019)*
a. Triage
b. Mitigation
c. Tagging
d. Surge capacity

17. Triage system is used for: *(Recent Question 2015)*
a. Burn
b. Earthquake
c. Polytrauma
d. Floods

■ BLUNT TRAUMA ABDOMEN

18. Most common organ involved in blunt injury to the abdomen: *(WB PG 2015, JIPMER 2011, 2014)*
a. Spleen
b. Liver
c. Intestines
d. Kidney

19. Babu is brought to the emergency as a case of road traffic accident. He is hypotensive. Most likely ruptured organ is:
a. Spleen
b. Mesentery *(All India 2001)*
c. Kidney
d. Rectum

20. A driver wearing seat belt applied brake suddenly to avoid accident. Most common organ injured in seat belt injury:
(AIIMS May 2013)
a. Liver
b. Spleen
c. Mesentery
d. Abdominal aorta

21. A male patient with blunt trauma abdomen is hemodynamically stable. What is the next line of management?
a. Observation *(All India 2008)*
b. Further imaging of abdomen
c. Exploratory laparotomy
d. Laparoscopy

22. Best diagnostic test in stable patient with blunt trauma abdomen is: *(Recent Question 2016, 2014; DNB 2012)*
a. CECT scan
b. MRI
c. DPL
d. FAST

23. A patient with blunt trauma of abdomen at 48 hours, USG shows normal, but patient had tenderness in left lumbar region. Best appropriate diagnosis is by:

(Recent Question 2018)

a. MCU
b. IVP
c. CECT abdomen
d. Repeat USG

24. Which of the following is not assessed in FAST?

(Recent Question 2015)

a. Right upper quadrant
b. Left upper quadrant
c. Hypogastrium
d. Sub-xiphoid area

25. Isolated splenic/hepatic injury in a child is most commonly managed by: *(Recent Question 2017)*

a. Conservative management
b. Laparotomy
c. Interventional
d. Splenectomy and liver packing

26. Which of the following is not scanned by FAST-USG?

(MCI June 2019)

a. Pericardium
b. Pleural cavity
c. Spleen
d. Liver

■ DAMAGE CONTROL SURGERY

27. Damage control surgery is: *(JIPMER 2014, AIIMS May 2013)*

a. Minimal intervention done to stabilize the patient and do the definitive surgery later
b. Maximum possible surgical intervention is done immediately
c. Done during triage procedure
d. Done to control damage during surgery

28. Where is the second step of damage control resuscitation carried out? *(AIIMS May 2018)*

a. In emergency
b. In ICU
c. In OT
d. Prehospital resuscitation

29. A trauma patient was brought to emergency. On evaluation, found to have metabolic acidosis and coagulopathy with liver and duodenal injury. Next step: *(Recent Question 2017)*

a. Damage control surgery
b. Liver repair
c. Whipples procedure
d. None of the above

■ ABDOMINAL COMPARTMENT SYNDROME

30. Abdominal compartment syndrome is characterized by the following except: *(UPSC 2007)*

a. Hypercarbia and respiratory acidosis
b. Hypoxia due to increased peak inspiratory pressure
c. Hypotension due to decrease in venous return
d. Oliguria due to ureter obstruction

31. Which of the following is best treatment for Grade II abdominal hypertension? *(Recent Question 2016)*

a. Laparotomy
b. Immediate decompression
c. Hypovolemic resuscitation
d. Normovolemic resuscitation

■ PENETRATING INJURIES

32. Organ most commonly damaged in penetrating injury of abdomen is: *(WBPG 2014, AIIMS Nov 94, Nov 95)*

a. Liver
b. Small intestine
c. Large intestine
d. Duodenum

33. A man comes to emergency with stab injury to left flank. He has stable vitals. What would be the next step in management: *(AIIMS Nov 2008)*

a. CECT
b. Diagnostic peritoneal lavage
c. Laparotomy
d. Laparoscopy

34. Which of the following is not done in case of puncture wound of left colon? *(Recent Question 2015)*

a. Primary suture
b. Hemicolectomy
c. Externalization
d. Resection and anastomosis

35. In the patient of penetrating injury to the abdomen with shock, next best step is: *(Recent Question 2017)*

a. USG
b. FAST
c. CT
d. Laparotomy

■ NECK INJURIES

36. Which of the following is used to define penetrating neck injury? *(AIIMS May 2009, All India 2008)*

a. 2 cm depth of wound
b. Injury to vital structures
c. Breach of platysma
d. Through and through wound

37. The probable cause of sudden death in a case superficial injury to neck is: *(DNB 2005)*

a. Injury to phrenic nerve
b. Air embolism through external jugular vein
c. Bleeding from subclavian artery
d. Injury to trachea

38. Zone of neck involving great vessels at thoracic inlet:

a. I
b. II   *(Recent Question 2016)*
c. III
d. IV

■ BLAST INJURIES

39. In a blast injury, which of the following organ is least vulnerable to the blast wave? *(AIIMS June 2003)*

a. GI tract
b. Lungs
c. Liver
d. Ear drum

40. Most common organ injured in underwater explosion:

a. TM
b. GIT   *(MHSSMCET 2009)*
c. Lungs
d. Heart

■ HEPATIC INJURIES

41. A 17-year-old boy is admitted to the hospital after a road traffic accident. Per abdomen examination is normal. After adequate resuscitation, his pulse rate is 80/min and BP is 110/70 mm Hg. Abdominal CT reveals 1 cm deep laceration in the left lobe of the liver extending from the done more than half way through the parenchyma. Appropriate management at this time would be: *(DPG 2011, UPSC 2005)*

a. Conservative treatment
b. Abdominal exploration and packing of hepatic wounds
c. Abdominal exploration and ligation of left hepatic artery
d. Left hepatectomy

■ SPLENIC INJURIES

42. A child presents in causality in stable condition after a blunt abdominal trauma associated with splenic trauma. Treatment of choice is:

(Recent Question 2016, AIIMS Nov 2000)

a. Observation
b. Splenectomy
c. Arterial embolization
d. Splenorrhaphy

43. Trauma to spleen in a stable patient is best diagnosed by:
    a. X-ray abdomen   *(MCI Sept 2005, March 2008)*
    b. USG
    c. CT scan
    d. Diagnostic peritoneal lavage

44. A 27-year-old patient presented with left sided abdominal pain 6 hours after RTA. He was hemodynamically stable and FAST positive. CT scan showed grade III splenic injury. What will be appropriate treatment? *(Recent Question 2015)*
    a. Splenectomy   b. Splenorrhaphy
    c. Splenic artery embolization
    d. Conservative management

■ STOMACH, DUODENUM AND PANCREATIC INJURIES

45. Which of the following statements related to gastric injury is not true?   *(All India 2007)*
    a. Mostly related to penetrating trauma
    b. Treatment is simple debridement and suturing
    c. Blood in stomach is always related to gastric injury
    d. Heals well and fast

■ CHEST TRAUMA

46. A patient died after a blunt trauma to chest. Most common cause of death in blunt trauma to chest is: *(Recent Question 2016)*
    a. Esophageal rupture
    b. Tracheo-bronchial rupture
    c. Pulmonary laceration
    d. Pneumothorax

47. Which of the following is most common cause of hypotension in fracture ribs (T10 -T12)?   *(AIIMS Nov 99, June 99)*
    a. Abdominal solid visceral organ injury
    b. Injury to aorta
    c. Inter costal artery damage
    d. Pulmonary contusion

48. Treatment of simple rib fracture include all of the following except: *(Recent Question 2015)*
    a. Analgesic   b. Physiotherapy
    c. Strapping   d. Early ambulation

49. Best approach in thoracic trauma is: *(Recent Question 2013)*
    a. Midline sternotomy
    b. Parasternal thoracotomy
    c. Anterolateral thoracotomy
    d. Posterolateral thoracotomy

50. The following patient has presented after blunt trauma to the chest. On examination crepitus is felt. The clinical diagnosis is?   *(MCI Dec 2018)*

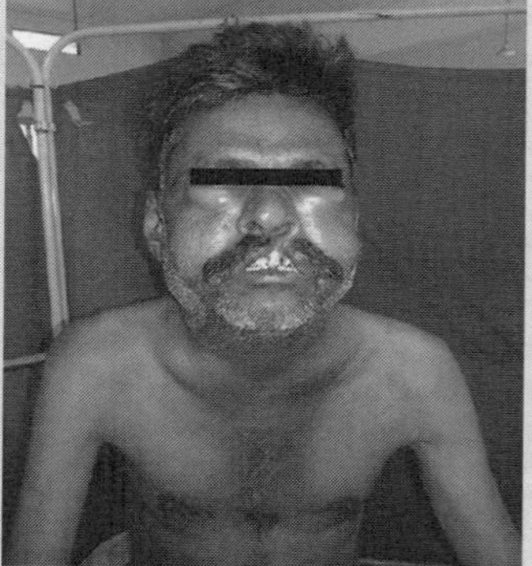

a. Subcutaneous emphysema
b. Gas gangrene
c. Acute tubercular necrosis
d. SVC syndrome

■ FLAIL CHEST

51. Management of flail chest with respiratory failure is:
    a. Chest tube drainage   *(DNB 2008, MCI Sept 2006)*
    b. Oxygen administration
    c. IPPV
    d. Internal operative fixation of the fractures segments

52. Simple rib fracture should be treated with all except: *(Recent Question 2014, MHPGMCET 2007)*
    a. Analgesics   b. Physiotherapy
    c. Early ambulation   d. Strapping of chest

53. Treatment of choice of flail chest is: *(Recent Question 2013)*
    a. External fixation of flail segment and mechanical ventilation
    b. Strapping
    c. O_2 administration
    d. Intrapleural local analgesia

■ DIAPHRAGMATIC INJURY

54. About diaphragmatic injury, true statement is:
    a. Treatment is conservative   *(AIIMS June 98)*
    b. Resolves spontaneously
    c. Left side is more common
    d. Associated with pneumothorax

■ HEAD INJURY

55. Prognosis in head injury is best given by:
              (All India 2007, AIIMS Nov 2006)
    a. Glasgow coma scale   b. Age of patient
    c. Mode of injury   d. CT head

56. Base of the skull fracture presents with involvement of the petrous temporal bone, which of the following important sign is seen?   *(UPPG 2007)*
    a. Subconjuctival hematoma
    b. CSF rhinorrhea
    c. Raccoon eyes
    d. Battle sign

57. Which of the following is commonest source of extradural hemorrhage?   *(AIIMS Nov 98, Feb 97, All India 96)*
    a. Middle meningeal artery
    b. Subdural venous sinus
    c. Charcot's artery
    d. Middle cerebral artery

58. Skull base fracture is associated with all of the following except: *(Recent Question 2017)*
    a. Racoon eyes   b. Hemiparesis
    c. CSF Rhino-otorrhea   d. Battle sign

59. Abbreviated injury scale score digit for head injury:
    a. 1   b. 2   *(Recent Question 2016)*
    c. 3   d. 4

60. SDH is caused by injury of: *(Recent Question 2016)*
    a. Middle meningeal artery
    b. Cortical veins
    c. Superficial temporal artery
    d. None

■ VASCULAR INJURIES

61. **During surgery, both femoral artery and femoral vein injured, next best step:** *(Recent Question 2017)*
    a. Ligate femoral vein & repair femoral artery
    b. Ligate femoral vein & femoral artery
    c. Ligate femoral artery & repair femoral vein
    d. None of the above

■ SEAT BELT INJURY

62. **Seat belt causes injury to:** *(MAHE 2004)*
    a. Duodenum
    b. Head injury due to wind screen
    c. Thorax   d. All of the above

63. **Seat belt injury leads to:** *(MCI June 2019)*
    a. Splenic laceration
    b. Splenic contusion
    c. Gut ischemia
    d. Mesenteric adenitis

■ MISCELLANEOUS

64. **Which one of the following is not a principle followed in the management of missile injuries?** *(UPSC 2004)*
    a. Excision of all dead muscles
    b. Removal of foreign bodies
    c. Removal of fragments of bone
    d. Leaving the wound open

65. **During reconstruction of an amputated limb which of the following is done first?** *(AIIMS Nov 2010)*
    a. Arterial repair   b. Venous repair
    c. Fixation of the bone   d. Nerve anastomoses

66. **In treatment of hand injuries, the greatest priority is:** *(MCI June 2018)*
    a. Repair to tendons   b. Repair of skin cover
    c. Repair of nerves   d. All of the above

67. **During resuscitation, artifacts of fractured ribs most commonly involve:** *(AIIMS May 2014)*
    a. 2nd–4th ribs   b. 3rd–5th ribs
    c. 4th–6th ribs   d. 5th–7th ribs

■ TRAUMA

1. Ans. d. Maintenance of airways
2. Ans. c. Airway
3. Ans. a. Airway maintenance
4. Ans. a. Log roll
5. Ans. b. Check carotid pulse
6. Ans. c. Maintaining permissible hypotension to avoid bleeding *(Ref: Schwartz 11/e p144, 10/e p98; Current Therapy of Trauma and Surgical Critical Care By Juan A. Asensio 2/e p602)*

   Balanced resuscitation in trauma management is maintaining permissible hypotension to avoid bleeding.

   Components of Damage Control Resuscitation
   - Permissive hypotension[Q]
   - Minimizing crystalloid-based resuscitation[Q]
   - Immediate release & administration of pre-defined blood products (red blood cells, plasma & platelets) in ratios similar to those of whole blood[Q].

7. Ans. b. 1:1:1 *(Ref: Sabiston 20/e p72; Schwartz 11/e p193, 10/e p98)*
8. Ans. a. Inability to speak
9. Ans. b. Tongue *(Ref: Bailey 27/e p355, 26/e p341)*

   "The mouth and nasal passages form part of the upper aero- digestive tract. Lacerations and fractures of the facial skeleton may give rise to immediate or delayed respiratory obstruction. Immediate obstruction may arise from inhalation of tooth fragments, accumulation of blood and secretions, and loss of control of the tongue in the unconscious or semiconscious patient." - Bailey 27/e p341

10. Ans. b. Airway, breathing and circulation *(Ref: Sabiston 20/e p413; Schwartz 11/e p184, 10/e p161; Bailey 27/e p323)*
11. Ans. d. Glasgow coma scale *(Ref: Bailey 27/e p323)*

■ TRAUMA SCORING SYSTEM

12. Ans. c. Pulse rate *(Ref: Sabiston 20/e p411; Trauma Manual by Moore and Mattox 4/e p6; The Trauma manual: Trauma and Acute Care Surgery 3/e p5)*
13. Ans. b. RTS + ISS + age
14. Ans. c. Neurogenic injury

■ TRIAGE

15. Ans. c. Yellow- Stable patients, observation *(Ref: Pediatric Emergency Medicine By Jill M. Baren (2008)/p1087)*
16. Ans. a. Triage *(Ref: Bailey 27/e p412, 413)*
17. Ans. c. Polytrauma

■ BLUNT TRAUMA ABDOMEN

18. Ans. a. Spleen *(Ref: Sabiston 20/e p435; Schwartz 11/e p277, 10/e p173-174; Bailey 27/e p313)*
19. Ans. a. Spleen
20. Ans. c. Mesentery *(Bailey 27/e p 106)*

    Most common organ injured in seat belt injury is Mesentery.

21. Ans. b. Further imaging of abdomen *(Ref: CSDT 12/e p228)*

    A **hemodynamically stable patient** after **blunt trauma abdomen** should need **further evaluation by imaging**. Imaging of the abdomen with Ultrasound (**FAST**) is the best **next line of investigation**.

22. Ans. a. CECT Scan
23. Ans. c. CECT abdomen
24. Ans. c. Hypogastrium
25. Ans. a. Conservative management *(Ref: Sabiston 20/e p433, 1896; Schwartz 11/e p225, 227, 10/e p206)*
26. Ans. b. Pleural cavity *(Ref: Bailey 27/e p372)*

■ DAMAGE CONTROL SURGERY

27. Ans. a. Minimal intervention done to stabilize the patient and do the definitive surgery later *(Ref: Sabiston 20/e p417; Schwartz 11/e p215, 10/e p192-195; Bailey 27/e p318, 319, 326, 327, 378-80)*
28. Ans. b. In ICU
29. Ans. a. Damage control surgery *(Ref: Sabiston 20/e p417; Schwartz 11/e p215, 10/e p192; Bailey 27/e p326)*

■ ABDOMINAL COMPARTMENT SYNDROME

30. Ans. d. Oliguria due to ureter obstruction   **31.** Ans. c. Hypovolemic resuscitation

■ PENETRATING INJURIES

32. Ans. a. Liver

33. Ans. a. CECT *(Ref: Sabiston 20/e p434; Washington Manual of Surgery 5/e p373)*

According to **EAST Guidelines "Current recommendations for nonoperative management** of **penetrating** trauma include use of **Triple Contrast CT** (IV, oral and rectal) and **serial examinations."**

34. Ans. b. Hemicolectomy   **35.** Ans. d. Laparotomy *(Ref: Sabiston 20/e p434)*

■ NECK INJURIES

36. Ans. c. Breach of platysma *(Ref: Sabiston 20/e p423; Schwartz 11/e p198-199, 10/e p197-200)*

37. Ans. b. Air embolism through external jugular vein *(Ref: Bailey 25/e p75, 76, 1381, 1382)*

> When **neck or chest veins are injured,** air may enter the veins and causes **immediate death due to air embolism.**

38. Ans. a. I *(Ref: Sabiston 20/e p423; Schwartz 11/e p198, 10/e p197-200)*

■ BLAST INJURIES

39. Ans. c. Liver *(Ref: Sabiston 20/e p594-595; Bailey 27/e p430)*   **40.** Ans. a. TM

■ HEPATIC INJURIES

41. Ans. a. Conservative treatment *(Ref: Sabiston 20/e p437-438; Bailey 27/e p 374)*

■ SPLENIC INJURIES

42. Ans. a. Observation   **43.** Ans. c. CT scan

44. Ans. d. Conservative management

■ STOMACH, DUODENUM AND PANCREATIC INJURIES

45. Ans. c. Blood in stomach is always related to gastric injury *(Ref: Sabiston 20/e p439; Schwartz 11/e p228-229, 10/e p207; Bailey 27/e p375)*

Blood in stomach is suggestive of injury to the stomach but it is not always due to stomach injury.

Blood in stomach may result from injury to adjacent gastrointestinal tract such as the esophagus or from stress ulcerations.

> **GASTRIC INJURIES**
>
> - **Gastric injuries** are **most commonly results from penetrating trauma**[Q].
> - **Most common treatment** of penetrating gastric injuries is **simple debridement** and **suturing**[Q].
> - **Stomach** has a **rich blood supply,** so healing in gastric injuries is good and poses no special problem.

■ CHEST TRAUMA

46. Ans. b. Tracheo-bronchial rupture

47. Ans. a. Abdominal solid visceral organ injury *(Ref: Sabiston 20/e p428; Schwartz 11/e p193, 10/e p625)*

> - **MC cause of hypotension in trauma** patients: **Hemorrhage**[Q]
> - **MC cause of shock** after trauma is **hypovolemia,** and there are **five places** that a patient **can lose large volume of blood:** **Externally,** the **chest,** the **abdomen,** the **retroperitoneum,** and into **muscle compartments (Blood on the floor and four more).**[Q]
> - **Fracture of lower ribs (T_9-T_{12})** are usually associated with **splenic** or **hepatic injuries**[Q]
> - **Fracture of upper ribs (T_1-T_3), clavicle** or **scapula** is usually associated with **major vascular injuries**[Q].

48. Ans. c. Strapping   **49.** Ans. c. Anterolateral thoracotomy

50. Ans. a. Subcutaneous emphysema *(Ref: Bailey 27/e p370)*

■ FLAIL CHEST

51. Ans. c. IPPV   **52.** Ans. d. Strapping of chest

53. Ans. a. External fixation of flail segment and mechanical ventilation

◼ DIAPHRAGMATIC INJURY

54. Ans. c. Left side is more common

◼ HEAD INJURY

55. Ans. a. Glasgow coma scale
56. Ans. a. Subconjunctival hematoma *(Ref: Harrison 20/e p3184; Sabiston 20/e p419)*
57. Ans. a. Middle meningeal artery *(Ref: Sabiston 20/e p417)*
58. Ans. b. Hemiparesis *(Ref: Schwartz 11/e p217, 10/e p1715-1716; Bailey 27/e p333)*
59. Ans. a. 1   60. Ans. b. Cortical veins

◼ VASCULAR INJURIES

61. Ans. a. Ligate femoral vein & repair femoral artery *(Ref: Sabiston 20/e p443, 444)*

◼ SEAT BELT INJURY

62. Ans. a. Duodenum   63. Ans. c. Gut ischemia *(Ref: Bailey 27/e p351, 1061)*

◼ MISCELLANEOUS

64. Ans. c. Removal of fragments of bone *(Ref: http://surgeryonline.wordpress.com/tag/missile-injuries/)*

MANAGEMENT OF MISSILE INJURIES

- In limb wounds, **exploration** is followed by **thorough wound excision**[Q], after which, with very few exceptions, the **wound should be left open**[Q].
- A minimal amount of skin edge (i.e. only that which has been contaminated) should be excised[Q] around the entrance and exit wounds.

> - **Foreign matter** should be **removed** from the wound[Q].
> - **Delayed primary closure** should follow **within 4-7 days** after injury[Q].

- Dead muscle that does not bleed or contract, is mushy in consistency or has an unhealthy colour must be excised. These criteria comprise is the '4 Cs' for **muscle excision (Colour, Contractility, Consistency, Capillary bleeding)**[Q]

> - **Bone shattered** by high-energy transfer will in many instances **still have attachment to periosteum or muscle**[Q].
> - Such fragments must not be discarded. Loss of bone may result in malunion (e.g. shortening) or nonunion[Q].

65. Ans. c. Fixation of the bone *(Ref: Master Techniques in Orthopedic Surgery Series by Moran and Cooney (2008)/487)*

Bone is the first structure to be fixed in hand injuries.

SEQUENCE OF REPAIR IN HAND INJURIES (BE FAN OF VEINS)

1. Bone shortening and stabilization/fixation[Q]Extensor tendon repair[Q]Flexor tendon repair[Q]
4. Arterial anastomoses[Q]Nerve repair[Q]Venous anastomosis[Q]
7. Skin/wound closure[Q]

66. Ans. a. Repair to tendons

SPINAL CORD INJURIES

- **High spinal cord injuries** can also **result in systemic hypotension** because of **loss of sympathetic tone**[Q].
- The patient will usually have **hypotension** and **relative bradycardia** and will show evidence **of good peripheral perfusion** on physical examination[Q].
- The term **neurogenic shock** is used but is somewhat of a **misnomer** because these patients are **typically hyperdynamic**, with **high cardiac output secondary to loss of sympathetic vascular tone**[Q].

Treatment

- **Hypotension associated with high spinal injury** can be **treated by** alpha-agonist **phenylephrine**[Q].

67. Ans. c. 4th–6th ribs *(Ref: https://storify.com/forensicmed/cardiopulmonary-resuscitation-related-rib-fracture)*

During resuscitation, artifacts of fractured ribs most commonly involve 4th – 6th ribs.

- **"The vast majority (90%+) of fractures occur in ribs 2 to 7**; *fractures in the bony parts of rib numbers* **1** *and* **8 to 10** *are possible but probably* **very rare**; *it is* **difficult to see** *how fractures can occur in rib numbers* **11** *and* **12** *following* **standard manual CPR.**" *- https://storify. com/forensicmed/cardiopulmonary-resuscitation-related-rib-fracture.*

Transplantation

HISTORY OF TRANSPLANTATION

History of Organ Transplantation	
First **Renal** transplantation	• **Murray**[Q] **(1954) in identical twins**
First **Liver** transplantation	• **Starzl**[Q] **(1963)**
First **Pancreas** transplantation	• **Kelly & Lillhei**[Q] **(1966)**
First **Heart** transplantation	• **Christian Barnard**[Q] **(1967)**
First **Lung** transplantation	• **Fritz Derom**[Q] **(1968)**
First **Islet cell** transplantation	• **Sutherland**[Q] **(1974)**
First **Heart & Lung** transplantation	• **Reitz & Shumway**[Q] **(1981)**
First **successful Intestinal** transplantation	• **Deltz**[Q] **(1988)**

TYPES OF GRAFT REJECTION

Types of Graft Rejection		
Hyperacute Rejection	**Acute (cellular) Rejection**	**Chronic Rejection**
• **Immediate** (within minutes to hours) **graft destruction** due to **ABO** or **pre-formed anti-HLA antibodies**[Q]. • Characterised by **intravascular thrombosis**[Q] • **Kidney transplants** are **particularly vulnerable**[Q] to hyperacute graft rejection • **Heart** and **liver transplants** are **relatively resistant**[Q].	• Occurs **during** the **first 6 months**[Q] • Most commonly presents **between 5-30**[Q] days after transplantation • **T-cell dependent,** characterized by **mononuclear cell infiltration**[Q] • Usually **reversible**[Q]	• Occurs **after** the **first 6 months**[Q] • **MC cause** of **graft failure**[Q] • **Non-immune factors** may contribute to pathogenesis • Characterized by **myointimal proliferation** in **graft arteries** leading to **ischemia** and **fibrosis**[Q]

Manifestations of Chronic Graft Rejection	
Kidney	• **Glomerular sclerosis & tubular atrophy**[Q]
Pancreas	• **Acinar loss & islet cell destruction**[Q]
Heart	• **Accelerated coronary artery disease** (Cardiac allograft vasculopathy[Q])
Liver	• **Vanishing bile duct syndrome**[Q]
Lungs	• **Obliterative bronchiolitis**[Q]

HLA MATCHING

HLA ANTIGENS

- In organ transplantation, **HLA-A, -B** and **-DR** are the **most important antigens** to take into account when matching donor and recipient in an attempt to reduce the risk of graft rejection
- **HLA matching** has a relatively small but **definite beneficial effect on renal allograft survival** (HLA-DR[Q] >HLA-B >HLA-A).
- Are the **MC cause of graft rejection**[Q]
- Their physiological function is to act as **antigen recognition units**
- Are **highly polymorphic** (amino acid sequence differs widely between individuals)
- **Anti-HLA antibodies** may cause **hyperacute rejection**[Q]

> - In the case of liver transplants, HLA matching **does not confer an advantage**[Q]
> - Although it is **beneficial in cardiac transplantation,** it is **not practicable because of the relatively small size of the recipient pool** and the **short permissible cold ischemic time**[Q].

■ TYPES OF GRAFT

Graft			
Autograft	**Isograft**	**Homograft (Allograft)**	**Heterograft (Xenograft)**
• Tissue transplanted **from one site to another** on the **same patient**[Q]	• **Transplant** from a genetically identical donor, such as an **identical twin**[Q]	• Transplant **from** individual of **same species**[Q]	• Transplant **from another species**[Q]

Xenograft	
Concordant Xenograft	**Discordant Xenograft**
• **Transplant between closely related species**[Q] • Example: **For humans, old world monkeys & apes** • Advantage: **Hyperacute rejections is not a threat**[Q] • **Disadvantages: Zoonotic transfer of disease** (Particularly retroviral transmission)	• Transplant **between distant related or divergent species**[Q] • Example: **For humans, new-world monkeys & other mammals** • For physiologic concern (organ size & availability), **pigs are preferred animal donor**[Q] • **Disadvantages: High risk of hyperacute rejection**[Q]

■ COMPLICATIONS OF IMMUNOSUPPRESSION

Complications of Immunosuppression		
Infection	**Malignancy**	**Non-Immune Side Effects**
• **High risk** of opportunistic infection **by viruses**[Q] • **Recipient derived infections**[Q] are **more common** than donor derived infections • **Risk of bacterial infection** is **highest during first month**[Q] of transplantation • **Risk of viral infection** is **highest during first 6 months**[Q] of transplantation; **MC problem is CMV**[Q] **Infection** • **Viral infection** may result from **reactivation of latent virus** or from **primary infection** • **Chemoprophylaxis** is important in **high risk patients** • **Pre-transplant vaccination** against community acquired infection should be considered	• **MC malignancy in transplant recipient: Skin cancer**[Q] **(SCC)** • **Increased risk of PTLD &** **Kaposi sarcoma**	• **Hypertension & chronic allograft nephropathy** caused by **calcineurin inhibitors**[Q] • **New onset diabetes** after transplant is associated with **tacrolimus or steroids**[Q] • **Hyperlipidemia, anemia & accelerated cardiovascular disease**[Q] • **Cardiovascular disease** is the **leading cause of death in transplant survivors**[Q]

Common Infections After Solid Organ Transplantation, by Site of Infection			
	Period after Transplantation		
Infected Site	**Early (<1 Month)**	**Middle (1-4 Months)**	**Late (>6 Months)**
Donor organ	Bacterial and fungal infections of the graft, anastomotic site, and surgical wound	**CMV infection**[Q]	**EBV infection**[Q] (may present in allograft organ)
Systemic	Bacteremia and candidemia (often resulting from central venous catheter colonization)	**CMV infection**[Q] (fever, bone marrow suppression)	**CMV infection**[Q], especially in patients given **early posttransplantation prophylaxis; EBV proliferative syndromes** (may occur in donor organs)
Lung	Bacterial aspiration pneumonia with prevalent nosocomial organisms associated with intubation and sedation (highest risk in lung transplantation)	*Pneumocystis infection*[Q]; CMV pneumonia[Q] **(highest risk in lung transplantation);** *Aspergillus* **infection**[Q] **(highest risk in lung transplantation)**	*Pneumocystis* **infection**[Q]; granulomatous lung diseases (nocardiae, reactivated fungal and mycobacterial diseases)
Kidney	Bacterial and fungal (*Candida*) infections (cystitis, pyelonephritis) associated with urinary tract catheters (highest risk in kidney transplantation)	**Renal transplantation: BK virus infection (associated with nephropathy**[Q]**);** JC virus infection	**Renal transplantation**: Bacteria (late urinary tract infections, usually not associated with bacteremia); **BK virus (nephropathy**[Q]**, graft failure, generalized vasculopathy)**
Liver and biliary tract	Cholangitis	**CMV hepatitis**[Q]	**CMV hepatitis**[Q]

Contd…

Contd...

Infected Site	Early (<1 Month)	Middle (1-4 Months)	Late (>6 Months)
Heart	–	*Toxoplasma gondii* infection[Q] (highest risk in heart transplantation)	*Toxoplasma gondii* infection[Q] (highest risk in heart transplantation)
Gastrointestinal tract	Peritonitis, especially after liver transplantation	Colitis secondary to *Clostridium difficile*[Q] infection (risk can persist)	Colitis secondary to **C. difficile** infection (risk can persist)
Central Nervous System	–	*Listeria* (meningitis); *T. gondii* infection	Listeria meningitis[Q]; Cryptococcus meningitis; Nocardia abscess; JC virus-associated PML

■ POST-TRANSPLANT LYMPHOPROLIFERATIVE DISORDER

POST-TRANSPLANT LYMPHOPROLIFERATIVE DISORDER (PTLD)

- PTLD is associated with **replication of EBV in B cells** induced by **enhanced immunosuppression**, primarily observed in patients who have received **more than one** course of polyclonal antilymphocyte globulin (**ALG**) or **monoclonal OKT3**[Q].

Clinical Features

- Clinical presentation of PTLD includes **fever, malaise** and **lymphadenopathy**[Q]

Diagnosis

- The **diagnosis** is made by **tissue biopsy**[Q].

Treatment

- **Polyclonal PTLD: Discontinuation of immunosuppression** and **antiviral therapy**[Q].
- **Monoclonal PTLD: Radiation, chemotherapy** and occasionally **surgical resection. Antibody against CD20**[Q] represents a novel approach in treating monoclonal PTLD with favorable outcome.

■ CLINICAL TESTING OF BRAINSTEM DEATH

CLINICAL TESTING FOR BRAINSTEM DEATH

- **Absence of cranial nerve reflexes:** (PCO)
  - **Pupillary** reflex[Q]
  - **Corneal** reflex[Q]
  - **Pharyngeal** (Gag) & **Tracheal** (Cough) reflex[Q]
  - **Oculovestibular (Caloric) reflex**[Q]
- **Absence of motor response:**
  - Absence of motor response **to painful stimuli applied to head & face plus**[Q]
  - Absence of motor response **within the cranial nerve distribution to adequate stimulation**[Q]
- **Absence of spontaneous respiration**[Q]

■ DONORS

ORGAN DONORS

- Organ donors are of two types: Dead or deceased donors & living donors

Dead or Deceased Donors	Living Donors

• **Brain dead donors** also known as **heart beating donors** or **donation after brain death**[Q] (DBD)
• **Cardiac or circulatory dead** also known as **non-heart beating donors** or **donation after circulatory death**[Q] (DCD)
	• Limited to donation of:
	  – Kidney[Q]
	  – Liver[Q]
	  – Lung lobe[Q]

Donation after Brain Death (DBD) Donors	Donation after Circulatory Death (DCD) Donors
• **Most deceased donors organs** are obtained from **patients with brain-stem death**[Q]. • **Brain death** occurs when **severe brain injury causes irreversible loss of capacity of consciousness combined with irreversible loss of capacity for breathing**[Q].	• Due to rising demand for organ transplantation, increase in the use of organs from DCD donors • **DCD donors** are grouped according to **Maastricht classification**[Q]

Contd...

Contd...

Maastricht Classification for Donation after Circulatory Death (DCD) Donors	
Category	**Description (DRACUIa)**
1	<u>D</u>ead on arrival at hospital[Q]
2	<u>R</u>esuscitation attempted without success[Q]
3	<u>A</u>waiting cardiac arrest after withdrawal of support[Q] (**Most DCD donors from Category 3[Q]**)
4	<u>C</u>ardiac arrest while brain dead[Q]
5	<u>C</u>ardiac arrest & <u>U</u>nsuccessful resuscitation in hospital[Q]

Uncontrolled Donors	Controlled Donors
• Includes category **1, 2 & 5**[Q] • **Warm ischemic time** is **longer & less predictable**[Q]	• Includes category **3 & 4**[Q] • Death results from **planned withdrawal of life-sustaining cardiorespiratory support**[Q] • **Most DCD donors** are from **controlled donors**[Q]

■ EXTENDED CRITERIA DONORS (ECD) FOR KIDNEY & LIVER TRANSPLANTATION

Extended Criteria Donors	
Kidney Transplant	**Liver Transplant**

• Donor **>60 years** of age[Q]
 • Donor age **50-59 years** with at least two of the following:
   – **Cerebrovascular accident** as cause of death[Q]
   – **Pre-existing hypertension**[Q]
   – Terminal serum **creatinine >1.5 mg/dL**[Q]
	• **Mild to moderate steatosis**[Q]
	 • **Hepatitis C positive**[Q]
	 • **Hepatitis B—core antibody positive**[Q]

■ ORGAN PRESERVATION SOLUTION

ORGAN PRESERVATION SOLUTION

• **Liver, pancreas and kidney** can be successfully preserved for **up to 2 days** by **flushing** the organ **with University of Wisconsin solution** and storing them at hypothermia (0-5°C)[Q].

UNIVERSITY OF WISCONSIN SOLUTION

• **UW solution:** Cationic composition (**high potassium** and **low sodium**) **mimics intracellular levels**[Q] to minimize diffusion down electrochemical gradients.
• UW solution (marketed as **Viaspan**) contains **high** level of **potassium** and **adenosine**[Q].

Special composition of UW solution	
Lactobionate and raffinose	• **Minimizes cell swelling**[Q]
Hydroxyethyl starch	• **Prevention of the extracellular space expansion**[Q]
Glutathione	• **Anti-oxidant**[Q]
Allopurinol	• **Free radical scavenger**[Q]
Adenosine	• **Precursor for energy metabolism**[Q]

■ MAXIMUM & OPTIMAL COLD STORAGE TIME

Maximum and Optimal Cold Storage Times		
Organ	**Optimal storage time (hours)**	**Safe maximum storage time (hours)**
Kidney	<18[Q]	36[Q]
Liver	<12	18
Pancreas	<10	18
Small intestine	<4	6
Heart	<3[Q]	6[Q]
Lung	<3[Q]	8

■ LIVER TRANSPLANTATION

LIVER TRANSPLANTATION

- **First liver transplantation** was done by **Starzl**[Q] in 1963, in **Denver, University of Colorado.**
- **MC cause of death in LT: Sepsis & sepsis-induced multiple organ failure**[Q]
- **Combined liver & heart transplantation** is done **in amyloidosis**[Q]
- **Combined liver & lung transplantation** is done in **cystic fibrosis**[Q]

Indications of Liver Transplantation	
MC indication of LT	• **HCV induced cirrhosis**[Q]
2nd MC indication of LT	• **Alcoholic liver disease**[Q]
MC indication of **pediatric LT**	• **Biliary atresia**[Q]
MC **metabolic disorder** requiring LT	• **Alpha-1 antitrypsin deficiency**[Q]
MC indication for LT **following acute liver failure**	• **Acetaminophen toxicity**[Q]

■ TYPES OF LIVER TRANSPLANTATION

Types of Liver Transplantation (LT)	
Orthotopic LT	• **Graft** is **placed at normal anatomical position** after recipient hepatectomy[Q]
Heterotopic LT	• **Graft** is placed **at an alternative site** rather than normal anatomical position[Q]
Auxiliary	• **Native liver remains in-situ** & whole or partial transplant is added[Q]
APOLT	• **Left lobe** of recipient liver is **excised** & donor liver occupies the vacated space[Q]
Auxiliary Heterotopic LT	• **Whole liver or lobe placed in subhepatic space**[Q]
Piggyback LT	• **Orthotopic transplant** that **preserves recipient IVC**[Q]
Split LT	• **Cadaveric donor liver** is **divided** & given to **two recipients**[Q]
Reduced LT	• **Graft** is **reduced to** a functional unit of **appropriate size for** the **recipient**[Q]

■ SEQUENCE OF ANASTOMOSIS IN ORTHOTOPIC LIVER TRANSPLANTATION (OLT)

SEQUENCE OF ANASTOMOSIS IN ORTHOTOPIC LIVER TRANSPLANTATION (SIPH-B)

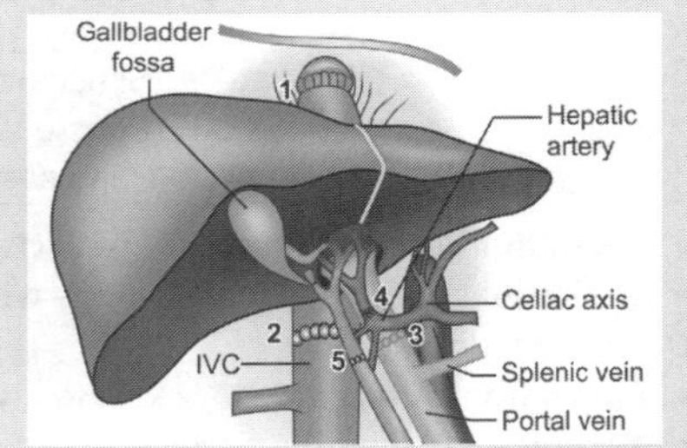

- 1. Supra hepatic IVC 2. Infra hepatic IVC 3. Portal vein 4. Hepatic artery 5. Bile duct[Q]
- **Preferred method of biliary drainage:**
  - **Direct end-to-end anastomosis** between donor & recipients bile duct[Q]
  - **Choledocho-choledochostomy** is **preferred over choledochojejunostomy**[Q]
- Indications of choledochojejunostomy:
  - **Diseased recipients extrahepatic bile duct**[Q]
  - **Significant recipient-donor duct size mismatch**[Q]

■ RENAL TRANSPLANTATION

RENAL TRANSPLANTATION

- **First RT** was performed by **Murray in 1954 in identical twins**[Q]

Indication of Renal Transplantation	
End Stage Renal Disease Caused By: (GD for HR POSt at 4 AM) • **G**lomerulonephritis[Q] • **D**iabetic nephropathy[Q] • **H**ypertensive nephrosclerosis[Q] • **R**enal vascular disease[Q]	• **P**olycystic kidney disease[Q] • **P**yelonephritis[Q] • **O**bstructive uropathy[Q] • **S**LE[Q] • **A**nalgesic nephropathy[Q] • **M**etabolic disease[Q] (**Oxalosis, amyloid**)

Contraindication of Renal Transplantation	
Absolute	**Relative**
• **Active malignant disease**[Q]	• Limited life expectancy
• **Active infection**[Q]	• History of non-adherence to medication regimen
• Unreconstructable **peripheral vascular disease**[Q]	• History of non-compliance with dialysis
• **Severe cardiac or pulmonary disease**[Q]	• Financial barrier
• **Active IV drug abuse**[Q]	• Renal disease with high recurrence rate
• Significant psychosocial barriers	• Morbid obesity

Contd…

Contd...

Procedure:
- **Renal graft** is placed in **iliac fossa in retroperitoneal position,** leaving the **native kidney in-situ**[Q]
- **Donor renal vein is anastomosed to external iliac vein**[Q]
- **Donor renal artery on Carrel's patch** (Small portion of surrounding aorta) of donor aorta is **anastomosed to external iliac artery**[Q]
- If **donor renal artery lacks aortic patch** (in cases of **living donor renal transplantation**), graft renal artery is anastomosed to **internal iliac artery**[Q]
- **Ureter** is kept reasonably short to avoid distal ischemia & **anastomosed to bladder by:**
  - **Lich-Gregoir Technique (Preferred**[Q]**):** Direct implantation of ureter into dome of bladder with mucosa to mucosal anastomoses followed by closure over ureter to create a short tunnel
  - **Lead-Better Politano technique**[Q]

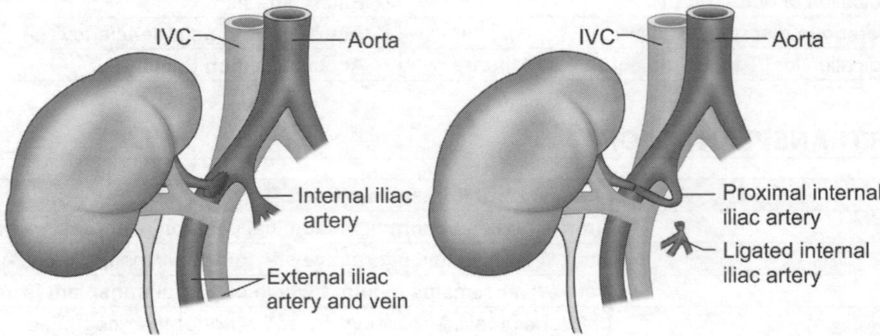

■ PANCREAS TRANSPLANTATION

PANCREAS TRANSPLANTATION (PT)

- **First PT** was performed by **Kelly & Lillhei**[Q] in 1996.

Types of Pancreas Transplantation
• **SPK** (Simultaneous Pancreas & Kidney) Transplantation: **80% cases**[Q]
• **PAK** (Pancreas after Kidney) Transplantation: **15% cases**
• **PTA** (Pancreas Transplantation alone): **8% cases** (usually done for brittle diabetes)

- **Indications of PT: Type-1 DM with clear C-peptide deficiency**[Q]
- **Indications of SPK: Insulin therapy with C-peptide level <2 ng/mL**[Q] or **insulin therapy with C-peptide level >2 ng/mL & BMI <28 kg/m²**

Donor Selection
- Organ from **younger, leaner & hemodynamically stable deceased donors are preferred**[Q].
- **Pancreas with significant steatosis** should be **avoided** because of postoperative complications (pancreatitis, peripancreatic fat necrosis, infection[Q]).

Contraindications for Procurement	
• **Type I DM**[Q]	• **Chronic pancreatitis**[Q]
• **Previous pancreatic surgery**[Q]	• **History of recent malignancy**[Q]

Procurement Principle, Preparation & Transplant:
- During the procurement **minimal handling of pancreas is optimal**[Q]
- **Pancreas & liver** are **removed en-bloc** to prevent increased warm ischemic times[Q]

Back-Table Preparation Includes
• Removal of spleen • Suture reinforcement of mesenteric root • Maintaining **at least 1 cm of portal vein**[Q] • Trimming excess distal & proximal duodenum • **Iliac artery** is used as **Y–graft**[Q] in which end-to-end anastomosis of **internal iliac artery to splenic artery** & **external iliac artery to SMA** is done[Q]

- **Pancreas transplant** is placed on the **right side**[Q] to prevent stretching of venous anastomosis.
- For **systemic venous drainage, portal vein** is **anastomosed to external iliac vein or common iliac vein or distal vena cava** in end-to-side fashion[Q]

Contd...

Contd…

- **Iliac artery graft** is sutured to **common iliac artery of recipient**[Q]
- **For portal drainage**, donor portal vein is **anastomosed to recipient proximal SMV**[Q].
- For **enteric drainage** of exocrine secretions, transplant **duodenal stump** is anastomosed side-to-side **to the recipient mid-jejunum**[Q].
- For **bladder drainage** of exocrine secretions, 4-5 cm cystostomy is made on anterior dome of bladder (**Duodenum is oriented inferiorly**[Q]).

- **In pancreas transplantation, enteric drainage & systemic venous drainage** is **most commonly done**[Q].
- For **bladder drainage**, graft should be oriented with **duodenum inferiorly**[Q]
- For **enteric drainage, duodenum can be superior or inferior**[Q]
- **Enteric drainage** is preferred over bladder drainage[Q]
- **Advantage of bladder drainage:** Allows **monitoring of urinary amylase level** as an **early sign of graft rejection**[Q]

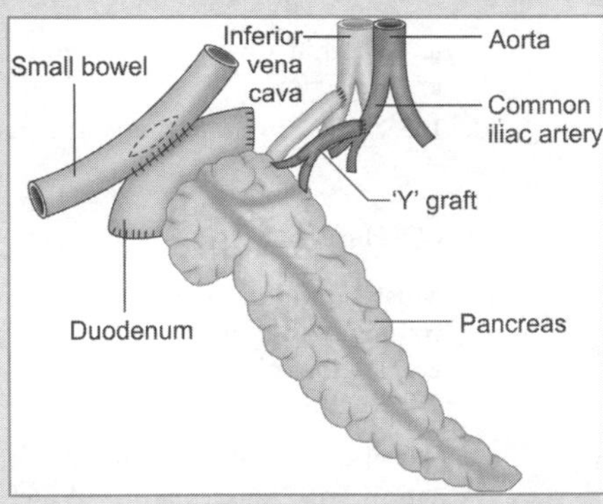

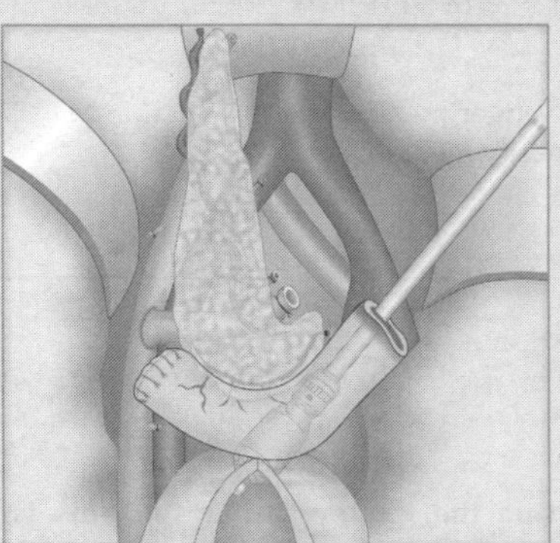

Multiple Choice Questions

■ FLUIDS USED IN TRANSPLANTATION

1. **Amputated digits are preserved:**
   (AIIMS GIS Dec 2011, All India 92)
   a. Cold saline
   b. Cold Ringer Lactate
   c. Plastic bag in ice
   d. Deep freezer

2. **Allopurinol is used in organ preservation as:**
   a. Antioxidant
   b. Preservative
   c. Free radical scavenger *(AIIMS May 2009)*
   d. Precursor for energy metabolism

■ GRAFT

3. **Kidney transplantation is an:**
   (DNB 2009, COMEDK 2006)
   a. Allograft
   b. Isograft
   c. Xenograft
   d. Synergic graft

4. **If mother is donating the kidney to her son, this is an example of:** *(Recent Question 2019, MCI June 2018)*
   a. Autograft
   b. Allograft
   c. Isograft
   d. Xenograft

5. **A kidney transplant between identical twins is an example of:** *(Recent Question 2017, COMEDK 2011)*
   a. Isograft
   b. Allograft
   c. Autograft
   d. Xenograft

6. **Concordant xenograft is:** *(Recent Question 2017)*
   a. Between closely related different species
   b. Between same species of different races
   c. Between same species
   d. Between non-identical twins

■ MATCHING AND GRAFT REJECTION

7. **Acute cellular rejection following solid organ transplantation occurs:** *(COMEDK 2011)*
   a. Within minutes to hours of transplantation
   b. Within 48 hours of transplantation
   c. Between 5 to 30 days of transplantation
   d. Beyond 30 days after transplantation

8. **Hyperacute rejection is due to:**
   (Recent Question 2016, AIIMS Nov 2012)
   a. Preformed antibodies
   b. Cytotoxic T-lymphocyte medicated injury
   c. Circulating macrophage mediated injury
   d. Endothelitis caused by donor antibodies

9. **Most important HLA for organ transplantation and tissue typing:** *(Recent Question 2016, MAHE 98)*
   a. HLA-A
   b. HLA-B
   c. HLA-C
   d. HLA-D

■ KIDNEY TRANSPLANTATION

10. **Commonest malignancy in renal transplant recipient is:**
    a. Skin cancer
    b. Renal cell carcinoma
    c. Non-Hodgkin's lymphoma
    d. Hodgkin's lymphoma *(AIIMS Nov 95)*

11. **Most common malignancy in post-transplant individuals:**
    a. PTLD *(Recent Question 2017)*
    b. Squamous cell carcinoma of skin
    c. Kaposi sarcoma
    d. CNS Lymphoma

12. **Principal cause of death in renal transplant patients:**
    (Recent Question 2016)
    a. Uremia
    b. Malignancy
    c. Rejection
    d. Infection

13. **Infection in renal transplant patient is usually caused by:**
    (Recent Question 2016)
    a. CMV
    b. HIV
    c. Herpes
    d. Salmonella

14. **Most common disease caused by CMV in a post renal transplant patients:** *(JIPMER 2011)*
    a. Pyelonephritis
    b. Meningitis
    c. Pneumonia
    d. GI ulceration

15. **An elderly male presents 2 months after renal transplantation with nephropathy. Which of the following can be a viral etiological agent?** *(AIIMS May 2014)*
    a. Polyoma virus BK
    b. Human herpes virus type 6
    c. Hepatitis C
    d. Human papilloma virus, high risk types

16. **All of the following are absolute contraindications for renal transplantation except:** *(Recent Question 2017)*
    a. Active infection
    b. Active malignancy
    c. Active drug abuse
    d. Reduced life expectancy

17. **In renal transplant, transplanted kidney is placed in:**
    (MCI Dec 2019, Recent Question 2018)
    a. Iliac fossa
    b. Subcostal area
    c. Renal fossa
    d. Loin

18. **Left kidney is preferred for transplantation because:**
    a. Longer renal vein *(Recent Question 2018)*
    b. Higher location
    c. Ease of surgery due to anatomical relations
    d. To prevent damage to liver

■ LIVER TRANSPLANTATION

19. **Most common indication of liver transplantation in children:**
    (Recent Question 2019)
    a. Biliary atresia
    b. Wilson's disease
    c. Hemochromatosis
    d. Primary biliary cirrhosis

20. **Auxiliary orthotopic liver transplant is indicated for:**
    a. Metabolic liver disease *(AIIMS May 2008)*
    b. As a standby procedure until finding a suitable donor
    c. Drug induced hepatic failure
    d. Acute fulminant liver failure for any cause

21. **All are scoring system used in liver transplant except:**
    (Recent Question 2016)
    a. CTP
    b. PELD
    c. MELD
    d. MPI

22. **Liver transplantation was first done by:** *(Recent Question 2014)*
    a. Starzl
    b. Huggins
    c. Carrel
    d. Christian Bernard

23. **Which of the following is not an indication for liver transplantation?** *(DNB 2002)*
    a. Fatty liver
    b. HIV
    c. Willson's disease
    d. Primary hyperoxaluria

24. **Most common indication for liver transplantation is:**
    a. HCV induced cirrhosis   *(Recent Question 2017)*
    b. HBV induced cirrhosis
    c. Primary sclerosing cholangitis
    d. HCC

■ PANCREAS TRANSPLANTATION

25. **Site of transplantation in islet cell transplant for diabetes mellitus:** *(Recent Question 2016)*
    a. Forearm muscles
    b. Pelvis
    c. Thigh
    d. Injected into the portal vein

■ SMALL INTESTINE TRANSPLANTATION

26. **Most common cause of death in intestinal transplant:** *(Recent Question 2017)*
    a. Sepsis
    b. Acute rejection
    c. PTLD
    d. GVHD

■ HEART TRANSPLANTATION

27. **Human heart transplant was first done by:**
    a. Christian Bernard   *(Recent Question 2017)*
    b. Roy Calne
    c. Sutherland
    d. Reitz and Norman Shumway

28. **Dr. Christian Bernard is associated with:** *(DNB 2009)*
    a. Heart transplant
    b. Renal transplant
    c. Liver transplant
    d. Hair transplant

■ LUNG TRANSPLANTATION

29. **Indications of lung transplantation:**
    a. COPD
    b. Alpha-1 antitrypsin deficiency
    c. Cystic fibrosis and brochiectasis
    d. All of the above

30. **Order of anastomosis in lung transplant:** *(Recent Question 2017)*
    a. Pulmonary artery, pulmonary vein, bronchus
    b. Pulmonary vein, bronchus, pulmonary artery
    c. Pulmonary vein, pulmonary artery, bronchus
    d. Pulmonary artery, bronchus, pulmonary vein

■ POST-TRANSPLANT INFECTIONS

31. **Post-transplant lymphoma is most commonly associated with:**
    a. EBV
    b. CMV   *(AIIMS May 2012)*
    c. Herpes simplex
    d. HHV-6

■ MISCELLANEOUS

32. **Commonest complication of immunosuppression is:** *(Recent Question 2016)*
    a. Malignancy
    b. Graft rejection
    c. Infection
    d. Thrombocytopenia

33. **Which of the following organs/tissues are presently not being used for organ/tissue transplantation?** *(All India 2011)*
    a. Blood vessels
    b. Lung
    c. Liver
    d. Urinary bladder

34. **Cold ischemic time of the kidney should be ideally below:**
    a. 2 hours
    b. 6 hours   *(DNB 2010)*
    c. 12 hours
    d. 24 hours

35. **Length of time for which an organ can be cold stored before transplantation is maximum with:** *(MHCET 2016)*
    a. Liver
    b. Pancreas
    c. Kidney
    d. Small intestine

36. **Best temperature to store the procured organ for transplantation is:** *(Recent Question 2017)*
    a. –2°C
    b. 0°C
    c. 4°C
    d. 6°C

37. **All of the following nerves are commonly used for grafting except:** *(Recent Question 2018)*
    a. Medial antebrachial cutaneous nerve
    b. Dorsal sensory branch of vagal nerve
    c. Musculocutaneous nerve
    d. Sural nerve

Explanations

■ FLUIDS USED IN TRANSPLANTATION

1. **Ans. c. Plastic bag in ice** (*Ref: Sabiston 20/e p1996; Schwartz 11/e p1938, 10/e p 1800*)

   - The **amputated digits** are **cleansed under saline solution**, **wrapped in saline moistened gauze**, and **placed in a plastic bag**[Q].
   - The **plastic bag containing the part** is then **placed on** (not packed in) a **bed of ice** in a suitable container[Q].
   - The amputated part should never be immersed in nonphysiological solution such as antiseptics or alcohol.

2. **Ans. c. Free radical scavenger** (*Ref: Schwartz 11/e p366-368, 10/e p 332; Bailey 27/e p1546*)

■ GRAFT

3. **Ans. a. Allograft** (*Ref: Schwartz 11/e p214, 220, 10/e p 266; Bailey 27/e p 1533*)

4. **Ans. b. Allograft**   5. **Ans. a. Isograft**

6. **Ans. a. Between closely related different species** (*Ref: Sabiston 20/e p631*)

   "Concordant Xenografts: Concordant xenografts refer to transplants between closely related species; for humans, these include Old World monkeys and apes. The critical element defining an animal as concordant is the assembly of carbohydrate antigens on the cell surface. Similar to humans, concordant species lack galactosyl transferase, and as a result, their carbohydrates are the typical blood group antigens and they lack the N-linked disaccharide galactose-α(1- 3)-galactose (α-Gal). Thus, the natural antibodies present in the circulation of potential human recipients can be predicted by straightforward blood group typing, thereby avoiding the problem of hyperacute rejection."-Sabiston 20/e p631

■ MATCHING AND GRAFT REJECTION

7. **Ans. c. Between 5 to 30 days of transplantation** (*Ref: Schwartz 11/e p358, 9/e p274-275; Bailey 27/e p 1533-1537*)

8. **Ans. a. Preformed antibodies**   9. **Ans. d. HLA-D** (*Ref: Bailey 27/e p 1534-1538*)

■ KIDNEY TRANSPLANTATION

10. **Ans. a. Skin cancer** (*Ref: Bailey 27/e p1542*)

11. **Ans. b. Squamous cell carcinoma of skin** (*Ref: Sabiston 20/e p629*)

12. **Ans. d. Infection** (*Ref: Campbell 10/e p1251-1253*)

MOST COMMON CAUSE OF DEATH IN RENAL TRANSPLANT PATIENTS

   - Heart disease[Q] >Infection[Q] >Stroke

13. **Ans. a. CMV**   14. **Ans. c. Pneumonia**

15. **Ans. a. Polyoma virus BK** (*Ref: Harrison 20/e p508*)

    Polyoma virus BK can be an etiological agent in an elderly male, who presents 2 months after renal transplantation with nephropathy.

16. **Ans. d. Reduced life expectancy** (*Ref: Sabiston 20/e p650*)

17. **Ans. a. Iliac fossa**

18. **Ans. a. Longer renal vein**

    The left kidney is preferred because of implantation advantage associated with a longer left renal vein making anastomosis easier.

■ LIVER TRANSPLANTATION

19. **Ans. a. Biliary atresia**

20. **Ans. a Metabolic liver disease, d. Acute fulminant liver failure for any cause** (*Ref: Blumgart 5/e p1689-1693*)

21. **Ans. d. MPI**

22. **Ans. a. Starzl**

23. **Ans. b. HIV**

24. **Ans. a. HCV induced cirrhosis** (*Ref: Sabiston 20/e p638*)

    "Chronic hepatitis C virus (HCV) infection is the most common indication for transplantation in the West at present."-Sabiston 20/e p638

1. **Ans. b. Fat embolism** *(Ref: Apley's 8/e p535-536, Rockwood 6/e p553)*
   - Discussed in chapter no. 29 Thorax and Lung.

2. **Ans. c. Within 24 hours** *(Ref: Bailey 27/e p19)*

Hemorrhage		
Primary Hemorrhage	**Reactionary Hemorrhage**	**Secondary Hemorrhage**
• Hemorrhage occurring **immediately as a result of an injury**[Q] (or **surgery**).	• Reactionary hemorrhage is delayed hemorrhage (**within 24 hours**[Q]) • Usually **caused by dislodgement of clot**[Q] by resuscitation, normalization of blood pressure and vasodilatation. • May result from **technical failure** such as **slippage of a ligature**[Q].	• Secondary hemorrhage is caused by **sloughing of** the **wall of a vessel.** • It usually occurs **7–14 days after injury**[Q] • **Precipitated by** factors such as **infection, pressure necrosis**[Q] (such as from a drain) or malignancy.

3. **Ans. b. Occurs 7-16 days after surgery**

4. **Ans. b. Pulmonary embolism** *(Ref: Harrison 19/e p1631; Sabiston 20/e p230, 294; Bailey 27/e p296, 986-91)*

5. **Ans. a. Pneumothorax** *(Ref: Complications in Anesthesiology by Kirby (2007)/169)*

6. **Ans. a. Radial** *(Ref: Lee Anesthesia 12/e p25)*

   - **Arterial puncture** and **cannulation** is performed to measure PaO_2, $PaCO_2$, SpO_2 and pH to clarify the **acid-base** and **electrolyte status.**
   - Any artery that can be compressed after puncture may be used (but **not end arteries**), usually the **radial**[Q] (**preferred**), brachial or femoral.

7. **Ans. b. Stopping aspirin for 7 days and then do surgery** *(Ref: www.facs.org › surgerynews › surgerynewsupdat 2012)*
   Aspirin should be **stopped 1 week before surgery**[Q].

8. **Ans. a. Thrombocytopenia** *(Ref: Schwartz 11/e p125, 10/e p90-91,1428)*

9. **Ans. a. Halothane** *(Ref: en.wikipedia.org/wiki/Halothane)*

   ### PHYSICAL PROPERTIES OF HALOTHANE

   - **No analgesia**[Q] and **least pungent (non-irritant)**[Q]
   - **Pleasant to smell**, so **excellent for induction in children**[Q]
   - Halothane has **highest fat/blood coefficient**[Q] 51 (can get deposited in adipose tissues after prolonged exposure)
   - **Trifluoroacetic acid** is a **metabolite** and **found in urine**[Q]

10. **Ans. a. IV antibiotics for 72 hours** *(Ref: Sabiston 20/e p223; Bailey 27/e p1266)*

Enhanced Recovery after Surgery (ERAS) Protocols (Fast Track Programs[Q])
• ERAS refers to **patient-centered, evidence-based, multidisciplinary team developed pathways** for a surgical specialty and facility culture **to reduce the patient's surgical stress response, optimize their physiologic function & facilitate recovery.** • These care pathways form an **integrated continuum**, as the patient moves **from home through the pre-hospital / preadmission, preoperative, intraoperative & postoperative phases** of surgery and home again.

Key Elements of an ERAS Program	
• Pre-admission counseling	• **Avoidance of opiate analgesia**[Q]
• **Avoidance of mechanical bowel preparation**[Q]	• Maintenance of perioperative temperature
• **Preoperative carbohydrate loading**[Q]	• Prevention of postoperative nausea and vomiting
• **Avoidance of preoperative dehydration**[Q]	• **Early mobilization**[Q]
• **No nasogastric tubes**[Q]	• **Early introduction of oral fluids/diets/ supplements**[Q]
• **Short, transverse incisions**[Q] (or laparoscopic procedure)	• **Early removal of urinary catheters**[Q]
• **Short-acting anaesthetic drugs**[Q]	• Continual audit of outcomes
• **Avoidance of perioperative fluid/salt overload**[Q]	
• **Thoracic epidurals**[Q]	

Robotics, Laparoscopy and Bariatric Surgery

■ LAPAROSCOPY

LAPAROSCOPY

- **Needle used** for pneumoperitoneum: **Veress needle**[Q]
- **Most commonly used gas**: CO_2[Q]
- **Flow of gas**: 1L/min[Q]
- **Intra-abdominal pressure maintained during laparoscopy**: 12-15 mm Hg[Q]
- **Trocar** is inserted **at** or **just below** the **umbilicus**[Q] penetrating **skin, superficial & deep fascia, fascia transversalis & parietal peritoneum.**[Q]
  - Post-laparoscopy **shoulder pain** is due to CO_2 **retention** causing **irritation of diaphragm &** referred pain to the **shoulder** through **phrenic nerve**[Q].

■ PNEUMOPERITONEUM

PNEUMOPERITONEUM

- Pneumoperitoneum can be created by **closed or open method.**

Closed Method	Open Method
• Uses **veress needle**[Q]	• Uses **Hasson cannula**[Q]
• **Low risk of bowel injury**[Q] due to presence of safety valve at tip	• **Low risk of major vessel injury**[Q]

■ GASES USED IN LAPAROSCOPY

GASES USED IN PNEUMOPERITONEUM

- **First pneumoperitoneum** was created by **filtered room air**[Q].
- CO_2 & N_2O are now **preferred** because of **increased risk of gas embolism with room air**[Q].
- CO_2: 200 times **more diffusible than** O_2, **rapidly cleared** from the body & lungs, **does not support combustion**[Q]
- N_2O: 68% as **rapidly absorbed in blood** as CO_2, have **mild analgesic effect**, used **for short operative procedures** like sterilization or drilling[Q].
- For prolonged laparoscopic procedures, N_2O should **not be preferred** because it **supports combustion** better than air[Q].

■ PHYSIOLOGICAL EFFECTS OF LAPAROSCOPY

Physiological Effects of Laparoscopy	
Cardiovascular	• ↑ Intra-abdominal pressure leads to ↑ CVP, ↑ PCWP, ↑SVR and ↑ MAP which further ↓ Preload and ↑ Afterload, ultimately decreasing cardiac output[Q].
Pulmonary	• Cephalad shift of diaphragm decreases FRC, chest wall compliance & tidal volume increasing the work of breathing[Q]. • Hypercapnia leading to increase in respiratory rate further adds to this.
Renal	• Increased IAP decreases renal flow, decreasing GFR & reduced urine output. • Raised pCO_2 leads to RAAS stimulation. No long term change in GFR/UO.
Gastrointestinal	• **Decreased perfusion to intestines & stomach** (as a result of increase IAP) **decreases pH** • Decreased portal and hepatic flow leads to elevation of LFTs
Peripheral vascular	• Incidence of DVT, PE is generally lower post-laparoscopic procedures probably secondary to improved prophylaxis • Risk is increased with longer procedures and reverse Trendelenburg position.

■ GAS EMBOLISM

GAS EMBOLISM

- **Most commonly** seen **during induction of pneumoperitoneum** at the time of insufflations of gas from **unintended insufflations of gas directly into an open vein**[Q].
- The more soluble a gas in the blood, the lower chances are for gas embolism.
- CO_2 is **preferred for pneumoperitoneum** as it is **highly soluble in blood** and is **rapidly eliminated**[Q].
- CO_2 **Embolism:** An **initial rise in ET-CO_2** due to **pulmonary excretion of absorbed CO_2** is followed by a **sudden decrease due to fall in cardiac output**[Q].

■ DAY CARE SURGERY

DAY CARE SURGERY OR AMBULATORY SURGERY

- Surgical procedures suitable for ambulatory surgery should be accompanied by **minimal postoperative physiologic disturbances** and an **uncomplicated recovery**[Q].
- The **primary predictors of prolonged stay** or **unanticipated admission after day-care surgery** are related to the **type of surgical procedure** and **associated complications** (e.g. **blood loss, incision pain, postoperative nausea** & **vomiting**)[Q]
- For **superficial procedures** (e.g. **mastectomy,**) **reductions in** both **cost** & **per-operative complications** have been observed when these procedures are performed on an **outpatient basis**[Q].

■ MINIMAL ACCESS SURGERY

Minimal Access Surgery (MAS) includes	
• **Laparoscopy**[Q]	• **Perivisceral endoscopy**[Q]
• **Thoracoscopy**[Q]	• **Arthroscopy & intra-articular**
• **Endoluminal endoscopy**[Q]	**joint surgery**[Q]

Advantages of Minimal Access Surgery (MAS)	
• **Decrease** in **wound size**[Q]	• **Improved mobility**[Q]
• **Reduction** in **wound infection, dehiscence, bleeding, herniation & nerve entrapment**[Q]	• Decreased wound trauma
	• **Decreased heat loss**[Q]
• **Decrease** in **wound pain**[Q]	• **Improved vision**[Q]
	• Faster recovery & shorter hospital stay

■ OBESITY & BMI

Category	BMI
Underweight	<18.5[Q]
Normal	18.5-24.9[Q]
Overweight	25.0-29.9[Q]
Obesity (Class I)	**30-34.9**[Q]
Severe obesity (Class II)	**35-39.9**[Q]
Morbid obesity (Class III)	**40-49.9**[Q]
Superobesity	**>50**[Q]

■ PATHOLOGIC CONSEQUENCES OF OBESITY

Pathologic Consequences of Obesity	
System	**Pathology**
Health	• **Increase in mortality**[Q]
Endocrine	• **Insulin resistance** and type 2 **diabetes mellitus**[Q]
Reproductive	• Male hypogonadism, gynecomastia, menstrual abnormalities, polycystic ovarian syndrome
Cardiovascular	• **Coronary disease,** congestive heart failure

Contd…

Contd…

Pathologic Consequences of Obesity	
System	**Pathology**
Pulmonary	• Obstructive sleep apnea, "obesity hypoventilation syndrome", **pulmonary hypertension, DVT & pulmonary embolism**[Q]
Heaptobiliary	• Nonalcoholic fatty liver disease, symptomatic **gallstones**
Bone, joint, and cutaneous disease	• Osteoarthritis, acanthosis nigricans, friability of skin, **venous stasis & ulcers**[Q]
Neurologic	• Carpal Tunnel syndrome, pseudotumor cerebri, stroke

Increased Cancer Risk in Obese Patients (PEEL CP GO KBC)		
• **Prostate**[Q]	• **Cervix**[Q]	• **Kidney**[Q]
• **Endometrial**[Q]	• **Pancreas**[Q]	• **Bile duct**[Q]
• **Esophagus**[Q]	• **Gallbladder**[Q]	• **Breast**[Q]
• **Liver**[Q]	• **Ovarian**[Q]	• **Colon & rectum**[Q]

■ BARIATRIC SURGERY

BARIATRIC SURGERY

- **Indication for Bariatric Surgery**
  - Patients that have a BMI of **35 Kg/m²** or more with **comorbidity**[Q]
  - Those with a BMI of **40 kg/m²** or greater regardless of comorbidity[Q]

Bariatric Operation	Mechanism of Action
• **Vertical banded gastroplasty** • Laparoscopic adjustable **gastric banding (Safest & reversible)**	• **Restrictive**[Q]
• Roux-en-Y gastric bypass (**RYGB**): MC performed procedure now-a-days	• **Largely Restrictive**[Q]/Mildly Malabsorptive
• **Bilopancreatic diversion** • **Duodenal switch**	• **Largely Malabsorptive**[Q]/Mildly Restrictive

VERTICAL BANDED GASTROPLASTY

- **Restrictive operation**: Restricts or decrease food intake[Q]
- **Upper stomach** near esophagus is **stapled vertically** to create a **small pouch along** the **lesser curvature of stomach**[Q]

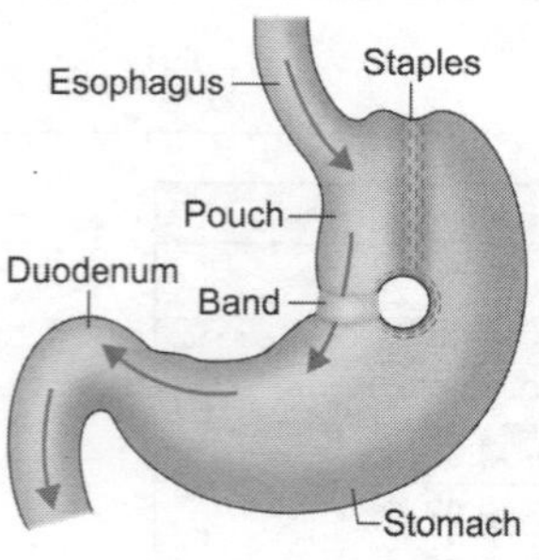

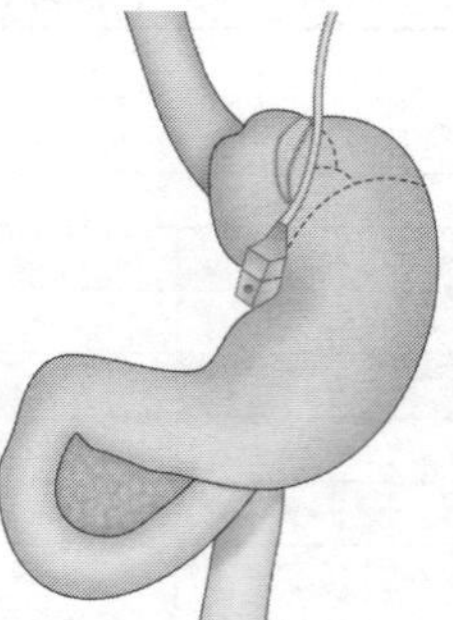

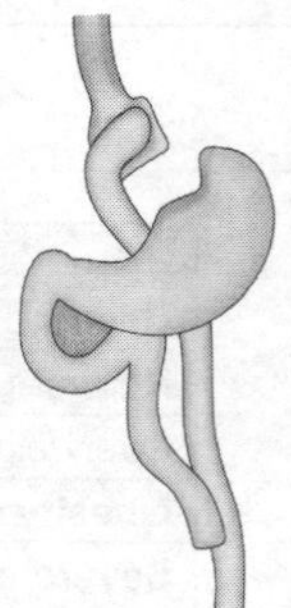

Vertical banded gastroplasty   Laparoscopic adjustable gastric banding   Roux-en-Y gastric bypass

LAPAROSCOPIC ADJUSTABLE GASTRIC BANDING

- **Least invasive, safest & reversible**[Q]
- Involves placement of **adjustable silicon band around the top part of stomach &** creates a **small stomach pouch**[Q]

ROUX-EN-Y GASTRIC BYPASS

- **Most commonly performed bariatric surgery worldwide**[Q]
- Upper part of stomach is separated from lower part & connected to Roux-limb of jejunum[Q]
- **Content of gastric pouch: 30-50 mL**[Q]; **Length of Roux-limb of jejunum: 70-100 cm**[Q]

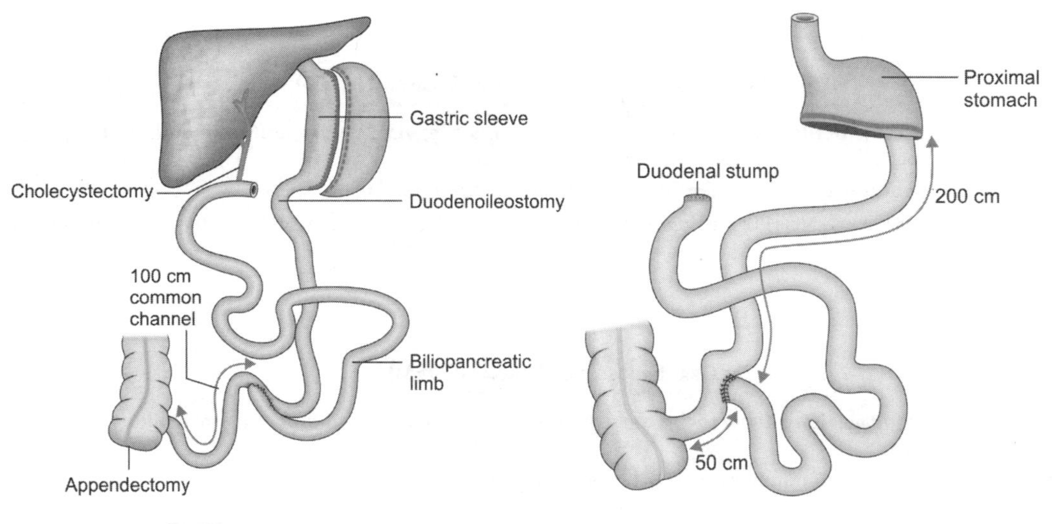

Duodenal Switch   **Biliopancreatic Diversion**

BILIOPANCREATIC DIVERSION

- When the bile is diverted from the intestinal tract so that only the **distal 50 to 100 cm** of **ileum** is **used for bile reabsorption**, the procedure is termed a biliopancreatic diversion.
- **Most effective bariatric surgery**[Q], especially valuable in patients with **severe morbid obesity** or in those who have **failed to maintain weight loss** following gastric bypass surgery or restrictive procedures[Q].
- **Main side effect** with BPD: Patients usually have an increase of **2-4 bowel movements**/day, which in general are **more malodorous**, suggesting fat malabsorption.

DUODENAL SWITCH OPERATION

- It involves a greater curvature **sleeve gastrectomy** with maintenance of the **continuity of** the antrum, pylorus and **first portion** of the duodenum.
- This allows for a **lower marginal ulcer** rate and a lower incidence of **dumping syndrome**.

Components of Duodenal Switch Operation	
• **Sleeve gastrectomy**[Q]	• **Cholecystectomy**[Q]
• **Duodenoileostomy**[Q]	• **Appendectomy**[Q]
• **Jejunoileal bypass**[Q]	

■ PERIOPERATIVE MORTALITY IN BARIATRIC SURGERY

PERIOPERATIVE MORTALITY IN BARIATRIC SURGERY

- **MC cause of death** within 30 days of bariatric surgery: **Pulmonary embolism**[Q] (36%) > **Cardiac complications** (24%) > **Anastomotic leaks** (20%)
- **MC cause of death** in **immediate postoperative period**: Peritonitis secondary to anastomotic leak[Q] (leak **most commonly** occurs at the **gastrojejunostomy**)

■ NEW GUIDELINES OF BARIATRIC SURGERY FOR ASIA

NEW GUIDELINES FOR ASIA

- **Overweight** if the BMI is **23 kg/m²** or more[Q] (International Standard is 25).
- **Obese** if the BMI is **25 kg/m²** or more[Q] (I.S. is 30).
- An Indian qualifies for **bariatric surgery** for obesity if the BMI is **32.5 kg/m²** (I.S. 35) **with comorbidity**[Q] or **37.5 kg/m²** without comorbidity (I.S. 40)[Q].

■ NOTES

Natural Orifice Transluminal Endoscopic Surgery (NOTES)

- **NOTES** is a technique whereby the **peritoneal cavity is entered endoscopically, via a natural orifice (mouth, rectum, vagina)** and the surgery is carried out using specialised endoscopic technology and techniques.

NOTES cholecystectomy & appendicectomy have been successfully carried out in humans.

- Additional procedures performed with NOTES: Staging of intra-abdominal malignancy, segmental colectomy, gastrojejunostomy

■ POEM

Per Oral Endoscopic Myotomy (POEM)

- POEM is the **application of esophageal myotomy to the concept of NOTES** by **submucosal tunneling** method[Q].
- Used for **treatment of achalasia**[Q]
- Involves creation of **long esophageal myotomy using flexible endoscope**[Q]

■ ROBOTIC SURGERY

Robotic Surgery

Da Vinci Robot
• It works on **"master-slave" principle**[Q].
• The **surgeon** inserts his hands into a **"master"** that translates motions of his hands into motions of the robotic arms and hand-like instruments. The surgeon acts as the "master" and the robot as the "slave" in this telerobotic "master-slave" system.
• It is commonly used for **prostatectomies, cardiac valve repair** and **gynecological Surgical procedures**[Q]

Multiple Choice Questions

◼ LAPAROSCOPY

1. **The intra-abdominal pressure during laparoscopy should be set between:** *(Recent Question 2017, DNB 2011, AIIMS Nov 2003)*
   a. 5-8 mm of Hg
   b. 10-15 mm of Hg
   c. 20-25 mm of Hg
   d. 30-35 mm of Hg

2. **Which gas is used in laparoscopy?**
   (Recent Question 2018, 2015, DNB 2012, AIIMS June 94)
   a. CO_2
   b. N_2O
   c. O_2
   d. N_2

3. **Shoulder pain post laparoscopy is due to:**
   (Recent Question 2014, AIIMS Nov 2007)
   a. Subphrenic abscess
   b. CO_2 retention
   c. Positioning of the patient
   d. Compression of the lung

4. **Advantage of minimal access surgery:** *(Recent Question 2016)*
   a. ↑ Heat loss
   b. Better hemostasis control
   c. Improved vision
   d. ↓ in wound pain

5. **Advantage of minimally invasive surgery over open surgery are all except:** *(Recent Question 2015)*
   a. Wide/better field of vision
   b. Less operative time
   c. Lest post-operative time
   d. Less post-operative morbidity

6. **During laparoscopy, the intra-abdominal pressure is:**
   (Recent Question 2014, MHSSMCET 2008)
   a. 5-10 mm Hg
   b. 12-15 mm Hg
   c. 15-20 mm Hg
   d. 20-25 mm Hg

◼ NOTES

7. **In surgical procedure NOTES, entry point is through:**
   (Recent Question 2015)
   a. Abdomen
   b. Umbilicus
   c. Mouth
   d. Axilla

8. **POEM is used for:** *(Recent Question 2018)*
   a. Achalasia cardia
   b. Cancer esophagus
   c. Diffuse esophageal spasm
   d. Nutcracker esophagus

◼ BARIATRIC SURGERY

9. **Physiological changes seen in laparoscopy include all except:** *(AIIMS May 2015)*
   a. Increased ICP
   b. Decreased FRC
   c. Increased CVP
   d. Increased pH

10. **All of the following are primarily restrictive operations for morbid obesity, except:** *(All India 2010)*
    a. Vertical band gastroplasty
    b. Duodenal switch operation
    c. Roux-en-Y operation
    d. Laparoscopic adjustable gastric banding

11. **Vertical banded gastroplasty also known as stomach stapling is done for:** *(DNB 2010)*
    a. Gastric carcinoma
    b. Achalasia cardia
    c. Perforated gastric ulcer
    d. Morbid obesity

12. **Bariatric surgery which results in maximum weight loss:** *(MHCET 2016)*
    a. Biliopancreatic diversion
    b. Gastric sleeve
    c. Gastric banding
    d. Gastric bypass

13. **Most commonly performed and acceptable method of bariatric surgery is:** *(AIIMS May 2015)*
    a. Biliopancreatic diversion
    b. Biliopancreatic diversion with ileostomy
    c. Laparoscopic gastric banding
    d. Roux-en-Y gastric bypass

14. **Bariatric surgery with maximum benefits and comorbidity reduction:** *(Recent Question 2017)*
    a. Roux-en-Y gastric bypass
    b. Laparoscopic sleeve gastrectomy
    c. Biliopancreatic diversion
    d. Laparoscopic adjustable gastric banding

◼ ROBOTIC SURGERY

15. **What is the name of most commonly used robot used for the given surgery?**
    a. PUMA 560
    b. DaVinci robot
    c. PROBOT
    d. ROBODOC

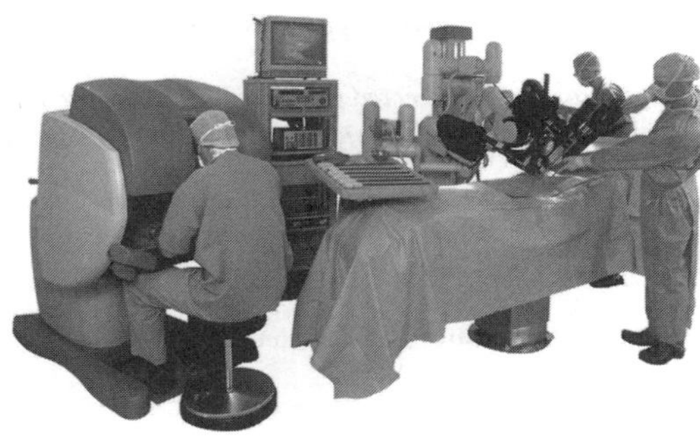

Explanations

■ LAPAROSCOPY

1. Ans. b. 10-15 mm of Hg *(Ref: Sabiston 20/e p394-396; Schwartz 11/e p456, 10/e p417)*
2. Ans. a. CO_2
3. Ans. b. CO_2 retention
4. Ans. c. Improved vision, d. ↓ in wound pain *(Ref: Bailey 27/e p105-108)*
5. Ans. b. Less operative time
6. Ans. b. 12-15 mm Hg

■ NOTES

7. Ans. c. Mouth *(Ref: Bailey 27/e p117)*
8. Ans. a. Achalasia cardia

■ BARIATRIC SURGERY

9. Ans. d. Increased pH *(Ref: Bailey 26/e p94; http://www.laparoscopyhospital.com/physiological-changes-laparoscopy.html)*
   Metabolic acidosis (decrease pH) from CO_2 absorption is the primary derangement with laparoscopy.
10. Ans. b. Duodenal switch operation
11. Ans. d. Morbid obesity
12. Ans. a. Biliopancreatic diversion
13. Ans. d. Roux-en-Y gastric bypass *(Sabiston 20/e p1169; Schwartz 11/e p1180, 10/e p1102-1103; Harrison 20/e p2849)*
    Most commonly performed and acceptable method of bariatric surgery is Roux-en-Y gastric bypass

    "The three restrictive-malabsorptive bypass procedures combine the elements of gastric restriction and selective malabsorption. These procedures are Roux-en-Y gastric bypass, biliopancreatic diversion, and biliopancreatic diversion with duodenal switch. Roux-en-Y is the most commonly undertaken and most accepted bypass procedure. It may be performed with an open incision or by laparoscopy."- Harrison 20/e p2849

14. Ans. a. Roux-en-Y gastric bypass *(Ref: Sabiston 20/e p1049, 1178)*

    "In appropriately selected patients, laparoscopic Roux-en-Y gastric bypass is the most durable method of weight loss and control of obesity-related comorbidities, including GERD."-Sabiston 20/e p1049

■ ROBOTIC SURGERY

15. Ans. b. DaVinci robot *(Ref: Sabiston 20/e p399)*

Sutures and Anastomoses

■ TYPES OF SUTURES

Suture Materials	
Absorbable	**Non-absorbable**

• These sutures **get absorbed** in the tissues either **by enzymatic digestion** or by **phagocytosis[Q]**.
1. **Natural absorbable:**
   – Plain & chromic **catgut[Q]**
2. **Synthetic absorbable: (PVD)**
   – <u>P</u>olydioxanone (PDS)[Q], <u>P</u>olyglycaprone
   – Polyglactin (<u>V</u>icryl)[Q]
   – Polyglycollic acid (<u>D</u>exon)[Q]
	• These sutures **remain in** the **tissues for indefinite period.**
	1. **Natural non-absorbable:**
	   – **Linen[Q]** – **Silk[Q]**
	2. **Synthetic non-absorbable: (PEN)**
	   – **<u>P</u>olypropylene (Prolene)[Q]**
	   – <u>P</u>olyester[Q] (ethibond)
	   – Monofilament polyamide (<u>E</u>thilon)[Q]
	   – <u>N</u>ylon[Q]

Depending upon Number of Strands	
Monofilament	**Polyfilament**
• Consist of **single strand[Q]** of fiber • Sutures are **smooth & strong[Q]** • Chances of **bacterial contamination is less[Q]** • **Knot tied** may become **loose[Q]** • Prolene, Ethilon, nylon	• Consist of **multiple strands[Q]** braided together • **Easier to handle** and **knot tied does not slip[Q]** • Bacteria may lodge in the crevices of the suture, so **not suitable in presence of infection[Q]** • <u>S</u>ilk, <u>l</u>inen, <u>p</u>olyglycollic acid (SLIP)

■ SUTURES: IMPORTANT POINTS

Suture	Types	Raw material	Tensile strength	Absorption rate
Silk	Braided or twisted **multifilament**; Coated (with wax or silicone) or uncoated	Natural protein Raw silk from silkworm	Loses 20% when wet; 80-100% lost by 6 months	Fibrous encapsulation in body at 2-3 weeks ; **Absorbed** slowly over **1-2 year[Q]**
Catgut	Plain	Collagen derived from healthy **sheep** or cattle	Lost within 7-10 days	**Phagocytosis** and **enzymatic degradation** within **7-10 days[Q]**
Catgut	**Chromic**	Tanned with **chromium salts** to **improve handling** and **resist degradation** in tissue[Q]	Lost within 21-28 days	Phagocytosis and enzymatic degradation **within 90 days**
Polyglactin (Vicryl)	Braided multifilament	Copolymer of **lactide & glycolide[Q]** in a ratio of 90:10, coated with polyglactin & calcium stearate	Approx, 60% remains at 2 weeks; 30% remains at 3 weeks	Hydrolysis minimal until 5-6 weeks; Complete absorption **60-90 days[Q]**
Polyglyconate	Monofilament Dyed or undyed	Copolymer of **glycolic acid** and **trimethylene carbonate[Q]**	Approx, 70% remains at 2 weeks; 55% remains at 3 weeks	Hydrolysis minimal until 8-9 weeks; Complete absorption **180 days[Q]**
Polyglycaprone (Monocryl)	Monofilament	Coplymer of **glycolide & caprolactone[Q]**	21 days maximum	**90-120 days[Q]**
Polyglycolic acid (Dexon)	Braided multifilament Dyed or undyed Coated or Uncoated	Polymer of **polyglycolic acid[Q]**	Approx, 40% remains at 1 week; 20% remains at 3 weeks	**Hydrolysis[Q]** minimal at 2 weeks; significant at 4 weeks; Complete absorption **60-90 days[Q]**
Polydioxanone (PDS)	Monofilament dyed or undyed	**Polyester polymer[Q]**	Approx, 70% remains at 2 weeks; 50% remains at 4 weeks; 14% remains at 8 weeks	**Hydrolysis** minimal at 90 days; Complete absorption **180 days[Q]**

■ PRINCIPLES OF SUTURING & ANASTOMOSES

WOUND CLOSURE & ANASTOMOSES

- As a general rule, **each suture** should be **separated by a gap** that is **twice** the **thickness of** the **skin**[Q].
- When **knots are cut short**, the **free ends** or 'ears' should be left **at least 1-2 mm** long[Q]. This is particularly important with **monofilament non-absorbables**[Q].

> - It has been suggested by **Jenkins** that a **suture length to wound length ratio** of **4:1** indicates the **optimum size of tissue bites** and of **suture spacing**[Q].

- **Anastomosis of vessels** was **pioneered by Carrel**[Q].
- **Elliptical incisions** must be **at least 3 times of the width** for the wound **to heal without tension**.
- **Length to width ratio: 3:1**

■ TYPES OF SURGICAL KNOTS

Square (Reef) Knot	Surgeons Knot	Granny (Pseudo-square) Knot
• Consist of **two throws** • **Crossing** is done **in each throw** • Secured knot	• Consist of **two throws** • **Two wraps** in **first throw** • **Crossing** occurs **in each throw**	• Consist of **two throws** • **Crossing does not occur** in any throw • **Not a secured knot**

■ SUTURING TECHNIQUES

SUTURING TECHNIQUES

1. **Simple Interrupted Suture:**
- **Needle** is **inserted at right angle, to the incision**
- Pass through the both aspects of suture line, & exit again at right angles
- **Each successive suture** should be **placed at twice the distance from edge of the wound**[Q].

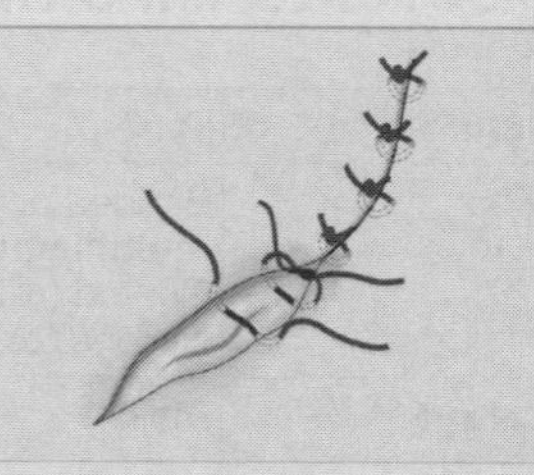

2. **Continuous Suture:**
- First suture is inserted in an identical manner to an interrupted suture
- Rest of the sutures is inserted in a continuous manner, until the far end of wound is reached.
- **At the far end** of the wound suture line should be **secured with Aberdeen knot**[Q] or by tying free end to the loop of cast suture.

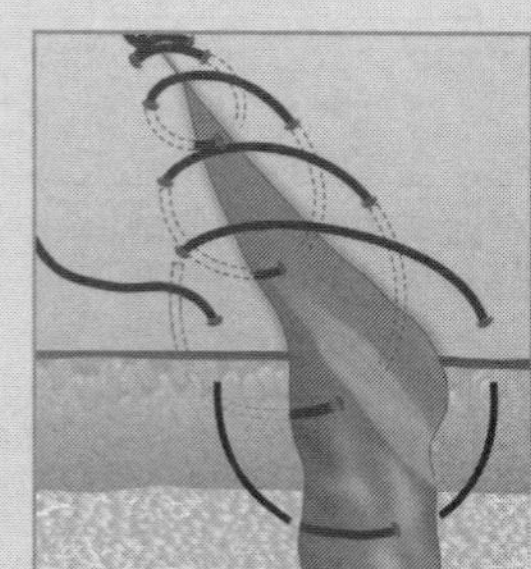

Aberdeen Knot
• Free end of suture is partially pulled through the final loop, several times before being pulled through a final time, completely, prior to cutting.

3. **Mattress Sutures:**
- Used to **produce eversion or inversion** of wound edges[Q]
- Useful in producing **accurate approximation of wound edges**, when the **edges are irregular in depth or disposition**[Q]

Contd...

Horizontal Mattress	Vertical Mattress
• Initial suture is inserted as for an interrupted suture but then **needle moves horizontally** & **traverses both edges** of the wound once again[Q]	• Initial suture is inserted as for an interrupted suture but then **needle moves vertically** & **traverses both edges** of wound once again[Q].

4. Subcuticular Suture:
- Used in **skin**, where **cosmetic appearance is important**[Q] & skin edges are approximated easily.
- **MC used suture is monocryl[Q]** (**polyglycaprone**[Q])

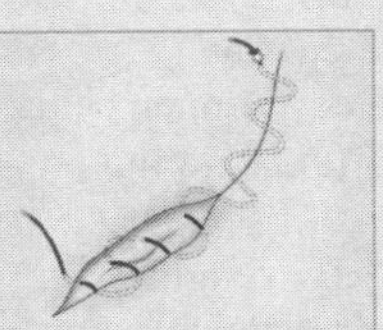

5. Purse String Suture:
- **Continuous stitch parallel to a circular wound is applied**[Q]
- Used for **hernia sac & appendectomy**[Q]

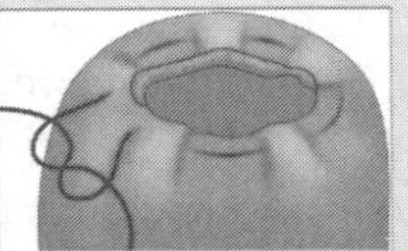

■ BOWEL ANASTOMOSES

BOWEL ANASTOMOSES

- **Lembert** described **seromuscular suture technique** for **bowel anastomosis** in 1826[Q].
- **Senn** advocated a **two-layer technique for closure**[Q].
- **Halsted** favoured a **one-layer extramucosal closure**[Q].
- **Connell** used a **single layer of interrupted sutures** incorporating all layers of the bowel[Q].
- **Kocher's method**, a **two layer anastomosis**, first a **continuous all-layer suture using catgut**, then an **inverting continuous** (or interrupted) **seromuscular layer** suture **using silk**, became the standard. There is evidence that **inversion is safest in bowel** (least likely to leak), although end-to-end staplers give an everted anastomosis without complication.
- The **single-layer extramucosal anastomosis**, advocated by **Matheson**[Q], causes the least tissue necrosis or luminal narrowing.
- The **Cheatle split** (making a **cut into the anti-mesenteric border**) may help to **enlarge the lumen of distal, collapsed bowel**[Q].
- **Bowel anastomotic leaks** are generally occur **on day 7**[Q].

■ VASCULAR ANASTOMOSES

VASCULAR ANASTOMOSES

- **Vascular anastomoses** require **more precision** than bowel anastomoses as they must be **immediately watertight**[Q] at the end of the operation when the clamps are removed.
- **Suture size depends on vessel calibre:**
  - 2/0 for **aorta**[Q]
  - 4/0 for **femoral artery**[Q]
  - 6/0 for **popliteal to distal arteries**[Q]
  - **Microvascular anastomoses** are made using a loupe and an interrupted suture down to **10/0 size**

- **Polypropylene-like sutures** with indefinite integrity give the **best results**[Q]
- **Intimal suture line** must be **smooth**[Q]
- **Knots** must be **secure**[Q]
- **Needle** must **pass from within outwards**[Q]

■ TISSUE GLUE

TISSUE GLUE

- **Tissue glue** is also available based upon a **solution of n-butyl- 2-cyanoacrylate monomer**[Q].
- When it is **applied to a wound, it polymerizes to form a firm adhesive bond**[Q]
- **Wound does need to be clean, dry, with near perfect hemostasis and under no tension**[Q].
- **Specific uses:** Closing a laceration on the forehead of a fractious child in Accident and Emergency thus dispensing with local anaesthetic and sutures.
- **Relatively expensive**, it is **quick to use, does not delay wound healing** and is associated with an **allegedly low infection rate**.

Multiple Choice Questions

■ SUTURES

1. Which of the following is a non-absorbable suture?
   (Recent Question 2016, All India 2008)
   a. Polypropylene
   b. Vicryl
   c. Catgut
   d. Polydioxanone

2. Catgut is prepared from submucosal layer of the intestine of: *(Bihar PG 2014, DNB 2005, 2000)*
   a. Cat
   b. Sheep
   c. Human being
   d. Rabbit

3. Which of the following is not absorbable suture?
   (DNB 2011, APPG 2008)
   a. Catgut
   b. Polyamide
   c. Polyglactin
   d. Polyester

4. Catgut is preserved in: *(Recent Question 2013)*
   a. Glutaraldehyde
   b. Isopropyl alcohol
   c. Iodine
   d. Cetrimide

5. After a midline laparotomy, you have been asked to suture the incision. What length of suture will you choose?
   (AIIMS Nov 2016)
   a. 2x incision length
   b. 4x incision length
   c. 6x incision length
   d. 8x incision length

6. Which of the following is the preferred suture material for vascular anastomosis? *(Recent Question 2017)*
   a. Non-absorbable, elastic
   b. Non-absorbable, non-elastic
   c. Absorbable, elastic
   d. Absorbable, non-elastic

7. Which the following statement is true about the given suture? *(Recent Question 2018)*

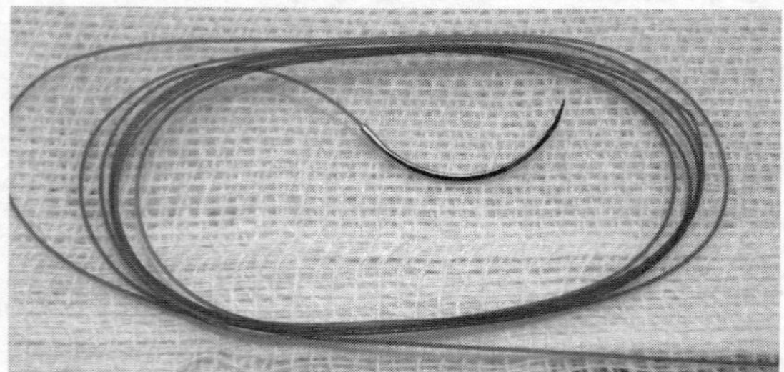

   a. It is less reactive
   b. Derived from cat gut mucosa
   c. It is absorbed by phagocytosis and enzymatic dehydration
   d. Made from rabbit gut

■ ANASTOMOSIS

8. In elliptical incisions, length to width ratio:
   (Recent Question 2017)
   a. 4:1
   b. 3:1
   c. 2:1
   d. 1:1

9. Length of suture required closing the incision to the wound length ratio: *(Recent Question 2017)*
   a. 4:1
   b. 3:1
   c. 2:1
   d. 1:1

10. Intestinal anastomosis strength is provided by:
    (JIPMER 2015)
    a. Mucosa
    b. Submucosa
    c. Serosa
    d. Muscularis mucosa

11. Tissue suturing glue contains: *(Recent Question 2015)*
    a. Cyanoacrylate
    b. Ethanolamine oleate
    c. Methacrylate
    d. Polychloroprene

■ MESH

12. Which of the following statement is incorrect about mesh?
    a. Mesh can shrink upto 50% *(Recent Question 2017)*
    b. Weight of light-weight mesh is < 40 gm/m²
    c. Weight of heavy-weight mesh is > 80 gm/m²
    d. Flat sheet meshes does not require fixation

13. What is the weight of low-weight mesh?
    (Recent Question 2017)
    a. <40 gm/m²
    b. <60 gm/m²
    c. <80 gm/m²
    d. <90 gm/m²

■ KNOTS

14. What is the name of this knot? *(Recent Question 2019)*

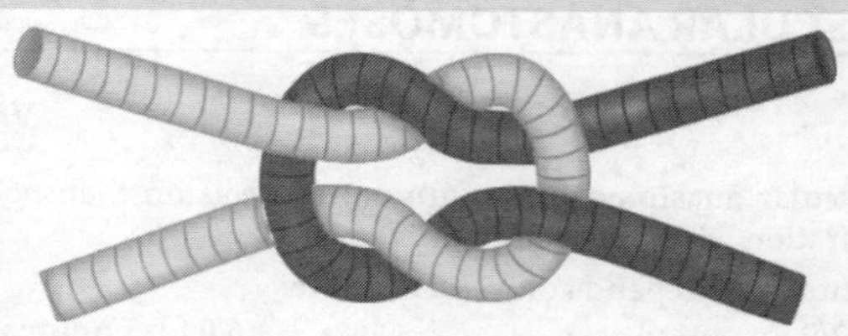

    a. Reef knot
    b. Granny knot
    c. Surgeon's knot
    d. Half-in-half knot

Explanations

■ SUTURES

1. **Ans. a. Polypropylene** *(Ref. Bailey 27/e p90)*
2. **Ans. b. Sheep** *(Ref. Bailey 27/e p93)*

SUTURES

- **John Hunter** discovered **catgut**[Q].
- **Plain catgut** is derived from **submucosa of sheep's intestine**[Q].
- **Plain catgut** loses **50% tensile strength in 3 days**[Q] and **all tensile strength in 15 days** & **absorbed in 60 days**[Q].
- **Isopropyl alcohol**[Q] is used as **preservative for packing catgut sutures.**

  > - **Vicryl** (Co-polymer of **glycolide** & **lactide**) maintains **tensile strength for 28-30 days**[Q] & gets **absorbed in 80-90 days (Delayed absorption)**[Q]
  > - **Vicryl** is used for **bile duct surgeries**[Q].

- **PDS** sutures exhibit the **lowest affinity to the adherence of E. coli** & **Staphylococcus aureus**; **Dexon sutures** exhibit the **highest affinity** to these species.
- **Polydioxanone (PDS)** undergoes **hydrolysis** & **complete absorption within 180 days.**
- **Raw material used in nylon suture:** Polyamide polymer
- **MC used for subcuticular suturing: Monocryl (Polyglycaprone)**[Q]
- **Work-Horse suture for general surgeries: Vicryl**[Q]

3. **Ans. d. Polyester**   4. **Ans. b. Isopropyl alcohol**   5. **Ans. b. 4x incision length**

6. **Ans. b. Non-absorbable, non-elastic** *(Ref: Bailey 27/e p99)*

"Vascular anastomosis: Non-absorbable monofilament suture material should be used, e.g. polypropylene." -Bailey 27/e p99

"Vascular anastomoses require an extremely accurate closure as they must be immediately watertight at the end of the operation when the vascular clamps are removed. In many cases, some form of prosthetic material or graft may be used which will never be integrated into the body tissues and so the integrity of the suture line needs to be permanent. For this reason, polypropylene is one of the best sutures as it is not biodegradable. It is used in its monofilament form, mounted on an atraumatic, curved, round-bodied needle. Knot security is important, and as polypropylene is monofilament and the anastomosis often depends on one final knot, several throws (between six and eight) of a well-laid reef knot are required. The suture line must be regular and watertight with a smooth intimal surface to minimise the risk of thrombosis and embolus, as well as to avoid any leakage." -Bailey 27/e p99

7. **Ans. c. It is absorbed by phagocytosis and enzymatic dehydration** *(Ref: Bailey 27/e p93)*

- *The given suture is catgut (absorbable suture), which is prepared from sheep gut and absorbed by phagocytosis and enzymatic dehydration.*

■ ANASTOMOSES

8. **Ans. b. 3:1** *(Ref: Bailey 27/e p85)*

*"Occasionally, it may be necessary to excise a skin lesion with a circular incision in an area when the direction of Langer's lines are not apparent. However, once the circular incision has been made, it can often be observed that the circular incision is converted to an ellipse thus indicating the lines of tension. This circular incision should then be formally converted into an elliptical incision, remembering the **rule of thumb that 'an elliptical incision must be at least three times as long as it is wide' for the wound to heal without tension.**" -Bailey 27/e p85*

9. **Ans. a. 4:1** *(Ref: Bailey 27/e p1041)*

"It has also been confirmed that the optimal ratio of suture length to wound length is 4:1 (Jenkins' rule). If less length than this is used, the suture bites are too far apart or too tight and the converse applies if more length than this is used." -Bailey 27/e p1041

10. **Ans. b. Submucosa**   11. **Ans. a. Cyanoacrylate** *(Ref; Bailey 27/e p96)*

■ MESH

12. **Ans. d. Flat sheet meshes does not require fixation** *(Ref: Bailey 27/e p1027)*
13. **Ans. a. <40 gm/m²** *(Ref: Bailey 27/e p1028)*

"The terms 'light, medium and heavy' are not precisely defined but meshes less than 40 g/m² are generally referred to as light and meshes more than 80 g/m² are heavy." -Bailey 27/e p1028

■ KNOTS

14. **Ans. b. Granny knot**

Sterilization and Infection

■ TECHNIQUES OF STERILIZATION

Techniques of Sterilization	
Steam (121°C for 15 minutes)	• Surgical instruments[Q]
Ethylene oxide	• **Heart lung machine**[Q], respirators, dental labs
Hot air oven	• **Glass syringe**[Q], test tubes, **flasks**[Q], cutting instruments
Irradiation **(gamma rays)**	• **Industrial packaging**[Q]
Paracetic acid (STERIS)	• **Flexible endoscopes**[Q]
Isopropyl alcohol	• **Clinical thermometer**[Q]
Beta propiolactone >Formaldehyde	• **Fumigation of OT, labs, wards**[Q]
2% Glutaraldehyde	• **Endoscope (cystoscope, bronchoscope)**[Q]
Autoclaving	• **Culture media, suture materials except catgut**[Q]

■ HOSPITAL ACQUIRED INFECTION

Hospital Acquired Infection (HAI)

- Infection that **follows surgery** or **admission to hospital**
- **Common HAI are:**

1. **Respiratory infections**[Q] (including ventilator-associated pneumonia)	**10–15%**
2. **UTI**[Q] (mostly related to urinary catheters)	**30–40% (MC)**[Q]
3. Bacteremia (mostly related to indwelling vascular catheters)	**10–15%**
4. **Surgical site infections**[Q]	**15–20% (2nd MC)**[Q]
5. **Antibiotic associated diarrhea**, caused by Clostridium difficile[Q]	**5–10%**

■ PREVENTIVE MEASURES FOR HOSPITAL ACQUIRED INFECTION

Preventive Measure for Hospital Acquired Infection

- **Isolation: Infective patients** must be isolated in **room with adequate ventilation** and **negative pressure**[Q]
- **Hospital staff:** Those who are suffering from skin disease, sore throat, common cold, ear infection diarrhea or dysentery and other infections ailments should be **kept away from work until complete cured**[Q].

  > - **Handwashing**[Q]: The **most common route of infection** is **via the hands**[Q]. Hands washing with soap and water may not be sufficient; a **suitable disinfectant must be employed** for handwashing[Q].

- **Dust control:** Hospital dust contains numerous bacteria and virus. Suppression of dust by **wet dusting** and **vacuum (negative pressure) cleaning**[Q] are important control measure.
- **Disinfection:** The article used by the patient as well as patient's urine, feces, sputum should properly disinfect. **Proper sterilization**[Q] of instrument should be enforced.
- **Control of droplet infection:** Use of **face masks**[Q], proper bad spacing, prevention of overcrowding and ensuring adequate lighting and ventilation are important control measure.
- **Nursing technique:** Barrier nursing and task nursing have also been recommended to minimize cross infection.
- **Administrative measures:** There should be a **hospital control infection committee**[Q] to form late policies regarding control of hospital acquired infection.

■ AREA OF CLEANING & DRAPING IN SURGERIES

Area of Cleaning & Draping in Surgeries	
Cranial surgery	• Depends upon surgeon
Thyroid or neck surgery	• **Chin to nipple** with shoulder & axilla[Q]
Eye surgery	• **Cut eyelashes** of affected eye
Nasal surgery	• No shaving unless with mustache
Ear surgery	• **Two & half inches around ear**[Q]
Chest surgery	• **Base of neck to waist, axilla & inner arm**[Q]
Abdominal & pelvic surgery	• **Nipple to symphysis pubis, vulva, perineum & thigh**[Q]
Kidney-anterior	• **Nipple to perineum**, side to side; supra scapular region to buttocks
Vaginal, scrotal, rectal surgery	• **Waist to perineum** plus **anterior & inner aspect of thigh**[Q] and 6 inches from groin; posterior-entire buttocks & anus
Lower extremities	• **Digits 2 inches above knee**, entire extremity and groin[Q]
Upper extremities	• **Distal arm 2 inches above elbow**, elbow up to axilla[Q]

■ PROPHYLACTIC ANTIBIOTICS

Prophylactic Antibiotics

- **Antibiotics** should be used **when local wound defenses** are **not established** (the decisive period).
- Ideally, **maximal blood** and **tissue levels** should be **present at the time** at which the **first incision** is made and before contamination occurs.

  - **IV** administration at **induction**[Q] **of anesthesia** is optimal.
  - If induction is not mentioned in the option go for **30 minutes** to **1 hour before surgery**[Q].

- In **long operations,** those involving the **insertion of a prosthesis,** when there is **excessive blood loss** or when **unexpected contamination** occurs, antibiotics may be **repeated 8 and 16 hours later**[Q].
- The use of the newer, **broad-spectrum antibiotics for prophylaxis should be avoided**[Q].
- **Benzylpenicillin**[Q] should be used if **Clostridium** gas gangrene infection is a possibility
- Patients with **heart valve** disease or a **prosthesis** should be **protected** from bacteremia caused by **dental work, urethral instrumentation or visceral surgery**[Q]

■ HOW TO AVOID SURGICAL SITE INFECTION?

Avoiding Surgical Site Infections

- **Staff** should **always wash their hands** between patients[Q]
- **Length of patient stay** should be **kept** to a **minimum**[Q]
- **Preoperative shaving** should be **avoided** if possible[Q]
- **Antiseptic skin preparation** should be standardized[Q]
- Attention to theatre technique and discipline[Q]
- **Avoid hypothermia** perioperatively and ensure **supplemental oxygenation** in recovery[Q]

■ SURGICAL SITE INFECTION

Surgical Site Infections

- A **major SSI** is defined as a **wound** that either **discharges significant quantities of pus spontaneously** or **needs a secondary procedure to drain it.** The patient may have **systemic signs** such as **tachycardia, pyrexia** and a **raised WBC count [systemic inflammatory response syndrome (SIRS)]**
- Minor wound infections may discharge pus or infected serous fluid but should not be associated with excessive discomfort, systemic signs or delay in return home
- The differentiation between major and minor and the definition of SSI is important in audit or trials of antibiotic prophylaxis.
- There are scoring systems for the severity of wound infection, which are particularly useful in surveillance and research.
- Examples are the **Southampton** and **ASEPSIS systems**[Q].

Southampton Wound Grading System	
Grade/Appearance	**Subtype/Appearance**
0: Normal healing[Q]	
I: Normal healing with mild bruising or erythema[Q]	• **Ia:** Some **bruising** • **Ib: Considerable bruising** • **Ic: Mild erythema**
II: Erythema plus other signs of inflammation[Q]	• **IIa:** At **one point** • **IIb: Around sutures** • **IIc: Along** wound • **IId: Around** wound
III: Clear or hemoserous discharge[Q]	• **IIIa:** At **one point** only (<2 cm) • **IIIb: Along** wound (>2 cm) • **IIIc: Large volume** • **IIId: Prolonged** (>3 days)
IV: Pus[Q]	• **IVa:** At **one point** only (<2 cm) • **IVb: Along** wound (>2 cm)
V: Deep or Severe	• Wound infection with or without tissue breakdown

ASEPSIS Wound Score	
Criterion	**Points**
Additional treatment[Q]	0
• Antibiotics for wound infection	10
• Drainage of pus under local anaesthesia	5
• Debridement of wound under general anaesthesia	10
Serous discharge[Q]	Daily 0–5
Erythema[Q]	Daily 0–5
Purulent exudate[Q]	Daily 0–10
Separation of deep tissues[Q]	Daily 0–10
Isolation of bacteria from wound[Q]	10
Stay as inpatient prolonged over 14 days as result of wound infection[Q]	5

■ WOUND DEHISCENCE

WOUND DEHISCENCE (BURST ABDOMEN)

- **Serous** or **serosanguinous discharge** from the wound is the **first sign**[Q] of dehiscence (Salmon fluid sign[Q])

  - **Most commonly** observed between 5th and 8th postoperative day[Q] (may occur at any time following wound closure)

- Wound dehiscence is **partial** or **total disruption** of any or all layers of the operative wound.
- **Extrusion** of **abdominal viscera** after rupture of all layers is known as **evisceration**[Q].

Management

- **Wound dehiscence** without evisceration: **Prompt elective closure**[Q] of the wound
- **Wound dehiscence with evisceration:**
  - Wound is **covered with moist towels**
  - Under GA, **any exposed bowel** or **omentum** is rinsed with RL containing **antibiotics** and then **returned to abdomen**
  - Previous sutures are removed, wound is reclosed (**Tension suturing**[Q])

Predisposing Factors for Wound Dehiscence

Local Risk Factors	Systemic Risk Factors

• **Inadequate closure** (**Most important**)[Q]
  – Use of **absorbable sutures**
  – **Multilayer closure** (single layer has lower incidence)
• **Midline** and **vertical incisions** are **more prone** than transverse incisions
• **Increased** intra-abdominal **pressure**
• **Deficient wound healing** due to:
  – **Infections**[Q], **Seroma**[Q], **Hematoma**[Q]
  – **Presence of drain**[Q]
	• **Old age**[Q]
	• **Obesity**[Q]
	• **Immunosuppression**[Q]
	• **Systemic diseases:**
	  – **Diabetes**[Q]
	  – **Uremia**[Q]
	  – **Jaundice, Sepsis**[Q]
	  – **Cancer**[Q]

■ SEPSIS, SEPTIC SHOCK & MODS

Condition	Definition	Criteria in 2016
Sepsis	• A life threatening **organ dysfunction** caused by a **dysregulated host response to infection**[Q]	• **Suspected** (or documented) **infection** and an **acute increase in ≥2** sepsis related organ failure assessment **(SOFA) points**[Q]
Septic Shock	• A subset of sepsis in which **underlying circulatory and cellular/metabolic abnormalities** lead to substantially **increased mortality risk**[Q]	• **Suspected** (or documented) **infection plus vasopressor therapy** needed to maintain **mean arterial pressure at ≥ 65 mm Hg**[Q] **& serum lactate > 2.0 mmol/L despite adequate fluid resuscitation**[Q]
SOFA score is a **24-point measure of organ dysfunction** that uses **six organ systems**[Q] (renal, cardiovascular, pulmonary, hepatic, neurologic, hematologic[Q]), where **0–4 points** are assigned **per organ system.**		

MULTIORGAN DYSFUNCTION SYNDROME (MODS)

- **Definition:** Simultaneous **presence of physiologic dysfunction** and/or **failure of two or more organs**[Q].
- Occurs in the setting of **severe sepsis**[Q], **shock** of any kind[Q], **severe inflammatory conditions** such as **pancreatitis**[Q] **& trauma**[Q].
- **Organ failure must persist beyond 24 hours**[Q]; mortality risk increases with accrual of failing organs[Q]; prognosis worsens with increased duration of organ failure[Q].

■ CELLULITIS

CELLULITIS

- It is **non-suppurative & invasive inflammation, spreading along** the **subcutaneous tissues** and **connective tissue planes** and across intercellular spaces[Q].
- The term is a misnomer, as the **lesion** is one of the **connective** and **interstitial tissue** and not of the cells.

> - MC causative organism: Streptococcus pyogenes[Q]

Pathology
- The **organism** usually gains **access through a wound** or **scratch or** following **surgical incision**[Q].
- There is **wide speared swelling** and **redness** at the area of inflammation, but without definite localization **blebs** and **bullae** form on the skin. **Central necrosis** may occur **at later stage**[Q].

Clinical Features
- There is varying degree of **fever** and **toxemia. Affected part** is very much **swollen** and **painful**[Q].
- **Diabetic individual** often suffer from cellulitis[Q]
- **Examination:** Affected part is warm, swollen and tender, there is **pitting edema** and **brawny induration. Surrounding lymph vessels** may be seen as **red streaks** due to lymphangitis[Q].

Treatment
- **Rest** and **elevation** of the part to reduce edema; Appropriate **antibiotic** preferably broad spectrum[Q]
- **Penicillin** is **still sensitive against streptococci**[Q]

> - **Failure** of inflammatory swelling **to subside after 48 to 72 hours** suggests that an **abscess** has developed. In that case **incision** and **drainage** of the pus should be accomplished[Q].

■ ERYSIPELAS

ERYSIPELAS

- This is a **sharply demarcated streptococcal infection** of the **superficial lymphatic vessels**, usually associated with **broken skin** on the face[Q].

Clinical Features
- Affected area is **erythematous** and **edematous.** Patient may be **febrile** and have a **leucocytosis**[Q].

Treatment
- Prompt administration of **broad-spectrum antibiotics after** swabbing the area for **culture and sensitivity** is usually all that is necessary.

■ CARBUNCLE

CARBUNCLE

- A **carbuncle** is an abscess larger than a boil, usually with one or more openings draining pus onto the skin.
- **Most commonly** caused by **Staphylococcus aureus**[Q]; **MC location: Nape of the neck**[Q].

Etiology
- **Triggers for carbuncle: Folliculitis, friction** from clothing or shaving, having the **hair pulled out,** generally **poor hygiene, poor nutrition** or **weakening of immunity**[Q].
- Persons with **diabetes**[Q] and **immune system diseases** are **more likely** to develop carbuncles.

Clinical Features
- **Carbuncle:** Made up of several skin boils, infected mass is filled with fluid, pus and dead tissues.
- It may be **red and irritated, grow very fast** and have a **white** or **yellow center**[Q].

Treatment
- **Proper excision by cruciate incision**[Q] will usually treat the condition effectively
- **Surgical incision** and **drainage** of **all suppurative collections** with **antibiotics**[Q].

■ NECROTIZING FASCIITIS

NECROTIZING FASCIITIS

- Necrotizing fasciitis is a **rapidly progressive bacterial infection** characterized by involvement and **necrosis of** the **subcutaneous tissue** and **fascia**, with typical **sparing of** the **underlying muscle**[Q].
- **MC site of infection: Lower extremities**[Q]
- May involve trunk, **perineum (Fournier's gangrene)** or head and neck and any other site.

Etiological Agents

- **MC single etiological agents: Group A beta hemolytic streptococci**[Q]

  > - More commonly, **necrotizing fasciitis** results from a **polymicrobial synergistic infection**[Q]

- Microorganism responsible: **Group A beta hemolytic streptococci** + Staphylococcus, E. coli, Pseudomonas, Proteus, Bacteroides/ Clostridium (**Anaerobes**)

Risk Factors for Necrotizing Fasciitis		
• **Diabetes**[Q]	• **Smoking**[Q]	• Peripheral vascular disease[Q]
• Pressure sores	• **Penetrating trauma**[Q]	• **Skin infection / damage**[Q]
• **Immunocompromised states**[Q]	• **Obesity**[Q]	(abrasions, bites, boils)
	• **IV drug abuse**[Q]	

Clinical Presentation

- **Pain** is the **most important presenting symptom**
- **Pain** is **disproportionately greater**[Q] than that expected from degree of cellulites present

  > - Without treatment **pain may decrease due to thrombosis of small blood vessels** and **destruction of peripheral nerves** (an **ominous sign**[Q])

- **Skin Features: Edema, erythema**[Q] (Infected area is red, hot, shiny, swollen and exquisitely tender)
- **Woody hard texture** to subcutaneous tissue
- **Skin vesicles/cutaneous bullae, soft tissue crepitus** due to **gas production**[Q] may be seen when necrotizing fasciitis is caused due to mixed flora but not due to group A streptococcus
- **Systemic features:** Fever, **hypotension**, tachycardia, progression to **septic shock, DIC** or **multiple organ failure**[Q]

Management

- This is a **surgical emergency** and **surgical debridement is mandatory**[Q]

  > - Treatment: **Urgent surgical debridement + IV fluids + Broad spectrum IV antibiotics + Supportive treatment**[Q]

- **Mortality rate** is nearly **100% without surgical debridement**[Q]
- **Hyperbaric oxygen** helps in **wound healing**[Q]

■ GAS GANGRENE

GAS GANGRENE

- Caused by **C. perfringens (Gram-positive, anaerobic, spore-bearing** bacilli are widely found in **soil** and **feces)**[Q].
- This is relevant to **military, traumatic surgery** and **colorectal operations**[Q].

Risk Factors
- **Immunocompromised, diabetics** or patients with **malignant disease**[Q]
- Wounds containing **necrotic** or **foreign material**, resulting in **anaerobic conditions**[Q]

Clinical Features
- **Severe local wound pain** and **crepitus (gas in the tissues**, which may also be **noted on plain radiographs)**[Q].
- The **wound produces** a **thin, brown, sweet smelling exudate**[Q], in which Gram staining will reveal bacteria.

  > - **Gas** and **smell** are **characteristic**[Q] (Myonecrosis)
  > - If septicemia occurs, **gas** may be **produced** in the other organ, notably the **liver** known as **'foaming liver'**[Q].

- **Edema** and **spreading gangrene** follow the release of **collagenase, hyaluronidase**, other proteases and **alpha toxin**[Q].
- **Early systemic complications** with **circulatory collapse** and **multi-organ failure**[Q] follow if prompt action is not taken

Treatment
- **Antibiotic prophylaxis** in patients at risk, especially when **amputations** are performed **for peripheral vascular disease with open necrotic ulceration**[Q].

  > - Once a **gas gangrene infection is established, large doses of IV penicillin** and **aggressive debridement** of affected tissues are required[Q].
  > - The use of **hyperbaric oxygen** is controversial.

- **Closure of traumatic wounds** or **compound fractures** should be **delayed for 5–6 days**[Q] until it is certain that these sites are free of infection.

  > - **Passive anti-gas gangrene serum** given IM or **in emergencies IV**[Q] used to be common practice in prophylaxis.

■ TETANUS

TETANUS

- Caused by **Clostridium tetani (anaerobic, terminal spore-bearing, Gram-positive** bacterium)[Q] following implantation into tissues or a wound
- **Spores** are widespread in **soil** and **manure**, and so the infection is **more common in traumatic civilian** or **military wounds.**

Clinical Features

- Signs and symptoms of tetanus are mediated by the release of the **exotoxin tetanospasmin,** which **affects myoneural junctions** and the **motor neurons** of the **anterior horn** of the spinal cord.
- **MC initial symptoms:** Trismus (lockjaw)[Q], **muscle pain** and **stiffness,** back pain, and difficulty swallowing.

  - A **short prodromal period,** which has a **poor prognosis,** leads to **spasms** in the distribution of the **short motor nerves of** the face followed by the **development of severe generalised motor spasms** including **opsithotonus, respiratory arrest** and **death**[Q].
  - A **longer prodromal period** of 4–5 weeks is **associated with a milder form of** the **disease**[Q].

- The **entry wound** may show a **localized small area of cellulitis**; exudate or aspiration may give a sample that can be stained to show the presence of Gram-positive rods.

  - **Risus sardonicus (sardonic grin**[Q]**):** Highly characteristic, abnormal, **sustained spasm of** the **facial muscles** that appears to **produce grinning**

Treatment

- **Prophylaxis with tetanus toxoid** is the **best preventative treatment**[Q].
- **Established infection: Minor debridement** of the wound with antibiotic **benzylpenicillin**[Q]
- **Relaxants** may also be required, and the patient may require **ventilation in severe forms,** which may be associated with a high mortality.
- **Anti-toxin using human immunoglobulin** for both **at-risk wounds** and **established infection**[Q].

■ TUBERCULOUS LYMPHADENITIS

TUBERCULOUS LYMPHADENITIS

- Most commonly affects **children** or **young adults**[Q], but can occur at any age.
- **Deep upper cervical nodes** are **most commonly affected**[Q], but there may be a widespread cervical lymphadenitis with many matting together.
- In most cases, the **tubercular bacilli gain entrance through** the **tonsil** of the corresponding side as the lymphadenopathy.
- Both **bovine**[Q] and **human tuberculosis** may be responsible.

Pathology

- In approximately **80% of patients,** the **tuberculous process is limited to the clinically affected group of lymph nodes**[Q], but a primary focus in the lungs must always be suspected.
- If **treatment** is **not instituted,** the **caseated node** may **liquefy** and **break down** with the formation of a **cold abscess**[Q] in the neck.

  - **Collar-stud abscess**[Q]**:** Pus is initially confined by the **deep cervical fascia,** but after weeks or months, this may **become eroded at one point, pus flows through the small opening** into the **space beneath the superficial fascia** known as 'collar-stud' abscess.

Treatment

- **Treatment: ATT**
- If an **abscess fails to resolve despite ATT: Excision of the abscess** and its surrounding **fibrous capsule** with the **relevant lymph nodes**[Q].

■ CHRONIC BURROWING ULCER

CHRONIC BURROWING ULCER (MELENEY GANGRENE)

- Caused by **synergistic infection** of Microaerophilic non-hemolytic Streptococci and aerobic hemolytic staphylococci.
- Also known as **burrowing phagedenic ulcer, Meleney's ulcer, progressive synergistic gangrene**
- Associated with the **formation of burrowing cutaneous fissures** and **sinus tracts** that open at distant sites. (**Meleney's burrowing ulcers**)

Multiple Choice Questions

■ STERILIZATION AND DISINFECTION

1. **Flexible endoscopes are best sterilized with:**
   (MHSSMCET 2008, MHPGMCET 2007)
   a. Formaldehyde b. Ethylene oxide
   c. Gamma irradiation d. Peracetic acid

2. **Best disinfectant for endoscope is:** *(JIPMER 2014, 2012)*
   a. Hypochlorite b. Formaldehyde
   c. Glutaraldehyde d. Chlorohexidine

3. **Blood spills in OT is cleaned with:**
   a. Phenol *(AIIMS Nov 2017, Recent Question 2017)*
   b. Alcohol
   c. Quarternary ammonium compound
   d. Chloride compounds

■ PREVENTION OF INFECTION AND PROPHYLAXIS

4. **Optional timing of administration of prophylactic antibiotic for surgical patients is:** *(APPG 2015)*
   a. At the induction of anesthesia
   b. Any time during the surgical procedure
   c. One hour after induction
   d. One hour prior to induction of anesthesia

5. **Preoperative shaving is ideally done at:** *(Recent Question 2016)*
   a. Evening before b. Morning of operation
   c. Just before operation d. At operation table

6. **In a surgical postoperative ward, a patient developed wound infection. Subsequently 3 other patients developed similar infections in the ward. What is the most effective way of preventing the spread of infection?** *(AIIMS Nov 2001)*
   a. Give IV antibiotics to all patients in the ward
   b. Proper hand washing of all ward personnel
   c. Fumigation of the ward
   d. Wash OT instruments with 1% perchlorate

7. **Which of the following is preferred for preoperative preparation?** *(Recent Question 2017)*
   a. On table clipping of hair
   b. Shaving of hair on the table
   c. Shaving of hair before entry to operation theatre
   d. Shaving of hair one day before surgery

8. **Prophylactic antibiotics to minimize surgical site infection are given:** *(MCI June 2019)*
   a. 60 minutes before skin incision
   b. 1-3 hours before skin incision
   c. At time of surgical incision
   d. Night before surgery for peaking of effect

■ SIRS AND MODS

9. **SIRS with established source of infection is known as:**
   a. Sepsis b. Severe sepsis
   c. Septic shock d. MODS

10. **Which of the following is not a component of SIRS (Systemic Inflammatory Response Syndrome)?** *(MCI Dec 2019)*
    a. Fever >38° or hypothermia <360°
    b. Tachycardia >90 beats/min
    c. Tachypnea >24 breaths/min
    d. Leucocytosis >12 × 10⁹/Litre or leukopenia <4 × 10⁹/Litre

11. **Indicator of hypoperfusion in severe sepsis:**
    (Recent Question 2016)
    a. Systolic BP <90 mm Hg b. Lactic acidosis
    c. Oliguria d. All of the above

12. **Q-SOFA score includes:** *(PGI May 2018)*
    a. Pulse rate b. Respiratory rate
    c. Systolic blood pressure d. Altered mental status
    e. Mean arterial pressure

13. **Characteristics of SIRS include all of the following except:**
    a. Leukocytosis b. Thrombocytopenia
    c. Infectious or non-infectious cause *(MCI June 2018)*
    d. Oral temperature more than 38°C

■ CELLULITIS AND PYOGENIC BACTERIAL INFECTION

14. **What is the most probable diagnosis based on the given image?** *(Recent Question 2017)*

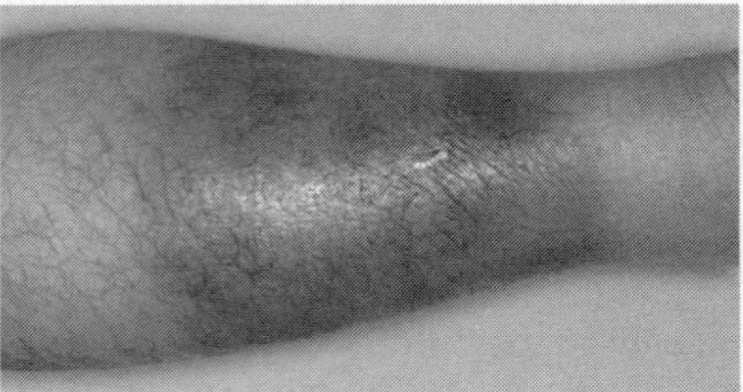

    a. Cellulitis b. Erysipelas
    c. Ecthyma d. Erythema nodosum

15. **Cellulitis is most commonly caused by:**
    (Recent Question 2014, MCI Sept 2008, 2010)
    a. Clostridia b. Staphylococci
    c. Streptococci d. H. influenza

16. **What is the most probable diagnosis based on the given image?** *(Recent Question 2017)*

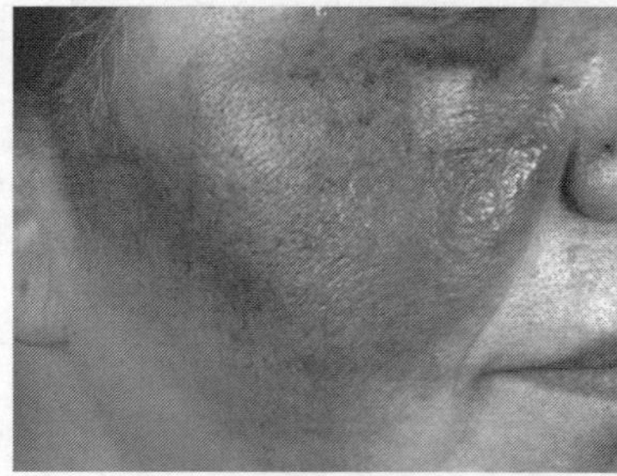

    a. Cellulitis b. Erysipelas
    c. Ecthyma d. Erythema nodosum

17. **A carbuncle is treated by:** *(UPSC 95)*
    a. Incision and drainage
    b. Cruciate incision and deroofing
    c. Antibiotics alone
    d. Wide excision

18. **Best management of contaminated wound with necrotic material:** *(Recent Question 2014, AIIMS Nov 2013)*
    a. Debridement b. Tetanus toxoid
    c. Gas gangrene serum
    d. Broad spectrum antibiotics

19. **A boil is due to staphylococcal infection of:** *(MCI June 2018)*
    - a. Hair follicle
    - b. Sweat gland
    - c. Subcutaneous tissue
    - d. Epidermis

20. **Cellulitis is:** *(MCI Dec 2019)*
    - a. Nonsuppurative and noninvasive
    - b. Suppurative and noninvasive
    - c. Nonsuppurative and invasive
    - d. Suppurative and invasive

■ GAS GANGRENE

21. **Hyperbaric oxygen is useful in:**
    (Recent Question 2014, PGI 88)
    - a. Tetanus
    - b. Gas gangrene
    - c. Frostbite
    - d. Vincent's angina

22. **Best way to prevent gas gangrene is:**
    - a. Immunoglobulins *(Recent Question 2013, AIIMS Nov 93)*
    - b. Hyperbaric oxygen
    - c. Proper wound debridement
    - d. Anti gas gangrene serum

23. **Hypotension in a cause of gas gangrene is best treated by:**
    (Recent Question 2016)
    - a. Ringer lactate
    - b. Normal saline
    - c. Plasma
    - d. Whole blood

24. **Treatment of contaminated wound in gas gangrene is:**
    - a. Debridement of wound *(Recent Question 2016)*
    - b. Systemic penicillin
    - c. Metronidazole administration
    - d. Peroxide dressings

25. **Foaming liver is seen in:** *(Recent Question 2016)*
    - a. Organophosphorus poisoning
    - b. Actinomycosis
    - c. Gas gangrene
    - d. Anthrax

26. **Treatment of contaminated wound of leg:**
    - a. Debridement and antibiotics *(Recent Question 2015)*
    - b. Hyperbaric oxygen
    - c. Amputation
    - d. None

■ TETANUS

27. **Tetanus is caused by:**
    - a. Cl. tetani
    - b. Cl. welchii
    - c. Cl. edematiens
    - d. Cl. septicum

28. **Period of onset in tetanus refers to the time between:**
    - a. First injury to spasm *(Karnataka 2006)*
    - b. First symptom to spasm
    - c. First spasm to deathd.Trismus to laryngeal spasm

■ TUBERCULOSIS

29. **Regarding tuberculous lymphadenitis, which is correct?**
    - a. Seen in children and young adults
    - b. Seen in the aged
    - c. History of contact or drinking infected milk
    - d. Mostly cervical
    - e. All are the correct

30. **Commonest cause of acute lymphadenitis in India:**
    - a. Barefoot walking
    - b. TB *(MAHE 2005)*
    - c. Staphylococcal skin infection
    - d. Lymphoma

31. **A 10 years old child with pain and mass in right lumbar region with no fever, with right hip flexed and X-ray shows spine changes. Most probable diagnosis is:**
    - a. Psoas abscess
    - b. Pyonephrosis
    - c. Retrocecal appendicitis *(AIIMS Nov 2017)*
    - d. Torsion of right undescended testis

32. **A 35-years-old lady has presented with a 6-month painless fluctuant, non-transilluminant swelling with a thin watery discharge-clinical diagnosis is?** *(MCI Dec 2018)*

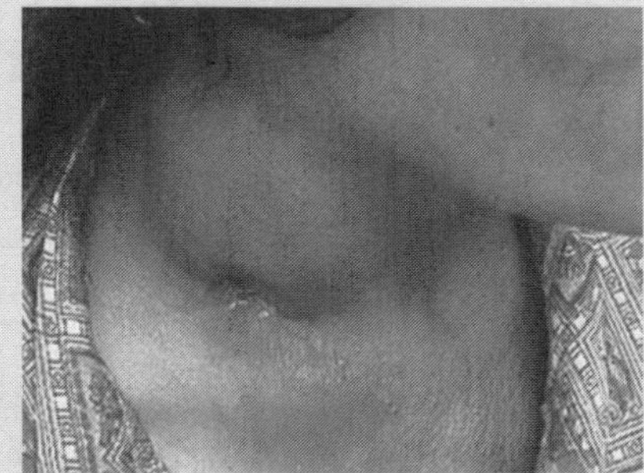

    - a. Branchial cyst
    - b. Secondaries
    - c. TB
    - d. Lymphoma

■ SYPHILIS

33. **Moth eaten alopecia is seen with:** *(Recent Question 2016)*
    - a. Leprosy
    - b. Syphilis
    - c. Fungal infection
    - d. Cylindroma

34. **Thymus gland abscess seen in congenital syphilis is called:**
    (Recent Question 2016)
    - a. Fouchier's abscess
    - b. Politzeri abscess
    - c. Douglas abscess
    - d. Dubois abscess

■ LEPROSY

35. **Globi is seen in leprosy:** *(Recent Question 2016)*
    - a. Tuberculoid
    - b. Lepromatous
    - c. Border line
    - d. Borderline tuberculoid

36. **Which of the following parts of the body is not affected by leprosy?** *(Recent Question 2016)*
    - a. Testes
    - b. Ovary
    - c. Nasal mucosa
    - d. Axilla

■ ACTINOMYCOSIS

37. **Most common form of actinomycosis is:**
    - a. Fascio cervical
    - b. Thoracic
    - c. Right iliac fossa
    - d. Liver

38. **A patient with a fistula and chronic pus discharge from lower face and mandible is most commonly suffering from:**
    (Recent Question 2016)
    - a. Dental cyst
    - b. Vincent's angina
    - c. Ludwig's angina
    - d. Actinomycosis

■ HIV AND COMPLICATIONS

39. **Which of the following is not the personal protective equipment?** *(Recent Question 2019)*
    - a. Gloves
    - b. Lab coat
    - c. Face shield
    - d. Goggles

40. **An intern while doing scalp suturing injured his index finger. Which of the following is not correct regarding the management?** *(Recent Question 2019)*
    - a. Should inform authorities
    - b. High risk of HIV transmission
    - c. Injuries during suturing is more common in non-dominant hand
    - d. The part should be washed under running tap water

■ ANTHRAX

41. Most common form of anthrax is: *(Recent Question 2016)*
   a. Wool sorters disease   b. Alimentary type
   c. Cutaneous type   d. None of the above

42. Malignant pustule occurs in: *(KGMC 2011)*
   a. Melanoma   b. Gas gangrene
   c. Ovarian tumour   d. Anthrax

■ HAND INFECTIONS

43. Most common hand infection is due to: *(DPG 2008)*
   a. E. coli   b. Staph. aureus
   c. Streptococcus   d. Pseudomonas

44. From the index finger infection goes to: *(AIIMS Nov 96)*
   a. Thenar space   b. Hypothenar space
   c. Mid-palmar space   d. Space of parona

45. Felon is: *(Recent Question 2015, DPG 2005)*
   a. Mid palmer space infection
   b. Terminal pulp space infection
   c. Infection of ulnar bursa
   d. Infection of radial bursa

46. Felon most commonly present at: *(Recent Question 2016)*
   a. Index finger   b. Ring finger
   c. Little finger   d. Middle finger

■ INTRA-ABDOMINAL INFECTIONS

47. Sub phrenic abscess, not seen is: *(DPG 2006)*
   a. Air fluid level
   b. Leucopenia
   c. More common on right side
   d. Associated with shoulder pain

48. Which of the following is the most pathognomonic sign of impending burst abdomen?   *(Recent Question 2015)*
   a. Fever   b. Shock
   c. Pain
   d. Serosanguinous discharge

49. True regarding wound dehiscence: *(Recent Question 2018)*
   a. If you suspect dehiscence, close with continuous suture of non-absorbable material
   b. Dehiscence happens on 2nd postoperative day
   c. The management of wound dehiscence depends on degree of evisceration and gangrenous bowel
   d. There will sudden gush of fluid just before the dehiscence

■ NOSOCOMIAL INFECTIONS

50. In a surgical patient, the causes of non-surgical infection:
   a. Lower RTI   *(DPG 2010, PGI June 2004)*
   b. Wound infection
   c. Clostridium difficile diarrhea
   d. UTI

51. Most common nosocomial infection:
   (Recent Question 2016, Bihar PG 2016)
   a. Surgical site infection
   b. Respiratory tract infection
   c. Urinary tract infection
   d. Skin & soft tissue infection

52. Most common organism responsible for UTI in hospital:
   (Recent Question 2017)
   a. E. coli   b. Klebsiella
   c. Proteus   d. Pseudomonas

53. Which of the following is not a hospital-acquired infection?
   (MCI Dec 2018)
   a. Surgical site infection   b. STD
   c. UTI   d. Pneumonia

■ HILTON'S METHOD

54. Hilton's method of treatment of an axillary abscess is advised because it: *(Karnataka 94)*
   a. Protects vital structure
   b. Ensures adequate drainage
   c. Hinders the spread of infection
   d. Allows local instillation of antibiotics

55. Hilton's method is best used in: *(Recent Question 2015)*
   a. Breast abscess   b. Axillary abscess
   c. Paronychia   d. Pulp abscess

■ MISCELLANEOUS

56. Chronic burrowing ulcer is caused by:
   (All India 2007, AIIMS May 2008)
   a. Microaerophilic streptococci
   b. Peptostreptococcus
   c. Streptococcus viridians
   d. Streptococcus pyogenes

57. Mycotic abscesses are due to: *(All India 2006)*
   a. Bacterial infection   b. Fungal infection
   c. Viral infection   d. Mixed infection

58. Golden period for treatment of open wound in hours:
   a. 4   b. 6
   c. 12   d. 24

59. Pyrexia due to wound infection commonly occurs after:
   a. Third post operation day   *(Recent Question 2017)*
   b. Fifth post operation day
   c. Seventh post operation day
   d. Second post operation day

60. Which of these scoring systems is helpful in assessing severity of wound infection and is used for research and surveillance?   *(AIIMS Nov 2016)*
   a. Southampton grading scale
   b. ASA classification
   c. Glasgow score
   d. APGAR

61. Long term diabetic patient with blisters walked barefoot few miles on hot sand. He presented with this clinical condition. What is the most probable diagnosis?   *(MCI Dec 2019)*

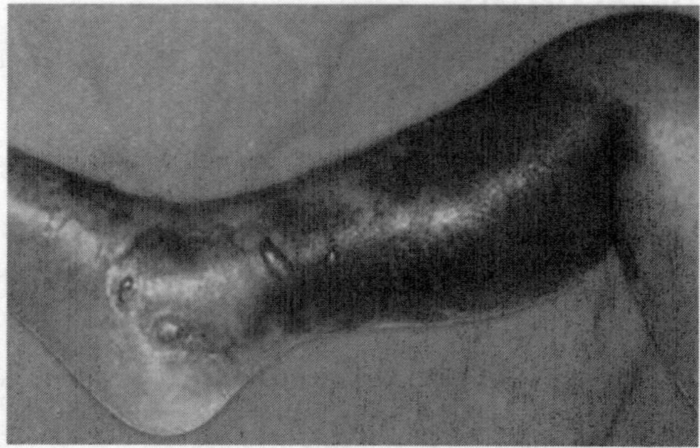

   a. Diabetic foot   b. Burn
   c. Necrotizing fasciitis   d. Gangrene

■ STERILIZATION AND DISINFECTION

1. Ans. d. Peracetic acid

2. Ans. c. Glutaraldehyde

3. Ans. d. Chloride compounds *(Ref: Infection Control in Clinical Practice By Jennie Wilson (2006)/p173)*

"High-concentration chlorine-releasing compounds provide the most economical and effective method of treating many spills, especially large spills of blood. Chlorine-releasing granules have the advantage of containing the spill rather than adding to it; they have a longer shelf-life than hypochlorite solutions and are more portable." -Infection Control in Clinical Practice By Jennie Wilson (2006)/p173

■ PREVENTION OF INFECTION AND PROPHYLAXIS

4. Ans. a. At the induction of anesthesia

5. Ans. c. Just before operation

6. Ans. b. Proper hand washing of all ward personnel

7. Ans. a. On table clipping of hair *(Ref: Sabiston 20/e p232, 286)*

"Preoperative skin shaving should be undertaken in the operating theatre immediately before surgery as the SSI rate after clean wound surgery may be doubled if it is performed the night before; minor skin injury enhances superficial bacterial colonisation. Cream depilation is messy and hair clipping is best, with the lowest rate of infection." -Bailey 27/e p52

8. Ans. a. 60 minutes before skin incision *(Ref: Bailey 27/e p1202)*

■ SIRS AND MODS

9. Ans. a. Sepsis

10. Ans. c. Tachypnea >24 breaths/ min *(Ref: Bailey 27/e p51)*

Systemic Inflammatory Response Syndrome (SIRS)   Mnemonic: THR Counts
Two or more of the following: • **Temperature** (core) **>38°C** or **<36°C**[Q]   • **Heart rate >90** beats/min[Q]   • **Respiratory rate >20**[Q] breaths/min for patients spontaneously ventilating or a **PaCO$_2$ <32** mm Hg[Q]   • **WBC count >12,000**[Q] cells/mm^3 or **<4000**[Q] cells/mm^3 or **>10% immature (band) cells** in the peripheral blood smear

11. Ans. d. All of the above

12. Ans. b. Respiratory rate, c. Systolic blood pressure, d. Altered mental status *(Ref: Schwartz 11/e p161)*

Quick Sequential Organ Failure Assessment (SOFA) Score	
qSOFA (Quick SOFA) Criteria	Points
Respiratory rate ≥22/min[Q]	1
Change in **mental status**[Q]	1
Systolic BP ≤100 mm Hg[Q]	1

Interpretation	
Score	Mortality
0	<1%
1	2-3%
≥2	≥10%

13. Ans. b. Thrombocytopenia

■ CELLULITIS AND PYOGENIC BACTERIAL INFECTION

14. Ans. a. Cellulitis *(Ref: Schwartz 11/e p524-525, 10/e p151; Bailey 27/e p596, 597)*

15. Ans. c. Streptococci

16. Ans. b. Erysipelas *(Ref: Schwartz 11/e p524, 10/e p151; Bailey 27/e p596, 597)*

Erysipelas can be differentiated from cellulitis by its characteristically raised, advancing edges and sharply demarcated borders, reflecting its more superficial nature. Cellulitis has no lymphatic component and exhibits indiscreet margins.

17. Ans. a. Incision and drainage, d. Wide excision *(Ref: Schwartz 11/e p524)*

18. Ans. a. Debridement

19. Ans. a. Hair follicle

20. Ans. c. Nonsuppurative and invasive *(Ref: Bailey 27/e p48)*

"Cellulitis is a non-suppurative, invasive infection of tissues, which is usually related to the point of injury. There is poor localisation in addition to the cardinal signs of spreading inflammation." - Bailey 27/e p48

■ GAS GANGRENE

21. Ans. b. Gas gangrene, c. Frostbite
22. Ans. c. Proper wound debridement
23. Ans. a. Ringer lactate
24. Ans. a. Debridement of wound, b. Systemic penicillin
25. Ans. c. Gas gangrene
26. Ans. a. Debridement and antibiotics

■ TETANUS

27. Ans. a. Cl. tetani *(Ref: Schwartz 11/e p208, 294, 10/e p186,264; Bailey 27/e p50, 417)*
28. Ans. b. First symptom to spasm

■ TUBERCULOSIS

29. Ans. a. Seen in children and young adults, c. History of contact or drinking infected milk, d. Mostly cervical *(Ref: Bailey 27/e p77, 757)*
30. Ans. c. Staphylococcal skin infection *(Ref: Sabiston 20/e p1860; Schwartz 11/e p1710, 10/e p1602; Bailey 27/e p996, 997)*

Acute Lymphadenitis

- **Enlarged tender lymph nodes** are usually the result of a **bacterial infection** (**staphylococcal**[Q] or **streptococcal**).
- **Treatment of** the **primary cause** (e.g., **otitis media** or **pharyngitis**) **with antibiotics** often is all that is necessary.
- **Fluctuant nodes: Incision** and **drainage**[Q]

31. Ans. a. Psoas abscess *(Ref: Harrison 20/e p958; Bailey 27/e p1065)*

"Patients with psoas abscesses frequently present with fever, lower abdominal or back pain, or pain referred to the hip or knee. CT is the most useful diagnostic technique." -Harrison 19/e p852

32. Ans. c. TB *(Ref: Bailey 27/e p78)*

■ SYPHILIS

33. Ans. b. Syphilis *(Ref: Rook's 7/e p30.1-30.30, 25.20-39)*
34. Ans. d. Dubois abscess

Dubois Abscesses

- An **abscess of** the **thymus** associated with **congenital syphilis**[Q]
- It can present with **chest pain** behind the sternum.

■ LEPROSY

35. Ans. b. Lepromatous *(Ref: Rooks 7/e p29.1-29.19)*

Type of leprosy	Characteristic feature	
Neuritic	• Slit smear negative[Q]	
TT	• Single skin lesion[Q]	• MC type in India and Africa[Q]
BT	• Satellite lesion[Q]	• MC type in South East Asia[Q]
BB>BL	• Inverted saucer lesion[Q]	
LL	• Subepidermal free zone[Q]	• Lozarine leprosy reaction[Q]
	• Globi[Q] are seen	• Leonine facies[Q]
	• Lucio phenomenon[Q]	

Leprosy

- **MC affected peripheral nerve** in leprosy: **Ulnar nerve**[Q]
- **Organ not involved** in leprosy: **Ovary**[Q]

36. Ans. b. Ovary

■ ACTINOMYCOSIS

37. Ans. a. Fascio cervical
38. Ans. d. Actinomycosis

■ HIV AND COMPLICATIONS

39. Ans. b. Lab coat
40. Ans. b. High risk of HIV transmission

■ ANTHRAX

41. **Ans. c. Cutaneous type** *(Ref: Harrison 20/e p936)*

ANTHRAX

- Caused by **Bacillus anthracis**[Q]
- Three major clinical forms: **Cutaneous**[Q] **(MC)**, gastrointestinal and inhalational

Risk Factors for Necrotizing Fasciitis	
Woolsorters' disease	• **Occupational hazard for people who sorted wool**[Q] • **Most dangerous form** of inhalational anthrax[Q]
Hide porter's disease	• Caused by **contact with contaminated hair, wool, hides** or **products made from them** **(Hide-porter's disease)**[Q]
Malignant pustule	• Commonly seen in **head and neck**[Q] • **Eschar stage** that appears 2-6 days after the hemorrhagic vesicle dries to become a **depressed black scab**[Q] surrounded by redness and extensive edema

42. **Ans. d. Anthrax**

■ HAND INFECTIONS

43. **Ans. b. Staph. aureus** *(Ref: Sabiston 20/e p2000-2001; Bailey 27/e p503-504)*
44. **Ans. a. Thenar space** *(Ref: BDC 4/e vol I/129; Keith and Moore 4/e p765)*
45. **Ans. b. Terminal pulp space infection** *(Ref: Bailey 27/e p503-504)*
46. **Ans. a. Index finger**

■ INTRA-ABDOMINAL INFECTIONS

47. **Ans. b. Leucopenia**

    Leucocytosis is seen in subphrenic abscess, not the leucopenia.
48. **Ans. d. Serosanguinous discharge**
49. **Ans. c. The management of wound dehiscence depends on degree of evisceration and gangrenous bowel**

■ NOSOCOMIAL INFECTIONS

50. **Ans. a. Lower RTI, c. Clostridium difficile diarrhea, d. UTI** *(Ref: Sabiston 20/e p322-323; Harrison 19/e p913-916)*
51. **Ans. c. Urinary tract infection:** *(Ref: Harrison 19/e p913)*

    MC Nosocomial infection: UTI (30–40%) > Surgical Site Infection (15–20%)[Q]

52. **Ans. a. E. coli** *(Ref: Bailey 27/e p1441)*

    "UTI: Escherichia coli is the most common organism followed by Proteus mirabilis, Staphylococcus epidermidis and Streptococcus faecalis." - Bailey 27/e p1441

53. **Ans. b. STD** *(Ref: Bailey 27/e p47)*

■ HILTON'S METHOD

54. **Ans. a. Protects vital structure** *(Ref: lessons4medicos.blogspot.com/.../hiltons-method-to-drain-abscesses.)*
55. **Ans. b. Axillary abscess**

■ MISCELLANEOUS

56. **Ans. a. Microaerophilic streptococci** *(Ref: Dorland's Medical Dictionary 28/e p1770, 1771; Bailey 27/e p5, 419, 597)*
57. **Ans. b. Fungal infection**   58. **Ans. a. 4**
59. **Ans. b. Fifth post operation day** *(Ref: Bailey 25/e p265)*
60. **Ans. a. Southampton grading scale** *(Ref: Bailey's 27/e p48)*

    Southampton grading is used for surgical site infections.
61. **Ans. c. Necrotizing fasciitis** *(Ref: Bailey 27/e p419)*

Fluid, Electrolyte and Nutrition

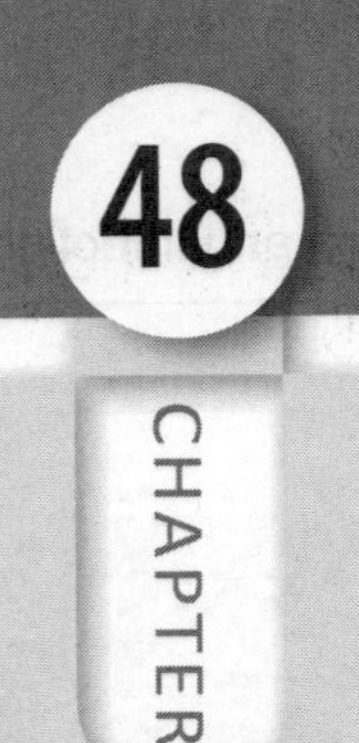

ADJUVANT NUTRITIONAL SUPPORT

ADJUVANT NUTRITIONAL SUPPORT

- Methods of adjuvant nutritional support: Enteral nutrition & total parenteral nutrition

ENTERAL NUTRITION

ENTERAL NUTRITION

- Enteral feeding means **delivery of nutrients into** the GIT[Q].
- The **alimentary tract** should be **used** whenever **possible**[Q].
- This can be achieved with oral supplements (sip feeding) or with a variety of **tube-feeding techniques delivering food into** the **stomach, duodenum** or **jejunum**[Q].

Advantages of Enteral route over Parenteral Route	
• **Maintains integrity** of **gastrointestinal tract**[Q] • **Reduces translocation of gut bacteria**[Q] that may lead to infection.	• **Reduces** the **levels of proinflammatory cytokines**[Q] generated by the gut that contribute to hypermetabolism.

ROUTES OF ENTERAL NUTRITION

ROUTES OF ENTERAL NUTRITION

- **Oral supplements** by mouth
- **Nasogastric tube/ Nasojejunal tube:** Nasojejunal tube is better due to low risk of aspiration[Q]
- **Feeding gastrostomy**
- **Feeding jejunostomy**

Gastrostomy	Jejunostomy
• Surgical technique of placing tube into stomach • Common techniques are: **Stamm**[Q], **Witzel**[Q] & **Janeway**[Q] • Now-a-days **percutaneous insertion under endoscopic control** known as **PEG**[Q] (**Percutaneous endoscopic gastrostomy**) is preferred • Three methods are used for PEG: **Push** technique, **pull** technique & **introducer** technique[Q]	• Usually **preferred over gastrostomy** due to **lower risk of aspiration**[Q] • Especially useful in **severe pancreatitis**[Q], in whom a degree of gastric outlet obstruction may present due to edematous head of pancreas[Q]

ENTERAL NUTRITION: INDICATIONS & CONTRAINDICATIONS

Enteral Nutrition

Indications	Contraindications
• **Protein-energy malnutrition** with **inadequate oral intake**[Q] • **Dysphagia** except for fluids[Q] • **Major trauma** (or **surgery**[Q]) when return to required dietary intake is prolonged • **Inflammatory bowel disease**[Q] • **Distal, low-output** (<200 mL/day) **enterocutaneous fistula**[Q] • To enhance adaptation after massive enterectomy	• **Small bowel obstruction or ileus**[Q] • **Severe diarrhea**[Q] • **Proximal small intestinal fistula**[Q] • **Severe pancreatitis**[Q]

■ COMPLICATIONS OF ENTERAL NUTRITION

Complications of Enteral Nutrition			
Tube-related	**Gastrointestinal**	**Metabolic**	**Infective**
• **Malposition**[Q] • **Displacement**[Q] • **Blockage**[Q] • **Breakage/leakage**[Q] • Local complications (e.g. **erosion of skin/mucosa**)[Q]	• **Diarrhea**[Q] • Bloating, nausea, vomiting • **Abdominal cramps**[Q] • Aspiration[Q] • **Constipation**[Q]	• **Electrolyte disorders**[Q] • **Vitamin, mineral, trace element deficiencies**[Q] • Drug interactions	• **Exogenous** (handling contamination) • **Endogenous** (patient)

■ TOTAL PARENTERAL NUTRITION (TPN)

TOTAL PARENTERAL NUTRITION (TPN)

- Provision of all nutritional requirements by means of IV route without use of GIT
- Routes of delivery: via **peripheral or central venous access**

Peripheral Parenteral Nutrition/PPN	Feeding via Central Venous Access
• Appropriate for **short-term feeding** of up to **2 weeks**[Q]. • Access can be achieved by: Catheter inserted into a **peripheral vein**[Q] and maneuvered into the central venous system [**peripherally inserted central venous catheter** (PICC) line] or by using a conventional **short cannula**[Q] in the wrist veins. • **PICC lines** have a **mean duration of survival** of **7 days**[Q]. • **Advantage: Avoids the complications** associated with **central venous administration**[Q] • **Disadvantage:** Development of **thrombophlebitis**[Q] • **Not indicated** if patients already have an **indwelling central venous line** or in those in whom **long-term feeding is anticipated.**	• Catheter can be inserted via the **subclavian** or **internal** or **external jugular vein.** • **Preferred access site for TPN: Subclavian vein**[Q] **> Internal jugular vein**[Q] **> Femoral vein**[Q] • Most ICU physicians and anesthetists favor **cannulation of internal** or **external jugular veins** as these vessels are easily accessible. **Disadvantage: Exit site** is situated inconveniently **on** the **side of** the **neck**, where **repeated movements** result in **disruption of dressing** with the **risk of sepsis**[Q] • **Infraclavicular subclavian**[Q] approach is **more suitable for feeding** as the catheter then lies flat on the chest wall, which optimizes nursing care. • For **longer term TPN Hickman lines**[Q] are **preferable (minimize line dislodgement** and **reduce** the possibility of line sepsis). • **Post-insertion chest X-ray** is **essential** before feeding is commenced **to confirm** the **absence of pneumothorax** and that the **catheter tip lies in** the **distal SVC to minimize** the risk of **central venous** or **cardiac thrombosis**[Q].

■ INDICATIONS OF TPN

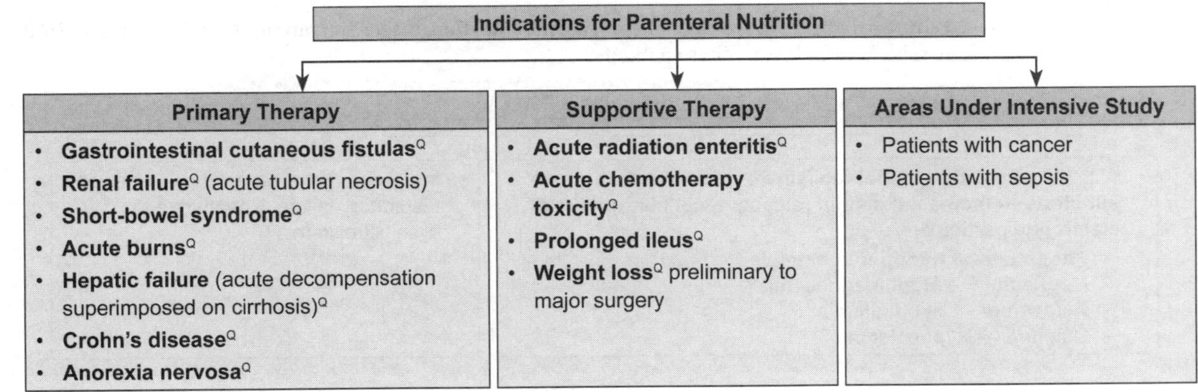

Indications for Parenteral Nutrition		
Primary Therapy	**Supportive Therapy**	**Areas Under Intensive Study**
• **Gastrointestinal cutaneous fistulas**[Q] • **Renal failure**[Q] (acute tubular necrosis) • **Short-bowel syndrome**[Q] • **Acute burns**[Q] • **Hepatic failure** (acute decompensation superimposed on cirrhosis)[Q] • **Crohn's disease**[Q] • **Anorexia nervosa**[Q]	• **Acute radiation enteritis**[Q] • **Acute chemotherapy toxicity**[Q] • **Prolonged ileus**[Q] • **Weight loss**[Q] preliminary to major surgery	• Patients with cancer • Patients with sepsis

■ TPN FORMULATIONS

TPN Formulations	
Solution with Lipids (3-in-1) **(60/20/20)[Q]**	**Solution without Lipids (2-in-1)** **(75/25)[Q]**
• Calories from **dextrose**: 55-60%	• Calories from **dextrose**: 75-80%
• Calories from **amino acids**: 20-25%	• Calories from **amino acids**: 20-25%
• Calories from **lipids**: 20%	

■ COMPLICATIONS OF TPN

COMPLICATIONS OF TPN

- MC complication of central venous catheterization (CVC): Catheter related sepsis[Q]
- Most dangerous complication following CVC: Pneumothorax[Q]

Complications of Parenteral Nutrition

Related to nutrient deficiency	Related to overfeeding	Related to sepsis	Related to line
• **Hypoglycemia[Q], hypocalcemia[Q], hypophosphatemia, hypomagnesemia** (refeeding syndrome) • **Chronic deficiency syndromes (essential fatty acids[Q], zinc[Q],** mineral and trace elements)	• **Excess glucose: hyperglycemia[Q], hyperosmolar dehydration[Q], hepatic steatosis[Q],** hypercapnia, increased sympathetic activity, fluid retention, **electrolyte abnormalities[Q]** • **Excess fat: hypercholesterolemia[Q]** and formation of lipoprotein X, hypertriglyceridemia[Q], hypersensitivity reactions • **Excess amino acids:** hyperchloremic **metabolic acidosis, hypercalcemia[Q],** aminoacidemia, uremia[Q]	• **Catheter-related sepsis[Q]** • **Increased risk of systemic sepsis[Q]**	• **On insertion: pneumothorax[Q], damage to adjacent artery[Q], air embolism,[Q] thoracic duct damage[Q],** cardiac perforation or tamponade, **pleural effusion,** hydromediastinum • **Long-term use: occlusion, venous thrombosis[Q]**

Electrolyte Abnormalities in TPN

• **Hyponatremia** and **hypernatremia[Q]**	• **Hypocalcemia** and **hypercalcemia[Q]**
• **Hypokalemia** and **Hyperkalemia[Q]**	• **High zinc** and low **zinc[Q]**
• **Hypophosphatemia** and **hyperphosphatemia[Q]**	• **High copper** and low **copper[Q]**
• **Hypomagnesemia** and **Hypermagnesemia[Q]**	• **Hyperchloremic metabolic acidosis[Q]**

■ REFEEDING SYNDROME

REFEEDING SYNDROME

- Potentially lethal condition
- Occur with **rapid & excessive feeding** of patients with **severe underlying malnutrition** due to: Starvation, alcoholism, delayed nutritional support, anorexia nervosa & massive weight loss in obese patients[Q]

Pathophysiology

• With refeeding, **shift in metabolism** from **fat to carbohydrate substrate** → **Increased insulin release** → **cellular uptake of electrolyte** particularly:
   – **Phosphate → Hypophosphatemia[Q]**
   – **Magnesium → Hypomagnesemia[Q]**
   – **Potassium → Hypokalemia[Q]**
   – **Calcium → Hypocalcemia[Q]**
	• Increased risk of arrhythmia, confusion, respiratory failure & death due to dyselectrolytemia[Q]

Contd...

Contd…

- Occur with **both enteral & TPN**; More common with **TPN**[Q]
- **Rate of feeding should begin slowly** to prevent metabolic changes[Q]

Treatment

- Treatment involves **matching intake with requirements**[Q]
- **Avoid over feeding**; Calorie delivery should be **increased slowly**[Q]
- Vitamin administration, especially **thiamine before initiation of feeding**[Q]
- **Hypophosphatemia & hypomagnesemia requires treatment**[Q]

■ COMPOSITION OF CRYSTALLOIDS & COLLOIDS

Composition of crystalloid and colloid solutions (mM/L)						
Solution	Na+	K+	Ca²⁺	Cl⁻	Lactate	Colloid
Hartmann's (RL)	130	4	< 2.7	109	28	
Normal saline (0.9% NaCl)	154			154		
Dextrose saline (4% dextrose in 0.18% saline)	30			30		
Gelofusine	150		< 1	150		Gelatin 4%
Hemacel	145	5.1	< 6.26	145		Polygelin 75 g/L
Hetastarch						Hydroxyethyl starch 6%
Lactated potassium saline injection (Darrow's solution)	121	35		103	53	

■ HEMODYNAMIC MONITORING

Hemodynamic Monitoring

Central Venous Pressure (CVP)

- **Measurement of CVP** and its response to a small fluid challenge may assist in **distinguishing cardiogenic shock** and Hypovolemic shock[Q].
- In **seriously ill patients**, the **CVP** is **not a reliable indicator of left ventricular function** because of the **wide disparity** that can exist **between left** and **right ventricular functions**[Q].

Pulmonary Capillary Wedge Pressure (PCWP)

- It is a **better indicator** for both **blood volume** and **left ventricular function** than CVP[Q].
- Obtained by **pulmonary artery flotation balloon catheter (Swan-Ganz)**[Q].
- Used to **differentiate left** and **right ventricular failure, pulmonary embolism, septic shock** and **ruptured mitral valve**[Q]
- **Accurate guide** to therapy with **fluids, inotropic agents** and **vasodilators**[Q].
- May also be used to **measure cardiac output** by thermodilution technique.

Multiple Choice Questions

■ ENTERAL NUTRITION

1. The length of the feeding tube to be inserted for transpyloric feeding is measured from the tip of: *(AIIMS Nov 2002)*
   a. Nose to the umbilicus
   b. Ear lobe to the umbilicus
   c. Nose to the knee joint
   d. Ear lobe to the knee joint

2. Not a contraindication of enteral nutrition: *(Punjab 2009)*
   a. Severe diarrhea
   b. Severe pancreatitis
   c. IBD
   d. Intestinal fistula

■ TOTAL PARENTERAL NUTRITION

3. Which of the following nutrients are not included in TPN? *(All India 2011)*
   a. Lipids
   b. Carbohydrates
   c. Proteins
   d. Fibers

4. Best vein for total parenteral nutrition is: *(MHPGMCET 2002, Recent Question 2017)*
   a. Subclavian vein
   b. Femoral vein
   c. Brachial vein
   d. Saphenous vein

5. Most common complication of parenteral nutrition includes all except: *(MCI Sept 2009)*
   a. Hyperglycemia
   b. Hyperkalemia
   c. Hyperosmolar dehydration
   d. Azotemia

6. Which is best method for supplementing nutrition in patients who have undergone massive resection of the small intestine is? *(MCI Sept 2009)*
   a. Parenteral
   b. Enteral
   c. Gastrostomy
   d. All of the above

7. All of the following are complications in a patient on total parenteral nutrition except: *(MCI Sept 2008)*
   a. Hypercholesterolemia
   b. Hyperglycemia
   c. Hypotriglyceridemia
   d. Hypophosphatemia

8. Which of the following is the most common complication of TPN? *(Recent Question 2016)*
   a. Catheter related complications
   b. Acidosis
   c. Acaculous cholecystitis
   d. Hypokalemia

9. Albumin infusion for parenteral use is restricted because:
   a. It is costly *(Recent Question 2015)*
   b. Carcinogenic
   c. Does not raise oncotic pressure
   d. All of the above

10. Following TPN, one expects weight gain after: *(Recent Question 2016)*
    a. 2 days
    b. 7 days
    c. 4 weeks
    d. 6 weeks

11. The minimum amount of proteins needed for positive nitrogen balance is: *(Recent Question 2016)*
    a. 20-30 gm/day
    b. 35-40 gm/day
    c. 50 gm/day
    d. 60 gm/day

12. Complication of total parenteral nutrition is: *(Recent Question 2013)*
    a. CHF
    b. Hypochloremia
    c. Metabolic acidosis
    d. Leukopenia

■ ELECTROLYTE ABNORMALITIES

13. Condition which does not cause metabolic acidosis: *(Recent Question 2016)*
    a. Renal failure
    b. Ureterosigmoidostomy
    c. Pancreatic or biliary fistula
    d. Pyloric stenosis

14. In post burn patient, true is: *(AIIMS June 94)*
    a. Hypokalemic alkalosis
    b. Hyperkalemic alkalosis
    c. Hyperkalemic acidosis
    d. Hypokalemic acidosis

15. Which of the following is not an important cause of hyponatremia? *(All India 2004)*
    a. Gastric fistula
    b. Excessive vomiting
    c. Excessive sweating
    d. Prolonged Ryle's tube aspiration

■ IV FLUIDS

16. The highest concentration of potassium is in:
    a. Plasma
    b. Isotonic saline
    c. Ringer lactate
    d. Darrow's solution

17. Low molecular weight dextran is contra indicated in:
    a. Fetal distress syndrome *(Recent Question 2016)*
    b. Cerebrovascular accident
    c. Electrical burns
    d. Thrombocytopenia

18. 10% dextrose is: *(DNB 2005)*
    a. Isotonic
    b. Hypotonic
    c. Hypertonic
    d. None

19. Sodium content of one liter of isotonic saline is: *(DNB 2011)*
    a. 140 mEq
    b. 154 mEq
    c. 40 mEq
    d. 70 mEq

20. Which among the following is best method to assess intake of fluid in polytrauma patient? *(PGI June 2006, AIIMS Nov 95, AIIMS Nov 94)*
    a. Urine output
    b. CVP
    c. Pulse
    d. BP

21. Which of the following is hypertonic? *(DNB 2009)*
    a. 5% dextrose
    b. 0.45% normal saline
    c. 0.9% normal saline
    d. 3% normal saline

22. Concentration of sodium in RL is: *(Recent Question 2013)*
    a. 154
    b. 120
    c. 130
    d. 144

■ MISCELLANEOUS

23. Insensible daily water loss is: *(Recent Question 2016)*
    a. 500-600 mL
    b. 800-1000 mL
    c. 1000-1500 mL
    d. 2000 mL

Explanations

■ ENTERAL NUTRITION

1. **Ans. b. Ear lobe to the umbilicus**

   - **Feeding tube length** is measured by following the normal route for the tube (Nasal ala → To ear lobe → To epigastrium)[Q]
   - The distance between the nasal ala and ear lobe is almost equal to the distance between the epigastrium and umbilicus, the length can be measured from **ear lobe to umbilicus**[Q].

2. **Ans. c. IBD**

■ TOTAL PARENTERAL NUTRITION

3. **Ans. d. Fibers** *(Ref: Bailey 27/e p286)*

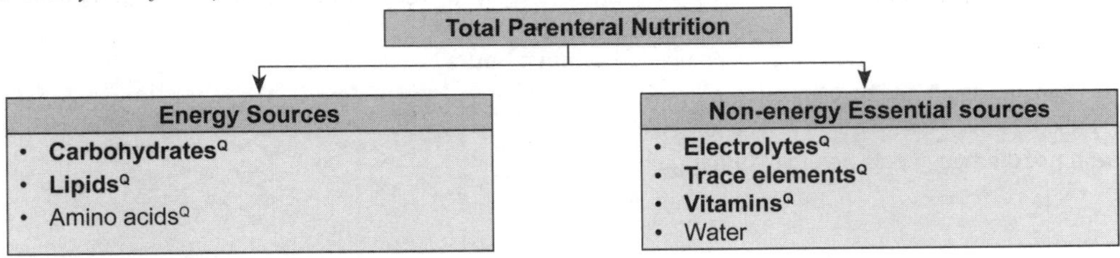

4. **Ans. a. Subclavian vein** *(Ref: Sabiston 20/e p118; Bailey 27/e p287)*

   - **Preferred** site for **central vein infusion: SVC**[Q]
   - **Preferred access site** for **TPN: Subclavian**[Q] > **Jugular** > **Femoral vein**

5. **Ans. None** *(Ref: CSDT 12/e p161)*   6. **Ans. a. Parenteral**   7. **Ans. c. Hypotriglyceridemia**

8. **Ans. a. Catheter related complications**

   - MC complication of central venous catheterization (CVC): Catheter related sepsis[Q]
   - Most dangerous complication following CVC: Pneumothorax[Q]

9. **Ans. a. It is costly**   10. **Ans. b. 7 days**

11. **Ans. d. 60 gm/day**   12. **Ans. c. Metabolic acidosis**

■ ELECTROLYTE ABNORMALITIES

13. **Ans. d. Pyloric stenosis**   14. **Ans. c. Hyperkalemic acidosis**

15. **Ans. c. Excessive sweating**

■ IV FLUIDS

16. **Ans. d. Darrow's solution** *(Ref: Bailey 27/e p281; www.idruginfo.com/?cat=drug...Darrow's%20Solution)*

17. **Ans. d. Thrombocytopenia**

   - **Dextran interferes with platelet function**[Q].

18. **Ans. c. Hypertonic**   19. **Ans. b. 154 mEq**

20. **Ans. a. Urine output**

21. **Ans. d. 3% normal saline** *(Ref: Fluids and Electrolytes by Lippincott Williams and Wilkins/55)*

Isotonic	Hypertonic	Hypotonic
Dextrose 5% in water	5% dextrose in half normal saline	0.45 normal saline
0.9% normal saline	5% dextrose in normal saline	
Ringer lactate	Dextrose 10% in water	

22. **Ans. c. 130**

■ MISCELLANEOUS

23. **Ans. b. 800-1000 mL** *(Ref: Bailey 25/e p226)*

Blood Transfusion

■ TRANSFUSION PROTOCOL

TRANSFUSION PROTOCOLS

- BT should commence within 30 minutes or removing blood bag from refrigerators because of increased risk of bacterial contamination[Q]
- **Whole blood or packed RBC** transfusion must be completed **within 4 hours**[Q]
- **Platelet and FFP** transfusion should be completed within **20 minutes**[Q]
- **Transfusion set** should have standard filter of **170 μm size**[Q]
- Usual **transfusion needle** size should be of **18-19 gauge**[Q]

■ CHARACTERISTICS OF SELECTED BLOOD COMPONENETS

Characteristics of Selected Blood Components			
Component	**Volume (mL)**	**Content**	**Clinical Response**
Whole Blood	450 mL ± 45	• No elements removed • Contains **RBCs, WBCs, plasma** and **platelets** (**WBCs** and **platelets** may be **non-functional**[Q])	• Not for routine use • Used for **acute massive bleeding, open heart surgery** and neonatal total exchange
Packed RBCs	180–200	• **RBCs** with variable **leukocyte** content and **small** amount of **plasma**	• Increase **Hb 1 gm/dL** and **hematocrit 3%**[Q]
Platelets	50–70	• 5.5×10^{10}/RD unit	• Increase platelet count **5000–10,000/μL**[Q]
FFP	200–250	• **Plasma proteins: Coagulation factors, proteins C and S, antithrombin**[Q]	• Increases **coagulation factors about 2%**
Cryoprecipitate	10–15	• Cold-insoluble plasma proteins, **fibrinogen, factor VIII, vWF**[Q]	• Topical fibrin glue, also **80 IU factor VIII**[Q]

■ ANTICOAGULANTS

Whole Blood	
Anticoagulant used	**Maximum storage**
ACD/CPD/CP2D	**21 days**[Q]
CPDA-1 (citrate phosphate dextrose adenine)	**35 days**[Q]
SAGM (saline adenine glucose mannitol	**42 days**[Q]

Actions of Ingredients of anticoagulant solution	
Glucose	• **ATP generation by glycolysis**[Q]
Adenine	• **Synthesis of ATP**[Q] • **Increases shelf life of RBC to 42 days**[Q]
Citrate	• **Prevents coagulation by chelating calcium**[Q]
Sodium diphosphate	• **Maintain optimum pH**[Q]

■ MASSIVE BLOOD TRANSFUSION

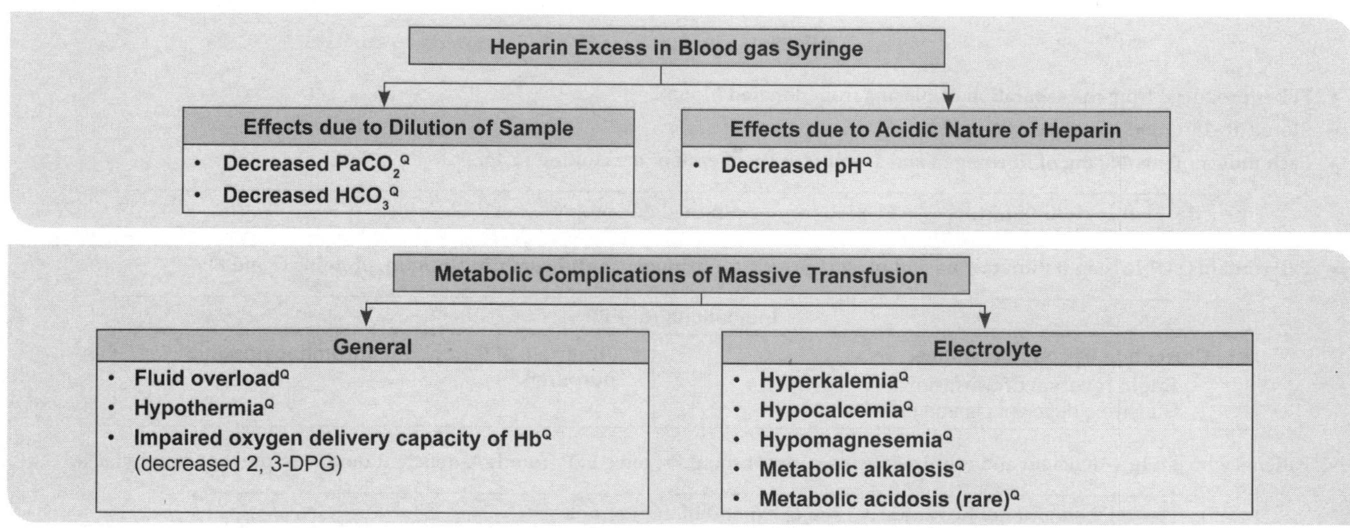

■ COMPLICATIONS OF BLOOD TRANSFUSION

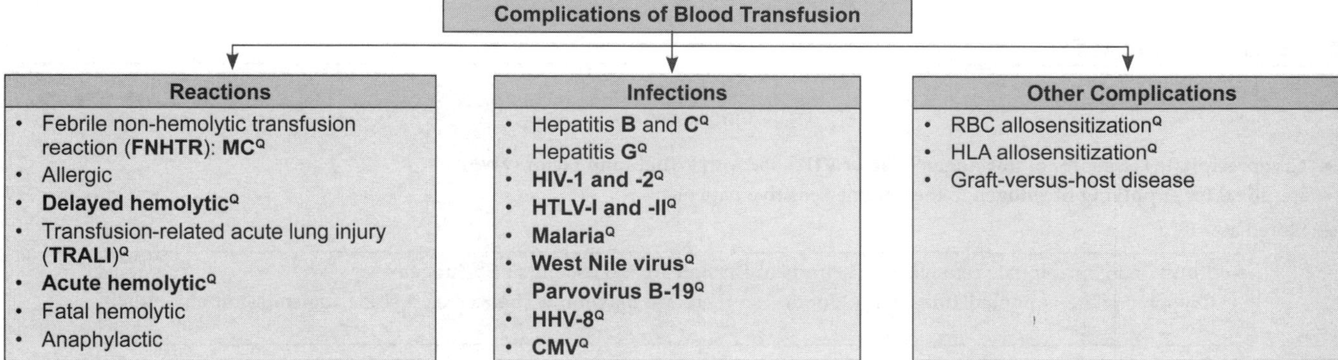

■ RED BLOOD CELLS

RED BLOOD CELLS

• **RBCs** are **stored at 1-6°C**[Q]; **Mean life** of **transfused RBCs is 35 days**[Q].

Anticoagulant used	Maximum storage
ACD/CPD/CP2D	21 days[Q]
CPDA-1	35 days[Q]

■ PLATELETS

PLATELET CONCENTRATES

• **Volume: 50 mL**[Q]
• Platelets are the **only blood products** which are **stored at room temperature, 20-24°C**[Q] (survival is 4-5 days)[Q].
• **1 unit of platelet** increases the count by **5000-10000**[Q].

> • The **threshold for prophylactic platelet transfusion** is **10,000/μL**[Q].
> • **For invasive procedures**, **50,000/μL** platelets is the usual target level.
> • Platelet count should be **1,00,000/μL** before accepting the patient **for surgery**.

• **Transfused platelets** generally **survive for 2-7 days** following transfusion.
• **ABO compatibility** is desirable but **not necessary**.

> • **Blood platelets in stored blood** are **non-functional after 24 hours**[Q].

■ FRESH FROZEN PLASMA

Fresh-frozen Plasma (FFP)

- FFP is produced from the **separation of plasma** from **donated blood**[Q].
- **Stored** at **-18°C** and has a **shelf life** of **1 year**[Q].
- **Each unit** contains **400 mg of fibrinogen** and **1 unit activity of each** of the **clotting factors**[Q].

> - **Most labile clotting factors** (**V and VIII**) may be **diminished**[Q] proportional to shelf life.

- FFP contains stable coagulation factors and plasma proteins: fibrinogen, antithrombin, albumin, proteins C and S[Q].

Indications for FFP

Indications for FFP	

• **Correction of coagulopathies:**
   – **Rapid reversal of warfarin**[Q]
   – Supplying deficient plasma proteins[Q]
	• Treatment of **thrombotic thrombocytopenic purpura**[Q]

- Patients who are **IgA-deficient** and **require plasma support** should receive **FFP** from IgA-deficient donors to prevent anaphylaxis.

> - **FFP should not be** routinely **used to expand blood volume**[Q].
> - **FFP:** An **acellular component** and **does not transmit intracellular infections**, e.g., CMV.

■ CRYOPRECIPITATE

Cryoprecipitate

- **Cryoprecipitate** is a source of **fibrinogen**[Q], **factor VIII**[Q] and **von Willebrand factor (vWF)**[Q].
- It is **ideal for supplying fibrinogen** to the volume-sensitive patient.
- Stored at ≤-18°C

> - **1 unit** of cryoprecipitate contains **80-145 units of Factor VIII** and **250 mg of fibrinogen**[Q].
> - Cryoprecipitate is **pooled from many donors**, so there are **maximum chances of disease transmission** among all blood products[Q].

- Cryoprecipitate may also **supply vWF** to patients with **dysfunctional (type II)** or **absent (type III) von Willebrand disease**.

■ DEXTRAN

Dextran

- It is a **polysaccharide polymer** of varying molecular weight producing an **osmotic pressure** similar to the plasma
- **Disadvantages:**
  - **It induces rouleaux of RBCs** and this **interferes with blood grouping** and **cross matching**[Q] procedures, hence need for a blood sample beforehand.
  - It **interferes with platelet function**, hence it is recommended that **total volume** of dextran **should not exceed 1000 mL**.

> - **LMW dextran (short acting) prevents sludging of RBCs in vessels** and **renal shut down in severe hypotension** and it is **less likely to induce rouleaux formation** than HMW dextran (long acting).

Multiple Choice Questions

■ BLOOD TRANSFUSION

1. MC blood transfusion reaction is: *(All India 2008)*
   a. Febrile non-hemolytic transfusion reaction
   b. Hemolysis
   c. Transmission of infections
   d. Electrolyte imbalance

2. Fresh hold blood transfusion is done with in how much time of collection? *(DNB 2006)*
   a. Immediately
   b. 1 hours
   c. 4 hours
   d. 24 hours

3. One unit of fresh blood arises the Hb% concentration by: *(All India 2003, DNB 2012)*
   a. 0.1 gm%
   b. 1 gm%
   c. 2 gm%
   d. 2.2 gm%

4. Which of the following is better indicator of need for transfusion? *(Recent Question 2016)*
   a. Urine output
   b. Hematocrit
   c. Colour of skin
   d. Clinical examination

5. Storage period of 35 days for blood is seen with: *(AIIMS Nov 2017)*
   a. CPD
   b. CPDA-1
   c. ACD
   d. CP2D

6. Massive blood transfusion is defined as:
   a. Whole blood volume in 24 hours *(Recent Question 2013)*
   b. Half blood volume in 24 hours
   c. 40% blood volume in 24 hours
   d. 60% blood volume in 24 hours

■ BLOOD TRANSFUSION COMPLICATIONS

7. All of the following are major complications of massive transfusion except: *(All India 2006)*
   a. Hypokalemia
   b. Hypothermia
   c. Hypomagnesaemia
   d. Hypocalcaemia

8. Massive transfusions results in: *(Recent Question 2016)*
   a. DIC
   b. Hypothermia
   c. Hypercalcemia
   d. Thrombocytopenia

9. Which of the following is not seen in massive blood transfusion? *(MCI June 2018)*
   a. DIC
   b. Hypothermia
   c. Hypercalcemia
   d. Thrombocytopenia

■ RED BLOOD CELLS

10. The maximum life of a transfused RBC is: *(Recent Question 2016)*
    a. One hour
    b. One day
    c. 15 days
    d. 50 days

■ PLATELETS

11. Platelets can be stored at: *(AIIMS Nov 2005)*
    a. 20-24°C for 5 days
    b. 20-24°C for 8 days
    c. 4-8°C for 5 days
    d. 4-8°C for 8 days

12. Blood platelets in stored blood do not remain functional after: *(Recent Question 2016)*
    a. 24 hours
    b. 48 hours
    c. 72 hours
    d. 96 hours

13. In a patient with thrombocytopenia, what is the target platelet count after transfusion to perform an invasive procedure? *(AIIMS May 2015)*
    a. 30,000
    b. 40,000
    c. 50,000
    d. 60,000

■ PLASMA

14. Stored plasma is deficient in: *(Recent Question 2016)*
    a. Factors 7 and 8
    b. Factors 2 and 5
    c. Factors 5 and 8
    d. Factors 7 and 9

15. Half life of factor VIII is: *(Recent Question 2016)*
    a. 4 hours
    b. 8 hours
    c. 34 hours
    d. 48 hours

16. Rosenthal's syndrome is seen in deficiency of factor:
    a. II
    b. V *(DNB 91)*
    c. IX
    d. XI

■ CRYOPRECIPITATE

17. Cryoprecipitate contains: *(MCI March 2009)*
    a. Factor II
    b. Factor V
    c. Factor VIII
    d. Factor IX

18. Cryoprecipitate is a rich source of: *(Recent Question 2016)*
    a. Thromboplastin
    b. Factor VIII
    c. Factor X
    d. Factor VII

19. Cryoprecipitate contains all except: *(MHCET 2016, AIIMS Nov 2007)*
    a. Factor VIII
    b. Factor IX
    c. Fibrinogen
    d. VWF

Explanations

■ BLOOD TRANSFUSION

1. Ans. a. Febrile non-hemolytic transfusion reaction *(Ref: Harrison 19/e p138e-3)*
2. Ans. d. 24 hours
3. Ans. b. 1 gm%
4. Ans. b. Hematocrit
5. Ans. b. CPDA-1 *(Ref: Wintrobe's 13/e p1278)*
6. Ans. a. Whole blood volume in 24 hours

■ BLOOD TRANSFUSION COMPLICATIONS

7. Ans. a. Hypokalemia
8. Ans. a. DIC; b. Hypothermia; d. Thrombocytopenia
9. Ans. c. Hypercalcemia *(Ref: Bailey 27/e p22)*

■ RED BLOOD CELLS

10. Ans. d. 50 days *(Ref: Schwartz 11/e p116, 10/e p1914-1915; Bailey 27/e p21)*

■ PLATELETS

11. Ans. a. 20-24° C for 5 days *(Ref: Harrison 18/e p953; Sabiston 19/e p588; Schwartz 11/e p120, 10/e p85; Bailey 27/e p21)*
12. Ans. a. 24 hours
13. Ans. c. 50,000 *(Bailey 26/e p23; Nelson 20/e p2374)*

■ PLASMA

14. Ans. c. Factors 5 and 8
15. Ans. b. 8 hours
16. Ans. d. XI

■ CRYOPRECIPITATE

17. Ans. c. Factor VIII *(Ref: Harrison 18/e p953; Sabiston 19/e p588; Schwartz 11/e p120, 10/e p73-75,1599; Bailey 26/e p21)*
18. Ans. b. Factor VIII
19. Ans. b. Factor IX

Shock

■ SHOCK

SHOCK

- Shock is a **clinical syndrome resulting from inadequate tissue perfusion**
- **Shock is MC cause of death among surgical patients**[Q]

Classification of Shock	
1. **Hypovolemic**[Q] **(MC type)**	4. Septic: **Hyperdynamic**[Q] **(early) & Hypodynamic**[Q] **(late)**
2. Traumatic	5. Neurogenic
3. Cardiogenic	6. Hypoadrenal

Monitoring in Shock
1. The best management of shock is done by putting pulmonary catheter. **PCWP is considered better guide than CVP for fluid titrations**[Q] as it can also determine left ventricular preload.
2. **Invasive arterial pressure** is **mandatory**[Q].
3. **Blood gas analysis**[Q]: There is **metabolic acidosis** in shock.
4. **Mixed venous oxygen saturation** is considered as **best guide for tissue perfusion** (i.e. cardiac output)
5. **Urine output** is **best clinical guide of tissue perfusion**[Q].

■ HYPOVOLEMIC SHOCK

HYPOVOLEMIC SHOCK

- **MC type of shock**[Q]
- Causes of **hypovolemic shock:**
  - **Blood loss**[Q] **(Trauma, bleeding)**
  - **Loss of plasma** due to **extravascular fluid seqestration in burns**[Q]
  - **Loss of body sodium & water** (diarrhea & vomiting[Q])

Pathophysiology of Hypovolemic Shock
• **↓ Intravascular volume → ↓ Venous return → ↓ Ventricular filling → ↓ Stroke volume → ↓ Cardiac output → Inadequate tissue perfusion & compensatory mechanism activation**[Q]
• **Inadequate tissue perfusion → Cold clammy skin; Oliguria → anuria; Drowsiness & confusion**[Q]
• **Inadequate tissue perfusion → Lactic acidosis**[Q] **→ Metabolic acidosis**[Q] **→ Tachypnea**[Q]
• **Compensatory mechanism activation**[Q] **→ Sympathetic stimulation**[Q] (↑Adrenaline & ↑Noradrenaline)

Sympathetic stimulation (↑ Adrenaline & ↑ Noradrenaline)	
• **Tachycardia**[Q] (↑Pulse rate)	• **Sweating**[Q]
• **Weak or thready pulse** (↑Total peripheral resistance)	• **Initially maintained BP** followed by **hypotension**

Contd…

Contd…

Four Classes of Hemorrhagic Shock (According to the ATLS course)				
	Class			
Parameter	I	II	III	IV
Blood loss (%)	0-15[Q]	15-30[Q]	30-40[Q]	>40[Q]
CNS	**Slightly** anxious	**Mildly** anxious	**Anxious** or confused	Confused or **lethargic**
Pulse (beats/min)	<100	>100	>120	>140
Blood pressure	Normal	Normal	**Decreased**[Q]	**Decreased**[Q]
Pulse pressure	Normal	**Decreased**	**Decreased**[Q]	**Decreased**[Q]
Respiratory rate	14-20/min	20-30/min	30-40/min[Q]	>35/min[Q]
Urine (mL/hr)	>30	20-30	5-15	Negligible[Q]
Fluid	Crystalloid[Q]	Crystalloid[Q]	Crystalloid + blood[Q]	Crystalloid + blood[Q]
Base deficit	0 to −2 mEq/L	−2 to −6 mEq/L	−6 to −10 mEq/L	−10 mEq/L or less

Clinical Features

- History of trauma, bleeding, burns, diarrhea & vomiting

Class I	Class II	Class III	Class IV
• Compensatory mechanism maintains cardiac output • **Compensated hypovolemic shock**[Q]	• **Hypoxemia**[Q] • **Hypotension**[Q] • **Generalized vasoconstriction** • **Urine output: 20-30 mL/hour**	• **Decompensated shock**[Q] (↓ CO, ↓ SBP) • **Hypotension**[Q] • **Tachycardia**[Q] (PR >120/min) • **Tachypnea**[Q] • **Urine output: 5-15 mL/hour**[Q] • Patient is **confused**[Q]	• **Refractory stage**[Q] • **Marked hypotension**[Q] • **Tachycardia & tachypnea**[Q] • **No urine output**[Q] • Patient is **comatose**[Q]

■ CARDIOGENIC SHOCK

CARDIOGENIC SHOCK

- **Impaired ability of the heart to pump blood**

Causes of Cardiogenic Shock	
Systolic dysfunction	• **Myocardial infarction**[Q] • **Myocardial depressants: Beta-blockers, calcium channel blockers, anti-arrhythmic**
Diastolic dysfunction	• **Ventricular hypertrophy**[Q]**; Restrictive cardiomyopathy**[Q]**; Cardiac tamponade**[Q]
Increased after load	• **Aortic stenoses**[Q]**; Malignant hypertension**[Q]
Valvular structural abnormalities	• **Papillary muscle rupture**[Q] • **Aortic & mitral regurgitation**[Q]
Arrhythmias[Q]	• Ventricular tachyarrhythmia

Pathophysiology of Cardiogenic Shock
• **Impaired pumping ability of left ventricle → ↓ Stroke volume & inadequate systolic emptying** • **↓ Stroke volume → ↓ Cardiac output → ↓ BP → ↓ Tissue perfusion**[Q] • **Inadequate systolic emptying → ↑ Left ventricular filling pressure (↑ preload) → ↑ Left atrial pressure → ↑ Pulmonary artery & capillary pressure → Pulmonary edema**[Q]

Clinical Features

- Clinical features vary depending on the cause:
  - **Signs of myocardial failure:** ↑ JVP, reduced pulse volume, hypotension, tachycardia, basal coarse crackles[Q]
  - **Obstructive (cardiac tamponade):** Muffled heart sounds, pulsus paradoxus[Q]
  - **Pulmonary embolism:** Sudden onset **dyspnea, tachypnea, tachycardia, hypotension, localized pleural rub**[Q], severe central chest pain in massive emboli
  - **Other signs: Cold clammy peripheries** with **pallor, peripheral & central cyanosis**[Q]

■ SEPTIC SHOCK

Septic Shock	
Definition	• A subset of sepsis in which **underlying circulatory and cellular/metabolic abnormalities** lead to substantially **increased mortality risk**[Q]
Criteria in 2016	• **Suspected** (or documented) **infection plus vasopressor therapy** needed to maintain **mean arterial pressure at ≥65 mm Hg**[Q] & **serum lactate >2.0 mmol/L despite adequate fluid resuscitation**[Q]

- Septic shock refers to **sepsis accompanied by hypotension** that **cannot be corrected by infusion of fluids**[Q]

- **Refractory septic shock:** Septic shock that lasts for **>1 hour** & **does not respond to fluid or pressure administration**

Pathophysiology of Septic Shock
• Initiated by **gram-negative (MC)** or gram-positive **bacteria**, fungi or virus
• **Cell wall** of organisms contain **endotoxins & exotoxins**
• **Endotoxins** → Release of **inflammatory mediators** → **Vasodilatation & ↑ capillary permeability** → Altered peripheral circulation & massive dilation → **Shock**[Q]
• **Infection** → Local inflammatory reaction → Release of inflammatory mediators → Systemic inflammatory response → Diffuse endothelial injury, vasodilatation & ↑ capillary permeability → Progressive vasodilatation & maldistribution of blood flow → Organ hypoperfusion → Multiple organ dysfunction syndrome[Q]

Clinical Features

- **Fever with chills & rigor, warm peripheries** due to vasodilatation[Q]
- **Bounding pulse, rapid capillary refilling & hypotension**[Q]
- Evidence of **infection at local site**[Q]

Treatment

- **First line of treatment: Aggressive volume expansion with crystalloids & restoration of arterial oxygenation with inspired oxygen &** frequently with mechanical ventilation are the **highest priorities**[Q].
- **Second line:** Ionotropic support with dopamine, norepinephrine, or vasopressin in presence of hypotension or dobutamine if arterial pressure is normal[Q].
- **High dose activated protein C**[Q] **(APC)** provides a **survival benefit in** patients with **severe sepsis & septic shock**
- **Plasma expanders** are useful as septic shock is associated with **peripheral vasodilatation causing reactive hypovolemia**[Q]
- **Antibiotics & surgical debridement or drainage** to control infection[Q]

■ NEUROGENIC SHOCK

- Result from **loss or suppression of sympathetic tone** → Massive vasodilatation in venous vasculature →↓Venous return → ↓ Cardiac output → Impaired tissue perfusion & cellular metabolism[Q]

Causes of Neurogenic Shock	
• **High cervical spinal cord injury**[Q]	• **Deep general anesthesia**[Q] (depress vasomotor tone)
• Inadvertent **cephalad migration of spinal** anesthesia[Q]	• **Devastating head injury**[Q]

Clinical Features

- **Paralysis below the level of lesion; Hypotension**[Q]
- **Bradycardia** due to **loss of sympathetic tone**[Q] → **Arterial & venous vasodilatation**[Q] → **Warm & dry skin**[Q]
- **Hypothermia**[Q]

Treatment

- Treatment involves a simultaneous approach to **relative hypovolemia** & to **loss of vasomotor tone.**
- **Excessive volumes of fluid**[Q] may be required to restore normal hemodynamics if given alone.
- Once hemorrhage has been ruled out, **norepinephrine** or a **pure alpha-adrenergic agent**[Q] **(phenylephrine)** may be necessary

■ HYPOADRENAL SHOCK

HYPOADRENAL SHOCK

- In the **stress or illness, surgery** or **trauma**, adrenal secretes increased amount of cortisol[Q]
- Unrecognized adrenal insufficiency complicates the host response to stress induced by **acute illness or major surgery** → **Hypoadrenal shock**[Q]

Causes of Hypoadrenal Shock
• **Chronic administration of high doses of exogenous glucocorticoids**[Q]
• **Adrenal insufficiency** secondary to: **Idiopathic atrophy**[Q]; Use of **etomidate**[Q] for intubation; **Tuberculosis**[Q], **Metastatic disease**[Q]; **Bilateral adrenal hemorrhage**[Q]; **Amyloidosis**[Q]

■ CHARACTERISTIC FEATURES OF VARIOUS TYPES OF SHOCK

Physiologic Characteristics of the Various Forms of Shock				
Type of Shock	**CVP and PCWP**	**Cardiac Output**	**SVR**	**Venous O_2 Saturation**
Hypovolemic	↓	↓	↑	↓
Cardiogenic	↑	↓	↑	↓
Septic				
Hyperdynamic	↑↓	↓	↓	↑
Hypodynamic	↑↓	↑	↑	↑↓
Traumatic	↓	↑↓	↑↓	↓
Neurogenic	↓	↓	↓	↓
Hypoadrenal	↑↓	↓	=↓	↓

■ PARAMETERS FOR SHOCK

Shock Index (SI)	Modified Shock Index (MSI)
• **SI is defined as heart rate divided by systolic BP**[Q]. • **Better marker for assessing severity of shock than heart rate & BP alone**[Q]. • Utility in **trauma patients, sepsis, obstetrics, myocardial infarction, stroke & other acute critical illnesses**[Q]. • **Correlated with need for interventions** such as blood transfusion & invasive procedures including operations. • SI is known as a **hemodynamic stability indicator**[Q]. • SI does **not take into account** the **diastolic BP**	• **MSI is defined as heart rate divided by mean arterial pressure**[Q]. • **High MSI** indicates a **value of stroke volume & low systemic vascular resistance, a sign of hypodynamic circulation**[Q]. • **Low MSI indicates a hyperdynamic state**[Q]. • **MSI** has been considered a **better marker than SI for mortality rate prediction**[Q].

PULSE RATE OVER PRESSURE EVALUATION (ROPE)

- ROPE = Pulse Rate/Pulse pressure = PR/(SBP–DBP)
- ROPE is useful in the **assessment of compensated hemorrhagic shock**.

■ DRUG OF CHOICE IN SHOCK

Drug of Choice in Shock	
Anaphylactic shock	• **Adrenaline**[Q]
Cardiogenic shock	• **Noradrenaline or dopamine**[Q]
Distributive shock	• **Noradrenaline or phenylephrine**[Q]
Hypovolemic shock	• **Crystalloids**[Q]
Shock with oliguria	• **Dopamine**[Q]
Hypoadrenal shock	• **Corticosteroids**[Q]
Septic shock	• **Broad-spectrum antibiotics**[Q]

■ SHOCK

1. **Shock is clinically best assessed by:** *(Recent Question 2016)*
   - a. Urine output
   - b. CVP
   - c. BP
   - d. Hydration

2. **Which of the following is true for shock?** *(MCI Sept 2005)*
   - a. Hypotension
   - b. Hypoperfusion to tissues
   - c. Hypoxia
   - d. All of the above

3. **Best guide for the management of resuscitation is:** *(AIIMS Nov 2017)*
   - a. CVP
   - b. Urine output
   - c. Blood pressure
   - d. Saturation of oxygen

4. **Modified shock index formula is:** *(AIIMS Nov 2017)*
   - a. Heart rate / Systolic BP
   - b. Heart rate / Diastolic BP
   - c. Heart rate/ Mean arterial pressure
   - d. Pulse rate/ Systolic BP

5. **First line of therapy in shock in the patients of trauma:** *(Recent Question 2017)*
   - a. Crystalloids
   - b. Colloids
   - c. Inotropes
   - d. Blood transfusion

6. **Optimum urine output in post-operative patient:** *(Recent Question 2017)*
   - a. 1 mL/min
   - b. 2 mL/min
   - c. 3 mL/min
   - d. 4 mL/min

7. **A patient came with profuse diarrhea and dehydration reaches OPD. For examination flow of fluids which cannula can be inserted:** *(AIIMS Nov 2018)*
   - a. Green
   - b. Blue
   - c. Grey
   - d. Violet

■ NEUROGENIC SHOCK

8. **Neurogenic shock is characterized by:** *(AIIMS May 2014)*
   - a. Hypertension and tachycardia
   - b. Hypertension and bradycardia
   - c. Hypotension and tachycardia
   - d. Hypotension and bradycardia

9. **A patient with spine, chest and abdominal injury in road traffic accident developed hypotension and bradycardia. Most likely reason is:** *(AIIMS Nov 2013)*
   - a. Hypovolemic shock
   - b. Hypovolemic + neurogenic shock
   - c. Hypovolemic + septicemic shock
   - d. Neurogenic shock

10. **Which of the following are true about neurogenic shock?** *(Recent Question 2016)*
    - a. Tachycardia
    - b. Cold and moist extremity
    - c. Due to parasympathetic blockade
    - d. Diagnosis of exclusion

■ HEMORRHAGIC SHOCK

11. **Hemorrhage leads to:** *(MCI Sept 2005)*
    - a. Septic shock
    - b. Neurogenic shock
    - c. Hypovolemic shock
    - d. Cardiogenic shock

12. **In traumatic cases, shock is most likely due to:** *(Recent Question 2016, DNB 2011, MCI Sept 2007)*
    - a. Injury to intra abdominal solid organ
    - b. Head injury
    - c. Septicemia
    - d. Cardiac failure

13. **Which of the following is ideal in moderate hemorrhagic shock?** *(Karnataka 2012, MCI Sept 2007)*
    - a. Dextrose
    - b. Ringer lactate
    - c. Blood
    - d. Dextran

14. **Blood loss in class II hemorrhagic shock is:** *(Recent Questions 2013)*
    - a. < 15%
    - b. 15-30%
    - c. 30-40%
    - d. >40%

15. **Amount of blood loss in class III hemorrhagic shock:** *(MCI Dec 2018)*
    - a. <15%
    - b. 15–30%
    - c. 30–40%
    - d. >40%

16. **Most common type of shock in emergency room is:** *(Recent Question 2013)*
    - a. Cardiogenic
    - b. Hypovolemic shock
    - c. Obstructive
    - d. Neurogenic

17. **Most common type of shock in surgical practice:** *(DNB 2014)*
    - a. Cardiogenic
    - b. Hypovolemic
    - c. Neurogenic
    - d. Septic shock

18. **Most common feature of polytrauma in pediatric age group is:** *(Recent Question 2015)*
    - a. Hypothermia
    - b. Hypovolemic shock
    - c. Hypotension
    - d. Hypoxemia

19. **In traumatic cases, shock is most likely due to:** *(MCI June 2018)*
    - a. Injury to intra-abdominal solid organ
    - b. Head injury
    - c. Septicemia
    - d. Cardiac failure

20. **In hypovolemic shock which organ should be assessed for determining under-perfusion?** *(MCI June 2019)*
    - a. Kidney
    - b. Heart
    - c. Lung
    - d. Liver

■ SEPTIC SHOCK

21. Plasma expanders are used in:
     (Recent Question 2013, DNB 2012)
     a. Septic shock
     b. Vasovagal shock
     c. Neurogenic shock
     d. Cardiogenic shock

22. All of the following are true about distributive shock except:
     a. Decreased venous return   *(Recent Question 2017)*
     b. Decreased cardiac output
     c. Decreased vascular resistance
     d. High mixed venous saturation

■ MISCELLANEOUS

23. Green coloured IV cannula, the size is: *(Recent Question 2015)*
     a. 18 Gauge
     b. 20 Gauge
     c. 22 Gauge
     d. 24 Gauge

24. In a patient with dehydration, which the following color intravenous cannula will you place for rapid fluid resuscitation?   *(AIIMS May 2016)*
     a. Grey
     c. Blue
     b. Pink
     d. Green

25. 22 Gauge IV cannula color is: *(AIIMS Nov 2017)*
     a. Green
     b. Grey
     c. Blue
     d. Pink

26. Oliguria is defined as: *(MCI June 2018)*
     a. Absence of urine production
     b. More than 900 mL of urine excreted in a day
     c. 600 mL to 700 mL of urine excreted in a day
     d. Less than 300 mL of urine excreted in a day

Explanations

■ SHOCK

1. **Ans. a. Urine output** *(Sabiston 20/e p554; Schwartz 11/e p152, 10/e p109-131; Bailey 27/e p17)*

SHOCK

- **Shock: Inadequate delivery of oxygen** and **nutrients** due to **poor tissue perfusion**[Q] to maintain normal tissue and cellular function
- **Mean arterial pressure <60 mm Hg** in previously normotensive patients
- **Systemic vascular resistance rises** leading to **decreased cutaneous blood flow**[Q] and **autoregulation** is **critical in sustaining cerebral** and **coronary blood flow**[Q].

Blalock Classification of Shock	
1. **Hypovolemic (MC)**[Q]	3. Cardiogenic
2. Vasogenic	4. Neurogenic

- **Shock is MC cause of death among surgical patients.**

2. **Ans. d. All of the above**

3. **Ans. b. Urine output** *(Ref: Sabiston 20/e p520; Schwartz 11/e p152, 10/e p169; Bailey 27/e p17)*

> *"Ultimately, the goal of treatment is to restore cellular and organ perfusion. Ideally, therefore, monitoring of organ perfusion should guide the management of shock. The best measures of organ perfusion and the best monitor of the adequacy of shock therapy remains the urine output."*
> *- Bailey 27/e p17*

4. **Ans. c. Heart rate/ Mean arterial pressure** *(Ref: Sabiston 20/e p52)*

5. **Ans. a. Crystalloids**

6. **Ans. a. 1 mL/min** *(Ref: Sabiston 20/e p520; Schwartz 11/e p152, 10/e p169; Bailey 27/e p17)*

> *"Urine output of more than 1 mL/kg is an adequate measure of renal perfusion in the absence of underlying renal disease."*
> *- Sabiston 20/e p520*

7. **Ans. c. Grey**

■ NEUROGENIC SHOCK

8. **Ans. d. Hypotension and bradycardia**

9. **Ans. d. Neurogenic shock** *(Ref: Harrison 19/e p1750)*

> A patient with **spine, chest and abdominal injury** in road traffic accident developed **hypotension** and **bradycardia**. Most likely reason is **neurogenic shock.**
> *"Neurogenic shock: In addition to **arteriolar dilation, venodilation** causes **pooling in the venous system**, which **decreases venous return and cardiac output.**" - Harrison 19/e p1750*

10. **Ans. d. Diagnosis of exclusion**

■ HEMORRHAGIC SHOCK

11. **Ans. c. Hypovolemic shock**

12. **Ans. a. Injury to intra-abdominal solid organs**

13. **Ans. b. Ringer lactate**

- Patients with **blunt trauma** and **hypovolemia** should be **examined first for intra-abdominal bleeding** even if there is no overt existence of abdominal trauma.[Q]

14. **Ans. b. 15-30%**

15. **Ans. c. 30-40%** *(Ref: Bailey 27/e p19)*

16. **Ans. b. Hypovolemic shock**

17. **Ans. b. Hypovolemic**
18. **Ans. b. Hypovolemic shock**
19. **Ans. a. Injury to intra-abdominal solid organ**
20. **Ans. a. Kidney** *(Ref: Bailey 27/e p17)*

■ SEPTIC SHOCK

21. **Ans. a. Septic shock**
22. **Ans. b. Decreased cardiac output** *(Ref: Sabiston 20/e p554; Bailey 27/e p13)*

"Distributive shock describes the pattern of cardiovascular responses characterising a variety of conditions, including septic shock, anaphylaxis and spinal cord injury. Inadequate organ perfusion is accompanied by vascular dilatation with hypotension, low systemic vascular resistance, inadequate afterload and a resulting abnormally high cardiac output."- Bailey 27/e p13

■ MISCELLANEOUS

23. **Ans. a. 18 Gauge**
24. **Ans. a. Grey** *(Ref: Bailey 25/e p29)*

    Grey cannula has the **large bore (16 G)** with **flow rate of 180 mL/min** and is the **preferred option for rapid fluid resuscitation** in patients with rehydration.

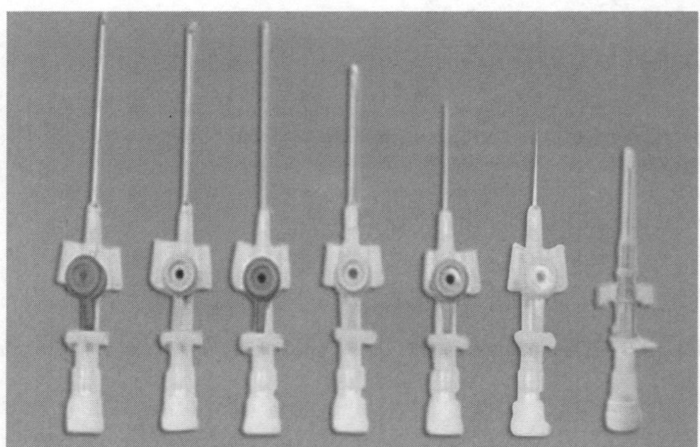

Color code	Gauge	External Diameter (mm)	Length (mm)	Flow Rate (ml/min)	Indications
Orange	14G	2.1	45	240	Trauma, surgical procedures
Grey	16G^Q	1.8	45	180^Q	Trauma, surgical procedures
Green	18G^Q	1.3	32/45	90^Q	Trauma, quick blood transfusion
Pink	20G^Q	1.1	32	60^Q	Normal IV or blood transfusion
Blue	22G^Q	0.9	25	36^Q	Children, older adults
Yellow	24G	0.7	19	20	Neonates, children, elderly
Violet	26G	0.6	19	13	Neonates

25. **Ans. c. Blue** *(Ref: Manual of ICU Procedures By Mohan Gurjar (2015)/p240)*
26. **Ans. d. Less than 300 mL of urine excreted in a day**

Miscellaneous

Multiple Choice Questions

1. **Referred pain from all of the following conditions may be felt along the inner side of right thigh, except:**
   a. Inflamed pelvic appendix *(All India 2006)*
   b. Inflamed ovaries
   c. Stone in pelvic ureter
   d. Pelvic abscess

2. **FNAC needle size:** *(AIIMS Nov 2007)*
   a. 18-22   b. 22-26
   c. 27-29   d. 16-18

3. **The most dangerous injury is:** *(Recent Question 2016)*
   a. Snake bite   b. Scorpion bite
   c. Wasp sting   d. Human bite

4. **The best site for intramuscular injection is:**
   a. Deltoid *(Recent Question 2016)*
   b. Anterolateral part of thigh
   c. Upper outer segment of buttocks
   d. Upper inner segment of buttocks

5. **Hereditary spherocytosis is transmitted as:**
   (Recent Question 2016)
   a. Autosomal dominant   b. Autosomal recessive
   c. X-linked dominant   d. X-linked recessive

6. **'Sterile needle test' helps in differentiating:** *(Gujrat 2014)*
   a. Healing process   b. Depth of burns
   c. Degenerative process   d. Infection

7. **Van Buchem's syndrome is characterized by all except:**
   a. Overgrowth *(Gujrat 2014)*
   b. Distortion of mandible
   c. Facial Palsy
   d. Increased acid phosphatase

8. **Quant's sign (a T-shaped depression in the occipital bone) may be present in:**
   (Gujrat 2014)
   a. Down's syndrome   b. Head injury
   c. Rickets   d. Scurvy

9. **Nezelof's syndrome is recurrent episodes of:** *(Gujrat 2014)*
   a. Appendicitis   b. Cholecystitis
   c. Intestinal obstruction   d. Pneumonia

10. **Usually employed technique for splanchnic block is:**
    (Recent Question 2016)
    a. Braun's method   b. Kappi's method
    c. Wending's method   d. None of the above

11. **Secondary amyloidosis occurs in:** *(Recent Question 2016)*
    a. Chronic osteomyelitis   b. Rheumatoid arthritis
    c. Leprosy   d. Syphilis

12. **Arrow headed finger on X-ray is suggestive of:**
    (Recent Question 2016)
    a. Acromegaly   b. Hyperparathyroidism
    c. Down's syndrome   d. Sarcoidosis

13. **A Seldinger needle is used for:** *(Recent Question 2016)*
    a. Liver biopsy   b. Suturing skin
    c. Arteriography   d. Lymphography

14. **A cricoid hook is used particularly:**
    a. In thyroidectomy *(Recent Question 2016; DNB 89)*
    b. In block dissection of the neck
    c. For retracting the superior laryngeal nerve
    d. In tracheostomy

15. **Not a premalignant ulcer:** *(Kerala 94)*
    a. Bazin's ulcer   b. Paget's disease of nipple
    c. Marjolin's ulcer   d. Lupus vulgaris

16. **A female patient complains of periumbilical pain and nausea particularly after taking food. The diagnosis is:** *(UPPG 95)*
    a. Meckel's diverticulum   b. Peptic ulcer syndrome
    c. Lactose intolerance   d. None

17. **Failure of migration of neural crest cells is seen in:**
    (Kerala 2001)
    a. Albinism   b. Congenital megacolon
    c. Odonotomes   d. Adrenal tumour

18. **The commonest symptom post operatively seen is:**
    a. Depression   b. Psychosis *(Kerala 97)*
    c. Euphoria   d. None of the above

19. **The most sensitive qualitative method for detection of air embolism is:** *(Gujrat 2014)*
    a. Doppler ultra sound   b. Elector cardiogram
    c. Arterial pressure
    d. End expiratory carbon dioxide content

20. **Fiberoptic endoscopy is contraindicated in:**
    a. Children *(Recent Question 2016)*
    b. Aneurysm of arch of aorta
    c. Cervical spondylosis
    d. Hemoptysis

21. **Who said these words: To study the phenomenon of disease without books is to sail an uncharted sea, while to study books without patients is not to go to sea at all?**
    (Karnataka 2004)
    a. Hamilton Bailey   b. Sir Robert Hutchison
    c. Sir William Osler   d. J.B. Murphy

22. **Lamina dura lining the alveolus is:** *(Karnataka 2002)*
    a. Cancellous bone   b. Ligament
    c. Dense cortical bone   d. Muscle

23. **Vidian neurectomy is indicated in:** *(MAHE 2005)*
    a. Glossopharyngeal neuralgia
    b. Trigeminal neuralgia
    c. Vasomotor rhinitis
    d. Atrophic rhinitis

24. **Orthobaric oxygen in used in:** *(MAHE 2005)*
    a. Carbon monoxide poisoning
    b. Ventilation failure
    c. Anaerobic infection
    d. Gangrene

25. **About congenital torticollis all are except:** *(AIIMS Nov 2006)*
    a. Always associated with breech extraction
    b. Spontaneous resolution in most cases
    c. 2/3rd cases have palpable neck mass at birth
    d. Uncorrected cases develop plagicephaly

26. **Dye used in chromoendoscopy for detection of cancer:**
    (AIIMS May 2009)
    a. Gentian violet
    b. Toluidine blue
    c. Hemotoxiline and eosine
    d. Methylene blue

27. **Smoking may be associated with all of the following cancer's except:**
    (All India 2009)
    a. CA Larynx
    b. CA Nasopharynx
    c. CA Bladder
    d. CA Esophagus

28. **Hutchinson and Pepper syndrome is a feature of:**
    (COMEDK 2004)
    a. Von Recklinghausen's
    b. Neuroblastoma
    c. Renal cell carcinoma
    d. Meningioma

29. **What is this sign called?** *(APPG 2016)*

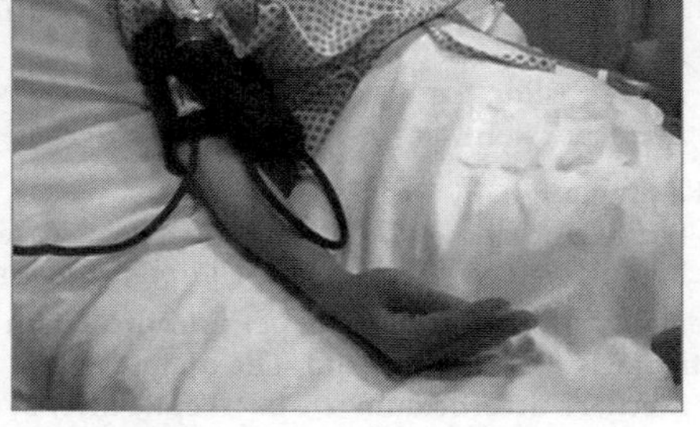

    a. Troisier sign
    b. Chvostek's sign
    c. Lhermitte's sign
    d. Trousseau's sign

30. **Not a submucosal lesion:** *(Punjab 2009)*
    a. Lipoma
    b. Ranula
    c. Carcinoid
    d. None

31. **Which of the following is the most commonly used 'fixative' in diagnostic pathology?** *(Recent Question 2016)*
    a. Formaldehyde
    b. Ethyl alcohol
    c. Mercuric chloride
    d. Picric acid

32. **Aflatoxins are produced by:** *(All India 2011)*
    a. Aspergillus flavus
    b. Aspergillus niger
    c. Aspergillus fumigates
    d. Candida

33. **Axillary abscess is safely drained by which approach?**
    (AIIMS May 2011)
    a. Medial
    b. Posterior
    c. Lateral
    d. Floor

34. **Topical mitomycin C is used in :** *(AIIMS May 2011)*
    a. Basal skull carcinoma
    b. Tracheal stenosis
    c. Skull base osteomyelitis
    d. Angiofibroma

35. **Potato nodes are feature of:** *(DNB 2010)*
    a. Sarcoidosis
    b. Tuberculosis
    c. Carcinoid
    d. Lymphoma

36. **Moures sign is seen in:** *(Recent Questions 2013)*
    a. Carcinoma
    b. Appendicitis
    c. Varicose vein
    d. Pancreatitis

37. **Choose the Wrong combination of cancer and its suspected carcinogen:** *(APPG 2016)*
    a. Tobacco - bladder
    b. Phenacetin - lung
    c. Arsenic - skin
    d. Vinyl chloride - liver

38. **French in Foley's catheter refers to:** *(AIIMS Nov 2017)*
    a. Outer circumference measurement
    b. Inner circumference measurement
    c. Diameter of catheter
    d. Lumen size

39. **In a preoperative patient surgical checklist, which of the following is not required?** *(AIIMS Nov 2017)*
    a. Oral consent
    b. Doctor's signature
    c. Site marking
    d. Confirming patient's identity

40. **In fasciotomy the layers that are opened are:**
    (Recent Question 2018)
    a. Skin, subcutaneous tissue and superficial fascia
    b. Skin, subcutaneous tissue alone cut
    c. Skin alone cut
    d. Skin, subcutaneous tissue, superficial fascia and deep fascia

41. **Correct procedure of inserting nasogastric tube is:**
    (MCI June 2019)
    a. Supine with neck flexed
    b. Supine with neck extended
    c. Sitting with neck flexed
    d. Sitting with neck extended

1. **Ans. d. Pelvic abscess**

2. **Ans. b. 22-26** *(Ref: www.ncbi.nlm.nih.gov/pubmed/17405171)*

   - **FNAC Needle Size: 21-25 guaze[Q]**

3. **Ans. a. Snake bite**   4. **Ans. c. Upper outer segment of buttocks**   5. **Ans. a. Autosomal dominant**

6. **Ans. b. Depth of burns** *(Ref: Sabiston 20/e p506; Schwartz 11/e p253, 10/c p 229, 230)*

   - **'Sterile needle test'** helps in **differentiating depth of burns.**

7. **Ans. b. Distortion of mandible** *(Ref: http://www.ncbi.nlm.nih.gov/pmc/articles/PMC1376897/)*

   ### VAN BUCHEM DISEASE

   - Van Buchem disease (**hyperostosis corticalis generalisata**) is an **autosomal recessive** disorder characterized by **hyperostosis of the skull, mandible, clavicles, ribs,** and **diaphyseal cortices** of the **long bones[Q].**
   - **Most striking clinical features** are the **enlargement of the jaw** and **thickness of the skull,** which may lead to **facial nerve palsy, hearing loss,** and **optic atrophy[Q].**

8. **Ans. c. Rickets** *(Ref: http://www.kmle.com/search.php?Search=Quant's%20s).*

   ### QUANT'S SIGN

   - A **T-shaped depression in** the **occipital bone** occurring in many cases of **rickets,** especially in **infants lying constantly in bed** with pressure on the **pressure on the occiput[Q].**

9. **Ans. d. Pneumonia**

   ### NEZELOF SYNDROME

   - **Nezelof syndrome** (also known as **"Thymic dysplasia with normal immunoglobulins"**)
   - An **autosomal recessive** congenital immunodeficiency condition due to underdevelopment of the thymus.
   - It causes **severe infections** and **malignancies[Q].**
   - **Treatment: Antimicrobial therapy, IV immunoglobulin, bone marrow transplantation,** thymus transplantation and thymus factors.

10. **Ans. a. Braun's method** *(Ref: Lee Anesthesia (2005)/449)*

    ### SPLANCHNIC BLOCK

    - **Splanchnic block** can be performed **from the front (Braun[Q],** Wendling), or **from behind (Kappis).**

11. **Ans. a. Chronic osteomyelitis, b. Rheumatoid arthritis, c. Leprosy** *(Ref: Harrison 20/e p805)*

    ### AMYLOIDOSIS

    - Amyloidosis is a pathological proteinaceous substance **deposited between cells[Q]** in various tissues and organs of the body in a variety of clinical settings.

    ### TYPES OF AMYLOID PROTEIN

    - **AL (Amyloid Light chain):**
      - This is **derived from plasma cells[Q]** and contains immunoglobulin light chains
      - Associated with **primary amyloidosis** and immunocyte dyscrasias with amyloidosis like **multiple myeloma[Q]**
    - **AA (Amyloid Associate protein):**
      - It is unique non-immunoglobulin protein synthesized by **reticuloendothelial cells of liver[Q].**
      - Associated with **secondary amyloidosis** and **reactive systemic amyloidosis[Q].**

      > - Chronic inflammatory conditions: Tuberculosis[Q], Bronchiectasis[Q], Osteomyelitis[Q]
      > - **Connective tissue disorders: Rheumatoid Arthritis (MC)[Q],** Ankylosing spondylitis[Q] and Primary biliary cirrhosis[Q]
      > - **Non immune derived tumors: Renal cell carcinoma[Q]** and Hodgkin's lymphoma[Q]

    - β_2**microalbumin (Aβ_2m): Hemodialysis associated amyloidosis[Q]**
    - β_2 **Amyloid protein: Senile cerebral[Q], Alzheimer's disease[Q]**
    - **Transthyretin (ATTR): Familial amyloidotic neuropathies[Q]** and Systemic senile amyloidosis[Q]

Contd…

Contd…

- Calcitonin associated amyloid (A cal): **Medullary CA thyroid**[Q]
- **Islet amyloid peptide (AIAPP): Type II DM**[Q]
- **Atrial natriuretic factor associated amyloid:** Isolated atrial Amyloidosis and Misfolded prion protein (PrPsc) disease

> - **Common Biopsy sites in Amyloidosis: Subcutaneous abdominal fat aspirate**[Q], **Rectum**[Q], **Skin**[Q], **Gingiva**[Q]

12. Ans. a. Acromegaly *(Ref: www.acromegalycommunity.com/blog)*

- **Arrow headed finger** on X-ray is suggestive of **Acromegaly**[Q].

13. Ans. c. Arteriography *(Ref: Sabiston 20/e p1787; Schwartz 10/e p1051; Bailey 25/e p903)*

Seldinger **needle** is **used for angiography** (arteriography).

ARTERIOGRAPHY

- **Aortic** and **lower extremity arteriograms** are generally performed **by needle puncture** of the **femoral**[Q] or **brachial arteries**[Q] followed by **guidewire placement** and **catheter insertion** using the **Seldinger technique**.

14. Ans. d. In tracheostomy
- A **cricoids hook** is **used in tracheostomy**[Q].

15. Ans. a. Bazin's ulcer

BAZIN DISEASE

- **Bazin disease** (or "**Erythema induratum**") is a **panniculitis** on the **back of the calves**[Q].
- It is now considered a **panniculitis** that is **not associated with a single defined pathogen**[Q]·
- It occurs **mainly in women**[Q], but is very rare now.

16. Ans. a. Meckel's diverticulum   **17. Ans. b. Congenital megacolon**

18. Ans. d. None of the above

POSTOPERATIVE PSYCHIATRIC SYMPTOMS

- **Delirium**[Q] **(20%)** >Depression (9%) >Dementia (3%) >Functional psychosis (2%).

19. Ans. d. End expiratory carbon dioxide content *(Ref: Schwartz 9/e p787-789)*

20. Ans. b. Aneurysm of arch of aorta
- **Fiberoptic endoscopy** is **contraindicated in aneurysm of arch of aorta**.

21. Ans. c. Sir William Osler

- **Sir William Osler:** "To study the phenomenon of disease without books is to sail an uncharted sea, while to study books without patients is not to go to sea at all"[Q]

22. Ans. c. Dense cortical bone

23. Ans. c. Vasomotor rhinitis *(Ref: www.ncbi.nlm.nih.gov/pubmed/16686388)*

- **Vidian neurectomy** is indicated **in** the cases of **vasomotor rhinitis** with **profuse secretion refractory to conservative treatment**[Q].

24. Ans. a. Carbon monoxide poisoning *(Ref: www.biomedsearch.com/searchlist.html?p=3101…txt=oxygen…)*
- Severe **carbon monoxide poisoning** treated by **hyperbaric oxygen therapy**[Q].

25. Ans. a. Always associated with breech extraction *(Ref: Bailey 27/e p582)*

TORTICOLLIS

- In torticollis the **head is tilted toward** and **rotated away from the tight sternocleidomastoid muscle**.
- **Congenital torticollis** is usually **secondary to intrauterine moulding** but may present with fixed **sternocleidomastoid contracture** or with a **palpable mass in the muscle**.
- **Most cases resolve with stretching** but, occasionally, **surgical release** of the sternocleidomastoid at one or both ends is needed.

26. Ans. d. Methylene blue

CHROMOENDOSCOPY

- **Chromoendoscopy: Dyes** are **instilled into the GIT at** the time of **visualization** with **fibre-optic endoscopy**[Q].
- **Chiefly enhance** the **characterization of tissues**[Q]
- **Detail achieved** can often **allow for identification of the tissue type** or **pathology**[Q]

Others

Section 10

Contd…

Stains used

- **Absorptive stains** have an affinity **for particular mucosal elements**, and include Lugol's iodine, methylene blue and **gentian violet[Q]**.

Lugol's iodine	• Specifically **stains non-keratinized squamous epithelium[Q]** • **Useful for** identifying **squamous tissue, squamous dysplasia & squamous cell carcinomas[Q]**.
Methylene blue	• Stains **absorptive epithelium[Q]** • Useful for **identifying** abnormality in **small intestine, colon & Barrett's esophagus[Q]** (intestinal metaplasia)

- **Contrast stains** are **not absorbed** but rather **provide contrast** by **permeating between irregularities in the mucosa to highlight irregularities**. The primary contrast stain is **indigo carmine[Q]**.

  > • **Chief use** of Indigo carmine: Identification of dysplastic cells in individuals with **chronic UC[Q]**.

- **Reactive stains** undergo an **observable change** due to a **chemical process** related to the function of the gastrointestinal tract. **Congo red** is used as a **test for achlorhydria in the stomach[Q]**, as it changes **colour from red to black** at a pH less than 3.

Uses of Chromoendoscopy

- Identification of **squamous cell carcinomas** or **dysplasia** of the esophagus[Q]
- Identification of **Barrett's esophagus & dysplasia[Q]**
- identification of **early gastric cancer[Q]**
- Characterization of **colonic polyps** & **colorectal cancer[Q]**
- In **screening for dysplasia** in individuals with **ulcerative colitis[Q]**.

27. **Ans. None** *(Ref: Harrison 20/e p3293)*

    Smoking may be associated with all of the above cancers.

Smoking Associated Cancers		
• **Lung[Q]** • **Nasopharynx, oropharynx hypopharynx** and **Larynx[Q]** • **Nasal cavity** and **paranasal sinuses[Q]**	• **Oral cavity[Q]** • **Esophagus[Q]** • **Stomach[Q]** • **Pancreas[Q]** • **Liver[Q]**	• **Kidney[Q]** • Ureter and **Urinary Bladder[Q]** • **Uterine Cervix[Q]** • Acute Myeloid Leukemia

- **Smoking** is **not associated with postmenopausal Breast cancer** and **endometrial cancer**.

28. **Ans. b. Neuroblastoma**

NEUROBLASTOMA

- **Hutchinson and Pepper syndrome** is **skull metastasis** seen in neuroblastoma[Q].

29. **Ans. d. Trousseau's sign**

30. **Ans. b. Ranula** *(Ref: Bailey 27/e p779)*

31. **Ans. a. Formaldehyde** *(Ref: Surgical Pathology by Rosai and Ackermann 9/e p27)*

FORMALIN

- **Formaldehyde** as a **buffered 10% aqueous solution (formalin[Q])** is the **fixative most commonly used** in **histology[Q]**
- In routine clinical diagnostics it **offers the best possible compromise** between a **simple** and a **reliable method** as well as **extremely good structural preservation[Q]**.

  > • The **strong cross-linking action** of formaldehyde is essential, **to protect the tissue from the aggressive effect of concentrated solvents** in the **course of fixation** and **embedding in paraffin[Q]**.

- **Fixation of tissue arrests** the **autolysis** and **putrefaction** and **stabilizes the cellular and tissue contents[Q]**

32. **Ans. a. Aspergillus flavus** *(Ref: Ananthnarayan 7/e p625)*
    - **Primary Aflatoxin Producing Fungi: Aspergillus flavus[Q]** and **Aspergillus parasiticus[Q]**

33. **Ans. d. Floor** *(Ref: BDC 4/e pI/58)*

AXILLARY ABSCESS

- An **axillary abscess** is **incised through** the **floor[Q]** of the axilla, midway between the anterior and posterior axillary folds, and nearer to the medial wall in order **to avoid injury to** the **main vessels running along the anterior, posterior** and **lateral walls.**

34. Ans. b. Tracheal stenosis *(Ref: Dhillon 3/e p67)*

- **Topical Mitomycin C** is the **drug of choice** used to aid the treatment of **laryngeal stenosis**[Q].
- **Topical Mitomycin C** can **inhibit fibroblast activity** and **restenosis**[Q].

35. Ans. a. Sarcoidosis *(Ref: Essentials of Chest Radiology by Janette Collins/165)*

SARCOIDOSIS

- **Sarcoidosis** is a systemic disease characterized by **non-caseating granulomas in multiple organs**
- In **90% of cases**, **symmetrical massive bilateral hilar lymphadenopathy** occur
- The **cardiac border (Potato nodes)** or lung involvement is present and can be revealed by chest X-ray or transbronchial biopsy

36. Ans. a. Carcinoma

- "In normal persons, a click is felt when larynx is moved from side to side over vertebral column, this is called laryngeal click (post cricoid crepitus) It is absent in post cricoid carcinoma" — Moure's sign.

37. Ans. b. Phenacetin - lung

38. Ans. c. Diameter of catheter *(Ref: The ICU Book By Paul L. Marino 3/e p108)*

"The size of vascular catheters is expressed in terms of outside diameter of the catheter. Two units of measurements are used to describe catheter size: a metric-based French size and a wire-based gauge size. The French size is a series of whole numbers that increases from zero in increments of 0.33 millimeters (e.g., a size 5 French catheter will have an outside diameter of $5 \times 0.33 = 1.65$ mm). The gauge size was introduced for solid wires and is an expression of how many wires can be placed side-by-side in a given space. The gauge size varies inversely with the diameter of the wire (or catheter)." -The ICU Book By Paul L. Marino 3/e p108

39. Ans. b. Doctor's signature *(Ref: Sabiston 20/e p232; Schwartz 11/e p404, 10/e p1969)*

Elements of the Surgical Safety Checklist		
Sign In	**Time-Out**	**Sign Out**
• Before induction of anesthesia, members of the team (at least the nurse and an anesthesia professional) state that the following have been done: • **Patient has verified his or her identity, surgical site & procedure and consent.** • The **surgical site is marked** or site marking is not applicable. • **Pulse oximeter** is on the patient & functioning. • All members of the team are aware of whether the patient has a **known allergy**. • **Patient's airway & risk of aspiration** have been evaluated, and appropriate equipment & assistance are available. • If there is a risk of blood loss of at least 500 mL (or 7 mL/kg body weight in children), appropriate access and fluids are available.	• Before skin incision, the entire team (nurses, surgeons, anesthesia professionals, and any others participating in the care of the patient) or specific members state aloud the following: • Team confirms that all team members have been introduced by name & role. • **Team confirms the patient's identity, surgical site & procedure.** • Team reviews the anticipated critical events. • Surgeon reviews critical and unexpected steps, operative duration & anticipated blood loss. • Anesthesia professionals review concerns specific to patient. • Nurses review confirmation of sterility, equipment availability, and other concerns. • **Team confirms that prophylactic antibiotics have been administered ≤60 minutes before incision is made or that antibiotics are not indicated.** • Team confirms that all **essential imaging results for correct patient are displayed in operating room.**	• Before the patient leaves the operating room, the following are done: • Nurse reviews the following aloud with the team: • **Name of procedure**, as recorded • That **needle, sponge, & instrument counts are complete** (or not applicable) • That specimen (if any) is correctly labeled, including patient's name • Whether there are any issues with equipment that need to be addressed • The surgeon, nurse & anesthesia professional review aloud the key concerns for the recovery and care of the patient.

40. Ans. d. Skin, subcutaneous tissue, superficial fascia and deep fascia *(Ref: Bailey 27/e p28)*

"Fasciotomy involves incising the deep muscle fascia and is best carried out via longitudinal incisions of skin, fat and fascia. The muscle will be then seen bulging out through the fasciotomy opening." -Bailey 27/e p28

41. Ans. c. Sitting with neck flexed

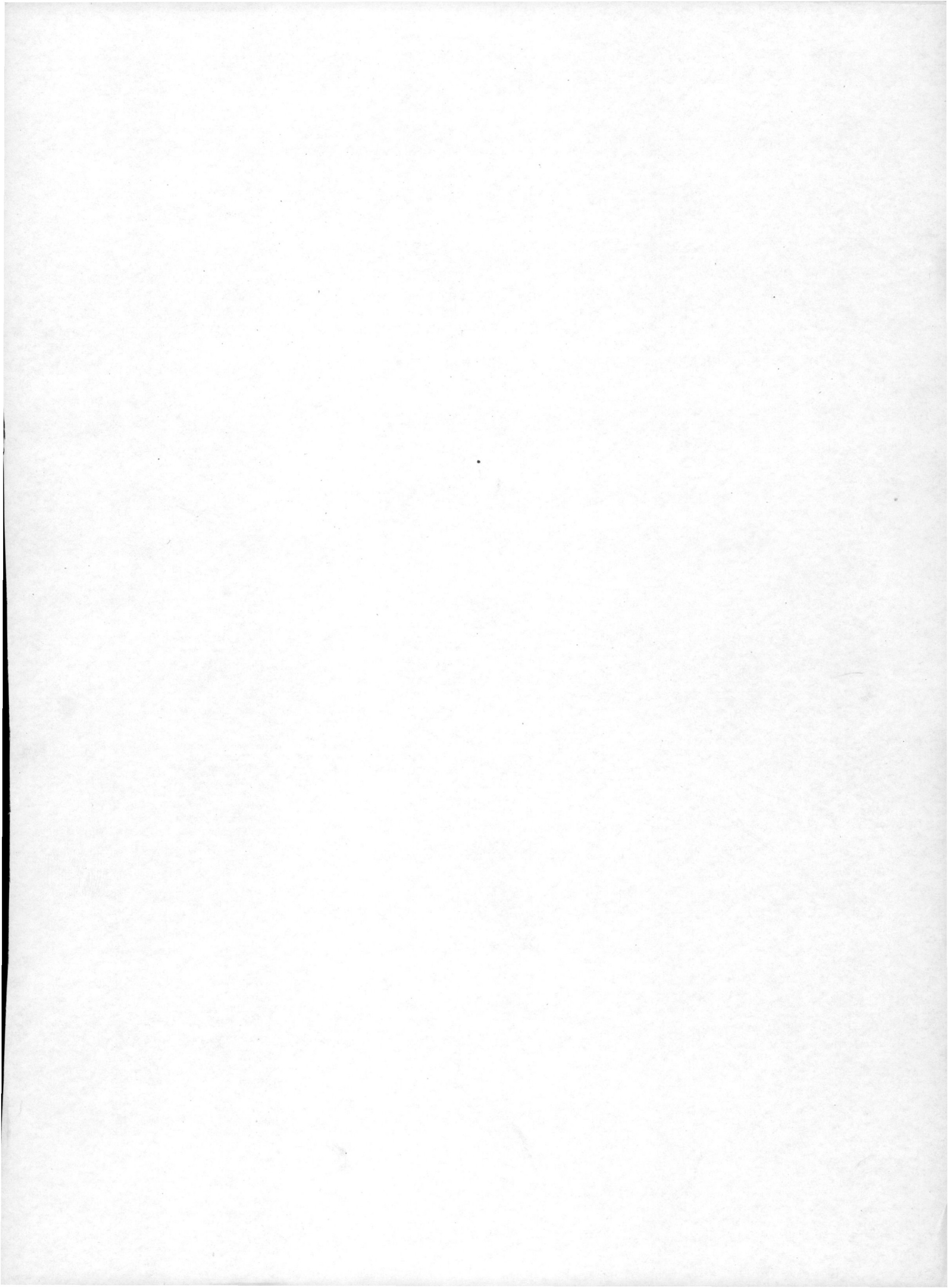